Stedman's

ORTHOPAEDIC & REHAB WORDS

INCLUDES

CHIROPRACTIC,

OCCUPATIONAL THERAPY,

PHYSICAL THERAPY, PODIATRIC

& SPORTS MEDICINE

FOURTH EDITION

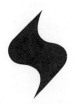

Stedman's
ORTHOPAEDIC & REHAB
WORDS

INCLUDES
CHIROPRACTIC, OCCUPATIONAL THERAPY,
PHYSICAL THERAPY, PODIATRIC,
& SPORTS MEDICINE

FOURTH EDITION

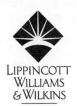

LIPPINCOTT
WILLIAMS
& WILKINS

Publisher: Rhonda M. Kumm, RN, MSN
Senior Manager: Julie K. Stegman
Senior Managing Editor: Nancy S. Wachter
Associate Managing Editor: Trista A. DiPaula
Art Program Project Manager: Jennifer Clements
Assistant Production Manager: Kevin Iarossi
Typesetter: Peirce Graphic Services, Inc.
Printer & Binder: Malloy Litho, Inc.

Printed in the United States of America

Fourth Edition, 2003

Library of Congress Cataloging-in-Publication Data

Stedman's orthopaedic & rehab words : includes chiropractic,
occupational therapy, physical therapy, podiatric, & sports medicine.--
4th ed.
    p. ; cm.
Developed from the database of Stedman's Medical dictionary, 27th ed.
and supplemented by terminology found in current medical literature.
Includes bibliographical references.
  ISBN 0-7817-3836-9 (alk. paper)
  1. Orthopedics--Terminology. 2. People with
disabilities--Rehabilitation--Terminology.
  [DNLM: 1. Orthopedic Procedures--Terminology--English. 2. Athletic
Injuries--Terminology--English. 3. Foot Diseases--Terminology--English.
4. Manipulation, Chiropractic--Terminology--English. 5. Physical
Therapy Techniques--Terminology--English. 6.
Rehabilitation--Terminology--English. WE 15 S812 2003] I. Title:
Stedman's orthopaedic and rehab words. II. Title: Orthopaedic & rehab
words. III. Stedman, Thomas Lathrop, 1853-1938. IV. Stedman, Thomas
Lathrop, 1853-1938. Medical dictionary.
  RD723 .S74 2003
  616.7'001'4--dc21

                                                                    2002034057
                                                                       03 04
                                              2 3 4 5 6 7 8 9 10

Contents

Contents

Acknowledgments

An important part of our editorial process is the involvement of medical transcriptionists—as advisors, reviewers, and/or editors.

We extend special thanks to Jeanne Bock, CSR, MT, and Kathryn C. Mason, CMT, for editing the manuscript, helping resolve many difficult questions, and contributing material for the appendix sections. We are grateful to our MT Editorial Advisory Board members, including Janice Deal, RN, BSN; Joann Grano, MTS; Diane Hernandez, CMT; Lana Hirschfield, MTS; Darcy Johnson; Beverly S. Oberline, CMT; and Jenifer Walker, MA, who were instrumental in the development of this reference. They recommended sources and shared their valuable judgment, insight, and perspective.

We also extend thanks to Jeanne Bock, CSR, MT, for working on the appendix. Additional thanks to Helen Littrell for performing the final prepublication review. Other important contributors to this edition include Robin Koza; Wendy Ryan, RHIT; and Sandra Wideburg, CMT.

And, as always, Barb Ferretti played an integral role in the process by reviewing the content files for format, updating the database, and providing a final quality check. Special thanks also goes to Kathy Cadle and Lisa Fahnestock for their assistance with the database work.

As with all our *Stedman's* word references, this resource incorporates the suggestions and expertise of our many contacts in the medical transcriptionist community. Thanks to all of our advisory board participants, reviewers, and editors; AAMT meeting attendees; and others who have written us with requests and comments—keep talking, and we'll keep listening.

Editor's Preface

We live in a fast-paced society. No American wants to be sidelined from life, whether by congenital conditions, work-related injuries, or those sustained in an accident. When the maladies are skeletal or muscular in nature, specialists in orthopaedics, podiatry, chiropractic, occupational therapy, and physical therapy are able to get those injured back to their lifestyle at a rapid pace. These medical specialists often work hand in hand to achieve such a goal. The compilation of terms found in this book provides one easy-to-use reference to meet the needs of medical language specialties as they relate to these specialties.

This newest edition of *Stedman's Orthopaedic & Rehab Words* has an extensive number of orthopaedic procedures, equipment, and techniques gleaned from medical journals, textbooks, and medical reports. Additionally we have included many new terms related to the specialties of podiatry, chiropractic, OT, and PT using the same types of resources.

You will find the appendix section in this book to be thorough and informational. We have included a variety of orthopaedic procedures in the sample reports section. The anatomical illustrations extensively cover bones, muscles, ligaments, tendons, and nerves involved in orthopaedic injuries. You will also find tables detailing the original and insertion points of muscles, ligaments and tendons, as well as their action or articulation.

I am thankful to Kathryn C. Mason, CMT for assisting in the editing of this manuscript and extend special thanks to Barb Ferretti, our skilled database editor. Thanks also to those of you who have sent in suggestions now incorporated into this resource.

Jeanne Bock, CSR, MT

Publisher's Preface

Stedman's Orthopaedic & Rehab Words, Fourth Edition, offers an authoritative assurance of quality and exactness to the wordsmiths of the healthcare professions—medical transcriptionists, medical editors and copyeditors, health information management personnel, court reporters, and the many other users and producers of medical documentation.

We have received many requests to update this title. As a result, we have published this new edition that includes orthopaedic, rehabilitation, chiropractic, occupational therapy, physical therapy, and sports medicine terminology. In this new edition, we have expanded all terminology, particularly in the areas of chiropractic and podiatric terminology. New to this edition is terminology relevant to sports medicine.

In *Stedman's Orthopaedic & Rehab Words, Fourth Edition,* users will find terms for protocols, diagnostic and therapeutic procedures, new techniques, lab tests, clinical research terms, as well as abbreviations with their expansions pertinent to orthopaedics, rehabilitation, occupational therapy, physical therapy, and sports medicine. The appendix sections provide anatomical illustrations with useful captions and labels; fracture illustrations; a table of muscles; a table of ligaments and tendons; style rules; professional organizations, associations, and titles; sample reports; common terms by procedure; and drugs by indication.

This compilation of more than 100,000 entries, fully cross-indexed for quick access, was built from a base vocabulary of approximately 66,000 medical words, phrases, abbreviations, and acronyms. The extensive A-Z list was developed from the database of *Stedman's Medical Dictionary, 27th Edition,* and supplemented by terminology found in current medical literature (see References on page xvi).

We at Lippincott Williams & Wilkins strive to provide you with the most up-to-date and accurate word references available. Your use of this word book will prompt new editions, which we will publish as often as updates and revisions justify. We welcome your suggestions for improvements, changes, corrections, and additions—whatever will make this *Stedman's* product more useful to you. Please complete the postpaid card in this book, and send your recommendations care of "Stedman's" at Lippincott Williams & Wilkins.

Explanatory Notes

Medical transcription is an art as well as a science. Both approaches are needed to correctly interpret the dictation of a physician, whose language is a product of education, training, and experience. This variety in medical language means that there are several acceptable ways to express certain terms, including jargon. *Stedman's Orthopaedic & Rehab Words, Fourth Edition,* provides variant spellings and phrasings for many terms. These elements, in addition to complete cross-indexing, make *Stedman's Orthopaedic & Rehab Words, Fourth Edition,* a valuable resource for determining the validity of terms as they are encountered.

Alphabetical Organization

Alphabetization of main entries is letter by letter as spelled, ignoring punctuation, spaces, prefixed numbers, or other characters. For example:

Nitalloy
2-nite
nitidus

Terms beginning or ending with Greek letters show the Greek letters spelled out and listed alphabetically. For example:

alpha, α
   a. antagonist

In subentry alphabetization, the abbreviated singular form or the spelled-out plural form of the noun main entry word is ignored.

Format and Style

All main entries are in **boldface** to expedite locating a sought-after term, to enhance distinction between main entries and subentries, and to relieve the textual density of the pages.

Irregular plurals and variant spellings are shown on the same line as the singular or preferred form of the word. For example:

nucleus, pl. nuclei
physial, physeal

Hyphenation

As a rule of style, multiple eponyms (e.g., Mears-Rubash approach) are hyphenated. Also, hyphens have been added between a manufacturer and one or more eponyms (e.g., Vital-Metzenbaum dissecting scissors). Please note that in many cases, hyphenation is a question of style, not of accuracy, and thus is a matter of choice.

Possessives

Possessive forms have been dropped in this reference for the sake of consistency and conformance with the guidelines of the American Association for Medical Transcription (AAMT) and other groups. Please note, however, that in many cases, retaining the possessive, like hyphenating, is a question of style, not of accuracy, and thus is a matter of choice. To form the possessive of a word, simply add the apostrophe or apostrophe "s" to the end of the word.

Cross-indexing

The word list is in an index-like main entry-subentry format that contains two combined alphabetical listings:

(1) A *noun* main entry-subentry organization, which is typical of the A-Z section of medical dictionaries like *Stedman's:*

Spenco
- S. arch support
- S. boot
- S. insole

spike
- ball-tip s.
- endplate s.
- heel s.

(2) An *adjective* main entry-subentry organization, which lists words and phrases as you hear them. The main entries are the adjectives or modifiers in a multiword term. The subentries are the nouns around which the terms are constructed and to which the adjectives or modifiers pertain:

physiologic
- p. barrier
- p. flatfoot
- p. motion

posttraumatic
- p. angulation
- p. apoplexy
- p. arthritis

This format provides the user with more than one way to locate and iden-
tify a multiword term. For example:

analysis
   postural a.

postural
   p. analysis

subscapular
   s. artery injury

injury
   subscapular artery i.

It also allows the user to see together all terms that contain a particular
descriptor, as well as all types, kinds, or variations of a noun entity. For
example:

motorized
   m. bur
   m. meniscal cutter
   m. reamer

scapular
   s. approximation test
   s. border
   s. dysfunction

Wherever possible, abbreviations are separately defined and cross-refer-
enced. For example:

SCD
   sequential compression device

sequential
   s. compression device (SCD)

device
   sequential compression d. (SCD)

References

In addition to the manufacturers' literature we gather at various medical meetings, scientific reports from hospitals, and the lists of our MT Editorial Advisory Board members (from their daily transcription work), we used the following sources for new terms in *Stedman's Orthopaedic & Rehab Words, Fourth Edition.*

Books

Adelaar RS. Complex Foot & Ankle Trauma. Philadelphia: Lippincott Williams & Wilkins, 1999.

Banks AS, Downey MS, Martin DE, Miller SJ. Foot and Ankle Surgery, 3rd Edition. Philadelphia: Lippincott Williams & Wilkins, 2001.

Blauvelt CT, Nelson FRT. A Manual of Orthopaedic Terminology, 6th Edition. Philadelphia: Mosby-Yearbook, 1998.

Bracker MD. The 5-Minute Sports Medicine Consult. Philadelphia: Lippincott Williams & Wilkins, 2001.

Brammer CM, Spires MC. Manual of Physical Medicine & Rehabilitation. Philadelphia: Hanley & Belfus, Inc., 2002.

Crim JR, Cracchiolo A, Hall RL. Imaging of the Foot and Ankle. Philadelphia: Lippincott Williams & Wilkins, 1996.

Dorland's Orthopedic Word Book for Medical Transcriptionists. Philadelphia: Saunders, 2002.

Drake E. Sloane's Medical Word Book, 4th Edition. Philadelphia: Saunders, 2001.

Lance LL. Quick Look Drug Book. Baltimore: Lippincott Williams & Wilkins, 2002.

Olson T. A.D.A.M. Student Atlas of Anatomy. Philadelphia: Lippincott Williams & Wilkins, 1996.

Orthopedic/Neurology Words and Phrases, 2nd Edition. Modesto, CA: Health Professions Institute, 2000.

Safran MR, McKeag DB, Van Camp SP. Manual of Sports Medicine. Philadelphia: Lippincott Williams & Wilkins, 1998.

Sponseller, PD, Frassica FJ, Wenz, JF. The 5-Minute Orthopaedic Consult. Philadelphia: Lippincott Williams & Wilkins, 2000.

Stedman's Medical Dictionary, 27th Edition. Baltimore: Lippincott Williams & Wilkins, 2000.

Stedman's Orthaedic & Rehab Words, 3rd Edition. Baltimore: Lippincott Williams & Wilkins, 1998.

Tessier C. The AAMT Book of Style. Modesto, CA: AAMT, 1995.

Vera Pyle's Current Medical Terminology, 8th Edition. Modesto, CA: Health Professions Institute, 2000.

Journals

ACSM's Health & Fitness Journal. Baltimore: Lippincott Williams & Wilkins, 1999–2000.

Chiropractic Products. Los Angeles: Medical World Communications, Inc., 2000.

Clinical Journal of Sports Medicine. Philadelphia: Lippincott Williams & Wilkins, 2001–2002.

Current Opinion in Orthopaedics. Philadelphia: Lippincott Willaims & Wilkins, 2001–2002.

Foot & Ankle International. Philadelphia: Lippincott Willaims & Wilkins, 1999–2002.

Journal of the American Association for Medical Transcription. Modesto, CA: American Association for Medical Transcription, 2000–2001.

Journal of Bone & Joint Surgery. Needham, MA: The Journal of Bone & Joint Surgery, Inc. 1999–2002.

Journal of Foot & Ankle Surgery. Park Ridge, IL: American College of Foot and Ankle Surgeons, 1999–2002.

Latest Word. Philadelphia: Saunders, 1999–2002.

O & P Almanac. Alexandria, VA: American Orthotic and Prosthetic Association, 1999–2000.

OrthoKinetic Review. Los Angeles: MWC/Allied Healthcare Group, 2001.

Perspectives on the Medical Transcription Profession. Modesto, CA: Health Professions Institute, 2001.

Physical Therapy Products. Los Angeles: MWC/Allied Healthcare Group, 1998–1999.

Podiatric Products. Los Angeles: MWC/Allied Healthcare Group, 1999–2000.

Sports Medicine Digest. Philadelphia: Lippincott Williams & Wilkins, 2001–2002.

Websites

http://physicaltherapy.about.com

http://www.accessdata.fda.gov/scripts/cdrh/cfdocs/cfTopic/MDA/mda-list.cfm?list+1

http://www.aaos.org

http://www.aota.org

http://www.aotf.org

http://www.apma.org

http://www.bonehome.com/Home/Topics/orthopedics/orthopedics.html

http://www.chiroweb.com

http://www.fda.gov

http://www.hpisum.com

http://www.mtdaily.com

http://www.mtdesk.com

http://www.mtmonthly.com

http://www.podiatrychannel.com

A
> A pin
> A wave

AA
> active-assistive

AAA
> antigen-extracted allogenic
> diagnostic arthroscopy, operative arthroscopy, and possible operative arthrotomy
>> AAA bone
>> AAA bone graft

AAD
> atlantoaxial dislocation

AAE
> active-assistive exercise

AAI
> activating adjusting instrument
> axial acetabular index

AAL
> anterior axillary line

AAOS
> American Academy of Orthopaedic Surgeons
>> AAOS acetabular abnormality classification
>> AAOS Knee Society Clinical Rating Score

AARF
> atlantoaxial rotatory fixation

AAROM
> active ankle joint complex range of motion
> active-assisted range of motion

Aarskog-Scott syndrome

AAS
> atlantoaxial subluxation

AAT
> animal-assisted therapy

AB/AD ratio

ABAQUS modeling program

abarthrosis

abarticular

abarticulation

abasia
> atactic a.

abasic

abatement

abatic

Abbe operation

Abbott
> A. brace
> A. gouge
> A. method
> A. operation

> A. posterior approach
> A. splint

Abbott-Carpenter posterior approach

Abbott-Fischer-Lucas hip arthrodesis

Abbott-Gill
> A.-G. epiphysial plate exposure
> A.-G. epiphysiodesis
> A.-G. osteotomy

Abbott-Lucas
> A.-L. arthrodesis
> A.-L. shoulder operation

Abbreviated Injury Scale (AIS)

ABC
> aneurysmal bone cyst

abdominal
> a. binder
> a. dressing
> a. flap
> a. lap pad
> a. muscle
> a. view

ABD pad

abduct

abducted thumb

abduction
> a. bolster
> a. brace
> a. contracture
> Cruiser hip a.
> a. cushion
> a. deformity
> a. external rotation test
> a. finger splint
> hinge a.
> hip a.
> a. hip orthosis
> a. humeral splint
> humerothoracic a.
> index finger a.
> a. knee separator
> a. load and shift test
> a. osteotomy
> a. pillow
> a. pillow cover splint
> a. sign
> a. stress test
> a. thumb splint
> a. traction technique
> a. wedge

abduction-external
> a.-e. rotation (AER)
> a.-e. rotation fracture

abductor
> a. digiti minimi (ADM)
> a. digiti minimi muscle

abductor *(continued)*
    a. digiti minimi nerve
    a. digiti minimi opponensplasty
    a. digiti quinti (ADQ)
    a. digiti quinti muscle
    a. digiti quinti opponensplasty
    a. digiti quinti tendon
    a. hallucis longus flap
    a. hallucis muscle
    a. hallucis oblique head
    a. hallucis tendon
    a. hallucis transverse head
    a. insufficiency
    a. lever arm
    a. lurch
    a. lurch gait
    a. mechanism
    a. pollicis brevis (APB)
    a. pollicis brevis muscle
    a. pollicis brevis tendon
    a. pollicis longus (APL)
    a. pollicis longus muscle
    a. pollicis longus tendon
    side-lying hip a.
    a. slide technique
abductor/adductor ratio
abductor-plasty
    flexor pollicis longus a.-p.
    Smith flexor pollicis longus a.-p.
abductory
    a. midfoot osteotomy
    a. wedge osteotomy
abductovalgus
    adolescent hallux a.
    hallux a. (HAV)
abductus
    digitus a.
    forefoot a.
    hallux a. (HA)
    interphalangeal a.
    metatarsus a.
    midfoot a.
    pes planovalgus a.
    pollex a.
Abernethy fascia
aberration
    hypokinetic a.
abet
ABG cement-free hip system
ability
    abstracting a.
    bathing and dressing a.
    conceptual a.
    constructional a.
    fluid absorption a.
    general a.
    positive a.

    self-help a.
    squatting a.
ablation
    cartilage a.
    cyst a.
    nerve rootlet a.
    radical nail bed a.
    surgical a.
    Zadik total nailbed a.
ablative
    a. arthroplasty
    a. laser therapy
    a. surgery
ablator
    Concept a.
Ableware Volumeter
abnormal
    a. fixation
    a. instantaneous axis of rotation
    A. Involuntary Movement Scale (AIMS)
    a. posterior talar process
    a. shoe wear
abnormality
    alignment a.
    biochemical a.
    bony a.
    bulbar a.
    cranial nerve a.
    cytoarchitectonic a.
    dislocation contour a.
    engulfment a.
    fibropathic a.
    frontal plane growth a.
    sensorineural a.
    soft tissue a.
    sonographic a.
    spinal cord injury without radiographic a. (SCIWORA)
    tissue texture a. (TTA)
    torsional a.
abouna splint
above
    a. elbow (AE)
    a. knee (AK)
above-elbow
    a.-e. amputation (AEA)
    a.-e. cast
above-knee
    a.-k. amputation (AKA)
    a.-k. prosthesis
    a.-k. suction enhancement system
abrader
    cartilage a.
Abraham-Pankovich tendo calcaneus repair
Abramson catheter

abrasion
    a. arthroplasty
    a. chondroplasty
    graft-bony tunnel wall a.
Abrikossoff tumor
abscess
    arthrifluent a.
    bone a.
    Brodie a.
    bursal a.
    button a.
    cold a.
    collar-button a.
    growth plate a.
    gummatous a.
    horseshoe a.
    hypostatic a.
    intraosseous a.
    ischiorectal a.
    lumbar a.
    metaphysial a.
    midpalmar a.
    ossifluent a.
    paraspinal a.
    paravertebral a.
    pelvic a.
    periarticular a.
    posterior pharyngeal a.
    Pott a.
    psoas a.
    retropharyngeal a.
    retrosternal a.
    sacrococcygeal a.
    serous a.
    soft tissue a.
    spinal a.
    subaponeurotic a.
    subcutaneous a.
    subfascial a.
    subgaleal a.
    subperiosteal a.
    subphrenic a.
    subplatysmal a.
    subungual a.
    supralevator a.
    suture a.
    syphilitic a.
    thecal a.
    traumatic a.
abscessogram
absconsio

absence
    limb a.
absent
    a. patella
    a. radius
    a. reflex
    a. spinous process
    a. tibia
    a. ulna
absolute
    A. absorbable screw
    a. refractory period
    a. scotoma
absorbable
    a. biomaterial
    a. collagen paste (ACP)
    a. polymeric pin
    a. polyparadioxanone pin
absorptiometry
    dual-energy x-ray a. (DEXA, DXA)
    dual-photon a. (DPA, DPX)
    peripheral dual-energy x-ray a. (pDXA)
absorption
    bone a.
    bony a.
    a. cavity
    energy a.
    lysosomal a.
    shock a.
absorptive dressing
abstracting ability
Abumi technique
abut
abutment
    calcaneofibular a.
    a. splint
    ulnocarpal a.
AC
    acromioclavicular
    AC joint
    AC joint separation
acampsia
acantha
acanthoma
    clear cell a.
    epidermolytic a.
acanthosis nigricans
acanthotic

NOTES

accelerated
    a. bone maturation
    a. chondral wear
acceleration
    angular a.
    swing-phase a.
    tibial a.
acceleration/deceleration injury
accelerator
    Bevatron a.
    linear a. (LINAC)
    Philips linear a.
    Siemens linear a.
accelerometer
    piezoelectric a.
acceptance
    weight a.
access
    eccentric a.
    southern a.
accessiflexor
accessory
    a. abductor hallucis
    a. atlantoaxial ligament
    Auto Glide walker a.
    a. bone
    a. cartilage
    a. collateral ligament
    a. communicating tendon
    a. digit
    a. epiphysis
    Isola spinal implant system a.
    a. lateral collateral ligament
    a. motion
    a. movement technique
    a. navicular
    a. navicular avulsion
    a. navicular cast
    a. navicular fracture
    a. nerve
    a. nerve injury
    a. ossicle
    a. ossicle fracture
    a. ossification center of calcaneus
    a. phalanx
    pneumatic drill a.
    portal a.
    a. portion
    a. sesamoid
    a. soleus
    a. soleus muscle
AccessTrainer exerciser
accident
    compensable a.
    motorcycle a. (MCA)
    motor vehicle a. (MVA)
    pedestrian a.
    vascular a.

acclimate
acclivity
accommodation
    a. curve
    a. reflex
accommodative
    a. brace
    a. equipment
    a. orthosis
    a. shoe
Accommodator arch support
accordion test
accoucheur hand
Accu-Back back support
Accucore II
Accu-Cut
    A.-C. osteotomy guide
    A.-C. osteotomy guide system
Accuflate tourniquet
Accu-Flo
    A.-F. polyethylene bur hole cover
    A.-F. silicone rubber bur hole
      cover
    A.-F. ultrafiltration system
Accugraft allograft
Acculength arthroplasty measuring
system
Accu-Line
    A.-L. dual pivot
    A.-L. femoral resector
    A.-L. guide
    A.-L. knee instrument
    A.-L. knee instrumentation
    A.-L. tibial resector
accumulation
    onset of blood lactate a. (OBLA)
AccuPressure heel cup
Accurate Surgical and Scientific
   Instruments Corporation (ASSI)
AccuSharp carpal tunnel release
   instrument
Accusway balance measurement system
AccuTread shoe
Accu-Tron microcurrent machine
Accuvac smoke evacuation attachment
ACDF
    anterior cervical diskectomy and fusion
Ace
    A. adherent bandage
    A. bandage reduction
    A. brace
    A. intramedullary (AIM)
    A. intramedullary femoral nail
      system
    A. pin
    A. screw
    A. Unifix fixation
    A. Unifix fixation apparatus

A. Unifix fixation device
A. wrap
Ace-Colles
   A.-C. external fixator
   A.-C. fixation
   A.-C. fracture frame
   A.-C. frame technique
   A.-C. half ring
Ace-Fischer
   A.-F. external fixator
   A.-F. fixation
   A.-F. fracture frame
   A.-F. ring frame
Ace/Normed osteodistractor
ACET
   aquatic cardiac evaluation and testing
   ACET system
acetabula (*pl. of* acetabulum)
acetabular
   a. allograft
   a. angle
   a. angle of Sharp
   a. augmentation graft
   a. bone
   a. branch
   a. cap
   a. cement compactor
   a. component
   a. component loosening
   a. cup
   a. cup arthroplasty
   a. cup holder
   a. cup peg drill guide
   a. cup positioner
   a. cup system
   a. cup template
   a. cyst
   a. depth to femoral head diameter
    (AD/FHD)
   a. dysplasia
   a. endoprosthesis
   a. expander
   a. extensile approach
   a. fossa
   a. gauge
   a. head index (AHI)
   a. head quotient
   a. index
   a. knee
   a. knife
   a. labrum

a. line
a. notch
a. osteolysis
a. posterior wall fracture
a. pressurizer
a. prosthesis
a. prosthetic interface
a. prosthetic liner
a. protrusio deformity
a. reamer
a. recess
a. reconstruction plate
a. rim
a. rim fracture
a. rim syndrome
a. roof
a. round chisel
a. seating hole
a. shelf osteotomy
a. slot
a. spacer
a. trial set
acetabulectomy
acetabuli
   arteria a.
   protrusio a.
acetabuloplasty
   Albee a.
   Pemberton a.
   posttraumatic degenerative disease
    Lance a.
   shelf a.
acetabulum, pl. **acetabula**
   deep-shelled a.
   dysplastic a.
   false a.
   floor of a.
   lip of a.
   malunited a.
   true a.
acetate
   compression-molded ethylene
    vinyl a. (CM EVA)
   ethylene vinyl a. (EVA)
   mafenide a.
   methylprednisolone a.
   triamcinolone a.
ACF
   anterior cervical fusion
ACFS
   anterior cervical plate fixation system

NOTES

ache
    a.'s and pains
    theater a.
acheiria
acheiropodia
achilleocalcaneal
    a.-plantar system
    a. vascular network
Achilles
    A. bulge sign
    A. esesthopathy
    A. heel pad
    A. jerk
    A. paratendinitis
    A. peritendinitis
    A. squeeze test
    A. tendinitis
    A. tendinopathy
    A. tendon (AT)
    A. tendon advancement
    A. tendon bursa
    A. tendon bursitis
    A. tendon enthesis
    A. tendon enthesis calcification
    A. tendon lengthening
    A. tendon pain
    A. tendon reflex
    A. tendon repair (ATR)
    A. tendon resurfacing
    A. tendon rupture (ATR)
    A. tendon shortening
    A. tendon taping technique
    A. tendon test
    A. tendon xanthoma
    A. tendon Z-lengthening
    A. tenotomy
Achillis
    tendo A.
achillobursitis
achillodynia
    Albert a.
achillogram
Achillon instrument guide
achillorrhaphy
achillotenotomy
    plastic a.
achillotomy
Achillotrain
    A. active Achilles tendon support
    Bauerfeind A.
aching pain
achondrogenesis
achondroplasia
achondroplastic
    a. dwarfism
    a. pelvis
    a. stenosis
achondroplasty

achromatopsia
Achterman-Kalamachi fibular hemimelia
ACI
    autologous chondrocyte implantation
acid
    polyglycolic acid-polylactic a.
    (PGA-PLA)
    self-reinforcing polylevolactic a.
    (SR-PLLA)
    a. treatment
acidosis
    lactic a.
acidosteophyte
Ackerman criteria for osteomyelitis
acknemia
ACL
    anterior cruciate ligament
    ACL drill
    ACL drill guide
    ACL graft
    ACL graft knife
    ACL guide set
    ACL Lite functional knee brace
    ACL reconstruction
    ACL repair
Acland
    A. clamp-applying forceps
    A. clamp approximator
    A. double-clamp approximator
    A. microvascular clamp
aclasia
aclasis
    diaphysial a.
    metaphysial a.
    tarsoepiphysial a.
aclastic
ACL-deficient knee
ACLR
    anterior capsulolabral reconstruction
acnemia
Acoma scanner
acorn
    Midas Rex a.
    a. reamer
Acor Quikform I, II shoe
acoustic myography
ACP
    absorbable collagen paste
    anterior cervical plate
AC-PC
    anterior commissure-posterior
    commissure
    AC-PC line
    AC-PC plane
ACPS
    acrocephalopolysyndactyly
acquired
    a. brain injury

a. clubfoot
a. digital fibrokeratoma
a. flatfoot
a. myopathy
a. tarsal coalition
a. thumb flexion contracture
a. torticollis

acquisita
myotonia a.

ACR
American College of Rheumatology
ACR classification

Acra-Cut wire pass drill
acral
a. digital fibrokeratoma
a. lentiginous melanoma

Acrel ganglion
acroarthritis
acroataxia
acrocephalopolysyndactyly (ACPS)
acrocephalosyndactylism
acrocephalosyndactyly
acrochordon
acrocontracture
acrocyanosis
acrodysesthesia
acrodysplasia
Acro-Flex artificial disk
acrokeratoelastoidosis
acrokinesia
acromacria
AcroMed
A. screw
A. VSP fixation system
A. VSP plate

acromegalic
a. arthralgia
a. arthritis
a. facies

acromegalogigantism
acromegaloidism
acromegaly
acromelia
acrometagenesis
acromial
a. angle
a. bone
a. profile
a. spur
a. spur index (ASI)

acromiale
os a.

acromioclavicular (AC)
a. arthroplasty
a. articulation
a. cyst
a. disk
a. injury classification
a. joint
a. joint dislocation
a. joint injury
a. joint repair
a. ligament
a. separation
a. sprain

acromiocoracoid ligament
acromiohumeral interval (AHI)
acromion
hooked a.
a. process

acromionectomy
Armstrong a.

acromionizer tip
acromioplasty
anterior a.
arthroscopic a.
decompressive a.
McLaughlin a.
McShane-Leinberry-Fenlin a.
Neer a.
Rockwood anterior a.

acromioscapular
acromyotonia
acromyotonus
acroosteolysis
frostbite a.

acroosteosclerosis
acropachy
acropachyderma
acroparalysis
acroparesthesia
Nothnagel a.
Schultze a.

acropathology
acropathy
amyotrophic a.
ulcerative mutilating a.

acropectorovertebral dysplasia
acrosclerosis
acrostealgia
acrosyndactyly
Apert a.

NOTES

7

Acrotorque hand engine
acrylic
> a. bar prosthesis
> a. bone cement
> a. cap splint
> a. implant material
> a. orthotic device
> a. template splint

Acryl-X orthopaedic cement removal system
ACS
> anterior compartment syndrome
> ACS Gemini prosthesis
> ACS Profile prosthesis
> ACS Star prosthesis

ACSM
> American College of Sports Medicine
> ACSM Guidelines for Exercise Testing and Prescription

act
> A. joint support
> A. knee support

ACTH
> adrenocorticotropic hormone

actinic keratosis
actinomycosis
action
> concentric muscle a.
> a. current
> double-pendulum a.
> eccentric muscle a.
> A. elbow wrap
> A. Jr. wheelchair
> a. line
> a. myoclonus
> a. potential (AP)
> A. thumb sling
> A. traction system
> a. tremor
> A. wrist wrap

activated partial thromboplastin time test (APTT)
activating adjusting instrument (AAI)
activation
> electromyographic a.
> a. force
> latency of a.
> order of a.
> volitional a.

activator
> tissue-type plasminogen a.

active
> A. ankle brace
> a. ankle joint complex range of motion (AAROM)
> A. Ankle support
> a. bending test
> a. contraction
> a. dorsiflexion
> a. electrode
> a. flexion
> a. hip movement
> a. insufficiency
> a. integral range of motion (AIROM)
> a. integral range of motion airplane brace
> a. knee extension (AKE)
> a. knee extension test
> a. mobility
> a. motion testing (AMT)
> a. movement testing
> a. muscle co-contraction
> a. and passive range of motion
> a. range of motion (AROM)
> a. range-of-motion exercise
> a. restraint
> a. sock
> a. splint
> A. support and brace
> a. treatment

active-assisted
> a.-a. range of motion (AAROM)
> a.-a. range-of-motion exercise

active-assistive (AA)
> a.-a. exercise (AAE)
> a.-a. motion therapy

active-release technique (ART)
activity
> a. adaptation
> a. analysis
> biphasic endplate a.
> a. configuration
> a. of daily living (ADL)
> discrete a.
> diversional a.
> endplate a.
> functional a.
> a. grading
> a. group
> high-altitude a.
> high-impact a.
> involuntary a.
> A. Loss Assessment (ALA)
> mechanoreceptor a.
> monophasic endplate a.
> motion a.
> motor a.
> opsonic a.
> physical a.
> pivoting and cutting a.
> pivot-sport a.
> purposeful a.
> push-pull a.
> spontaneous a.
> sudomotor a.

a. synthesis
a. training (AT)
volitional a.
voluntary a.

Activity-Lite knee brace
activity-pattern analysis
Activ slideboard
actomyosin
actual leg length test
actuator
NYU-Hosmer electric elbow and prehension a.
ACU-derm wound dressing
AcuDriver osteotome
ACU-dyne antiseptic
Acufex
A. alignment guide
A. ankle distractor
A. arthroscopic instrument
A. arthroscopic instrumentation
A. bioabsorbable fixation device
A. bioabsorbable Suretac suture
A. bioabsorbable suture anchor
A. convex rasp
A. curette
A. curved basket forceps
A. distractor pin
A. double-lumen arthroscopic cannula
A. drill
A. drill-guide
A. Edge
A. gouge
A. grasper
A. knee laxity arthrometer
A. mallet
A. meniscal basket
A. meniscal stitcher
A. microsurgical rear-entry to front-entry femoral guide system
A. microsurgical tendon stripper
A. MosaicPlasty instrument
A. nerve hook
A. osteotome
A. probe
A. rotary biting basket forceps
A. rotary punch
A. scissors
A. tensiometer
A. T-Fix suture anchor
A. tibial guide
AcuFix anterior cervical plate system

Acuforce 7.0 therapy tool
Acu-Magnet therapy
AcuMatch
A. A, L, M Series acetabular component
A. integrated hip system
A. M Series modular femoral hip prosthesis
Acumed
A. great toe system
A. suture anchor
Acumeter
acupoint
Acupoint stimulator
AcuPressor myotherapy tool
acupressure
Neiguan point a.
Acu-Pressure slipper
acupuncture
Korean hand a.
Acuson imaging system
AcuSpark piezoelectric device
Acustar surgical navigation system
acute
a. angular kyphosis
a. avulsion fracture
a. brachial radiculitis
a. calcific tendinitis
a. exertional compartment syndrome (AECS)
a. foot strain
a. gout
a. hematogenous arthritis
a. hematogenous osteomyelitis (AHO)
a. inflammatory demyelinating polyradiculoneuropathy (AIDP)
a. inflammatory polyradiculopathy
a. ischemic contracture
a. low back syndrome
a. pain
a. phase rehabilitation
a. progressive myositis
a. reflex bone atrophy
a. repetitive seizure (ARS)
a. spinal arthritis
a. stretch injury
a. transverse myelitis
a. traumatic hemarthrosis
a. traumatic lesion
a. whiplash

NOTES

Acutrak
 A. screw system
 A. small bone fixation system
Acu-Treat electroacupuncture
AcuVibe massager
adactylous
adactyly, adactylia
 partial a.
Adair
 A. breast clamp
 A. screw compressor
Adair-Dighton syndrome
ADAM
 amniotic deformity, adhesion, mutilation
Adam
 A. and Eve rib belt splint
 A. sign
Adamantiades-Behçet syndrome
adamantinoma
 a. of long bone
 tibial a.
Adamkiewicz artery
Adams
 A. forward-bending test
 A. hip operation
 A. position test
 A. procedure
 A. saw
 A. scoliosis test
 A. splint
 A. transmalleolar arthrodesis
 A. view
Adapta physical therapy table
adaptation
 activity a.
 high-altitude a.
adapted stroller
adapter, adaptor
 Christmas tree a.
 chuck a.
 Collet screwdriver a.
 French a.
 Grace plate 4-hole a.
 Hudson chuck a.
 Jacobs chuck a.
 Lloyd a.
 Mayfield a.
 SACH foot a.
 Smith-Petersen nail with Lloyd a.
 Trinkle brace and a.
 Trinkle chuck a.
Adapteur multifunctional drill guide
Adaptic
 A. crown
 A. dressing
 A. gauze
 A. pack

 A. packing
 A. sponge
adaptive equipment
adaptor (*var. of* adapter)
Adcon adhesive control gel
Adcon-L anti-adhesion barrier gel
Add-A-Clamp
 Hex-Fix A.-A.-C.
adducent
adduct
adducta
 coxa a.
adducted thumb
adduction
 a. contracture
 a. deformity
 Edgarton-Grand thumb a.
 a. fracture
 a. load and shift test
 a. osteotomy
 a. sign
 a. stress to finger
 a. stress test
 a. traction technique
adduction-internal rotation deformity
adductocavus
 metatarsus a.
adductor
 a. aponeurosis
 a. hallucis longus
 a. hallucis muscle
 a. hallucis tendon
 a. hamstring tightness
 a. hiatus
 a. longus muscle rupture
 a. magnus
 a. magnus adductor flap
 a. muscle group
 a. origin
 a. pollicis brevis tendon
 a. pollicis muscle
 a. pollicis paralysis
 a. pollicus
 a. reflex
 a. sweep of thumb
 a. tendon and lateral capsular
  release
 a. tenotomy
 a. tenotomy and obturator
  neurectomy (ATON)
 a. tubercle
 a. tuberosity
adductovarus
 a. deformity
 forefoot a.
 metatarsus a.
adductus
 compensated metatarsus a.

congenital metatarsus a.
digitus a.
dynamic metatarsus a.
forefoot a.
metatarsus a. (MTA)
metatarsus primus a. (MPA)
midfoot a.
pes equinovarus a.
simple metatarsus a.
true metatarsus a. (TMA)
Adelaar-Williams-Gould ten-point scale
Adelmann operation
A-delta fiber
adenoma
papillary a.
adenomyosis
adenosine thallium scan
AD/FHD
acetabular depth to femoral head
diameter
adherence
skin a.
adherent
a. profundus tendon
Tuf-Skin tape a.
adhesion
bandlike a.
capsular a.
fibrous a.
filmy a.
a. formation
intraarticular a.
subacromial bursal a.
subdeltoid bursal a.
adhesion/cohesion mechanism
adhesive
APR cement fixation a.
a. arachnoiditis
Aron Alpha a.
benzoin a.
Biobrane a.
a. capsulitis
Coe-pak paste a.
Coverlet a.
Cover-Roll gauze a.
cyanoacrylate a.
a. drape
a. dressing
fibrin glue a.
Histoacryl glue a.
hydroxyapatite a.
Implast a.

ligand a.
LLPS hydroxyapatite a.
medical a.
methyl methacrylate a.
a. neuralgia
Orthomite II a.
Palacos cement a.
Simplex cement a.
a. strapping
Superglue a.
Surfit a.
Surgical Simplex P a.
a. tenosynovitis
T-Stick a.
Zimmer low-viscosity a.
ADI
atlantodens interval
adiabatic fast passage
adipofascial flap
adipose
a. ligament
a. tissue
adiposus
panniculus a.
ADJ
adjustable dynamic joint
adjoining pedicle
adjunct
walking a.
adjunctive screw fixation
Adjustaback wheelchair backrest system
adjustability
3D positional a.
adjustable
A. Advanced Reciprocating Gait
Orthosis (ARGO)
a. aiming apparatus
a. aiming device
a. angle guide
a. brace
a. cane
a. cane board
a. dynamic joint (ADJ)
A. Leg and Ankle Repositioning
Mechanism (ALARM)
a. nail
a. pedicle connector
a. postoperative protective prosthetic
socket (APOPPS)
a. splint
a. two-point caliper sensory
assessment device

NOTES

Adjusta-Wrist
    A.-W. hinge
    A.-W. splint
adjusting table
adjustive
    a. thrust
    a. treatment
adjustment
    atlas a.
    chiropractic spinal a.
    a. equipment
    figure-eight a.
    general a.
    manual a.
    osseous a.
    psychological a.
    set-hold a.
    specific a.
    a. of spine
    toggle-recoil a.
    vectored a.
    vertebral a.
adjuvant chemotherapy
adjuvant-induced arthritis (AIA)
ADK
    automated disposable keratome
Adkins
    A. spinal arthrodesis
    A. spinal fusion
ADL
    activity of daily living
    adrenoleukodystrophy
    extended ADLs
    hierarchical scales of ADLs
    ADL index
    indices of ADLs
    instrumental ADLs
    Northwick Park Index of
      Independence in ADL
ADM
    abductor digiti minimi
adolescent
    a. back pain
    a. condylar blade plate
    a. hallux abductovalgus
    a. idiopathic scoliosis (AIS)
    a. kyphosis
    A. and Pediatric Pain Tool
      (APPT)
    A. and Pediatric Pain Tool Scale
    a. rigid foot
    a. round back
    a. scoliosis
    a. tibia vara
adolescentium
    apophysitis tibialis a.
ADQ
    abductor digiti quinti

adrenal
    a. cortex
    a. disorder
adrenergic vagal function
adrenocorticotropic hormone (ACTH)
adrenoleukodystrophy (ADL)
ADROM
    ankle dorsiflexion range of motion
adromia
Adson
    A. cerebellar retractor
    A. clip-introducing forceps
    A. conductor
    A. drill guide
    A. drill guide forceps
    A. enlarging bur
    A. hemilaminectomy retractor
    A. hypophysial forceps
    A. laminectomy chisel
    A. maneuver
    A. perforating bur
    A. periosteal elevator
    A. rongeur
    A. saw guide
    A. sign
    A. spiral drill
    A. suction tube
    A. test
    A. twist drill
    A. wire saw
Adson-Rogers perforating drill
ADT
    anterior drawer test
adult
    a. acquired flatfoot
    a. gait
    a. rickets
    a. scoliosis
    a. scoliosis surgery
adult-acquired flatfoot deformity
advance
    A. PS total knee prosthesis
    A. PS total knee system
advanced
    A. mobile-bearing knee implant
    a. mobile-bearing prosthesis
advancement
    Achilles tendon a.
    Atasoy V-Y a.
    calcaneonavicular ligament-tibialis
      posterior tendon a.
    Chandler patellar a.
    en bloc a.
    a. flap
    a. flap graft
    frontoorbital a.
    heel cord a. (HCA)
    Johnson pronator a.

A

Lloyd-Roberts-Swann trochanteric a.
Maquet a.
Murphy Achilles tendon a.
Murphy heel cord a.
patellar a.
plantar calcaneonavicular ligament-tibialis posterior tendon a.
profundus a.
tendon a.
tongue-in-groove a.
trochanteric a.
vastus medialis a. (VMA)
Wagner profundus a.
Wagner trochanteric a.

advancer
Advanta Orthopaedics
Advantim
    A. revision knee system
    A. total knee prosthesis
    A. total knee system
    A. unconstrained prosthesis
adventitia
adventitial
    a. forceps
    a. scissors
adventitious
    a. bursa
    a. movement
adversive attack
advisor
    Schwinn Fitness A.
Advocate electric flexion distraction table
AE
  above elbow
    AE amputation
AE1, AE3 antibody
AEA
  above-elbow amputation
Aeby muscle
AECS
  acute exertional compartment syndrome
AEP
  auditory evoked potential
Aequalis
    A. head
    A. humeral prosthesis
    A. reamer
    A. shoulder prosthesis
    A. stem
    A. system

AER
  abduction-external rotation
aerate
aeration
aerobic
    a. bacterium
    a. capacity
    a. cellulitis
    a. conditioning
    a. conditioning functional assessment
    a. exercise
    a. infection
    a. walking
aerobics
    karate-inspired a.
AerobiCycle
  Universal A.
Aerodyn orthotic
aeroplane splint
Aeroplast dressing
Aesculap
    A. ABC cervical plating system
    A. bipolar cautery
    A. bipolar cautery forceps
    A. clamp
    A. drill
    A. headholder
    A. saw
Aesculap-PM noncemented femoral prosthesis
aesthesiometer
AF
  antifungal
  arcuate fasciculus
affection
  patellar a.
afferent
    a. fiber
    a. nerve impulse
AFI total hip replacement prosthesis
AFO
  ankle-foot orthosis
    articulated AFO
    AFO brace sock
    AFO molded
    AFO pediatric brace
    AFO posterior leaf-spring
    sliding AFO
    AFO standard shell
    Type C-50, C-90 AFO
A-Force dorsal night splint

NOTES

A-frame
    A-f. notch
    A-f. orthosis
afterdrop
afterpotential
    negative a.
    positive a.
AG
  antigravity
AGC
  anatomically graduated component
    AGC Biomet total knee system
    AGC femoral prosthesis
    AGC knee prosthesis
    AGC knee replacement system
    AGC tibial prosthesis
AGE
  angle of greatest extension
age
    bone a.
    Greulich-Pyle bone a.
    skeletal a. (SA)
age-associated degenerative change
Agee
    A. carpal tunnel release system
    A. endoscope
    A. external fixator
    A. force-couple splint reduction
    A. four-pin fixation device
    A. WristJack external fixator
    A. WristJack fracture reduction system
Agency for Healthcare Research and Quality (AHCPR)
agenesis
    Bayne classification of radial a.
    caudal spinal a.
    lumbar a.
    odontoid a.
    radial a.
    sacral a.
agenetic fracture
agent
    Albunex ultrasound imaging a.
    alpha-adrenergic blocking a.
    anabolic a.
    antiosteoclastic a.
    antipyretic a.
    cellulose hemostatic a.
    chondroprotective a.
    chymopapain blocking a.
    contrast a.
    enzymatic debriding a.
    fibrinolytic a.
    keratolytic a.
    mechanical a.
    nociceptor a.
    phlogistic a.
    physical a.
    thermal a.
    uricosuric a.
    water-soluble contrast a.
AGF
  angle of greatest flexion
aggressive
    a. infantile fibromatosis
    a. solitary plasmacytoma
    a. tumor
agility
    a. drill
    A. total ankle system
agitans
    paralysis a.
Agliette
    A. measurement
    A. supracondylar osteotomy
Agnew splint
agnosia
    finger a.
agonist
    gamma-aminobutyric acid a.
    a. muscle
agonist-antagonist
agonistic muscle
agraphia
AHCPR
  Agency for Healthcare Research and Quality
    AHCPR guidelines for treatment of acute low back pain
Ahern trochanteric débridement
AHI
  acetabular head index
  acromiohumeral interval
  Arthritis Helplessness Index
Ahlback change
AHO
  acute hematogenous osteomyelitis
AHP
  American Hand Prosthetics
    AHP digital prosthesis
AHSC
  Arizona Health Science Center
    AHSC elbow prosthesis
AHSC-Volz
    AHSC-V. elbow prosthesis
    AHSC-V. hinge
AIA
  adjuvant-induced arthritis
aid
    Carex ambulatory a.
    erogenic a.
    extension a.
    mobility a.
    Ortho-Turn transfer a.
    prosthetic speech a.

sock a.
speech a.
StraddleSitter seating a.
Turn-Easy transfer a.
ultrasonic mobility a.
walking a.

AIDP
acute inflammatory demyelinating
polyradiculoneuropathy

AIIS
anterior inferior iliac spine
AIIS avulsion fracture

AIM
Ace intramedullary
AIM continuous passive motion
AIM CPM
AIM femoral nail system

aimer
Arthrotek femoral a.
tibial a.

aiming
a. bow
a. guide

AIMS
Abnormal Involuntary Movement Scale
Alberta Infant Motor Scale
Arthritis Impact Measurement Scale

ainhum
Ainslie acrylic splint
Ainsworth modification of Massie nail
air
a. arthrography
a. band
a. bed
a. bicycle
A. Castaway
a. compression osteotome
a. contrast
a. cylinder
A. DonJoy patellofemoral brace
a. drill
a. embolism
a. flow mat
a. inflation system
a. myelography
a. plasma spray (APS)
a. pressure splint
a. sinus
a. splint
A. Townsend brace
a. walker

Air-Back spinal system

airborne bacterium
Aircast
A. ankle brace
A. Cryo/Cuff
A. Cryo/Cuff brace
A. fracture brace
A. Knee System
A. leg brace
A. pneumatic air stirrup
A. Pneumatic Air Stirrup brace
A. pneumatic walker
A. Rolimeter
A. Swivel-Strap
A. Swivel-Strap brace
A. walking brace

air-contrast study
air-driven
a.-d. bur
a.-d. oscillating saw

Air-Drop chiropractic table
Air-Dyne bicycle
Airex
A. balance pad
A. mat

AirFlex carpal tunnel splint
Air-Flex chiropractic table
air-flow enclosure
Airfoam splint
AirGEL ankle brace
Air-Limb
Airlite
A. alignable ankle block
A. prosthesis

AirLITE support pad
AIROM
active integral range of motion

airplane
a. cast
a. shears
a. splint
a. splint orthosis
a. splint shoulder brace

air-powered cutting drill
Airprene
A. Action knee brace
A. hinged knee prosthesis

Air-Soft Splint
AirStance pylon
Air-Stirrup ankle training brace
Airtrac ambulatory cervical/lumbar traction system
airway management akathisia

NOTES

AIS
    Abbreviated Injury Scale
    adolescent idiopathic scoliosis
Aitken
    A. classification of epiphysial
      fracture
    A. epiphysial fracture classification
    A. femoral deficiency
AJ
    ankle jerk
AJC
    ankle joint complex
AK
    above knee
    applied kinesiology
    AK prosthesis
AKA
    above-knee amputation
akathisia
    airway management a.
AKE
    active knee extension
    AKE test
Akin
    A. bunionectomy
    A. operation
    A. procedure
    A. proximal phalangeal osteotomy
akinesia amnestica
aknemia
Akron midtarsal osteotomy
Akros
    A. extended care mattress
    A. pressure mattress
AkroTech mattress
ALA
    Activity Loss Assessment
ala, pl. **alae**
    a. ilii
    sacral a.
**AlamarBlue osteoblast proliferation
assay**
Alanson amputation
alar
    a. bone
    a. cartilage
    a. chest
    a. creaking
    a. crease
    a. dysgenesis
    a. ligament
    a. plate
    a. rim
    a. scapula
    a. screw
    a. spine
alaria

ALARM
    Adjustable Leg and Ankle Repositioning
      Mechanism
alarm cushion
alata
    scapula a.
Albee
    A. acetabuloplasty
    A. bone graft
    A. drill
    A. hip arthrodesis
    A. lumbar spinal fusion
    A. olive-shaped bur
    A. operation
    A. orthopaedic table
    A. osteotome
    A. shelf procedure
Albee-Compere fracture table
Albee-Delbert operation
Albers-Schönberg
    A.-S. disease
    A.-S. marble bone
Albert
    A. achillodynia
    A. disease
    A. knee operation
Alberta Infant Motor Scale (AIMS)
Albinus muscle
Albrecht bone
Albright
    A. disease
    A. dystrophy
    A. hereditary osteodystrophy
    A. syndrome
    A. synovectomy
Albright-Chase arthroplasty
Albright-McCune-Sternberg syndrome
Albunex ultrasound imaging agent
Alcock canal
alcohol
    a. cauterization
    a. fat embolism syndrome
    a. injection
    a. neurolysis
alcoholic neuropathy
Alcon
    A. Closure System
    A. Instrument Delivery System tray
Alden CDI orthotic
aldolase
aldose reductase inhibitor
Alexander
    A. chisel
    A. costal osteotome
    A. costal periosteotome
    A. gouge
    A. periosteal elevator
    A. rasp

A. technique
A. view
Alexander-Farabeuf
A.-F. periosteotome
A.-F. rasp
alexia
Alexian Brothers overhead frame
algesimeter
Aly a.
Björnström a.
Alginate dressing
algiomotor
algiomuscular
AlgiSite Alginate wound dressing
algodystrophy syndrome
AlgoMed infusion system
algometer
algoneurodystrophy
algorithm
injury a.
Tile polytrauma a.
AliCool splint spray
AliCork Foot Orthosis
AliDeep massage cream
alien hand sign
aligner
Charnley femoral inlay a.
femoral a.
patellar a.
tibial a.
alignment
a. abnormality
anatomic a.
angular a.
atlantoaxial a.
colinear a.
dynamic a.
extramedullary a.
foot a.
a. of fracture fragment
a. guide
a. guide rod
a. index
integrity and a.
a. measurement
optimal a.
patellar a.
patellofemoral a.
a. pin
poor a.
rotational a.
static a.

talocrural a.
tibiofemoral a.
toe a.
torsional a.
transfemoral a.
a. of vertebral bodies
AliMed
A. Conductive Patient Shifter
A. diabetic night splint
A. hemi arm sling
A. insert
A. putty
A. sensor floor mat
A. turnbuckle elbow splint
A. wrist/thumb support
AliMed-Freedom arthritis support
alimentary osteopathy
Aliplast
A. blank
A. custom-molded foot orthosis
A. insole
A. pad
Alisoft splinting material
AliStrap
Alivium
A. implant metal
A. implant metal prosthesis
alkaline phosphatase
alkaloid
Alkphase-B immunoassay
ALL
anterior longitudinal ligament
all-alumina socket
Allen
A. arthroscopic elbow positioner
A. arthroscopic knee positioner
A. arthroscopic wrist positioner
A. Diagnostic Module
A. hand/arm surgery table
A. head screwdriver
A. maneuver
A. open reduction of calcaneal
   fracture
A. reduction
A. shoulder arthroscopy
A. shoulder/wrist arthroscopy
   traction system
A. sign
A. stirrup
A. test
A. wrench
Allen-Brown prosthesis

NOTES

Allender vertical laminar flow room
Allen-Ferguson Galveston pelvic fixation
Allen-Kocher clamp
allergenic arthritis
Allevyn
    A. Island dressing
    A. wound dressing
Allgöwer
    A. apparatus
    A. stitch
    A. suture technique
Alliance rehabilitation system
alligator
    a. bone-reduction forceps
    a. grasping forceps
all-inside repair
Allis
    A. clamp
    A. maneuver
    A. sign
    A. test
    A. tissue forceps
Allman
    A. acromioclavicular injury
      classification
    A. modification of Evans ankle
      reconstruction
all-median nerve hand
AlloAnchor RC allograft device
allodynia
    heat a.
Allofit acetabular cup system
Allofix
    A. freeze-dried bone
    A. freeze-dried cortical bone pin
allogenic, allogeneic
    antigen-extracted a. (AAA)
    a. bone graft
    a. lyophilized bone graft implant
      material
allograft
    Accugraft a.
    acetabular a.
    bone a.
    bone-tendon-bone a.
    a. bone vise
    a. coronary artery disease
    femoral cortical ring a.
    femoral diaphysial a.
    freeze-dried cancellous a.
    fresh frozen a.
    HTO wedge human donor tissue a.
    a. iliac bone
    intercalary diaphysial a.
    large composite a.
    a. ligament replacement
    MTE a.
    napkin ring calcar a.

    osteoarticular a.
    osteochondral a.
    a. reconstruction of fibular
      collateral ligament
    Red Cross freeze-dried a.
    shell a.
    tendon-bone a.
    a. transplantation
allograft-host junction
AlloGrip bone vice
AlloGro bone graft material
alloimplant
AlloMatrix
    A. bone graft putty
    A. injectable putty
allopathic medicine
alloplastic
    a. graft
    a. material
Allo-Pro hip system
all-or-none law
alloy
    cobalt-based a.
    cobalt-chromium a.
    Eligoy metal a.
    stainless steel a.
    Ti-Nidium a.
    titanium a.
    Vitallium a.
    Wood a.
All Poly Deltafit keel
all-polyethylene socket
Allport retractor
All-Purpose
    A.-P. Boot (APB)
All-Tronics scanner
all-ulnar nerve hand
Allurion foot prosthesis
Alm wound retractor
Alouette
    A. amputation
    A. operation
ALP
    ankle ligament protector
    ALP Plus ankle brace
Alpers syndrome
alpha
    a. antagonist
    A. Chymar
    a. chymotrypsin
    A. cushion liner
    A. flat sheet
    a. index
    A. suction attachment block kit
alpha-adrenergic blocking agent
alpha-a$_2$-plasmin inhibitor
alphabet board

alpha-BSM
> a.-BSM bone repair material
> a.-BSM bone substitute material

alphaprodine

AlphaStar table

alpha-sympathomimetic

Alphatec
> A. mini lag-screw system
> A. small fragment system

ALPS
> anterior locking plate system
> Amset ALPS
> ALPS EasyLiner

ALPSA
> anterior labrum periosteal sleeve avulsion
> ALPSA lesion

Alps CustomPro custom liner

ALRI
> anterolateral rotary instability
> ALRI test

ALS
> amyotrophic lateral sclerosis
> anterolateral sclerosis

Alsberg
> A. angle
> A. triangle

alta
> A. advance tibial/humeral rod
> A. cancellous screw
> A. CFX reconstruction od
> A. condylar buttress plate
> A. cortical screw
> A. cross-locking screw
> A. distal fracture plate
> A. lag screw
> A. modular trauma system
> patella a.
> A. supracondylar screw
> A. tibial-humeral rod
> A. tibial nail
> A. transverse screw

altered
> a. intervertebral mechanics
> a. regional mechanics
> a. sensation

alternating
> a. pressure pad
> a. range of motion (ARM)

alternative
> graft material a.
> a. medicine

altitude syndrome

altitudinal anopsia

Alumafoam splint

alumina
> a. bioceramic joint replacement
> a. cemented total hip prosthesis
> a. ceramic

alumina-alumina total hip replacement prosthesis

alumina-on-alumina prosthesis

aluminum
> a. bridge splint
> a. contouring template set
> a. fence splint
> a. finger cot splint
> a. foam splint
> a. hand splint
> implant alloy a.
> a. master rod
> a. oxide arthroplasty material
> a. oxide ceramic coating
> a. toxicity
> a. wire splint

Alvarado
> A. collateral ligament protector
> A. knee holder
> A. legholder
> A. Orthopedic Research

Alvar condylar bolt

alveolar
> a. bone fracture
> a. osteitis
> a. rhabdomyosarcoma
> a. soft-part sarcoma
> a. supporting bone ankle bone

Aly algesimeter

ALZET continuous infusion osmotic pump

Alznner orthotic

amalgam

AMBI
> AMBI compression hip screw system
> AMBI fixation
> AMBI hip screw
> AMBI wrist brace

ambidextrous

AMBRI
> atraumatic, multidirectional, bilateral rehabilitation inferior
> AMBRI procedure

ambulate with assistance

NOTES

ambulation
    assisted a.
    brace-free a.
    crutch a.
    functional a.
    a. index
    prosthetic a.
    a. skills
    a. training orthosis
ambulator
    Apex a.
    A. biomechanical footwear
    A. Bio-Rocker sole
    A. Chukka Boot
    A. conform footwear
    A. H1200 healing shoe
ambulatory
    a. function
    A. shoe
    a. status
    a. traction
AMC total wrist prosthesis
AMD
    arthroscopic microdiskectomy
    articular motion device
AME
    American Medical Electronics
    Austin Medical Equipment
    AME bone growth stimulator
    AME microcurrent TENS unit
    AME pin site shield
amebiasis
Amefa Flatware
amelanotic
amelia
    brachial a.
    complete a.
amenorrhea
    athletic a.
    exercise-induced a.
American
    A. Academy of Orthopaedic Surgeons (AAOS)
    A. Academy of Orthopaedic Surgeons classification of acetabular deficiency
    A. Academy of Orthopaedic Surgeons/Hip Society questionnaire
    A. Academy of Orthopedic Surgeons Pediatrics Outcomes Instrument
    A. Board of Certification of Orthotics and Prosthetics
    A. Board of Physical Therapy Specialists
    A. Chiropractic College of Radiology adjusting table
    A. College of Rheumatology (ACR)
    A. College of Sports Medicine (ACSM)
    A. Hand Prosthetics (AHP)
    A. Heyer-Schulte chin prosthesis
    A. Heyer-Schulte-Hinderer malar prosthesis
    A. Heyer-Schulte Radovan tissue expander prosthesis
    A. Joint Commission on Cancer staging systems
    A. Knee Society
    A. Knee Society score
    A. leech
    A. Medical Electronics (AME)
    A. Musculoskeletal Tumor Society rating scale
    A. Orthopaedic Association (AOA)
    A. Orthopaedic Foot and Ankle Society (AOFAS)
    A. Orthopaedic Foot and Ankle Society Ankle-Hindfoot Scale
    A. Rheumatism Association (ARA)
    A. Rheumatism Association classification
    A. Seating Access-O-Matic bed
    A. Shoulder and Elbow Surgeons rating
    A. Shoulder and Elbow Surgeons scale
    A. shoulder and elbow system (ASES)
    A. Society of Anesthesiologists physical status classification system
    A. Society for Testing and Materials (ASTM)
    A. Spinal Cord Injury Association classification
    A. Spinal Injury Association (ASIA)
    A. Spinal Injury Association impairment scale
AMFH
    angiomatoid malignant fibrous histiocytoma
Amfit
    A. custom orthosis
    A. digitizer
    A. orthotic
Amico drill
Amigo mechanical wheelchair
amikacin
aminoglycoside
aminoglycoside-impregnated methyl methacrylate bead
aminophylline

Amipaque contrast medium
AMK
    anatomic modular knee
        AMK fixed bearing knee system
        AMK total knee system
        AMK unconstrained prosthesis
AML
    anatomic medullary locking
        AML Plus prosthesis
        AML socket
        AML Tang femoral prosthesis
        AML total hip prosthesis
        AML total hip system
        AML trial hip component
AM-MI orthopaedic table
amnestica
    akinesia a.
**amniotic deformity, adhesion, mutilation
  (ADAM)**
amorphous eosinophilic material
Amoss sign
amphiarthrodial disk
amphiarthrosis
amphidiarthrodial joint
Amplatz anchor system
amplifier
    Omniace RT3200N
    electromyographic a.
amplitude
    high velocity low a.
amplitude-summation
    a.-s. interferential current
    a.-s. interferential current therapy
    (ASICT)
Ampoxen sling
amputation
    above-elbow a. (AEA)
    above-knee a. (AKA)
    AE a.
    Alanson a.
    Alouette a.
    Anderson a.
    aperiosteal a.
    BE a.
    Béclard a.
    below-elbow a. (BEA)
    below-knee a. (BKA)
    Berger interscapular a.
    Bier a.
    bilateral a.
    bloodless a.
    border ray a.

Boyd ankle a.
Bunge a.
Burgess below-knee a.
button toe a.
Callander a.
Carden a.
central ray a.
cervix a.
Chopart hindfoot a.
cinematic a.
cineplastic a.
circular open a.
circular supracondylar a.
closed flap a.
coat-sleeve a.
complete a.
consecutive a.
a. in contiguity
a. in continuity
corporectomy a.
cutaneous a.
diaclastic a.
Dieffenbach a.
digital a.
disarticular a.
double-flap a.
dry a.
Dupuytren a.
eccentric a.
elliptical a.
end-bearing a.
excentric a.
Farabeuf a.
femoral head a.
fingertip a.
fishmouth a.
flap a.
flapless a.
forearm a.
forefoot digital a.
forequarter a.
Gordon-Taylor hindquarter a.
great toe a.
Gritti a.
Gritti-Stokes a.
guillotine a.
Guyon a.
Hancock a.
hand a.
Hey a.
hindquarter a.
immediate a.

NOTES

amputation *(continued)*
    incomplete a.
    index-ray a.
    interilioabdominal a.
    interinnominoabdominal a.
    intermediary a.
    intermediate a.
    interpelviabdominal a.
    interphalangeal a.
    interscapular a.
    interscapulothoracic forequarter a.
    intrapyretic a.
    Jaboulay a.
    kineplastic a.
    King-Steelquist hindquarter a.
    Kirk distal thigh a.
    knee disarticulation a.
    a. knife
    Krukenberg a.
    Langenbeck a.
    Larrey a.
    Le Fort a.
    linear a.
    Lisfranc a.
    lower extremity a. (LEA)
    Mackenzie a.
    Maisonneuve a.
    major a.
    Malgaigne a.
    McKittrick transmetatarsal a.
    mediotarsal a.
    metacarpal a.
    middle finger a.
    midthigh a.
    Mikulicz-Vladimiroff a.
    minor a.
    mixed a.
    modified Boyd a.
    multiple ray a.
    musculocutaneous a.
    nonreplantable a.
    oblique a.
    one-stage a.
    open a.
    osteoplastic a.
    oval a.
    partial hand a.
    pathologic a.
    periosteoplastic a.
    phalangophalangeal a.
    Pirogoff a.
    primary a.
    provisional a.
    pulp a.
    quadruple a.
    racket a.
    ray a.
    rectangular a.
    replantable a.
    a. retractor
    Ricard a.
    a. saw
    secondary a.
    semicircular flap a.
    shoulder a.
    Sorondo-Ferré hindquarter a.
    spontaneous a.
    Stokes a.
    a. stump
    a. stump neuroma
    subastragalar a.
    subperiosteal a.
    supracondylar a.
    supramalleolar open a.
    Syme ankle disarticulation a.
    tarsal a.
    tarsometatarsal a.
    tarsotibial a.
    Teale a.
    tertiary a.
    through-the-knee a.
    toe a.
    transcarpal a.
    transcondylar a.
    transfemoral a.
    transfixation a.
    transhumeral a.
    transiliac a.
    translumbar a.
    transmetacarpal a.
    transmetatarsal a. (TMA)
    transpelvic a.
    transphalangeal a.
    transtibial a.
    transverse a.
    traumatic a.
    traverse a.
    Tripier a.
    Vladimiroff-Mikulicz a.
    Wagner modification of Syme a.
    Wagner two-stage Syme a.

amputation-related bone pain

amputee
    a. athlete
    a. cushion
    transfemoral a.

Amrex
    A. muscle stimulator
    A. SynchroSonic muscle
      stimulation-ultrasound
    A. therapeutic ultrasound

AMS
    antimigration system
    AMS intramedullary fixation

Amset
    A. ALPS

A

A. ALPS anterior locking plate system
A. R-F fixation system
A. R-F rod
A. R-F screw

Amspacher-Messenbaugh
A.-M. closing wedge osteotomy
A.-M. technique

Amstutz
A. cemented hip prosthesis
A. femoral component
A. reattachment
A. resurfacing
A. resurfacing operation
A. resurfacing technique
A. total hip replacement

Amstutz-Wilson osteotomy

AMT
active motion testing

AMX knee brace
amyloid neuropathy
amyloidosis
beta-2-microglobulin a.
skeletal a.

amyoplasia congenita
amyostasia
amyostatic
amyosthenia
amyosthenic
amyotaxy
amyotonia
a. congenita
Oppenheim a.

amyotrophia
amyotrophic
a. acropathy
a. lateral sclerosis (ALS)

amyotrophy
Aran-Duchenne a.
diabetic a.
hemiplegic a.
neuralgic a.
neuritic a.
primary progressive a.
progressive nuclear a.
progressive spinal a.
syphilitic a.

amyous

ANA
antinuclear antibody

anabolic agent

anaerobic
a. bacterium
a. cellulitis
a. exercise
a. infection
a. osteomyelitis
a. threshold (AT)

anal
a. reflex
a. triangle
a. wink

analgesia
patient-controlled a. (PCA)

analgesic
nonnarcotic a.

analgia

analog
a. neurotrophic factor
visual a. scale

analogous signal detector

analysis, pl. **analyses**
activity a.
activity-pattern a.
bioelectrical impedance a. (BIA)
biomechanical a.
cerebrospinal fluid a.
chiropractic a.
computerized musculoskeletal a.
deformity a.
DeLee radiographic a.
EMED gait a.
footprint a.
force plate foot a.
Fourier a.
frequency a.
F-Scan foot pressure a.
gait a.
high-resolution a.
job task a. (JTA)
Khan-Lewis phonological a.
kinetic gait a.
lateral flexion dynamic visual a.
muscle a.
occipital-fiber a.
peak-pressure a.
pedobarographic a.
plumb-line a.
postural a.
roentgen stereophotogrammetric a. (RSA)
spinal a.
three-dimensional a.

NOTES

23

analysis *(continued)*
    trapezius fiber a.
    video-dimensional a. (VDA)
    video-gate a.

analyzer
    Arthrodial Protractor range-of-
      motion a.
    CA-6000 spine motion a.
    Elite Plus motion a.
    Futrex body fat a.
    Metrecom spinal a.
    NordicTrack Motion A.
    Pediatric Ultrasound Bone A.
    Sam Jr. posture a.
    Stride A.
    Tanita Professional Body
      Composition A.

Anametric
    A. total knee prosthesis
    A. total knee system

anaphylaxis
    exercise-induced a.
    latex a.

anapophysis

anarrhexis

anastomosis, pl. **anastomoses**
    extradural a.
    fishmouth a.
    flexor tendon a.
    gastrointestinal a., pl. anastomoses
      (GIA)
    intradural a.
    Ma-Griffith end-to-end a.
    Ma-Griffith tendon a.
    Martin-Gruber a.
    microvascular surgical a.
    peroneus brevis to longus a.
    Riche-Cannieu a.

anatomic
    a. alignment
    a. axis
    a. barrier
    a. fracture reduction principle
    a. hook
    a. insertion
    a. intermetatarsal angle
    a. landmark
    a. leg length inequality
    a. medullary locking (AML)
    a. medullary locking hip system
    a. modular knee (AMK)
    a. neck fracture
    a. nerve trunk
    a. plane
    porous-coated a. (PCA)
    a. porous replacement (APR)
    a. porous replacement hemispheric
      acetabular component

    A. Precoat hip prosthesis
    a. reduction
    a. short leg
    a. snuffbox
    a. surface prosthesis

anatomical
    a. classification system of Severin
    a. vertical

anatomically
    a. based exercise system
    a. graduated component (AGC)

anatomopathological study

Anatomotor traction/massage table

anatomy
    cervicothoracic pedicle a.
    cross-sectional a.
    Daseler-Anson classification of
      plantaris muscle a.
    designed after natural a. (DANA)
    developmental a.
    dorsalis pedis artery a.
    neurovascular a.
    pedicle a.

anchor
    Acufex bioabsorbable suture a.
    Acufex T-Fix suture a.
    Acumed suture a.
    Anchorlok soft tissue a.
    Anspach suture a.
    Arthrex bone a.
    Arthrex TwistLoc suture a.
    AxyaWeld bone a.
    Bio-Anchor suture a.
    Bio-FASTak a.
    Biologically Quiet Mini-Screw
      suture a.
    Biomet bone a.
    Bio-Phase suture a.
    BioROC a.
    BioSphere suture a.
    Bone Bullet suture a.
    Bone Button orthopaedic suture a.
    buttress and button a.
    Catera suture a.
    Corkscrew suture a.
    CurvTek drill bone a.
    E-Z ROC a.
    FASTak suture a.
    FASTIN suture a.
    FASTIN threaded a.
    GII Snap-Pak a.
    GLS suture a.
    Harpoon suture a.
    a. hole
    Howmedica bone a.
    implantable bone a.
    Innovasive bone a.
    intraosseous suture a.

Isola spinal implant system a.
Linvatec bone a.
MicroLite suture a.
Mini Bio-Phase suture a.
Mini GLS a.
Mini-Revo Screws suture a.
Mini-ROC a.
Mitek absorbable a.
Mitek bone a.
Mitek FASTIN threaded a.
Mitek GII easy a.
Mitek GL a.
Mitek knotless a.
Mitek ligament a.
Mitek micro a.
Mitek Mini GLS a.
Mitek Panalok RC a.
Mitek rotator cuff a.
Mitek Tacit threaded a.
Ogden bone a.
Orthofix Ogden a.
Panalok absorbable a.
PLA a.
a. plate
PLLA a.
Revo suture a.
ROC a.
RotorloC absorbable rotator cuff
    suture a.
a. screw
Sherlock threaded suture a.
a. splint
Stealth a.
suture a.
Tacit threaded a.
Therap-Loop door a.
traction a.
UltraFix MicroMite suture a.
UltraFix RC suture a.
UltraSorb suture a.
Wright Medical bone a.
Zimmer-Statak a.
anchorage-dependent growth
anchoring
    a. hole
    a. peg
    a. point
    a. tendon
Anchorlok
    A. soft tissue anchor
    A. soft tissue suture anchor system
anchovy procedure

ancient tuberculous arthritis
ancillary muscle group
anconeal
anconeus
    a. arthroplasty
    a. muscle
anconitis
anconoid
Anderson
    A. acetabular prosthesis
    A. amputation
    A. ankle fusion
    A. distractor
    A. fixation apparatus
    A. fixation device
    A. leg-lengthening apparatus
    A. leg-lengthening device
    A. medial-lateral grind test
    A. modification of Berndt-Harty
        classification
    A. operation
    A. pin fixation
    A. screw placement technique
    A. splint
    A. system
    A. tibial lengthening
    A. tibial pseudarthrosis
        classification
    A. traction
**Anderson-D'Alonzo odontoid fracture
    classification**
Anderson-Fowler
    A.-F. anterior calcaneal osteotomy
        pes planus
    A.-F. calcaneal displacement
        osteotomy
    A.-F. procedure
Anderson-Green growth prediction
Anderson-Hutchins
    A.-H. operation
    A.-H. technique
    A.-H. unstable tibial shaft fracture
Anderson-Neivert osteotome
Andersson hip status system
André Thomas sign
Andrews
    A. anterior instability test
    A. gouge
    A. iliotibial band reconstruction
    A. iliotibial band tenodesis
    A. lateral tenodesis
    A. osteotome

NOTES

Andrews *(continued)*
    A. spinal surgery frame
    A. SST-3000 spinal surgery table
    A. technique
anemia
    blood loss a.
    Fanconi a.
    foot-strike hemolysis a.
    iron-deficiency a.
    sickle-cell a.
    sports a.
anergy
aneroid gauge
anesthesia
    ankle block a.
    Bier block a.
    bulbar a.
    compression a.
    continuous intravenous regional a.
      (CIVRA)
    crash induction of a.
    digital block a.
    dissociative a.
    epidural a.
    field block a.
    gauntlet a.
    general endotracheal a.
    glove a.
    glove-and-stocking a.
    graded spinal a.
    hypotensive a.
    inhalation a.
    intrathecal a.
    intravenous block a.
    intravenous regional a. (IVRA)
    local standby a.
    lumbar a.
    Madajet XL local a.
    Mayo block a.
    patient-controlled a. (PCA)
    peripheral nerve block a.
    regional a.
    ring block a.
    saddle block a.
    short-acting block a.
    spinal a.
    supraclavicular brachial block a.
    tactile a.
    thermal a.
    toe block a.
anesthetic
    foot a.
aneurysm
    arterial a.
    benign bone a.
    brachial artery a.
    clavicular fracture a.

    false a.
    Park a.
aneurysmal bone cyst (ABC)
aneurysmorrhaphy
angel
    a. wing
    a. wing guide
Angell
    A. James dissector
    A. James hypophysectomy forceps
Anghelescu sign
angina cruris
angioblastoma
angiodysplasia
angioendotheliomatosis
angiofibroblastic
    a. hyperplasia tendinosis
    a. proliferation
angiofibroma
angiogram
    biplane a.
angiography
    digital subtraction a. (DSA)
    spinal cord a.
    vertebral a.
angiokeratoma
    diffuse a.
angioleiomyoma
angiolipoma
angioma
    cirsoid a.
angiomatoid malignant fibrous
   histiocytoma (AMFH)
angiomatosis
    skeletal-extraskeletal a.
angiosarcoma
angiosclerotica
    dysbasia a.
    myasthenia a.
angiospasm
angiotropic lymphoma
angle
    acetabular a.
    acromial a.
    Alsberg a.
    anatomic intermetatarsal a.
    antegonial a.
    anteroposterior talocalcaneal a.
      (APTC)
    antetorsion a.
    arch a.
    articular facet a.
    articular set a.
    Baumann a.
    Beatson combined ankle a.
    bimalleolar a.
    Böhler calcaneal a.
    Böhler lumbosacral a.

Bowman a.
Bragg a.
C a.
calcaneal inclination a.
calcaneal pitch a. (CPA)
calcaneal-second metatarsal angle inclination a.
calcaneoplantar a.
calcaneotibial a.
capital epiphysial a.
capitolunate a.
carrying a.
CCD a.
CE a.
center-edge a.
central collodiaphysial a.
cervicothoracic pedicle a.
Citelli a.
Clarke arch a.
Cobb scoliosis a.
Codman a.
condylar a.
condylar plateau a. (CPA)
congruence a.
a. of convergence
costal a.
costolumbar a.
costophrenic a.
costosternal a.
costovertebral a. (CVA)
craniofacial a.
cuboid abduction a.
cuboid declination a.
declination a.
a. of declination
distal articular set a. (DASA)
distal metatarsal articular a. (DMAA)
a. of divergence
dorsiflexion a. (DFA)
dorsoplantar talometatarsal a.
dorsoplantar talonavicular a.
Drennan metaphysial-epiphysial a.
elevation a.
Engel a.
Euler a.
eulerian a.
facet a.
femoral-trunk a.
femorotibial a. (FTA)
Ferguson sacral base a.
a. finder

finger a.
first–fifth intermetatarsal a.
first–second intermetatarsal a.
flexion a.
foot a.
foot progression a. (FPA)
Fowler-Philip a.
functional intermetatarsal a.
a. of gait
Garden a.
Gissane a.
gonial a.
a. of greatest extension (AGE)
a. of greatest flexion (AGF)
hallux valgus a. (HVA)
hallux valgus interphalangeus a.
head-shaft a.
Hibbs metatarsocalcaneal a.
Hilgenreiner a.
hip joint a. (HJA)
humeroulnar a.
inclination a.
a. of incongruity
increased carrying a.
inferior a.
intermetatarsal a. (IMA)
intrascaphoid a.
a. isometric testing
Kite a.
Konstram a.
kyphotic a.
Laurin lateral patellofemoral a.
Levine Drennan a.
Lisfranc articular set a. (LASA)
Lovibond a.
Ludovici a.
Ludwig a.
lumbosacral joint a.
mandibular a.
manubriosternal a.
a. of Mary
Meary metatarsotalar a.
medial proximal tibial a.
mediolateral radiocarpal a.
Merchant congruence a.
metaphysial-diaphysial a.
metaphysial-epiphysial a.
metatarsal phalangeal fifth a.
metatarsocalcaneal a.
metatarsocuneiform a.
metatarsotalar a.
metatarsus adductus a.

NOTES

angle *(continued)*
metatarsus primus declination a.
Mikulicz a.
navicular to first metatarsal a.
neck-shaft a. (NSA)
negative congruence a.
neutral a.
occipitocervical a.
Pauwels a.
pedicle axis a.
pelvic a.
pelvic-femoral a.
physial a.
plantar metatarsal a.
popliteal a.
proximal articular facet a.
proximal articular set a. (PASA)
Q a.
quadriceps a.
quadriceps neutral a. (QNA)
radiocarpal a.
resting forefoot supination a.
a. of retroversion
rib-vertebral a.
sacral base a.
sacrofemoral a.
sacrohorizontal a.
sacrovertebral a.
sagittal pedicle a.
salient a.
scapholunate a.
set a.
Sharp acetabular a.
slip a.
Southwick lateral slip a.
spinographic a.
a. splint
sternoclavicular a.
subscapular a.
sulcus a.
talar axis–first metatarsal base a.
   (TAMBA)
talar declination a.
talar-tilt a.
talocalcaneal a.
talocrural a.
talometatarsal a.
talonavicular a.
tarsometatarsal a.
thigh-foot a. (TFA)
a. of thoracic inclination
tibiofemoral a. (TFA)
tibiotalar a.
toe-out a.
a. of torsion
Toygar a.
transverse pedicle a.
tuber a.

tuber-joint a.
tuberosity joint a.
ulnohumeral a.
valgus a.
varus MTP a.
a. of Wiberg
Wiberg center edge a.
Wiberg fracture a.
Wiltze a.

angled
a. arthroscope
a. awl
a. bearing insert
a. blade plate fixation
a. DeBakey clamp
a. dissector
a. jaw rongeur
a. Lowman-type bone clamp
a. pituitary rongeur
a. probe
a. rasp
a. Scoville curette

angled-down forceps

angled-up forceps

angry backfiring C nociceptor

angular
a. acceleration
a. alignment
a. bone rongeur
a. curvature
a. deviation
a. displacement
a. elevator
a. hinge clamp
a. momentum
a. motion
a. position
a. process of orbit
a. spine
a. tilt
a. velocity

angulated fracture

angulation
anterior a.
apex anterior a.
apex dorsal a.
apex posterior a.
cephalic a.
a. deformity
degrees of valgus a.
degrees of varus a.
forefoot a.
kyphotic a.
limb length a.
a. motion
a. osteotomy
plantar a.
posttraumatic a.

radius of a.
screw a.
spinal a.
valgus a.
varus-valgus a.
angulatory malunion
Angus-Cowell scale
anhidrosis, anidrosis
anhydrous ethanol
animal-assisted therapy (AAT)
animal beanbag exerciser
anion transport inhibitor
anisomelia
anisospondyly
anisotropy
Ank-L-Aid brace
ankle
a. arthrodesis
a. arthrography
a. arthroplasty
a. arthroscopy
autologous reverse graft to a.
a. block
a. block anesthesia
a. bone
Buechel-Pappas total a.
a. clonus
a. clonus test
a. contracture orthosis
C Stance a.
a. disarticulation
disk of a.
a. disk device
a. disk training
a. dislocation
a. dorsiflexion range of motion (ADROM)
a. dorsiflexion test
a. effusion
a. equinus
a. eversion
a. exercise machine
a. exerciser
footballer's a.
fused a.
a. fusion
a. guard
a. hitch
a. immobilizer
a. impingement
a. infectious arthritis
a. inferior transverse ligament

a. injury
a. instability
internal fixation compression arthrodesis of the a.
a. inversion-eversion range of motion
Irvine a.
A. Isolator
A. Isolator ankle rehabilitator
A. Isolator foot and ankle exerciser
a. jerk (AJ)
a. jerk reflex
a. joint
a. joint complex (AJC)
a. joint leg-curl
a. laxity
a. ligament protector (ALP)
a. ligament protector brace
a. loose body
a. magnet
a. mortise
a. mortise diastasis
a. mortise fracture
a. mortise widening
Multi Axis A.
neuropathic a.
New Jersey a.
a. orthosis (AO)
a. osteoarthritis
a. osteomyelitis
a. prosthesis
a. reconstruction
a. rehab pump
R-HAB lighter weight a.
a. rheumatoid arthritis
Rincoe human action bionic a.
a. scoring system of Baird and Jackson
snowboarder's a.
a. sprain
a. stability
a. stabilizer
a. stabilizing orthosis (ASO)
a. stabilizing orthosis support
a. stirrup brace
a. systolic pressure
tailor's a.
a. traction bandage
transmalleolar a.
USMC multiaxis a.

NOTES

ankle *(continued)*
    a. weight
    Wiltse osteotomy of a.
ankle-brachial pressure ratio
ankle-foot
    a.-f. electrogoniometer
    a.-f. orthosis (AFO)
    a.-f. orthosis brace sock
    a.-f. orthotic splint
    a.-f. plastic orthosis
ankle-hindfoot scale
ankle-level arteriotomy
ankle-pump exercise
AnkleTough
    A. ankle rehabilitation system
    A. Rehab System
ankylodactylia
ankylodactyly
ankylopoietic
ankylose
ankylosing
    a. hyperostosis
    a. spinal hyperostosis
    a. spinal stenosis
    a. spondylitis
ankylosis
    artificial a.
    bony a.
    capsular a.
    carpal bone fracture a.
    extraarticular a.
    extracapsular a.
    false a.
    fibrous a.
    intracapsular a.
    ligamentous a.
    operative a.
    partial a.
    shoulder a.
    spurious a.
    true a.
    unsound a.
    vertebral a.
ankylotic
anlage
    cartilaginous a.
    fibular a.
    radial head a.
    ulnar a.
ANNA-DOTE Positioning Support
Annandale operation
Ann Arbor double towel clamp
anneal
annular *(var. of* anular)
annulare
    limbus a.
    subcutaneous granuloma a.
annulotomy

annulus *(var. of* anulus)
anodal block
anomalous
    a. fibular nutrient artery
    a. insertion
anomaly
    congenital a.
    facet a.
    hand a.
    Kimerle a.
    Poland a.
    root a.
    vertebral abnormality, anal
      imperforation, tracheoesophageal
      fistula, and radial, ray, or
      renal a.'s (VATER)
    vertebral segmentation a.
anonychia
anopsia
    altitudinal a.
anoscope
anosteoplasia
anoxia
anserine
    a. bursa
    a. bursitis
anserinus
    pes a.
Anspach
    A. Cement Eater
    A. cementome
    A. 65K Universal instrument
      system
    A. power drill
    A. reamer
    A. suture anchor
antagonist
    alpha a.
    opiate receptor a.
    opioid a.
    reversal of a. (ROA)
antagonistic
    a. muscle
    a. reflex
antalgic
    a. gait
    a. lean
    a. limp
anteater nose
antebrachial
    a. cutaneous nerve
    a. fascia
    a. fascial graft
antebrachium
antecedent sign
antecubital fossa
anteflex
anteflexion

antegonial angle
antegrade
- a. femoral nail
- a. method
- a. nailing

antegrade/retrograde compression nail
antenatal dislocation
antenna procedure
Antense antitension device
anterior
- a. acromioplasty
- a. acromioplasty approach
- a. acute flexion elbow splint
- a. angulation
- a. ankle impingement
- a. ankle shift operation
- a. aspiration
- a. atlantooccipital membrane
- a. atlantoodontoid interval
- a. axillary approach
- a. axillary line (AAL)
- a. bending moment
- a. calcaneal osteotomy
- a. calcaneal process fracture
- a. capsule
- a. capsulectomy
- a. capsulolabral reconstruction (ACLR)
- a. capsulotomy
- a. cavus
- a. cervical body fusion
- a. cervical cord syndrome
- a. cervical diskectomy and fusion (ACDF)
- a. cervical fascia
- a. cervical fusion (ACF)
- a. cervical plate (ACP)
- a. cervical plate fixation system (ACFS)
- a. cervicothoracic junction surgery
- a. collateral ligament
- a. column disruption
- a. column fracture
- a. column osteosynthesis
- a. column of spine
- a. commissure-posterior commissure (AC-PC)
- a. compartment
- a. compartment syndrome (ACS)
- a. construct
- a. cord compression
- a. cord impingement
- a. corpectomy
- a. correction
- a. cortex penetration
- a. cruciate
- a. cruciate deficit knee
- a. cruciate ligament (ACL)
- a. cruciate sprain
- a. curvature
- a. distraction instrumentation
- a. drainage
- a. drawer sign
- a. drawer stress radiograph
- a. drawer test (ADT)
- a. epineurotomy
- a. equinus
- a. extensile approach
- a. fiber-region
- a. fibular ligament
- a. foot draw sign
- a. forceps
- a. glenoid labrum
- a. glide
- a. heel
- a. hiatal sign
- a. hip dislocation
- a. hip release
- a. horn
- a. horn cell
- a. horn meniscal tear
- a. horn of spinal cord
- a. humeral line
- a. iliofemoral technique
- a. impingement spur
- a. inferior iliac spine (AIIS)
- a. innominate
- a. innominate rotation
- a. internal fixation
- a. internal fixation device
- a. joint impingement
- a. jugular vein
- a. Kostuik-Harrington distraction system
- a. kyphosis
- a. labrum periosteal sleeve avulsion (ALPSA)
- a. locking plate system (ALPS)
- a. longitudinal ligament (ALL)
- a. long toe flexor
- a. lower cervical spine surgery
- a. lumbar interbody fusion
- a. lumbar vertebral interbody fusion

NOTES

31

anterior *(continued)*
- a. maxillary spine
- a. medial ankle ligament
- a. meniscofemoral ligament
- a. metallic fixation
- a. metatarsal arch
- a. myocutaneous flap
- a. neutralization
- a. oblique ligament (AOL)
- a. oblique meniscal tear
- a. occipitocervical arthrodesis
- a. occipitocervical spine
- a. pelvic tilt
- a. plate fixation
- a. plate system (APS)
- a. portal
- a. and posterior (AP)
- a. and posterior fusion
- a. pronator teres
- a. quadriceps musculocutaneous flap technique
- a. quadrilateral triplane frame
- a. radial collateral artery
- a. recurrent tibial artery
- a. retroperitoneal decompression
- a. retroperitoneal flank approach
- a. sacrococcygeal ligament
- a. sacroiliac joint plate
- a. sacroiliac ligament
- a. screw fixation
- a. shear
- a. shin splint
- a. short-segment stabilization
- a. shoulder dislocation
- a. shoulder instability
- a. shoulder release
- a. sliding tibial graft
- a. slot graft arthrodesis
- a. soft tissue impingement
- a. spinal artery
- a. spinal fixation
- a. spinal fusion
- a. spinal line
- a. spinocerebellar tract
- a. spinothalamic tract
- a. spurring
- a. stabilization procedure
- a. sternoclavicular joint
- a. sternomastoid approach
- a. superior iliac spine (ASIS)
- a. surgical exposure
- a. talar translation (ATT)
- a. talofibular ligament (ATFL)
- a. talofibular ligament rupture
- a. talofibular sprain
- a. talotibial ligament
- a. talus shift
- a. tarsal resection
- a. tarsal tendinitis
- a. thoracic nerve
- a. tibial artery
- a. tibial compartment syndrome
- a. tibial fasciocutaneous flap
- tibialis a.
- a. tibial margin
- a. tibial nerve
- a. tibial nerve dermatome
- a. tibial sign
- a. tibial spine
- a. tibial tendon
- a. tibial tubercle
- a. tibiofibular ligament
- a. tibiotalar fascicle (ATTF)
- a. tibiotalar ligament
- a. transfer
- a. translation
- a. transthoracic approach
- a. triangle
- a. upper spine
- a. view
- a. Zielke instrumentation

anterior-inferior
- a.-i. capsular ligament dysfunction
- a.-i. compression
- a.-i. dislocation
- a.-i. fusion
- a.-i. glide
- a.-i. movement
- a.-i. tibiofibular ligament

anterior-posterior
- a.-p. compression (APC)
- a.-p. fusion with SSI
- a.-p. glide
- a.-p. listhesis
- a.-p. movement

anterocentral arthroscopic portal
anterodistal
anteroinferior
- a. glenohumeral ligament
- a. portal
- a. spondylolisthesis

anterolateral
- a. approach
- a. capsule
- a. compression fracture
- a. decompression
- a. dislocation
- a. drainage
- a. femorotibial ligament tenodesis
- a. fragment
- a. impingement syndrome
- a. portal
- a. raphe
- a. release
- a. rotary instability (ALRI)

a. rotary knee instability
a. sclerosis (ALS)
anterolateral-anteromedial rotary instability
anterolisthesis
anteromedial
a. bundle
a. capsule
a. drainage
a. glenohumeral ligament
a. humeral head defect
a. incision
a. portal
a. retropharyngeal approach
a. rotary instability
a. tubercle transfer
anteromedial-posteromedial rotary instability
anteroposterior (AP)
a. control orthosis
a. lateral sway
a. stress test
a. talocalcaneal angle (APTC)
a. talocalcaneal divergence
a. tilt
a. translation
anteroproximal
anterosuperior (AS)
a. external ilium movement (ASEx)
a. glenohumeral ligament
a. iliac spine graft
a. ilium major
a. internal ilium movement (ASIn)
anteroventral
antetorsion
a. angle
femoral a.
anteversion
a. determination
femoral a. (FA)
femoral head/neck a.
neutral a.
a. syndrome
anthropometric
a. caliper
a. measurement
a. measuring tape
a. method
a. total hip (ATH)
anthropometry
antibacterial pillow
antibiosis

antibiotic
a. bead pouch
a. and saline solution
antibiotic-impregnated
a.-i. bead
a.-i. polymethyl methacrylate
antibody
AE1, AE3 a.
antihistocompatibility a.
antinuclear a. (ANA)
anticavitation drill
anticentromere
anticoagulant
lupus a.
a. therapy
anticoagulation
prophylactic a.
anticonvulsant therapy
antidecubitus
a. mattress
a. pad
antidromic stimulation
antiembolic
a. position
a. stockings
antiemetic
antifungal (AF)
antigen
antiproliferating cell nuclear a.
carcinoembryonic a. (CEA)
HLA-B27 blood a.
human leukocyte a. (HLA)
human lymphocyte a. (HLA)
transplantation a.
antigen-extracted
a.-e. allogenic (AAA)
a.-e. allogenic bone
antiglide plate
antigravity (AG)
antihistocompatibility antibody
antiinflammatory medication
antimigration system (AMS)
antinuclear
a. antibody (ANA)
a. antibody test
antiosteoclastic agent
antiproliferating cell nuclear antigen
antiprotrusio cage
antipyretic agent
antirotation
a. cable (ARC)
a. device

NOTES

antiseptic
    ACU-dyne a.
    colored a.
    a. solution
Antishear gel sheet
antishock garment
Anti-Shox
    A.-S. foot cushion
    A.-S. heel cup
    A.-S. orthosis
    A.-S. sports orthotic
antistreptolysin-O titer (ASOT)
antitension line
antithrombin III
antithrombotic therapy
antithrust seat
antitipper wheelchair
antitoxin
antituberculosis drug
antivibration glove
anular, annular
    A1–A4 a. pulley
    a. cartilage
    congenital a. band
    a. constricting band syndrome
    a. fiber
    a. fibrosis
    a. groove
    a. injury
    a. ligament
    a. ligament entrapment
    a. ligament of radius
    a. periradial recess
anulospiral ending of muscle spindle
anulus, annulus
    a. fibrosus
anvil
    a. bone
    Bunnell a.
    a. sign
    a. test
any-angle splint
AO
    ankle orthosis
    atlantooccipital
    AO ankle fracture classification
    AO brace
    AO cancellous screw
    AO classification of ankle fracture
    AO compression
    AO compression apparatus
    AO condylar blade plate
    AO contoured T plate
    AO contouring apparatus
    AO cortex screw
    AO drill bit
    AO dynamic compression plate

    AO dynamic compression plate construct
    AO external fixation
    AO femoral distractor
    AO fixateur interne
    AO fixateur interne instrumentation
    AO fracture pattern
    AO group
    AO group shoulder arthrodesis
    AO guidepin
    AO hook plate
    AO internal fixator
    AO lag screw
    AO minifragment set
    AO notched instrumentation
    AO plate bender
    AO procedure
    AO pseudoisochromatic color plate test
    AO reconstruction plate
    AO reduction forceps
    AO screw fixation
    AO semitubular plate
    AO slotted medullary nail
    AO small fragment plate
    AO spinal internal fixation
    AO spongiosa screw
    AO spoon plate
    AO surgical technique
    AO tap
    AO tension band
AOA
    American Orthopaedic Association
    AOA cervical immobilization brace
    AOA halo cervical traction
AO-ASIF
    Arbeitsgemeinschaft für Osteosynthesefragen-Association for the Study of Internal Fixation
    AO-ASIF compression plate
    AO-ASIF compression technique
    AO-ASIF fixateur interne
    AO-ASIF orthopaedic implant
    AO-ASIF screw
AOFAS
    American Orthopaedic Foot and Ankle Society
    AOFAS Hallux Rating system
    AOFAS Lesser Metatarsophalangeal-Interphalangeal Scale (LMIS)
    AOFAS score
AOL
    anterior oblique ligament
AP
    action potential
    anterior and posterior
    anteroposterior
    AP fusion

AP nail
AP supine view
AP translatory motion
aparthrosis
APB
abductor pollicis brevis
All-Purpose Boot
APB Hi All-Purpose Boot
APC
anterior-posterior compression
APD
automated percutaneous diskectomy
ape hand
apelike hand
aperiosteal amputation
Apert
A. acrosyndactyly
A. disease
A. syndrome
aperta
spina bifida a.
aperture pad
apex, pl. **apices**
A. ambulator
A. Ambulator shoe
a. anterior angulation
a. dorsal angulation
A. Energetics
a. of head of patella
A. insole
a. patellae
A. pin
a. plantar deformity
a. posterior angulation
A. Universal Drive and Irrigation System
a. vertebra
Apfelbaum mirror
aphalangia
complete a.
congenital a.
partial a.
aphasia
Broca a.
Wernicke a.
apical
a. axis guide
a. corn
a. dental ligament
a. distraction
a. lordotic view
a. segment

a. stitch
a. vertebra
apices (*pl. of* apex)
APL
abductor pollicis longus
APL Plus ankle brace
APLD
automated percutaneous lumbar diskectomy
Apley
A. compression test
A. distraction test
A. examination
A. grinding test
A. knee test
A. maneuver
A. scratch test
A. traction
apocope
apodia
Apofix cervical instrumentation
Apollo
A. DXA bone densitometry system
A. hip prosthesis
A. hip system
A. hot/cold Pak
A. knee prosthesis system
A. TM electric flexion table
A. total knee system
aponeurectomy
aponeurorrhaphy
aponeurosis
adductor a.
digital a.
meniscal a.
palmar a.
plantar a.
quadriceps a.
a. of tendon
woven gastrocnemius a.
aponeurositis
aponeurotic
a. band
a. fibroma
a. lengthening
a. reflex
a. triangle
a. troika
aponeurotome
aponeurotomy
apophysial, apophyseal
a. complex

NOTES

35

apophysial *(continued)*
    a. fracture
    a. joint
    a. joint osteophyte
apophysis, pl. **apophyses**
    calcaneus a.
    iliac a.
    medial epicondylar a.
    slipped vertebral a.
    spinal process a.
    vertebral ring a.
apophysitis
    calcaneal a.
    iliac a.
    a. tibialis
    a. tibialis adolescentium
apoplexy
    delayed a.
    posttraumatic a.
APOPPS
    adjustable postoperative protective
    prosthetic socket
apparatus
    Ace Unifix fixation a.
    adjustable aiming a.
    Allgöwer a.
    Anderson fixation a.
    Anderson leg-lengthening a.
    AO compression a.
    AO contouring a.
    Axer compression a.
    Bassett electrical stimulation a.
    Benedict-Roth a.
    Bovie electrocautery a.
    Buck convoluted traction a.
    Buck Redi-Traction a.
    Calandruccio triangular
      compression a.
    Cameron fracture a.
    Charnley centering a.
    Charnley compression a.
    compression a.
    coracoclavicular fixation a.
    coring a.
    CPM a.
    DeWald spinal a.
    Deyerle fixation a.
    driver tunnel locator a.
    electrocautery a.
    electronic bone stimulation a.
    a. extensor
    external skeletal fixation a.
    fixating a.
    four-bar external fixation a.
    Fox internal fixation a.
    Georgiade visor halo fixation a.
    Giliberty a.
    Golgi a.

    halo vest a.
    Hamilton a.
    Hare a.
    hinged-distraction a.
    Hoffmann-Vidal external fixation a.
    Ilizarov a.
    internal fixation a.
    isokinetic joint a.
    isokinetic resistance a.
    Kinetron muscle strengthening a.
    Kirschner a.
    Kronner external fixation a.
    Küntscher traction a.
    leg-holding a.
    McLaughlin osteosynthesis a.
    Mueller compression a.
    nail plate a.
    Nauth traction a.
    Neufeld a.
    optoelectric measuring a.
    optoelectric signal detection a.
    Orthofix a.
    Parham-Martin fracture a.
    Philips Angiodiagnostics 96 a.
    Quengel a.
    Rancho anklet foot control a.
    Redi-Trac traction a.
    Rezaian external fixation a.
    rod-mounted targeting a.
    Roger Anderson external fixation a.
    Sayre suspension a.
    snap-fit a.
    Southwick pin-holding a.
    spine a.
    subneural a.
    Sutter-CPM knee a.
    Taylor a.
    Telectronics electrical stimulation a.
    triplanar protractor a.
    Vidal-Adrey modified Hoffman
      external fixation device a.
    Volkov-Oganesian external
      fixation a.
    Volkov-Oganesian-Povarov hinged
      distraction a.
    Wagner external fixation a.
    Wagner leg-lengthening a.
    Wagner-Schanz screw a.
    Zickel medullary a.
    Zickel supracondylar fixation a.
    Zimmer electrical stimulation a.
appearance
    bat-wing a.
    bone-within-bone a.
    crabmeat-like a.
    horseshoe a.
    mop-end a.
    spongy a.

appendage clamp
appendiceal retractor
appendicular
    a. bone mass measurement
    a. skeletal muscle (ASM)
    a. skeleton
Applause Super-Hemi wheelchair
apple-shape body
appliance (*See* device, orthosis)
    DeWald spinal a.
    Jobst a.
application
    cast a.
    cold a.
    controlled force a.
    diversified-type force a.
    force a.
    frame a.
    Harrington rod instrumentation
      force a.
    heat a.
    ice a.
    Isola spinal implant system a.
    Kumar a.
    paraffin wax therapeutic a.
    paraspinal rod a.
    traction a.
    a. of traction device
    transverse fixator a.
applicator
    infrared a.
applied
    a. kinesiology (AK)
    a. load
applier
    bayonet clip a.
    bulldog clamp a.
    clip a.
    Ligaclip a.
    Mayfield miniature clip a.
    Mayfield temporary aneurysm
      clip a.
    mini a.
    surgical staple a.
    Vari-Angle clip a.
apposing articular surface
apposition
    axonal a.
    bayonet a.
    bone-to-bone a.
    facet a.
appositional growth

apprehension
    a. shoulder
    a. sign
    a. test
apprentice kyphosis
approach
    Abbott-Carpenter posterior a.
    Abbott posterior a.
    acetabular extensile a.
    anterior acromioplasty a.
    anterior axillary a.
    anterior extensile a.
    anterior retroperitoneal flank a.
    anterior sternomastoid a.
    anterior transthoracic a.
    anterolateral a.
    anteromedial retropharyngeal a.
    Aufranc lateral a.
    Avila a.
    axillary a.
    Bailey-Badgley anterior cervical a.
    Banks-Laufman a.
    Bennett posterior shoulder a.
    Berger-Bookwalter posterior a.
    Bosworth a.
    Boyd a.
    Boyd-Sisk a.
    Brackett-Osgood posterior a.
    Brodsky-Tullos-Gartsman a.
    Broomhead medial a.
    Brown lateral a.
    Bruner a.
    Bruser lateral a.
    Bryan-Morrey extensive posterior a.
    Callahan and Scuderi a.
    Campbell posterior shoulder a.
    Campbell posterolateral a.
    Carnesale acetabular extensile a.
    Carroll a.
    Cave hip a.
    Cave knee a.
    cervical a.
    Charnley-Müller lateral a.
    Cloward cervical disk a.
    Codman saber-cut shoulder a.
    Colonna-Ralston medial a.
    combined anterior and posterior a.
    combined low cervical and
      transthoracic a.
    Coonse-Adams knee a.
    costotransversectomy a.
    Cozen transverse a.

NOTES

approach *(continued)*
Cubbins shoulder a.
curved a.
Darrach-McLaughlin a.
de Andrade and MacNab
anterior a.
de Boer lateral a.
deltoid-splitting shoulder a.
deltopectoral a.
Dickinson a.
dorsal finger a.
dorsal midline a.
dorsalward a.
dorsolateral a.
dorsomedial a.
dorsoplantar a.
dorsoradial a.
dorsorostral a.
dorsoulnar a.
Downey modification of Fowler-
Philip a.
Duran a.
DuVries a.
extended iliofemoral a.
extensile a.
extrabursal a.
extraperitoneal a.
extrapharyngeal a.
Fahey a.
Fernandez extensile anterior a.
Fowler-Philip a.
Gallie a.
Gatellier-Chastang posterolateral a.
Gibson a.
Gordon a.
Guleke-Stookey a.
Hardinge femoral a.
Hardinge lateral a.
Harmon cervical a.
Harmon modified posterolateral a.
Harris anterolateral a.
Harris lateral a.
Hay lateral a.
Henderson posterolateral a.
Henderson posteromedial a.
Henry anterior strap a.
Henry anterolateral a.
Henry extensile a.
Henry posterior interosseous
nerve a.
Henry radial a.
Hirschhorn compression a.
Hoffmann a.
Hoppenfeld-DeBoer a.
Hoppenfeld lateral a.
Horwitz ankle fusion a.
Howorth a.
iliofemoral a.

ilioinguinal acetabular a.
inguinal a.
Insall anterior a.
intraforaminal a.
ipsilateral a.
Jones and Brackett anterior a.
keyhole a.
Kikuchi-MacNap-Moreau a.
Kocher curved L a.
Kocher-Gibson posterolateral a.
Kocher-Langenbeck a.
Kocher lateral J a.
Koenig-Schaefer medial a.
Langenbeck anteromedial a.
lateral deltoid splitting a.
lateral Gatellier-Chastung a.
lateral J a.
lateral Kocher a.
lateral Ollier a.
lateral parapatellar a.
Lazepen-Gamidov anteromedial a.
Leslie-Ryan anterior axillary a.
Letournel-Judet a.
long deltopectoral a.
low cervical a.
Ludloff medial a.
Mayo a.
McAfee a.
McConnell extensile a.
McConnell median and ulnar
nerve a.
McFarland-Osborne lateral a.
McLaughlin a.
McWhorter posterior shoulder a.
Mears-Rubash a.
medial parapatellar capsular a.
midlateral a.
midline medial a.
Minkoff-Jaffe-Menendez posterior a.
Mize-Bucholz-Grogen a.
Moore posterior a.
Moore-Southern a.
Murphy lateral a.
neurodevelopmental a.
Ollier arthrodesis a.
Ollier lateral a.
oropharyngeal a.
Osborne posterior a.
palmar a.
paramedian a.
pararectus a.
paraspinal a.
patella turndown a.
Perry extensile anterior a.
Phemister posteromedial a.
plantar a.
Pogrund lateral a.
posterior costotransversectomy a.

posterior inverted U a.
posterior midline a.
posterior occipitocervical a.
posterior transolecranon a.
posterolateral a.
posteromedial a.
proprioceptive neuromuscular
  facilitation a.
proximal interphalangeal joint a.
proximal metatarsal a.
pulp a.
Putti posterior a.
Radley-Liebig-Brown a.
Reinert acetabular extensile a.
retroperitoneal a.
retropharyngeal a.
Roberts a.
Roos a.
Rowe posterior shoulder a.
saber-cut a.
sacral a.
sacroiliac a.
screw-plate a.
Senegas hip a.
sensorimotor stimulation a.
Shoemaker lateral a.
Sir Henry Platt transverse a.
Smith-Petersen a.
Smith-Petersen-Cave-Van Gorder
  anterolateral a.
Smith-Robinson cervical disk a.
Somerville anterior a.
Southwick-Robinson anterior
  cervical a.
Spetzler anterior transoral a.
split-heel a.
split patellar a.
stabilization a.
sternum-splitting a.
subclavicular a.
supraclavicular a.
surgical a.
Swedish a.
Thompson anterolateral a.
Thompson anteromedial a.
Thompson-Henry a.
Thompson posterior radial a.
thoracic a.
thoracoabdominal a.
thoracolumbar retroperitoneal a.
thoracotomy a.
thumb metacarpophalangeal joint a.

transacromial a.
transaxillary a.
transbrachioradialis a.
transcalcaneal a.
transclavicular a.
transfibular a.
transolecranon a.
transpedicular a.
transperitoneal a.
transsternal a.
transthoracic a.
transtrochanteric a.
transverse a.
triradiate acetabular extensile a.
triradiate transtrochanteric a.
trivector retaining a.
unilateral sacroiliac a.
volar a.
volarward a.
Wadsworth posterolateral a.
Wagner a.
Wagoner posterior a.
Watson-Jones anterior a.
Watson-Jones lateral a.
Wilson a.
Wiltberger anterior cervical a.
Wiltse a.
Wiltse-Spencer paraspinal a.
Yee posterior shoulder a.
Young medial a.
zigzag a.
Z-plasty a.

approximator
Acland clamp a.
Acland double-clamp a.
Bruni-Wayne clamp a.
Bunke-Schulz clamp a.
clamp a.
double-clamp a.
Henderson clamp a.
hook a.
Ikuta clamp a.
Iwashi clamp a.
Kleinert-Kutz clamp a.
Lalonde tendon a.
Lemmon sternal a.
rib a.
sternal a.
Van Beek nerve a.

APPT
Adolescent and Pediatric Pain Tool

NOTES

APR
anatomic porous replacement
APR acetabular prosthesis
APR cement fixation
APR cement fixation adhesive
APR femoral prosthesis
APR I femoral stem
APR hip stem
APR II hip system
APR II prosthesis
APR total hip system

apraxia
dressing a.

apraxic gait

Aprema III device

ApriVera skin and hair cleanser

APRL
Army Prosthetics Research Laboratory
APRL hand prosthesis
APRL prosthetic hook

apron
quadriceps a.

apropulsive gait

APS
air plasma spray
anterior plate system
APS Hi-Lo electric lift table

APTC
anteroposterior talocalcaneal angle

APTT
activated partial thromboplastin time test

APU brace

aqua
a. PT dry physiotherapy
a. PT water massage
A. Spray
A. Spray wet nail débridement
system
A. Thermassage

Aqua-Cel heating pad system

Aquaciser
A. hydrodynamic measurement
system
A. pool
A. 100R underwater treadmill
system

Aquaflex gel pad

AquaJogger buoyancy belt

AquaMED
A. dry hydrotherapy
A. dry hydrotherapy equipment

AquaMotion pool

**Aquanex hydrodynamic measurement
system**

Aquaphor gauze dressing

Aquaplast
A. splint
A. splinting material

AquaSens fluid monitoring system

AquaShield
A. orthopaedic cast cover
A. reusable cast cover

Aquasonic Transmission Gel

Aquasorb hydrogel wound dressing

Aquatech cast pad

aquatherapy

Aquatherm bed pad

aquatic
a. cardiac evaluation and testing
(ACET)
a. exercise
a. exercise program
a. rehabilitation
a. stabilization program
a. therapy pool

Aqua-Trainer

Aquatrek device

Aquatrend water workout station

Aqua/Whirl bath

ARA
American Rheumatism Association
ARA Test

arabinoside

arachidonic

arachnodactyly

arachnoid

arachnoiditis
adhesive a.

arachnoid-shape Beaver blade

Arafiles
A. elbow arthrodesis
A. elbow prosthesis

Aran-Duchenne
A.-D. amyotrophy
A.-D. disease

Arbeitsgemeinschaft
A. für Osteosynthesefragen-
Association for the Study of
Internal Fixation (AO-ASIF)
A. für Osteosynthesefragen-Danis-
Weber ankle fracture classification
A. für osteosynthesefragen
procedure
A. für Osteosynthesfragen-Morscher
plate
A. für Osteosynthesfragen-stopped
drill guide

ARC
antirotation cable

arc
carpal a.
flexion-extension a.
Leksell stereotactic a.
monosynaptic reflex arc
stereotactic a.
a. of motion

painful a.
reflex a.
shoulder ROM a.
arcade
a. of Frohse
Frohse ligamentous a.
a. of Struthers
superficialis a.
Arcelin view
arch, pl. **arches**
a. angle
anterior metatarsal a.
a. binder
a. of bone
carpal a.
cervical a.
a. cookie
coracoacromial a.
a. cushion
deep a.
fallen a.
a. of foot
a. fracture
a. of Frohse
Hapad metatarsal a.
Hapad scaphoid a.
Hillock a.
a. index
ischiopubic a.
Langer axillary a.
a. loading
longitudinal plantar a.
medial longitudinal a.
palmar a.
a. peak area
plantar arterial a.
posterior a.
Roman a.
a. and slouch position
superficial palmar a.
a. support
vertebral a.
archer's shoulder
arch-height
a.-h. index
a.-h. ratio
Archimedean drill
architectural alterations of bone
architecture
bony a.
foot a.

Arch-Lok
Swede-O A.-L.
archplasty
arch-up test
Archxerciser
arciform
Arco classification
ArCom processed polyethylene
Arctic Blaze hot/cold pack
arcuate
a. complex
a. fasciculus (AF)
a. foramen
a. movement
a. osteotomy
a. popliteal ligament
arcuatus
pes a.
arcus
area
arch peak a.
Broca a.
dorsolumbar a.
odontoid-axial a.
Patrick trigger a.
performance a.
pressure-sensitive a.
puboischial a.
pump bump a.
a. scar
thenar a.
trapezial a.
areflexia
detrusor a.
areola of bone
Arglaes film dressing
ARGO
Adjustable Advanced Reciprocating Gait
Orthosis
Ariat shoe
Ariel computerized exercise system
Arizona
A. ankle brace
A. Health Science Center (AHSC)
A. Health Science Center-Volz
elbow prosthesis
A. Health Sciences Center-Volz
hinge
A. universal leg support
ARM
alternating range of motion

NOTES

ARM *(continued)*
ARM method of physical examination

arm
abductor lever a.
articulating a.
a. band
a. board
a. cuff
a. cylinder cast
a. drift
a. elevator sling
flail a.
a. flap
a. fossa test
grenade thrower's a.
a. heel-strike synchrony
a. holder
lever a.
Leyla a.
linebacker's a.
moment a.
MonitorMate monitor a.
outrigger a.
Popeye a.
a. positioner
a. skate
a. swathe
tackler's a.
Utah artificial a.
wringer a.
Yasargil Leyla retractor a.
armboard
armchair splint
Armistead
A. technique
A. ulnar lengthening
A. ulnar lengthening operation
Armstrong
A. acromionectomy
A. plate
Army
A. bone gouge
A. osteotome
A. Prosthetics Research Laboratory (APRL)
Army-Navy retractor
Arnold
A. lumbar brace
A. nerve
Arnold-Chiari
A.-C. deformity
A.-C. malformation
A.-C. syndrome
AROM
active range of motion
Aron Alpha adhesive
Aronson-Prager technique

arrest
epiphysial a.
greater trochanteric apophysial a.
growth a.
Shapiro classification of mechanisms of growth a.
arrow
A. absorbable meniscal repair device
Biofix meniscus a.
Bionx a.
meniscal a.
A. pin clasp
ARS
acute repetitive seizure
ARS disorder
ART
active-release technique
ArtAssist arterial assist device
arteria acetabuli
arterial
a. aneurysm
a. flap
a. gas embolism
a. occlusion sign
a. oxygen saturation
a. ring
a. spasm
a. trauma
arteriogram
arteriography
femoral a.
magnetic resonance a.
peripheral a.
spinal a.
vertebral a.
arteriosclerosis obliterans
arteriotomy
ankle-level a.
arteriovenous
a. fistula (AVF)
a. malformation
arteritis
artery
Adamkiewicz a.
anomalous fibular nutrient a.
anterior radial collateral a.
anterior recurrent tibial a.
anterior spinal a.
anterior tibial a.
ascending cervical a.
axillary a.
basilic a.
brachial a.
carotid a.
cephalic a.
cervical a.

circumflex iliac a.
circumflex scapular a.
collateral a.
common carotid a.
common iliac a.
deep circumflex iliac a.
deltoid a.
digital a.
dorsal digital a. (DDA)
dorsal metatarsal a.
epiphysial a.
facial a.
femoral circumflex a.
fibular plantar marginal a.
first dorsal metacarpal a.
first dorsal metatarsal a. (FDMA)
first plantar metatarsal a. (FPMA)
genicular a.
geniculate a.
gluteal a.
hypogastric a.
iliac a.
iliofemoral flap a.
iliolumbar a.
inferior thyroid a.
intercostal a.
intermetatarsal a.
internal carotid a.
internal iliac a.
interosseous a.
lateral calcaneal a.
lateral plantar a.
lingual a.
medial geniculate a.
medial plantar a.
metaphysial a.
metatarsal a.
middle sacral a.
nutrient a.
obturator a.
paramalleolar a.
perforating a.
peripheral a.
peroneal a.
persistent sciatic a.
plantar a.
plantar digital a. (PDA)
plantar metatarsal a.
popliteal a.
posterior inferior cerebellar a.
  (PICA)
posterior radial collateral a.

posterior tibial a.
princeps pollicis a.
profunda brachii a.
pudendal a.
radial a.
radicular a.
retinacular a.
sacral a.
saphenous a.
second metatarsal a.
spinal a.
subclavian a.
superficial circumflex iliac a.
superficial femoral a. (SFA)
superficial temporal a.
superior laryngeal a.
superior thyroid a.
supraclavicular fossa a.
tarsal canal a.
tarsal sinus a.
thoracoacromial a.
thrombosis radial a.
tibial a.
ulnar a.
vertebral a.
volar digital a.
Arth-Aid Joint Formula
arthralgia
acromegalic a.
intermittent a.
migratory a.
nonspecific a.
periodic a.
subtalar a.
temporomandibular joint a.
arthrectomy
arthrempyesis
Arthrex
A. arthroscopy instrument
A. bone anchor
A. coring reamer
A. femoral guide
A. instruments and systems
A. meniscal dart
A. meniscal dart gun
A. sheathed interference screw
A. tibial guide
A. TwistLoc suture anchor
A. zebra pin
arthrifluent abscess
arthritic
a. ankle joint narrowing

NOTES

arthritic *(continued)*
- a. atrophy
- a. deterioration
- a. shoe
- a. talonavicular change

arthritis, pl. **arthritides**
- acromegalic a.
- acute hematogenous a.
- acute spinal a.
- adjuvant-induced a. (AIA)
- allergenic a.
- ancient tuberculous a.
- ankle infectious a.
- ankle rheumatoid a.
- assignment criteria for rheumatoid a.
- atrophic a.
- bacterial a.
- Bekhterev a.
- calcaneocuboid joint a.
- cervical a.
- Charcot a.
- chronic absorptive a.
- chronic villous a.
- chylous a.
- crystal-induced a.
- cystic rheumatoid a.
- a. deformans
- degenerative a. (DA)
- enteropathic a.
- erosive a.
- filarial a.
- A. Foundation
- fungal a.
- gonococcal septic a.
- gouty a.
- A. Helplessness Index (AHI)
- hemophilic a.
- hypertrophic a.
- hypotrophic a.
- A. Impact Measurement Scale (AIMS)
- A. Impact Measurement Scale classification
- infectious a.
- inflammatory bowel disease associated a.
- Jaccoud a.
- juvenile chronic a.
- juvenile-onset rheumatoid a.
- juvenile rheumatoid a. (JRA)
- Lyme disease a.
- Marie-Strümpell a.
- midfoot a.
- migratory a.
- monoarticular septic a.
- a. mutilans
- mutilans rheumatoid a.
- mycobacterial a.
- navicular a.
- neonatal septic a.
- neuropathic a.
- New York diagnostic criteria for rheumatoid a.
- a. nodosa
- nonarticular a.
- ochronotic a.
- oligoarticular a.
- pantalocrural a.
- pantrapezial a.
- patellofemoral a.
- pauciarticular a.
- periosteal a.
- peritrapezial a.
- pisotriquetral a.
- polyarticular juvenile rheumatoid a.
- postinfectious a.
- postmenopausal a.
- posttraumatic a.
- primary degenerative a.
- proliferative a.
- psoriatic a.
- pyogenic a.
- A. Quality of Life Scale
- radiocarpal a.
- reactive a.
- rheumatoid a. (RA)
- robust rheumatoid a.
- sarcoid a.
- septic a.
- seronegative rheumatoid a.
- seropositive rheumatoid a.
- silicone a.
- a. sock
- spinal a.
- staphylococcal a.
- subtalar joint a.
- suppurative a.
- tendon bowing in a.
- tibiotalar a.
- Tom Smith a.
- traumatic a.
- tuberculous a.
- vertebral a.
- viral-associated a.
- WHO/LAR Response Criteria for Rheumatoid A.

arthritis-associated psoriasis
ArthroCare
- A. arthroscopic system
- A. electrode
- A. wand

arthrocele
arthrocentesis
arthrochalasis
arthrochondritis

arthroclasia
arthrodesed digit
arthrodesis
Abbott-Fischer-Lucas hip a.
Abbott-Lucas a.
Adams transmalleolar a.
Adkins spinal a.
Albee hip a.
ankle a.
anterior occipitocervical a.
anterior slot graft a.
AO group shoulder a.
Arafiles elbow a.
arthroscopic subtalar a.
atlantoaxial a.
Baciu-Filibiu dowel ankle a.
Baciu-Filibiu transmalleolar a.
Badgley a.
Barrasso-Wile-Gage a.
Barr-Record ankle a.
Batchelor-Brown extraarticular
  subtalar a.
beak modification with triple a.
Benyi modification of Lambrinudi
  triple a.
bimalleolar approach to ankle a.
Blair ankle a.
Blair anterior a.
Blair-Morris-Dunn-Hand ankle a.
Blair tibiotalar a.
Bosworth femoroischial a.
Brett a.
Brewster triple a.
Brittain ischiofemoral a.
Brockman-Nissen a.
Brooks atlantoaxial a.
calcaneocuboid distraction a.
  (CCDA)
calcaneopelvic a.
calcaneotibial a.
Campbell-Akbarnia a.
Campbell posterior a.
Campbell-Rinehard-Kalenak
  anterior a.
Carceau-Brahms ankle a.
Carroll a.
cervical a.
Chandler a.
Chapchal knee a.
Charcot hip a.
Charnley ankle a.
Charnley compression a.

Charnley-Houston shoulder a.
Chuinard-Peterson ankle a.
Chuinard-Peterson anterior a.
closing wedge a.
Cloward cervical a.
combined resection arthroplasty
  and a.
Compere-Thompson a.
compression a.
cone a.
coracoclavicular a.
cuneiform joint a.
Davis a.
Dennyson-Fulford extraarticular
  subtalar a.
distal fibulotalar a.
distraction bone block a.
distraction-compression bone
  graft a.
distraction subtalar a.
double a.
dowel a.
Dunn-Brittain triple a.
Dunn triple a.
Elmslie triple a.
Enneking knee a.
excisional a.
extension injury posterior
  atlantoaxial a.
extraarticular a.
failed triple a.
fibulotalar a.
first cuneiform joint a.
first cuneiform-navicular joint a.
first metatarsal-first cuneiform a.
flat-cut a.
flexion injury posterior
  atlantoaxial a.
fused a.
Gallie ankle a.
Gallie atlantoaxial a.
Gant hip a.
Garceau-Brahms a.
Gill a.
Gill-Stein a.
Gissane a.
glenohumeral a.
Goldner spinal a.
Graham ankle a.
Grice extraarticular subtalar a.
Grice-Green extraarticular
  subtalar a.

NOTES

45

arthrodesis *(continued)*
    Guttmann subtalar a.
    Haddad-Riordan a.
    hallux interphalangeal joint a.
    hallux rigidus a.
    Harris-Beath a.
    Heiple a.
    Henderson a.
    Hibbs a.
    hindfoot a.
    Hoke triple a.
    Horwitz-Adams a.
    Horwitz transmalleolar a.
    Hunt-Thompson pantalar a.
    Ilizarov ankle a.
    interbody a.
    intercarpal a.
    internal fixation compression a.
    interphalangeal a.
    intertransverse process a.
    intraarticular a.
    Johannson-Barrington a.
    John C. Wilson a.
    joint a.
    Kapandji-Sauvé a.
    Key intraarticular knee a.
    Kickaldy-Willis a.
    knee a.
    Kostuik-Alexander a.
    Küntscher modified knee a.
    Lambrinudi triple a.
    Lapidus modified a.
    lesser tarsal a.
    limited intertarsal a.
    Lionberger-Bishop-Tullos anterior a.
    Lipscomb metatarsophalangeal a.
    Lipscomb modified McKeever a.
    Lisfranc a.
    Lord total hip a.
    Lucas-Murray knee a.
    lunotriquetral a.
    Mann-Coughlin a.
    Mann modified McKeever a.
    Mann-Thompson-Coughlin a.
    Marcus-Balourdas-Heiple
      transmalleolar a.
    McKeever metatarsophalangeal a.
    metatarsocuneiform a.
    metatarsophalangeal joint a.
    midcarpal a.
    midfoot a.
    Millender-Nalebuff wrist a.
    Moberg a.
    modified Boyd ankle a.
    modified Lapidus a.
    Morris-Hand-Dunn anterior a.
    Mueller a.
    Nalebuff a.

    Naughton-Dunn triple a.
    naviculocuneiform joint a.
    nonfused a.
    occipitocervical a.
    panastragaloid a.
    pantalar a.
    paraarticular a.
    Podiatry Institute procedures for
      ankle a.
    Pontenza a.
    posterior atlantoaxial a.
    Potter a.
    Pridie ankle a.
    primary subtalar a.
    Pritchett-Mallin-Matthews a.
    Putti knee a.
    radiocarpal a.
    resection a.
    Richards a.
    Richardson subtalar a.
    Robinson-Riley cervical a.
    Robinson-Smith spinal a.
    Robinson spinal a.
    Ryerson triple a.
    salvage a.
    scaphocapitolunate a. (SCL)
    scaphotrapeziotrapezoid a.
    scapulothoracic a.
    Schneider hip a.
    Scranton transmalleolar a.
    a. screw
    Seoffert triple a.
    shoulder a.
    Shriver-Johnson interphalangeal a.
    Siffert-Forster-Nachamie a.
    Simmons spinal a.
    sliding a.
    Smith-Robinson interbody a.
    Soren a.
    Spier elbow a.
    spinal a.
    Staples elbow a.
    Stark a.
    Steindler elbow a.
    Stewart-Harley transmalleolar
      ankle a.
    stone a.
    subtalar a.
    talar triple a.
    talonavicular a.
    tarsal a.
    tarsometatarsal truncated-wedge a.
    thoracoscapular a.
    tibiocalcaneal a.
    tibiotalar joint primary a.
    tibiotalocalcaneal a.
    transfibular a.
    transmalleolar ankle a.

triple a.
triquetrum-lunate a.
triscaphe a.
Trumble a.
truncated tarsometatarsal wedge a.
Uematsu shoulder a.
ulnocarpal a.
Watson-Jones a.
Whitecloud-LaRocca cervical a.
White posterior a.
Wilson cone a.
Wilson-Johansson-Barrington cone a.
Wolf blade plate ankle a.
arthrodial
a. articulation
a. cartilage
a. protractor
A. Protractor range-of-motion
   analyzer
arthrodiastasis
arthrodynia
arthrodysplasia
arthroempyesis
arthroendoscopy
arthroereisis
Maxwell-Brancheau a. (MBA)
peg-in-hole a.
staple a.
subtalar a.
arthrofibrosis
Arthrofile orthopaedic rasp
Arthro-Flo
A.-F. arthroscopic irrigation system
A.-F. irrigator
Arthroforce III hand instrument
arthrogenic gait
arthrogenous
arthrogram
double-contrast a.
Gordon-Broström single-contrast a.
joint a.
nuclear a.
saline-enhanced MR a.
single-contrast a.
**arthrographic capsular distension and
   rupture technique**
arthrography
air a.
ankle a.
contrast a.
coronal computed tomographic a.
   (CCTA)

double-contrast a.
joint a.
magnetic resonance a.
opaque a.
osteochondral fracture a.
arthrogryposis
a. multiplex congenita
myopathic a.
neurogenic a.
arthrogrypotic clubfoot
arthrokatadysis
arthrokinematic
arthrokleisis
arthrolith
arthrolithiasis
arthrology
Arthro-Lok system of Beaver blade
arthrolysis
arthromeningitis
arthrometer
Acufex knee laxity a.
Genucom a.
joint a.
KT-1000 joint a.
KT-1000/Jr a.
KT-1000 knee ligament a.
KT-2000 knee ligament a.
KT-1000/s surgical a.
a. measurement
Medmetric knee ligament a.
Medmetric KT-1000 knee laxity a.
Robinson a.
stress-testing a.
Stryker knee laxity a.
a. test
a. testing
arthrometric knee laxity measurement
arthrometry
arthroncus
arthroneuralgia
arthronosos
arthroonychodysplasia syndrome
arthroophthalmopathy
hereditary progressive a.
arthroosteoonychodysplasia
arthropathic
arthropathology
arthropathy
Charcot a.
crystal-induced a.
crystal-related a.
cuff-tear a.

NOTES

arthropathy *(continued)*
    degenerative vertebral a.
    diabetic a.
    dislocating a.
    disuse a.
    gonococcal a.
    Heberden a.
    hemodialysis-related a.
    hemophilic a.
    inflammatory a.
    Jaccoud a.
    joint a.
    long-leg a.
    midfoot a.
    neuropathic a. (NA)
    neuropathic spinal a.
    ochronotic a.
    palindromic a.
    pyrophosphate a.
    sacroiliac joint a.
    seronegative a.
    SLE a.
    static a.
    stationary a.
    tabetic a.
arthrophyte
arthroplasty
    ablative a.
    abrasion a.
    acetabular cup a.
    acromioclavicular a.
    Albright-Chase a.
    anconeus a.
    ankle a.
    Ashworth hand a.
    Ashworth implant a.
    Aufranc cup a.
    Aufranc-Turner a.
    Austin Moore a.
    autogenous interpositional
      shoulder a.
    Bankart a.
    Bechtol a.
    Bigliani/Flatow total shoulder a.
    bipolar hip a.
    Bosworth a.
    Bowers radial a.
    Brain a.
    Breslow a.
    Bryan a.
    a. bur
    Campbell interpositional a.
    Campbell resection a.
    capitellocondylar total elbow a.
    capsular interposition a.
    carpometacarpal a.
    Carroll and Taber a.

Castle-Schneider resection
  interposition a.
a. cement
cemented total hip a.
cementless surface replacement a.
  (CSRA)
cementless total hip a.
Charcot a.
Charnley low-friction a.
Charnley-Müller a.
Charnley total hip a.
Clayton forefoot a.
Clayton resection a.
Colonna trochanteric a.
condylar implant a.
constrained ankle a.
constrained shoulder a.
convex condylar-implant a.
Coonrad-Morrey total elbow a.
Coonrad total elbow a.
Cracchiolo forefoot a.
Cracchiolo-Sculco implant a.
Crawford-Adams acetabular cup a.
Cubbins a.
cuff-tear a.
cup a.
Dewar-Barrington a.
distraction a.
DuVries a.
Eaton implant a.
Eaton volar plate a.
Eden-Hybbinette a.
elbow a.
Ewald capitellocondylar total
  elbow a.
Ewald-Walker kinematic knee a.
excision a.
extensor brevis a.
failed implant a.
fascial a.
finger joint a.
forefoot a.
four-in-one a.
Ganley modification of Keller a.
gap a.
Girdlestone resection a.
Global total shoulder a.
Gore-Tex interpositional a.
a. gouge
Green a.
Gristina-Webb total shoulder a.
Gunston a.
Gustilo-Kyle cementless total hip a.
Harrington total hip a.
Head hip a.
Helal flap a.
hemijoint a.
hemiresection interposition a.

hip a.
Hungerford-Krackow-Kenna knee a.
hydroxyapatite-coated ankle a.
ICLH double cup a.
implant a.
Inclan-Ober a.
Inglis triaxial total elbow a.
Insall-Burstein-Freeman knee a.
interphalangeal a.
interpositional a.
ipsilateral total elbow a.
ipsilateral total shoulder a.
Irvine ankle a.
Jaccoud a.
Johnson resection a.
Jones resection a.
Kates forefoot a.
Keller-Brandes resection a.
Keller-Lelièvre a.
Keller-Mann resection a.
Keller-Mayo diabetic foot a.
Keller-Regnauld a.
Keller resection a.
knee a.
Kocher-McFarland hip a.
Koenig metatarsophalangeal joint a.
Kutes a.
Lacey rotating hinge a.
Larmon forefoot a.
laser image custom a. (LICA)
Magnuson-Stack a.
Mann-DuVries a.
Mann resection a.
Mark II Sorrells hip a.
Matchett-Brown hip a.
Mayo ankle a.
Mayo resection a.
Mayo-Stone-Valenti hallux
  limitus/rigidus a.
Mayo total elbow a.
McAtee-Tharias-Blazina a.
McKee-Farrar total hip a.
McLaughlin a.
Memford-Gurd a.
metacarpophalangeal joint a.
metatarsophalangeal a.
Meuli a.
Millender a.
Miller-Galante knee a.
mobile-bearing knee a.
modified Keller resection a.

modified mold and surface
  replacement a.
mold acetabular a.
monospherical total shoulder a.
Morrey-Bryan total elbow a.
mosaic a.
Mould a.
Mueller hip a.
Mumford-Gurd a.
Nara a.
NEB a.
Neer unconstrained shoulder a.
Neviaser a.
New England Baptist hip a.
Nicola a.
Niebauer trapeziometacarpal a.
noncemented total hip a.
Post total shoulder a.
press-fit condylar knee a.
primary a.
A. Products Consultants foot and
  legholder
prosthetic a.
Putti-Platt a.
Regnauld modification of Keller a.
resection a.
revision hip a.
Robinson a.
rotator cuff tear a.
Sauvé-Kapandji a.
Schlein elbow a.
Schrock a.
Scott a.
semiconstrained total elbow a.
shoulder a.
Silastic lunate a.
silicone implant a.
silicone rubber a.
silicone wrist a.
Smith-Petersen cup a.
Speed a.
Stanmore shoulder a.
Steffee thumb a.
surface replacement hip a.
Sutter silicone metacarpophalangeal
  joint a.
Swanson convex condylar a.
Swanson interpositional wrist a.
Swanson metatarsophalangeal
  joint a.
Swanson PIP joint a.
Swanson radial head implant a.

NOTES

arthroplasty *(continued)*

Swanson silicone wrist a.
tendon interposition a.
Thackray low friction a.
Thompson a.
total ankle a. (TAA)
total articular replacement a.
  (TARA)
total articular resurfacing a.
  (TARA)
total elbow a.
total hip a. (THA)
total joint a. (TJA)
total knee a. (TKA)
total patellofemoral joint a.
total shoulder a.
total wrist a.
triaxial total elbow a.
Trillat a.
Tupper a.
UCLA anatomic shoulder a.
ulnar hemiresection interposition a.
unconstrained shoulder a.
unicompartmental knee a. (UKA)
Vainio a.
Valenti a.
Van Ness rotational a.
Vitallium cup a.
volar plate a.
Volz total wrist a.
Wilson-McKeever a.
Woodward a.

arthropneumoradiography
arthropneumoroentgenography
arthropneumotography
Arthropor

A. acetabular cup
A. II acetabular prosthesis
A. cup pad
A. cup prosthesis
A. oblong cup for acetabular
  defect
A. II porous socket

ArthroProbe

A. arthroscopic laser
Contact A.
A. laser system

arthropyosis
arthrorheumatism
arthrorisis
arthroscintigraphy
arthrosclerosis
arthroscope

angled a.
Baxter angled a.
Citscope disposable a.
Dyonics a.
Eagle straight-ahead a.

fiberoptic a.
GoldenEye a.
O'Connor operating a.
Panoview a.
Sapphire View a.
Storz oblique a.
Stryker viewing a.
triangulation technique for a.
Trio a.
Wolf a.

arthroscopic

a. abrasion chondroplasty
a. acromioplasty
a. augmentation
a. Bankart repair
a. cannula
a. cheilectomy
a. coplaning
a. débridement
a. drilling
a. entry portal
a. examination
a. grabber
a. knife
a. knot
a. laser instrument
a. laser surgery
a. leg holder
a. legholder
a. meniscectomy
a. microdiskectomy (AMD)
a. monopolar thermal stabilization
  forefoot compression sleeve
a. mosaicplasty
a. osteotome
a. probe
a. pump
a. punch
a. scissors
a. screw fixation
a. shaver
a. shaving
a. sheath
a. shield
a. subtalar arthrodesis
a. synovectomy
a. tourniquet
a. transglenoid suture stabilization
  procedure
a. transhumeral reconstruction

arthroscopically

a. assisted anterior cruciate
  ligament reconstruction
a. assisted synovectomy

arthroscopy

Allen shoulder a.
ankle a.
a. basket forceps

calcaneonavicular joint a.
diagnostic and operative a. (DOA)
electrothermal a.
extraarticular a.
Gillquist a.
a. grasping forceps
Hawkeye suture needle for a.
knee a.
laser a.
lateral hip a.
metacarpophalangeal a.
midcarpal a.
operative a.
radiocarpal a.
Ringer a.
second-look a.
wrist a.
**arthroscopy-assisted patellar tendon
substitution**
ArthroSew arthroscopic suturing device
arthrosis
Charcot a.
crystal-induced a.
cystic a.
a. deformans
a. deformity
degenerative a.
Eaton CMC a. (stages I–IV)
end-stage a.
Malleoloc anatomic ankle a.
posttraumatic a.
primary cystic a.
subtalar a.
trapezial a.
uncovertebral a.
Arthrosol dressing
arthrosteitis
arthrostomy
arthrosynovitis
Arthrotek
A. calibrated cylinder
A. Ellipticut hand instrumentation
A. femoral aimer
A. tibial fixation device
arthrotome
arthrotomy
diagnostic arthroscopy, operative
arthroscopy, and possible
operative a. (AAA)
Magnuson-Stack shoulder a.
medial parapatellar a.
operative a.

parapatellar a.
subtalar a.
arthrotropic
ArthroWand
CAPS A.
A. device
A. tool
arthroxerosis
arthroxesis
articular
a. block
a. blockage
a. bone lamella
a. bone tubercle
a. capsule
a. cartilage
a. cartilage autograft
a. cartilage autografting
a. cartilage lesion
a. cortex
a. crepitus
a. defect
a. disk
a. facet
a. facet angle
a. fragment
a. gout
a. insert
a. instability
a. labrum
a. mass separation
a. mass separation fracture
a. motion device (AMD)
a. nerve
a. pillar
a. pillar fracture
a. process
a. set angle
a. strain
a. structure
a. surface
articular-ligamentous system
articulated
a. AFO
a. chin implant
a. external fixator
a. skeleton
a. tension device
articulate minifixator
articulating
a. arm
a. bone end

NOTES

articulatio humeri
articulation
    acromioclavicular a.
    arthrodial a.
    atlantoaxial a.
    calcaneocuboid a.
    calcaneonavicular a.
    carpal a.
    carpometacarpal a.
    carporadial a.
    chondrosternal a.
    Chopart a.
    condylar a.
    congruent a.
    coracoclavicular a.
    costocentral a.
    costosternal a.
    costovertebral a.
    coxofemoral a.
    DIP a.
    a. disturbance
    ellipsoidal a.
    false a.
    a. of foot
    Goldman-Fristoe test of a.
    hinge a.
    humeroradial a.
    humeroulnar a.
    iliosacral a.
    immovable a.
    incongruent a.
    incudomalleolar a.
    intercarpal a.
    intermetacarpal a.
    interphalangeal a.
    Lisfranc joint a.
    manipulation of a.
    metacarpophalangeal a.
    metatarsocuneiform a.
    occipitocervical a.
    patellofemoral a.
    phalangeal a.
    PIP a.
    a. of pisiform bone
    plane-type acromioclavicular a.
    proximal radioulnar a.
    radiocapitellar a.
    radiocarpal a.
    radiohumeral a.
    radioscaphoid a.
    radioulnar a.
    sacrococcygeal a.
    sacroiliac a.
    scapuloclavicular a.
    slightly movable a.
    sternochondral a.
    sternoclavicular a.
    subtalar a.

    superior tibial a.
    talocalcaneonavicular ligament a.
    talofibular a.
    talonavicular a.
    tarsometatarsal a.
    tibiofemoral a.
    tibiofibular a.
    transverse tarsal a.
    trochoid a.
    ulnolunate a.
    ulnotriquetrum a.
    Vermont spinal fixator a.
    zygapophysial a.
articulatory
    a. procedure
    a. skill
    a. tic
artifact
    electric a.
    friction a.
    movement a.
    a. on x-ray
    shock a.
    stimulus a.
artifactual
artificial
    a. ankylosis
    a. fat pad
    a. joint implant
    a. leech
    a. ligament
    a. limb
    a. vertebral body
Artisan cement system
Artscan 200 arthroscopic cartilage
  stiffness testing device
arum fixation pin
arytenoid cartilage
arytenoidectomy
arytenoiditis
arytenoidopexy
AS
    anterosuperior
    AS ilium
    AS subluxation
ascending cervical artery
ascension
    A. MCP total joint replacement
    A. PIP total joint replacement
Ascent total knee system
Asch
    A. forceps
    A. splint
ascites
    chylous a.
ASE
    axilla, shoulder, elbow
    ASE bandage

aseptic
- a. fashion
- a. felon
- a. loosening
- a. necrosis

ASES
American shoulder and elbow system
- ASES shoulder score

ASEx
anterosuperior external ilium movement
- ASEx ilium
- ASEx subluxation

Asher physical build assessment technique

Ashhurst
- A. fracture classification system
- A. leg splint
- A. sign

Ashhurst-Bromer ankle fracture classification

Ashworth
- A. hand arthroplasty
- A. implant arthroplasty
- A. scale
- A. score of muscle spasticity

ASI
acromial spur index

ASIA
American Spinal Injury Association
- ASIA impairment scale
- ASIA impairment scale for classification of spinal cord injury

Asics GEL-MC shoe

ASICT
amplitude-summation interferential current therapy

ASIF
Association for the Study of Internal Fixation
- ASIF broad dynamic compression bone plate
- ASIF cancellous screw
- ASIF chisel
- ASIF cortical screw
- ASIF malleolar screw
- ASIF right-angle blade plate
- ASIF screw fixation operation
- ASIF screw fixation technique
- ASIF screw pin
- ASIF system
- ASIF T-plate
- ASIF twist drill

ASIn
anterosuperior internal ilium movement
- ASIn ilium
- ASIn subluxation

ASIS
anterior superior iliac spine

Asissto-Seat
- Maddapult A.-S.

Aslan endoscopic scissors

ASM
appendicular skeletal muscle

Asnis
- A. III cannulated screw
- A. 2 guided-screw system
- A. pin
- A. pinning
- A. technique

ASO
ankle stabilizing orthosis
- ASO ankle brace
- ASO support

ASOT
antistreptolysin-O titer

aspect
- dorsal a.
- laminar cortex posterior a.
- medial a.
- posterolateral a.
- volar a.

Aspen
- A. cervical collar
- A. CTO
- A. electrocautery

aspergillosis infection

aspirated fat

aspiration
- anterior a.
- bone marrow a.
- joint a.
- lateral a.
- medial a.
- a. needle biopsy

aspirator
- Cavitron ultrasonic surgical a.
- Sonocut ultrasonic a.

assay
- AlamarBlue osteoblast proliferation a.
- cefazolin a.
- chemiluminescent microtiter protein kinase activity a.

NOTES

assay *(continued)*
- deoxypyridinoline crosslinks urine a.
- enzyme-linked immunosorbent a.
- microtiter protein kinase a.
- osteoblast proliferation fluorometric a.
- Pyrilinks-D urine a.
- radioisotope clearance a.
- vitamin D receptor gene serum a.

assembly
- foot-ankle a.
- Massie nail a.
- multiple hook a.
- nail a.
- nail-screw sideplate a.
- proximal drill-guide a.

assessment
- Activity Loss A. (ALA)
- aerobic conditioning functional a.
- BFM arm impairment a.
- body composition a.
- Brief Test of Head Injury A.
- Brunnstrom-Fugl-Meyer impairment a.
- closed-chain functional a.
- environmental a.
- ergonomic a.
- functional capacity a.
- home a.
- impairment a.
- isokinetic a.
- Jebsen a.
- a. for limiting condition
- Moire topographic scoliosis a.
- motor function a.
- Musculoskeletal Function A. (MFA)
- neurologic a.
- overuse injury a.
- pressure ulcer a.
- rehabilitation a.
- return-to-play injury a.
- return-to-play musculoskeletal a.
- Rivermead Motor A.
- SCATBI A.
- Short Musculoskeletal Function A. (SMFA)
- Tinetti gait a.
- vascular a.
- vocational a.

ASSI
- Accurate Surgical and Scientific Instruments Corporation
- ASSI coagulator
- ASSI wire-pass drill

assignment criteria for rheumatoid arthritis

assimilation
- atlantooccipital a.
- a. pelvis

ASSIST
- Thera-Band ASSIST

assist
- Elite posterior spring a.
- first dorsal interosseous a.
- knee extension a.
- thumb interphalangeal extension a.

assistance
- ambulate with a.

assistant
- A. Free calibrated femoral tibial spreader
- A. Free foot/ankle support
- A. Free long prong collateral ligament retractor
- A. Free self-retaining hip surgery retractor system
- A. Free Shubbs short prong collateral ligament retractor
- A. Free Stulberg leg positioner
- A. Free wide PCL retractor

assisted ambulation

assistive
- a. movement
- a. technology device (ATD)

Assmann disease

associated myofascial trigger point

association
- American Orthopaedic A. (AOA)
- American Rheumatism A. (ARA)
- American Spinal Injury A. (ASIA)
- Japanese Orthopedic A. (JOA)
- A. Research Circulation Osseous classification system
- A. for the Study of Internal Fixation (ASIF)

astasia

astasia-abasia gait

astereognosis

asterixis

asthenia

asthenic

asthma
- exercise-induced a.

ASTM
- American Society for Testing and Materials
- augmented soft tissue mobilization
- ASTM augmented soft tissue mobilization
- ASTM designation of Biophase

Aston
- A. cartilage reduction
- A. patterning

astragalar bone

astragalectomy
astragalocalcaneal bone
astragalocalcanean
astragalocrural bone
astragaloid bone
astragaloscaphoid bone
astragalotibial bone
astragalus
    aviator's a.
    a. bone
Astralac needle
Astroturf toe
asymmetric
    a. incurvatum reflex
    a. skin fold
    a. subtalar joint development
    a. tonic neck reflex (ATNR)
    a. wear
asymmetrical growth
asymmetry
    interinnominate a.
    pure limb apraxia limb a.
asyndesis
asyndetic communication
asynergia
asynergic
AT
    Achilles tendon
    activity training
    anaerobic threshold
atactic abasia
Atak knee brace
Atasoy
    A. triangular advancement flap
    A. volar V-Y flap
    A. V-Y advancement
    A. V-Y technique
Atasoy-Kleinert flap
Atasoy-type flap for nail injury repair
Atavi atraumatic spine fusion system
atavicus
    metatarsus primus a.
atavistic
    a. cuneiform
    a. epiphysial
    a. foot
ataxia
    Bruns a.
    cerebellar a.
    equilibratory a.
    Friedreich a.
    hereditary spinocerebellar a.

    limb a.
    locomotor a.
    spinocerebellar a.
    traumatic brain injury-related a.
    vestibulocerebellar a.
ataxiadynamia
ataxia-telangiectasia
ataxic
    a. cerebral palsy
    a. gait
ataxy
ATD
    assistive technology device
atelectasis
    plate-like a.
    pulmonary a.
ateliotic dwarfism
atelocollagen gel
atelomyelia
atelopodia
atelorachidia
Aten olecranon screw
ATFL
    anterior talofibular ligament
ATH
    anthropometric total hip
atherosclerosis
atherostenosis
athetoid cerebral palsy
athetosis
athetotic
athlete
    amputee a.
    high-power a.
    single-organ a.
    weekend a.
athlete's
    a. foot
    a. heart
    a. pseudoanemia
athletic
    a. amenorrhea
    a. brace
    a. heart syndrome
    a. injury
    a. shoe carbon fiber plate
    a. trainer
Atkin epiphysial fracture
Atkinson endoprosthesis
Atlanta
    A. brace orthosis
    A. hip brace

NOTES

atlantal transverse ligament
Atlanta-Scottish
    A.-S. Rite abduction orthosis
    A.-S. Rite brace
Atlantic
    A. overlap brace
    A. rim brace
Atlantis cervical plate system
atlantoaxial
    a. alignment
    a. arthrodesis
    a. articulation
    a. dislocation (AAD)
    a. fracture-dislocation
    a. fusion
    a. impaction
    a. instability
    a. interval
    a. joint
    a. lesion
    a. ligament
    a. luxation
    a. rotary displacement
    a. rotatory fixation (AARF)
    a. rotatory subluxation
    a. separation
    a. stabilization
    a. subluxation (AAS)
atlantodens interval (ADI)
atlantooccipital (AO)
    a. anterior membrane
    a. assimilation
    a. disability
    a. fusion
    a. joint
    a. joint dislocation
    a. junction
    a. ligament
    a. subluxation
atlantoodontoid
    a. interspace
    a. joint
atlas
    A. adjustable stand
    a. adjustment
    A. cable system
    a. fracture
    a. laterality
    A. modular humeral prosthesis
    A. orthogonal percussion instrument
    a. vertebral subluxation complex
atlas-axis
    a.-a. complex
    a.-a. movement
atlas-dens interval
ATNR
    asymmetric tonic neck reflex

ATODC
    atraumatic osteolysis of distal clavicle
ATON
    adductor tenotomy and obturator
    neurectomy
atonia
atony
atopic dermatitis
ATO walker
ATR
    Achilles tendon repair
    Achilles tendon rupture
    ATR brace
atracurium besylate
Atra-Grip clamp
atraumatic
    a. forceps
    a., multidirectional, bilateral
      rehabilitation inferior (AMBRI)
    a., multidirectional, bilateral
      rehabilitation inferior (capsular
      shift)
    a. multidirectional instability
    a. necrosis
    a. needle
    a. osteolysis of distal clavicle
      (ATODC)
atretic
atrophic
    a. arthritis
    a. fracture
    a. muscular paralysis
    a. neuroarthropathy
    a. nonunion
atrophica
    myotonia a.
atrophy
    acute reflex bone a.
    arthritic a.
    Charcot-Marie a.
    Charcot-Marie-Tooth a.
    cortical a.
    Cruveilhier a.
    disuse a.
    Duchenne muscular a.
    Erb a.
    familial spinal muscular a.
    fascioscapulohumeral muscular a.
    fat pad a.
    Fazio-Londe a.
    gauntlet a.
    Hoffmann muscular a.
    inactivity a.
    infantile progressive spinal
      muscular a.
    juvenile muscular a.
    Kienböck a.

Kugelberg-Welander juvenile spinal
  muscle a.
muscular a.
myopathic a.
neurogenic a.
neurotrophic a.
peroneal muscular a.
progressive muscular a. (PMA)
quadriceps a.
scapular peroneal a.
scapulohumeral a.
spinal cord a.
spinal muscular a. (SMA)
spinal muscular a. (type I–III)
Sudeck a.
thenar a.
thigh a.
traction a.
Vulpian a.
Vulpian-Bernhardt spinal
  muscular a.
Werdnig-Hoffmann spinal
  muscular a.
Zimmerlin a.

ATT
anterior talar translation
ATT-300 LAT traction table
attachment
Accuvac smoke evacuation a.
capsular a.
femoral a.
fibrous a.
ligamentous a.
muscle-tendon a.
muscular a.
osseous a.
Pearson splint a.
PRAFO PKA KAFO a.
pyramid a.
splint a.
tendinous a.
tendon-bone a.
tendon-to-bone a.
Thomas splint with Pearson a.
a. versatility
attack
adversive a.
drop a.
Attenborough total knee prosthesis
attenuate

attenuation
bone ultrasound a. (BUA)
a. of tendon
ATTF
anterior tibiotalar fascicle
Atton disease
attrition
a. rupture of tendon
a. of tendon
attritional perforation
atypical dislocation
auditory evoked potential (AEP)
Aufranc
A. awl
A. cobra hip prosthesis
A. cobra retractor
A. concentric hip mold
A. cup arthroplasty
A. gouge
A. lateral approach
A. modification of Smith-Petersen
  cup
A. osteotome
A. periosteal elevator
A. reamer
Aufranc-Turner
A.-T. acetabular cup
A.-T. arthroplasty
A.-T. cemented hip prosthesis
A.-T. femoral component
A.-T. operation
A.-T. stem
Aufricht glabellar rasp
auger
augmentation
arthroscopic a.
bladder a.
extraarticular a.
fascial flap a.
hamstring ligament a.
iliotibial band graft a.
Leach-Schepsis-Paul a.
slotted acetabular a.
synthetic a.
augmented
a. reconstruction
a. repair
a. soft tissue mobilization (ASTM)
Augustine boat nail
AuRA cemented total hip system
Aussies-Isseis unstable scoliosis
austenitic stainless steel

NOTES

Austin
A. bunionectomy
A. chevron osteotomy fixation
A. Medical Equipment (AME)
A. Moore arthroplasty
A. Moore chisel
A. Moore extractor
A. Moore femoral head prosthesis
A. Moore hemiarthroplasty
A. Moore hook
A. Moore impactor
A. Moore pin
A. Moore rasp
A. Moore reamer
A. osteotomy
Austin-Akin bunionectomy
auto
A. Glide walker accessory
A. Suture stapler
autoamputation
autochthonous graft
autocinesis
autoclave
autocompression plate
autodistractor
autoerythrophagocytosis
Autoflex II, III CPM unit
autofusion
autogéné
Soudre a.
Autogenesis automator for Ilizarov screw
autogenic
autogenous
a. bone slurry
a. cancellous bone graft
a. cartilage transplantation
a. fat
a. fibular graft
a. iliac bone
a. interpositional shoulder arthroplasty
a. meniscal cartilage replantation
a. osteocartilage transfer
a. patellar ligament graft
a. patellar tendon reconstruction
a. semitendinosus-gracilis graft
autograft
articular cartilage a.
bone-patellar tendon-bone a.
a. bridge
cartilage a.
free revascularized a.
patellar bone-tendon-bone a.
Russell fibular head a.
autografting
articular cartilage a.
impaction cancellous a.

autoimmunization
surgical a.
Auto-Implant
A.-I. operation
A.-I. procedure
autologous
a. blood
a. blood transfusion
a. cancellous bone graft
a. chondrocyte implantation (ACI)
a. cultured chondrocyte
a. reverse graft
a. reverse graft to ankle
a. traction
automated
a. disposable keratome (ADK)
a. percutaneous diskectomy (APD)
a. percutaneous lumbar diskectomy (APLD)
a. shaver
automatic
a. neonatal walking reflex
a. screwdriver
a. staple
Automator device
autonomic
a. dysreflexia
a. nervous system
autonomous zone
Autophor
A. ceramic total hip prosthesis
A. femoral prosthesis
autoplastic graft
auto-reinforced polyglycolide rod
autosomal dominant mild short limb dwarfism
autotome drill
autotraction
autotransfusion suction
Autovac autotransfusion canister
Auvard clamp
A-V
A-V Impulse foot pump
A-V Impulse system
A-V Impulse System foot pump DVT prophylaxis device
A-V Impulse System foot wrap DVT prophylaxis device
Avanta
A. MCP joint implant finger prosthesis
A. metacarpophalangeal implant prosthesis
avascular
a. fragment
a. necrosis (AVN)
a. necrosis of the femoral head (AVNFH)

a. nonunion
a. sequestrum
average evoked response
Averett hip prosthesis
Averill
A. press fit prosthesis
A. total hip replacement
AVF
arteriovenous fistula
aviator's astragalus
Avila
A. approach
A. operation
A. technique
Avitene
A. flour dressing
A. microfibrillar collagen
A. pack
AVN
avascular necrosis
AVNFH
avascular necrosis of the femoral head
avoidance gait
avulse
avulsed ligament
avulsion
accessory navicular a.
anterior labrum periosteal sleeve a. (ALPSA)
bony a.
chemical nail a.
a. chip fracture
coracoid tip a.
digitorum brevis a.
a. fragment
a. injury
isolated a.
labral a.
ligament a.
nail a.
a. of nail plate
a. stress fracture
syndesmotic a.
a. technique
tibial tubercle a.
tubercle a.
awakening trauma
awareness
body a.
kinesthetic a.
sensory a.

awl
angled a.
Aufranc a.
bone a.
Carter Rowe a.
curved a.
DePuy a.
Ender a.
Ferran a.
Küntscher a.
Mark II Kodros radiolucent a.
pointed a.
reaming a.
rectangular a.
Rush pin reamer a.
square-shaped a.
Stedman a.
Swanson lunate a.
Swanson scaphoid a.
T-handled a.
Zelicof orthopedic a.
Zuelzer a.
Axel wire twister
Axer
A. compression apparatus
A. compression device
A. lateral opening wedge osteotomy
A. operation
A. varus derotational osteotomy
Axer-Clark procedure
axes (*pl. of* axis)
axial
a. acetabular index (AAI)
a. calcaneal projection
a. calcaneus view
a. compression
a. compression injury
a. compression load
a. compression principle
a. compression screw
a. compression test
a. fixation
a. gripping strength
a. instability
a. loading
a. loading injury
a. loading of spine
a. load teardrop fracture
a. load test
a. manual traction test
a. musculature

NOTES

axial (continued)
a. neuritis
a. pattern flap
a. pin technique
a. plane
a. plane angular deformity
biomechanics
a. plate
a. resistance exerciser
a. rotation
a. sesamoid projection
a. sesamoid view
a. spinal system
a. stiffness
a. traction
axilla, pl. **axillae**
a., shoulder, elbow (ASE)
a., shoulder, elbow bandage
axillary
a. approach
a. artery
a. block
a. contracture
a. crutch
a. flap
a. lateral view
a. nerve
a. nerve injury
a. region
a. vein
Axiom
A. modular knee system
A. total knee
A. total knee system
axis, pl. **axes**
anatomic a.
A. ankle brace
bimalleolar-foot a.
a. bone
cardinal axes X,Y,Z
distal reference a. (DRA)
femoral shaft a.
A. fixation system
flexion a.
flexion-extension a.
foot-thigh a.
a. guide
hypothalamic-pituitary-adrenal a.
hypothalamoneurohypophysial a.
(HNA)

interepicondylar a.
leg a.
long a.
longitudinal a.
longitudinal midtarsal joint a.
(LMJA)
mechanical a.
metatarsal a.
mid-diaphysial a.
oblique midtarsal joint a. (OMJA)
proximal reference a. (PFA)
ray a.
a. of rib motion
rotation a.
a. of rotation
single a.
spinal a.
subtalar joint a. (SJA)
a. traction
transcondylar a. (TCA)
transepicondylar a.
transmalleolar a. (TMA)
transverse a.
vertical a.
weightbearing a.
X a.
Y a.
Z a.
axis-altering arthroereisis device
axle lock and bumper
axon
a. reflex
a. reflex test
a. response
axonal
a. apposition
a. degeneration
a. injury
axonotmesis
Axxess spinal cord stimulation lead
AxyaWeld
A. bone anchor
A. bone anchor system
A. instrument
A. J-tip suture welding system
Ayers needle holder
Ayres tactile discrimination
azotemic osteodystrophy

BA

bioactive

BA bone cement

Baastrup

B. disease

B. syndrome

Babcock

B. forceps

B. stainless steel wire

B. wire-cutting scissors

Babinski

B. percussion hammer

B. reflex

B. sign

B. test

Babinski-Fröhlich syndrome

Babinski-Nageotte syndrome

baby

b. Kocher clamp

b. Lane forceps

b. Satinsky clamp

BacFix system

bacille Calmette-Guérin (BCG)

bacitracin

b. solution

Baciu-Filibiu

B.-F. dowel ankle arthrodesis

B.-F. transmalleolar arthrodesis

back

adolescent round b.

b. brace

B. Bubble gravity traction unit

B. Bull lumbar support cushion

B. Bull lumbar support system

b. creaking

b. crease

b. exercise

b. flexion

B. Hammer muscle stimulator

hollow b.

b. manipulation

old man's b.

b. pain

poker b.

b. range of motion (BROM)

b. range-of-motion device

b. range-of-motion instrument

B. Revolution Stick

B. Revolution Stick exercise

B. Revolution System

B. Revolution traction/exercise unit

rigid round b.

saddle b.

B. Seat torso-wrap brace

B. Shu paraspinal point

B. Specialist chiropractic table

B. Specialist electric table

B. Specialist manual table

static b.

b. strain

b. support

sway b.

B. Trainer spinal exercise system

backache

Backbar device

backboard splint

backcutting osteotome

BackCycler continuous passive motion device

Back-Ease aromatherapy hot/cold pack

backfilling

bone substitute b.

backfire fracture

backfiring

Backhaus

B. towel clamp

B. towel forceps

Backhaus-Jones towel clamp

Backhaus-Kocher towel clamp

Back-Huggar

Bodyline B.-H.

B.-H. lumbar support

B.-H. lumbar support cushion

Backjoy seat

back-knee deformity

Backnobber II massage tool

backout

screw b.

backpack

b. palsy

b. paralysis

backside wear

backstroke

The B.

BackStrong lumbar extension machine

BackThing lumbar support

BackTracker

backward

b. bending

b. curvature

backward-cutting knife

Bacon

B. bone rongeur

B. rasp

bacterial

b. arthritis

b. culture

b. flora

bacterium, pl. **bacteria**

aerobic b.

bacterium *(continued)*
  airborne b.
  anaerobic b.
bacteruria
Bac-Track
badger leg
Badgley
  B. arthrodesis
  B. combination procedure
  B. iliac wing resection
  B. laminectomy retractor
  B. operation
  B. plate
  B. resection of iliac wing
  B. technique
Bado classification
Bad Wildungen Metz spine system
BAEP
  brainstem auditory evoked potential
BAER
  brainstem auditory evoked response
Baer
  B. bone-cutting forceps
  B. bone rongeur
  B. rib shears
bag
  B. Bath
  containment b.
  Infusible pressure infusion b.
  Versi-Splint carry b.
Bagby angled compression plate
bag-of-bones technique
Bahler hinge
Bahnson appendage clamp
Bailey
  B. bur
  B. conductor
  B. drill
  B. duckbill clamp
  B. rib contractor
  B. rib spreader
  B. saw guide
  B. wire saw
Bailey-Badgley
  B.-B. anterior cervical approach
  B.-B. cervical spine fusion
  B.-B. technique
Bailey-Cowley clamp
Bailey-Dubow
  B.-D. nail
  B.-D. osteotomy
  B.-D. rod
  B.-D. technique
Bailey-Gibbon rib contractor
Bailey-Gigli saw guide
Bailey-Morse clamp
bail-lock
  b.-l. brace

b.-l. knee joint
b.-l. knee joint orthosis
baja
  patella b.
BAK
  BAK fusion cage
  BAK interbody fusion system
  BAK/Proximity interbody fusion
  implant
  BAK/T thoracic interbody fusion
  system
Baker
  B. Achilles tendon lengthening
  procedure
  B. cyst
  B. lateral semitendinosus transfer
  B. patellar advancement operation
  B. technique
  B. trabecular traction
  B. translocation operation
Baker-Hill osteotomy
baker's leg
Balacescu closing wedge osteotomy
Balacescu-Golden technique
balance
  b. beam scale
  b. board
  b. board training
  b. bridge
  column b.
  dynamic standing b.
  electrolyte b.
  fluid b.
  B. hip prosthesis
  B. Master
  B. Master rehabilitation evaluation
  B. Master training and assessment
  system
  nitrogen b.
  b. pad
  b. padding orthosis
  postural b.
balanced
  b. forearm
  b. forearm orthosis (BFO)
  b. hemivertebra
  b. skeletal traction
  b. splint
  b. suspension
  b. suspension traction
balancing
  Chopart amputation with tendon b.
Baldan fracture splint
Baldwin
  B. Bowers radioulnar joint
  operation
  B. Bowers radioulnar joint repair

Balfour
- B. clamp
- B. self-retaining retractor

Balkan
- B. beam
- B. femoral splint
- B. fracture frame

ball
- b. bearing
- Body B.
- Bouncewell medicine b.
- b. bur
- Burst Resistance Fitness B.
- cold-weld femoral b.
- b. dissector
- ExerFlex b.
- b. extractor
- Finger Fitness Spring B.
- Fitness B.
- b. of foot
- Gertie b.
- Gripp squeeze b.
- b. guidepin
- gym b.
- Gymnastik b.
- Gymnic Plus exercise b.
- hand exercise b.
- Jurgan pin b.
- B. knee lock
- Ledraplastic exercise b.
- massage b.
- medicine b.
- New Versaback gym b.
- PhysioGymnic exercise b.
- Physio-Roll VisuaLiser exercise b.
- b. reamer
- R-Value exercise b.
- Silastic b.
- Slo-Mo b.
- squeeze b.
- Swiss b.
- Thera-Band exercise b.
- Theragym b.
- Vari-Firm Medicine B.
- vestibular b.

ball-and-socket
- b.-a.-s. ankle prosthesis
- b.-a.-s. giant pseudarthrosis
- b.-a.-s. giant pseudoarthritis
- b.-a.-s. joint
- b.-a.-s. trochanteric osteotomy

Ballantine
- B. clamp
- B. hemilaminectomy retractor

Ballenger
- B. periosteotome
- B. swivel knife

Ballenger-Hajek chisel
ballistic injury
balloon-assisted, endoscopic, retroperitoneal, gasless (BERG)
ballottable
ballottement test
ball-peen splint
ballpit
ball-point guidepin
ball-tip
- b.-t. guidepin
- b.-t. spike

ball-tipped Küntscher guide
ball-valve tumor
balmoral laced shoe
balneotherapy
Baló sclerosis
balsa wood filler block
Baltimore
- B. Therapeutic Equipment (BTE)
- B. Therapeutic Equipment Work Simulator

Bamberger-Marie
- B.-M. disease
- B.-M. syndrome

bamboo spine
Bamby clamp
banana
- b. Beaver blade
- b. finger extension splint
- b. knife

Bancroft sign
band
- air b.
- AO tension b.
- aponeurotic b.
- arm b.
- big b.
- Broca diagonal b.
- calf b.
- Can-Do Exercise B.
- congenital fibrous b.
- conjoined lateral b.
- constriction b.
- deossification b.
- distal thigh b.

NOTES

band *(continued)*
    exercise b.
    external b.
    fascial b.
    fibrous b.
    Fit-Lastic therapy b.
    GelBand arm b.
    Gennari b.
    iliopatellar b.
    iliotibial b. (ITB)
    internal b.
    Jobst air b.
    lateral b.
    M b.
    palpable b.
    Parham b.
    Parham-Martin b.
    Partridge b.
    patellar b.
    PDS b.
    pelvic b.
    periosteal b.
    pretendinous b.
    proximal thigh b.
    REB b.
    REP Bands exercise b.
    Resist-A-Band exercise b.
    Resist-A-Tube exercise b.
    rigid metal pelvic b.
    sagittal b.
    scar b.
    Simonart b.
    subsurface white b.
    taut b.
    tennis elbow arm b.
    b. tenodesis
    tension b.
    trochanteric b.
    True Blue exercise b.
    b. wire
    Xercise b.
    Z b.
bandage
    Ace adherent b.
    ankle traction b.
    ASE b.
    axilla, shoulder, elbow b.
    Barton b.
    capeline b.
    Champ elastic b.
    circular b.
    Comperm tubular elastic b.
    compression b.
    Conco elastic b.
    cotton elastic b.
    cravat b.
    demigauntlet b.
    Desault wrist b.

Dressinet netting b.
E Cotton b.
Elastic Foam b.
Elastomull elastic gauze b.
Elastoplast b.
Esmarch b.
Fabco gauze b.
fiberglass b.
figure-of-eight b.
Flex-Foam b.
flexible b.
Flexilite conforming elastic b.
Flex-Master b.
Fractura Flex b.
B. Gard cast protector
gauntlet b.
Gibney fixation b.
Gibson b.
gum rubber Martin b.
Hamilton b.
Helenca b.
Heliodorus b.
Hippocrates b.
Hueter b.
Hydron Burn B.
immobilizing b.
immovable b.
Kerlix b.
Kling elastic b.
Martin sheet rubber b.
Medi-Band b.
MPM b.
Nu Gauze b.
oblique b.
Orthoflex elastic plaster b.
Ortho-Trac adhesive skin
    traction b.
Ortho-Vent b.
Pavlik b.
plaster of Paris b.
PLAST-O-FIT thermoplastic b.
polyurethane b.
Redigrip pressure b.
replantation b.
restrictive b.
Ribble b.
Richet b.
Robert Jones b.
roller b.
Sayre b.
scarf b.
Scultetus b.
Shur-Band self-closure elastic b.
Silesian b.
sling-and-swathe b.
spica b.
spiral b.
starch b.

stockinette b.
Thera-Boot b.
triangular b.
Tricodur compression support b.
Tricodur Epi compression b.
Tricodur Omos compression b.
Tricodur Talus compression b.
Tru-Support EW b.
Tru-Support SA b.
TubeGauz b.
Tubigrip b.
tubular elastic b.
Velpeau b.
Webril b.

Bandi patellofemoral score
Band-It
B.-I. magnetic elbow support
B.-I. tennis elbow strap
bandlike
b. adhesion
b. pain
bandy-leg
Bane
B. bone rongeur
B. rongeur forceps
Bane-Hartmann bone rongeur
banjo
b. cast
b. splint
b. traction
bank
bone b.
B.'s bone graft
Bankart
B. arthroplasty
B. fracture
B. operation
B. procedure
B. reconstruction
B. retractor
B. shoulder dislocation
B. shoulder lesion
B. shoulder prosthesis
B. shoulder repair
B. shoulder repair set
B. tack
Bankart-Putti-Platt operation
banked bone
Banks-Laufman
B.-L. approach

B.-L. incision
B.-L. technique
Bannon-Klein implant
bantam
B. CDH prosthesis
B. wire-cutting scissors
BAP
Behavioral Assessment of Pain
BAPS
Biomechanical Ankle Platform System
BAPS Ankle System
BAPS board
bar
Bill b.
b. bolt fixation
bony b.
broomstick b.
calcaneonavicular b.
cartilaginous b.
congenital b.
cross b.
Denis Browne b.
derotator b.
distraction b.
b. drill
b. excision
Fillauer b.
Gerster traction b.
grab b.
intramedullary b.
Leyla b.
Livingston intramedullary b.
longitudinal spinal b.
lumbrical b.
medial talocalcaneal b.
metatarsal flatfoot b.
MT b.
opponens b.
patellar b.
physial b.
posterior thigh b.
quad b.
b. resection
rigid b.
rocker b.
screw alignment b.
b. section
side-cutting Swanson b.
spacer b.
spondylotic b.

NOTES

bar *(continued)*
Sports-Grip B.
spreader b.
stabilizing b.
stall b.
Stephen spreader b.
tarsal b.
Thera-P exercise b.
Thornton b.
Tommy trapeze b.
torsion b.
traction b.
trapeze b.
unsegmented vertebral b.
valgus b.
Zielke derotator b.
bar-and-shoe orthosis
Bárány-Nylen maneuver
barbed
b. broach
b. staple
barbell
Spring angled adjustable b.
barber chair position
barber-pole
b.-p. fashion
b.-p. vein graft
barbotage
Barbour
B. cervical fixation
B. technique
Bard clamp
Bardeen primitive disk
Bardeleben
B. bone-holding forceps
B. rasp
Bardenheuer
B. extension
B. incision
Bard-Parker
B.-P. blade
B.-P. handle
B.-P. knife
B.-P. scalpel
Bareskin knee positioner
barked injury
Barker operation
Barkow ligament
bar-like ventral defect
Barlow
B. cruciform infant splint
B. hip instability test
B. maneuver
B. provocative test
B. sign
Barnes curve
barognosis
Baron suction tube

barotrauma
middle-ear b.
pulmonary b.
Barouk
B. button space
B. cannulated bone screw
B. microscrew with shortening
osteotomy
B. microstaple
B. spacer
Barr
B. anterior transfer
B. bolt
B. bolt nail
B. hook
B. open reduction and internal
fixation
B. pin
B. tendon transfer operation
B. tibial fracture fixation
Barraquer needle holder
Barrasso-Wile-Gage arthrodesis
barrel
b. bur
b. chest
b. crawl
b. guide
guide b.
b. plate
sideplate b.
barreled sideplate
Barre-Lieou syndrome
barrel-stave osteotomy
barrier
anatomic b.
blood-brain b. (BBB)
Capset calcium sulfate bone
graft b.
elastic b.
B. lower extremity sheet
motion b.
pathologic b.
physiologic b.
side-bending b.
b. technique
Barr-Record ankle arthrodesis
Barsky
B. cleft closure
B. macrodactyly reduction
B. operation
B. procedure
B. technique
Barsony-Polgar syndrome
Barsony-Teschendorf syndrome
Barthel ADL index
Bartlett
B. nail fold

B. nail fold excision
B. procedure
bar-to-bar clamp
Barton
   B. bandage
   B. fracture
   B. sling
   B. tongs
   B. traction handle
Barton-Cone
   B.-C. tongs
   B.-C. tong traction
Bart-Phumphery syndrome
Barwell operation
basal
   b. block cervical saddle
   b. bone
   b. chevron osteotomy
   b. closing wedge osteotomy
   b. extension
   b. joint
   b. metabolic rate (BMR)
   b. neck
   b. neck fracture
base
   Dycal b.
   b. of finger
   b. of fingernail
   b. of gait
   metacarpal b.
   b. osteotomy
   plantar lateral b.
   Profix nonporous tibial b.
   b. of skull (BOS)
   b. of support
   b. wedge osteotomy
   b. wedge osteotomy/bunionectomy
baseball
   b. finger
   b. finger fracture
   b. finger splint
   b. pitcher's elbow
   b. shoulder
   b. stitch
   b. suture
baseline
   B. Bubble inclinometer
   b. capacity evaluation
   B. dynamometer
   b. view
basement membrane
base-of-the-neck osteotomy

basic
   b. calcium phosphate crystal
      deposition disease
   B. I, II cranial adjusting procedure
   b. hand splint
   b. lamella
   b. multicellular remodeling unit
   b. technique
basilar
   b. bone
   b. cartilage
   b. closing wedge metatarsal
      osteotomy
   b. crescentic osteotomy
   b. femoral neck fracture
   b. impression
   b. invagination
   b. plantarflexory metatarsal
      osteotomy
   b. region
   b. vertebra
Basile hip screw
basilic artery
basioccipital
basivertebral
basket
   Acufex meniscal b.
   b. forceps
   b. rongeur
   rotary b.
   Schutte shovelnose b.
   b. stockinette
   walker b.
basketball foot
basket-weave ankle taping
Basmajian technique
basocervical fracture
basograph
Basser syndrome
Bassett
   B. electrical stimulation apparatus
   B. electrical stimulation device
   B. electrical stimulation system
   B. sign
Basswood splint
Batchelor
   B. plaster
   B. plaster hip spica cast
   B. plate
Batchelor-Brown extraarticular subtalar
   arthrodesis

B

NOTES

Batch-Spittler-McFaddin
    B.-S.-M. knee disarticulation
    B.-S.-M. technique
Bateman
    B. femoral neck prosthesis
    B. finger prosthesis
    B. hemiarthroplasty
    B. shoulder operation
    B. UPF II bipolar knee system
    B. UPF II bipolar prosthesis
    B. UPF prosthesis
    B. UPF II shoulder prosthesis
bath
    Aqua/Whirl b.
    Bag B.
    contrast b. (CB)
    Dickson paraffin b.
    galvanic b.
    hot and cold contrast b.
    hot water b.
    mud pack b.
    Para-Care paraffin therapy b.
    paraffin b. (PB)
    whirlpool b. (WPB)
bathing and dressing ability
Bathlifter
    Leo B.
batrachian
    b. gait
    b. posture
Batson
    vein of B.
    B. vertebral brain system
battery
    Rand Functional Limitations B.
    Rand Physical Capacities B.
battery-driven hand drill
battery-pack Osteo-Stim bone stimulator
battery-powered instrument
batting
    Dacron b.
battledore incision
Battle sign
bat-wing appearance
Batzdorf
    B. cervical wire passer
    B. cervical wire twister
Bauerfeind
    B. Achillotrain
    B. ankle brace
    B. Comprifix knee brace
    B. Malleolic Ankle Orthosis
    B. silicone heel pad
    B. SofSpot Heel Cup
    B. support
Bauer-Jackson classification

Bauer-Tondra-Trusler
    B.-T.-T. operation
    B.-T.-T. technique
Baumann angle
Baumgaertel and Gotzen calcaneal fracture reduction technique
Baumgard-Schwartz
    B.-S. tennis elbow operation
    B.-S. tennis elbow technique
Baumrucker clamp irrigator
Bavarian splint
Baxter
    B. angled arthroscope
    B. nerve release
    B. personal Von-Loc ice pack
Baxter-D'Astous procedure
Bayley Scales of Infant Development
Baylor
    B. adjustable cross splint
    B. metatarsal splint
Bayne
    B. classification of radial agenesis
    B. radial agenesis classification
    B. ulnar ray deficiency classification
Bayne-Klug centralization
bayonet
    b. apposition
    b. clip applier
    b. dislocation
    b. fracture position
    b. knife
    b. leg
    b. nonunion
    b. osteotome
    b. position of fracture
    b. rongeur
    b. saw
    b. sign
    b. spacer
bayonet-point wire
Bazooka support surface
BBB
    blood-brain barrier
BBC
    biceps, brachialis, coracobrachialis
    BBC muscles
BB to MM
    belly button to medial malleolus
    BB to MM examination
BCG
    bacille Calmette-Guérin
BDD
    blistering distal dactylitis
BDH
    biologically designed hip
    BDH prosthesis

BE
below elbow
BE amputation
BEA
below-elbow amputation
beach chair position
beachcomber
The B. prosthetic foot
B. waterproof prosthesis
bead
aminoglycoside-impregnated methyl
methacrylate b.
antibiotic-impregnated b.
copolymer starch copolymer b.
gentamicin b.
metallic b.
methyl methacrylate b.
b. pouch
Septobal b.
targeting b.
bead-blasted prosthesis
beaded
b. guidewire
b. hip pin
b. reamer guidepin
b. transfixion wire
beaded-pin wrench
bead-loaded wire
beak
b. fingernail
b. fracture
b. ligament
metacarpal b.
b. modification with triple
arthrodesis
b. nail
talar b.
beaked
b. cervicomedullary junction
b. pelvis
beaking
b. of head of talus
b. joint
talar b.
beaklike osteophyte formation
Beall-Webel-Bailey technique
Beals
B. syndrome
B. test
beam
Balkan b.

load b.
primary x-ray b.
beanbag
bearing
ball b.
pretibial b. (PTB)
radial b.
spinal load b.
Steinmann pin with ball b.
ulnar b.
unipolar b.
bearing-seating forceps
bear's paw hand
Beasley-Babcock forceps
Beath
B. bone intramedullary peg
B. needle
B. pin
B. view
Beatson combined ankle angle
Beaty lateral release
Beaufort seating orthosis
Beau line
Beaver
B. blade handle
B. cataract knife
B. discission blade
B. keratome blade
B. saw
Beaver-DeBakey
B.-D. blade
B.-D. knife
Beaver-tail rasp
Bebax
B. Bootie
B. orthosis
B. shoe
Bechterew
B. disease
B. test
Bechtol
B. acetabular component
B. arthroplasty
B. hip prosthesis
B. screw
B. shoulder prosthesis
B. system prosthesis
Beckenbaugh
B. correction
B. technique
Becker
B. brace

NOTES

Becker *(continued)*
- B. hand prosthesis
- B. 655 motion control limiter
- B. muscular dystrophy (BMD)
- B. orthopaedic spinal system (BOSS)
- B. orthopaedic spinal system orthotic device
- B. orthopaedic thermoformable ankle system
- B. screwdriver
- B. technique
- B. tendon repair
- B. variant of Duchenne dystrophy

Becker-type tardive muscular dystrophy
Beckman retractor
Beck-Steffee total ankle prosthesis
Béclard amputation
Becton
- B. open reduction
- B. technique

bed
- air b.
- American Seating Access-O-Matic b.
- BioDyne b.
- bone graft b.
- Borg-Warner orthopaedic b.
- Burke Bariatric b.
- Cardiopulmonary Paragon 8500 b.
- Carrom orthopaedic b.
- Chick-Foster orthopedic b.
- circle b.
- CircOlectric b.
- Clinitron air b.
- b. cradle
- DMI orthopedic b.
- Flexicair b.
- FluidAir b.
- Foster b.
- fracture b.
- Gatch b.
- Goodman orthopedic b.
- Hausted orthopedic b.
- high-air-loss b.
- high muscular resistance b.
- Hill-Rom orthopedic b.
- hi-lo rehab b.
- Hollywood b.
- Inland Super Multi-Hite orthopedic b.
- Inter-Royal frame orthopedic b.
- Joerns orthopedic b.
- Keane Mobility b.
- KinAir b.
- Lapidus b.
- low-air-loss b.
- Magnum 800 b.

- Medicus b.
- Mega-Air b.
- Mega Tilt and Turn b.
- b. mobility skill
- nail b.
- obese b.
- orthopaedic b.
- Plastizote foot b.
- b. rest
- Restcue b.
- b. rest-related deconditioning
- b. of rib
- ROHO b.
- Roto-Rest b.
- Simmons Multi-Matic orthopedic b.
- Simmons Vari-Hite orthopedic b.
- skeletal b.
- Skytron b.
- SMI 3000, 5000 b.
- Smith-Davis Converta-Hite orthopedic b.
- Spa B.
- Stryker b.
- Superior Sleeprite Hi-Lo orthopedic b.
- Swinger car b.
- Thera Pulse b.
- Tilt and Turn Paragon b.
- Ultraflex orthopedic b.
- b. wedge

Bed-Bar support rail
Bednar tumor
bedroom fracture
bed-to-chair transfer
Beebe wire-cutting scissors
beefburger procedure
Beery Visual Motor Integration Test
Beeson
- B. cast spreader
- B. plaster spreader

bee venom therapy
Beevor sign
behavior
- compensatory b.
- occupational b.

behavioral
- B. Assessment of Pain (BAP)
- B. Assessment of Pain Questionnaire
- b. mapping

Behçet syndrome
Behr syndrome
Beighton hypermobility syndrome criteria
Bekhterev
- B. arthritis
- B. deep reflex
- B. disease

B. rheumatoid spondylitis
B. sitting test
Bekhterev-Mendel reflex
Bekhterev-Strümpell spondylitis
Belcher clamp
bell
Hydro-Tone B.
B. palsy
b. rasp
B. suture
B. table
Bell-Dally cervical dislocation
Bellemore-Barrett closing wedge osteotomy
Bell-Tawse
B.-T. open reduction
B.-T. open reduction technique
B.-T. procedure
Bellucci alligator scissors
belly
b. button to medial malleolus (BB to MM)
b. button to medial malleolus examination
muscle b.
belly-press test
Belos compression pin
below
b. elbow (BE)
b. knee (BK)
below-elbow
b.-e. amputation (BEA)
b.-e. prosthesis
below-knee
b.-k. amputation (BKA)
b.-k. prosthesis
b.-k. suspension
b.-k. walking cast
belt
AquaJogger buoyancy b.
Carabelt therapeutic b.
cast b.
Cool-Flex A/K suspension b.
gait b.
Meek pelvic traction b.
pelvic traction b.
Posey b.
Reed cast b.
rib b.
sacroiliac b.
Schiek B.
seat b.

Serola sacroiliac b.
SI b.
Silesian b.
Soma sacroiliac stabilization b.
Spine Power pelvic stabilizer b.
S'port Max sacroiliac b.
Sports Plus II back b.
TES b.
Thera-Band Aqua B.
Tri-Flex auxiliary suspension b.
waist suspension b.
WRUN-N equipment reflective safety b.
bench
Ensolite padded transfer b.
b. examination
Invacare vinyl transfer b.
Paramount 3-Way Press B.
pelvic b.
b. test
Winco Adjusting B.
bend
deep knee b. (DKB)
sitting side b.
standing side b.
Bend-A-Boot foot splint
bender
AO plate b.
Bunnell knuckle b.
cast b.
DePuy rod b.
French rod b.
Luque rod b.
plate b.
rod b.
Rush b.
bender's
Knuckle B.
bending
backward b.
cantilever b.
forward b.
b. fracture
ipsilateral side b.
lateral b.
b. load
rod b.
side b.
b. strength
b. stress
b. toward the side of injury
Bendixen-Kirschner traction

NOTES

benediction
    b. attitude sign
    b. posture
Benedict-Roth apparatus
benefit
    pedal disability b.
    Viscolas heel pain and
      disability b.
Benefoot & Birkenstock orthotic sandal
benign
    b. bone aneurysm
    b. chondroblastoma
    b. congenital myopathy
    b. cortical defect
    b. fasciculation
    b. hypermobile joint syndrome
    b. subsidence
    b. tumor
Benink tarsal index
Bennett
    B. basic hand dislocation
    B. basic hand fracture
    B. basic hand splint
    B. bone retractor
    B. comminuted fracture
    B. elevator
    B. fracture-dislocation
    B. fracture of thumb
    B. lesion
    B. nail biopsy
    B. orthosis
    B. pain model
    B. posterior shoulder approach
    B. quadriceps plastic operation
    B. quadriceps plastic procedure
    B. thumb fracture classification
    B. tibial retractor
bent
    b. nail
    B. operation
bent-knee
    b.-k. cast
    b.-k. syndrome
Bentson procedure
Benyi modification of Lambrinudi triple arthrodesis
benzoin
    b. adherent tape
    b. adhesive
    tincture of b.
BeOK hand exercise putty
Berens
    B. muscle clamp
    B. muscle clamp forceps
    B. osteotomy

BERG
    balloon-assisted, endoscopic,
      retroperitoneal, gasless
    BERG lumbar interbody fusion
Berg balance test
Berger
    B. capsulodesis
    B. exercise
    B. interscapular amputation
    B. operation
    B. paresthesia
Berger-Bookwalter posterior approach
Bergman mallet
Bergstrom
    B. cannula
    B. needle
Berke clamp
Berliner percussion hammer
Berman-Gartland
    B.-G. metatarsal osteotomy
    B.-G. procedure
Berman-Moorhead metal locator
Bermuda spica cast
Berndt
    B. classification
    B. hip ruler
Berndt-Hardy classification of transchondral fracture
Bernese periacetabular osteotomy
Bernhard clamp
Berstein cast table
Bertin
    B. bone
    B. hip retractor
    B. ligament
Bertolotti syndrome
Besnier rheumatism
Bestfoam insole
besylate
    atracurium b.
Betadine
    B. dressing
    B. scrub solution
    B. soak
    B. soap
Betadine-soaked pledget
beta-endorphin
    plasma b.-e.
beta-2-microglobulin
    b.-2-m. amyloidosis
    b.-2-m. deposition
Beta Pile II, III splint strap
beta-sympathomimetic
Bethesda bone
Bethune
    B. clamp
    B. periosteal elevator
    B. rib shears

Bethune-Coryllos rib shear
Bevatron accelerator
bevel
beveled chisel
bevel-point Rush pin
Bevin shoe
Beyer rongeur
Beyer-Stille bone rongeur
BFM
    Brunnstrom-Fugl-Meyer
      BFM arm impairment assessment
      BFM impairment
BFO
    balanced forearm orthosis
      BFO Kit
      BFO Orthosis
B.H. Moore procedure
BIA
    bioelectrical impedance analysis
Bi-Angular shoulder prosthesis
biarticular
    b. bone-cutting forceps
    b. bone shears
biarticulate
bias-cut
    b.-c. stockinette
    b.-c. tape
biaxial
    b. flap
    b. joint
    B. Weave composite prosthesis
BICAP
    Bipolar Circumactive Probe
      BICAP cautery
bicapsular
bicentric prosthesis
biceps
    b., brachialis, coracobrachialis
    (BBC)
    b. brachialis muscle transfer
    b. brachialis tendon
    b. brachii muscle
    b. brachii tendon
    b. elevator
    b. femoris
    b. femoris muscle
    b. femoris tendon
    b. interval lesion (BIL)
    b. jerk (BJ)
    b. jerk reflex test
    b. reflex
    b. tendinitis

Bichat ligament
bicipital
    b. bursitis
    b. groove
    b. muscle
    b. rib
    b. sulcus
    b. syndrome
    b. tendinitis
    b. tendon
    b. tenosynovitis
    b. tuberosity
    b. tuberosity view
Bickel
    B. intramedullary nail
    B. intramedullary rod
    B. legholder
Bickel-Moe procedure
bicolumn fracture
bicompartmental
    b. implant
    b. knee implant prosthesis
    b. replacement of knee
    b. soft tissue sarcoma
biconcave
    b. deformity
    b. vertebra
bicondylar
    b. ankle prosthesis
    b. graft
    b. knee prosthesis
    b. tibial plateau
    b. T-shaped fracture
    b. Y-shaped fracture
Bicon-Plus Cup
bicorrectional Austin osteotomy
bicortical
    b. iliac bone
    b. iliac bone graft
    b. ilial strip graft
    b. screw
    b. screw fixation
bicycle, bike
    air b.
    Air-Dyne b.
    b. brace
    b. ergometer
    b. ergometry
    b. exerciser
    FES exercise b.
    b. injury

NOTES

bicycle *(continued)*
    Monark b.
    New Schwinn 900 b.
    New Schwinn elliptical b.
    recumbent b.
    Schwinn Air-Dyne b.
    Schwinn Spinner b.
    Schwinn 900 stationary b.
    b. spoke fracture
BID
    bilateral interfacetal dislocation
bidirectional traction
Bielschowsky head tilt test
Bielschowsky-Jansky disease
Bier
    B. amputation
    B. amputation saw
    B. block
    B. block anesthesia
    B. lumbar puncture needle
    B. operation
bifid
    b. condyle
    b. foot
    b. graft
    b. hook
    b. spinous process
    b. thumb
    b. thumb deformity
bifida
    spina b.
bifilar needle recording electrode
biflanged drill
Bi-Flex
bifocal manipulative with distraction jing
biframed distraction technique
bifrontal incision
bifurcate
    b. ligament
    b. navicular
bifurcated
    b. bladeplate
    b. vein graft for vascular reconstruction
bifurcation osteotomy
bifurcatum
    ligamentum b.
big
    b. band
    b. toe test
Bigelow
    B. crural
    B. iliopectineal
    B. ligament
    B. maneuver
    B. septum

Bigliani/Flatow
    B./F. complete shoulder
    B./F. total shoulder arthroplasty
biglycan
bike *(var. of* bicycle)
Bike ankle brace
BIL
    biceps interval lesion
bilateral
    b. acute radicular syndrome
    b. amputation
    b. arm raise back exercise technique
    b. chronic radicular syndrome
    b. frame
    b. hemiplegia
    b. heterotopic ossification
    b. interfacetal dislocation (BID)
    b. lateral fusion
    strength test eccentric b.
    b. talocalcaneal coalition
    b. variable screw placement system
    b. V-Y Kutler flap
Bilhaut-Cloquet procedure
Bill bar
bilobed
    b. digital neurovascular island flap
    b. skin flap
bilocular joint
Bilos
    B. pin
    B. pin extractor
bimalleolar
    b. angle
    b. ankle fracture
    b. approach to ankle arthrodesis
bimalleolar-foot axis
Bi-Metric
    B.-M. hip prosthesis
    B.-M. Interlok femoral prosthesis
    B.-M. porous primary femoral prosthesis
Bindegewebsmassage
binder
    abdominal b.
    arch b.
    cloth b.
    Dale abdominal b.
    Helenca b.
    sacroiliac b.
    Scultetus b.
binding
    biologic b.
bind wire
Bing-Horton syndrome
binocular loupe

bioabsorbable
    b. material
    b. tack repair
Bio-Absorbable interference screw
BioAction great toe implant
bioactive (BA)
    b. bone cement
    b. implant
Bio-Anchor suture anchor
Bio-Boot
Biobrane
    B. adhesive
    B. glove
BioCast wrist/hand orthosis
bioceramic implant material
biochemical
    b. abnormality
    b. marker
Bio-Chromatic hand prosthesis
Bioclad with pegs reinforced acetabular prosthesis
Bioclusive select transparent film dressing
biocompatibility
    implant b.
biocompatible
BioCompression Pneumatic Sleeve
Biocoral
Bio-Corkscrew
    headed B.-C.
biocorrosion
BioCuff
    B. C bioresorbable cannulated screw
    B. C bioresorbable spike washer implant
biodegradable
    b. calcium phosphate cement
    b. fixation device
    b. fixation instrumentation
    b. implant
    b. plate
    b. surgical tack
    b. synthetic polymer
Biodel implant
Bio-Dermal hydrogel kit
Biodex
    B. Balance System
    B. cycle ergometer
    B. Gait Trainer
    B. isokinetic dynamometer
    B. isokinetic testing machine

    B. Multi-Joint System 3 MVP
    B. target balance trainer
    B. test
    B. Unweighing Support System
    B. Unweighing System partial weight therapy
Biodynamic Molding System
BioDyne bed
bioelectric
    b. phenomenon
    b. potential
bioelectrical
    b. impedance
    b. impedance analysis (BIA)
    b. repair of delayed union or nonunion
bioenergy imbalance syndrome (BIS)
Bio-FASTak
    B.-F. anchor
    B.-F. suture
biofeedback-assisted method
Biofeedback 5DX
BioFit Press-Fit acetabular prosthesis
Biofix
    B. absorbable fixation
    B. absorbable fixation system
    B. arrow gun
    B. biodegradable implant
    B. meniscus arrow
    B. system pin
BIOflex
    B. Magnet Back Support
    B. magnetic counterforce brace
    B. medical magnet
    B. orthotic
Bio Flote air flotation system
Biofoot orthotic
Bio-Form glove
Bio-Gel decubitus pillow
Bioglass prosthesis
Bio-Groove
    B.-G. acetabular prosthesis
    B.-G. Macrobond HA femoral prosthesis
bioimplant
    OrthoBlast osteoinductive b.
Bio-Interference
    B.-I. screwdriver
    B.-I. tibial screw
biokinetic remediation
Biokinetics pedobarograph
BioKnit garment electrode

NOTES

Biolectron bone growth stimulator
biologic
- b. binding
- b. dressing
- b. fixation
- b. fracture management

biologically
- b. designed hip (BDH)
- B. Quiet interference screw
- B. Quiet Mini-Screw suture anchor
- B. quiet stapler

Biolox
- B. ceramic coating

biomagnet
biomaterial
- absorbable b.
- carbon-based b.
- ceramic b.
- collagen-based b.
- PGA-PLA b.
- polymethylmethacrylate b.

biomechanical
- b. analysis
- B. Ankle Platform System (BAPS)
- b. control
- b. factor
- b. failure of implant
- b. frame of reference
- b. integrity
- b. principle
- b. stress
- b. testing

biomechanics
- axial plane angular deformity b.
- bone b.
- distraction instrumentation b.
- Dwyer instrumentation b.
- gait b.
- impact b.
- posterior fixation system b.
- propulsion b.
- soft tissue b.
- walking b.

biomedium
- Dynafill graft b.

BioMed TENS unit
Biomet
- B. acetabular cup
- B. AGC knee prosthesis
- B. ankle arthrodesis nail
- B. Ascent total knee
- B. bone anchor
- B. button
- B. cement-removal hand chisel
- B. custom implant
- B. fracture brace
- B. hip prosthesis

- B. M2A metal-on-metal hip articulation system
- B. MARS acetabular component
- B. Maxim knee system
- B. revision acetabular component
- B. revision hip stem
- B. revision knee system
- B. Second Assistant knee positioner
- B. shoulder component
- B. staple
- B. total toe prosthesis
- B. Ultra-Drive cement remover
- B. Ultra-Drive ultrasonic revision system

biometal
Biometric prosthesis
Bio-Modular
- B.-M. shoulder prosthesis
- B.-M. total shoulder system

Bio-Moore endoprosthesis
bionic
- Rincoe human action b. (R-HAB)

Bionicare 1000 stimulator system
Bionx
- B. absorbable cannulated screw
- B. arrow
- B. self-reinforced PLLA smart screw
- B. servohydraulic testing machine

Bio-Oss synthetic bone
Biophase
- ASTM designation of B.
- B. implant metal
- B. implant metal prosthesis

Bio-Phase suture anchor
biophysics
- chiropractic b. (CBP)

bioplastic
BioPolyMeric graft
BioPro ceramic TARA head
bioprosthesis
- bovine collagen b.

biopsy (Bx)
- aspiration needle b.
- Bennett nail b.
- bone b.
- bone marrow b.
- b. cannula
- channel-and-core b.
- closed core needle b.
- cone bone b.
- core needle b.
- Dunn b.
- excisional b.
- forage core b.
- b. forceps
- Fosnaugh nail b.

freehand CT-guided b.
incisional b.
lumbar spine b.
Michele vertebral b.
needle b.
open b.
percutaneous core bone b.
punch b.
Scher nail b.
spinal infection b.
synovial b.
thoracic spine b.
trephine needle b.
Turkel bone b.
ultrasound-guided echo b.
ultrasound-guided stereotactic b.
Valls-Ottolenghim-Schajowicz
   needle b.
Zaias nail b.
BioRCI screw
bioresorbable
   b. drug delivery system
   b. pin
BioROC anchor
Bio-R-Sorb resorbable poly-L-lactic acid ministaple
BioScrew absorbable interference screw
Biosensor biomechanical testing system
BioSkin
   B. DP wrist support
   B. Q knee brace
BioSole GEL orthotic
BioSorbFX SR self-reinforced plate and screw
BioSorb suture
BioSphere
   B. suture anchor
   B. suture anchor implant
BioStinger low profile fixation device
BioStop G bone cement restrictor
Biosyn synthetic monofilament suture
Biotens neurostimulator
Biotex
   B. implant metal
   B. implant metal prosthesis
biothesiometer testing
Biothotic
   B. foot orthosis
   B. orthotic
   B. orthotic mold
Biotone Polar lotion
Bio-Wick sock

BioWrap lumbosacral/sacral support
bipartita
   patella b.
bipartite
   b. fracture
   b. ossification
   b. patella
   b. scaphoid
   b. tibial sesamoid
bipedal walking
bipedicle dorsal flap
biphasic
   b. action potential
   b. endplate activity
   b. waveform
bipivotal hinge knee brace
biplanar
   b. fixator
   b. radiography
biplane
   b. angiogram
   b. Dwyer osteotomy
   b. roentgenogram
   b. trochanteric osteotomy
biplaning of osteotomy
bipolar
   b. acetabular cup
   b. cauterization
   b. cautery
   B. Circumactive Probe (BICAP)
   b. coagulator
   b. femoral component
   b. femoral head prosthesis
   b. forceps
   b. hip arthroplasty
   b. hip arthroplasty component
   b. hip replacement prosthesis
   b. IF waveform
   b. needle recording electrode
   b. prosthetic cup
   b. release
   b. stimulating electrode
   b. vertebral traction
Bircher
   B. bone-holding clamp
   B. cartilage clamp
   B. meniscotome
   B. meniscus knife
Bircher-Ganske cartilage forceps
Bircher-Weber technique
birdcage splint
Bird & Cronin wrist brace

NOTES

birefringent lipid crystals in tendinitis
Birkenstock
B. Blue Footbed arch support
B. high-flange arch support
B. shoe
birth
b. fracture
b. injury
b. trauma
BIS
bioenergy imbalance syndrome
bisacromial
Bischof myelotomy
bisector line
Bishop
B. bone clamp
B. chisel
B. classification
B. gouge
B. saw
Bishop-Black tendon tucker
Bishop-DeWitt tendon tucker
Bishop-Peter tendon tucker
bit
AO drill b.
cannulated drill b.
b. drill
drill b.
femoral drill b.
Gore b.
hip fracture compaction drill b.
Howmedica Microfixation System
drill b.
Leibinger Micro System drill b.
Luhr Microfixation System drill b.
Storz Microsystems drill b.
Synthes Microsystems drill b.
biter
Stille bone b.
suction b.
bite sign
bivalved
b. cylinder cast
b. pancake plaster hand cast
bivalve overlap brace
bizarre
b. high-frequency discharge
b. parosteal osteochondromatous
proliferation (BPOP)
b. repetitive discharge
b. repetitive potential
BJ
biceps jerk
Björk
B. prosthesis
B. rib drill
Björnström algesimeter

BK
below knee
BK mole syndrome
BK prosthesis
BKA
below-knee amputation
black
b. heel syndrome
B. Max mid size knee component
B. peroneal tendon sheath injection
B. rasp
B. repair
B. technique
Black-Broström staple technique
Blackburn
B. technique
B. traction
Blackburne ratio
Blackburn-Peel
B.-P. measurement
B.-P. ratio
black-dot heel
bladder
b. augmentation
b. dysfunction
b. injury
neurogenic b.
blade
arachnoid-shape Beaver b.
Arthro-Lok system of Beaver b.
banana Beaver b.
Bard-Parker b.
Beaver-DeBakey b.
Beaver discission b.
Beaver keratome b.
cartilage shaver b.
Caspar b.
cast b.
chisel b.
Curdy b.
curved meniscotome b.
discission knife Beaver b.
Dynagrip handle of b.
Dyonics arthroscopic b.
Field b.
Gigli saw b.
Hebra b.
Hibbs b.
hook b.
Incisor arthroscopic b.
K b.
keratome Beaver b.
knife b.
Merlin arthroscopy b.
mini-meniscus b.
3M Maxi Driver b.
notchplasty b.
Paufique b.

b. plate
b. plate driver
b. plate fixation
PowerCut drill b.
resector b.
retrograde Beaver b.
retrograde meniscal b.
rosette Beaver b.
shoulder b.
sickle-shape Beaver b.
side-cutting b.
Smillie-Beaver b.
Superblade b.
Swann-Morton surgical b.
Synovator arthroscopic b.
synovectomy b.
Taylor spinal retractor b.
Temperlite saw b.
Tiger b.
triradial resector b.
Zimmer-Gigli saw b.
bladeplate
bifurcated b.
b. construct
fixed-angle AO b.
blade-point retractor
blade-spike retractor
Blair
B. ankle arthrodesis
B. ankle fusion
B. anterior arthrodesis
B. chisel
B. elevator
B. knife
B. procedure
B. saw guide
B. talar body fusion blade plate
B. technique
B. tibiotalar arthrodesis
B. tibiotalar arthrodesis blade plate
Blair-Brown skin graft
Blair-Morris-Dunn-Hand ankle arthrodesis
Blair-Omer rerouting
Blajwas-Schwartz-Marcinko irrigation drainage system
Blalock clamp
Blanchard
B. traction device
B. traction device blade plate
blank
Aliplast b.

implant b.
Nickelplast b.
Plastazote b.
Blanke inverted tibialis posterior tendon orthotic
blanket
Hollister Hot/Ice knee b.
Rowe b.
blastomycosis
North American b.
blastomycotic osteomyelitis
Blatt
B. capsulodesis
B. procedure
Blatt-Ashworth procedure
Blauth knee prosthesis
Blazina
B. prosthesis
B. tendinopathy
BLE
both lower extremities
bleb capsulodesis
Bleck
B. iliopsoas recession
B. metatarsus adductus classification
B. method
B. recession technique
Bledsoe
B. cast brace
B. fracture brace
B. knee brace
B. leg brace
bleeding
b. bone
b. point
blennorrhagica
keratoderma b.
blind
b. anchorage hole
b. medullary nail
b. medullary nailing
blink
b. reflex
b. response
Bliskunov implantable femoral distractor
blister
bone b.
b. of bone
B. Film dressing
fracture b.
blistering distal dactylitis (BDD)
Blix contractile force curve

NOTES

79

bloc
    en b.

Bloch equation

block
    Airlite alignable ankle b.
    ankle b.
    anodal b.
    articular b.
    axillary b.
    balsa wood filler b.
    Bier b.
    bone and limb growth velocity
      ratios bone b.
    Boyd posterior bone b.
    brachial plexus b.
    Campbell posterior bone b.
    common peroneal nerve b.
    conduction b.
    condyle b.
    cutting b.
    depolarization b.
    differential spinal b.
    digital nerve b.
    facet joint b.
    femoral nerve b.
    field b.
    filler b.
    B. fixator
    forefoot nerve b.
    four-in-one cutting b.
    functional grip pushup b.
    ganglion b.
    ganglionic b.
    Gill posterior bone b.
    graduated-height b.
    hand b.
    Hara infiltration b.
    Howard bone b.
    iliac crest bone b.
    Inclan posterior bone b.
    intercostal nerve b.
    interscalene b.
    joint b.
    Kohs b.
    lumbar sympathetic b.
    Mayo nerve b.
    median nerve b.
    metacarpal b.
    metatarsal b.
    Mikhail bone b.
    motor point b.
    musculocutaneous nerve b.
    nerve root b.
    neurolytic b.
    neuromuscular b.
    b. osteotomy
    parasacral b.
    paravertebral b.
    patellar tendon bone b.
    PED b.
    pelvic b.
    perineural b.
    peripheral nerve b.
    plantar V infiltration b.
    plexus b.
    popliteal sciatic nerve b.
    posterior bone b.
    presacral b.
    pudendal b.
    push-up b.
    Putti posterior bone b.
    recurrent median nerve b.
    regional b.
    sacral b.
    sacroiliac b.
    scalene b.
    sciatic leg b.
    S-cutting b.
    sphenopalatine ganglion b.
    spinal cord b.
    Steinberg infiltration b.
    stellate sympathetic ganglion b.
    Styrofoam filler b.
    subarachnoid b.
    sympathetic b.
    b. test
    tibial cutting b.
    transsacral b.
    two-point nerve b.
    ulnar nerve b.
    b. vertebra
    vertebral b.

blockade
    central neural b.
    popliteal fossa neural b.
    sympathetic b.

blockage
    articular b.
    extensor tendon b.

blocker
    b. exostosis
    hook b.

blood
    autologous b.
    b. cast
    b. culture
    b. flow
    b. loss
    b. loss anemia
    b. pool phase
    b. pressure
    b. pressure monitor (BPM)
    b. pressure monitoring
    b. supply
    b. transfusion
    b. vessel tumor

b. viscosity
b. volume pulse (BVP)
blood-borne infection
blood-brain barrier (BBB)
bloodless
b. amputation
b. field
bloody effusion
bloom
B. splint
B. syndrome
Bloomberg sign
Bloom-Raney
B.-R. modification
B.-R. modification of Smith-Robinson technique
blot test
Blount
B. anvil retractor
B. blade plate
B. bone spreader
B. brace
B. disease
B. displacement osteotomy
B. epiphysiodesis
B. fracture staple
B. knee retractor
B. knife
B. laminar spreader
B. osteotome
B. splint
B. stapling
B. technique for osteoclasis
B. tracing technique
Blount-Barber disease
Blount-Schmidt Milwaukee brace
blow-in fracture
blow-out fracture
B&L pinch gauge
Blucher
B. laced shoe
blue
B. Brand Therapy Putty
b. foot syndrome
B. Line orthotic
methylene b.
b. toe syndrome
Blumensaat line
Blumenthal bone rongeur
Blumer shelf
Blundell-Jones
B.-J. hip osteotomy

B.-J. operation
B.-J. technique
B.-J. varus osteotomy
blunt
b. arthroscopic cannula
b. caliper
b. dissection
b. forceps
b. hook
b. hook dissector
b. nose hemostat
b. obturator
b. pressure testing
b. stylet
b. tapered T-handled reamer
b. trocar
blunt-tip
b.-t. iris scissors
b.-t. probe
BMC
bone mineral content
BMD
Becker muscular dystrophy
bone mineral density
BME
brief maximal effort
BMI
body mass index
BMP
bone marrow pressure
bone morphogenetic protein
BMP cabling and plating system
BMR
basal metabolic rate
Bo
Tae Bo
board
adjustable cane b.
alphabet b.
arm b.
balance b.
BAPS b.
broad-based cane b.
English cane b.
Euroglide MKII slide b.
Flexisplint flexed arm b.
glider cane b.
grid maze b.
Hadfield hand b.
hand b.
J b.
Lowman balance b.

B

NOTES

board *(continued)*
    manipulation b.
    memory b.
    powder b.
    quad b.
    Rock ankle exercise b.
    rocker b.
    Rock & Roller exercise b.
    spine b.
    b. splint
    Spri Xercise b.
    Steffensmeier b.
    string drawing b.
    Tegtmeier hand b.
    transfer b.
    vertical foot b.
    Visual Neglect B.
    wobble b.
    Yucca b.
BoarderAnkle brace
boat nail
Bobath technique
Bobechko
    B. sliding barrel hook
    B. spreader
bob and weave
Bock
    B. knee prosthesis
    B. nerve
Bodenstab tourniquet
Bodnar retractor
body, pl. **bodies**
    alignment of vertebral bodies
    ankle loose b.
    apple-shape b.
    B. Armor short leg walker
    B. Armor walker cast
    artificial vertebral b.
    b. awareness
    B. Ball
    cartilaginous loose b.
    b. cast syndrome
    b. composition
    b. composition assessment
    fibrous loose b.
    foreign b. (FB)
    B. Gard neoprene support
    B. Glove orthopaedic product
    intraarticular loose b.
    b. jacket
    b. jacket cast
    Kelvin b.
    b. logic rehabilitation system
    loose joint b.
    b. mass index (BMI)
    B. Master
    B. Masters MD 510 hi-lo pulley
        system

    Maxwell b.
    b. mechanics
    B. Mechanics Evaluation Checklist
    melon-seed b.
    navicular b.
    newtonian b.
    Ortho-Mold lumbar b.
    B. Oscillation Integrates
        Neuromuscular Gain (BOING)
    osteocartilaginous loose b.
    osteochondrotic loose b.
    pear-shaped b.
    B. Pedistal
    pedunculated loose b.
    Renaut b.
    B. Response system
    rice b.
    b. righting reflex
    rigid b.
    b. of scapula
    b. side integration
    B. Sport ankle brace
    B. Sticks massager
    b. sway
    talar b.
    Verocay b.
    b. of vertebra
    vertebral b.
    b. weight
    b. weight/composition
    winterize b.
BodyBilt chair
Bodyblade
bodyCushion
    SwimEx aquatic therapy b.
body-exhaust suit
BodyIce
    B. cold pack
    B. cold pack wrap
Bodyline
    B. Back-Huggar
    B. sleeper mattress overlay
    B. Sports Brace
Bodynapper Comfort Pillow
body-powered prosthetic device
Body-Solid exercise equipment
bodywork
Boeck sarcoid
bogginess
boggy
    b. consistency
    b. swelling
    b. synovitis
Böhler
    B. brace
    B. calcaneal angle

B. calcaneal fracture reduction
technique
B. calcaneal view
B. cast breaker
B. clamp
B. extension bow
B. fracture frame
B. guideline
B. lumbosacral angle
B. lumbosacral view
B. nail
B. pin
B. reducing frame
B. skintight cast
B. stirrup
B. tongs
B. tong traction
B. wire splint
Böhler-Braun
B.-B. frame
B.-B. leg sling
B.-B. splint
Böhler-Knowles hip pin
Böhler-Steinmann
B.-S. pin
B.-S. pin holder
Bohlman
B. anterior cervical vertebrectomy
B. cervical fusion technique
B. pin
B. triple-wire fusion
B. triple-wire technique
Boies forceps
BOING
Body Oscillation Integrates
Neuromuscular Gain
Boitzy open reduction
Bold compression screw
Boldrey brace
Bolero lift bath trolley
Bolin wedge filter system
bollard device
Bollinger knee brace
Boloxie OT Prehension Game
bolster
abduction b.
cotton b.
finger b.
knee b.
padded b.
roll control b.
rubber b.

Telfa b.
tie-over b.
bolt
Alvar condylar b.
Barr b.
bone lock b.
cannulated b.
connecting b.
b. cutter
DePuy b.
Fenton tibial b.
fixation b.
b. fixation
Hardinge expansion b.
Harris b.
Herzenberg b.
hexhead b.
Holt b.
Hubbard b.
Hubbard-Nylok b.
Moreira b.
No-Lok b.
Norman tibial b.
Recon proximal drill guide b.
Richmond b.
slotted b.
solid hex b.
tibial b.
transfixion b.
trochanteric b.
Webb-Andreesen condylar b.
Webb stove b.
Wilson b.
wire fixation b.
Zimmer tibial b.
Boltzmann distribution
bolus
bombardment by nociceptor
Bombelli-Mathys-Morscher hip prosthesis
Bombelli-Morscher femoral component
Bond arm splint
Bondek suture
bonding
Poly-Lock b.
bone
AAA b.
b. abscess
b. absorption
accessory b.
acetabular b.
acromial b.
adamantinoma of long b.

NOTES

83

bone *(continued)*
- b. age
- b. age according to Greulich and Pyle
- b. age ratio
- alar b.
- Albers-Schönberg marble b.
- Albrecht b.
- Allofix freeze-dried b.
- b. allograft
- allograft iliac b.
- alveolar supporting bone ankle b.
- ankle b.
- antigen-extracted allogenic b.
- anvil b.
- arch of b.
- architectural alterations of b.
- areola of b.
- articulation of pisiform b.
- astragalar b.
- astragalocalcaneal b.
- astragalocrural b.
- astragaloid b.
- astragaloscaphoid b.
- astragalotibial b.
- astragalus b.
- b. autogenous graft
- autogenous iliac b.
- b. awl
- axis b.
- b. bank
- banked b.
- basal b.
- basilar b.
- Bertin b.
- Bethesda b.
- bicortical iliac b.
- b. biomechanics
- Bio-Oss synthetic b.
- b. biopsy
- b. biopsy needle
- bleeding b.
- b. blister
- blister of b.
- b. block fusion
- b. block graft
- b. block procedure
- b. in bone finding
- Bonfiglio b.
- b. borer
- b. bowing
- breast b.
- bregmatic b.
- Breschet b.
- bridging b.
- brittle b.
- b. bruise
- b. bruise sign

- B. Bullet suture anchor
- bundle b.
- b. bur
- B. Button orthopaedic suture anchor
- cadaver b.
- calcaneal b.
- calcaneocuboid b.
- Calcitite b.
- b. callus
- calvarial free b.
- cancellated b.
- cancellous versus cortical b.
- candle wax appearance of b.
- cannon b.
- capitate b.
- carpal b.
- cavalry b.
- b. cement
- central b.
- cervical vertebral b.
- chalky b.
- chevron b.
- b. chip
- b. chip graft
- b. chisel
- coalition of b.
- coccygeal b.
- coffin b.
- collar b.
- compact b.
- b. conduction threshold
- cone and socket b.
- continuity of b.
- convoluted b.
- b. core
- coronary b.
- corticocancellous b.
- costal b.
- coxal b.
- cranial b.
- b. crisis
- cuboid b.
- cuneiform b.
- b. curette
- b. cyst
- b. cyst excision
- b. cyst fracture probability
- b. cyst treatment
- dead b.
- b. debris
- b. defect
- demineralized b.
- dense b.
- b. densitometry
- b. density
- b. density and arthritis testing system

b. density study
b. deposition
b. depression
dermal b.
b. destructive process
detritus b.
b. development
dimple the b.
b. disease
disorganized b.
b. dissection
b. dollop
b. dowel
b. drill set
Durapatite b.
b. dysplasia
eburnated b.
ectocuneiform b.
ectopic b.
elbow b.
b. elevator
enchondral b.
enchondroma of b.
b. end
endochondral b.
entocuneiform b.
entrapped plantar b.
eosinophilic granuloma of b.
epactal b.
epipteric b.
exercise b.
exoccipital b.
b. extension clamp
b. extractor
femoral b.
b. femoral plug
fibular b.
b. file
b. fixation surface coating
flank b.
b. flap fixation plate
flat b.
Flower b.
fourth turbinated b.
fovea centralis b.
b. fragment
fragmental b.
freshening of b.
frontal b.
fusiform periosteal new b.
Goethe b.
b. gouge

b. graft bed
b. graft collapse
b. graft decompression
B. Grafter instrument
b. graft extrusion
b. graft incorporation
b. graft placement
b. graft punch
b. graft repair
b. graft shoe horn
greater multangular b.
great toe b.
b. growth
growth center of b.
b. growth stimulator
hamate b.
b. hand drill
b. harvesting
b. healing
heterotopic b.
highest turbinated b.
b. holder
b. hole punch
hollow b.
b. hook
hooked b.
hook of hamate b.
humeral b.
hydroxyapatite b.
hyoid b.
hyperplastic b.
b. hypertrophy
iliac b.
immature b.
b. impactor
b. implant
b. implant material
incarial b.
incisive b.
incomplete fracture of b.
b. infarct
b. infarction
infected b.
b. infection
b. ingrowth
innominate b.
intermaxillary b.
interparietal b.
Interpore b.
b. interstice
intrachondrial b.
irregular b.

NOTES

bone *(continued)*
    ischial b.
    b. island
    b. isograft
    ivory b.
    jugal b.
    Kiel b.
    knuckle b.
    Krause b.
    lacrimal b.
    b. lacuna
    lamellar b.
    lamellated b.
    laminar b.
    b. lavage
    lenticular b.
    lesser multangular b.
    b. and limb growth velocity ratios
      bone block
    b. liner
    b. lock bolt
    long axis of b.
    b. loss
    lunate b.
    lunocapitate b.
    luxated b.
    lyophilization of b.
    malar b.
    b. mallet
    marble b.
    b. marrow
    b. marrow aspiration
    b. marrow biopsy
    b. marrow edema
    b. marrow embolism
    b. marrow graft
    b. marrow pressure (BMP)
    b. marrow stimulating technique
    b. marrow tumor
    b. matrix
    b. maturation
    b. maturity
    b. meal
    medial metacarpal b.
    membranous b.
    mesocuneiform b.
    b. metabolic unit
    metacarpal b.
    metatarsal b.
    b. mill
    b. mineral content (BMC)
    b. mineral density (BMD)
    b. mineralization isotope
    morcellized b.
    b. morphogenetic protein (BMP)
    b. mortise
    b. mulch screw
    multangular b.

navicular b.
b. necrosis
necrotic b.
b. neoplasm
newly woven b.
Nicoll b.
nonlamellar b.
nonlamellated b.
occipital b.
omovertebral b.
orbitosphenoidal b.
osteoclast-mediated b.
osteonal lamellar b.
osteopenic b.
osteoporotic b.
pagetoid b.
palatine b.
parietal b.
particle of b.
b. paste
b. pathology
b. peg
b. peg epiphysiodesis
b. pegging
b. peg graft
perilesional b.
periosteal new b.
petrosal b.
petrous temporal b.
phalangeal b.
ping-pong b.
Pirie b.
pisiform b.
B. Plast bone replacement material
b. plate selection
b. plombage
b. plug cutter
b. plug extractor
b. plug setter
porotic b.
postulnar b.
preinterparietal b.
primary lymphoma of b. (PLB)
primitive b.
b. production
b. prosthesis
pterygoid b.
pubic b.
b. punch forceps
b. punch rongeur
quadripartite b.
radial b.
raw b.
b. reamer
b. remodeling
b. remodeling unit
replacement b.
b. resection

B

b. resorption
b. resurfacing
resurrection b.
rider's b.
Riolan b.
rudimentary b.
sacral b.
b. saw
b. scan
scaphoid b.
b. scintigraphy
b. sclerosis
sclerotic b.
b. screw depth gauge
b. screw ruler gauge
b. screw targeter
scroll b.
semilunar b.
b. sequestrum
sesamoid b.
b. setting
b. shaft
b. shaft fracture
shank b.
shin b.
short b.
shoulder b.
b. sialoprotein
b. skid
sliver of b.
b. slurry
b. spacer
b. spicule
spike of b.
splint b.
spongy b.
b. spreader
b. spur
squamooccipital b.
squamous-type b.
b. staple system
b. stock
b. strength
stump of b.
subchondral b.
subcoracoid b.
subperiosteal new b.
b. substance
b. substitute
b. substitute backfilling
supernumerary b.
supraoccipital b.

suprasternal b.
b. surface lesion
b. survey
sutural b.
b. suture fixation
b. suturing wire chisel-tip wire
synthetic b.
talonavicular b.
b. tamp
tarsal b.
temporal b.
thoracic b.
three-cornered b.
tibia b.
trabecular b.
b. transfer
trapezium b.
trapezoid b.
b. trephine
triangular wrist b.
tripartite b.
triquetrum b.
b. trough
b. tuberculoma
tumor-bearing b.
b. tunnel
tympanic b.
ulna b.
ulnar sesamoid b.
ulnar styloid b.
b. ultrasound attenuation (BUA)
unciform b.
uncinate b.
vascular bundle implantation
  into b.
vascular metaphysial b.
vesalian b.
Vesalius b.
vomer b.
b. wax
b. wax gelatin sponge
b. wedge
whettle b.
b. wire guide
wormian b.
woven b.
xiphoid b.
zygomatic b.
bone-biting forceps
bone-breaking forceps
bone-cement interface
bone-cutting forceps

NOTES

bone-forming
    b.-f. sarcoma bone imaging
    b.-f. tumor
bone-graft plug
bone-grasping forceps
bone-holding
    b.-h. clamp
    b.-h. forceps
    b.-h. instrumentation
bone-implant interface
bone-ingrowth fixation
bonelet
Boneloc cement
bonemeal tablet
bone-nibbling rongeur
bone-patellar
    b.-p. ligament-bone (BPB)
    b.-p. tendon-bone (BPB, BPTB)
    b.-p. tendon-bone autograft
    b.-p. tendon-bone preparation
bone-peg interface
BonePlast bone void filler
bone-remodeling
bone-screw interface strength
BoneSource hydroxyapatite cement
bone-specific alkaline phosphatase
  (BSAP)
bone-splitting forceps
bone-tendon
    b.-t. exposure
    b.-t. graft
    b.-t. graft material
bone-tendon-bone
    b.-t.-b. allograft
    b.-t.-b. graft
bone-to-bone
    b.-t.-b. apposition
    b.-t.-b. graft
bone-within-bone appearance
Bonferroni correction
Bonfiglio
    B. bone
    B. bone graft
    B. bone replacement material
    B. modification
    B. modification of Phemister
      technique
Bonfiglio-Bardenstein technique
Bonner position
bonnet
    gluteal b.
Bonney clamp
Bonney-Kessel dorsiflexionary tilt-up
  osteotomy
Bonola technique
bony
    b. abnormality
    b. absorption

    b. ankylosis
    b. architecture
    b. avulsion
    b. bar
    b. bridge
    b. bridge resection
    b. consolidation
    b. crepitus
    b. deformity
    b. demineralization
    b. distal end
    b. eburnation
    b. element destruction
    b. encroachment
    b. erosion
    b. excrescence
    b. exostosis
    b. fossa
    b. hallux limitus
    b. interface
    b. landmark
    b. lesion
    b. mass
    b. metastasis
    b. necrosis and destruction
    b. osteophyte
    b. overgrowth
    b. pelvis
    b. procedure
    b. purchase
    b. reabsorption
    b. semicircular canal
    b. sequestrum
    b. skeleton
    b. slurry leakage
    b. spurring
    b. tenderness
    b. union
Boo-Boo Pacs
Book Butler book-grip device
boomerang wrist support
boot
    All-Purpose B. (APB)
    Ambulator Chukka B.
    APB Hi All-Purpose B.
    b. brace
    Bunny b.
    cast b.
    Chukka b.
    clamshell AFO b.
    compression b.
    Cryo/Cuff b.
    derotation b.
    external sequential pneumatic
      compression b.
    fluid barrier b.
    fracture b.
    gelatin compression b.

Gibney b.
Hang Ups gravity b.
Heelift suspension b.
Heel-Up Boot suspension b.
Jobst b.
Junod b.
L'Nard b.
Markell brace b.
Markell open-toe b.
Moon b.
Multi Podus b.
pneumatic compression b.
Primer modified Unna b.
quadriceps De Lorme b.
RIK FootHugger fluid heel b.
rocker b.
sequential pneumatic compression b.
SlimLine cast b.
Sorrel-type snowboard b.
Spenco b.
Unna paste b.
Venodyne b.
weight b.
Wilke b.
b. wrap
booth
B. test
B. wire osteotomy
bootie
Bebax B.
boot-top
b.-t. fracture
b.-t. laceration
Boplant
B. Surgibone
B. Surgibone bovine bone
substitute
Bora
B. centralization
B. operation
B. technique
borazone blade cutting machine
Borchardt olive-shaped bur
Borchgrevin traction
Borden-Spencer-Herman osteotomy
border
cryptotic medial b.
lateral acromial b.
medial b.
b. ray
b. ray amputation
scapular b.

scapulovertebral b.
superior b.
vertebral b.
bore needle
borer
bone b.
cork b.
Borge clamp
Borggreve
B. limb rotation
B. method
Borggreve-Hall technique
Borg scale
Borg-Warner orthopaedic bed
boring pain
BOS
base of skull
Bose
B. nail fold excision
B. procedure
BOSS
Becker orthopaedic spinal system
boss
carpal b.
carpometacarpal b.
bosselated
bosselation
bossing
frontal b.
Bostick staple
Boston
B. bivalve cast
B. brace thoracolumbosacral
orthosis
B. Classification System
B. elbow system
B. LINAC
B. overlap brace
B. postoperative hip orthosis
B. scoliosis brace
B. soft body jacket
B. soft corset
B. thoracic brace
B. thoracic splint
Bosworth
B. approach
B. arthroplasty
B. bone peg insertion
B. coracoclavicular screw
B. crown drill
B. femoroischial arthrodesis
B. femoroischial transplant

NOTES

Bosworth *(continued)*
    B. femoroischial transplantation
    B. fracture
    B. lumbar spinal fusion
    B. screwdriver
    B. shelf operation
    B. shelf procedure
    B. spine plate
    B. splint
    B. technique
    B. tendo calcaneus repair
Bosworth-type reverse plasty
both
    b. lower extremities (BLE)
    b. upper extremities (BUE)
both-bone fracture
both-column fracture
botryoid sarcoma
bottle sign
bottom
    hoof b.
    weaver's b.
Bottoms-Up posture system
Bouchard
    B. node
    B. nodule
    B. sign
bouche de tapir
bougie needle
bounce home test
Bouncewell medicine ball
bouncing
    ligamentous b.
Bourgery ligament
Bourneville disease
boutonnière
    b. deformity
    b. hand dislocation
    b. splint
Bouvier maneuver
Bovie
    B. cauterization
    B. cautery
    B. coagulating unit
    B. electrocautery apparatus
    B. electrocautery device
    B. knife
    underwater B.
bovine
    b. collagen
    b. collagen bioprosthesis
    b. collagen graft
    b. collagen implant
    b. collagen material prosthesis
bow
    aiming b.
    B. & Arrow cannulated drill guide
    Böhler extension b.

    cupid's b.
    extension b.
    Framer finger extension b.
    Kirschner wire traction b.
    maximum radial b.
    posterior b.
    posteromedial b.
    Schwarz finger extension b.
    traction b.
Bowden cable suspension system
bowed leg
bowel
    neurogenic b.
    b. training
Bowen
    B. chisel
    B. osteotome
    B. periosteal elevator
    B. suture drill
Bowen-Grover meniscotome
Bowers
    B. radial arthroplasty
    B. technique
bowing
    bone b.
    congenital posteromedial b.
    b. deformity
    b. fracture
    lateral b.
    tibial b.
Bowlby arm splint
bowl curette
bowleg
    b. brace
    b. deformity
bowler's thumb
Bowman
    B. angle
    B. disk
    B. muscle
bowstring
    b. sign
    b. tear
    b. test
bow-tie sign
box
    b. and block test of arm disability
    BTE Bolt B.
    b. chisel
    b. curette
    fracture b.
    high toe b.
    ligamentous b.
    b. osteotome
    sit-and-reach b.
    toe b.
    wide toe b.
box-end wrench

boxer's
    b. elbow
    b. fracture
    b. knuckle
    b. punch
boxwood mallet
Boyd
    B. ankle amputation
    B. approach
    B. classification
    B. communicating perforation vein
    B. dual-onlay bone graft
    B. formula
    B. hip disarticulation
    B. Modification of the Tardieu
      spastic measurement scale
    B. operation
    B. perforator
    B. podiatry chair
    B. posterior bone block
    B. side plate
    B. type II fracture
Boyd-Anderson
    B.-A. biceps tendon repair
    B.-A. technique
Boyd-Bosworth procedure
Boyd-Griffin trochanteric fracture
  classification
Boyd-Ingram-Bourkhard treatment
Boyd-McLeod
    B.-M. procedure
    B.-M. tennis elbow technique
Boyd-Sisk
    B.-S. approach
    B.-S. posterior capsulorrhaphy
    B.-S. procedure
Boyer degenerative joint disease
  grading system
Boyes
    B. brachioradialis transfer technique
    B. muscle clamp
    B. test
    B. transfer
Boyes-Goodfellow hook
Boyle-Davis retractor
Boyle-Thompson tendon transfer
Boytchev procedure
Bozzini light conductor
BPB
    bone-patellar ligament-bone
    bone-patellar tendon-bone
      BPB autologous graft

BPM
    blood pressure monitor
      Laserflo BPM
BPOP
    bizarre parosteal osteochondromatous
      proliferation
BPTB
    bone-patellar tendon-bone
      BPTB graft
BPTI
    brachial plexus traction injury
brace
    Abbott b.
    abduction b.
    accommodative b.
    Ace b.
    ACL Lite functional knee b.
    Active ankle b.
    active integral range of motion
      airplane b.
    Active support and b.
    Activity-Lite knee b.
    adjustable b.
    AFO pediatric b.
    Aircast ankle b.
    Aircast Cryo/Cuff b.
    Aircast fracture b.
    Aircast leg b.
    Aircast Pneumatic Air Stirrup b.
    Aircast Swivel-Strap b.
    Aircast walking b.
    Air DonJoy patellofemoral b.
    AirGEL ankle b.
    airplane splint shoulder b.
    Airprene Action knee b.
    Air-Stirrup ankle training b.
    Air Townsend b.
    ALP Plus ankle b.
    AMBI wrist b.
    AMX knee b.
    Ank-L-Aid b.
    ankle ligament protector b.
    ankle stirrup b.
    AO b.
    AOA cervical immobilization b.
    APL Plus ankle b.
    APU b.
    Arizona ankle b.
    Arnold lumbar b.
    ASO ankle b.
    Atak knee b.
    athletic b.

NOTES

B

brace *(continued)*
    Atlanta hip b.
    Atlanta-Scottish Rite b.
    Atlantic overlap b.
    Atlantic rim b.
    ATR b.
    Axis ankle b.
    back b.
    Back Seat torso-wrap b.
    bail-lock b.
    Bauerfeind ankle b.
    Bauerfeind Comprifix knee b.
    Becker b.
    bicycle b.
    Bike ankle b.
    BIOflex magnetic counterforce b.
    Biomet fracture b.
    BioSkin Q knee b.
    bipivotal hinge knee b.
    Bird & Cronin wrist b.
    bivalve overlap b.
    Bledsoe cast b.
    Bledsoe fracture b.
    Bledsoe knee b.
    Bledsoe leg b.
    Blount b.
    Blount-Schmidt Milwaukee b.
    BoarderAnkle b.
    Bodyline Sports B.
    Body Sport ankle b.
    Böhler b.
    Boldrey b.
    Bollinger knee b.
    boot b.
    Boston overlap b.
    Boston scoliosis b.
    Boston thoracic b.
    bowleg b.
    Brite-Life wrist b.
    Buck knee b.
    cable-twister b.
    cage-back b.
    Caligamed b.
    caliper b.
    Callender derotational b.
    Camp b.
    Cam Walker ankle b.
    Cam Walker leg b.
    Can Am b.
    canvas b.
    Capener b.
    Carpal Lock CTS b.
    Carpal Lock wrist b.
    carpenter's b.
    CASH b.
    Castaway leg b.
    Cast Boot polypropylene hip
      abduction b.

    Castiglia ankle b.
    Centec Formfit ankle b.
    Centec Propoint knee b.
    cervical collar b.
    chairback b.
    Charleston nighttime bending b.
    Charleston scoliosis b.
    Charnley b.
    Cheetah ankle b.
    CHH cervical b.
    Chopart b.
    CI functional knee b.
    Cinch Lock CTS b.
    Cincinnati ACL b.
    clamshell b.
    Clinch Lock CTS wrist b.
    CM-Band 505N b.
    CM-Band silicone rubber b.
    Cole hyperextension b.
    collar b.
    Combined Instabilities functional
      knee b.
    contraflexion b.
    controlled-motion b.
    controlled position b. (CPB)
    Cook walking b.
    cool CPB b.
    Cooper ankle b.
    Counter Rotation System b.
    Count'R-Force arch b.
    cowhorn b.
    CRM rehab b.
    CRS b.
    Cruiser hip abduction b.
    CTi b.
    CTi2 knee b.
    Cunningham b.
    custom-fitted b.
    cutout patellar b.
    Dalco Astro ankle b.
    Darco back b.
    DarcoGel ankle b.
    Defiance functional knee b.
    Dennison cervical b.
    DePuy fracture b.
    derotation b.
    3D fracture walker b.
    dial-lock b.
    DonJoy ALP b.
    DonJoy four-point Super Sport
      knee b.
    DonJoy Gold Point knee b.
    DonJoy Opal knee b.
    DonJoy Quadrant shoulder b.
    DonJoy Universal ankle b.
    donut support b.
    dorsiflexion stop b.
    double Becker ankle b.

B

double-upright short leg b.
b. drill
drop-foot b.
drop-lock knee b.
Drytex RocketSoc ankle b.
Duncan shoulder b.
Dura-Flex back b.
dynamic abduction b.
dynamic hinge elbow fracture b.
Easy Lok ankle b.
Easy-On elbow b.
eclipse ankle b.
Eclipse Gel ankle b.
economy ROM b.
EconoSoc ankle b.
Edge knee b.
elastic-hinge knee b.
elastic knee sleeve b.
Elite knee b.
English b.
Equalizer cast b.
Exotec b.
felt b.
figure-of-eight b.
Fisher b.
Flagg fiberglass knee b.
Flex Foam b.
flexor-hinge hand-splint b.
FlexTech knee b.
FLOAM ankle stirrup b.
Florida back b.
Florida cervical b.
Florida contraflexion b.
Florida extension b.
Florida hyperextension b.
Florida J-24, J-35, J-45, J-55 b.
Florida post-fusion b.
Florida spinal b.
foot-ankle b.
footdrop b.
Forrester cervical collar b.
four-point IROM b.
four-point SuperSport functional
  knee b.
four-poster cervical b.
Frazer wrist b.
Friedman b.
functional fracture b.
furniture b.
Futuro wrist b.
Galveston metacarpal b.

Generation II Unloader ADJ
  knee b.
Generation II Unloader Select
  knee b.
Genutrain knee b.
GII Unloader ADJ knee b.
Gillette b.
GLS b.
GoldPoint ACL functional knee b.
GoldPoint hinged knee b.
GoldPoint PCL functional knee b.
Goldthwait b.
Guilford cervical b.
halo b.
hand b.
H buttress support
  patellofemoral b.
head b.
Hennessy knee b.
Hessing b.
high-Knight b.
high-tide walking b.
Hilgenreiner b.
hinged knee b.
Hi-Top foot/ankle b.
Hoke lumbar b.
horseshoe patellofemoral b.
Hudson-Jones knee-cage b.
Hudson TLSO b.
hyperextension b.
Ilfeld b.
InCare b.
Inner Lok ankle b.
internal tibial torsion b.
Intrepid functional knee b.
I-Plus system humeral fracture b.
I-Plus system ulnar fracture b.
ischial weightbearing leg b.
IsoDyn knee b.
J-45 contraflexion b.
Jewett-Benjamin cervical b.
Jewett contraflexion b.
Jewett hyperextension b.
Jewett postfusion b.
J-59 Florida b.
J-35 hyperextension b.
Jones b.
J-55 postfusion b.
Juzo b.
Kallassy b.
Key wrist b.

NOTES

brace *(continued)*

Kicker Pavlik harness hip abduction b.
King cervical b.
Kleinert postoperative traction b.
Klengall b.
Klenzak spring b.
Kling cervical b.
knee cage b.
knee MD b.
KneeRanger hinged knee b.
Knight back b.
Knight-Taylor thoracic b.
knock-knee b.
Korn Cage knee b.
KS 5 ACL b.
KSO b.
Küntscher-Hudson b.
Kydex b.
kyphosis b.
lace-on b.
lace-up RocketSoc ankle b.
lacing ankle b.
lateral buttress support J patellofemoral b.
leaf-spring b.
LeCocq b.
leg b.
Legend ACL functional knee b.
Legend PCL functional knee b.
Lenox Hill derotational knee b.
Lenox Hill Spectralite knee b.
Lerman hinge b.
Liberty CMC thumb b.
ligamentous control b.
limb b.
Lofstrand b.
long arm b.
long leg hinged b.
Lorenz b.
Lovitt-Uhler modification of Jewett post-fusion b.
low-tide walking b.
LSU reciprocation-gait orthosis b.
lumbar b.
lumbosacral b.
Lyman-Smith toe drop b.
MacAusland lumbar b.
Magnetic Support b.
M-Brace knee b.
McClintoch b.
McCollough internal tibial torsion b.
McDavid knee b.
McKee b.
MCL b.
McLight PCL b.
MC walker b.

MD b.
Medical Design b.
Medipedic Multicentric knee b.
Metcalf spring drop b.
Miami fracture b.
Miami TLSO scoliosis b.
b. migration
Milwaukee scoliosis b.
Minerva cervical b.
MKS II knee b.
Monarch knee b.
Moon Boot b.
Mooney b.
MTA b.
Mueller ATF ankle b.
Mueller hinged knee b.
Mueller Lite ankle b.
Mueller orthopedic shoulder b.
Mueller Ultralite b.
Mueller wrap-around knee b.
Multi-Lig knee b.
Multi-Lock knee b.
Murphy b.
Nakamura b.
neck b.
neoprene wrist b.
Nevin ankle b.
New England scoliosis b.
Newington b.
Newport MC hip orthosis b.
Nextep knee b.
night b.
nonweightbearing b.
Northville b.
no-stretch RocketSoc b.
OAdjuster knee b.
OA knee b.
OAsys knee b.
offloading knee b.
Omni knee b.
Opiela b.
Oppenheim b.
Orbital shoulder stabilizer b.
Orthomedics b.
Ortho-Mold spinal b.
Orthoplast fracture b.
Orthotech Controller knee b.
Osgood-Schlatter knee b.
OS-5/Plus 2 knee b.
OsteoArthritic knee b.
osteoarthritis padded night sleeve b.
out-of-cast ankle b.
outside-the-boot b.
oyster-shell b.
Palumbo dynamic patellar b.
Palumbo stabilizing b.
pantaloon b.

Got a Good Idea for STEDMAN'S?

Help us keep STEDMAN'S products fresh and up-to-date with new words and new ideas! How can we make your STEDMAN'S product the best medical word reference possible? Do we need to add or revise any items? Is there a better way to organize the content? What other medical references can Stedman's provide?

Fill in the spaces provided with your thoughts and recommendations and drop the card in the mailbox (postage-paid) or visit us at **www.stedmans.com** to submit your ideas. Feel free to e-mail us with your suggestions at **stedmans@LWW.com**. Please be specific! You're our most important contributor, and we want to know what's on your mind.

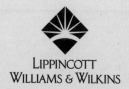

Please tell us a little about yourself.

Name/Title: _____

Company: _____

Address: _____

City/State/Zip: _____

Day Telephone No.: _____

E-mail Address: _____

Terms to be revised:

CURRENT TERM	SUGGESTED REVISION
_____	_____
_____	_____
_____	_____

New terms/words you would like us to add:

_____

_____

_____

Which of the following *Stedman's Word Book* titles need to be revised?

	NOT NECESSARY TO REVISE				REVISE NOW!
Stedman's Equipment Words	1	2	3	4	5
Stedman's OB-GYN Words	1	2	3	4	5
Stedman's Pediatric Words	1	2	3	4	5
Stedman's Endocrinology Words	1	2	3	4	5
Stedman's Cardio/Pulm Words	1	2	3	4	5

Others: _____

Additional ideas, suggestions, & comments:

_____

_____

_____

May we quote you? ☐ Yes ☐ No

All done? Great, just drop this card in the mail. OR visit us at **www.stedmans.com** and click on the "Got a Good Idea?" link.

Thank You!

ORTHO 738369

BUSINESS REPLY MAIL

FIRST CLASS   PERMIT NO. 724   BALTIMORE, MD

POSTAGE WILL BE PAID BY ADDRESSEE

ATTN: JULIE STEGMAN
LIPPINCOTT WILLIAMS & WILKINS
351 WEST CAMDEN STREET
BALTIMORE MD   21201-2436

Parachutist ankle b.
patellar stabilizing b. (PSB)
patellar tendon-bearing b.
patellofemoral b.
Patten-Bottom-Perthes b.
pediatric PRAFO b.
pelvic b.
performer ultralight knee b.
Perlstein b.
PFT traction b.
Phelps b.
Philadelphia Plastizote cervical b.
piano-wire dorsiflexion b.
Playmaker functional knee b.
PlayTuf knee b.
PMT halo system b.
Pneu Knee b.
Pneu-trac neck b.
Polaris knee rehab b.
Power Play knee b.
PPG-AFO b.
PPG-TLSO b.
Pro-8 ankle b.
Procase Ankle-Lock b.
progressive resistance b.
Proline Stomatex shoulder b.
PTB b.
PTS knee b.
Push medical b.
Quadrant advanced shoulder b.
QualCare knee b.
Raney flexion jacket b.
range of motion b.
ratchet-type b.
reamer b.
Rebel knee b.
Rehab TROM b.
Rhino Triangle polypropylene hip
  abduction b.
Richie b.
rigid postoperative b.
RocketSoc ankle b.
Rolyan TakeOff Sprint b.
Rolyan tibial fracture b.
ROM knee b.
ROM walker b.
Saltiel b.
Sarmiento fracture b.
SAS II b.
Sawa shoulder b.
Schanz collar b.
SCOI shoulder b.

scoliosis overlap b.
Scottish Rite b.
Selectively Lockable knee b.
semirigid ankle b.
Seton hip b.
short arm b.
short leg caliper b.
short leg double-upright b.
short leg walking b.
shoulder subluxation inhibitor b.
six-point knee b.
SmartBrace b.
SmartWrap elbow b.
Smedberg b.
snap-lock b.
SofTec rigid b.
SOMI b.
Speed b.
Spinal Technology bivalve
  TLSO b.
SpineCor nonrigid b.
Sports-Caster I, II knee b.
SSI b.
Stardox wrist b.
Stealth knee b.
Stille b.
Stimprene electrotherapy b.
stirrup b.
stop action b.
straight walker b.
Strap Lok ankle b.
Stromgren ankle b.
Stubbs 4-way clavicle b.
Sully shoulder stabilizer b.
Sure Step ankle b.
Swede-O Ankle Loc b.
Swede-O-Universal b.
Swivel-Strap ankle b.
Taylor back b.
Taylor-Knight b.
Taylor spine b.
telescoping b.
Teufel cervical b.
Teurlings wrist b.
Thermoskin b.
Thomas cervical collar b.
Thomas walking b.
thoracolumbar standing orthosis b.
TLSO b.
toe-drop b.
Tomasini b.
Toronto b.

NOTES

brace *(continued)*
    total anatomical hinge knee b.
    Townsend Rebel convertible b.
    Tracker knee b.
    Tri-angle shoulder abduction b.
    Trinkle b.
    TROM knee b.
    Tru-Fit b.
    turnbuckle ankle b.
    turnbuckle knee b.
    two-poster b.
    UBC b.
    UCLA functional long leg b.
    Ultrabrace b.
    underarm b.
    unilateral calcaneal b. (UCB)
    University of British Columbia b.
    Unloader ADJ Unloader b.
    Unloader Bi-ComPF knee b.
    Unloader Express Unloader b.
    Unloader Select Unloader b.
    Unloader Spirit knee b.
    Value Walker b.
    Varney acromioclavicular b.
    Verlow b.
    Victorian b.
    von Lackum transection shift
     jacket b.
    walking b.
    Warm Springs b.
    Watco b.
    weightbearing b.
    Wheaton Pavlik Harness b.
    Wilke boot b.
    Williams b.
    Wilmington scoliosis b.
    Wright Universal b.
    Yale b.
    Zimmer reamer b.
    Zinco Air Cam b.
    Zinco Airprene b.
    Zinco Cam Walker b.
    Zinco Castaway D b.
    Zinco Hi-Top b.
    Zinco Minerva cervical b.
    Zinco Multi-Lig knee b.
    Zinco Pin Cam Walker b.
brace/corset
    Hoke lumbar b./c.
brace-free ambulation
bracelet
    Nussbaum b.
    Q-Ray b.
    b. test
braceRAP
brace-type reamer
brachia (*pl. of* brachium)

brachial
    b. amelia
    b. artery
    b. artery aneurysm
    b. artery injury
    b. neuralgia
    b. neuritis
    b. plexopathy
    b. plexus
    b. plexus block
    b. plexus injury
    b. plexus neuropathy
    b. plexus palsy
    b. plexus paralysis
    b. plexus repair
    b. plexus tendon
    b. plexus tension test
    b. plexus traction injury (BPTI)
brachialgia
brachialis
    b. muscle
    b. tendon
brachiocephalic vein
brachiocrural
brachiocubital
brachiocyllosis
brachiocyrtosis
brachiogram
brachioradialis
    b. flap
    b. muscle
    b. reflex
    b. tendon
    b. transfer
    b. transfer for wrist extension
brachium, pl. **brachia**
brachybasia
brachybasocamptodactyly
brachybasophalangia
brachycnemic
brachydactylia
brachydactyly
brachykerkic
brachymelia
brachymesophalangia
brachymetacarpalia
brachymetacarpia
brachymetapody
brachymetatarsia
brachyphalangia
brachypodous
brachyskelic
brachyskelous
brachystasis
brachytelephalangia
bracing
    cast b.

fracture b.
postoperative b.
bracket
longitudinal epiphysial b.
bracketed splint
Brackett-Osgood posterior approach
Brackett-Osgood-Putti-Abbott
B.-O.-P.-A. operation
B.-O.-P.-A. technique
Brackett osteotomy
Bradford
B. fracture frame
B. fusion
**Bradley femoral canal preparation
scraper**
Brady
B. balanced-suspension splint
B. leg splint
bradycinesia
Brady-Jewett technique
bradykinesia
bradykinin
bradymetatarsalgia
Bragard
B. reinforcement
B. sign
B. test
Bragg angle
Bragg-peak photon-beam therapy
Brahms
B. foot operation
B. procedure
braid
carbon fiber lamination b. (CFLB)
braided suture
Brailsford disease
brain
B. arthroplasty
B. reflex
brainstem
b. auditory evoked potential
(BAEP)
b. auditory evoked response
(BAER)
transtentorial b.
brake
b. lever extension
b. phenomenon
Braly-Bishop-Tullos decompression
branch
acetabular b.
calcaneal b.

digital b.
distal communicating b. (DCB)
dorsal ulnar cutaneous b.
interosseous b.
motor b.
posterior interosseous b.
proper digital nerve b.
proximal communicating b. (PCB)
superior laryngeal nerve external b.
thenar b.
branched calculus
brand
B. tendon-holding forceps
B. tendon passer
B. tendon-passing forceps
B. tendon stripper
B. tendon transfer technique
Brannock
B. Device shoe sizer
B. foot measuring device
Brannon-Wickström technique
Brant aluminum splint
Brantigan cage
Brantigan-Voshell procedure
brassiere
Jobst b.
Brattström condylar height ratio
Braun
B. frame
B. procedure
B. shoulder tenotomy
B. skin graft
Braun-Yasargil right-angle clip
breach
naviculocuneiform b.
break
b. point
b. screw extractor
b. test
breakable screw breaker
breakage
pedicle screw b.
screw b.
tack b.
breakaway
b. lap cushion
b. pin
b. weakness
breakdancer's thumb
breakdown
skin b.

NOTES

97

breaker
    Böhler cast b.
    breakable screw b.
    cast b.
    Wolfe-Böhler cast b.
breast
    b. bone
    chicken b.
    funnel b.
    pigeon b.
    B. Vest Exu-Dry one-piece wound
        dressing
breastbone
breaststroker's knee
Breck
    B. pin
    B. pin cutter
bregma
bregmatic
    b. bone
    b. bone Brissaud scoliosis
bregmatomastoid suture
Bremer
    B. AirFlo halo vest
    B. halo cervical traction
    B. Halo Crown cervical collar
    B. halo system
Breschet bone
Breslow
    B. arthroplasty
    B. classification of melanoma
Brett
    B. arthrodesis
    B. osteotomy
Brett-Campbell tibial osteotomy
Breuerton view
breve
    vinculum b.
brevicollis
breviflexor
brevis
    abductor pollicis b. (APB)
    extensor carpi radialis b. (ECRB)
    extensor digitorum b. (EDB)
    extensor pollicis b. (EPB)
    flexor digitorum b. (FDB)
    flexor digitorum quinti b. (FDQB)
    flexor hallucis b. (FHB)
    flexor pollicis b. (FPB)
    peroneus b. (PB)
    b. release
Brewster triple arthrodesis
Brickner position
bridge
    autograft b.
    b. back exercise technique
    balance b.
    bony b.

    b. graft
    B. Hip system
    iliac crest b.
    b. of meniscus
    osseous b.
    physial b.
    b. plate
    b. plate fixation
    skin b.
    tarsal b.
    tendon-bone b.
bridging
    b. bone
    b. callus
    b. of defect
    heterotrophic ossification b.
    myocardial b.
    b. osteophyte
bridle
    b. posterior tibial tendon transfer
        operation
    B. procedure
brief
    b. maximal effort (BME)
    b., small, abundant, polyphasic
        potential (BSAPP)
    b., small, abundant potential
        (BSAP)
    B. Test of Head Injury (BTHI)
    B. Test of Head Injury
        Assessment
Brigham prosthesis
Brighton electrical stimulation system
brim
    pelvic b.
    proximal medial b.
    quadrilateral b.
brisement
    b. forcé
    b. therapy
Brissaud
    B. scoliosis
    B. syndrome
Bristow
    B. operation
    B. periosteal elevator
    B. procedure
    B. rasp
    B. shoulder reconstruction
Bristow-Helfet procedure
Bristow-Latarjet procedure
Bristow-May procedure
Brite-Life wrist brace
British test
Brittain
    B. chisel
    B. ischiofemoral arthrodesis
    B. operation

brittle
 b. bone
 b. bone disease
 b. bone failure
 b. nail
broach
 barbed b.
 cemented b.
 cementless b.
 Charnley femoral b.
 chipped-tooth b.
 drilling b.
 b. extractor
 femoral prosthesis b.
 Harris b.
 Koenig metatarsal b.
 Mittlemeir b.
 orthopaedic b.
 root canal b.
 smooth b.
 square-hole b.
 Swanson metatarsal b.
 Zimmer femoral canal b.
broad
 b. AO dynamic compression plate
 b. foot
 b. thumb–big toe syndrome
broad-based
 b.-b. cane
 b.-b. cane board
 b.-b. gait
Broadbent-Woolf four-limb Z-plasty
broad-toed shoe
Broberg-Morrey
 B.-M. elbow function scale
 B.-M. fracture
Broca
 B. aphasia
 B. area
 B. convolution
 B. diagonal band
Brockman
 B. foot operation
 B. incision
 B. procedure
Brockman-Nissen arthrodesis
Broden
 B. stress examination
 B. stress radiography
 B. view
Brodie
 B. abscess

 B. bursa
 B. disease
 B. knee
 B. ligament
Brodsky-Tullos-Gartsman approach
BROM
 back range of motion
bromidrosis, bromhidrosis
 plantar b.
Brooke Army Hospital splint
Brooker
 B. classification of heterotopic ossification I–IV
 B. double-locking unreamed tibial nail
 B. femoral nail
 B. frame
 B. heterotopic bone formation classification
 B. wire
Brooker-Wills nail
Brooks
 B. atlantoaxial arthrodesis
 B. cervical fusion
 B. cervical fusion operation
 B. shoe
 B. technique
Brooks-Gallie
 B.-G. cervical fusion
 B.-G. cervical operation
Brooks-Jenkins
 B.-J. atlantoaxial fusion
 B.-J. atlantoaxial fusion technique
 B.-J. cervical fusion
 B.-J. cervical operation
Brooks-Jones tendon transfer
Brooks-Seddon
 B.-S. pectoralis major tendon transfer
 B.-S. tendon transfer
 B.-S. transfer technique
Brooks-type fusion
Broomhead medial approach
broomstick
 b. bar
 b. cast
 b. curl-up
Brophy periosteal elevator
Broström
 B. injection technique
 B. lateral ankle ligament repair

B

NOTES

Broström (*continued*)
    B. ligament reconstruction
    B. procedure
Broström-Gould ankle instability operation
Broughton-Olney-Menelaus tibial diaphysial shortening
Browlift bone bridge system
brown
    B. dermatome
    b. fat tumor
    B. fibular transfer
    B. knee approach operation
    B. knee joint reconstruction
    B. lateral approach
    B. periosteotome
    B. rasp
    B. technique
    B. tissue forceps
    b. tumor of hyperparathyroidism
    B. two-portal carpal tunnel release
Brown-Adson forceps
Brown-Cushing forceps
Browne splint
Brown-Mueller T-fastener set
Brown-Roberts-Wells (BRW)
    B.-R.-W. stereotactic had frame
Brown-Séquard
    B.-S. lesion
    B.-S. syndrome
brucellosis
    spinal b.
Bruce protocol
Bruck disease
Brudzinski
    B. reflex
    B. sign
Bruening chisel
Bruening-Citelli rongeur
Bruger
    cul-de-sac of B.
Bruininks-Oseretsky Test of Motor Proficiency
bruisability
bruise
    bone b.
    reticular bone b.
Bruner
    B. approach
    B. incision
Brunhilde strain
Bruni-Wayne clamp approximator
Brunner
    B. modified incision
    B. palmar incision
    B. rib shears

Brunn plaster shears
Brunnstrom-Fugl-Meyer (BFM)
    B.-F.-M. impairment assessment
Bruns
    B. ataxia
    B. bone curette
    B. gait apraxia Bruns syndrome
Brunswick-Mack rotating drill
Bruser
    B. lateral approach
    B. skin incision
    B. technique
brush
    Cohort bone b.
    delta b.
    Plak-Vac oral suction b.
    b. test
brush-evoked pain testing
bruxism
BRW
    Brown-Roberts-Wells
    BRW head ring halo
Bryan
    B. arthroplasty
    B. procedure
    B. total knee implant prosthesis
Bryan-Morrey
    B.-M. extensive posterior approach
    B.-M. technique
Bryant
    B. line
    B. sign
    B. traction
    B. triangle
BSAP
    bone-specific alkaline phosphatase
    brief, small, abundant potential
BSAPP
    brief, small, abundant, polyphasic potential
BTE
    Baltimore Therapeutic Equipment
    BTE Assembly Tree
    BTE Bolt Box
    BTE dynamic lift
    BTE Work Simulator
BTHI
    Brief Test of Head Injury
BUA
    bone ultrasound attenuation
bubbly bone lesion
buccinator
    b. muscle
    b. myomucosal flap
Buchanan disease
Buch-Gramcko gouge

Buchholz
B. acetabular cup
B. prosthesis
buck
b. bone curette
B. convoluted traction apparatus
B. convoluted traction device
B. extension
B. extension splint
B. fascia
B. femoral cement restrictor inserter
B. knee brace
B. method
B. neurological hammer
B. operation
B. percussion hammer
B. periosteal elevator
B. plug
B. Redi-Traction apparatus
B. traction
B. traction splint
B. traction stockinette
bucket
Denis Browne b.
kick b.
Lenox b.
bucket-handle
b.-h. fracture
b.-h. fragment
b.-h. plica
b.-h. rib
b.-h. rib motion
b.-h. tear
Buck-Gramcko
B.-G. pollicization
B.-G. technique
buckle
b. fracture
wire-fixation b.
Buckley chisel
buckling
plantar b.
reverse b.
Bucky
B. diaphragm
B. view
B. x-ray tray
Bucy-Frazier suction cannula
bud
limb b.

buddy
b. splint
b. strap
b. taping
Budge
ciliospinal center of B.
Budin
B. hammertoe splint
B. joint
B. toe splint
Budin-Chandler
B.-C. anteversion determination
B.-C. method
Budlinger-Ludlof-Laewen disease
BUE
both upper extremities
BUE strength
Buechel-Pappas
B.-P. total ankle
B.-P. total ankle prosthesis
B.-P. total ankle replacement
B.-P. total ankle replacement system
Buerger-Allen exercise
buffalo hump
buffing sponge
Buford complex
Bugg-Boyd technique
buggy
cruiser b.
Maclaren mobile b.
Buhl spirometer
Builder Grip hand exerciser
build-up
Elevations shoe b.-u.
buildup (noun)
build up (verb)
bulb
b. dynamometer
irrigation b.
b. neuroma
b. suture
b. and thumb screw valve
bulbar
b. abnormality
b. anesthesia
bulbocavernosus reflex
bulge
disk b.
bulging disk
bulk graft

NOTES

101

bulky hand dressing
bulla, pl. **bullae**
   hemorrhagic b.
bulldog
   b. clamp
   b. clamp applier
   b. clamp-applying forceps
bullet
   b. driver
   b. stretching
bullosa
   epidermolysis b.
Bullseye femoral guide
bull's eye shoulder
bump
   Haglund b.
   hip b.
   inion b.
   pump b.
   runner's b.
bumper
   axle lock and b.
   b. cast
   dorsiflexion b.
   flexion b.
   b. fracture
   b. wedge
Buncke
   B. technique
   B. transfer
bundle
   anteromedial b.
   b. bone
   cleidoepitrochlear b.
   b. dressing
   b. function
   interdigital nerve b.
   intermediate b.
   medial neurovascular b.
   b. nailing
   neurovascular b.
   posterolateral b.
   superior gluteal neurovascular b.
   b. suture
bundle-nailing method
Bunge amputation
bunion
   b. complex
   b. deformity
   b. dissector
   dorsal b.
   b. formation
   juvenile b.
   b. shield
   tailor's b.
bunionectomy
   Akin b.
   Austin b.

Austin-Akin b.
b. capsular closure
chevron b.
closing wedge osteotomy b.
DuVries-Mann modified b.
Hauser b.
Hohmann b.
Joplin b.
Juvara b.
juvenile b.
Kelikian modified Z b.
Keller b.
Kreuscher b.
Lapidus b.
Ludloff b.
Mann b.
Mayo b.
McBride b.
McKeever b.
Mitchell b.
modified Hohmann b.
modified Mau b.
modified McBride b.
osteotomy b.
Reverdin b.
Reverdin-Green b.
Reverdin-Laird b.
Reverdin-McBride b.
short Z b.
Silver b.
Stone b.
supratubercular wedge osteotomy b.
tailor's b.
tricorrectional b.
Wilson b.
Wu b.
Z b.
bunionette
   b. deformity
   b. excision
   tailor's b.
bunionette-hallux valgus-splayfoot complex
bunion-hallux valgus complex
bunk
   b. bed fracture
   b. bed injury
Bunker footpiece
Bunke-Schulz clamp approximator
Bunnell
   B. active hand and finger splint
   B. anvil
   B. atraumatic technique
   B. bone drill
   B. crisscross suture
   B. digital exertion measurer
   B. dissecting probe
   B. dressing

B. figure-eight suture
B. finger extension splint
B. finger loop
B. forwarding probe
B. gutter splint
B. hand drill
B. knuckle bender
B. knuckle-bender splint
B. modification of Steindler flexorplasty
B. opponensplasty
B. outrigger splint
B. posterior tibial tendon transfer
B. posterior tibial tendon transfer operation
B. pullout wire
B. reverse knuckle bender splint
B. safety-pin splint
B. solution
B. stitch
B. technique of pulley reconstruction
B. tendon needle
B. tendon passer
B. tendon repair
B. tendon stripper
B. tendon suturing technique
B. tendon transfer technique
B. test
B. wire pull-out suture
B. zigzag fashion
Bunnell-Littler test
Bunnell-Williams procedure
bunny
B. boot
B. boot foot splint
bur, burr
Adson enlarging b.
Adson perforating b.
air-driven b.
Albee olive-shaped b.
arthroplasty b.
Bailey b.
ball b.
barrel b.
bone b.
Borchardt olive-shaped b.
Burwell b.
Caparosa b.
carbide b.
coarse carbide cone b.
coarse-olive b.

cone b.
conical b.
crosscut b.
Cushing b.
cutting b.
cylindrical b.
decortication b.
dental b.
D'Errico enlarging drill b.
D'Errico perforating drill b.
diamond b.
Doyen cylindrical b.
Doyen spherical b.
b. drill
Dyonics arthroplasty b.
enlarging b.
Fantastic Burr nail b.
fine olive b.
finish b.
fissure b.
flame-tip b.
Hall b.
high-speed b.
high-torque b.
b. hole
Hudson bone b.
Hudson brace with b.
large-nail spicule b.
Lindeman b.
Lindermann b.
long coarse b.
long-stemmed powered b.
McKenzie enlarging b.
medium carbide cone b.
medium fine b.
Midas Rex b.
motorized b.
new happy b.
old smoothie b.
olive-shaped b.
orthopaedic b.
Ossotome b.
paronychia b.
pear b.
perforating b.
pilot b.
Podi-Burr nail b.
power b.
right-ankle b.
Rosen b.
Rotablator rotating b.
rotary b.

NOTES

bur *(continued)*
    round b.
    Shannon 44 b.
    short coarse b.
    short fine b.
    side-cutting b.
    small nail spicule b.
    smoothie junior b.
    spherical b.
    Stille b.
    three-in-one diamond b.
    water-cooled power b.
    Zimmer rotary b.
Burch-Greenwood tendon tucker
Burch-Schneider antiprotrusio cage
bur-down technique
Burford-Finochietto rib spreader
Burford rib spreader
Burgess
    B. below-knee amputation
    B. technique
buried K-wire fixation in digital fusion
Burke
    B. Bariatric bed
    B. test
Burkhalter
    B. modification of Stiles-Bunnell
    technique
    B. transfer technique
Burkhalter-Reyes method phalangeal
   fracture
burn
    B. bench test
    b. boutonnière deformity
    b. contracture
    irrigation b.
    mafenide acetate for b.
    plaster cast application b.
    b. syndactyly
Burner phenomenon
Burnham
    B. finger splint
    B. thumb splint
    B. view
burning
    b. foot
    b. pain
    paroxysmal b.
burning-feet syndrome
burn-related pigmentation change
Burns
    B. disease
    B. ligament
    B. plate
Burns-Haney incision
Burow
    B. skin flap technique
    B. triangle

burr *(var. of* bur)
Burrows technique
Burrow triangle
bursa, pl. **bursae**
    Achilles tendon b.
    adventitious b.
    anserine b.
    Brodie b.
    calcaneal b.
    deltoid b.
    Fleischmann b.
    infrapatellar b.
    intermetatarsal b.
    intermetatarsophalangeal b.
    ischiogluteal b.
    Luschka b.
    Monro b.
    no-name, no-fame b.
    olecranon b.
    patellar b.
    pisiform b.
    pre-Achilles b.
    prepatellar b.
    radial b.
    radiohumeral b.
    retro-Achilles b.
    retrocalcaneal b.
    rider's b.
    sacral b.
    scapulohumeral b.
    subacromial b.
    subacromiodeltoid b.
    subdeltoid b.
    subtendinous iliac b.
    subtendinous prepatellar b.
    synovial b.
    trochanteric b.
    ulnar b.
    Voshell b.
bursal
    b. abscess
    b. cyst
    b. débridement
    b. flap
    b. fluid
    b. inflammation
    b. projection
    b. sac
    b. synovitis
    b. tissue
bursata
    exostosis b.
bursectomy
bursitis
    Achilles tendon b.
    anserine b.
    bicipital b.
    calcaneal b.

B

calcific b.
cubital b.
Duplay b.
hip b.
iliopectineal b.
iliopsoas b.
infracalcaneal b.
infrapatellar b.
intermetatarsal b.
intermetatarsophalangeal b.
intertubercular b.
ischial b.
ischiogluteal b.
lateral premalleolar b.
medial gastrocnemius b.
olecranon b.
patellar b.
pelvic region b.
pes anserine b.
pigmented villonodular b.
postcalcaneal b.
pre-Achilles b.
prepatellar b.
pyogenic b.
radiohumeral b.
retrocalcaneal b.
scapulothoracic b.
semimembranosus b.
septic b.
subacromial b.
subcalcaneal b.
subdeltoid b.
subgluteal b.
subscapularis b.
tarsal navicular b.
tibial collateral ligament b.
Tornwaldt b.
trochanteric b.
tuberculous trochanteric b.
bursocentesis
bursography
Mikasa subacromial b.
subacromial b.
bursolith
bursopathy
bursotomy
burst
b. fracture
b. injury
B. Resistance Fitness Ball

bursting dislocation
burst-type laceration
Burton-Pelligrini excising trapezium
Burton sign
Burwell-Scott modification of Watson-Jones incision
Busenkell posterior hip retractor
bushing
guide b.
Uniflex drill b.
Busquet disease
Butler
B. fifth toe operation
B. procedure to correct overlapping toes
butterfly
B. cushion
B. cushion with strap
b. fracture
b. fracture fragment
b. vertebra
butterfly-shaped monoblock vertebral plate
buttocks
heart-shaped b.
b. pad
button
b. abscess
Biomet b.
Charnley suture b.
collared b.
Drummond b.
Hewson ligament b.
b. hook
ligament b.
padded b.
patellar b.
periosteal b.
polyethylene b.
pull-out b.
b. sequestrum
Silastic b.
B. Spacer
subdural b.
b. suture
b. toe amputation
Wisconsin b.

NOTES

buttonhole
- b. deformity
- b. fracture
- b. rupture

buttress
- b. and button anchor
- OMNI pretibial b.
- b. pad
- b. pie plate
- pretibial b. (PTB)
- rotator cuff b. (RCB)
- b. thread screw

buttressed hook

buttressing in internal fixation

buttress-type plate

butyrophenone

BVP
- blood volume pulse

Bx
- biopsy

Byars mandibular prosthesis

bypass
- dorsal pedal b.
- extended tibial in situ b.
- femoral above-knee popliteal b.
- femorodistal b.
- popliteus b.
- b. surgery

C

C angle
C clamp
C knife
C sign
C Stance ankle
C washer

C-2

C-2 hip system
C-2 OsteoCap hip prosthesis

C1–C3 cruciate pulley
CA-5000 drill-guide isometer
CA-6000 spine motion analyzer
cable

antirotation c. (ARC)
c. cerclage method
chrome-cobalt c.
Dall-Miles c.
Dwyer scoliosis c.
fiberoptic c.
FlexStrand c.
Gallie fusion-using c.
Howmedica cerclage c.
interspinous c.
liquid c.
c. nerve graft
scoliosis correction with Dwyer c.
Songer c.
c. suspension system
c. tensioner
titanium c.
twister c.

cable-hook compression instrumentation
Cable-Ready cable grip system
cable-twister

c.-t. brace
c.-t. orthosis

Cabot

C. leg splint
C. posterior splint

Cacchione syndrome
cacomelia
CAD

coronary artery disease
CAD femoral stem prosthesis

cadaver

c. bone
c. bone graft

cadaveric knee
CAD/CAM

computer-assisted design-controlled
alignment method
CAD/CAM prosthesis

cadence of gait

Cadenza

C. girdle
C. panty

CAECS

chronic anterior exertional compartment
syndrome

café au lait spot
Caffey

C. disease
C. hyperostosis
C. syndrome

Caffey-Kenny disease
Caffey-Silverman syndrome
Caffinière trapeziometacarpal prosthesis
cage

antiprotrusio c.
BAK fusion c.
Brantigan c.
Burch-Schneider antiprotrusio c.
carbon-fiber-composite c.
carbon-fiber-reinforced c.
elastic knee c.
fusion c.
Harms c.
InterFix RP threaded spinal
fusion c.
InterFix titanium threaded spinal
fusion c.
lumbar intersomatic fusion
expandable c. (LIFEC)
Moss c.
Novus LC threaded interbody
fusion c.
Novus LT titanium threaded
interbody fusion c.
osseocartilaginous thoracic c.
protrusio c.
Pyramesh c.
Ray TFC threaded fusion c.
rib c.
SL c.
stereolithography c.
Swedish knee c.
threaded fusion c. (TFC)

cage-back brace
CAH

Camber axis hinge

Cairns hemostatic forceps
Calandriello

C. hip reduction
C. procedure

Calandruccio

C. cemented hip prosthesis
C. clamp
C. II compression device

C

Calandruccio (*continued*)
   C. external fixation system
   C. fixation
   C. impaction screw-plate
   C. nail
   C. side plate
   C. technique
   C. triangular compression apparatus
   C. triangular compression fixation
     device
calcaneal
   c. apophysitis
   c. avulsion fracture
   c. axial view
   c. bone
   c. bone graft
   c. branch
   c. bursa
   c. bursitis
   c. compartment pressure
     measurement
   c. displaced fracture
   c. distraction
   c. facet
   c. fat pad
   c. fracture reduction
   c. gait
   c. gait pattern
   c. inclination angle
   c. L osteotomy
   c. malunion
   c. neck lengthening
   c. nerve
   c. pin
   c. pin traction
   c. pitch
   c. pitch angle (CPA)
   c. pseudocyst
   c. region
   c. resection
   c. sliding corrective osteotomy
   c. spreader
   c. spur
   c. spur cookie orthosis
   c. spur pad in shoe
   c. spur syndrome
   c. stance
   c. sulcus
   c. tendon
   c. tenodesis
   c. tuberosity
   c. type I–III fracture
   c. valgus
   c. varus
   c. Y plate
calcaneal-second metatarsal angle
   inclination angle
calcanectomy

calcanei (*pl. of* calcaneus)
calcaneoapophysitis
calcaneoastragaloid ligament
calcaneocavovarus deformity
calcaneocavus
   c. deformity
   c. foot
   talipes c.
calcaneoclavicular ligament
calcaneocuboid (CC)
   c. articulation
   c. bone
   c. coalition
   c. distraction arthrodesis (CCDA)
   dorsal c. (DCC)
   c. joint
   c. joint arthritis
   c. joint nutcracker injury
   c. ligament
   long c. (LCC)
   short c. (SCC)
   c. subluxation
calcaneocuboideum
calcaneodynia
calcaneofibular
   c. abutment
   c. ligament (CFL)
   c. sprain
calcaneonavicular
   c. articulation
   c. bar
   c. bar resection
   c. bar section
   c. coalition
   c. joint
   c. joint arthroscopy
   c. ligament
   c. ligament-tibialis posterior tendon
     advancement
calcaneopelvic arthrodesis
calcaneoplantar angle
calcaneoscaphoid
calcaneotibial
   c. angle
   c. arthrodesis
   c. fusion
   c. ligament
calcaneovalgocavus
calcaneovalgus
   c. deformity
   c. flatfoot
   c. foot
   talipes c.
calcaneovarus
   c. deformity
   talipes c.
calcaneus, pl. calcanei
   accessory ossification center of c.

c. apophysis
c. deformity
displaced intraarticular c.
distal c.
c. excursion
pes c.
sulcus calcanei
talipes c.
tendo c.
c. tongue fracture
tuberosity of c.
White-Kraynick tendo c.

calcanodynia
calcar

c. collar
c. femorale development
c. pedis
c. pivot
pivot of c.
c. planer
c. reamer
c. replacement
c. replacement femoral prosthesis
c. replacement stem

calcareous deposit
calcidiol test
calcific

c. bursitis
c. density
c. deposit
c. spur
c. tendinitis
c. tendinosis

calcificans

chondrodystrophia c.

calcification

Achilles tendon enthesis c.
eggshell-like c.
falx c.
c. of falx
flocculent focus of c.
focal c.
heterotopic c.
juvenile intervertebral disk c. (JIDC)
paraarticular c.
periarticular c.
provisional c.
soft tissue c.
supraspinatus c.

calcified

c. cartilage
c. osteoid

calcify
calcifying aponeurotic fibroma
calcinosis

c. circumscripta
c., Raynaud, esophageal motility disorders, sclerodactyly, telangiectasia (CREST)
tumoral c.

calciphylaxis
Calcitite

C. bone
C. graft
C. graft material

calcium

c. alginate dressing
c. deposit
c. gout
c. hydroxyapatite
c. oxalate deposition
c. phosphate
c. phosphate ceramic
c. pyrophosphate dihydrate deposition (CPPD)
c. pyrophosphate dihydrate deposition disease
serum c.
c. sulfate ceramic

calcodynia
calculus, pl. **calculi**

branched c.
hemic c.
staghorn c.

Caldani ligament
Caldwell-Coleman

C.-C. flatfoot operation
C.-C. flatfoot technique

Caldwell-Durham

C.-D. tendon operation
C.-D. tendon transfer

Caldwell hanging cast
calf, pl. **calves**

c. band
c. bone dowel
c. circumference
football c.
gnome's c.
c. hypertension
c. raise back exercise

C

NOTES

calf *(continued)*
    c. shell
    c. squeeze test
calibrated
    c. clubfoot splint
    c. guidepin
    c. guide wire
    c. monofilament
    c. pin
    c. pin guide
    c. probe
calibration curve
calibrator
    screw depth c.
California soft spinal system (CASS)
Caligamed
    C. ankle orthosis
    C. brace
caliper
    anthropometric c.
    blunt c.
    c. brace
    Digimatic c.
    Harpenden c.
    Lafayette skinfold c.
    Lange skinfold c.
    Mitutoyo digital c.
    c. orthosis
    c. rib movement
    skinfold c.
    Thomas walking c.
    Townley femur c.
    Vernier c.
    weight-relieving c.
Callahan
    C. extension of cervical injury
    C. fusion technique
    C. method
    C. and Scuderi approach
Callander amputation
Callaway test
Calleja exercise
Callender
    C. derotational brace
    C. technique hip prosthesis
callosal lesion
callosity
    metatarsal c.
    plantar c.
    shearing c.
callotasis
callous
    c. bone union
    c. formation
callus
    bone c.
    bridging c.
    central c.

    definitive c.
    c. distraction
    c. distraction procedure
    elephant-foot c.
    ensheathing c.
    florid c.
    fracture c.
    horse's foot c.
    intermediate c.
    irritation c.
    c. massage
    medullary c.
    myelogenous c.
    permanent c.
    pinch c.
    provisional c.
    shearing c.
    temporary c.
    c. weld
Calmette-Guérin
    bacille C.-G. (BCG)
Calnan-Nicolle
    C.-N. finger implant
    C.-N. finger prosthesis
    C.-N. metatarsophalangeal prosthesis
    C.-N. synthetic joint prosthesis
calor
Caltagirone chisel
calvarial
    c. free bone
    c. free bone graft
Calvé-Legg-Perthes syndrome
Calvé-Perthes disease
calves *(pl. of* calf)
Calypso lift
CAM
    complimentary alternative medicine
    computer-assisted myelography
    controlled ankle motion
Cam
    C. Lock knee joint
    C. Walker ankle brace
    C. Walker ankle walker
    C. Walker leg brace
Camber axis hinge (CAH)
cambium layer
camelback sign
camera
    DyoCam 550 arthroscopic video c.
    DyoCam arthroscopic view c.
    Endius spinal endoscopic c.
    gamma c.
    Saticon tube c.
    Sony CCD/RGB DXC-151 color video c.
    Stryker c.
    Vidicon vacuum chamber pickup tube for video c.

Cameron
- C. femoral component removal
- C. fracture apparatus
- C. fracture device

Cameron-Haight periosteal elevator

Camino catheter technique

Camitz
- C. opponensplasty
- C. technique
- C. tendon transfer

camouflage prosthesis

camp
- C. brace
- C. corset
- C. Diversity arthritis program

Campbell
- C. ankle operation
- C. ankle procedure
- C. cannulated screw
- C. corset
- C. gouge
- C. interpositional arthroplasty
- C. ligament
- C. nerve root retractor
- C. onlay bone graft
- C. osteotome
- C. periosteal elevator
- C. posterior arthrodesis
- C. posterior bone block
- C. posterior shoulder approach
- C. posterolateral approach
- C. reamer
- C. resection arthroplasty
- C. rongeur
- C. screw fixation
- C. technique
- C. tibial osteotomy
- C. traction splint
- C. transfer
- C. triceps reflection

Campbell-Akbarnia
- C.-A. arthrodesis
- C.-A. procedure

Campbell-Goldthwait procedure

Campbell-Rinehard-Kalenak anterior arthrodesis

camper
- C. chiasma
- C. fascia

camplodactyly

camptocormia

camptodactyly

camptomelia

camptomelic dwarfism

camptospasm

CamStar
- C. exercise machine
- C. power leg press

Canadian
- C. Academy of Sports Medicine emergency kit
- C. crutch
- C. hip disarticulation prosthesis
- C. Knee Orthosis
- C. Occupational Performance Measure

Canakis beaded hip pin

canal
- Alcock c.
- bony semicircular c.
- carpal c.
- cartilage c.
- central c.
- cerebrospinal c.
- cervical c.
- Civinini c.
- cortical bone primary c.
- Dorello c.
- Dupuytren c.
- femoral medullary c.
- c. finder
- Guyon c.
- haversian c.
- humeral c.
- Hunter c.
- hydrops c.
- iliac c.
- c. innominate osteotomy
- intersacral c.
- intramedullary c.
- Kanavel c.
- lumbar c.
- marrow c.
- medullary c.
- narrowing of spinal c.
- Recklinghausen c.
- Richet tibial-astragalocalcaneal c.
- sacral c.
- spinal cord c.
- talar c.
- tarsal c.
- tibial medullary c.
- tibioastragalocalcaneal Richet c.
- tight spinal canal trefoil c.

NOTES

canal *(continued)*
    vertebral c.
    Volkmann c.
Canale
    C. osteotomy
    C. technique
    C. view
Canale-Kelly
    C.-K. talar neck fracture
    C.-K. talar neck fracture
      classification
    C.-K. view
canaliculus, pl. **canaliculi**
canal-to-calcar isthmus ratio
Can Am brace
Canavan disease
Canavan-van Bogaert-Bertrand disease
cancellated bone
cancellectomy
cancellous
    c. bone carrier
    c. bone screw
    c. chip
    c. chip bone graft
    c. insert
    c. insert graft
    c. morselized bone graft
    c. pin
    c. surface
    c. versus cortical bone
cancer treatment-related lymphedema
Candela SPTL laser
candle wax appearance of bone
Can-Do Exercise Band
cane
    adjustable c.
    broad-based c.
    Double Duty c.
    English c.
    glider c.
    MAFO c.
    offset c.
    quad c.
    single-point c.
    small-base quad c.
    Thera c.
    tripod c.
Canfield shoe
canister
    Autovac autotransfusion c.
cannon
    c. bone
    C. Law of Denervation
      Supersensitivity
cannula
    Acufex double-lumen
      arthroscopic c.
    arthroscopic c.

    Bergstrom c.
    biopsy c.
    blunt arthroscopic c.
    Bucy-Frazier suction c.
    Concept c.
    Dyonics c.
    Endotrac c.
    Eriksson muscle biopsy c.
    inflow c.
    large-bore inflow c.
    large egress c.
    McCain TMJ c.
    microirrigating c.
    outflow c.
    self-sealing c.
    small egress c.
    suction c.
    suprapatellar c.
    c. system
    Teflon c.
    zone-specific c.
cannulated
    c. bolt
    c. cancellous lag screw
    c. cortical step drill
    c. drill bit
    c. drill point
    c. expulsion piston
    c. guided hip screw system
    c. Henderson reamer
    c. hip screw
    c. nail
    C. Plus screw system
    c. reaming technique
    c. screwdriver
    c. wrench
cannulation
    unilateral pedicle c.
canted finger hook
cantilever
    c. bending
    c. external fixator
canvas brace
CAOS
    computer-assisted orthopedic surgery
caoutchouc pelvis
cap
    acetabular c.
    Carnation corn c.'s
    cartilaginous c.
    Cloward drill guard c.
    digit c.
    flexor c.
    nerve c.
    plaster toe c.
    plastic end c.
    Silipos mesh c.
    c. splint

toe c.
Zang metatarsal c.
Zimmer tibial nail c.
capacitive
c. coupling
c. sensor
capacity
aerobic c.
exercise c.
forced vital c.
physical work c. (PWC)
cap-and-anchor plate
Caparosa
C. bur
C. wire crimper
CAPE
Clifton Assessment Procedures for the
Elderly
continuous anatomical passive exerciser
capeline bandage
Capello
C. press-fit prosthesis
C. slim-line abduction pillow
C. technique
C. total hip replacement
Capener
C. brace
C. coil splint
C. finger splint
C. gouge
C. lateral rhachotomy
capillary
c. fracture
c. hemangioma
c. ischemia
c. refill
c. refill, sensation, motor function,
temperature (CSMT)
c. refill time
CAPIS
CAPIS bone plate system
CAPIS screw
CAPIS screw assortment tray
CAPIS screwdriver
capital
c. crescentic shelf osteotomy
c. epiphysial angle
c. epiphysis (CE)
c. femoral epiphysis
c. fragment
c. ligament
capitate bone

capitate-hamate joint
capitate-lunate
c.-l. instability
c.-l. joint
capitellar
c. fracture
c. osteochondritis
capitellocondylar
c. total elbow arthroplasty
c. unconstrained elbow prosthesis
capitellum
Hahn-Steinthal fracture of c.
Kocher-Lorenz fracture of c.
capitolunate angle
capitular
c. epiphysis
c. process
capitulum fracture
Caplan syndrome
capped elbow
Caprolactam suture
CAPS
CAPS ArthroWand
CAPS ArthroWand device
**Capset calcium sulfate bone graft
barrier**
capsular
c. adhesion
c. ankylosis
c. attachment
c. flap
c. imbrication
c. imbrication procedure
c. incision
c. interposition arthroplasty
c. layer
c. length insufficiency
c. ligament
c. plication
c. reefing
c. release
c. shift
c. shift procedure
c. strap
c. support tissue
capsular-ligamentous tension
capsular-shift reconstruction
capsule
anterior c.
anterolateral c.
anteromedial c.
articular c.

NOTES

113

capsule *(continued)*
    dorsal c.
    elbow c.
    facet c.
    fibrous c.
    c. formation
    Gerota c.
    joint c.
    medial talonavicular c.
    meniscofemoral c.
    meniscotibial c.
    metatarsophalangeal joint c.
    midlateral c.
    midmedial c.
    plantar c.
    posterior c.
    posterolateral c.
    posteromedial c.
    c. repair
    suprasellar c.
    talonavicular c.
    trapeziometacarpal c.
    volar c.
    wrist c.
capsulectomy
    anterior c.
    circumferential c.
    silhouette c.
capsulitis
    adhesive c.
    dorsal carpal c.
    glenohumeral adhesive c.
capsulodesis
    Berger c.
    Blatt c.
    bleb c.
    dorsal c.
    intercarpal ligament c.
    Zancolli flexion c.
capsulolabral complex
capsuloligamentous
    c. complex
    c. mechanism
    c. system
    c. tissue
capsuloperiosteal
    c. envelope
    c. flap
capsuloplasty
    Zancolli c.
capsuloputaminal infarction
capsuloputaminocaudate infarction
capsulorrhaphy
    Boyd-Sisk posterior c.
    electrothermally assisted c. (ETAC)
    laser-assisted c.
    medial c.
    open-staple c.

    pants-over-vest c.
    posterior c.
    Rockwood posterior c.
    Roux-duToit staple c.
    staple c.
    c. staple
    thermal c.
    Tibone posterior c.
capsulotomy
    anterior c.
    Curtis PIP joint c.
    dorsal transverse c.
    dorsolateral and medial c.
    dorsoplantar c.
    linear c.
    L-shaped c.
    medial V-Y c.
    metatarsophalangeal c.
    posterior c.
    stereotaxic anterior c.
    subtalar c.
    talonavicular c.
    transmetatarsal c.
    transverse c.
    T-shaped c.
    V c.
    vertical c.
CAQ
    Clinical Analysis Questionnaire
Carabelt
    C. lower back support
    C. therapeutic belt
carbide bur
CarboFlex odor-control dressing
carbohydrate oxidation
CarboJet lavage
carbon
    C. Copy II Foot prosthesis
    C. Copy high performance foot
      prosthesis
    C. Copy HP foot prosthesis
    C. Copy II Light Foot
    C. Copy II Light prosthesis
    c. dioxide laser
    c. fiber fixator
    c. fiber graft
    c. fiber half ring
    c. fiber lamination braid (CFLB)
    c. fiber-reinforced plate
    c. fiber-reinforced polyethylene
    c. implant
    C. Monotube long bone fracture
      external fixation system
    pyrolytic c.
    c. steel drill point
carbon-based biomaterial
carbon-fiber-composite cage
carbon-fiber-reinforced cage

carbon-tungsten rasp
CARBONX active heel
Carboplast
    C. II composite
    C. II sheeting
    C. II sheet orthotic material
Carborundum grinding wheel
Carceau-Brahms ankle arthrodesis
carcinoembryonic antigen (CEA)
carcinogen
    chemical c.
carcinoma
    clear cell c.
    joint verrucous c.
carcinomatous myopathy
Carcon stent
Carden amputation
cardiac
    c. output
    c. precautions
cardinal axes X,Y,Z
cardioboxing
CardioKarate
CardioKickboxing
cardiomyopathy
    dilated c.
    hypertrophic c.
    nonspecific c.
    right ventricular c.
Cardiopulmonary Paragon 8500 bed
Cardona keratoprosthesis prosthesis
care
    corrective spinal c.
    Miami Acute C. (MAC)
    palliative c.
    postoperative wound c.
    rehabilitation c.
Caregiver Strain Index (CSI)
Carex ambulatory aid
car hand control
caries sicca
carinatum
    pectus c.
Carleton spot
Carl P. Jones traction splint
C-arm
    C-a. fluoroscopy
    C-a. fluoroscopy unit
    C-a. image intensifier
Carman meniscus sign
Carmody-Batson operation
Carmody perforator drill

Carnation corn caps
Carnesale
    C. acetabular extensile approach
    C. hip approach operation
    C. technique
Carnesale-Stewart-Barnes
    C.-S.-B. classification of hip
        dislocation
    C.-S.-B. hip dislocation
        classification
Carolina rocker
Carolon AFO sock
carotid
    c. artery
    c. artery compression
    c. sheath
    c. vein
carpal
    c. arc
    c. arch
    c. articulation
    c. bone
    c. bone fracture ankylosis
    c. bone stress fracture
    c. boss
    c. canal
    C. Care carpal tunnel exerciser
    C. Care exercise
    C. Care rehabilitative program
    c. coalition
    c. compression test
    c. dislocation
    c. height ratio
    c. instability
    c. instability dissociation (CID)
    c. instability nondissociative (CIND)
    c. ligament
    C. Lock cock-up splint
    C. Lock CTS brace
    C. Lock wrist brace
    C. Lock wrist splint
    c. lunate implant prosthesis
    c. navicular fracture
    c. pedal spasm
    c. row
    c. scaphoid
    c. scaphoid bone fracture
    c. scaphoid implant prosthesis
    c. scaphoid screw
    c. sulcus
    c. synovectomy
    C. Trac traction

C

NOTES

carpal (continued)
    C. Trac traction device
    c. tunnel (CT)
    c. tunnel decompression (CTD)
    c. tunnel glove
    c. tunnel release (CTR)
    c. tunnel stretch
    C. Tunnel Stretch exerciser
    c. tunnel surgery relief kit
    c. tunnel syndrome (CTS)
    c. tunnel syndrome injection
      therapy
    c. tunnel view
carpal-intercarpal joint
Carpal-Lock wrist support
carpal-metacarpal
carpectomy
    distal row c.
    Omer-Capen c.
    proximal row c.
carpenter's
    c. brace
    c. knee
Carpenter syndrome
carpet-layer's knee
carpi (pl. of carpus)
carpometacarpal (CMC)
    c. arthroplasty
    c. articulation
    c. boss
    c. fracture-dislocation
    c. joint
    c. joint dislocation
    c. joint fracture
    c. joint radiography
    c. ligament
carpophalangeal joint
carporadial articulation
carposcope
carprofen
carpus, pl. **carpi**
    complex instability of c. (CIC)
    carpi radialis brevis tendon
    carpi radialis longus tendon
Carrel
    C. method
    C. patch
    C. suture
    C. treatment
Carrell
    C. fibular substitution
    C. fibular substitution technique
    C. resection
Carrell-Girard screw
Carrie car seat
carrier
    cancellous bone c.
    Cave-Rowe ligature c.

    clamp c.
    double-headed stereotactic c.
    Finochietto clamp c.
    ligature c.
    Yasargil ligature c.
Carrington Dermal wound gel
Carroll
    C. approach
    C. arthrodesis
    C. bone-holding forceps
    C. dressing forceps
    C. hand retractor
    C. periosteal elevator
    C. skin hook
    C. and Taber arthroplasty
    C. tendon-pulling forceps
    C. tendon retriever
    C. test
    C. tissue forceps
Carroll-Bennett retractor
Carroll-Bunnell drill
Carroll-Legg
    C.-L. osteotome
    C.-L. periosteal elevator
Carroll-Smith-Petersen osteotome
Carrom orthopaedic bed
Carr-Purcell-Meiboom-Gill sequence
Carr-Purcell sequence
carrying
    c. angle
    c. angle of forearm
Carstan reverse wedge osteotomy
cart
    Harloff c.
Cartam-Treander reverse wedge
  osteotomy
Carter
    C. elevation pillow
    C. foam pillow
    C. immobilization cushion
    C. mycetoma
    C. Rowe awl
    C. splint
Carter-Rowe
    C.-R. shoulder score
    C.-R. view
Carter-Wilkinson criteria for
  hypermobility syndrome
Carticel cartilage-cell culturing service
cartilage
    c. ablation
    c. abrader
    accessory c.
    alar c.
    anular c.
    arthrodial c.
    articular c.
    arytenoid c.

c. autograft
basilar c.
calcified c.
c. canal
c. cell
circumferential c.
c. clamp
condylar c.
connecting c.
costal c.
cricoid c.
cryopreserved c.
degenerated c.
diarthrodial c.
eburnation of c.
elastic c.
c. elastic pullover kneecap splint
ensiform c.
falciform c.
fibroelastic c.
fibrous c.
floating c.
c. forceps
free flap of c.
glenoid c.
c. graft
c. healing
hyaline c.
c. hypertrophy
c. implant
interarticular c.
interosseous c.
intervertebral c.
c. knife
c. lacuna
loose c.
nonossified tarsal navicular c.
c. oligomeric matrix protein
  (COMP)
patellofemoral groove c.
physial c.
pitted c.
quadrangular c.
roughened c.
c. scissors
scored c.
semilunar c.
c. shaver blade
shelling off of c.
slipping rib c.
c. space
c. stripper

c. synovium
tendon c.
thyroid c.
triradial c.
triradiate c.
c. volume
yellow c.
cartilage-hair hypoplasia (CHH)
cartilaginous
c. anlage
c. bar
c. cap
c. cap of phalangeal head
c. coalition
c. degeneration
c. disk
c. glenoid labrum
c. growth plate
c. hallux limitus
c. hamartoma
c. hypertrophy
c. joint
c. lesion
c. loose body
c. metaplasia
c. navicular
c. ossification
c. ring
c. spur
c. tissue
c. tumor
cartwheel fracture
Cartwright implant
cascade
clotting c.
C. Up and About system
Cascading Tower Technology
Casey pelvic clamp
CASH
cruciform anterior spinal hyperextension
CASH brace
CASH thoracolumbosacral orthosis
CASP
contoured anterior spinal plate
Caspar
C. alligator forceps
C. anterior cervical plating
  technique
C. anterior instrumentation
C. blade
C. cervical plate

NOTES

Caspar *(continued)*
C. cervical screw
C. retractor
Caspari
C. arthroscopic portal
C. repair
C. shuttle
C. suture punch
CASS
California soft spinal system
Casselberry suture punch
casserian muscle
Casser perforated muscle
cast
above-elbow c.
accessory navicular c.
airplane c.
c. application
arm cylinder c.
banjo c.
Batchelor plaster hip spica c.
below-knee walking c.
c. belt
c. bender
bent-knee c.
Bermuda spica c.
bivalved cylinder c.
bivalved pancake plaster hand c.
c. blade
blood c.
Body Armor walker c.
body jacket c.
Böhler skintight c.
c. boot
C. Boot polypropylene hip
  abduction brace
Boston bivalve c.
c. bracing
c. breaker
broomstick c.
bumper c.
Caldwell hanging c.
circular c.
Comfort C.
corrective c.
Cotrel scoliosis c.
cotton c.
c. cover
C. Cozy
C. Cozy toe covering
c. cushion
Cutter c.
c. cutter
cylinder walking c.
double hip spica c.
EDF scoliosis c.
elbow c.
Equalizer short leg walking c.

c. equipped with rubber pedestal
extension body c.
fiberglass c.
figure-of-eight c.
flexion body c.
Fractura Flex c.
full thumb spica c.
gaiter c.
C. Gard cast protector
gauntlet c.
gel c.
Gelocast c.
gravity equinus c.
groin-to-ankle c.
gutter c.
Gypsona c.
halo c.
handshake c.
hanging arm c.
Hexcelite c.
hinged cylinder c.
hip spica c.
hyperextension c.
c. immobilization
c. immobilizer
inhibitive c.
intermediate c.
intern's triangle in hip spica c.
Jones compression c.
Kite clubfoot c.
Kite metatarsal c.
c. knife
leg walking c.
light c.
c. liner
localizer c.
long arm c. (LAC)
long arm finger c.
long bent-knee leg c.
long leg c. (LLC)
long leg walking c. (LLWC)
long leg weightbearing c.
  (LLWBC)
Lorenz c.
Lovell clubfoot c.
MaxCast c.
medial malleolus c.
3M fiberglass c.
Minerva c.
modified Cotrel c.
Moe modified Cotrel c.
Mooney c.
Munster c.
negative impression c.
Neufeld c.
nonwalking c.
O'Donoghue cotton c.
one-half spica c.

one and one-half spica c.
onlay bone graft c.
Orfizip knee c.
Orfizip wrist c.
Orthoplast slipper c.
outrigger c.
c. padding
pantaloon spica c.
pantaloon walking c.
patellar dislocation c.
patellar tendon weightbearing c.
petaling the c.
Petrie spica c.
plaster of Paris c.
plastic c.
polyurethane c.
pontoon spica c.
POP c.
PTB c.
quadriceps femoris muscle c.
Quengel c.
removable c.
c. removal
rigid below-the-knee c.
Risser localizer scoliosis c.
Risser turnbuckle c.
Sarmiento short leg patellar
  tendon-bearing c.
Sbarbaro spica c.
Schmeisser spica c.
scoliosis c.
semirigid fiberglass c. (SRF)
serial wedge c.
c. shoe
short arm c. (SAC)
short arm fiberglass c.
short arm gauntlet c.
short arm navicular c. (SANC)
short leg c. (SLC)
short leg plaster c.
short leg walking c. (SLWC)
short walking c.
shoulder spica c.
single-leg spica c.
skin-tight c.
slipper c.
c. sock
spica c.
sugar-tong c.
c. syndrome
c. table

c. tape
three-finger spica c.
three-point pressure c.
thumb spica c.
toe spica c.
toe-to-groin c.
toe-to-midthigh c.
tone-inhibiting leg c.
total contact c.
traction c.
turnbuckle c.
underarm c.
univalve c.
Unna boot c.
Velpeau c.
c. walker
walking boot c.
warm-and-form c.
c. wedge
wedging c.
well-leg c.
c. window
windowed c.
c. with dorsal toe plate extension
c. with volar toe plate extension
zipper c.
castaway
  Air C.
  C. ankle walker
  C. leg brace
  C. leg walker
  US Manufacturing Air C.
Castech extremity support
Castiglia ankle brace
casting
  foam c.
  intermittent c.
  negative c.
  postoperative c.
  serial c.
  total contact c. (TCC)
Castle procedure
**Castle-Schneider resection interposition
  arthroplasty**
Castroviejo
  C. bladebreaker knife
  C. needle holder
  C. trephine
CAT
  computerized axial tomography
Catagni criteria

NOTES

119

catapophysis
catastrophic deterioration
cat-back
    rachitic c.-b.
CAT-CAM
    contoured adduction trochanteric-
    controlled alignment method
catch and clunk test
catching sensation
catch-up clunk
category
    Functional Ambulation c. (FAC)
    Westin-Turco c.
Catera suture anchor
Cateye Ergociser
Cathcart Orthocentric hip prosthesis
cathepsin
catheter
    Abramson c.
    condom c.
    c. entrapment
    c. kinking
    Mentor Self-Cath soft c.
    Simpson arthrectomy c.
    tracer c.
    wicking c.
cathode
Catlin amputating knife
Caton method
Cat's Paw Exerciser
Catterall
    C. classification
    C. hip score
cauda
    c. equina
    c. equina compression
    c. equina syndrome
caudad anterior mold
caudal
    c. lamina resection
    c. retinaculum
    c. spinal agenesis
    c. translation
    c. vertebra
caudalward
caudocephalad
caudocranial
causalgia
causalgic pain
cauterization
    alcohol c.
    bipolar c.
    Bovie c.
    phenol c.
    unipolar c.
cautery
    Aesculap bipolar c.
    BICAP c.

    bipolar c.
    Bovie c.
    chemical c.
    Concept hand-held c.
    intraarticular c.
    Mira c.
    monopolar c.
    slow c.
    unipolar c.
cavalry bone
cavalryman's osteoma
Cavanaugh-Rogers footprint classification
cave
    C. hip approach
    C. knee approach
    C. operation
cavern chordoma
cavernous
    c. hemangioma
    c. lymphangioma
Cave-Rowe
    C.-R. ligature carrier
    C.-R. shoulder dislocation operation
    C.-R. shoulder dislocation technique
Cavin osteotome
cavitary
    c. defect
    c. deficiency
    glenoid c.
cavitation
    joint c.
    manual c.
Cavitron ultrasonic surgical aspirator
cavity
    absorption c.
    cotyloid c.
    glenoid c.
    idiopathic bone c.
    joint c.
    marrow c.
    Meckel c.
    medullary c.
    saclike c.
    synovial c.
cavoequinovarus
cavovalgus
    pes c.
    talipes c.
cavovarus
    c. deformity
    c. foot
    pes c.
    talipes c.
cavus
    anterior c.
    combined c.
    c. foot
    c. foot deformity

C. foot support
forefoot c.
global c.
hindfoot c.
lesser tarsus c.
local c.
metatarsus c.
midfoot c.
pes c.
posttraumatic c.
c. posture
pronated pes c.
rigid foot c.
talipes c.

CAWO
closing abductory-wedge osteotomy
CB
contrast bath
C-bar orthosis
CBP
chiropractic biophysics
CBP technique
CBWO
closed base wedge osteotomy
CC
calcaneocuboid
coracoclavicular
CC joint
CC ligament
CC Rider closed-chain rehabilitation
system
CCD
central collodiaphysial
CCD angle
CCDA
calcaneocuboid distraction arthrodesis
CCF
compound comminuted fracture
C-clamp
Fukushima C-c.
CCN
cervical cord neurapraxia
CCPQ
Children's Comprehensive Pain
Questionnaire
CCS
chronic compartment syndrome
CCTA
coronal computed tomographic
arthrography
C-D
Cotrel-Dubousset

C-D fixation device
C-D hook
C-D instrumentation
C-D instrumentation device
C-D instrumentation fixation
strength
C-D instrumentation rigidity
C-D rod insertion
C-D screw modification
CDH
congenital dislocation of hip
congenital dysplasia of hip
CDH cup inserter
CDH Precoat Plus hip prosthesis
CDP
computerized dynamic posturography
CE
capital epiphysis
CE angle
CEA
carcinoembryonic antigen
Cebotome
C. bone cement drill
C. osteotome
Cedell fracture
Cedell-Magnusson
C.-M. arthritis classification
C.-M. classification of arthritis on
x-ray
cefamandole
cell
anterior horn c.
cartilage c.
chondrosarcoma c.
c. cushion
dorsal horn c.
endothelial c.
mesenchymal c.
osteoclastic giant c.
osteogenic c.
osteoprogenitor c.
Schwann c.
squamous c.
synovial stromal c.
c. therapy
cell-mediated immunity
cellular
c. immunity
c. periosteal osteocartilaginous mass
c. response to implant material
c. schwannoma

NOTES

C

121

cellulitis
    aerobic c.
    anaerobic c.
celluloid implant material
cellulose
    c. hemostatic agent
    Oxycel oxidized c.
CEM
    central extensor mechanism
cement
    acrylic bone c.
    arthroplasty c.
    BA bone c.
    bioactive bone c.
    biodegradable calcium phosphate c.
    bone c.
    Boneloc c.
    BoneSource hydroxyapatite c.
    c. centralizer
    centrifugation of c.
    CMW bone c.
    c. compactor
    c. curette
    DePuy CMW type-1 bone c.
    c. disease
    doughy c.
    Duall #88 c.
    C. Eater
    C. Eater drill
    Endurance bone c.
    Howmedica c.
    hydroxyapatite-coated porous alumni c.
    Implast bone c.
    c. injection gun
    c. interface
    Ketac c.
    key the c.
    c. line
    low viscosity bone c.
    c. mantle
    c. mantle grade classification
    master c.
    methyl methacrylate c.
    Norian SRS c.
    Orthocomp c.
    orthopaedic c.
    Orthoset radiopaque bone c.
    Osteobond copolymer bone c.
    Palacos radiopaque bone c.
    c. patty
    c. plug
    PMMA bone c.
    polymerization of bone c.
    polymethyl methacrylate bone c.
    pressurized c.
    Pronto c.

    prosthetic antibiotic-loaded acrylic c. (PROSTALAC)
    Protoplast c.
    c. pump
    radiopaque bone c.
    c. removal
    removal of excess c.
    residual c.
    c. restrictor
    c. restrictor inserter
    Simplex P bone c.
    c. spacer inserter
    c. spatula
    SRS injectable c.
    surface c.
    Surgical Simplex P radiopaque bone c.
    c. syringe
    VersaBond medium viscosity bone c.
    Zimmer bone c.
    Zimmer low-viscosity c.
cemental fracture
cement-bone interface
cemented
    c. broach
    c. component
    c. total hip arthroplasty
cementing fibroma
cementless
    c. broach
    c. disease
    c. femoral component
    c. fixation
    c. prosthesis
    c. Sportono (CLS)
    c. surface replacement arthroplasty (CSRA)
    c. technique
    c. total hip arthroplasty
    c. total hip replacement
cementome
    Anspach c.
cement-removal hand chisel
cement-wedge sign
cenesthopathy
Centec
    C. Formfit ankle brace
    C. Propoint knee brace
center
    Arizona Health Science C. (AHSC)
    c. of axial rotation
    central micturition c.
    c. of gravity (CG, COG)
    c. for independent living (CIL)
    Louisiana State University Medical C. (LSUMC)
    c. of mass

Midwest Regional Spinal Cord
   Injury C.
ossification primary c.
ossification secondary c.
pontine micturition c.
Veterans Administration
   Prosthetic C. (VAPC)
center-edge
   c.-e. angle
   c.-e. angle of Wiberg
centering
   c. drill
   c. hole
Centinela supraspinatus test
central
   c. bone
   c. callus
   c. canal
   c. canal stenosis
   c. collodiaphysial (CCD)
   c. collodiaphysial angle
   c. column
   c. cord
   c. cord syndrome
   c. core disease
   c. deficiency
   c. disk protrusion
   c. dislocation
   c. electromyography
   c. extensor mechanism (CEM)
   c. fiber-region
   c. heel pad syndrome
   c. herniation
   c. herniation syndrome
   c. horn
   c. micturition center
   c. necrosis
   c. nervous system (CNS)
   c. neural blockade
   c. physiolysis
   c. polydactyly
   c. posterior-anterior pressure
   c. ray
   c. ray amputation
   c. segment
   c. slip
   c. slip sparing technique
   c. spine spondylosis
   c. splitting technique
   c. talus fracture
   c. transpatellar tendon portal
Centralign precoat hip prosthesis

centralization
   Bayne-Klug c.
   Bora c.
   Manske-McCarroll-Swanson c.
   c. of radius operation
   tendon c.
centralizer
   cement c.
   PMMA c.
centralizing rod
centrifugation of cement
centrifuged methyl methacrylate
centromedullary
   c. nail
   c. nailing
centronuclear myopathy
centrosclerosis
cephalad
   c. anterior mold
   c. translation
cephalic
   c. angulation
   c. artery
   c. vein
cephalocaudad
cephalocaudal
cephalomedullary nail fracture
cephaloscapular projection
ceramic
   c. acetabular cup
   alumina c.
   c. biomaterial
   calcium phosphate c.
   calcium sulfate c.
   c. femoral head prosthesis
   c. implant
   c. ossicular prosthesis
   resorbable c.
   c. vertebral spacer
ceramic-on-ceramic bearing surface
Ceramion prosthesis
**Ceraver Osteal knee replacement
   system**
cerclage
   Dall-Miles cable c.
   c. fibreux
   Howmedica c.
   c. wire
   c. wire fixation
   c. wire inserter
   c. wire twister
cerclaged component

C

NOTES

cerebella (*pl. of* cerebellum)
cerebellar
    c. ataxia
    c. function test
    c. gait
    c. retractor
cerebellopontine angle tumor
cerebellum, pl. cerebella
cerebral
    c. palsy (CP)
    c. palsy-related dystonia
cerebroside reticulocytosis
cerebrospinal
    c. canal
    c. fluid (CSF)
    c. fluid analysis
Ceres' Secret aloe vera gel
Cerva Crane halter
cervical
    c. acceleration/deceleration syndrome
    c. AOA halo traction
    c. approach
    c. arch
    c. artery
    c. arthritis
    c. arthrodesis
    c. canal
    c. chair
    c. collar
    c. collar brace
    c. compaction test
    c. cord neurapraxia (CCN)
    c. corpectomy
    c. cushion
    c. Derifield procedure
    electromyocardiography
    c. disk
    c. disk disease
    c. diskectomy
    c. disk excision
    c. diskography
    c. disk surgery
    c. dorsal glide
    c. dorsal outlet syndrome
    c. drill
    c. extension strength
    c. fascia
    c. fracture tongs
    c. general rotation
    c. halter traction
    c. hypolordosis
    c. interbody fusion
    c. joint
    c. laminectomy punch
    c. ligament of tarsal sinus
    c. lordosis
    c. mallet
    c. manual traction

    c. microtrauma
    c. midline disk herniation
    c. mover ligament
    c. myofascial pain
    c. nerve root encroachment
    c. nerve root injection
    c. nerve root injury
    c. oblique facet wiring
    c. orthosis (CO)
    c. outlet
    c. plate
    c. plexus
    c. punch forceps
    c. radiculitis
    c. radiculopathy
    c. range-of-motion device
    c. range-of-motion instrument
    (CROM)
    c. region
    c. rib
    c. rib syndrome
    c. roll
    c. rongeur
    c. root
    c. rotation in extension
    c. saddle
    c. screw insertion technique
    c. sidegliding test
    c. sleep pillow
    c. specific rotation in flexion
    c. spinal cord
    c. spinal injury
    c. spine (C-spine)
    c. spine decompression
    c. spine extension injury
    c. spine internal fixation
    c. spine kyphotic deformity
    c. spine laminectomy
    c. spine posterior fusion
    c. spine posterior ligament
    disruption
    c. spine screw-plate fixation
    c. spine stabilization
    c. spine trauma
    c. spondylolysis
    c. spondylosis
    c. spondylotic myelopathy
    c. spondylotic myelopathy fusion
    technique
    c. spondylotic myelopathy
    vertebrectomy
    c. stairstep
    c. stenosis
    c. support
    c. sympathectomy
    c. sympathetic chain location
    c. synostosis
    c. tension myositis (CTM)

c. thoracic orthosis
c. triangle
c. trochanteric displaced fracture
c. trochanteric fracture
c. vertebra
c. vertebral bone
cervicalgia
cervical/lumbar hammer
cervicitis
cervicoaxillary
cervicobrachial
cervicobrachialgia
cervicocranial
cervicodorsal
cervicoencephalic syndrome
cervicogenic
c. headache
c. syndrome
cervicooccipital fusion
cervicoplasty
cervicoscapular
cervicothoracic
c. curve
c. jacket
c. junction
c. junction stabilization
c. junction surgery
c. orthosis (CTO)
c. pedicle anatomy
c. pedicle angle
c. transition
cervicothoracolumbosacral orthosis (CTLSO)
cervicotrochanteric
Cervifix system
Cervitrak device
cervix amputation
CES
cranial electrical stimulation
Cestan-Chenais syndrome
CFL
calcaneofibular ligament
CFLB
carbon fiber lamination braid
C-Flex supine cervical traction
CFS
contoured femoral stem
CFS hip prosthesis
CG
center of gravity
C-guide
screw placement C-g.

CH
coracohumeral
CH ligament
Chaddock
C. reflex
C. sign
C. test
Chadwick-Bentley classification
CHAG
coralline hydroxyapatite Goniopora
CHAG bone graft substitute material
chain
closed c.
closed kinetic c. (CKC)
kinetic c.
paravertebral sympathetic c.
pelvic kinematic c.
c. reaction exercise
sympathetic c.
wheelchair c.
chair
BodyBilt c.
Boyd podiatry c.
cervical c.
dynamic integrated stabilization c. (DISC)
ergonomically correct c.
EZ Rider support c.
Gardner c.
Hogg c.
Invacare padded shower c.
Kaleidoscope c.
Orthokinetics travel c.
Pogon c.
Portal Pro 2 treatment c.
sit/stand c.
STC 900-series travel c.
Vess c.
chairback
c. brace
c. lumbosacral orthosis
ChairCiser adjustable exerciser
Chalet frame
chalk-stick fracture
chalky bone
chamber
monoplace hyperbaric c.
multiplace hyperbaric c.
Portable Topical Hyperbaric Oxygen Extremity C.
Pudenz flushing c.

NOTES

Chamberlain line
Chambers
    C. osteotomy
    C. procedure
chamfer
    c. cut
    c. cut jig
    c. reamer
chamfered cylinder acetabular
  component
champ
    C. CTS cold therapy wrap
    C. elastic bandage
    C. Insulated Propac II
champagne bottle leg
champion
    C. Power Sox
    C. Trauma Score (CTS)
Championnière bone drill
Chance
    C. fracture thoracolumbar spine
    C. vertebral fracture
Chandler
    C. arthrodesis
    C. bone elevator
    C. disease
    C. felt collar splint
    C. hip fusion
    C. knee retractor
    C. patellar advancement
    C. procedure
    C. spinal perforating forceps
    C. tendon transfer
    C. unreamed interlocking tibial nail
change
    age-associated degenerative c.
    Ahlback c.
    arthritic talonavicular c.
    burn-related pigmentation c.
    Charcot c.
    degenerative arthritic c.
    diurnal c.
    Fairbanks c.
    Iowa degenerative c.
    kinematic gait pattern c.
    neuromuscular gait pattern c.
    sarcomatous c.
    therapeutic lifestyle c. (TLC)
    trophic c.
Chang-Miltner incision
channel
    interosseous anastomosing c.
    tibial c.
channel-and-core biopsy
Chapchal knee arthrodesis
Chaput
    C. fracture
    C. fragment

    C. method
    C. tubercle
characteristic
    electrooptical c. (EOC)
    receiver operating c.
Charcot
    C. arthritis
    C. arthropathy
    C. arthroplasty
    C. arthrosis
    C. change
    C. chondroma
    C. collapse
    C. deformity
    C. degeneration
    C. disruption
    C. foot
    C. gait
    C. hip arthrodesis
    C. joint
    C. joint disease
    C. neuroarthropathy
    C. restraint orthotic walker
    (CROW)
    C. spine
    C. syndrome
    C. triad
Charcot-Marie atrophy
Charcot-Marie-Tooth (CMT)
    C.-M.-T. atrophy
    C.-M.-T. disease
    C.-M.-T. Evaluation
charger view
Charles Bonnet syndrome
Charleston
    C. nighttime bending brace
    C. scoliosis brace
charley horse
Charlie Chaplin gait
Charnley
    C. acetabular cup
    C. acetabular cup prosthesis
    C. ankle arthrodesis
    C. ankle fusion procedure
    C. arthrodesis clamp
    C. bone clamp
    C. bone curette
    C. brace
    C. brace handle
    C. cemented prosthesis
    C. centering apparatus
    C. centering drill
    C. centering ring
    C. classification of function
    C. compression
    C. compression apparatus
    C. compression arthrodesis
    C. compression clamp

C. compression-type knee fusion
C. deepening reamer
C. expanding reamer
C. external fixation clamp
C. external fixation device
C. femoral broach
C. femoral condyle drill
C. femoral condyle radius gauge
C. femoral inlay aligner
C. femoral inlay guillotine
C. femoral prosthesis neck punch
C. femoral prosthesis pusher
C. flat-back femoral component
C. foam suture pad
C. functional classification
C. and Henderson extraarticular
  fusion
C. and Henderson intraarticular
  fusion
C. hip score
C. horizontal retractor
C. Howorth Exflow system
C. implant
C. incision
C. initial incision retractor
C. introducer
C. knee retractor
C. laminar flow room
C. low-friction arthroplasty
C. low-friction hip prosthesis
C. narrow-stem component
C. offset-bore cup
C. pain and function grading scale
C. pilot drill
C. pin
C. pin clamp
C. pin retractor
C. rasp
C. self-retaining retractor
C. socket gauge
C. standard-stem component
C. starting drill
C. suction drain
C. suture button
C. taper reamer
C. template
C. tibial onlay jig
C. total hip arthroplasty
C. total hip prosthesis
C. total hip replacement
C. total hip system
C. towel

C. trochanter holder
C. trochanter reamer
C. wire-holding forceps
C. wire passer
C. wire tightener
Charnley-Hastings prosthesis
Charnley-Houston shoulder arthrodesis
Charnley-Merle
  C.-M. D'Aubigné disability grading
    scale
  C.-M. D'Aubigné disability grading
    system
Charnley-Müller
  C.-M. arthroplasty
  C.-M. hip prosthesis
  C.-M. lateral approach
Charriere
  C. amputation saw
  C. bone saw
CHART
  Craig Handicap Assessment and
    Reporting Technique
chart
  Reality Orientation C.
  sclerotome pain c.
Chassaignac
  C. axillary muscle
  C. tubercle
Chatfield-Girdlestone splint
Chattanooga
  C. balance system Checkrein
    deformity
  C. traction
  C. traction device
**Chatzidakis hinged Vitallium implant
  prosthesis**
chauffeur's fracture
Chaves muscle transfer
Chaves-Rapp
  C.-R. muscle transfer
  C.-R. muscle transfer technique
  C.-R. paralysis
CHD
  congenital hip dysplasia
  CHD prosthesis
check
  Derifield pelvic leg c.
  head c.
  shoulder-to-head c.
  c. socket
Checkerboard wheelchair cushion

NOTES

checklist
    Body Mechanics Evaluation C.
    Low Back Pain Symptom C.
    McGill pain c.
    Ways of Coping c.
checkrein
    c. deformity
    c. ligament
    c. procedure
cheese-grater hemispherical reamer
Cheetah ankle brace
cheilectomy
    arthroscopic c.
    dorsal c.
    first MTP c.
    Garceau c.
    Mann-Coughlin-DuVries c.
    Sage c.
    Sage-Clark c.
cheilotomy
cheiralgia paresthetica
cheirarthritis
cheiroarthropathy
cheirobrachialgia
cheirognostic
cheiromegaly
cheiroplasty
cheiropodalgia
cheirospasm
chelation therapy
chemical
    c. carcinogen
    c. cautery
    c. matrixectomy
    c. nail avulsion
    c. neurolysis
    c. sympathectomy
chemiluminescent microtiter protein kinase activity assay
chemonucleolysis
    chymopapain c.
    double-needle c.
chemosterilized graft
chemosurgery
    phenol c.
chemotherapy
    adjuvant c.
    neoadjuvant c.
chemotherapy-related neuropathy
Cherf
    C. cast stand
    C. legholder
cherry
    C. drill
    C. osteotome
    C. screw extractor
    C. tong traction
    C. traction tongs

Cherry-Austin drill
Cherry-Kerrison laminectomy rongeur
chest
    alar c.
    barrel c.
    cobbler c.
    c. contusion
    c. expansion test
    flat c.
    foveated c.
    funnel c.
    keeled c.
    paralytic c.
    phthinoid c.
    pigeon c.
    pterygoid c.
    c. roll
    c. tube
chest-band transmitter
chevron
    c. bone
    c. bunionectomy
    c. fusion
    c. hallux valgus correction
    c. incision
    c. laceration
    c. modification of the Mitchell osteotomy
    c. osteotomy with rigid screw fixation
    c. procedure
    c. technique
chevron-Akin double osteotomy
Cheyne periosteal elevator
CHH
    cartilage-hair hypoplasia
    CHH cervical brace
chi
    tai c.
Chiari
    C. formation
    C. innominate osteotomy
    C. malformation
    C. shelf procedure
    C. technique
Chiari-Foix-Nicolesco syndrome
Chiari-Salter-Steel pelvic osteotomy
chiasma
    Camper c.
Chiba spinal system
Chick
    C. CLT operating frame
    C. CLT operating table
    C. fracture table
    C. nail
chicken breast
Chick-Foster orthopedic bed
Chick-Langren orthopedic table

Chiene test
chilblain
Child Development Inventory
children
    Total Knee for C.
children's
    C. Comprehensive Pain
      Questionnaire (CCPQ)
    C. Hospital hand drill
    C. Hospital screwdriver
    c. mat
Childress
    C. ankle fixation
    C. ankle fixation technique
    C. duck waddle test
Chinese
    C. fingertrap suture
    C. flap
    C. medicine
    C. red line sign
chin-to-chest test
chip
    bone c.
    cancellous c.
    c. fracture
    c. graft
Chippaux-Smirak arch index
chipped-tooth broach
chirarthritis
ChiroFlow adjustable back support
Chiro-Manis chiropractic table
chiropodalgia
chiropodical
chiropodist
chiropody
chiropractic
    c. adjustment procedure
    c. analysis
    c. biophysics (CBP)
    c. joint manipulation
    c. laser nonsurgical face lift
    c. lesion
    c. manipulative reflex technique
      (CMRT)
    c. manual manipulation
    c. manual manipulation of spine
    c. mattress
    c. spinal adjustment
    sports c.
    c. thermography
    c. x-ray film
chiropractor

chiropraxis
Chiroslide Jamar Hand Dynamometer
chirospasm
Chirotech x-ray system
chirurgicum mallei
chisel
    acetabular round c.
    Adson laminectomy c.
    Alexander c.
    ASIF c.
    Austin Moore c.
    Ballenger-Hajek c.
    beveled c.
    Biomet cement-removal hand c.
    Bishop c.
    c. blade
    Blair c.
    bone c.
    Bowen c.
    box c.
    Brittain c.
    Bruening c.
    Buckley c.
    Caltagirone c.
    cement-removal hand c.
    Cinelli-McIndoe c.
    Cloward spinal fusion c.
    cold c.
    Converse c.
    Cottle c.
    Dautrey c.
    D'Errico lamina c.
    c. elevator
    Fomon c.
    c. fracture
    Freer c.
    gold-paneled c.
    Hajek c.
    Harmon c.
    Hibbs c.
    hollow c.
    Kerrison c.
    Lambert-Lowman c.
    laminectomy c.
    Lexer c.
    Lowman c.
    Lowman-Hoglund c.
    Lucas c.
    Magnum c.
    Martin cartilage c.
    meniscotomy c.

NOTES

chisel *(continued)*
    Metzenbaum c.
    Meyerding c.
    Miles bone c.
    Moore prosthesis-mortising c.
    mortising c.
    Oratec c.
    orthopaedic c.
    Partsch c.
    Passow c.
    Pick c.
    Puka c.
    Schwartze c.
    seating c.
    Sheehan c.
    Simmons c.
    Smillie cartilage c.
    Smillie meniscectomy c.
    Smith-Petersen c.
    square-hollow c.
    Stille bone c.
    straight c.
    swan-neck c.
    Trautmann c.
    U.S. Army bone c.
    West bone c.
    White c.
chisel-edge elevator
chisel-tip wire
chloramphenicol osteomyelitis
chloride
    polyvinyl c. (PVC)
Cho
    C. anterior cruciate ligament
      reconstruction
    C. tendon technique
choked disk
choke syndrome
cholinergic vagal function
cholinesterase inhibitor
chondral fragment
chondralgia
chondrectomy
chondrification
chondritis
chondroblast
chondroblastic sarcoma
chondroblastoma
    benign c.
    humeral c.
chondrocalcinosis
chondroclast
chondrocyte
    autologous cultured c.
    hypertrophic c.
chondrodiastasis
chondrodynia

chondrodysplasia
    genotypic c.
    hereditary deforming c.
    hyperplastic c.
    McKusick-type metaphysial c.
    metaphysial c.
    c. punctata
    rhizomelic-type c.
chondrodystrophia calcificans
chondrodystrophy
chondroepiphysis
chondroepiphysitis
chondrofibroma
chondrogenesis
chondrography
chondroid syringoma
chondroitin
chondrolipoma
chondrolysis
chondroma
    Charcot c.
    extraskeletal c.
    joint c.
    juxtacortical c.
    periosteal c.
    synovial c.
chondromalacia
    c. patellae
    patellar c.
chondromalacic
chondromatosis
    Henderson-Jones c.
    synovial c.
chondromatous hamartoma
chondrometaplasia
chondromyofibroma
chondromyoma
chondromyxofibroma
chondromyxoid fibroma
chondromyxoma
chondromyxosarcoma
chondronecrosis
chondroosseous
    c. growth
    c. spur
chondroosteodystrophy
chondropathology
chondropathy
chondrophyte
chondroplastic
    c. dwarfism
    c. myotonia
chondroplasty
    abrasion c.
    arthroscopic abrasion c.
    c. knife
chondroporosis
chondroprotective agent

chondrosarcoma
c. cell
clear cell c.
dedifferentiated c.
differentiated c.
extracortical c.
extraskeletal c.
juxtacortical c.
mesenchymal c.
myxoid c.
parosteal c.
periosteal c.
pseudocapsule c.
chondrosarcomatosis
chondrosis
chondrosteoma
chondrosternal articulation
chondrosternoplasty
chondrotomy
chondrotrophic
chondroxiphoid
chonechondrosternon
Chopart
C. amputation with tendon balancing
C. ankle dislocation
C. articulation
C. brace
C. hindfoot amputation
C. joint line
C. midtarsal joint
C. operation
C. osseous joint injury
C. partial foot prosthesis
Cho-Pat
C.-P. Achilles tendon strap
C.-P. Dual Action Knee Strap
C.-P. elbow strap
C.-P. ITB Strap
C.-P. knitted compression support
choppy sea sign
chordoblastoma
chordocarcinoma
chordoma
cavern c.
sacrococcygeal c.
chordosarcoma
chordotomy
choreatic gait
choreiform
choristoma

Chow
C. endoscopic carpal tunnel release
C. transbursal carpal tunnel release technique
Choyce MK II keratoprosthesis prosthesis
CHPS
chronic heel pain syndrome
Chrisman-Snook
C.-S. ankle technique
C.-S. reconstruction
C.-S. reconstruction of ankle ligament
C.-S. tenodesis
C.-S. weave procedure
Christensen interlocking nail
Christiani maneuver
Christiansen hip prosthesis
Christmas
C. tree adapter
C. tree reamer
chromatography
high-performance liquid c. (HPLC)
high-pressure liquid c. (HPLC)
chromatolysis
chrome
cobalt c.
c. cobalt screw
chrome-cobalt cable
chromium-cobalt-alloy implant
chromium-cobalt mesh
chromomycosis
chronaxie, chronaxy
chronic
c. absorptive arthritis
c. Achilles tendinitis
c. ankle sprain
c. anterior exertional compartment syndrome (CAECS)
c. compartment syndrome (CCS)
c. foot sprain
c. functional instability
c. heel pain syndrome (CHPS)
c. hemorrhagic villous synovitis
c. intractable benign pain syndrome (CIBPS)
c. lateral ankle instability
c. low back pain (CLBP)
c. microtraumatic soft tissue injury
c. musculoskeletal pain syndrome (CMPS)
c. periostalgia

NOTES

chronic *(continued)*
    c. purulent synovitis
    c. recurrent ankle joint dislocation
    c. rheumatism
    c. sclerosing osteomyelitis of Garré
    c. subtalar joint pain
    c. tophaceous disease
    c. tophaceous gout
    c. traumatic encephalopathy (CTE)
    c. villous arthritis
    c. whiplash
chronotropic impairment
CHSD
    congenital hyperphosphatasemic skeletal dysplasia
chuck
    c. adapter
    c. drill
    gold-handled c.
    hand c.
    Jacobs c.
    pin c.
    Steinmann pin with pin c.
    T-handle Zimmer c.
    three-jaw c.
Chuinard autogenous bone graft
Chuinard-Peterson
    C.-P. ankle arthrodesis
    C.-P. ankle fusion
    C.-P. anterior arthrodesis
Chukka boot
chylothorax
chylous
    c. arthritis
    c. ascites
    c. leakage
Chymar
    Alpha C.
CI
    confidence interval
    CI functional knee brace
CIBPS
    chronic intractable benign pain syndrome
CIC
    complex instability of carpus
Cica-Care wound dressing
cicatricial scoliosis
cicatrix, pl. **cicatrices**
cicatrization
Cicherelli bone rongeur
CID
    carpal instability dissociation
Cierny-Mader technique
ciguatera
CIL
    center for independent living
ciliospinal center of Budge

cinch
    C. instant suction B.K. prosthesis
    joint c.
    C. Lock CTS brace
Cincinnati
    C. ACL brace
    C. incision
    C. Knee Rating System
    C. knee scoring questionnaire
    C. technique
CIND
    carpal instability nondissociative
cinearthrography
    triple-injection c.
cinefluoroscopy
Cinelli-McIndoe chisel
Cinelli osteotome
cine-magnetic resonance imaging (cine-MRI)
cinematic amputation
cinematographic gait study
cine-MRI
    cine-magnetic resonance imaging
cineplastic amputation
cineplastics
cineradiography
cine view
cingulotomy, cingulumotomy
Cintor
    C. bone rongeur
    C. knee prosthesis
CIQ
    Community Integration Questionnaire
circle
    c. bed
    c. draw test
CircOlectric
    C. bed
    C. frame
CircPlus bandage/wrap system
Circul'Air shoe process system
circular
    c. bandage
    c. cast
    c. external fixator
    c. fixation
    c. fixation device
    c. laminar hook with offset top
    c. open amputation
    c. saw
    c. supracondylar amputation
    c. wire
    c. wire fixator
circulation
    collateral c.
    extraosseous c.
    femoral c.

intraosseous c.
perichondral c.
Circulator boot system
circulatory embarrassment
circumduction maneuver
circumductor table
circumference
calf c.
pelvic c.
circumferential
c. capsulectomy
c. cartilage
c. dedicated knee coil
c. dressing
c. fracture
c. grommet
c. lamella
c. ligamentous sleeve
c. release
c. release of clubfoot
c. wire
c. wire-loop fixation
c. wiring
circumflex
c. iliac artery
c. scapular artery
circumscribed
circumscribing incision
circumscripta
calcinosis c.
Dubreuilh melanosis c.
Cirrus
C. composite prosthetic foot
C. foot prosthesis
C. foot prosthetic
cirsoid angioma
Citanest
Citelli
C. angle
C. punch forceps
Citscope disposable arthroscope
Civinini
C. canal
C. ligament
C. process
C. spine
CIVRA
continuous intravenous regional
anesthesia
CKC
closed kinetic chain

CKCE
closed kinetic chain exercise
CKS
Continuum knee system
CKS implant
CKS knee system
Claiborne external fixator
clamp
Acland microvascular c.
Adair breast c.
Aesculap c.
Allen-Kocher c.
Allis c.
angled DeBakey c.
angled Lowman-type bone c.
angular hinge c.
Ann Arbor double towel c.
appendage c.
c. approximator
Atra-Grip c.
Auvard c.
baby Kocher c.
baby Satinsky c.
Backhaus-Jones towel c.
Backhaus-Kocher towel c.
Backhaus towel c.
Bahnson appendage c.
Bailey-Cowley c.
Bailey duckbill c.
Bailey-Morse c.
Balfour c.
Ballantine c.
Bamby c.
Bard c.
bar-to-bar c.
Belcher c.
Berens muscle c.
Berke c.
Bernhard c.
Bethune c.
Bircher bone-holding c.
Bircher cartilage c.
Bishop bone c.
Blalock c.
Böhler c.
bone extension c.
bone-holding c.
Bonney c.
Borge c.
Boyes muscle c.
bulldog c.
C c.

NOTES

C

clamp *(continued)*

Calandruccio c.
c. carrier
cartilage c.
Casey pelvic c.
Charnley arthrodesis c.
Charnley bone c.
Charnley compression c.
Charnley external fixation c.
Charnley pin c.
Clevis c.
Cooley graft c.
Cooley iliac c.
Cooley multipurpose angled c.
Cooley multipurpose curved c.
Dandy c.
Davidson muscle c.
Demel wire c.
Demos tibial artery c.
Diethrich bulldog c.
Dingman bone and cartilage c.
disposable muscle biopsy c.
dissecting c.
distraction c.
Doctor Collins fracture c.
double c.
Edna towel c.
exclusion c.
extension bone c.
femoral c.
Ferguson bone c.
c. fixator
c. forceps
Frazier-Adson osteoplastic flap c.
Frazier-Sachs c.
Freeman c.
Friedrich c.
Friedrich-Petz c.
full-curved c.
Gerster bone c.
Goodwin bone c.
Greenberg c.
Halifax interlaminar c.
Harrington hook c.
Harrington rod c.
hemostat c.
hemostatic thoracic c.
Hex-Fix Universal swivel c.
Hey Groves c.
Hoen c.
Hoffmann ligament c.
c. holder
hook c.
Hugh Young pedicle c.
iliac c.
c. insert
interlaminar c.
Jackson bone c.

Jackson bone-extension c.
Jackson bone-holding c.
Jacobson bulldog c.
Jameson muscle c.
Jarit anterior resection c.
Jarit cartilage c.
Jarit meniscal c.
Jarit small bone-holding c.
Johns Hopkins bulldog c.
Jones thoracic c.
Jones towel c.
Kantrowitz thoracic c.
Kelly c.
Kern bone-holding c.
Kocher c.
Lahey c.
Lalonde dynamic compression
  bone c.
Lalonde oblique fracture large
  bone c.
Lalonde oblique fracture medium
  bone c.
Lalonde oblique metacarpal fracture
  bone c.
Lalonde small bone c.
Lambert-Lowman bone c.
Lambotte bone-holding c.
Lamis patellar c.
Lane bone-holding c.
Lewin bone-holding c.
ligament c.
lobster-type c.
Locke bone c.
locking c.
Lowman bone-holding c.
Lowman-Gerster bone c.
Lowman-Hoglund c.
Lulu c.
Malis hinge c.
Martin cartilage c.
Martin meniscal c.
Martin muscular c.
Masterson curved c.
Masterson pelvic c.
Masterson straight c.
Mastin muscular c.
Matthew cross-leg c.
Mayo c.
medial malleolar/small bone
  fragment c.
meniscal c.
metal c.
microvascular c.
miniature multipurpose c.
mini-Ullrich bone c.
Mitchel-Adam multipurpose c.
Mixter ligature-carrier c.
Mixter right-angle c.

mosquito c.
Moynihan towel c.
multipurpose angled c.
multipurpose curved c.
muscle biopsy c.
muscular c.
Naraghi-DeCoster reduction c.
osteoplastic flap c.
padded c.
Parham-Martin bone-holding c.
patellar cement c.
patellar reduction c.
Pean c.
pedicle c.
pelvic C-c.
Pemberton spur-crushing c.
phalangeal c.
pin c.
pin-to-bar c.
point-of-reduction c.
Price muscular biopsy c.
ratchet c.
Rayport muscular biopsy c.
reamer c.
Richards bone c.
rod c.
rubber shod c.
Rumel myocardial c.
Rumel rubber c.
Rumel thoracic c.
Rush bone c.
saddle c.
Schlein c.
Seidel bone-holding c.
self-retaining c.
Semb bone-holding c.
sesamoid c.
single c.
Slocum meniscal c.
Smith bone c.
Southwick c.
speed-lock c.
sponge c.
spur-crushing c.
stainless steel c.
Steinhauser bone c.
Steri-Clamp c.
swivel c.
towel c.
trochanter-holding c.
Ulrich bone-holding c.
Universal wire c.

Verbrugge bone c.
Vermont spinal fixator c.
vessel c.
VSF c.
Walton cartilage c.
Walton meniscal c.
Wells pedicle c.
Wester meniscal c.
West Shur cartilage c.
wire-tightening c.
Wylie lumbar bulldog c.
X c.
Zimmer cartilage c.

clamping mechanism
clamshell
    c. AFO boot
    c. brace
    c. prosthesis
Clancy
    C. cruciate ligament reconstruction
    C. lateral compartment
    C. ligament technique
    C. patellar tendon graft
Clancy-Andrews reconstruction
Clanton
    C. turf toe
    C. turf toe grading system
Clark
    C. classification of melanoma
    C. pectoralis major transfer
    C. sign
    C. transfer technique
Clarke
    C. arch angle
    C. patellar compression test
Clark-Southwick-Odgen modification
Clarus SpineScope
clasp
    Arrow pin c.
    EPI Sport epicondylitis c.
clasped
    c. thumb
    c. thumb deformity
classification
    AAOS acetabular abnormality c.
    ACR c.
    acromioclavicular injury c.
    Aitken epiphysial fracture c.
    Allman acromioclavicular injury c.
    American Rheumatism
      Association c.

C

NOTES

classification *(continued)*

American Spinal Cord Injury Association c.
Anderson-D'Alonzo odontoid fracture c.
Anderson modification of Berndt-Harty c.
Anderson tibial pseudarthrosis c.
AO ankle fracture c.
Arbeitsgemeinschaft für Osteosynthesfragen-Danis-Weber ankle fracture c.
Arco c.
Arthritis Impact Measurement Scale c.
Ashhurst-Bromer ankle fracture c.
Bado c.
Bauer-Jackson c.
Bayne radial agenesis c.
Bayne ulnar ray deficiency c.
Bennett thumb fracture c.
Berndt c.
Bishop c.
Bleck metatarsus adductus c.
Boyd c.
Boyd-Griffin trochanteric fracture c.
Brooker heterotopic bone formation c.
Burwell-Charnley fracture reduction c.
Canale-Kelly talar neck fracture c.
Carnesale-Stewart-Barnes hip dislocation c.
Catterall c.
Cavanaugh-Rogers footprint c.
Cedell-Magnusson arthritis c.
cement mantle grade c.
Chadwick-Bentley c.
Charnley functional c.
Clatter c.
Codman c.
Colonna hip fracture c.
Colton c.
Copeland-Kavat metatarsophalangeal dislocation c.
CP Sports Balance C.
Crowe congenital hip dysplasia c.
Danis-Weber fracture c.
D'Antonio acetabular c.
Darrow pain c.
Daseler-Anson plantaris muscle anatomy c.
Deknatel suture c.
DeLee c.
Denis Browne sacral fracture c.
Denis Browne spinal fracture c.
Denis compression fracture c.
Denis seat-belt injury c.

Devas stress fracture c.
Dias-Tachdijian physial injury c.
Dickhaut-DeLee discoid meniscus c.
Dorr bone c.
Durie and Salmon c.
Dyck-Lambert c.
Eckert-Davis c.
Edwards and Lee tibiofibular diastasis and syndesmotic injury c.
Ellis c.
Enneking c.
Epstein hip dislocation c.
Epstein-Thomas c.
Essex-Lopresti calcaneal fracture c.
Estok and Harris c.
Evans intertrochanteric fracture c.
femoral fracture following total hip replacement c.
Ficat and Arlet osteonecrosis c.
Ficat femoral head osteonecrosis c.
Ficat stage of avascular necrosis c.
Fielding femoral fracture c.
Fielding-Magliato subtrochanteric fracture c.
Flatt c.
floating knee fracture c.
fracture c.
Fränkel neurologic deficit c.
Franz-O'Rahilly c.
Freeman calcaneal fracture c.
Fries score for rheumatoid arthritis c.
Frykman distal radius fracture c.
Garden femoral neck fracture c.
Gartland humeral supracondylar fracture c.
Gartland Universal radial fracture c.
Gertzbein seat-belt injury c.
Graf c.
Grantham femur fracture c.
Greenfield spinocerebellar ataxia c.
Gumley seat beat injury c.
Gustilo-Anderson open fracture c.
Gustilo-Anderson tibial plafond fracture c.
Gustilo puncture wound c.
Gustilo tibial fracture c.
Hahn-Steinthal capitellum fracture c.
Hannover c.
Hansen fracture c.
Hardcastle c.
Hardy-Clapham sesamoid c.
Hawkins talar fracture c.
Henderson c.
Herbert-Fisher fracture system c.

Herbert scaphoid bone fracture c.
Herndon hip c.
Herring lateral pillar c.
Heyman hip c.
Hoaglund-States c.
Hohl-Luck tibial plateau fracture c.
Hohl-Moore c.
Hohl tibial condylar fracture c.
Holdsworth spinal fracture c.
Hughston Clinic injury c.
Ideberg glenoid fracture c.
Ingram-Bachynski hip fracture c.
Insall patellar injury c.
Jahss ankle dislocation c.
Jahss metatarsophalangeal joint
    dislocation c.
Janis tibialis posterior tendon
    dysfunction c.
Jeffery radial fracture c.
Jensen-Michelsen intertrochanteric
    hip fracture c.
Johansson fracture c.
Johner-Wruhs tibial fracture c.
Johnson-Boseker scale c.
Johnson-Jahss posterior tibial
    tendon tear c.
Johnson and Strom tibialis
    posterior tendon dysfunction c.
Jones-Barnes-Lloyd-Roberts c.
Jones congenital tibial deficiency c.
Jones diaphysial fracture c.
Judet epiphysial fracture c.
Jupiter and Belsky phalanx
    fracture c.
Kalamchi c.
Kalamchi-Dawe congenital tibial
    deficiency c.
Kelikian nail deformity c.
Kellam-Waddel c.
Key-Conwell pelvic fracture c.
Kilfoyle humeral medial condylar
    fracture c.
King thoracic scoliosis c.
Kocher c.
Kocher-Lorenz capitellum
    fracture c.
Kostuik-Errico spinal stability c.
Kümmel ulnar ray deficiency c.
Kuwada Achilles tendon injury c.
Kyle fracture c.
Kyle-Gustilo c.
Kyle-Gustilo-Premer c.

LaGrange humeral supracondylar
    fracture c.
Langenskiöld c. (stage I–VI)
lateral condylar fracture c.
Lauge-Hansen ankle fracture c.
Letournel-Judet acetabular
    fracture c.
Leung thumb loss c.
Lichtman aseptic necrosis c.
Lindell c.
Lloyd-Roberts-Catterall-Salamon c.
load-sharing c.
Macewen c.
MacNichol-Voutsinas c.
Mason radial head fracture c.
Mast-Spieghel-Pappas c.
Mathews olecranon fracture c.
Mayo carpal instability c.
Mayo elbow fracture c.
Mazur ankle elevation c.
McDermott radiological c.
McLain-Weinstein spinal tumor c.
Melone distal radius fracture c.
Merland perimedullary arteriovenous
    fistula c.
Meyers-McKeever tibial fracture c.
Milch condylar fracture c.
Milch elbow fracture c.
Minaar coalition c.
modified Frankel c.
modified Sillence c.
Moore tibial plateau fracture c.
MRC muscle function c.
Mueller femoral supracondylar
    fracture c.
Mueller humerus fracture c.
Mueller tibial fracture c.
Neer femur fracture c.
Neer-Horowitz humerus fracture c.
· Neer humerus fracture c.
Neer shoulder fracture c.
Neviaser frozen shoulder c.
Newman radial neck and head
    fracture c.
New York diagnostic criteria c.
Nicoll c.
Nurick spondylosis c.
O'Brien radial fracture c.
Oden peroneal tendon
    subluxation c.
Ogden epiphysial fracture c.
Ogden fracture c.

NOTES

classification *(continued)*

Ogden knee dislocation c.
Olerud and Molander fracture c.
O'Rahilly limb deficiency c.
ordinal c.
Orthopaedic Trauma Association c.
osteoarthritis grading c.
Outerbridge c.
Ovadia-Beals tibial plafond
  fracture c.
Paley c.
Palmer triangular fibrocartilage
  complex lesion c.
Papavasiliou olecranon fracture c.
Pauwels femoral neck fracture c.
Pennal c.
peripheral nerve tumor c.
pilon fracture c.
Pipkin posterior hip dislocation c.
Pipkin subclassification of Epstein-
  Thomas c.
Poland epiphysial fracture c.
pressure ulcer c.
Pritsch talar osteochondroma c.
Prosthetic Problem Inventory
  Scale c.
Quénu-Küss tarsometatarsal
  injury c.
Quinby pelvic fracture c.
Ranawat c.
Ratliff avascular necrosis c.
Regnauld hallux rigidus c.
Riordan club hand c.
Riseborough-Radin intercondylar
  fracture c.
Rockwood c.
Rowe calcaneal fracture c.
Rowe-Lowell fracture-dislocation c.
Rowe-Lowell hip dislocation c.
Ruedi-Allgower c.
Russe c.
Russell-Taylor c.
Rüter c.
Sage-Salvatore acromioclavicular
  joint injury c.
Saha shoulder muscle c.
Sakellarides calcaneal fracture c.
Salter epiphysial fracture c.
Salter-Harris-Rang epiphysial
  fracture c.
Salter-Harris tibial-fibular injury c.
Salter-Thompson c.
Sanders CT C.
Sanders intraarticular calcaneal
  fracture c.
scalar c.
Schatzker tibial plateau fracture c.

Seddon c.
Seinsheimer femoral fracture c.
Severin c.
Shapiro c.
Shelton femoral fracture c.
Sillence osteogenesis imperfecta c.
Singh osteoporosis c.
Sorbie calcaneal fracture c.
Speed radial head fracture c.
Stahl Kienbock disease c.
Steinbrocker rheumatoid arthritis c.
Steinert epiphysial fracture c.
Stelling and Tucker polydactyly c.
Steward-Milford fracture c.
Stulberg hip c.
Sunderland c. of nerve injury
Swanson c.
Tachdjian c.
talocalcaneal index c.
Thomas c.
Thompson-Epstein c.
Three Color Concept of Wound c.
tibial tuberosity fractures in
  children c.
Tile c.
Torg c.
Torode-Zieg c.
Toronto pelvic fracture c.
Tronzo intertrochanteric fracture c.
Trunkey fracture c.
Tscherne c.
Tscherne-Gotzen tibial fracture c.
Universal distal radius fracture c.
Universal Spine C.
Venn-Watson c.
Vostal radial fracture c.
Wagner c.
Waldenström c.
walking footprints c.
Warren-Marshall c.
Wassel thumb duplication c.
Watanabe discoid meniscus c.
Watson-Jones navicular fracture c.
Watson-Jones spinal fracture c.
Watson-Jones tibial fracture c.
Weber-Danis ankle injury c.
Weber fracture c.
Weiland c.
Weissman c.
Wiberg patellar c.
Wiley-Galey c.
Winquist femoral shaft fracture c.
Winquist-Hansen femoral fracture c.
Winquist-Hansen fracture
  comminution c.
Young pelvic fracture c.
Zickel c.

Zlotsky-Ballard acromioclavicular
injury c.
Zwipp c.
Clatter classification
Claude syndrome
claudication
intermittent c. (IC)
jaw c.
neurogenic c. (NC)
claudicatory
clavicectomy
clavicle
atraumatic osteolysis of distal c.
(ATODC)
c. excision
floating c.
intraarticular c.
c. orthosis
c. pin
tuberosity of c.
weightlifter's c.
clavicotomy
clavicular
c. birth fracture
c. cross splint
c. epiphysis
c. fracture aneurysm
c. notch
claviculectomy
clavipectoral
c. fascia
c. triangle
clavus foot
claw
c. finger
c. foot
c. hand
c. toe
clawed
c. hallux
c. pedicle hook
clawfoot
c. contracture
c. deformity
clawhand
c. deformity
c. sign
clawing
toe c.
clawtoe deformity
claw-type basic frame
clay shoveler's fracture

Clayton
C. forefoot arthroplasty
C. greenstick splint
C. osteotome
C. procedure
C. procedure with panmetatarsal
head resection
C. prosthesis
C. resection arthroplasty
Clayton-Fowler technique
CLBP
chronic low back pain
cleanser
ApriVera skin and hair c.
wound c.
cleansing
pressure ulcer c.
Cleanwheel
C. disposable neurological pinwheel
C. presterilized disposable device
clear
c. cell acanthoma
c. cell carcinoma
c. cell chondrosarcoma
c. cell sarcoma
c. space measurement
Clearfix screw
Clearpro suction socket
cleavage
c. fracture
horizontal c.
c. lesion
c. line
c. tear
Cleeman sign
cleft
c. closure
c. foot
c. foot deformity
gluteal c.
c. of Hahn
Hahn c.
c. hand
c. hand deformity
intergluteal c.
interinnominoabdominal c.
retropharyngeal fascial c.
c. spine
c. spinous process
venous c.
c. vertebra
vertebral column c.

NOTES

clefting of meniscus
C-Leg System artificial leg
cleidagra
cleidal
cleidarthritis
cleidocostal
cleidocranial
    c. dysostosis
    c. dysplasia
cleidoepitrochlear bundle
cleidomastoid
Cleland ligament
clenched
    c. fist syndrome
    c. fist view
Cleveland
    C. bone-cutting forceps
    C. bone rongeur
Cleveland-Bosworth-Thompson technique
Clevis clamp
CLI
    critical limb ischemia
click
    hip c.
    Mulder c.
    Ortolani c.
    c. sign
clicker
    compression c.
Clifton Assessment Procedures for the Elderly (CAPE)
climber
    Fitstep II stair c.
    Sprint C.
clinarthrosis
Clinch Lock CTS wrist brace
clinical
    C. Analysis Questionnaire (CAQ)
    c. bone sonometer
    c. diagnosis
    c. examination
    c. trial
Clinisert mattress
Clinitron air bed
clinodactyly
clinotherapy
clip
    c. applier
    Braun-Yasargil right-angle c.
    c. gauge
    Khodadad c.
    Michel c.
    palmar c.
    towel c.
    Weck c.
clip-applying forceps
clip-bending forceps
clip-cutting forceps

clip-introducing forceps
clivus
clock
    c. balance test
    shoulder c.
clog
    Hollander c.
    Markell Mobility Health C.'s
    wooden postoperative c.'s
clonus
    ankle c.
    drawn ankle c.
    patellar c.
    persistent c.
    sustained ankle c.
    three-beat c.
    transient c.
    unsustained c.
closed
    c. ankle fracture
    c. base wedge osteotomy (CBWO)
    c. chain
    c. core needle biopsy
    c. Cotrel-Dubousset hook
    c. dislocation
    c. drainage system
    c. femoral diaphysial shortening
    c. flap amputation
    c. indirect fracture
    c. intramedullary osteotomy
    c. irrigation
    c. kinetic chain (CKC)
    c. kinetic chain exercise (CKCE)
    c. kinetic chain injury
    c. kinetic chain progressive-resistance exercise
    c. Küntscher nail
    c. Küntscher nailing
    c. loop EndoButton
    c. manipulative maneuver
    c. medullary nailing
    c. pinning
    c. pseudarthrosis
    c. reduction (CR)
    c. reduction of fracture
    c. rupture
    c. soft tissue injury
    c. suction irrigation
    c. surgery
    c. transverse process TSRH hook
    c. treatment
    c. unlocked nail
    c. wedge osteotomy/bunionectomy
    c. wound
closed-chain
    c.-c. exercise
    c.-c. functional assessment
Close Encounter nut

Closer stapler
closing
    c. abductory-wedge osteotomy (CAWO)
    c. base wedge
    c. base-wedge osteotomy
    voluntary c. (VC)
    c. wedge arthrodesis
    c. wedge greenstick dorsal proximal metatarsal osteotomy
    c. wedge manipulation and reapplication of plaster
    c. wedge osteotomy bunionectomy
clostridial
    c. infection
    c. myonecrosis
    c. myositis
closure
    Barsky cleft c.
    bunionectomy capsular c.
    cleft c.
    delayed primary c. (DPC)
    epiphysial c.
    myofascial c.
    physial c.
    premature c.
    primary c.
    secondary c.
    skin c.
    SureClosure c.
    visual c.
    wound c.
clot
    exogenous fibrin c.
    fibrin c.
cloth
    c. binder
    c. tape occlusion method of Litt
clotheslining
clothespin spinal fusion graft
clotting
    c. cascade
    c. disorder
Cloutier unconstrained knee prosthesis
cloven-hoof fracture of finger
cloverleaf
    c. condylar plate fixation
    c. deformity
    c. Küntscher nail
    c. met foot pad
    c. pattern
    c. pin

    c. pin extractor
    c. plate
Cloward
    C. anterior spinal fusion
    C. back fusion
    C. blade retractor
    C. bone graft impactor
    C. cervical arthrodesis
    C. cervical disk approach
    C. cervical drill
    C. cervical drill guard
    C. cervical drill tip
    C. depth gauge
    C. disk rongeur
    C. dowel cutter
    C. dowel ejector
    C. drill guard cap
    C. drill guide
    C. drill shaft
    C. fusion diskectomy
    C. fusion diskography
    C. hammer
    C. intervertebral disk rongeur
    C. operation
    C. osteophyte elevator
    C. periosteal elevator
    C. spinal fusion chisel
    C. spinal fusion osteotome
    C. spreader
    C. surgical saddle
    C. technique
Cloward-Cone curette
Cloward-English laminectomy rongeur
Cloward-Harper laminectomy rongeur
cloxacillin
CLS
    cementless Sportono
    CLS hip system
club
    c. foot
    c. hand
clubbed
    c. finger
    c. nail
    c. toe
clubfoot
    acquired c.
    arthrogrypotic c.
    circumferential release of c.
    c. deformity
    extrinsic c.
    intrinsic c.

NOTES

clubfoot *(continued)*
 c. release
 resistant c.
 c. splint
clubhand
 c. deformity
 radial c.
 ulnar c.
clumsy
 c. gait
 c. hand dysarthria
 c. hand syndrome
cluneal nerve
clunk
 catch-up c.
 spontaneous wrist c.
 c. test
Clutton joint
Clyburn
 C. Colles fracture fixator
 C. external fixator
Clyde Mood scale
CM
 combined mechanical
  CM EVA
CMAP
 compound muscle action potential
 compound muscle-motor action potential
CM-Band
 CM-B. 505N brace
 CM-B. silicone rubber brace
CMC
 carpometacarpal
  CMC fusion
  CMC joint
  CMC splint
CME-MRI
 contrast medium-enhanced magnetic
  resonance imaging
CML prosthesis
CMO hydrocollator
CMPS
 chronic musculoskeletal pain syndrome
CMRT
 chiropractic manipulative reflex
  technique
CMT
 Charcot-Marie-Tooth
  CMT disease
  CMT Evaluation
CMW
  CMW bone cement
  CMW cement gun
cnemial
cnemis
cnemitis
CNS
 central nervous system

CO
 cervical orthosis
coach's finger
coagulated plasma
coagulating forceps
coagulation
 c. disorder
 disseminated intravascular c. (DIC)
 c. factor
 c. necrosis
coagulative necrosis
coagulator
 ASSI c.
 bipolar c.
 Concept bipolar c.
 Malis CMC-II bipolar c.
 Polar-Mate c.
coalescence
coalition
 acquired tarsal c.
 bilateral talocalcaneal c.
 c. of bone
 calcaneocuboid c.
 calcaneonavicular c.
 carpal c.
 cartilaginous c.
 complete c.
 congenital complete subtalar c.
 cubonavicular c.
 fibrous talocalcaneal c.
 incomplete c.
 interphalangeal c.
 lunatotriquetral c.
 Minaar classification of c.
 multiple tarsal c.'s
 naviculocuneiform c.
 nonosseous tarsal c.
 osseous c.
 subtalar c.
 talocalcaneal c.
 tarsal c.
 c. view
coapt
coaptation
 c. plate
 c. splint
coarse carbide cone bur
coarse-olive bur
coated implant
coating
 aluminum oxide ceramic c.
 Biolox ceramic c.
 bone fixation surface c.
 cobalt-chrome powder c.
 Porocoat porous c.
 porous c.
 sintering of cobalt-chrome
  powder c.

coat-sleeve amputation
coaxial needle electrode
Coballoy
    C. implant metal
    C. implant metal prosthesis
    C. twist drill
cobalt
    c. chrome
    c. implant
cobalt-based alloy
cobalt-chrome
    c.-c. powder coating
    c.-c. power sintering
cobalt-chromium
    c.-c. alloy
    c.-c. head
    c.-c. implant
    ion-bombarded c.-c.
    smooth c.-c.
cobalt-chromium-alloy prosthesis
cobalt-chromium-molybdenum (Co-Cr-Mo)
cobalt-chromium-tungsten-nickel (Co-Cr-W-Ni)
Coban
    C. elastic dressing
    C. elastic wrap
Cobb
    C. attachment for Albee-Compere fracture table
    C. curette
    C. gauge
    C. method
    C. method for measuring scoliosis
    C. osteotome
    C. periosteal elevator
    C. scoliosis angle
    C. scoliosis measuring technique
    C. spinal gouge
    C. syndrome
    technique of C.
    C. tibialis posterior tendon dysfunction procedure
cobbler chest
Coblation spinal surgery system
cobra
    C. Master
    c. retractor
cobra-design femoral component
cobra-head plate
coccidioidomycosis
coccyalgia

coccydynia
coccygalgia
coccygeal
    c. bone
    c. joint
    c. sinus
    c. spine
    c. vertebra
coccygectomy
coccygerector
coccygodynia
coccygotomy
coccyodynia
coccyx fracture
cockade sign
Cockayne syndrome
cocked-half flap
Cocke maxillectomy
Cockett communicating perforating veins
cocking injury
Cocklin toe operation
cock-robin head tilt
cock-up
    c.-u. arm splint
    c.-u. deformity
    c.-u. deformity of toe
    c.-u. hand splint
    c.-u. splint orthosis
    c.-u. wrist splint
    c.-u. wrist support
co-contraction
    active muscle c.-c.
    c.-c. exercise
Co-Cr-Mo
    cobalt-chromium-molybdenum
    Co-Cr-Mo alloy implant metal
    Co-Cr-Mo alloy prosthesis
    Co-Cr-Mo pin
Co-Cr-W-Ni
    cobalt-chromium-tungsten-nickel
    Co-Cr-W-Ni alloy implant metal
    Co-Cr-W-Ni alloy prosthesis
codfish
    c. deformity
    c. vertebra
Codivilla
    C. bone graft
    C. extension
    C. operation
    C. tendon lengthening
    C. tendon lengthening technique

NOTES

Codman
C. ACP system
C. angle
C. anterior cervical plating system
C. classification
C. exercise
C. saber-cut shoulder approach
C. sign
C. Ti-frame posterior fixation
system
C. triangle
C. tumor
C. wire-passing drill
Codman-Harper laminectomy rongeur
Codman-Kerrison laminectomy rongeur
Codman-Leksell laminectomy rongeur
Codman-Schlesinger cervical
laminectomy rongeur
coefficient of friction
Coe-pak
C.-p. paste
C.-p. paste adhesive
coffin bone
Coffin-Lowry syndrome
Cofield
C. shoulder prosthesis
C. technique
C. total shoulder system
CoFilm dressing
Co-Flex adherent wrap
COG
center of gravity
Cogent
C. light
C. LightWear headlight
C. XL illuminator
cogwheel
c. gait
c. rigidity
c. sign
Cohen
C. periosteal elevator
C. rongeur
cohesion
glenohumeral joint c.
cohort
C. anterior plate system
C. bone brush
C. bone screw
C. spinal impactor
c. study
C. Ti-spacer
COI
combination of isotonics
coil
circumferential dedicated knee c.
coilette
FLX flexible treatment c.

coin
fracture en c.
Coker-Arnold collar
ColBenemid
Colclough laminectomy rongeur
cold
c. abscess
c. application
c. chisel
c. compressive dressing
c. injury
c. intolerance
c. laser
c. laser treatment
c. pack
c. pad
c. pressor test
c. rolled rod
c. therapy
c. weld
cold-curing polymer
Coldflo cold therapy and sequential
compression
Coldhot pack
cold-mold prosthesis
cold-weld
c.-w. femoral ball
c.-w. femoral prosthesis
Cole
C. fracture frame
C. hyperextension brace
C. hyperextension frame
C. operation
C. osteotomy
C. osteotomy for midfoot deformity
C. procedure
C. technique
C. tendon fixation
Coleman
C. flatfoot technique
C. lateral block test
C. plasty
colinear alignment
colistin
collagen
Avitene microfibrillar c.
bovine c.
c. fiber
microcrystalline c.
c. scaffold
c. vascular disease (CVD)
collagen-based biomaterial
collagenous schwannoma
Collagraft bone graft matrix
collapse
bone graft c.
Charcot c.
exercise-associated c.

exercise-induced c.
foot c.
hindfoot-midfoot c.
hyperthermic exercise-associated c.
neuropathic c.
scapholunate advanced c. (SLAC)
scapholunate arthritis c. (SLAC)
vertebral body c.
collapsible
c. internal fixation device
c. pin
collapsing pes valgo planus
collar
Aspen cervical c.
c. bone
c. brace
Bremer Halo Crown cervical c.
calcar c.
cervical c.
Coker-Arnold c.
Cowboy C.
c. and crown scissors
c. and cuff
dynamization c.
Exo-Static cervical c.
foam c.
Forrester-Brown c.
Georgiade visor cervical c.
hard c.
Headmaster c.
Houston halo traction cervical c.
implant c.
Lerman-Minerva c.
Lewin c.
MAC cervical c.
Marlin cervical c.
Mayo rigid cervical c.
Mayo-Thomas c.
Miami Acute cervical c.
Miami J cervical c.
molded Thomas c.
myocervical c.
periosteal bone c.
Philadelphia cervical c.
Philadelphia rigid c.
pillow c.
plastic c.
Plastizote cervical c.
Pneu-trac cervical c.
2+2 Rehab C.
rigid c.
Schanz c.

serpentine foam c.
soft c.
Thomas rigid c.
Tuxedo c.
wire frame c.
collar-and-cuff sling
collar-button abscess
collar-calcar support femoral prosthesis
collared
c. button
c. femoral head
c. press-fit femoral stem implantation
collarless
c. polished taper
c., polished, tapered (CPT)
c. stem
collateral
c. artery
c. circulation
c. fibular ligament
c. ligament instability
c. ligament laxity
c. ligament rupture
c. radial ligament
c. tibial ligament
c. ulnar ligament
collectomy
shortening c.
college
C. Park TruStep foot
C. Park TruStep foot prosthesis
Colles
C. fascia
C. fracture
C. ligament
C. splint
Collet
C. screwdriver adapter
tibial C.
colli
fibromatosis c.
pterygium c.
collicular fracture
colliculus
posterior c.
Collier sign
collimation
Collimator
Multileaf C.
C. plugging pattern

NOTES

145

Collin
    C. amputating knife
    C. osteoclast
Collins
    C. dynamometer
    C. rib shears
Collis
    C. broken femoral stem technique
    C. retractor
    C. TDR instrument
Collis-Dubrul femoral stem removal
Collison
    C. body drill
    C. cannulated hand drill
    C. plate
    C. screw
    C. screwdriver
    C. tap drill
Collis-Taylor retractor
collodiaphysial
    central c. (CCD)
collodion dressing
colloid solution
colocutaneous fistula
Colonna
    C. hip fracture classification
    C. shelf operation
    C. trochanteric arthroplasty
Colonna-Ralston
    C.-R. incision
    C.-R. medial approach
color
    digital c.
    c. duplex imaging
color-coded therapy putty
colored antiseptic
Colpacs pack
Coltart
    C. calcaneotibial fusion
    C. fracture
    C. fracture technique
Colton classification
Columbus
    C. McKinnon assist for lifting or transfer
    C. McKinnon Hugger device
column
    c. balance
    central c.
    contrast c.
    radial c.
    spinal c.
    ulnar c.
    vertebral c.
comb
    toe c.
Combat Task Test

CombiDERM nonadhesive absorbent dressing
Combi Multi-Traction System
combination
    film-screen c.
    Grafton bone matrix/marrow c.
    Isola spinal implant system plate-rod c.
    c. of isotonics (COI)
    c. of isotonics technique
    jab and hook punch c.
combined
    c. ankle and knee motion gait determinant
    c. anterior and posterior approach
    c. cavus
    c. cavus deformity
    c. curve
    c. fixation device
    c. flexion-distraction injury and burst fracture
    c. flexion phenomenon
    C. Instabilities functional knee brace
    c. instability
    c. low cervical and transthoracic approach
    c. magnetic field system
    c. mechanical (CM)
    c. nerve palsy
    c. radial-ulnar-humeral fracture
    c. resection arthroplasty and arthrodesis
    c. scintigraphy
    c. stenosis
Comed postoperative shoe
Comet fragment
Comfeel Ulcus occlusive dressing
Comforfoam splint
comfort
    C. Ag prosthetic sock
    C. Cast
    C. Cast stirrup
    C. Club tub pillow
    C. Cool neoprene support
    c. level
    C. Rite footwear
    C. Take-Along wheelchair cushion
    C. wrist immobilizer
comforter
    Thermo hand c.
    Thermo knee c.
Comf-Orthotic
    C.-O. 3/4-length insole
    C.-O. sports replacement insole
    C.-O. wool felt insole
Comfortseat
    Flo-Fit C.

Comfort-U total body pillow
ComfortWalk
    C. foot system
    C. prosthetic foot
Comfy
    C. Elbow Orthosis
    C. elbow splint
    C. Knee Orthosis
    C. toilet lift seat
    C. walker
command
    C. hip instrumentation system
    C. instrument system surgical
    instrument
    C. joint replacement instrument
    system
comma sign
commemorative sign
comminuted
    c. bursting fracture
    c. intraarticular fracture
    c. teardrop fracture
comminution
commissural myelorrhaphy
commissure
    anterior commissure-posterior c.
    (AC-PC)
committee
    Fitness Safety Standards C.
    International Knee
      Documentation C. (ICD, IKDC)
    Policy and Review C. for Human
    Research
common
    c. carotid artery
    c. digital nerve
    c. dural sac
    c. extensor tendon
    c. iliac artery
    c. iliac vein
    c. peroneal nerve
    c. peroneal nerve block
    c. peroneal nerve paralysis
    c. peroneal nerve syndrome
communicans
    Gray ramus c.
communicating hydrosyringomyelia
communication
    asyndetic c.
communis
    extensor digitorum c. (EDC)
    flexor digitorum c. (FDC)

community
    C. Integration Questionnaire (CIQ)
    c. rehabilitation
Comolli sign
COMP
    cartilage oligomeric matrix protein
compact
    c. bone
    c. osteoma
compaction
    C. pliers
    vertical sacral c.
compactor
    acetabular cement c.
    cement c.
company
    United States Manufacturing C.
    (USMC)
comparative radiographic examination
comparison
compartment
    anterior c.
    Clancy lateral c.
    deep posterior c.
    dorsal c.
    fascial c.
    c. fasciotomy
    interosseous c.
    lateral c.
    medial c.
    Mueller lateral c.
    osteofascial c.
    patellofemoral c.
    plantar c.
    posterior c.
    posterolateral c.
    posteromedial c.
    superficial posterior c.
    c. syndrome
compartmental
    C. II knee prosthesis
    c. pressure
compass
    C. hinge
    C. Hinge external fixator
    C. stereotactic system
Compeed protective dressing
compensable accident
compensated
    c. metatarsus adductus
    c. talipes equinus
compensation reaction

NOTES

compensatory
- c. basilar osteotomy
- c. behavior
- c. curve
- c. deformity
- c. hypermobility
- c. lordosis
- c. movement
- c. scoliosis
- c. structural subluxation
- c. wedge

Compere
- C. fixation wire
- C. lengthening
- C. operation
- C. osteotome
- C. threaded pin

Compere-Thompson arthrodesis
Comperm tubular elastic bandage
complement
complete
- c. amelia
- c. amputation
- c. aphalangia
- c. coalition
- c. dislocation
- c. fracture
- c. paraxial hemimelia
- c. phocomelia
- c. subtalar release (CSR)
- c. syndactyly

complex
- c. acetabular reconstruction
- ankle joint c. (AJC)
- apophysial c.
- arcuate c.
- atlas-axis c.
- atlas vertebral subluxation c.
- Buford c.
- bunion c.
- bunionette-hallux valgus-splayfoot c.
- bunion-hallux valgus c.
- capsulolabral c.
- capsuloligamentous c.
- Edinger-Westphal c.
- Eisenmenger c.
- epiphysial c.
- fabellofibular c.
- femur button graft c.
- femur-fibular-ulna c.
- fibrocartilage c.
- foot-ankle c.
- forearm c.
- c. fracture
- c. fracture dislocation
- gastrocnemius-soleus c.
- Ghon-Sachs c.

hallux valgus-metatarsus primus varus c.
- hindfoot joint c.
- c. instability of carpus (CIC)
- knee c.
- lateral quadruple c.
- ligament-bone c.
- ligamentous c.
- Lisfranc joint c.
- lumbopelvic c.
- lymphedema c.
- medial quadruple c.
- c. meniscal tear
- c. motor unit action potential
- occipitoatlantoaxial joint c.
- plantar capsuloligamentous c.
- postural c.
- quadruple c.
- Ranke c.
- c. regional pain syndrome (CRPS)
- c. repetitive discharge
- semimembranosus c.
- shoulder c.
- c. skewfoot
- soleus c.
- spinal cord-meningeal c.
- spring ligament c.
- c. syndactyly
- talocalcaneonavicular c.
- three-joint c.
- tibiocalcaneal joint c.
- trialkylphosphine gold c.
- triangular fibrocartilage c. (TFC, TFCC)
- vertebral subluxation c. (VSC)
- zygomatic-malar c. (ZMC)

compliant
- C. prestress prosthetic bone implant device
- c. prestress system (CPS)

complicated
- c. complex syndactyly
- c. dislocation
- c. fracture

complication
- intraoperative c.
- neurologic c.
- neurovascular c.
- postoperative c.
- pulmonary c.
- urologic c.

complimentary alternative medicine (CAM)
component
- acetabular c.
- AcuMatch A, L, M Series acetabular c.
- AML trial hip c.

Amstutz femoral c.
anatomically graduated c. (AGC)
anatomic porous replacement
   hemispheric acetabular c.
Aufranc-Turner femoral c.
Bechtol acetabular c.
Biomet MARS acetabular c.
Biomet revision acetabular c.
Biomet shoulder c.
bipolar femoral c.
bipolar hip arthroplasty c.
Black Max mid size knee c.
Bombelli-Morscher femoral c.
cemented c.
cementless femoral c.
cerclaged c.
chamfered cylinder acetabular c.
Charnley flat-back femoral c.
Charnley narrow-stem c.
Charnley standard-stem c.
cobra-design femoral c.
custom-designed swan-neck
   femoral c.
Definition PM femoral implant c.
DePuy trispiked acetabular c.
dorsi stop c.
Duramer polyethylene c.
Durasul prosthetic c.
energy conservation walking c.
femoral c.
fluid controlled   c.
c. of gait
glenoid c.
Gustilo-Kyle femoral c.
Harris-Galante hip replacement
   acetabular c.
Harris-Galante I porous-coated
   acetabular c.
head-neck c.
Healey revision acetabular c.
Hoffmann II compact external
   fixation c.
humeral c.
hybrid fixation of hip
   replacement c.
Infinity femoral c.
internal rotary component of
   force c.
keel of glenoid c.
kinesiopathologic c.
large-head humeral c.
Lubinus acetabular c.

MARS revision acetabular c.
Meridian ST femoral implant c.
metal-backed acetabular c.
Metasul hip joint c.
modular large-head c.
monoblock femoral c.
Morse taper lock of modular hip
   implant c.
Neer II humeral c.
neuromuscular c.
NexGen c.
Ogee acetabular c.
Osteolock acetabular c.
Osteolock HA femoral c.
Osteonics Omnifit-HA c.
performance c.
polyethylene liner implant c.
porous cementless c.
porous-coated c.
posterior c.
postural c.
press-fit femoral c.
Profix porous femoral c.
progression walking c.
prosthesis c.
quadrant sparing acetabular c.
   (QSAC)
Reliance CM femoral implant c.
roof-reinforcement ring hip
   arthroplasty c.
sensory c.
Smith & Nephew reflection
   acetabular cup implant c.
Springlite II foot c.
Springlite G foot c.
S-ROM modular femoral c.
standing stability walking c.
sternal attachment c.
straight stem femoral c.
structural c.
c. subsidence
sympathetic c.
Taperloc femoral c.
Tharies femoral resurfacing c.
Tharies hip c.
thoracic extension c.
Ti-Bac acetabular c.
tibial c.
c. trial
trial femoral c.
Tri-Con c.
Tricon-M c.

NOTES

component *(continued)*
    Ultima C femoral c.
    uncemented femoral c.
    Universal radial c.
    V40 femoral head implant c.
    Vitalock cluster acetabular c.
    Vitalock solid-back acetabular c.
    wheel chair seating c.
    Zimmer NexGen LPS knee
      femoral c.

composite
    Carboplast II c.
    c. defect
    E-A-R specialty c.
    c. fracture
    c. free tissue transfer
    c. groin fascial free flap
    c. joint
    c. knee score
    c. material
    c. rib graft
    c. skin graft
    c. spring elastic splint
    void metal c. (VMC)

composition
    body c.

compound
    c. comminuted fracture (CCF)
    c. dislocation
    Hurler-Scheie c.
    c. joint
    c. mixed nerve action potential
    c. motor nerve action potential
    c. muscle action potential (CMAP)
    c. muscle-motor action potential
      (CMAP)
    OCT c.
    c. sensory nerve action potential
    c. shattered elbow

compression
    c. anesthesia
    anterior cord c.
    anterior-inferior c.
    anterior-posterior c. (APC)
    AO c.
    c. apparatus
    c. arthrodesis
    axial c.
    c. bandage
    c. boot
    carotid artery c.
    cauda equina c.
    Charnley c.
    c. clicker
    Coldflo cold therapy and
      sequential c.
    cord c.
    disk c.

    c. dressing
    duodenal c.
    dynamic c. (DC)
    elastic c.
    c. fracture
    c. glove
    c. Harrington instrumentation
    Harrington rod instrumentation c.
    c. hip screw
    c. hook
    c. inserter-extractor
    c. instrumentation posterior
      construct
    interfragmentary c.
    intermittent impulse c.
    intermittent pneumatic c.
    ischemic c.
    c. lag screw
    lateral c. (LC)
    c. load
    c. loading
    lower nerve root c.
    lower sacral nerve root c.
      (LSNRC)
    median nerve c.
    c. molding
    napkin ring c.
    nerve root c.
    neuraxial c.
    c. overload
    c. paralysis
    c. pattern
    c. plate
    c. plate fixation
    c. plating
    pneumatic pedal c.
    c. rod
    c. rod treatment
    c. screw-plate device
    c. sideplate
    c. sleeve shin splint
    spinal cord c.
    c. spring
    static c.
    c. stockings
    c. strain
    c. syndrome
    c. technique
    c. test
    c. testing
    c. therapy
    c. ultrasonography
    c. ultrasound
    c. U-rod instrumentation
    vasopneumatic intermittent c.
    venous c.
    vertebral c.
    vertical c.

C

c. wire
c. wiring
compression-molded
c.-m. ethylene vinyl acetate (CM EVA)
c.-m. prosthesis
compression-plus-torque cervical injury
compressive
c. centripetal wrapping
c. extension
c. flexion
c. flexion injury
c. hyperextension injury
c. internal fixating device
c. neuropathy
compressor
Adair screw c.
screw c.
Comprifix
C. active ankle support
C. ankle splint
compromise osteotomy
Compro Plus Knee support
Compton clavicle pin
Compudriver digital torque-meter
computed tomography (CT)
computer-assisted
c.-a. design/computer-assisted manufacturing prosthesis
c.-a. design-controlled alignment method (CAD/CAM)
c.-a. myelography (CAM)
c.-a. orthopedic surgery (CAOS)
c.-a. percutaneous internal fixation
computerized
c. axial tomography (CAT)
c. dynamic posturography (CDP)
c. isokinetic dynamometer
c. musculoskeletal analysis
Conaxial ankle prosthesis
concave
c. articular surface
c. loading socket
c. rod
concave-surface reamer
concavity
flexural c.
glenoid c.
concavoconcave
concavoconvex
concealed straight leg raising test

concentrate
platelet c.
concentric
c. bilateral isokinetic
c. contraction
c. function
c. isokinetic leg press exercise
c. lamella
c. loading
c. muscle action
c. needle electrode
c. plantar flexion peak torque newton-meter
c. reduction
c. work
concept
C. ablator
C. arthroscopy power system
C. beach chair shoulder positioning system
C. bipolar coagulator
C. cannula
Eftekhar c.
C. hand-held cautery
hinge axis c.
juvenile hinge axis c.
Klein-Vogelbach functional movement c.
one wound-one scar c.
C. Precise ACL guide system
C. rotator cuff repair system
C. II rowing ergometer
C. self-compressing cannulated screw system
C. Sterling arthroscopy blade system
three-column c.
C. two-pin passer
conceptual ability
concise
C. cementing sculp
C. compression hip screw
C. compression hip screw system
C. side plate
Conco elastic bandage
concomitant
concretion
concurrent force system
concussion
sideline assessment of c. (SAC)
concussor
condensing osteitis

NOTES

condition
    assessment for limiting c.
    degenerative spine c.
    dysvascular c.
    limiting c.
    sterile c.
    tumorous c.
conditioned stimulus (CS)
conditioner
    Shuttle cardiomuscular c.
conditioning
    aerobic c.
    Musculoskeletal Evaluation,
      Rehabilitation and C. (MERAC)
    work c.
condom catheter
conduction
    c. block
    c. time
    c. velocity
    c. velocity test
    volume c.
conductive Hydrogel wound dressing
conductor
    Adson c.
    Bailey c.
    Bozzini light c.
    light c.
conduit
    Neurotube bioabsorbable nerve c.
condylar
    c. angle
    c. articulation
    c. cartilage
    c. compression fracture
    c. cuff
    c. femoral fracture
    c. implant
    c. implant arthroplasty
    c. plate
    c. plateau angle (CPA)
    c. screw fixation
    c. split fracture
    total c. III (TC-III, TCP III)
condyle
    bifid c.
    c. block
    femoral c.
    flare of the c.
    humeral c.
    lateral femoral c.
    lateral tibial c.
    medial femoral c.
    medial humeral c.
    medial/lateral femoral c.
    occipital c.
    odontoid c.
    tibial c.
    volar c.
condylectomy
    DuVries phalangeal c.
    DuVries plantar c.
    phalangeal c.
    plantar c.
condylocephalic
    c. nail
    c. nailing
condyloid
    c. joint
    c. process
condylotomy
cone
    c. arthrodesis
    c. bone biopsy
    c. bur
    C. checkers game
    cutting c.
    hand c.
    Posey Palm C.
    prosthetic c.
    C. ring curette
    c. and socket bone
    C. splint
    stacking c.
    C. suction biopsy curette
coned-down view
Cone-Grant technique
confidence interval (CI)
configuration
    activity c.
    Cotrel-Dubousset hook claw c.
    Dudley J. Morton foot c.
    triangular base transverse bar c.
confinement
    wheelchair c.
confirmatory testing
confluent
confocal microscopy
Conform dressing
confrontational test
congenita
    amyoplasia c.
    amyotonia c.
    arthrogryposis multiplex c.
    dyskeratosis c.
    fragilitas ossium c.
    luxatio coxae c.
    myotonia c.
    osteogenesis imperfecta c. (OIC)
    pachyonychia c.
    paramyotonia c.
congenital
    c. anomaly
    c. anular band
    c. aphalangia

c. atlantoaxial instability
c. atonic pseudoparalysis
c. band syndrome
c. bar
c. clasped thumb
c. complete subtalar coalition
c. convex pes plano valgus
c. dislocation of hip (CDH)
c. dysplasia of hip (CDH)
c. dystrophy
c. fibrous band
c. flatfoot
c. fracture
c. general fibromatosis
c. hemivertebra
c. hip dislocation
c. hip dysplasia (CHD)
c. hip subluxation
c. hyperphosphatasemic skeletal
   dysplasia (CHSD)
c. hypotonia
c. kyphosis (type I, II)
c. laxity of ligament
c. limb deficiency
c. limb disorder
c. lymphedema
c. metatarsus adductus
c. myotonia
c. osteochondroma
c. patella dislocation
c. plexopathy
c. posteromedial bowing
c. predisposition
c. pseudoarthritis
c. radioulnar synostosis
c. ring
c. rocker-bottom flatfoot
c. scapular elevation
c. scoliosis
c. spondylolisthesis
c. stenosis
c. talipes equinovarus
c. tibial pseudarthrosis
c. torticollis
c. trigger digit
c. trigger finger
c. ulnar drift
c. vertical talus (CVT)
c. vertical talus foot deformity
c. wry neck
congenitally short limb

congestion
   flap c.
   intraosseous vascular c.
congestive heart failure
congruence
   c. angle
   joint c.
   patellofemoral c.
congruent
   c. articulation
   c. metatarsophalangeal joint
   c. reduction
congruous cup-shaped reamer
conical
   c. bur
   c. nut wrench
   c. obturator
   c. reamer
conical-point wire
conjoined
   c. gastrocnemius soleus fascial slip
   c. lateral band
   c. tendon
conjugated
Conley pin
connecting
   c. bolt
   c. cartilage
   c. plate
connection
   Martin-Gruber c.
   Riche-Cannieu c.
   vincula longa c.
connective
   c. tissue
   c. tissue disease
   c. tissue massage (CTM)
   c. tissue plasticity
connector
   adjustable pedicle c.
   domino spinal instrumentation c.
   intrinsic transverse c.
   longitudinal member to anchor c.
   longitudinal member to longitudinal
      member c.
   pedicle c.
   tandem c.
   transverse c.
Connolly
   C. procedure
   C. technique
Conn operation

C

NOTES

153

conoid
- c. ligament
- c. process
- c. tubercle

conoidal ankle prosthesis

conoideum

Conrad-Bugg
- C.-B. trapping
- C.-B. trapping of soft tissue

Conrad-Frost Achilles tenotomy procedure

Conradi
- C. disease
- C. syndrome

consecutive
- c. amputation
- c. dislocation

conservative
- c. management
- c. therapy

Conserve hip system

consideration
- return-to-play c.

consistency
- boggy c.
- doughy c.

console compression garment

consolidated graft

consolidation
- bony c.
- delayed c.
- fracture line c.
- premature c.

constancy
- form c.

constant
- c. direct current stimulator
- c. massive motion
- C. and Murley shoulder scoring system
- c. tension splint

constant-friction knee

constant-touch perception

ConstaVac
- C. autoreinfusion system
- C. drainage

constellation of clinical findings

constitutional stenosis

constrained
- c. ankle arthroplasty
- c. condylar knee
- c. hinged knee prosthesis
- c. nonhinged knee prosthesis
- c. shoulder arthroplasty

constriction
- c. band
- c. band syndrome

- hourglass c.
- c. ring

constrictive edema

construct
- anterior c.
- AO dynamic compression plate c.
- bladeplate c.
- compression instrumentation posterior c.
- disease c.
- double-rod c.
- Edwards modular system bridging sleeve c.
- Edwards modular system compression c.
- Edwards modular system distraction-lordosis c.
- Edwards modular system kyphoreduction c.
- Edwards modular system neutralization c.
- Edwards modular system rod sleeve c.
- Edwards modular system scoliosis c.
- Edwards modular system spondylar c.
- Edwards modular system standard sleeve c.
- hook-to-screw L4-S1 compression c.
- iliosacral and iliac fixation c.
- pedicle screw c.
- c. pedicle screw-laminar claw c.
- posterior c.
- rod-hook c.
- screw-to-screw compression c.
- segmental compression c.
- single-rod c.
- triplane c.
- TSRH double-rod c.
- upper cervical spine anterior c.
- upper cervical spine posterior c.
- Wiltse system double-rod c.
- Wiltse system H c.
- Wiltse system single-rod c.

Constructa-Foam

constructional ability

contact
- C. ArthroProbe
- c. force
- c. healing
- c. laser delivery system
- c. manipulation
- manual c.
- c. point
- c. shield
- C. SPH cups system
- standing knee bend PSIS-sacrum c.

contained
    c. disk herniation
    c. herniated disk
container
    Quickbox c.
containment bag
content
    bone mineral c. (BMC)
context
    performance c.
contiguity
    amputation in c.
contiguous
    c. articular surface
    c. vertebral structure
continuity
    amputation in c.
    c. of bone
    neuroma in c.
    synthesis of c.
continuous
    c. anatomical passive exerciser (CAPE)
    c. cryotherapy
    c. intravenous regional anesthesia (CIVRA)
    c. passive motion (CPM)
    c. passive motion machine
    c. wave arthroscopy pump
continuum
    C. bipolar acetabular head
    C. elliptical acetabular cup
    c. hip stem
    C. knee system (CKS)
    C. knee system implant
    C. polyethylene acetabular cup
    C. P/S total knee
    C. total knee base plate
    C. unconstrained prosthesis
contour
    C. DF-80 total hip operation
    double hump c.
    C. internal prosthesis
    patellar c.
    polyethylene proximal brim in quadrilateral c.
    spinal c.
    Wiberg type II patellar c.
contoured
    c. adduction trochanteric-controlled alignment method (CAT-CAM)
    c. anterior spinal plate (CASP)

    c. anterior spinal plate drill guide
    c. anterior spinal plate technique
    c. felt padding
    c. femoral stem (CFS, CSF)
    c. T-plate plate
    c. washer
contract
    Contract Relax Agonist c. (CRAC)
contractile force curve
contractility
    muscle c.
contraction
    active c.
    concentric c.
    detrusor c.
    direct c.
    eccentric c.
    extrafusal fiber c.
    c. fasciculation
    isometric c.
    isotonic c.
    lengthening c.
    maintained c.
    maximal voluntary c. (MVC)
    muscular c.
    reflex muscular c.
    repeated quick stretch superimposed upon an existing c. (RQS-SEC)
    shortening c.
    tetanic c.
    c. tremor
    c. type
    volitional c.
contractor
    Bailey-Gibbon rib c.
    Bailey rib c.
    Lemmon rib c.
    rib c.
    Sellors rib c.
contract-relax technique
contracture
    abduction c.
    acquired thumb flexion c.
    acute ischemic c.
    adduction c.
    axillary c.
    burn c.
    clawfoot c.
    c. deformity
    digital c.
    Dupuytren c.
    equinus c.

C

NOTES

contracture *(continued)*
    established c.
    c. exercise
    extension c.
    external rotation c.
    fixed flexion c. (FFC)
    flexion, abduction, external
      rotation c.
    flexor digitorum longus tendon c.
    flexor hallucis tendon c.
    forearm c.
    gastrocnemius soleus c.
    hip flexor c.
    intrinsic c.
    ischemic c.
    knee c.
    lumbrical intrinsic c.
    metacarpophysial joint extension c.
    muscle c.
    opposition c.
    paralytic c.
    pelvic flexion c. (PFC)
    postpoliomyelitic c.
    pronation c.
    quadriceps c.
    rectus femoris c.
    retropatellar fat pad c.
    rotational c.
    shoulder c.
    Skoog procedure for release of
      Dupuytren c.
    soft tissue c.
    spastic intrinsic c.
    supination c.
    valgus c.
    varus c.
    Volkmann c.
    web c.
    wrist c.
contraflexion brace
contraindication
    stretching c.
contralateral
    c. foot
    c. hypoplastic/agenetic pedicle
    c. pain
    c. sign
    c. spondylolysis
    c. straight leg raising
    c. straight leg raising test
contrast
    c. agent
    air c.
    c. arthrography
    c. bath (CB)
    c. column
    c. medium-enhanced magnetic
      resonance imaging (CME-MRI)

contrecoup
    c. contusion
    fracture by c.
    c. fracture
    c. injury
control
    biomechanical c.
    car hand c.
    3D positional c.
    Dupaco knee c.
    evaluation, prediction, intervention,
      and c. (EPIC)
    exsanguination tourniquet c.
    habitual c.
    hip joint aspiration under
      fluoroscopic c.
    maximum c. (MC)
    monitored anesthesia c. (MAC)
    motion c.
    postural c.
    pronation c.
    pronation/spring c. (PSC)
    rotary c.
    swing-phase c.
    Total Environment C. (TEC)
    tourniquet c.
    trunk c.
    verticality c.
    voluntary c. (VC)
controlled
    c. ankle motion (CAM)
    c. ankle walker
    c. comminuted fracture
    c. force application
    c. position brace (CPB)
    c. rotational osteotomy
controlled-motion brace
controller
    shoulder c.
    C. shoulder orthosis
contusion
    chest c.
    contrecoup c.
    coup c.
    cuff c.
    hip pointer c.
    muscle c.
    osteochondral c.
    pelvic region c.
    quadriceps c.
    rib c.
    rotator cuff c.
conus medullaris syndrome
conventional
    c. cutting needle
    c. osteosarcoma
    c. silicone elastomer (CSE)
    c. single-axis knee prosthesis

c. technique
c. tomography
convergence
angle of c.
c. facilitation
c. projection
Converse
C. chisel
C. periosteal elevator
C. splint
conversion
Tilt-In-Space wheelchair c.
Convery polyarticular disability index
convex
c. condylar-implant arthroplasty
c. fusion
c. pes valgus
c. rasp
c. rod
convexity
distal ulnar c.
left lumbar c.
c. of the spine
ulnar c.
convoluted bone
convolution
Broca c.
Conyers technique
Cook-Gordon mechanism
cookie
arch c.
c. cutter
Gelfoam c.
metatarsal c.
navicular shoe c.
scaphoid shoe c.
shoe c.
Cooksey-Cawthorne exercise
Cook walking brace
cool
c. CPB brace
c. IROM splint
c. pack
c. pack cryotherapy
c. TROM splint
Cool-Aid continuous controlled cold therapy
Cooley
C. graft clamp
C. iliac clamp
C. multipurpose angled clamp
C. multipurpose curved clamp

C. rib retractor
C. rib shears
Cooley-Baumgarten wire twister
Cool-Flex A/K suspension belt
cooling machine
CoolSorb absorbent cold transfer dressing
Coombs bone biopsy system
Coonrad
C. hinged prosthesis
C. semiconstrained elbow prosthesis
C. total elbow arthroplasty
Coonrad-Morrey
C.-M. elbow prosthesis
C.-M. total elbow arthroplasty
Coonse-Adams
C.-A. knee approach
C.-A. quadricepsplasty
C.-A. technique
Cooper
C. ankle brace
C. reduction
Coopercare Lastrap support wrap
Coopernail sign
Coopervision irrigation/aspiration handpiece
coordinate
C. complete revision knee system
c. system X,Y,Z
coordinated mobility
coordination
muscular c.
Copeland-Howard
C.-H. scapulothoracic fusion
C.-H. shoulder operation
C.-H. shoulder procedure
Copeland humeral resurfacing head
Copeland-Kavat
C.-K. classification of metatarsophalangeal dislocation
C.-K. metatarsophalangeal dislocation classification
Copenhagen Stroke study
Coping Strategies Questionnaire (CSQ)
coplaning
arthroscopic c.
copolymer
c. ankle-foot orthosis
LactoSorb resorbable c.
c. orthotic material
c. starch copolymer bead

NOTES

copper
> c. deficiency syndrome
> c. mallet

copropraxia

coracoacromial
> c. arch
> c. ligament
> c. ligament transfer
> c. process

coracobrachialis
> biceps, brachialis, c. (BBC)

coracobrachial muscle

coracoclavicular (CC)
> c. arthrodesis
> c. articulation
> c. distance
> c. fixation apparatus
> c. joint
> c. ligament
> c. screw fixation
> c. suture fixation
> c. technique

coracohumeral (CH)
> c. ligament

coracoid
> c. fracture
> c. impingement syndrome
> c. notch
> c. process
> c. tip avulsion
> c. tuberosity

coracoiditis

coracoradialis

coracoulnaris

Coraderm dressing

Corail
> C. HA-coated stem
> C. HA-coated stem hip implant
> C. hip system
> C. press-fit prosthesis

coralline hydroxyapatite

Corbett bone rongeur

cord
> anterior horn of spinal c.
> central c.
> cervical spinal c.
> c. compression
> digital c.
> heel c.
> lateral c.
> MGHL c.
> natatory c.
> c. portion
> pretendinous c.
> retrovascular c.
> space available for the c. (SAC)
> spinal c.
> Sport C.

> tenodesis of the heel c.
> tethered spinal c.
> vocal c.

Cordase injectable collagenase

cordate pelvis

cordiform pelvis

Cordis implantable drug reservoir device

cordlike structure

Cordon-Colles fracture splint

cordotomy

cord-traction syndrome

core
> c. biopsy obturator
> bone c.
> c. decompression
> c. decompression of femoral head
> c. drilling procedure
> C. Hibak Rest
> C. Lobak Rest
> C. Max-Relax Cushion
> c. needle biopsy
> C. Reflex wrist support
> C. Sitback Rest
> C. Slimrest
> c. suture
> C. Universal elastic knee support
> C. Universal elbow support
> C. Universal rib support

Corfit System 7000 Series Lumbosacral Support

coring
> c. apparatus
> c. device

Corin hip arthroplasty system

cork
> c. borer
> sheet c.

corkscrew
> c. femoral head extractor
> C. Parachute
> C. rotator cuff repair system
> C. suture anchor

corn
> apical c.
> end c.
> hard c.
> interdigital c.
> Lister c.
> neurovascular c.
> plantar c.
> soft c.
> web c.

Cornelia de Lange syndrome

corner
> c. fracture
> c. fragment

c. of knee
posteromedial c.
corneum
stratum c.
cornuate navicular
cornuradicular zone
Cornwall hip fracture study
coronal
c. computed tomographic
arthrography (CCTA)
c. plane
c. plane correction
c. plane deformity
c. plane deformity sagittal
translation
c. split fracture
c. tilting
coronary
c. artery disease (CAD)
c. bone
c. ligament
coronoid
c. line
c. process
c. process fracture
corpectomy
anterior c.
cervical c.
c. model
vertebral body c.
corporectomy amputation
corporotransverse
c. inferior ligament
c. superior ligament
correction
anterior c.
Beckenbaugh c.
Bonferroni c.
chevron hallux valgus c.
coronal plane c.
cubitus varus c.
frontal plane c.
hallux varus c.
Johnson-Spiegl hallux varus c.
Kilsyn-Evans principle of frontal
plane c.
King type IV curve posterior c.
kyphosis c.
loss of c.
mechanism of c.
neuromechanical c.
phalangeal malunion c.

rotational c.
Ruiz-Mora c.
scoliosis c.
somatovisceral c.
Steel c.
V-Y plasty c.
corrective
c. cast
c. lengthening osteotomy
c. orthosis
c. shoe
c. soft dressing
c. spinal care
c. therapy
corrosion
crevice c.
fretting c.
metal implant c.
corrugated reamer
corset
Boston soft c.
Camp c.
Campbell c.
dorsal lumbar c.
elastic ankle c.
c. front
Hoke lumbar c.
Kampe c.
leather ankle c.
lumbodorsal support c.
lumbosacral c.
soft c.
surgical c.
c. suspension
thigh c.
thoracolumbar c.
Warm 'n' Form lumbosacral c.
cortex, pl. **cortices**
adrenal c.
articular c.
femoral c.
lateral c.
c. screw
vertebral body anterior c.
cortical
c. atrophy
c. bone graft
c. bone modeling
c. bone primary canal
c. bone remodeling
c. bone screw
c. cancellous screw

NOTES

cortical (continued)
    c. débridement
    c. defect
    c. desmoid
    c. desmoid tumor
    c. destruction
    c. fibrous dysplasia
    c. fracture
    c. fragment
    c. index
    c. lucency
    c. perforation
    c. pin
    c. plasticity
    c. plate
    c. step drill
    c. strut graft
    c. thickening
    c. thickness
    c. thumb
    c. window
    c. windowing
corticalization
cortices (pl. of cortex)
corticocancellous
    c. bone
    c. bone graft
    c. bone strip
    c. chip graft
corticosteroid
    depot c.
    postoperative c.
    c. therapy (CS)
corticosteroid-induced avascular necrosis
corticotomy
    DeBastiani c.
    Ilizarov c.
    percutaneous c.
    c. of proximal tibia
COR/T implant
cortisone
corundum ceramic implant material
Coryllos-Doyen periosteal elevator
Coryllos rasp
cosmesis
    foot c.
    poor c.
    scarring c.
cosmetically acceptable foot
Cosmolon closure for splint
costal
    c. angle
    c. bone
    c. cartilage
    c. notch
    c. periosteotome
costalgia
costectomy

Costen syndrome
costocentral articulation
costochondral
    c. joint
    c. junction of ribs
costochondritis
costoclavicular
    c. ligament
    c. maneuver
    c. space
    c. syndrome
    c. syndrome test
costocoracoid
costogenic
costoinferior
costolumbar angle
costophrenic angle
costopleural
costoscapular
costoscapularis
costosternal
    c. angle
    c. articulation
costosternoplasty
costotransversarium
costotransverse
    c. joint
    c. ligament
costotransversectomy
    c. approach
    Seddon dorsal spine c.
    c. technique
costovertebral
    c. angle (CVA)
    c. angle tenderness (CVAT)
    c. articulation
    c. joint
costoxiphoid
cot
    finger c.
Cotrel
    C. pedicle screw
    C. pedicle screw fixation strength
    C. pedicle screw rigidity
    C. scoliosis
    C. scoliosis cast
    C. traction
Cotrel-Dubousset (C-D)
    C.-D. derotation operation
    C.-D. dynamic transverse traction device
    C.-D. hook claw configuration
    C.-D. hook-rod
    C.-D. pedicle screw instrumentation
    C.-D. rod
    C.-D. rod flexibility
    C.-D. spinal instrument
Cotting ingrown nail procedure

Cottle
- C. chisel
- C. mallet
- C. osteotome
- C. rasp
- C. saw

Cottle-MacKenty
- C.-M. elevator
- C.-M. rasp

cotton
- C. ankle fracture
- C. ankle instability test
- c. bolster
- c. cast
- c. cast padding
- c. dressing
- c. elastic bandage
- C. fibular bone hook test
- C. procedure
- C. reduction of elbow dislocation
- c. roll
- c. sheet wadding
- c. suture

Cotton-Berg syndrome
cottonloader position
cottonoid patty
cotyloid
- c. cavity
- c. notch

cotyloplasty technique
cotylosacral
Couch-Derosa-Throop transfer
cough
- c. fracture
- c. test

Coulter counter
council
- Medical Research C. (MRC)

counseling
- rehabilitation c. (RC)

count
- instrument, sponge, and needle c.
- lymphocyte c.
- platelet c.
- potassium-40 c.
- white blood cell c.

counter
- Coulter c.
- extended medial shoe c.
- heel c.
- c. nutation
- c. rotating saw

C. Rotation System (CRS)
C. Rotation System brace
c. sink
counterbalance
counterclockwise
counterextension
counterforce strap
counterrotational splint
countersinking osteotomy
countersink screw head
countersunk
countertraction splint
counterweight
Count'R-Force arch brace
coup contusion
coupled
- c. discharge
- c. motion

coupler
- Ferrier c.

coupling
- capacitive c.

Couvelaire incision
Covaderm Plus adhesive barrier dressing
Coventry
- C. distal femoral osteotomy
- C. proximal tibial osteotomy
- C. screw
- C. staple
- C. vagal osteotomy

cover
- Accu-Flo polyethylene bur hole c.
- Accu-Flo silicone rubber bur hole c.
- AquaShield orthopaedic cast c.
- AquaShield reusable cast c.
- cast c.
- Dryspell cast c.
- ShowerSafe waterproof cast and bandage c.
- soft cosmetic c.
- Springlite polyolefin BK c.
- Springlite polyurethane AK, BK conical c.

coverage
- skin c.

covering
- Cast Cozy toe c.
- epineural c.
- fascial sheath c.

NOTES

161

coverlet
    C. adhesive
    C. adhesive surgical dressing
    C. Strips wound dressing
Cover-Roll
    C.-R. adhesive gauze dressing
    C.-R. gauze
    C.-R. gauze adhesive
Covertell composite secondary dressing
Cowboy Collar
Cowden syndrome
Cowen-Loftus toe-phalanx
  transplantation
cowhorn brace
Co-Wrap dressing
coxa, pl. coxae
    c. adducta
    c. plana
    c. senilis
    c. valga
    c. vara
    c. vara deformity pelvic
      radiotherapy
coxal bone
coxalgia
coxalgic pelvis
coxankylometer
coxarthria
coxarthritis
coxarthrocace
coxarthropathy
coxarthrosis
    end-stage c.
Cox flexion-distraction technique
coxitic scoliosis
coxitis
coxodynia
coxofemoral
    c. articulation
    c. joint
coxotomy
coxotuberculosis
Cozen
    C. test
    C. transverse approach
Cozen-Brockway
    C.-B. technique
    C.-B. Z-plasty
cozy
    Cast C.
CP
    cerebral palsy
    CP Sports Balance Classification
CP2 inflatable cold pack
CPA
    calcaneal pitch angle
    condylar plateau angle

CPB
    controlled position brace
CPM
    continuous passive motion
      AIM CPM
      CPM apparatus
      CPM device
      CPM exerciser machine
CPPD
    calcium pyrophosphate dihydrate
    deposition
CPS
    compliant prestress system
cps, c/sec
    cycle per second
CPT
    collarless, polished, tapered
      CPT hip system
      CPT prosthesis
CR
    closed reduction
crab gait
crabmeat-like appearance
CRAC
    Contract Relax Agonist Contract
Cracchiolo
    C. forefoot arthroplasty
    C. procedure
Cracchiolo-Sculco
    C.-S. implant arthroplasty
    C.-S. implant operation
crack
    c. fracture
    hairline c.
cracking
    environmental stress c.
    c. of joint
    stress-corrosion c.
cradle
    c. arm sling
    bed c.
    Posey bed c.
Crafoord thoracic scissors
Craig
    C. abduction splint
    C. Handicap Assessment and
      Reporting Technique (CHART)
    C. pin
    C. pin remover
    C. vertebral biopsy set
Craig-Scott orthosis
Cramer wire splint
cramp
    c. discharge
    heat c.
    muscle c.
    muscular c.

cramping
    heat c.
Cram test
Crane
    C. mallet
    C. osteotome
    C. shoulder exercise
cranial
    c. bone
    c. electrical stimulation (CES)
    c. helmet
    c. Jacobs hook
    c. nerve abnormality
    c. tongs
cranial-sacral respiratory mechanism (CRSM)
cranioacromial
craniocaudal glide
craniocervical plate
craniofacial
    c. angle
    c. dysjunction fracture
craniomandibular dysfunction
craniosacral
    c. table
    c. therapy (CST)
    c. therapy technique
craniospinal trauma
craniotabes
craniovertebral
crank
    c. frame retractor
    c. table
    c. test
crankshaft phenomenon
crash induction of anesthesia
craterization
cravat bandage
Crawford
    C. head frame
    C. incision
    C. low lithotomy crutch
    C. L-shaped osteotomy
    C. small parts dexterity test
Crawford-Adams
    C.-A. acetabular cup
    C.-A. acetabular cup arthroplasty
    C.-A. pin
Crawford-Marxen-Osterfeld technique
crawl
    barrel c.

C-reactive protein
creaking
    alar c.
    back c.
    distal medial c.
    flexion c.
    infragluteal c.
    metatarsophalangeal c.
    palmar c.
    PIP flexion c.
    popliteal flexion c.
    skin c.
    thenar c.
    ulnar c.
    wrist c.
cream (*See also* creme)
    AliDeep massage c.
    Diapedic foot c.
    Free-Up massage c.
    Thera-Gesic c.
crease
    alar c.
    back c.
    distal palmar c. (DPC)
    flexor skin c.
    infragluteal c.
    metatarsophalangeal c.
    palmar c.
    popliteal c.
    skin c.
    thenar palmar c. (TPC)
creation
    kyphosis c.
    lordosis c.
Credé maneuver
Credo operation
Creed dissector
creep
    viscoelastic c.
    web space c.
creeping substitution
Crego
    C. femoral osteotomy
    C. hip reduction
    C. periosteal elevator
    C. retractor
    C. tendon transfer technique
Crego-McCarroll
    C.-M. pin
    C.-M. traction
cremasteric reflex

C

NOTES

creme (*See also* cream)
crepitans
    peritendinitis c.
    tenalgia c.
    tenosynovitis c.
crepitant
crepitation
    patellofemoral c.
crepitus
    articular c.
    bony c.
crescent
    C. Complete Sleeper pillow
    C. memory pillow
    c. sign
crescentic
    c. base wedge osteotomy
    c. base wedge
      osteotomy/bunionectomy
    c. basilar first metatarsal osteotomy
    c. calcaneal osteotomy
    c. rupture
    c. saw
    c. shelf osteotomy (CSO)
Crescent-Pillo pillow
crescent-shaped
    c.-s. fibrocartilaginous disk
    c.-s. osteotomy
CREST
    calcinosis, Raynaud, esophageal motility
    disorders, sclerodactyly, telangiectasia
    CREST syndrome
crest
    c. buttress pad
    iliac c.
    neural c.
    palpation of iliac c.
    c. sign
    c. sign side
    toe c.
cretinism
crevice corrosion
crick in the neck
cricoid
    c. cartilage
    c. ring
cricopharyngeal sphincter muscle
cricothyroid membrane
Crile
    C. forceps
    C. gasserian ganglion knife and
      dissector
    C. head traction
    C. hemostat
    C. knife
Crile-Wood needle holder
crimped Dacron prosthesis

crimper
    Caparosa wire c.
    pin c.
    Simmons c.
    washer c.
    wire c.
crisis, pl. crises
    bone c.
crispation
criteria, sing. criterion
    Beighton hypermobility syndrome c.
    Catagni c.
    Garcia wrist laxity c.
    Harris c.
    Hodgkinson acetabular component
      loosening c.
    Insall c.
    Kellgren degenerative disk
      disease c.
    Mackinnon-Dellon c.
    Mulholland and Gunn c.
    New York diagnostic c.
    Rome c.
    Salter c.
    Severin hip c.
    White and Panjabi cervical
      spine c.
Criticaid lotion
critical
    c. limb ischemia (CLI)
    c. load
CRM
    CRM cup
    CRM rehab brace
    CRM stem
    CRM system
crochet
    main en c.
CROM
    cervical range-of-motion instrument
Crosby reduction
cross
    c. bar
    c. friction
    c. leg pain
cross-arm flap
cross-bracing
    spinal rod c.-b.
    Wiltse system c.-b.
crosscut
    c. bur
    c. saw
crossed
    c. adductor reflex
    c. extensor reflex
    c. flexor reflex
    c. intrinsic transfer

c. Kirschner wire
c. straight leg raising (CSLR)

cross-extremity flap
cross-finger flap
cross-friction massage
crosshead displacement
crossing
nerve c.

cross-leg
c.-l. flap
c.-l. Patrick maneuver

cross-legged gait
crosslink
Edwards modular system rod c.
free pyridinium c.
Galveston fixation with TSRH c.
c. plate
c. plate size
pyridinium collagen c. (PYD)
pyridinoline collagen c. (PYD)
TSRH c.

crossover
femoral-femoral c.
c. second toe
c. syndrome
c. test

crossover-toe deformity
cross-screw fixation
cross-sectional anatomy
cross-slot screwdriver
cross-table
c.-t. lateral radiograph
c.-t. lateral view (CTLV)

crossunion
crotch strap
crouch gait
Crouzon syndrome
CROW
Charcot restraint orthotic walker

Crowe
C. congenital hip dysplasia
classification
C. congenital hip dysplasia
classification system
C. hip scale
C. pilot point
C. pilot point on Steinmann pin
C. subluxation
C. tip pin
C. (type I–IV) congenital hip
dysplasia

crown
Adaptic c.
c. and collar scissors
c. drill
c. drill screw
Unitek steel c.

CRPS
complex regional pain syndrome

CRS
Counter Rotation System
CRS brace
CRS Tibial Torsion System

CRSM
cranial-sacral respiratory mechanism

crucial angle of Gissane
cruciate
anterior c.
c. condylar knee system
c. condylar unconstrained prosthesis
c. fashion
c. head bone screw
c. ligament
c. ligament laxity
c. ligament reconstruction
c. ligament rupture
c. paralysis
posterior c.
c. punch

cruciate-retaining prosthesis
cruciate-sacrificing prosthesis
cruciform
c. anterior spinal hyperextension
(CASH)
c. anterior spinal hyperextension
orthosis
c. head bone screw
c. screwdriver
c. tibial base plate

cruiser
c. buggy
C. hip abduction
C. hip abduction brace

crural
Bigelow c.
c. fascia

cruris
angina c.
tinea c.

crush
c. fracture
c. injury
c. syndrome

NOTES

C

crushed eggshell fracture
crushing osteochondritis
crutch
    c. ambulation
    axillary c.
    c. and belt femoral closed nail
    c. and belt femoral closed nailing
    Canadian c.
    Crawford low lithotomy c.
    EuroCuff forearm c.
    Hardy aluminum c.
    iWALKfree hands-free c.
    Lofstrand c.
    c. palsy
    c. paralysis
    platform c.
    c. walking
    weightbearing c.
Crutchfield
    C. bone drill
    C. drill point
    C. hand drill
    C. operation
    C. pin
    C. skeletal tong traction
Crutchfield-Raney
    C.-R. drill
    C.-R. tongs
Cruveilhier
    C. atrophy
    C. disease
    C. joint
    C. ligament
    C. paralysis
cryoanalgesia
Cryo/Cuff
    Aircast C.
    C. ankle dressing
    C. boot
    C. compression support
    C. Knee Compression Dressing
      System
Cryocup ice massager
cryogenic denervation
cryohypophysectomy
cryoprecipitate
cryopreserved cartilage
cryosurgery
cryotherapy
    continuous c.
    cool pack c.
    liquid nitrogen c.
    c. rehabilitation
    verruca c.
cryptococcal infection
cryptococcosis
cryptopodia
cryptotic medial border

cry reflex
crystal
    C. adjusting table
    monosodium urate c.
    C. polymer gel
    uric acid c.
crystal-induced
    c.-i. arthritis
    c.-i. arthropathy
    c.-i. arthrosis
    c.-i. synovitis
crystalloid solution
crystal-related
    c.-r. arthropathy
    c.-r. joint disease
CS
    conditioned stimulus
    corticosteroid therapy
CSE
    conventional silicone elastomer
c/sec (var. of cps)
    cycle per second
CSF
    cerebrospinal fluid
    contoured femoral stem
      CSF prosthesis
C-shaped
    C-s. foot
    C-s. plate
CSI
    Caregiver Strain Index
CSLR
    crossed straight leg raising
CSMT
    capillary refill, sensation, motor function,
      temperature
CSO
    crescentic shelf osteotomy
CSQ
    Coping Strategies Questionnaire
CSR
    complete subtalar release
      McKay-Simons CSR
CSRA
    cementless surface replacement
      arthroplasty
CST
    craniosacral therapy
CT
    carpal tunnel
    computed tomography
      CT scan
CT-based CAD/CAM revision femoral
  implant
CTD
    carpal tunnel decompression
    cumulative trauma disorder

CTE
    chronic traumatic encephalopathy
C-Tek anterior cervical plate system
CTi2 knee brace
CTi brace
CTLSO
    cervicothoracolumbosacral orthosis
        CTLSO orthosis
CTLV
    cross-table lateral view
CTM
    cervical tension myositis
    connective tissue massage
CTO
    cervicothoracic orthosis
        Aspen CTO
CTR
    carpal tunnel release
CTS
    carpal tunnel syndrome
    Champion Trauma Score
        CTS gauge
        CTS Gripfit splint
Cubbins
    C. arthroplasty
    C. bone screwdriver
    C. incision
    C. open reduction
    C. operation
    C. screw
    C. shoulder approach
    C. shoulder dislocation technique
cube
    Temper Foam c.
CUBEx multifunctional step
cubital
    c. bursitis
    c. joint
    c. nerve
    c. process
    c. tunnel
    c. tunnel splint
    c. tunnel syndrome
cubiti (*pl. of* cubitus)
cubitocarpal
cubitoradial
cubitus, pl. **cubiti**
    patella cubiti
    c. pseudovarus
    c. recurvatum
    c. valgus

    c. varus
    c. varus correction
cuboid
    c. abduction angle
    c. bone
    c. decancellation
    c. declination angle
    c. fracture
    c. fusion
    c. notch
    c. sulcus
    c. syndrome
    c. wedge osteotomy
cuboidal tuberosity
cuboid-calcaneal osteotomy
cuboideonavicular ligament
cubonavicular
    c. coalition
    c. joint
cucullaris muscle
cucumber heel
Cuda shaver
cuff
    arm c.
    collar and c.
    condylar c.
    c. contusion
    c. of fascia
    hand c.
    joint distraction c.
    leather c.
    C. Link orthopedic device
    musculotendinous c.
    pneumatic tourniquet c.
    push c.
    Push-Ease Quad C.
    c. resection
    rotator c. (RC)
    shoulder c.
    Steri-Cuff disposable tourniquet c.
    supracondylar c.
    suprapatellar c. (SPC)
    c. suspension
    thigh c.
    Western Ontario Rotator C. (WORC)
cuff-tear
    c.-t. arthropathy
    c.-t. arthroplasty
cuing strategy
cul-de-sac of Bruger
Culler hook

NOTES

167

Culley ulnar splint
culture
    bacterial c.
    blood c.
    urine c.
    wound c.
Cummins procedure
cumulative trauma disorder (CTD)
cuneiform
    atavistic c.
    c. bone
    c. fracture
    c. injury
    c. joint
    c. joint arthrodesis
    c. mortise
    c. osteotomy
cuneiform-first metatarsal exostosis
cuneocuboid
cuneometatarsal joint
cuneonavicular
    c. joint
    c. ligament
cuneoscaphoid
Cuniard and Campell technique
cuniculatum
    epithelioma c.
Cunningham brace
cup
    AccuPressure heel c.
    acetabular c.
    Anti-Shox heel c.
    c. arthroplasty
    Arthropor acetabular c.
    Aufranc modification of Smith-
      Petersen c.
    Aufranc-Turner acetabular c.
    Bauerfeind SofSpot Heel C.
    Bicon-Plus C.
    Biomet acetabular c.
    bipolar acetabular c.
    bipolar prosthetic c.
    Buchholz acetabular c.
    ceramic acetabular c.
    Charnley acetabular c.
    Charnley offset-bore c.
    c. and cone method
    Continuum elliptical acetabular c.
    Continuum polyethylene
      acetabular c.
    Crawford-Adams acetabular c.
    CRM c.
    custom-made acetabular c.
    DePuy bipolar c.
    DePuy Tri-Lock interlocking
      acetabular c.
    Essential Energy C.
    Flo-Trol drinking c.

Ganz c.
Gemini c.
Hallister heel c.
Harris-Galante acetabular c.
Hedrocel c.
heel c.
c. holder
c. holder handle
Integrity acetabular c.
Interseal acetabular c.
jumbo acetabular c.
Kennedy spillproof c.
Laing concentric hip c.
Lineage acetabular c.
Lord c.
low-profile c.
Luck hip c.
McKee-Farrar acetabular c.
metal-backed acetabular c.
migration of acetabular c.
monolithic A1203 c.
Mueller c.
multipolar bipolar c.
NEB acetabular c.
New England Baptist acetabular c.
oblong polyethylene acetabular c.
Opti-Fix II acetabular c.
Osteonics acetabular c.
patella c.
plastic heel c.
Polysorb heel c.
porous-coated acetabular c.
c. positioner
PQ Premium heel c.
press-fit c.
prosthesis c.
c. reamer
Reflection I, V, and FSO
  acetabular c.
Restoration GAP acetabular c.
retroversion of acetabular c.
Riecken PQ premium heel c.
screw-in ceramic acetabular c.
Silipos Silicone Wonder C.
Smith-Petersen c.
Sorbothane II heel c.
S-ROM acetabular c.
S-ROM Super C.
trial acetabular c.
TuliGel heel c.
Tuli Pro Heel C.
Tuli rubber heel c.
University of California
  Biomechanics Laboratory heel c.
Wonder-Cup heel c.
Wonder-Spur heel c.
Wonderzorb heel c.

ZTT I, II c.
ZTT acetabular c.
cup-and-ball osteotomy
cup-cement interface
cupid's
c. bow
c. bow contour sign
cup-on-cup arthroplasty of the hip
cupped
c. curette
c. grasping forceps
curb tenotomy
Curdy blade
curettage
excision and c.
curette, curet
Acufex c.
angled Scoville c.
bone c.
bowl c.
box c.
Bruns bone c.
buck bone c.
cement c.
Charnley bone c.
Cloward-Cone c.
Cobb c.
Cone ring c.
Cone suction biopsy c.
cupped c.
curved c.
Daubenspeck bone c.
Dawson-Yuhl-Cone c.
Epstein c.
Faulkner c.
fine c.
fine-angled c.
fine bone c.
Gillquist suction c.
Halle bone c.
Hardy hypophysial c.
Hatfield bone c.
hex handle c.
Hibbs c.
hypophysial c.
Innomed bone c.
Jansen bone c.
Kerpel bone c.
Kerrison c.
Kevorkian c.
Lempert bone c.
long c.

Magnum c.
Malis c.
Martini bone c.
mastoid c.
McCain TMJ c.
McElroy c.
meniscal c.
Meyhoeffer bone c.
Microsect c.
Moe bone c.
orthopaedic c.
oval curved-cup c.
Piffard c.
ring c.
Schede bone c.
Scoville c.
short c.
Spratt bone c.
Spratt mastoid c.
Statak c.
stout-neck c.
straight c.
T-handle c.
Volkmann bone c.
Walker ruptured disk c.
Whitney single-use plastic c.
Williger bone c.
curl
dynamic trunk c.
neutral wrist c.
reverse wrist c.
seated hamstring c.
trunk c.
wrist c.
curl-up
broomstick c.-u.
curly
c. toe
c. toe deformity
current
action c.
amplitude-summation interferential c.
cutting c.
direct c.
interferential c.
low-frequency alternating c. (LFAC)
Currey model
Curry
C. hip nail
C. walking splint
Curschmann-Steinert disease

NOTES

Curtin
    C. incision
    C. plantar fibromatosis excision
Curtis
    C. PIP joint capsulotomy
    C. technique
Curtis-Fisher knee technique
curvature
    angular c.
    anterior c.
    backward c.
    dorsal kyphotic c.
    humpbacked spinal c.
    lateral c.
    posterior c.
    Pott spinal c.
    spinal c.
curve
    accommodation c.
    Barnes c.
    Blix contractile force c.
    calibration c.
    cervicothoracic c.
    combined c.
    compensatory c.
    contractile force c.
    displacement c.
    double major spinal c.
    double thoracic c.
    flattening of normal lordotic c.
    fractional c.
    full c.
    Hadley S-c.
    King type thoracic and lumbar c.
      (type I–IV)
    kyphotic c.
    length-tension c.
    load-deflection c.
    load-deformation c.
    load-displacement c.
    lordotic c.
    low single thoracic c.
    lumbar lordotic c.
    major c.
    c. measurement
    minor c.
    nonstructural c.
    normal lordotic c.
    c. pattern
    primary c.
    c. progression
    c. progression in scoliosis
    right thoracic c.
    rigid c.
    scoliotic c.
    severe rigid thoracic c.
    specific c.
    standardized growth c.

    strain-stress c.
    strength c.
    strength-duration c.
    stress-strain c.
    structural c.
    tension c.
    thoracic c.
    thoracolumbar c.
    torque c.
curved
    c. approach
    c. awl
    c. basket forceps
    c. bone rongeur
    c. curette
    c. gouge
    c. incision
    c. Küntscher nail system
    c. Mayo scissors
    c. meniscotome
    c. meniscotome blade
    c. osteotome
    c. osteotomy
    c. passer
    c. periosteal elevator
    c. retractor
curvilinear
    c. chin implant
    c. incision
CurvTek
    C. drill bone anchor
    C. TSR bone drill
Cushing
    C. bur
    C. disk rongeur
    C. dural hook
    C. flat drill
    C. Little Joker elevator
    C. perforator drill
    C. periosteal elevator
    C. retractor
    C. saw guide
    C. syndrome
Cushing-Gigli saw guide
Cushing-Hopkins periosteal elevator
cushion
    abduction c.
    alarm c.
    amputee c.
    Anti-Shox foot c.
    arch c.
    Back Bull lumbar support c.
    Back-Huggar lumbar support c.
    breakaway lap c.
    Butterfly c.
    Carter immobilization c.
    cast c.
    cell c.

cervical c.
Checkerboard wheelchair c.
Comfort Take-Along wheelchair c.
Core Max-Relax C.
Disc-O-Sit Jr. c.
Dry Flotation wheelchair c.
Easy Up c.
EcstaSeat seat c.
enhancer c.
FB cast c.
foam c.
foot c.
gel c.
Gel-Foam Ultra-Wedge c.
Geo-Matt contour c.
C. Grip Flatware
Healthier seating c.
c. heel
heel c.
Hudson Hydrofloat C.
hydro c.
hydrofloat c.
Invacare Comfort-Mate extra c.
invalid c.
Isch-Dish Plus c.
J2 c.
Jay basic c.
Jay Combi c.
Jay Rave c.
Jay Triad c.
Jay Xtreme c.
laptop c.
latex c.
lumbar support c.
MaxiFloat wheelchair c.
Pediplast c.
PERI-COMFORT c.
pommel c.
Posture Curve lumbar c.
Posture Wedge seat c.
pressure c.
pressure-relief c.
Prop'r Toes hammertoe c.
Quadtro c.
ring c.
ROHO Pack-It c.
saddle c.
Sat-A-Lite contoured wedge seat c.
Shockmaster heel c.
c. shoe liner
Sit-Straight wheelchair c.
Skil-Care c.

Sorbothane heel c.
Temper Foam c.
T-Foam c.
T-Gel c.
trilaminate c.
Vac-Lok immobilization c.
Viscoheel K heel c.
Viscoheel N c.
Viscoheel SofSpot viscoelastic
   heel c.
Viscolas heel c.
ViscoSpot heel c.
wheelchair c.
Y B Sore c.
cushioned shoe insert
cushion-throat wire cutter
Custodis implant
custom
   c. implant
   c. prosthesis
   c. rasp
**custom-designed swan-neck femoral
   component**
custom-fitted brace
custom-made
   c.-m. acetabular cup
   c.-m. insert
   c.-m. shoe
custom-molded shoe
custom-threaded prosthesis
cut
   chamfer c.
   freehand c.
   horizontal gantry c.
   jack upper c.
   notch c.
   Z-step c.
cutaneous
   c. amputation
   c. axon reflex
   c. distribution
   c. flap
   c. graft
   c. horn
   c. icing
   c. maceration
   c. nerve
   c. neuroma
   c. pressure threshold
cut-back zone
Cutinova
   C. cavity dressing

NOTES

Cutinova *(continued)*
    C. foam dressing
    C. thin dressing
cutout
    c. knee support
    c. patellar brace
    c. table
cut-out shoe
cutter
    bolt c.
    bone plug c.
    Breck pin c.
    C. cast
    cast c.
    Cloward dowel c.
    cookie c.
    cushion-throat wire c.
    diamond pin c.
    double-action c.
    end c.
    c. guide
    Hefty-bite pin c.
    Horsley bone c.
    Howmedica Microfixation System
     plate c.
    C. implant
    Jarit pin c.
    Kalish Duredge wire c.
    Kirschner wire c.
    Kleinert-Kutz bone c.
    Leibinger Micro System plate c.
    Luhr Microfixation System plate c.
    Martin diamond wire c.
    Midas Rex bone c.
    milling c.
    motorized meniscal c.
    M-Pact cast c.
    multiaction pin c.
    multiple action c.
    pin c.
    plug c.
    Redi-Vac cast c.
    rib c.
    Rochester harvest bone c.
    Rochester recipient bone c.
    Roos rib c.
    side c.
    side-cut pin c.
    Sklar pin c.
    Spartan jaw wire c.
    Storz Microsystems plate c.
    Synthes Microsystems plate c.
    toothed c.
    wire c.
    Wister wire/pin c.
cutting
    c. block
    c. bur

    c. cone
    c. current
    c. current knife
    c. forceps
    c. jig
    c. needle
    c. shaver
    c. weight
CVA
    costovertebral angle
    CVA Sling
CVAT
    costovertebral angle tenderness
CVD
    collagen vascular disease
CVT
    congenital vertical talus
C-wire inserter
cyanoacrylate
    c. adhesive
    c. glue
cyanocobalamin
cyanosis
cybernetics
Cybex
    C. back rehabilitation equipment
    C. cycle ergometer
    C. device
    C. I, II+ exercise system
    C. II isokinetic dynamometer
    C. II, II+ isokinetic exerciser
    C. 340 isokinetic rehabilitation and
     testing system
    C. isokinetic test
    C. machine
    C. tester
    C. testing
    C. Torso Rotation Testing and
     Rehabilitation Unit
    C. training system
    C. Trunk Extension Flexion unit
cycle
    Ergociser exercise c.
    c. ergometer
    Exer-Pedic c.
    gait c.
    c. per second (cps, c/sec)
    Power Trainer c.
    recumbent c.
    Saratoga c.
    Schwinn bi-directional Windjammer
     upper body c.
    c. time
    upper body c.
    walking c.
cyclic loading
cycling
    studio c.

cyclooxygenase product
cyclops
    c. formation
    c. lesion
    c. syndrome
cyclosporin A
cyclothymia
cylinder
    air c.
    Arthrotek calibrated c.
    Feldenkrais c.
    c. walking cast
cylindrical
    c. autologous dowel graft
    c. bur
    c. dowel
    c. osteotomy
    c. sleeve
cyma line
Cyriax
    C. evaluation
    C. technique
cyst
    c. ablation
    acetabular c.
    acromioclavicular c.
    aneurysmal bone c. (ABC)
    Baker c.
    bone c.
    bursal c.
    expansile c.
    ganglion c.

    giant popliteal synovial c.
    inclusion c.
    c. index
    juxtaarticular bone c.
    lipid inclusion c.
    meniscal c.
    mucous c.
    myxoid c.
    porencephalic c.
    postfracture c.
    rheumatoid c.
    sacral c.
    simple bone c.
    solitary bone c.
    subarticular c.
    subchondral bone c.
    synovial c.
    tibiofibular c.
    traumatic bone c.
    unicameral bone c.
cystic
    c. arthrosis
    c. bone lesion
    c. defect
    c. disease
    c. hygroma
    c. osteomyelitis
    c. rheumatoid arthritis
    c. tumor
cytoarchitectonic abnormality
cytotoxic drug

C

NOTES

3D
    three-dimensional
        3D fracture walker brace
        3D plate
        3D positional adjustability
        3D positional control
D/3
    distal third
DA
    degenerative arthritis
d'accoucheur
    main d.
Dacron
        D. batting
        D. graft
        D. polyester
        D. stent
        D. suture
        D. synthetic ligament material
Dacron-impregnated silicone rod
dactylalgia
dactylitis
    blistering distal d. (BDD)
    tuberculous d.
dactylocampsis
dactylocampsodynia
dactylodynia
dactylogryposis
dactylospasm
DAF
    dynamic axial fixator
Dafilon suture
Dagrofil suture
DAI
    diffuse axonal injury
Daily Adjusted Progressive Resistance Exercise (DAPRE)
Dakin tubing
Dalco Astro ankle brace
Dale
        D. abdominal binder
        D. first rib rongeur
Dallas grading system
Dall-Miles
        D.-M. cable
        D.-M. cable cerclage
        D.-M. cable/crimp cerclage system
        D.-M. cable grip system
        D.-M. cerclage wire
DALYs
    Disability Adjusted Life Years
damage
    physial d.
D'Ambrosia test
damp heat

DANA
    designed after natural anatomy
    DANA shoulder prosthesis
dance
    high-impact aerobic d. (HIAD)
    low-impact aerobic d. (LIAD)
    d. medicine
dancer's
    d. foot
    d. fracture
    d. pad
dancing
    d. bear gait
    d. bear syndrome
dandy
    D. clamp
    D. maneuver
Dandy-Walker deformity
dangling foot
Daniel iliac bone graft
Danis-Weber
    D.-W. classification of ankle injury
    D.-W. classification of malleolar fracture
    D.-W. fracture classification
Danniflex CPM exerciser
Dansko shoe
D'Antonio acetabular classification
DAPRE
    Daily Adjusted Progressive Resistance Exercise
    DAPRE strength training
Darco
        D. back brace
        D. foot splint
        D. medical surgical shoe and toe alignment splint
        D. moldable insole
        D. Podospray
        D. surgical shoe
        D. Wedge shoe
DarcoGel ankle brace
Darrach
        D. periosteal elevator
        D. procedure
        D. resection
        D. retractor
Darrach-Hughston-Milch fracture
Darrach-McLaughlin
        D.-M. approach
        D.-M. shoulder technique
Darrow pain classification
dart
    Arthrex meniscal d.

D

Das
D. Gupta procedure
D. Gupta scapular excision
D. Gupta scapulectomy
DASA
distal articular set angle
Dasco Pro angle finder
Daseler-Anson
D.-A. classification of plantaris muscle anatomy
D.-A. plantaris muscle anatomy classification
DASH
Disabilities of the Arm, Shoulder, and Hand
DASH scale
dashboard
d. dislocation
d. fracture
d. knee injury
DataHand system
DATT
deep anterior tibiotalar
DATT ligament
Daubenspeck bone curette
D'Aubigne
D. femoral prosthesis
D. femoral reconstruction
D. hip status system
D. patellar transplant
D. resection reconstruction
D'Aubigne-Postel postoperative function score
Dautrey
D. chisel
D. osteotome
Davey-Rorabeck-Fowler decompression technique
David
D. drainage
D. Letterman sign
Davidson muscle clamp
Davidson-Sauerbruch-Doyen periosteal elevator
Davies-Colley operation
Davis
D. arthrodesis
D. drainage technique
D. dura dissector
D. fusion
D. law
D. metacarpal splint
D. muscle-pedicle graft
D. percussion hammer
D. pin
D. saw guide
D. series
Dawbarn sign

Dawson-Yuhl
D.-Y. gouge
D.-Y. impactor
D.-Y. osteotome
D.-Y. periosteal elevator
D.-Y. rongeur forceps
D.-Y. suction tube
Dawson-Yuhl-Cone curette
Dawson-Yuhl-Kerrison rongeur forceps
Dawson-Yuhl-Key elevator
Dawson-Yuhl-Leksell rongeur forceps
DAW Strap-Pad
day
D. fixation device
D. fixation pin
D. fixation staple
d. treatment rehabilitation
Daytona cervical orthosis
DBM
demineralized bone matrix
DBS
deep bonding system
Denis Browne splint
DC
dynamic compression
DCB
distal communicating branch
DCC
dorsal calcaneocuboid
DCC ligament
DC-101 chiropractic table
D-Core support pillow
DCP
dynamic compression plate
DCS
dorsal column stimulator
Dynamic condylar screw
DCS pin
DDA
dorsal digital artery
DDD
degenerative disk disease
DDH
developmental dislocated hip
developmental dysplasia of the hip
DDH orthosis
DDP
dual drop pelvis
DDP table
de
de Andrade and MacNab anterior approach
de Barsy syndrome
de Boer lateral approach
de Kleyn position
de Kleyn test
de La Caffinière trapeziometacarpal prosthesis

de Lange syndrome
De Mayo hip positioner
de Morgan spot
de Quervain disease
de Quervain fracture
de Quervain injury
de Quervain stenosing tenosynovitis
de Quervain syndrome
de Quervain tendinitis
dead
d. arm syndrome
d. ball exercises
d. bone
d. lift
d. space
deafferentation pain
deafness
lentigines (multiple),
electrocardiographic abnormalities,
ocular hypertelorism, pulmonary
stenosis, abnormalities of
genitalia, retardation of growth,
and d. (sensorineural)
(LEOPARD)
d., onychoosteodystrophy, mental
retardation (DOOR)
Dean
D. bone rongeur
D. scissors
Deane unconstrained knee prosthesis
death
exercise-induced sudden d.
quadrant of d.
Deaver retractor
DeBakey prosthesis
DeBastiani
D. corticotomy
D. distractor
D. external fixator
D. femoral lengthening
D. fixation
D. technique
debonded femoral stem prosthesis
debonding
débridement
Ahern trochanteric d.
arthroscopic d.
bursal d.
cortical d.
diagnostic arthroscopy and d.
exploration and d.
irrigation and d. (I&D)

Magnuson d.
d. patella
debris
bone d.
fibrin d.
joint d.
loose d.
metallic d.
particulate wear d.
polyethylene d.
polymeric d.
pulvinar fibrofatty d.
tissue d.
wear d.
debris-incited osteolysis
debris-induced osteolysis
debris-retaining reamer
Debrunner kyphometer
debulking
d. procedure
Tsuge d.
deburring
decalcification
decancellation
cuboid d.
decerebrate posture
dechondrification
deciduous
Decker rongeur
deck plate
declination
angle of d.
d. angle
decompression
anterior retroperitoneal d.
anterolateral d.
bone graft d.
Braly-Bishop-Tullos d.
carpal tunnel d. (CTD)
cervical spine d.
core d.
d. equipment
extensive posterior d.
d. fasciotomy
foot d.
foramen magnum d.
fracture d.
lateral d.
leg d.
lumbar spine d.
Mubarak-Hargens d.
nerve root d.

NOTES

decompression *(continued)*
  posterior nerve d.
  posterolateral d.
  retroperitoneal d.
  d. rhachotomy
  sacral spine d.
  spinal d.
  subacromial d.
  d. technique
  thoracic spine d.
  thoracolumbar spine d.
  vertebral body d.
decompressive
  d. acromioplasty
  d. laminectomy
  d. osteotomy
deconditioned foot
deconditioning
  bed rest-related d.
  stroke-related d.
  d. syndrome
decorticate posture
decortication
  d. bur
  d. technique
decremental response
DeCube mattress
Decubitene oxygenated oil
decubitus
  d. position
  d. ulcer
decussation
dedifferentiated chondrosarcoma
Dee
  D. elbow hinge
  D. totally constrained elbow
    prosthesis
deep
  d. anterior tibiotalar (DATT)
  d. arch
  d. bonding system (DBS)
  d. circumflex iliac artery
  d. delayed infection
  d. fascia
  d. friction massage
  d. heat modality
  d. iliac dissection
  d. intracompartmental soft tissue
    sarcoma
  d. knee bend (DKB)
  d. lateral femoral notch sign
  d. peroneal nerve
  d. posterior compartment
  d. posterior tibiotalar (DPTT)
  d. retractor
  d. stroking and kneading massage

  d. tendon reflex (DTR)
  d. venous thrombosis (DVT)
  d. venous thrombosis prophylaxis
  d. wound infection
deepening reamer
deepithelialized rectus abdominis muscle
  (DRAM)
deep-shelled acetabulum
Deerfield test
deer tick disease
defect
  anteromedial humeral head d.
  Arthropor oblong cup for
    acetabular d.
  articular d.
  bar-like ventral d.
  benign cortical d.
  bone d.
  bridging of d.
  cavitary d.
  composite d.
  cortical d.
  cystic d.
  developmental d.
  diaphysial d.
  femoral condylar d.
  fibrous cortical d.
  fibrous metaphysial d.
  fusiform d.
  impression d.
  Klippel-Feil segmentation d.
  mapping the d.
  metaphysial fibrous d.
  metaphysial fibrous cortical d.
  neural tube d.
  nonsubperiosteal cortical d.
  d. nonunion
  osseous d.
  osteoarticular d.
  osteochondral d.
  pars d.
  posterior superior humeral head d.
  radial ray d.
  reverse Hill-Sachs d.
  segmental bone d.
  segmentation d.
  skeletal d.
  step d.
  subcortical d.
  subperiosteal cortical d.
  tibial d.
  triangular d.
  trochlear d.
  unremodeled d.
defervesce
Defiance functional knee brace

deficiency
Aitken femoral d.
American Academy of Orthopaedic Surgeons classification of acetabular d.
cavitary d.
central d.
congenital limb d.
factor VIII, IX d.
focal d.
Jones classification of congenital tibial d.
Kalamchi-Dawe classification of congenital tibial d.
long bone d.
longitudinal d.
magnesium d.
proximal femoral focal d.
proximal focal femoral d. (PFFD)
radial d.
segmental d.
skeletal limb d.
tibial longitudinal d.
transverse d.
vitamin C, D, K d.

deficient
d. knee
d. spinous process

deficit
executive function d.
motor d.
motor function d.
neurologic d.
perception d.
proprioceptive d.
sensorimotor d.
sensory d.
somatosensory d.

Definition PM femoral implant component

definitive
d. callus
d. cerclage wire
d. stabilization

deformability

deformans
arthritis d.
arthrosis d.
malum d.
osteitis d.
osteoarthritis d.
osteochondrodystrophia d.

Paget osteitis d.
spondylitis d.

deformation
elastic d.
plastic d.
stem d.

deformity
abduction d.
acetabular protrusio d.
adduction d.
adduction-internal rotation d.
adductovarus d.
adult-acquired flatfoot d.
d. analysis
angulation d.
apex plantar d.
Arnold-Chiari d.
arthrosis d.
back-knee d.
biconcave d.
bifid thumb d.
bony d.
boutonnière d.
bowing d.
bowleg d.
bunion d.
bunionette d.
burn boutonnière d.
buttonhole d.
calcaneocavovarus d.
calcaneocavus d.
calcaneovalgus d.
calcaneovarus d.
calcaneus d.
cavovarus d.
cavus foot d.
cervical spine kyphotic d.
Charcot d.
Chattanooga balance system Checkrein d.
checkrein d.
clasped thumb d.
clawfoot d.
clawhand d.
clawtoe d.
cleft foot d.
cleft hand d.
cloverleaf d.
clubfoot d.
clubhand d.
cock-up d.
codfish d.

NOTES

deformity *(continued)*
Cole osteotomy for midfoot d.
combined cavus d.
compensatory d.
congenital vertical talus foot d.
contracture d.
coronal plane d.
crossover-toe d.
curly toe d.
Dandy-Walker d.
digital d.
digitus flexus d.
dinner fork d.
DISI d.
double corn d.
dynamic digital d.
elevatus d.
equinocavovarus d.
equinovalgus d.
equinovarus hindfoot d.
equinus d.
Erlenmeyer flask d.
eversion-external rotation d.
extension d.
femoral head d.
finger d.
fishtail d.
fixed d.
flat back d.
flatfoot d.
flexion-internal rotational d.
flexion valgus d.
foot d.
forefoot abduction d.
fracture d.
garden spade d.
genu valgum d.
genu varum d.
gunstock d.
Haglund foot d.
hallux limitus d.
hallux valgus d.
hallux varus d.
hammer toe d.
hatchet-head d.
Hibbs extensor tendon transfer
 cavus d.
Hill-Sachs d.
hindfoot d.
hollow foot clawfoot d.
hook-nail d.
hourglass d.
humpback d.
hyperextension d.
Ilfeld-Holder d.
internal rotation d.
intrinsic minus d.
intrinsic plus d.

J-hook d.
joint d.
Kelikian classification of nail d.
Kirner d.
knock-knee d.
kyphotic d.
lobster-claw d.
lumbar spine kyphotic d.
Madelung d.
mallet finger d.
mallet toe d.
medial ray adduction d.
metatarsus adductus d.
metatarsus primus varus d.
metatarsus varus d.
Michal d.
multiplanar d.
neuropathic foot d.
oblique osteotomy for tibial d.
one-plane d.
pannus d.
pencil and cup d.
pes arcuatus clawfoot d.
pes cavus clawfoot d.
pes planovalgus d.
pes planus d.
pes valgo planus d.
planovalgus d.
plantar flexion-inversion d.
posttraumatic spinal d.
procurvatum d.
protrusio d.
pseudoboutonnière d.
pseudo-Hurler d.
pump bump d.
rearfoot d.
recurvatum angulation d.
reduction d.
rheumatoid d.
rigid equinovarus d.
rigid flatfoot d.
rockerbottom flatfoot d.
rotational d.
round shoulder d.
saber shin d.
sagittal d.
scaphoid humpback d.
seal-fin d.
shepherd's crook d.
silver-fork d.
skeletal d.
skewfoot d.
spastic hindfoot valgus d.
spastic thumb-in-palm d.
spinal coronal plane d.
spine d.
splayfoot d.
split-hand d.

split-nail d.
Sprengel d.
S-shaped d.
static foot d.
subcondylar d.
supination d.
swan-neck finger d.
talipes cavus d.
talus foot d.
thoracic spine kyphotic d.
thoracic spine scoliotic d.
three-plane d.
thumb d.
thumb-in-palm d.
torsional d.
triphalangeal thumb d.
turned-up pulp d.
two-plane d.
ulnar deviation d.
ulnar drift d.
valgus heel d.
varus hindfoot d.
Velpeau d.
vertical talus foot d.
volar angulation d.
Volkmann clawhand d.
windblown d.
windswept d.
wrist d.
Zancolli procedure for clawhand d.
Z foot d.
zigzag compensatory d.

deformity/instability
spinal d./i.
Defourmentel bone rongeur
Dega pelvic osteotomy
degenerated cartilage
degeneration
axonal d.
cartilaginous d.
Charcot d.
disk d.
endoneurium d.
fascicular d.
fibrinoid d.
immobilization d.
joint d.
Kirkaldy-Willis three phases of d.
mucoid d.
Regnauld-type great toe d.
retrograde d.

rotator cuff d.
spinal d.
spinocerebellar d.
wallerian d.
wear-and-tear d.
Zenker d.
degenerative
d. arthritic change
d. arthritis (DA)
d. arthrosis
d. disk disease (DDD)
d. disorder
d. joint disease (DJD)
d. lumbar scoliosis
d. lumbar spine fusion
d. meniscus
d. osteoarthritis
d. spine condition
d. spondylolisthesis
d. spondylosis
d. spondylosis decompression and fusion
d. spur
d. spurring
d. stenosis
d. tear
d. vertebral arthropathy
degloving
d. injury
phalangeal d.
d. procedure
degradable polyglycolide rod
degree
d.'s of freedom (DOF)
d. of separation
d.'s of valgus angulation
d.'s of varus angulation
degrees-of-freedom joint motion
dehiscence
prosthesis d.
wound d.
Zuckerkandl d.
Dejerine
D. disease
D. percussion hammer
D. sign
Dejerine-Davis percussion hammer
Dejerine-Sottas
D.-S. disease
D.-S. syndrome

D

NOTES

Deknatel
 D. orthopedic autotransfusion
 system
 D. suture classification
delamination
DeLaura knee prosthesis
DeLaura-Verner knee prosthesis
delay
 sensory d.
delayed
 d. apoplexy
 d. bone imaging
 d. bone maturation
 d. consolidation
 d. femoral osteotomy
 d. fracture union
 d. graft
 d. onset
 d. open reduction
 d. primary closure (DPC)
 d. primary repair
 d. reflex
 d. response
delayed-onset muscle soreness
Delbet splint
DeLee
 D. classification
 D. radiographic analysis
Delitala
 D. T-nail nail
 D. T-pin
Delore method
DeLorme exercise
Delrin-handle bone saw
Delrin joint
delta
 d. brush
 d. femoral nail
 d. frame
 d. phalanx
 d. receptor
 D. Recon nail
 D. Recon proximal drill guide
 d. rod
 d. tibial nail
 D. walker
Deltafit Keel
Delta-Lite
 D.-L. casting tape
 D.-L. FlashCast
Delta-Rol cast padding
deltoid
 d. artery
 d. bursa
 d. fascia
 d. flap
 d. insertion
 d. ligament

 d. ligament tear
 d. muscle
 d. origin
 d. reflex
 d. region
 d. sprain
Deltoid-Aid arm support
deltoid-splitting
 d.-s. incision
 d.-s. shoulder approach
deltopectoral
 d. approach
 d. flap
 d. groove
 d. interval
deltotrapezius fascial ligament
deluxe
 d. FIN pin
 d. FIN pin inserter
demand
 motion d.
 specific adaptation to imposed d.
 (SAID)
demarcation
 line of d.
Demariniff protractor
DeMartel wire saw
DeMartel-Wolfson clamp holder
DeMayo suture passer
Demel wire clamp
dementia
Demianoff sign
demigauntlet bandage
demineralization
 bony d.
demineralized
 d. bone
 d. bone graft
 d. bone matrix (DBM)
Demos tibial artery clamp
DeMuth hip screw
demyelination
dendritic synovitis
denervation
 cryogenic d.
 d. disease
 d. potential
 d. procedure
 d. supersensitivity
Denham
 D. external fixation
 D. external fixation device
 D. pin
Denis
 D. Browne bar
 D. Browne bar foot orthosis
 D. Browne bucket
 D. Browne clubfoot splint

D. Browne hip splint
D. Browne sacral fracture
  classification
D. Browne spinal fracture
  classification
D. Browne splint (DBS)
D. Browne talipes hobble splint
D. Browne three-column model
D. Browne three-column spine
  theory
D. Browne tray
D. compression fracture
  classification
D. seat-belt injury classification
D. spinal fracture
Dennison cervical brace
**Dennyson-Fulford extraarticular subtalar
  arthrodesis**
DENS
  direct electrical nerve stimulation
dens
  d. anterior screw fixation
  d. fracture
  d. x-ray view
dense bone
densitometry
  bone d.
  dual photon d. (DPD)
  fracture site nonunion Norland
    bone d.
  photon d.
  scanning d.
  video d. (VD)
density
  bone d.
  bone mineral d. (BMD)
  calcific d.
  fiber d.
  lumbosacral junction bone d.
  proton d.
dental
  d. bur
  d. drill
  d. mirror
  d. pick
dentate
  d. fracture
  d. ligament
dentinogenesis imperfecta
Denuce
  quadrate ligament of D.
denudation

denude
deodorant
  Deoshoes d.
Deoshoes deodorant
deossification band
deoxypyridinoline crosslinks urine assay
DePalma
  D. hip prosthesis
  D. modified patellar technique
  D. staple
  D. staple procedure
dependent edema
depolarization block
depolymerization
  increased d.
  unbalanced d.
deposit
  calcareous d.
  calcific d.
  calcium d.
  gouty tophaceous d.
  rotator cuff calcified d.
  tophaceous d.
deposition
  beta-2-microglobulin d.
  bone d.
  calcium oxalate d.
  calcium pyrophosphate dihydrate d.
    (CPPD)
  hemosiderin d.
  pseudotumorous mucin d.
depot corticosteroid
depressed
  d. fracture
  d. reflex
depression
  bone d.
  d. of fragment
  Hamilton Rating Scale for D.
  postactivation d.
depth
  d. caliper-meter stick method
  d. gauge
  d. inlay shoe
  D. orthopedic shoe
  wire penetration d.
depth-check drill
DePuy
  D. acetabular liner
  D. acetabular lining
  D. aeroplane splint
  D. AML hip

D

NOTES

DePuy *(continued)*
    D. AML Porocoat stem prosthesis
    D. any-angle splint
    D. awl
    D. bipolar cup
    D. bolt
    D. calcar grinder
    D. CMW type-1 bone cement
    D. coaptation splint
    D. drill
    D. femoral acetabular overlay
    guide
    D. fracture brace
    D. graft preparation table
    D. halter
    D. hip prosthesis with Scuderi
    head
    D. interference screw
    D. LCS mobile-bearing knee
    D. open-spindle splint
    D. open-thimble splint
    D. orthopedic implant
    D. pin
    D. plate
    D. rainbow frame
    D. rasp
    D. reamer
    D. reducing frame
    D. rocking leg splint
    D. rod bender
    D. rolled Colles splint
    D. screwdriver
    D. support
    D. Tri-Lock interlocking acetabular
    cup
    D. trispiked acetabular component
DePuy-Pott splint
derangement
    Hey internal d.
    internal d.
    joint internal d.
    structural d.
    d. syndrome
    vertebral d.
derby
    d. hat fracture
    D. nail
Derifield pelvic leg check
dermabrader
Dermagraft
Dermagran
    D. hydrophilic gauze dressing
    D. ointment wound dressing
dermal
    d. bone
    d. fasciectomy
    d. fibromatosis

    d. interposition splint
    d. sinus
DermaSite dressing
**DermaTemp infrared thermographic
sensor**
dermatitis, pl. **dermatitides**
    atopic d.
    shoe d.
dermatoarthritis
dermatocele
dermatofibroma
dermatofibrosarcoma protuberans
dermatogenic torticollis
dermatolymphangitis
dermatomal
    d. pain
    d. pattern
dermatome
    anterior tibial nerve d.
    Brown d.
    d. mapping
    mechanical d.
    Padgett electric d.
    Reese d.
    sacral d.
    Stryker d.
    Zimmer d.
dermatomyositis
dermatosensory evoked potential
dermatosis, pl. **dermatoses**
    juvenile plantar d.
Derma-Wand germicidal lamp
Dermiflex dressing
dermodesis
    resection d.
dermographia
dermometer
dermomyotome
Dero hole-in-one prosthetic sock
DeRosa-Graziano step-cut osteotomy
derotate
derotation
    d. boot
    d. brace
    oblique osteotomy with d.
derotational
    d. osteotomy
    d. pin
    d. reflex
derotator
    d. bar
    d. splint
DeRoyal LMB finger splint
D'Errico
    D. enlarging drill bur
    D. lamina chisel
    D. perforating drill

D. perforating drill bur
D. retractor
Desault
D. fracture
D. sign
D. wrist bandage
D. wrist dislocation
Deschamps needle
Descot fracture
designed after natural anatomy (DANA)
DesignLine orthotic
desirudin
desk
Posture-Rite lap d.
Desk-rest arm support
desktop therapy portal
desmalgia
desmectasis
desmitis
desmocytoma
desmodynia
desmoid
cortical d.
d. fibroma
d. lesion
periosteal d.
d. tumor
desmoma
desmopathy
desmoplasia
desmoplastic fibroma
desmopressin
desmorrhexis
desmosis
desmotomy
Desormaux endoscope
desquamation
Destot sign
destruction
bony element d.
bony necrosis and d.
cortical d.
geographic d.
localized bone d.
moth-eaten d.
pantalocrural arthritic d.
destructive
d. articular lesion
d. bone disease
d. joint disease
desyndactylization
Weinstock d.

detector
analogous signal d.
Isometer bone graft placement
site d.
deterioration
arthritic d.
catastrophic d.
determinant
combined ankle and knee motion
gait d.
knee flexion during stance phase
motion gait d.
pelvic rotation motion gait d.
pelvic shift motion gait d.
pelvic tilt motion gait d.
determination
anteversion d.
Budin-Chandler anteversion d.
fusion limit d.
leg length d.
skin blood flow d.
transcutaneous oxygen tension d.
Whitesides tissue pressure d.
detritus
d. bone
hyaline cartilage d.
detrusor
d. areflexia
d. contraction
d. hyperreflexia
detrusor-sphincter synergia
Deune knee prosthesis
Deutschländer disease
Devas stress fracture classification
development
asymmetric subtalar joint d.
Bayley Scales of Infant D.
bone d.
calcar femorale d.
motor d.
postural d.
reflex d.
developmental
d. anatomy
d. coxa vara
d. defect
d. dislocated hip (DDH)
d. dislocated hip orthosis
d. dyscalculia
d. dysplasia of the hip (DDH)
d. hip dysplasia
Deverle fixation

D

NOTES

deviation

angular d.
gait d.
lateral d.
proximal set angle d.
radial d.
rotary d.
standard d.
ulnar d.

device

Ace Unifix fixation d.
acrylic orthotic d.
Acufex bioabsorbable fixation d.
AcuSpark piezoelectric d.
adjustable aiming d.
adjustable two-point caliper sensory
assessment d.
Agee four-pin fixation d.
AlloAnchor RC allograft d.
Anderson fixation d.
Anderson leg-lengthening d.
ankle disk d.
Antense antitension d.
anterior internal fixation d.
antirotation d.
application of traction d.
Aprema III d.
Aquatrek d.
Arrow absorbable meniscal
repair d.
ArtAssist arterial assist d.
ArthroSew arthroscopic suturing d.
Arthrotek tibial fixation d.
ArthroWand d.
articular motion d. (AMD)
articulated tension d.
Artscan 200 arthroscopic cartilage
stiffness testing d.
assistive technology d. (ATD)
Automator d.
A-V Impulse System foot pump
DVT prophylaxis d.
A-V Impulse System foot wrap
DVT prophylaxis d.
Axer compression d.
axis-altering arthroereisis d.
Backbar d.
BackCycler continuous passive
motion d.
back range-of-motion d.
Bassett electrical stimulation d.
Becker orthopaedic spinal system
orthotic d.
biodegradable fixation d.
BioStinger low profile fixation d.
Blanchard traction d.
body-powered prosthetic d.
bollard d.

Book Butler book-grip d.
Bovie electrocautery d.
Brannock foot measuring d.
Buck convoluted traction d.
Calandruccio II compression d.
Calandruccio triangular compression
fixation d.
Cameron fracture d.
CAPS ArthroWand d.
Carpal Trac traction d.
C-D fixation d.
C-D instrumentation d.
cervical range-of-motion d.
Cervitrak d.
Charnley external fixation d.
Chattanooga traction d.
circular fixation d.
Cleanwheel presterilized
disposable d.
collapsible internal fixation d.
Columbus McKinnon Hugger d.
combined fixation d.
Compliant prestress prosthetic bone
implant d.
compression screw-plate d.
compressive internal fixating d.
Cordis implantable drug
reservoir d.
coring d.
Cotrel-Dubousset dynamic transverse
traction d.
CPM d.
Cuff Link orthopedic d.
Cybex d.
Day fixation d.
Denham external fixation d.
Deyerle fixation d.
Deyo d.
Disk-Criminator nerve stimulation
measuring d.
distal targeting d.
DressFlex orthotic d.
Dr. Grip writing d.
Dunn fracture d.
Dwyer d.
dynamic transverse traction d.
Easy-Pull sock aide d.
EBI d.
Edwards modular system sacral
fixation d.
Elbow-Up Protector elbow
suspension d.
Electronics electrical stimulation d.
Encore Orthopedics d.
EndoPearl bioabsorbable d.
EndoPearl fixation d.
Evershears surgical instrument d.
Exeter intramedullary bone plug d.

EX-FI-RE external fixation d.
E-Z Flex jaw exercising d.
EZ-Trac orthopedic suspension d.
FastOut d.
fixation d.
FootFlex performance stretching d.
forearm lift assist adjustable
  spring-loaded d.
four-bar external fixation d.
Fox internal fixation d.
fracture fixation d.
Fromm triangle orthopedic d.
GAIT spacer d.
Georgiade fixation d.
Giliberty d.
Golgi d.
Graftmaster d.
Grip-Ease d.
halo-gravity traction d.
halo vest d.
Hare splint d.
Harrington fixation d.
Harrington-Kostuik distraction d.
Harrington rod instrumentation
  distraction outrigger d.
Harris-Aufranc d.
Heyer-Schulte antisiphon d.
Hoffmann mini-lengthening
  fixation d.
Hoffmann-Vidal external fixation d.
hot/ice cold therapy cooler
  therapy d.
Ikuta fixation d.
Ilizarov d.
implantable bone anchor d.
inductive coupling d.
Innovasive d.
Insta-Nerve d.
intraarticular cautery d.
Intracell mechanical muscle d.
Intracell myofascial trigger-point d.
InvertaChair traction d.
isometric d.
JACE W550 CPM d.
JAS elbow motion d.
Kaneda distraction d.
Kendrick extrication d. (KED)
Kennedy ligament augmenting d.
Kerboull acetabular reinforcement d.
Kessler fixation d.
Kin-Con d.
kinetic rehab d. (KRD)

Kirschner d.
Knott rod distraction d.
KRD L2000 rehab d.
Kronner external fixation d.
Kuhlman cervical traction d.
Küntscher traction d.
Lawrence d.
Legasus support CPM d.
leg-holding d.
leg-lengthening d.
Leinbach d.
Leksell adapter to Mayfield d.
LifeGait partial weightbearing
  therapy d.
ligament augmentation d. (LAD)
Link Orthopaedics d.
LiteGait partial weight-bearing gait
  therapy d.
Luque fixation d.
Mayo elbow distraction d.
McAtee compression screw d.
McKeever patellar resurfacing d.
McLaughlin osteosynthesis d.
MediRule II measuring d.
Merry Walker ambulation d.
MicroFET2 muscle testing d.
Mobilimb CPM d.
Mueller fixation d.
muscle and neurological stimulation
  electrotherapy d.
MyoTrac d.
nail-bending d.
nail plate d.
Nauth traction d.
Necktrac traction d.
Neufeld d.
Neuro-Aide testing d.
newer-generation d.
notcher d.
Ogden Anchor soft tissue d.
Ommaya reservoir d.
Omni-Flexor d.
Oppociser exercise d.
Oratec d.
Original Jacknobber II muscle-
  massage d.
Orthofix external fixation d.
Orthofix ISKD d.
Ortholav irrigation and suction d.
orthotic d.
OssaTron noninvasive extracorporeal
  shock wave therapy d.

NOTES

device *(continued)*

OsteoAnalyzer d.
OsteoView x-ray d.
Oxford uncompartmental d.
Parham-Martin fracture d.
passive motion d.
passive positioning d.
PDN d.
peg d.
pegboard lateral positioning d.
Percuss-O-Matic jackhammer d.
Pivot Pole walking d.
Plastizote orthotic d.
PlexiPulse intermittent pneumatic
   compression d.
PLM d.
pneumatic external compression d.
PodoFlex reflexology d.
Polar Care 500 cryotherapy d.
posterior reduction d. (PORD)
PPT orthotic d.
Pressure-Specified Sensory D.
pronation spring-control d.
Pronex patient controlled pneumatic
   traction d.
prosthetic disk nucleus d.
ProTrac measurement d.
pulsatile pneumatic plantar-
   compression d.
pyrolytic carbon d.
Quartzo d.
Quengel d.
QuickTack d.
Rancho ankle foot control d.
Redi-Trac traction d.
Reichert-Mundinger stereotactic d.
Rezaian external fixation d.
Rezaian interbody d.
Richards lag screw d.
RMC knee replacement d.
ROC anchoring d.
Rochester bone trephine d.
rod distraction d.
rod-mounted targeting d.
Roeder manipulative aptitude
   test d.
Roger Anderson compression d.
Roger Anderson external
   fixation d.
Roger Anderson stabilization d.
RollerBack self-massage d.
Rolz d.
rope stretching d.
rotation d.
Safe-T mate anti-rollback d.
SAFHS ultrasound d.
Scully Hip S'port hip d.
sequential compression d. (SCD)

Servox d.
Sgarlato d.
shear-off d.
Sleeper Gripper prosthetic d.
sliding fixation d.
sliding nail d.
Slot distraction d.
snap-fit d.
Sock-Assist d.
Sofamor spinal d.
SOLEutions custom orthotic d.
SOLEutions Prefab orthotic d.
Sorbothane orthotic d.
Southwick pin-holding d.
Spenco orthotic d.
Sport-Rite Olympian d.
Sport-Rite Runner d.
sports terminal d.
SporTX stimulation d.
StairClimber assist d.
Statak soft tissue attachment d.
Stellbrink fixation d.
Stone clamp-locking d.
Stress-Ray varus-valgus d.
Stryker knee joint laxity d.
STx lumbar traction d.
STx Saunders lumbar disc d.
Sukhtian-Hughes fixation d.
SuperQuad assistive d.
Suretac bioabsorbable shoulder
   fixation d.
Sutter d.
Sutter-CPM knee d.
Tacticon peripheral neuropathy
   screening d.
Tekscan in-shoe monitoring d.
Telectronics electrical stimulation d.
Tenderlett d.
terminal d. (TD)
T-Fix absorbable meniscal repair d.
ThermaStim muscle warming d.
thermocouple skin temperature d.
The Rope stretch-and-traction d.
The Rope stretching d.
Thumper d.
toe-straight d.
transpedicularly implanted anterior
   spinal support d.
transverse loading d.
d. for transverse traction (DTT)
triangular compression d.
TriggerWheel d.
TSRH corkscrew d.
TSRH mini-corkscrew d.
Valenti arthroereisis d.
VariFix spinal implant d.
VariGrip spinal implant d.

Vidal-Adrey modified Hoffmann
external fixation d.
Viladot arthroereisis d.
visor halo fixation d.
Volkov-Oganesian elbow
distraction d.
Volkov-Oganesian external
fixation d.
voluntary closing terminal d.
voluntary opening terminal d.
Wagner distraction d.
Wagner external fixation d.
Wagner-Schanz screw d.
Walk-Rite d.
Wanger leg lengthening d.
Wasserstein fixation d.
wood probe reflexology d.
Wrist Pro wrist support d.
Xercise Band exercise d.
Xercise tube resistive d.
XTB knee extension d.
Zickel supracondylar d.
Zielke distraction d.
Zimmer electrical stimulation d.
Zimmer orthopedic d.
Zipper antidisconnect d.

devitalized
d. bone graft
d. portion
d. tissue

DeWald
D. spinal apparatus
D. spinal appliance

Dewar
D. posterior cervical fixation
procedure
D. posterior cervical fusion
D. posterior cervical fusion
technique

Dewar-Barrington
D.-B. arthroplasty
D.-B. clavicular dislocation
technique

Dewar-Harris
D.-H. paralysis
D.-H. shoulder technique

DEXA
dual-energy x-ray absorptiometry
DEXA scan

Dexon suture
dexterity
finger d.

dextran prophylaxis
dextrorotary scoliosis
dextrorotoscoliosis
dextroscoliosis scoliosis
Deyerle
D. drill
D. femoral fracture technique
D. fixation apparatus
D. fixation device
D. interlocking screw
D. II pin
D. plate
D. punch
D. sciatic tension test

Deyo device
DFA
dorsiflexion angle
D-Foam
DFS
distraction-flexion stage
DH pressure relief walker
DHS
dynamic hip screw
Diab-A-Foot
D.-A.-F. protection system
D.-A.-F. rocker insole
Diab-A-Pad insole
Diab-A-Sheet
Diab-A-Sheets shoe insert
Diab-A-Sole
D.-A.-S. flat insole
D.-A.-S. molded insole
Diab-A-Thotics orthotic
diabetic
d. amyotrophy
d. arthropathy
d. Charcot foot
D. Diagnostic insole
D. D-Sole foot orthosis
d. femoral mononeuropathy
d. neuropathy
d. neurotrophic ulcer
d. orthosis kit
d. polyradiculopathy
d. pressure relief shoe
D. Quality of Life
d. sock

diaclasis
diaclastic amputation
diacondylar fracture
diadochokinesia
diagnosis, pl. **diagnoses**

D

NOTES

diagnosis *(continued)*
    clinical d.
    differential d.
    palpatory d.
diagnostic
    d. arthroscopy and débridement
    d. arthroscopy, operative
      arthroscopy, and possible
      operative arthrotomy (AAA)
    d. imaging
    d. and operative arthroscopy
      (DOA)
    d. strategy
diagonal stretch
diagram
    free body d.
dial
    d. pelvic osteotomy
    d. periacetabular osteotomy
    d. test
dial-lock
    d.-l. brace
    d.-l. orthosis
diameter
    acetabular depth to femoral
      head d. (AD/FHD)
    horizontal pedicle d.
    lumbar spine pedicle d.
    neck d.
    orthonormal d.
    pedicle d.
    sagittal pedicle d.
    sagittal spinal canal d.
    thoracic spine pedicle d.
    transpedicular fixation effective
      pedicle d.
    transverse pedicle d.
    vertical pedicle d.
diametral
diametric pelvic fracture
diamond
    D. biomechanical table
    d. bur
    d. fraise
    d. high-speed drill
    d. inlay bone graft
    D. nail
    d. pin cutter
    d. point needle
    d. rasp
    d. tip wire
Diamondback
    D. 1100 recumbent stepper
    D. 1100 self-generated stepper
    D. 100 upright stepper
Diamond-Gould
    D.-G. reduction syndactyly
    D.-G. syndactyly operation

diamond-point wire double-strand wire
diamond-shaped medullary nail
diapedesis
Diapedic foot cream
diaphragm
    Bucky d.
    urogenital d.
diaphysectomy
diaphyses (*pl. of* diaphysis)
diaphysial, diaphyseal
    d. aclasis
    d. defect
    d. dysplasia
    d. fracture
    d. osteotomy
    d. plating
    d. sclerosis
    d. tuberculosis
diaphysial-epiphysial fusion
diaphysis, pl. **diaphyses**
    femoral d.
diaplasis
diaplastic
diarthrodial
    d. cartilage
    d. joint
diarthrosis
Dias-Giegerich
    D.-G. fracture technique
    D.-G. open reduction
Dias-Tachdijian physial injury
    classification
diastasis
    ankle mortise d.
    d. fibula
    frank d.
    interosseous d.
    latent d.
    pubic d.
    symphysis pubis d.
    syndesmotic d.
    tibiofibular d.
    tibiotalar d.
diastatic fracture
diastematomyelia
diastrophic
    d. dwarfism
    d. dysplasia
diathermy
    Magnatherm SSP pulse
      shortwave d.
    microwave d. (MWD)
    pulsed d.
    shortwave d. (SWD)
diathesis
    Dupuytren d.
Diaz disease

DIC
disseminated intravascular coagulation
Dick AO fixateur interne
Dickhaut-DeLee discoid meniscus classification
Dickinson
D. approach
D. calcaneal bursitis technique
Dickinson-Coutts-Woodward-Handler osteotomy
Dickson
D. geometric osteotomy
D. muscle transfer
D. operation
D. paraffin bath
D. paralysis
D. transplant technique
Dickson-Diveley
D.-D. foot operation
D.-D. procedure
dicondylar fracture
Didiee view
Dieffenbach
D. amputation
D. operation
die punch fracture
diet
Gerson d.
gouty d.
tea-and-toast d.
d. therapy
training d.
very low calorie d. (VLCD)
dietary
d. modification
d. protein
d. reference intake (DRI)
Diethrich bulldog clamp
difference
differential
d. diagnosis
d. spinal block
temperature d. (TD)
differentiated chondrosarcoma
differentiation failure
diffuse
d. angiokeratoma
d. axonal injury (DAI)
d. fasciitis
d. idiopathic skeletal hyperostosis (DISH)

d. idiopathic skeletal hyperostosis syndrome
d. infantile fibromatosis
d. pigmented villonodular synovitis (DPVNS)
digastric muscle
DiGeorge syndrome
Digi-Flex
D.-F. finger exerciser
D.-F. hand exerciser
Digikit finger tourniquet
Digimatic caliper
Digi Sleeve stockinette dressing
digit
accessory d.
arthrodesed d.
d. cap
congenital trigger d.
flail d.
infantile trigger d.
multiple d.'s
replantation of amputated d.
sausage d.
d. splint
supernumerary d.
trigger d.
d. tube
d. wrap
Digit-Aide fifth toe splint
digital
d. amputation
d. aponeurosis
d. artery
d. artery of foot
d. artery protection
D. Biofeedback System
d. block anesthesia
d. blood perfusion
d. branch
d. branch of plantar nerve
D. Care kit
d. color
d. contracture
d. cord
d. deformity
d. edge-detection
d. extensor mechanism
d. extensor tendon
d. flexor tendinitis
d. flexor tendon
d. flexor tendon sheath
d. formula

D

NOTES

digital (continued)
  d. impaction
  d. joint
  d. nail
  d. nerve block
  d. pad
  d. palpation
  d. photoplethysmography
  d. plethysmography
  d. prosthesis
  d. reflex
  d. response test
  d. self-retaining retractor
  d. shortening
  d. subtraction angiography (DSA)
  d. theca
  d. tourniquet
  d. vibrogram
digiti quinti proprius tendon
digitizer
  Amfit d.
  Metrecom d.
digitorum
  d. brevis avulsion
  d. communis tendon
digitus
  d. abductus
  d. adductus
  d. flexus deformity
  d. medius
  d. minimus
  d. primus
  d. valgus
  d. varus
Di Guglielmo disease
dilated cardiomyopathy
dilator
  Eder-Puestow metal olive d.
  lacrimal duct d.
  vessel d.
Dillwyn-Evans
  D.-E. osteotomy
  D.-E. resection
dilutional pseudoanemia
dimelia
  ulnar d.
dimension
  D. hip prosthesis
  D. hip system
Dimension-C femoral stem prosthesis
diminished sensation
Dimon-Hughston
  D.-H. fracture fixation
  D.-H. intertrochanteric osteotomy
  D.-H. technique
Dimon osteotomy
dimple
  d. the bone

pilonidal d.
  d. sign
ding foot
Dingman
  D. bone and cartilage clamp
  D. bone-holding forceps
  D. mouth gag
  D. osteotome
dinner fork deformity
diode
  infrared light-emitting d.
diorthosis
DIP
  distal interphalangeal
  DIP articulation
  DIP fusion
  DIP joint
diparesis
  spastic d.
diphasic
DIPJ
  distal interphalangeal joint
diplegia
  spastic d.
diplegic foot
diplomyelia
diploscope
dipropionate
dipyridamole
  d. handgrip test
  d. thallium imaging
direct
  d. contraction
  d. current
  d. current electrotherapy
  d. electrical nerve stimulation
    (DENS)
  d. fracture
  d. injury elbow dislocation
  d. lateral portal
  d. vertex impact
direct-impact prosthesis
director
  grooved d.
disability
  D. Adjusted Life Years (DALYs)
  D.'s of the Arm, Shoulder, and
    Hand (DASH)
  D.'s of Arm, Shoulder and Hand
    questionnaire
  D.'s of the Arm, Shoulder, and
    Hand scale
  atlantooccipital d.
  box and block test of arm d.
  Oswestry Low Back Pain D.
  permanent d.
  permanent partial d. (PPD)
  permanent and total d. (PTD)

reversible ischemic neurologic d. (RIND)
d. scale
secondary d.
tapping test of arm d.
disappearing bone disease
disarticular amputation
disarticulation
ankle d.
Batch-Spittler-McFaddin knee d.
Boyd hip d.
elbow d. (ED)
joint d.
Lisfranc d.
Mazet knee d.
metatarsophalangeal joint d.
sacroiliac d.
shoulder d. (SD)
wrist d. (WD)
DISC
dynamic integrated stabilization chair
disc (*var. of* disk)
discectomy (*var. of* diskectomy)
discharge
bizarre high-frequency d.
bizarre repetitive d.
complex repetitive d.
coupled d.
cramp d.
double d.
d. frequency
grouped d.
multiple d.
myokymic d.
myotonic d.
neuromyotonic d.
paired d.
pseudomyotonic d.
repetitive d.
triple d.
waning d.
disci (*pl. of* discus)
discission knife Beaver blade
discitis (*var. of* diskitis)
discogenic (*var. of* diskogenic)
discogram (*var. of* diskogram)
discography (*var. of* diskography)
discoid lateral meniscus
discoligamentous injury
discometry (*var. of* diskometry)
discontinuity
pelvic d.

discopathogenic
discopathy
traumatic cervical d.
Disc-O-Sit Jr. cushion
discotome (*var. of* diskotome)
discrepancy
leg length d. (LLD)
limb length d.
discrete activity
discrimination
Ayres tactile d.
right/left d.
sharp/dull d.
two-point d.
Weber static two-point d.
discus, pl. **disci**
disease
Albers-Schönberg d.
Albert d.
Albright d.
allograft coronary artery d.
Apert d.
Aran-Duchenne d.
Assmann d.
Atton d.
Baastrup d.
Bamberger-Marie d.
basic calcium phosphate crystal deposition d.
Bechterew d.
Bekhterev d.
Bielschowsky-Jansky d.
Blount d.
Blount-Barber d.
bone d.
Bourneville d.
Brailsford d.
brittle bone d.
Brodie d.
Bruck d.
Buchanan d.
Budlinger-Ludlof-Laewen d.
Burns d.
Busquet d.
Caffey d.
Caffey-Kenny d.
calcium pyrophosphate dihydrate deposition d.
Calvé-Perthes d.
Canavan d.
Canavan-van Bogaert-Bertrand d.
cement d.

NOTES

disease *(continued)*
    cementless d.
    central core d.
    cervical disk d.
    Chandler d.
    Charcot joint d.
    Charcot-Marie-Tooth d.
    chronic tophaceous d.
    CMT d.
    collagen vascular d. (CVD)
    connective tissue d.
    Conradi d.
    d. construct
    coronary artery d. (CAD)
    Cruveilhier d.
    crystal-related joint d.
    Curschmann-Steinert d.
    cystic d.
    deer tick d.
    degenerative disk d. (DDD)
    degenerative joint d. (DJD)
    Dejerine d.
    Dejerine-Sottas d.
    denervation d.
    de Quervain d.
    destructive bone d.
    destructive joint d.
    Deutschländer d.
    Diaz d.
    Di Guglielmo d.
    disappearing bone d.
    double Charcot d.
    Duchenne d.
    Duchenne-Aran d.
    Duplay d.
    Dupuytren d.
    Eddowes d.
    Ehlers-Danlos d.
    Ehrenfeld d.
    Emery-Dreifuss d.
    Engelmann d.
    Engel-Recklinghausen d.
    Erb-Landouzy d.
    Erdheim-Chester d.
    Erichsen d.
    facet joint d. (FJD)
    fascioscapulohumeral muscle
      atrophy d.
    Felix d.
    fibromuscular d.
    Forestier d.
    Freiberg d.
    Freiberg-Kohler d.
    Friedreich d.
    Garré d.
    Garrod d.
    Gaucher d.
    glenohumeral joint d.

    Gorham d.
    Grisel d.
    Gumboro d.
    Haas d.
    Haglund d.
    handcuff d.
    Hand-Schüller-Christian d.
    Hansen d.
    Heberden d.
    Henderson-Jones d.
    hereditary neuropathic d.
    Hoffa d.
    Hoffa-Kastert d.
    Hospital for Joint D. (HJD)
    Hurler d.
    hydroxyapatite deposition d.
    hypophosphatemic bone d.
    ischemic leg d.
    ischemic limb d. (ILD)
    Iselin d.
    Jaffe d.
    Jansen d.
    Jüngling d.
    Kashin-Bek d.
    Kienböck d.
    Koehler d.
    Köhler d.
    Köhler-Pellegrini-Stieda d.
    König d.
    Kugelberg-Welander d.
    Kümmell d.
    Kümmell-Verneuil d.
    Lance d.
    Larsen d.
    Larsen-Johansson d.
    Ledderhose d.
    lederhosen d.
    Legg-Calvé-Perthes d. (LCPD)
    Legg-Calvé-Waldenström d.
    Legg-Perthes d.
    Leri d.
    Leri-Weill d.
    Lichtman d.
    Lobstein d.
    Lyme d.
    MacLean-Maxwell d.
    Maffucci d.
    Marie-Bamberger d.
    Marie-Charcot-Tooth d.
    Marie-Strümpell d.
    Maroteaux-Lamy d.
    marrow d.
    Martin d.
    Mauclaire d.
    McArdle d.
    metabolic bone d.
    metastatic d.
    Meyer-Betz d.

milk-alkali d.
mini-core d.
mixed connective tissue d.
modified Kienböck d.
Moeller-Barlow d.
Morquio d.
Morquio-Ullrich d.
Morton d.
motor neuron d.
Mouchet d.
Munchmeyer d.
National Institute of Arthritis and
  Musculoskeletal and Skin D.'s
  (NIAMS)
neurogenic d.
neuromuscular d.
neuropathic joint d.
oligoarticular d.
Ollier d.
Oppenheim d.
Osgood-Schlatter d.
Otto d.
Paas d.
Paget d.
Panner d.
Parkinson d.
Pauzat d.
Pellegrini d.
Pellegrini-Stieda d.
peripheral arterial occlusive d.
  (PAOD)
peripheral vascular d. (PVD)
peripheral vascular obstructive d.
Perrin-Ferraton d.
Perthes d.
Poncet d.
Pott d.
Poulet d.
Preiser d.
pseudo-Pott d.
Pyle d.
Quervain d.
quiet hip d.
Raynaud d.
Recklinghausen d.
Reiter d.
rheumatoid d.
Roussy-Lévy d.
Rust d.
Schanz d.
Scheuermann d.
Schlatter d.

Schlatter-Osgood d.
Schmid d.
Schmorl d.
senile hip d.
Sever d.
Silfverskiöld d.
Sinding-Larsen-Johansson d.
skeletal hypoplasia d.
Steinert d.
steroid-induced bone d.
Still d.
Strümpell d.
Strümpell-Marie d.
Sudeck d.
Swediauer d.
synovial d.
Talma d.
Taratynov d.
Thiemann d.
Thomsen d.
thromboembolic d. (TED)
Trevor d.
upper motor neuron d.
Van der Hoeve d.
Van Neck d.
venous thromboembolic d. (VTED)
Volkmann d.
von Recklinghausen d.
Voorhoeve d.
Vrolik d.
Wagner d.
Waldenström d.
Wegner d.
Werdnig-Hoffmann d.
Wohlfart-Kugelberg-Welander d.
Woringer-Kolopp d.
Ziehen-Oppenheim d.
disease-modifying antirheumatologic drug
  (DMARD)
DISH
    diffuse idiopathic skeletal hyperostosis
    DISH syndrome
dishpan fracture
DISI
    distal intercalated segment instability
    dorsal intercalated segment instability
    dorsiflexed intercalated segment
      instability
    DISI collapse pattern
    DISI deformity
disk, disc
    Acro-Flex artificial d.

NOTES

195

disk *(continued)*
    acromioclavicular d.
    amphiarthrodial d.
    d. of ankle
    articular d.
    Bardeen primitive d.
    Bowman d.
    d. bulge
    bulging d.
    cartilaginous d.
    cervical d.
    choked d.
    d. compression
    contained herniated d.
    crescent-shaped fibrocartilaginous d.
    d. degeneration
    d. diffusion method
    d. diffusion test
    d. electrode
    Engelmann d.
    d. excision
    excision of intervertebral d.
    extruded d.
    d. extrusion
    fibrocartilaginous d.
    fixation d.
    d. forceps
    d. fragment
    frayed d.
    d. grabber
    hard d.
    herniated d.
    herniated intervertebral d. (HID)
    d. herniation
    I d.
    interarticular d.
    intermediate d.
    interpubic d.
    intervertebral d.
    intraarticular d.
    isotropic d.
    J d.
    d. lesion
    locking d.
    lumbar d.
    massive herniated d.
    noncontained d.
    d. plication
    d. pressure
    d. prolapse
    protruding d.
    d. protrusion
    Q d.
    d. rongeur
    ruptured d.
    sequestered d.
    sequestrated d.
    slipped d.

    d. space
    d. space saline acceptance test
    sternoclavicular d.
    swollen d.
    d. syndrome
    thin d.
    transverse d.
    vacuum d.
    Z d.
Diskard head halter
Disk-Criminator
    D.-C. nerve stimulation measuring
      device
    D.-C. sensory testing
diskectomy, discectomy
    automated percutaneous d. (APD)
    automated percutaneous lumbar d.
      (APLD)
    cervical d.
    Cloward fusion d.
    laminotomy and d.
    microlumbar d. (MLD)
    microsurgical d. (MSD)
    partial d.
    PercScope percutaneous d.
    percutaneous lumbar d.
    Robinson anterior cervical d.
    SMALL fluoroscopic d.
    Smith-Robinson anterior cervical d.
    Williams d.
    Wiltse d.
    d. with Cloward fusion
diskitis, discitis
    juvenile d.
diskogenic, discogenic
    d. neck pain
diskogram, discogram
    d. needle
diskography, discography
    cervical d.
    Cloward fusion d.
    lumbar d.
    microlumbar d.
    Williams d.
diskometry, discometry
diskotome, discotome
    Pheasant d.
dislocated
    d. knee
    d. patella
dislocating arthropathy
dislocatio erecta
dislocation
    acromioclavicular joint d.
    ankle d.
    antenatal d.
    anterior hip d.
    anterior-inferior d.

anterior shoulder d.
anterolateral d.
d. of articular process
atlantoaxial d. (AAD)
atlantooccipital joint d.
atypical d.
Bankart shoulder d.
bayonet d.
Bell-Dally cervical d.
Bennett basic hand d.
bilateral interfacetal d. (BID)
boutonnière hand d.
bursting d.
Carnesale-Stewart-Barnes
  classification of hip d.
carpal d.
carpometacarpal joint d.
central d.
Chopart ankle d.
chronic recurrent ankle joint d.
closed d.
complete d.
complex fracture d.
complicated d.
compound d.
congenital hip d.
congenital patella d.
consecutive d.
d. contour abnormality
Copeland-Kavat classification of
  metatarsophalangeal d.
Cotton reduction of elbow d.
dashboard d.
Desault wrist d.
direct injury elbow d.
divergent elbow d.
dorsal perilunate d.
dorsal transscaphoid perilunar d.
elbow d.
facet d.
d. factor
fracture d.
frank d.
gamekeeper's thumb d.
glenohumeral joint d.
habitual d.
Hill-Sachs shoulder d.
hip d.
incomplete d.
interphalangeal joint d.
intraarticular d.
irreducible fracture d.

isolated d.
Jahss classification of ankle d.
joint d.
Kienböck d.
knee d.
Kocher reduction of shoulder d.
ligamentous anterior d. (LAD)
Lisfranc d.
lumbosacral d.
lunate d.
luxatio erecta shoulder d.
medial swivel d.
metacarpophalangeal d.
metatarsophalangeal joint d.
Meyn reduction of elbow d.
milkmaid's elbow d.
Monteggia d.
Nélaton ankle d.
neuropathic joint d.
occipitoatlantal d.
old unreduced d.
open d.
Osborne-Cotterill elbow d.
Otto pelvis d.
Palmer transscaphoid perilunar d.
panclavicular d.
parachute jumper's d.
Pare elbow d. reduction
partial d.
patellar intraarticular d.
pathologic d.
perilunar transscaphoid d.
perilunate carpal d.
peroneal d.
phalangeal d.
posterior facet d.
posterior hip d.
posterior shoulder d.
posteromedial d.
prenatal d.
primitive d.
proximal tibiofibular joint d.
radial head d.
radiocarpal d.
radioulnar d.
recent d.
recurrent patellar d.
retrosternal d.
sacroiliac d.
shoulder d.
simple d.
Smith d.

D

NOTES

dislocation *(continued)*
    spontaneous hyperemic d.
    sternoclavicular joint d.
    subastragalar d.
    subcoracoid shoulder d.
    subglenoid shoulder d.
    subspinous d.
    subtalar joint d.
    superior d.
    swivel d.
    talar d.
    talonavicular d.
    tarsal d.
    tarsometatarsal d.
    temporomandibular joint d.
    teratologic d.
    tibialis posterior d.
    tibiofibular joint d.
    transscaphoid perilunate d.
    traumatic d.
    triquetrolunate d.
    unilateral interfacetal d.
    unreduced d.
    volar semilunar wrist d.
dislodgment
    hook d.
disorder
    adrenal d.
    ARS d.
    clotting d.
    coagulation d.
    congenital limb d.
    cumulative trauma d. (CTD)
    degenerative d.
    gait d.
    mixed connective tissue d.
    motor speech d.
    movement d.
    muscle d.
    myeloproliferative d.
    neurogenic d.
    neurologic d.
    neuromuscular junction d.
    nontotal-contact d.
    patellofemoral d.
    peripheral neurocompressive d.
    progressive neurologic d.
    recurrent d.
    repetitive strain d.
    repetitive stress d.
    repetitive trauma d. (RTD)
    retrocalcaneal d.
    rheumatoid d.
    rheumatologic d.
    spastic d.
    tendon d.
    trophic joint d.
    vasomotor d.

disorganized bone
disparity
    limb-length d.
dispenser
    Jet Vac cement d.
dispersion
    temporal d.
displaced
    d. intraarticular calcaneus
    d. intraarticular fracture
    d. pilon fracture
    d. vertebra
displacement
    angular d.
    d. anterior cavus V osteotomy
    atlantoaxial rotary d.
    crosshead d.
    d. curve
    Ellis-Jones peroneal tendon d.
    fracture fragment d.
    interregional d.
    lateral rotary d.
    Laurin lateral patella d.
    left-right leg d.
    load-to-grip d.
    medial d.
    oblique d.
    peroneal tendon d.
    posterior facet d.
    rotary d.
    tendon d.
    translational d.
    traumatic d.
    Y-axis translatory d.
display
    head-mounted d. (HMD)
    high-definition video d.
disposable
    d. muscle biopsy clamp
    d. one-piece osteotome
Disposatrode disposable electrode
disproportionate dwarfism
disrelationship
    persistent occiput/atlas d.
disruption
    anterior column d.
    cervical spine posterior ligament d.
    Charcot d.
    end-stage d.
    facet capsule d.
    fibular joint d.
    forefoot d.
    interosseous ligament d.
    joint d.
    lateral compartment d.
    ligamentous d.
    medial compartment d.
    pedicle cortex d.

physial d.
sesamoid d.
skeletal d.
talocalcaneal ligament d.

dissecans
osteochondritis d. (OCD, OD)

dissecting
d. clamp
d. probe
d. scissors

dissection
blunt d.
bone d.
deep iliac d.
extracapsular d.
field of d.
fingertip d.
Pack-Ehrlich deep iliac d.
sharp d.
subligamentous d.
subperiosteal d.

dissector
Angell James d.
angled d.
ball d.
blunt hook d.
bunion d.
Creed d.
Crile gasserian ganglion knife and d.
Davis dura d.
dura d.
Effler-Groves d.
Freer d.
golf stick d.
grooved d.
Hajek-Ballenger d.
hand d.
hockey stick d.
joker d.
Kidner d.
Kocher d.
Lewin bunion d.
McDonald d.
Penfield 4 d.
sesamoidectomy d.
transsphenoidal d.
West hand d.

disseminated
d. intravascular coagulation (DIC)
d. pigmented villonodular synovitis

dissociation
carpal instability d. (CID)
hypnotic d.
lunotriquetral d.
d. movement
radioulnar d.
scapholunate d.
scapulothoracic d.

dissociative anesthesia

distal
d. articular set angle (DASA)
d. biceps brachii tendon rupture
d. bone end
d. calcaneus
d. clavicular excision
d. communicating branch (DCB)
d. compression test
d. concave articular surface
d. dystrophy
d. femoral cutting guide
d. femoral epiphysial fracture
d. femoral resection
d. femur
d. fibula
d. fibulotalar arthrodesis
d. forearm
d. fragment
d. humeral epiphysis
d. humeral fracture
d. humerus
d. intercalated segment instability (DISI)
d. interlocking
d. interphalangeal (DIP)
d. interphalangeal joint (DIPJ)
d. intrinsic release
d. latency
d. locking
d. locking screw
d. L osteotomy
d. medial creaking
d. metaphysis
d. metatarsal articular angle (DMAA)
d. neurolysis
d. oblique sliding osteotomy
d. palmar crease (DPC)
d. parabola toe length
d. phalanx (DP)
d. phocomelia
d. radial fracture
d. radioulnar joint (DRUJ)

D

NOTES

distal *(continued)*
   d. radioulnar joint prosthesis
   d. radioulnar joint stabilization
   d. radius
   d. realignment
   d. reference axis (DRA)
   d. row carpectomy
   d. segment weight
   d. soft tissue release (DSTR)
   d. star pad
   d. targeting
   d. targeting device
   d. thigh band
   d. third (D/3, distal/3)
   d. third of shaft
   d. tibia
   d. tibial epiphysial injury
   d. tibial physis
   d. tibiofibular fusion
   d. tibiofibular joint
   d. transfer
   d. tuberosity of finger
   d. tuberosity of toe
   d. tuft
   d. ulna
   d. ulnar convexity
   d. Wagner femoral metaphysial
      shortening
distal/3
   distal third
distalward
distance
   coracoclavicular d.
   focal film d.
   fulcrum d.
   protrusion d.
distension
distolateral
distoocclusal
distortion
   multisegmental spinal d.
   sacral base d.
   structural intersegmental d.
distraction
   apical d.
   d. arthroplasty
   d. bar
   d. bone block arthrodesis
   calcaneal d.
   callus d.
   d. clamp
   fixed d.
   flexion d.
   d. force
   d. of fracture
   fracture fragment d.
   Guhl d.
   halo-cast d.

halo-femoral d.
halo-pelvic d.
d. histogenesis
d. hook
d. injury
d. instrumentation
d. instrumentation biomechanics
joint d.
d. laminoplasty
d. lengthening
longitudinal d.
manipulation with d.
Monticelli-Spinelli d.
d. osteogenesis
physial d.
d. pin
d. rod
d. screw
slow d.
small step d.
spinal d.
d. subtalar arthrodesis
d. technique
d. test
distraction-compression
   d.-c. bone graft arthrodesis
   d.-c. scoliosis treatment
distraction-flexion stage (DFS)
distractive
   d. extension
   d. flexion
   d. motion
distractor
   Acufex ankle d.
   Anderson d.
   AO femoral d.
   Bliskunov implantable femoral d.
   DeBastiani d.
   femoral d.
   hook d.
   Ilizarov d.
   intramedullary skeletal kinetic d.
     (ISKD)
   joint d.
   Kessler metacarpal d.
   Mark II distal femur d.
   Monticelli-Spinelli d.
   Mueller d.
   Orthofix M-100 d.
   Pinto d.
   Santa Casa d.
   turnbuckle d.
   Wagner d.
distribution
   Boltzmann d.
   cutaneous d.
   stocking-glove d.
   stress d.

disturbance
articulation d.
gait d.
pain-related sleep d.
disuse
d. arthropathy
d. atrophy
d. osteoporosis
diurnal
d. change
d. variation in straight leg raising
divergence
angle of d.
anteroposterior talocalcaneal d.
divergent elbow dislocation
diversified
D. chiropractic manipulative therapy
d. manipulation
diversified-type force application
diversional activity
divided navicular
division
Swafford-Lichtman d.
divisionary line
divot sign
Dix-Hallpike maneuver
DJD
degenerative joint disease
DKB
deep knee bend
D-L internal fixator
DMAA
distal metatarsal articular angle
DMARD
disease-modifying antirheumatologic
drug
DMI orthopedic bed
DOA
diagnostic and operative arthroscopy
Doane knee retractor
Doctor Collins fracture clamp
documented pseudarthrosis
Dodd perforator
DOF
degrees of freedom
doffing
donning and d.
d. prosthesis
dog-ear repair
dogleg fracture

dolichostenomelia
doll
d. eye sign
Lizzie d.
D. trochanteric reattachment
D. trochanteric reattachment
technique
dollar
d. sign
d. sign side
dollop
bone d.
dolorimeter
dolorosus
hallux d.
dome
d. fracture
Maquet d.
d. plunger
d. proximal tibial osteotomy
shoulder d.
talar d.
weightbearing acetabular d.
dome-shaped osteotomy
dominance
hand d.
left-hand d.
right-hand d.
domino spinal instrumentation connector
Donaghy angled suture needle holder
Donati suture
DonJoy
D. ALP brace
D. four-point Super Sport knee
brace
D. Gold Point knee brace
D. knee splint
D. Opal knee brace
D. Quadrant shoulder brace
D. Ultrasling shoulder immobilizer
D. Universal ankle brace
D. wrist splint
donning
d. and doffing
d. prosthesis
donning-doffing skill
donor
d. site
d. team
donut support brace

D

NOTES

DOOR
  deafness, onychoosteodystrophy, mental
    retardation
  DOOR syndrome
Doppler
  D. ankle systolic pressure
  D. pulse evaluation
  D. scope
  D. study
  D. technique
  D. ultrasound
  D. ultrasound flowmeter
Dorello canal
Dorr
  D. bone classification
  D. ratio
Dorrance
  D. hand prosthesis
  D. procedure
dorsal
  d. arch of wrist
  d. aspect
  d. bunion
  d. calcaneocuboid (DCC)
  d. capsule
  d. capsulodesis
  d. carpal capsulitis
  d. cheilectomy
  d. columella implant
  d. column stimulator (DCS)
  d. column stimulator implant
  d. compartment
  d. cross-finger flap
  d. cutaneous nerve
  d. digital artery (DDA)
  d. drainage
  d. drawer test
  d. extension block splint
  d. finger approach
  d. glide
  d. hood
  d. horn cell
  d. intercalated segment instability
    (DISI)
  d. interosseous muscle
  d. kyphotic curvature
  d. linear incision
  d. lithotomy position
  d. longitudinal incision
  d. lordosis
  d. lumbar corset
  d. malalignment
  d. metatarsal artery
  d. midline approach
  d. neuroma
  d. pedal bypass
  d. pedal pulse
  d. perilunate dislocation

  d. planar x-ray
  d. point
  d. radial slope
  d. rami
  d. recumbent position
  d. reflex
  d. ridge
  d. root entry zone (DREZ)
  d. root ganglion (DRG)
  d. root ganglionectomy
  d. scapular nerve
  d. skin
  d. subcutaneous nerve transposition
  d. synovectomy
  d. tenosynovectomy
  d. toe plate extension
  d. translation
  d. transscaphoid perilunar
    dislocation
  d. transverse capsulotomy
  d. transverse incision
  d. ulnar cutaneous branch
  d. venous arch of hand
  d. vertebra
  d. wing
  d. wing fracture
  d. wire-loop fixation
  d. wrist splint
  d. wrist splint with outrigger
dorsalgia
dorsalia
dorsalis
  d. pedis artery anatomy
  d. pedis fasciocutaneous flap
  d. pedis pulse
  tabes d.
dorsal-V osteotomy
dorsalward approach
Dorsey screw-holding screwdriver
dorsi
  elastofibroma d.
  d. jam syndrome
  latissimus d.
  osteochondritis deformans
    juvenilis d.
  d. stop component
dorsiflexed
  d. intercalated segment instability
    (DISI)
  d. metatarsal
dorsiflexion
  active d.
  d. angle (DFA)
  d. assist ankle joint ankle-foot
    orthosis
  d. bumper
  d. flexion
  d. foot splint

d. metatarsal osteotomy
passive d.
resisted d.
d. stop brace
d. stress ankle x-ray
d. view
dorsiflexion-eversion test
dorsiflexion-plantar flexion position
dorsiflexor gait
dorsiflexory wedge osteotomy
Dorsiwedge night splint
dorsodynia
dorsolateral
d. approach
d. and medial capsulotomy
dorsolumbar area
dorsomedial
d. approach
d. cutaneous nerve
d. incision
dorsoplantar
d. approach
d. capsulotomy
d. projection
d. radiographic view
d. talometatarsal angle
d. talonavicular angle
dorsoradial
d. approach
d. ligament (DRL)
dorsorostral approach
dorsoulnar approach
dorsum of hand
double
d. arthrodesis
d. Becker ankle brace
d. bent Hohmann acetabular
retractor
d. binocular operating microscope
d. camelback sign
d. Charcot disease
d. clamp
d. Cobra plate
d. contrast arthrotomography of
shoulder
d. corn deformity
d. crush syndrome
d. discharge
d. drape
D. Duty cane
D. Duty cane reacher
d. flexion wave

d. fracture
d. hemiplegia
d. hip spica cast
d. hump contour
d. incision
d. inflow cannula system
d. jointed
d. leg raise test
d. major curve pattern
d. major curve scoliosis
d. major spinal curve
d. osteotomy
d. pearl-face hip joint
d. portal technique
d. right-angle suture
d. simultaneous sensory stimulation
d. support time
d. tendon transfer
d. thoracic curve
d. thoracic curve scoliosis
d. tourniquet
d. Zielke instrumentation
double-action
d.-a. ankle joint
d.-a. bone-cutting forceps
d.-a. cutter
d.-a. rongeur
double-arc sign
double-cannula system
double-clamp approximator
double-contrast
d.-c. arthrogram
d.-c. arthrography
d.-c. study
double-ended
d.-e. nail
d.-e. right-angle retractor
double-flap amputation
double-flexion knee motion
double-headed stereotactic carrier
double-hollow nail
double-hook Lovejoy retractor
double-H plate
double-incision fasciotomy
double-leg stance phase of gait
double-looped
d.-l. gracilis graft
d.-l. semitendinous and gracilis
hamstring graft knee
reconstruction technique
double-L spinal rod
double-needle chemonucleolysis

D

NOTES

double-occlusal splint
double-open hook
double-pendulum action
double-pronged skin hook
double-ring frame
double-rod
    d.-r. construct
    d.-r. technique
double-sharp forceps
double-stem
    d.-s. silicone implant
    d.-s. silicone lesser MP joint
double-step gait
double-stranded wire double-twisted
  wire
doublet
double-tap gait
double-threaded Herbert screw
double-thumb thrust
double-upright short leg brace
Double-Z rhombic skin flap
doughnut
    d. headrest
    d. ring
doughy
    d. cement
    d. consistency
Douglas skin graft
Dow
    D. Corning titanium hemi-implant
    D. Corning Wright finger joint
    prosthesis
dowager's hump
dowel
    d. arthrodesis
    bone d.
    d. bone graft
    calf bone d.
    cylindrical d.
    graft d.
    d. graft technique
    d. grip
    iliac crest d.
    d. spinal fusion
    threaded cortical d.
doweled
doweling
    d. spondylolisthesis
    d. spondylolisthesis technique
down
    D. epiphysial knife
    D. syndrome
down-angle hook
downbiting rongeur
Downey
    D. hemilaminectomy retractor

    D. modification of Fowler-Philip
    approach
    D. texture discrimination test
Downey-McGlamery procedure
Downey-Rubin overlapping toe repair
  procedure
downgoing toes
Downing
    D. cartilage knife
    D. staple
downsized circular laminar hook
Doyan periosteal elevator
Doyen
    D. bone mallet
    D. costal rasp
    D. cylindrical bur
    D. cylindrical drill
    D. rib elevator
    D. rib rasp
    D. spherical bur
Dozier radiolucent Bennett retractor
DP
    distal phalanx
    Springlite Advantage DP
DPA
    dual-photon absorptiometry
DPB
    dynamic pedobarography
DPC
    delayed primary closure
    distal palmar crease
DPD
    dual photon densitometry
DPTT
    deep posterior tibiotalar
    DPTT ligament
DPVNS
    diffuse pigmented villonodular synovitis
DPX
    dual-photon absorptiometry
Dr.
    Dr. Grip writing device
    Dr. Joseph's diabetic foot kit
    Dr. Joseph's Original Footbrush
    Dr. Kho's CMC Support
DRA
    distal reference axis
drafting
    overlay d.
Dragstedt skin graft
drag-to gait
drain
    Charnley suction d.
    fishmouth d.
    Hemovac Hydrocoat d.
    Heyer-Schulte wound d.
    Jackson-Pratt d.
    Nélaton rubber tube d.

open fracture wound d.
Penrose d.
polyethylene d.
PVC d.
rubber d.
Shirley d.
Silastic d.
subcutaneous d.
Surgivac d.
Wound-Evac d.

drainage
anterior d.
anterolateral d.
anteromedial d.
ConstaVac d.
David d.
dorsal d.
ilium d.
incision and d. (I&D)
infusion-aspiration d.
Klein d.
lateral d.
medial d.
Ober posterior d.
open d.
pelvic d.
posterior d.
posterolateral d.
posteromedial d.
suction d.

draining infected nonunion
DRAM
deepithelialized rectus abdominis muscle
DRAM flap

drape
adhesive d.
double d.
fenestrated d.
foot d.
incise d.
isolation d.
lint-free d.
Loban adhesive d.
3M skin d.
NeuroDrape surgical d.
Opmi microscopic d.
Opraflex d.

draped out
drawer
flexion-rotation-d. (FRD)
d. sign
d. test

drawing
pain d.
preoperative d.
drawn ankle clonus
dream
D. Pillow
D. Ride car seat
Drennan
D. metaphysial-epiphysial angle
D. posterior transfer
DressFlex
D. orthotic
D. orthotic device
Dressinet netting bandage
dressing
abdominal d.
absorptive d.
ACU-derm wound d.
Adaptic d.
adhesive d.
Aeroplast d.
Alginate d.
AlgiSite Alginate wound d.
Allevyn Island d.
Allevyn wound d.
d. apraxia
Aquaphor gauze d.
Aquasorb hydrogel wound d.
Arglaes film d.
Arthrosol d.
Avitene flour d.
Betadine d.
Bioclusive select transparent
film d.
biologic d.
Blister Film d.
Breast Vest Exu-Dry one-piece
wound d.
bulky hand d.
bundle d.
Bunnell d.
calcium alginate d.
CarboFlex odor-control d.
Cica-Care wound d.
circumferential d.
Coban elastic d.
CoFilm d.
cold compressive d.
collodion d.
CombiDERM nonadhesive
absorbent d.
Comfeel Ulcus occlusive d.

NOTES

dressing *(continued)*

Compeed protective d.
compression d.
conductive Hydrogel wound d.
Conform d.
CoolSorb absorbent cold transfer d.
Coraderm d.
corrective soft d.
cotton d.
Covaderm Plus adhesive barrier d.
Coverlet adhesive surgical d.
Coverlet Strips wound d.
Cover-Roll adhesive gauze d.
Covertell composite secondary d.
Co-Wrap d.
Cryo/Cuff ankle d.
Cutinova cavity d.
Cutinova foam d.
Cutinova thin d.
Dermagran hydrophilic gauze d.
Dermagran ointment wound d.
DermaSite d.
Dermiflex d.
Digi Sleeve stockinette d.
dry sterile d. (DSD)
DuoDerm d.
Eakin cohesive seal d.
Elastikon d.
Elastomull d.
Elastoplast d.
Ensure-It d.
Epigard d.
Esmarch d.
Exu-Dry wound d.
Fabco gauze d.
felt d.
figure-of-eight d.
fixed d.
Flexderm wound d.
Flexigrid d.
Flexinet d.
fluff d.
Fuller shield d.
Furacin gauze d.
FyBron d.
gauze d.
Geliperm d.
Gelocast Unna boot compression d.
Glasscock ear d.
Granuflex d.
hydrocolloid occlusive d.
Hydrocol wound d.
Hydrogel wound d.
Inerpan flexible burn d.
Intact d.
IntraSite d.
J&J ulcer d.
Jones d.

Kaltostat d.
Kelikian foot d.
Kerlix d.
Kling adhesive d.
Koch-Mason d.
Kollagen d.
LYOfoam C d.
LYOfoam wound d.
Medi-Rip d.
Microfoam d.
Mills d.
modified Robert Jones d.
moleskin strip d.
Mother Jones d.
neoprene d.
nonadherent gauze d.
N-Terface d.
Nu Gauze d.
NutraFill hydrophilic d.
NutraStat wound d.
OASIS wound d.
occlusive d.
O'Donoghue d.
Omniderm d.
Opraflex d.
OpSite wound d.
Orthoflex d.
Orthoplast d.
OsmoCyte Island wound-care d.
Owen gauze d.
palm-to-axilla d.
Panogauze Hydrogel wound d.
patch d.
pledget d.
Polyderm hydrophilic polyurethane
  foam d.
PolyMem wound care d.
polymeric d.
Polyskin d.
polyurethane foam d. (PFD)
PolyWic d.
pressure ulcer d.
Primaderm d.
Primapore wound d.
ProCyte transparent d.
Profore wound d.
PVD d.
RepliCare wound d.
Reston d.
Restore CalciCare d.
rigid d.
Robert Jones d.
Schanz d.
Scherisorb d.
semirigid postoperative d.
Setopress d.
SignaDRESS hydrocolloid d.
Silastic gel d.

silk mesh gauze d.
SkinTemp collagen skin d.
sling d.
Sof-Rol d.
soft bulky d.
Sof-Wick d.
Spenco Second Skin d.
stent d.
sterile dry d. (SDD)
d. stick
Stimson d.
SuperSkin thin film d.
Surgilast tubular elastic d.
Suture-Self d.
Synthaderm d.
Tegaderm d.
Telfa gauze d.
THINSite d.
Toe-Aid d.
toe-to-groin modified Jones d.
transparent adhesive d.
Tricodur Epi compression d.
Tricodur Omos compression d.
Tricodur Talus compression d.
Tubex gauze d.
Tubigrip d.
Ultec thin d.
Uniflex d.
Velpeau d.
Vi-Drape d.
Vigilon d.
Webril d.
wet-to-dry d.
wide-mesh petroleum gauze d.
Xeroform gauze d.

Dreyer formula
Dreyfus
D. prosthesis forceps
D. prosthesis placement instrument
DREZ
dorsal root entry zone
DREZ lesion
DREZ modification of Eriksson
technique
DREZ procedure
DRG
dorsal root ganglion
DRI
dietary reference intake
Driessen hinged plate
drift
arm d.

congenital ulnar d.
leg d.
osseous d.
pronator d.
radial d.
ulnar d.

drill
ACL d.
Acra-Cut wire pass d.
Acufex d.
Adson-Rogers perforating d.
Adson spiral d.
Adson twist d.
Aesculap d.
agility d.
air d.
air-powered cutting d.
Albee d.
Amico d.
Anspach power d.
anticavitation d.
Archimedean d.
ASIF twist d.
ASSI wire-pass d.
autotome d.
Bailey d.
bar d.
battery-driven hand d.
biflanged d.
bit d.
d. bit
d. bit fracture
Björk rib d.
bone hand d.
Bosworth crown d.
Bowen suture d.
brace d.
Brunswick-Mack rotating d.
Bunnell bone d.
Bunnell hand d.
bur d.
cannulated cortical step d.
Carmody perforator d.
Carroll-Bunnell d.
Cebotome bone cement d.
Cement Eater d.
centering d.
cervical d.
Championnière bone d.
Charnley centering d.
Charnley femoral condyle d.
Charnley pilot d.

NOTES

drill *(continued)*
    Charnley starting d.
    Cherry d.
    Cherry-Austin d.
    Children's Hospital hand d.
    chuck d.
    Cloward cervical d.
    Coballoy twist d.
    Codman wire-passing d.
    Collison body d.
    Collison cannulated hand d.
    Collison tap d.
    cortical step d.
    crown d.
    Crutchfield bone d.
    Crutchfield hand d.
    Crutchfield-Raney d.
    CurvTek TSR bone d.
    Cushing flat d.
    Cushing perforator d.
    dental d.
    depth-check d.
    DePuy d.
    D'Errico perforating d.
    Deyerle d.
    diamond high-speed d.
    Doyen cylindrical d.
    driver nail d.
    Elan d.
    Elan-E power d.
    extractor nail d.
    fingernail d.
    Fisch d.
    flat d.
    Galt hand d.
    Gates-Glidden d.
    glenoid d.
    Gray bone d.
    d. guard
    d. guide
    d. guide forceps
    Hall air d.
    Hall-Dundar d.
    Hall Micro-Aire d.
    Hall power d.
    Hall stepdown d.
    Hall Versipower d.
    Hamby twist d.
    hand d.
    hand-operated d.
    Harold Crowe d.
    Harris-Smith anterior interbody d.
    Hewson d.
    high-speed twist d.
    hip fraction compaction d.
    d. hole
    hollow mill d.
    Hudson bone d.
    Hudson brace d.
    initiator d.
    intramedullary d.
    Jacobs chuck d.
    Jordan-Day d.
    Kerr electro-torque d.
    Kerr hand d.
    Kirschner bone d.
    Kirschner wire d.
    Kodex d.
    Küntscher d.
    Lentulo spiral d.
    Loth-Kirschner d.
    Luck bone d.
    Lusskin bone d.
    Macewen d.
    Magnuson twist d.
    Mathews hand d.
    Mathews load d.
    McKenzie bone d.
    McKenzie perforating twist d.
    Michelson-Sequoia air d.
    Micro-Aire d.
    Midas Rex d.
    mini-Stryker power d.
    Minos air d.
    Mira d.
    Modny d.
    Moore bone d.
    nail d.
    Neil-Moore perforator d.
    Neurain d.
    Neurairtome d.
    nippers nail d.
    Orthairtome II d.
    Osseodent surgical d.
    Osteone air d.
    Patrick d.
    Pease bone d.
    pencil-tip d.
    penetrating d.
    Penn finger d.
    perforating twist d.
    perforator d.
    pilot d.
    d. pin
    pistol-grip hand d.
    Podospray podiatry d.
    d. point
    Portmann d.
    power d.
    pronator d.
    Ralks bone d.
    Ralks fingernail d.
    Raney bone d.
    Raney perforator d.
    retention d.
    rib d.

Rica bone d.
Richards Lovejoy bone d.
Richards pistol-grip d.
Richmond subarachnoid twist d.
Richter bone d.
right-angle dental d.
scissors nail d.
Shea d.
Sherman-Stille d.
Sklar bone d.
d. sleeve
Smedberg hand d.
Smedberg twist d.
SMIC sternal d.
Smith automatic perforated d.
spiral d.
Spirec d.
step d.
step-down d.
Stille bone d.
Stille hand d.
Stille-Sherman bone d.
Stiwer hand d.
Stryker d.
Surgairtome air d.
surgical orthopedic d.
suture hole d.
Synthes d.
tap d.
Thornwald antral d.
Toti trephine d.
Treace stapes d.
trephine d.
Trinkle bone d.
Trinkle power d.
Trinkle Super-Cut twist d.
Trowbridge-Campau bone d.
Trow Bridge triple-speed d.
twist d.
Ullrich d.
Uniflex calibrated step d.
union broach retention d.
Universal two-speed hand d.
Vitallium d.
Warren-Mack rotating d.
wire d.
Wolferman d.
Wullstein d.
Xomed d.
Zimmer Cebotome bone cement d.
Zimmer hand d.

Zimmer-Kirschner hand d.
Zimmer Universal d.
drill-guide
Acufex d.-g.
drilling
arthroscopic d.
d. broach
excision, curettage and d. (ECD)
d. jig
percutaneous transmalleolar d.
retrograde d.
d. technique
drill-tipped guidewire
D-ring strap
drip-suck irrigation
drive
Jacobs chuck d.
worm d.
drive-extractor
driver
blade plate d.
bullet d.
Eby band d.
femoral head d.
Flatt d.
graft d.
Hall d.
Harrington hook d.
Jewett d.
Ken d.
Kirschner wire d.
Küntscher nail d.
K-wire d.
Linvatec d.
Lloyd nail d.
Massie d.
Maxi-Driver d.
McReynolds d.
Micro Series wire d.
Milewski d.
Moore d.
Moore-Blount d.
nail d.
d. nail drill
Neufeld d.
Nystroem nail d.
Nystroem-Stille d.
Orthairtome wire d.
ParaMax angled d.
plate d.
polyethylene-faced d.
prosthesis d.

NOTES

driver *(continued)*
    Pugh d.
    Rush d.
    Sage d.
    Schneider nail d.
    Sharbaro d.
    staple d.
    supine position d.
    surgical pin d.
    Sven-Johansson d.
    Teflon-coated d.
    tibial d.
    trial d.
    d. tunnel locator apparatus
    wire d.
    Zimmer Orthair ream d.

driver-bender-extractor
    Rush d.-b.-e.

driver-extractor
    Hansen-Street d.-e.
    Ken d.-e.
    McReynolds d.-e.
    Sage d.-e.
    Schneider d.-e.

drivethrough sign

DRL
    dorsoradial ligament

dromedary gait

droopy shoulder syndrome

drop
    d. attack
    d. finger
    foot d.
    d. shoulder
    wrist d.
    d. wrist splint

drop-arm
    d.-a. sign
    d.-a. test

drop-entry (closed body) hook

drop-foot
    d.-f. brace
    d.-f. gait
    d.-f. redression stockings
    d.-f. splint

dropfoot

drop-lock
    d.-l. knee brace
    d.-l. ring

dropped
    d. foot
    d. hallux

drug
    antituberculosis d.
    cytotoxic d.
    disease-modifying
      antirheumatologic d. (DMARD)

    National Collegiate Athletic
      Association prohibited d.
    nonsteroidal antiinflammatory d.
      (NSAID)
    slow-acting antirheumatic d.
      (SAARD)

drug-induced myotonia

drug-related hydantoin syndrome

DRUJ
    distal radioulnar joint
    DRUJ instability
    DRUJ prosthesis

drummer-boy palsy

Drummond
    D. button
    D. and Hastings cuboid extrusion
      injury
    D. hook
    D. hook holder
    D. spinal instrumentation
    D. spinous wiring technique
    D. wire

drumstick finger

drunken sailor gait

dry
    d. amputation
    D. Flotation wheelchair cushion
    d. gangrene
    d. heat therapy
    d. hydrotherapy
    d. infected nonunion
    d. joint
    d. necrosis
    d. sterile dressing (DSD)
    d. synovitis

Dryspell cast cover

Drytex RocketSoc ankle brace

DSA
    digital subtraction angiography

DSD
    dry sterile dressing

DSIS
    dynamic stabilizing innersole system
    DSIS orthotic

D-Soles
    D-S. insole
    D-S. orthotic

DSTR
    distal soft tissue release

DTR
    deep tendon reflex

DTT
    device for transverse traction
    DTT implant
    DTT system

dual
    d. compression scoliosis treatment
    d. drop pelvis (DDP)

d. nerve root suction retractor
d. onlay cortical bone graft
d. photon densitometry (DPD)
d. photon densitometry test
d. photon densitometry test for osteoporosis
d. pin redresser
d. plate
D. Range Limiter System
d. square-ended Harrington rod

dual-energy x-ray absorptiometry (DEXA, DXA)

Duall #88 cement

dual-lock
d.-l. total hip prosthesis
d.-l. total hip replacement system

dual-photon
d.-p. absorptiometry (DPA, DPX)
d.-p. electrospinal orthosis

Dubreuilh
D. melanosis circumscripta
melanosis circumscripta preblastomatosis of D.

Duchenne
D. disease
D. muscular atrophy
D. muscular dystrophy

Duchenne-Aran disease

Duchenne-Erb palsy

duckbill
d. elevator
d. rongeur

duck-waddle
d.-w. gait
d.-w. test

duck waddle

duct
thoracic d.

ductility

Dudley J. Morton foot configuration

Dugas test

Duhot line

dull aching pain

dumbbell
d. tumor
d. wagon

Dumon-Gilliard prosthesis introducer

Duncan
D. loop
D. prone rectus test
D. shoulder brace

Duncan-Lovell modification

Dunlop-Shands view

Dunlop traction

Dunn
D. biopsy
D. fracture device
D. hip operation
D. multiple comparison test
D. osteotomy
D. technique
D. triple arthrodesis

Dunn-Brittain
D.-B. foot stabilization
D.-B. foot stabilization technique
D.-B. triple arthrodesis

Dunn-Hess trochanteric osteotomy

Duo-Cline Dual Support contoured bed wedge

Duocondylar knee prosthesis

duodenal compression

DuoDerm dressing

Duo-Drive screw

Duo-Lock hip prosthesis

duopatellar unconstrained prosthesis

Duo-trac traction machine

Dupaco
D. knee control
D. knee prosthesis

Dupel BLUE iontophoresis electrode

Duplay
D. bursitis
D. disease
D. syndrome

duplex
d. Doppler ultrasonography
d. ultrasound

duplicate
d. sternum
d. thumb

duplicated metacarpal

duplication
Marks-Bayne technique for thumb d.
symmetric thumb d.
thumb d.
Wassel type IV thumb d.

duPont Bunion Rating Score

Dupont distal humeral plate system

Dupré muscle

Dupuytren
D. amputation
D. canal
D. contracture

NOTES

D

Dupuytren *(continued)*
    D. contracture release
    D. diathesis
    D. disease
    D. exostosis
    D. fascia
    D. fasciitis
    D. fibromatosis
    D. fracture
    D. hydrocele
    D. and Langer skin tension line
    D. operation
    D. sign
    D. splint
    D. suture

dura
    d. dissector
    d. hook
    d. mater
    d. mater graft

DuraBoot orthosis

Duracon
    D. knee implant
    D. prosthesis

Dura-Flex back brace

Dura-Kold reusable compression ice wrap

dural
    d. ectasia
    d. elevator
    d. ligament
    d. repair

Duraleve custom molded foot orthotic

Durallium implant

Duraloc
    D. acetabular cup system
    D. acetabular liner
    D. prosthesis

duralumin

Duramer polyethylene component

Duran
    D. approach
    D. passive mobilization

Duran-Houser
    D.-H. protocol
    D.-H. wrist splint

Durapatite
    D. bone
    D. bone replacement material
    D. implant

DuraPrep

Dura-Soft soft-compression reusable ice or heat wrap

Dura-Stick adhesive electrode

Durasul
    D. head system
    D. polyethylene

    D. polyethylene, high wear resistant acetabular insert
    D. prosthetic component

Duraval Hook & Loop strap material

Duray-Reed gouge

Durham
    D. flatfoot operation
    D. plasty
    D. procedure for flatfoot

Durie and Salmon classification

Durkan
    D. carpal compression test
    D. CTS gauge

durometer

durum
    heloma d. (HD)
    osteoma d.

dust
    nail d.

Dutchman's roll

duToit shoulder staple

Duval elevator

Duverney fracture

DuVries
    D. approach
    D. arthroplasty
    D. deltoid ligament reconstruction technique
    D. hammertoe repair
    D. incision
    D. modified McBride hallux valgus operation
    D. phalangeal condylectomy
    D. plantar condylectomy
    D. procedure
    D. technique for overlapping toe

DuVries-Mann modified bunionectomy

Dvorak test

DVT
    deep venous thrombosis
    Flowtron DVT
    DVT prophylaxis

dwarfism
    achondroplastic d.
    ateliotic d.
    autosomal dominant mild short limb d.
    camptomelic d.
    chondroplastic d.
    diastrophic d.
    disproportionate d.
    Langer mesomelic d.
    Laron d.
    metatropic d.
    micromelic d.
    phocomelic d.
    Pott d.
    proportionate d.

Russell-Silver d.
short-limb d.

dwarf pelvis

Dwyer

D. calcaneal osteotomy
D. clawfoot operation
D. correction of scoliosis
D. device
D. incision
D. instrumentation biomechanics
D. procedure
D. scoliosis cable
D. spinal instrumentation
D. spinal mechanical stapler
D. spinal screw
D. tensioner

Dwyer-Hall plate

Dwyer-Wickham electrical stimulation system

DXA

dual-energy x-ray absorptiometry
DXA scan

Dycal base

Dycem roll matting

Dyck-Lambert classification

Dycor

D. Geriatric ADL single axis foot prosthesis
D. prosthetic foot

dye

methylene blue d.
d. punch injury

dye-punch fracture

Dyggve-Melchior-Clausen syndrome

dying bug exercise

Dyke-Davidoff-Masson syndrome

Dyna-Disc

Exertools D.-D.
D.-D. gymball

DynaDisc exercise equipment

DYNAfabric material

Dynafill graft biomedium

DynaFix external fixation system

DynaFlex

D. Gyro exerciser
D. multilayer compression system

DynaGraft implant

Dynagrip

D. blade handle
D. handle of blade

DynaHeat hot pack

Dyna knee splint

Dyna-Lok

D.-L. pedicle screw system
D.-L. plating system

dynametric testing

dynamic

d. abduction brace
d. alignment
d. axial fixator (DAF)
d. canal glide
d. compression (DC)
d. compression plate (DCP)
d. compression plate fixation
d. compression plate instrumentation
D. condylar screw (DCS)
d. condylar screw fixation
d. condylar screw tap
d. digital deformity
D. digit extensor tube
d. double tendon replacement
D. Edge rehabilitation equipment
D. elbow orthosis
d. electromyography
d. external fixation
d. fault
d. footprint
D. foot stabilizer
d. friction
d. gait
d. hallux varus
d. hammertoe
d. hinge elbow fracture brace
d. hip screw (DHS)
d. integrated stabilization chair (DISC)
d. joint force
D. knee orthosis
d. listing
d. listing nomenclature
d. locking nail
d. lumbar stabilization
d. magnetic resonance imaging
d. metatarsus adductus
d. motion x-ray
d. movement
d. MRI
d. muscle transfer
d. pedobarography (DPB)
d. pedodynographic finding
d. repair
d. splint
d. splinting
d. stability index

NOTES

D

dynamic *(continued)*
    d. stabilization trainer
    d. stabilizing innersole system
      (DSIS)
    d. standing balance
    d. stress x-ray view
    d. stump exercise
    d. traction method
    d. transverse traction device
    d. trunk curl
    D. wrist orthosis
dynamics
    foot d.
dynamization collar
dynamometer
    Baseline d.
    Biodex isokinetic d.
    bulb d.
    Chiroslide Jamar Hand D.
    Collins d.
    computerized isokinetic d.
    Cybex II isokinetic d.
    electromechanical d.
    hand grip d.
    handheld d. (HHD)
    Harpenden d.
    Isobex d.
    Jamar hydraulic hand d.
    Lido isokinetic d.
    orthopaedic d.
    Smedley d.
    Spark handheld d.
    squeeze d.
dynamometry
    isokinetic d.
    tip-pinch d.
DynaPak electrode kit
Dynaphor iontophoresis
Dynaplex knee prosthesis
DynaPrene splinting thermoplastic
Dynasplint
    D. knee extension
    D. knee extension unit
    D. shoulder system
DynaSport athletic tape
Dynatron
    D. 50, 125, 525 electrotherapy
    D. Mini 2000 electrotherapy
    D. 2000 muscle test
    D. TX 900 electrotherapy
DyoCam
    D. 550 arthroscopic video camera
    D. arthroscopic view camera
Dyonics
    D. arthroplasty bur
    D. arthroscope
    D. arthroscopic blade
    D. cannula

    D. Golden Retriever magnet
    D. shaver
dysarthria
    clumsy hand d.
    spinal d.
dysarthrosis
    patellofemoral d.
dysbaric
    d. osteonecrosis
    d. oxygen
dysbasia
    d. angiosclerotica
    d. lordotica progressiva
dyscalculia
    developmental d.
dyschondroplasia
    Ollier d.
dyschondrosteosis
dyscollagenosis
dyscrasia
    plasma cell d.
dyscrasic fracture
dysdiadochokinesia
dysesthesia
dysfunction
    anterior-inferior capsular ligament d.
    bladder d.
    craniomandibular d.
    endothelial d.
    extensor mechanism d.
    facet joint d.
    flexor hallucis longus d. (FHLD)
    joint d.
    mechanical d.
    motor d.
    neuroarticular d.
    painful minor intervertebral d.
      (PMID)
    patellofemoral d. (PFD)
    pelvic pain and organic d.
    pilomotor d.
    posterior tibial tendon d. (PTTD)
    posttraumatic sacroiliac d.
    scapular d.
    segmental d.
    somatic d.
    sympathetic d.
    d. syndrome
dysgenesis
    alar d.
    epiphysial d.
dyshidrosis, dyshydrosis
dyskeratosis congenita
dyskinesia
    d. intermittens
    positional d.
    poststatic d. (PSDK)
    retrolisthesis positional d.

dyskinetic cerebral palsy
dysmetria
  lower limb d.
  truncal d.
dysnomia
dysostosis
  cleidocranial d.
  Jansen metaphysial d.
  Schmid metaphysial d.
  Spahr metaphysial d.
dysplasia
  acetabular d.
  acropectorovertebral d.
  bone d.
  cleidocranial d.
  congenital hip d. (CHD)
  congenital hyperphosphatasemic
    skeletal d. (CHSD)
  cortical fibrous d.
  Crowe (type I–IV) congenital
    hip d.
  developmental hip d.
  diaphysial d.
  diastrophic d.
  dyssegmental d.
  epiarticular osteochondromatous d.
  epiphysial d.
  faciodigitogenital d.
  femoral head d.
  fibrous d.
  focal fibrocartilaginous d.
  foot d.
  d. of hip
  Holt-Oram d.
  intracortical fibrous d.
  Meyer d.
  Mondini d.
  monostotic fibrous d.
  multiple epiphysial d.
  Namaqualand hip d.
  oculoauriculovertebral d.
  osteofibrous d.
  patellofemoral d.
  polyostotic fibrous d.
  progressive diaphysial d.
  rhizomesomelic bone d.
  skeletal d.
  Sponastrine d.
  spondyloepiphysial d.
  Streeter d.
  vertebral (defects), (imperforate)
    anus, tracheoesophageal (fistula),

  radial and renal (d.) anomalies
    (VATER)
dysplastic
  d. acetabulum
  d. fibula
  d. nevus syndrome
  d. spondylolisthesis
  d. tibia
dysponetic
dysraphism
  spinal d.
dysreflexia
  autonomic d.
dyssegmental dysplasia
dysstasia
dysstatic
dyssynergia
dystaxia
dystelephalangy
dystonia
  cerebral palsy-related d.
  focal d.
  d. lenticularis
  d. musculorum
  torsion d.
dystopia
  shoulder d.
dystrophic
  d. gait
  d. nail
  d. toenail
dystrophica
  myotonia d.
dystrophinopathy
dystrophy
  Albright d.
  Becker muscular d. (BMD)
  Becker-type tardive muscular d.
  Becker variant of Duchenne d.
  congenital d.
  distal d.
  Duchenne muscular d.
  Emery-Dreifuss d.
  Erb muscular d.
  fascioscapulohumeral muscular d.
  Fröhlich adiposogenital d.
  Gowers muscular d.
  humeroperoneal muscular d.
  juvenile muscular d.
  Kiloh-Nevin ocular form of
    progressive muscular d.
  Landouzy-Dejerine d.

D

NOTES

dystrophy *(continued)*
    Leyden-Möbius muscular d.
    limb-girdle muscular d.
    muscular d. (MD)
    myotonic muscular d.
    osseous d.
    pelvofemoral muscular d.
    posttraumatic d.

    progressive muscular d. (PMD)
    pseudohypertrophic d.
    reflex neurovascular d.
    reflex sympathetic d. (RSD)
    sex-linked muscular d.
    sympathetic reflex d.
dysvascular condition

E-2
    E-2 foot prosthesis
    E-2 hydrocollator heating unit
EACS
    exertional anterior compartment
    syndrome
EADL
    extended activities of daily living
eagle
    e. beak bone-cutting forceps
    E. straight-ahead arthroscope
Eagle-Barrett syndrome
Eakin cohesive seal dressing
Earle sign
EARLY
    ergonomic assessment of risk and
    liability
Early Fit night splint
E-A-R specialty composite
earth electrode
EAS
    endoskeletal alignment system
EAST
    external rotation-abduction stress test
Easton cock-up splint
East-West retractor
Eastwood technique
easy
    E. Access foot splint
    E. Lok ankle brace
    E. Up cushion
EasyAnchor
    GII E.
EasyLiner
    ALPS E.
Easy-On elbow brace
Easy-Pull sock aide device
Easyslide sliding mat
EasyStand 6000 glider
EasyStep pressure relief walker
eater
    Anspach Cement E.
    Cement E.
    Zimmer Cibatome cement e.
Eaton
    E. closed reduction
    E. CMC arthrosis (stages I–IV)
    E. implant arthroplasty
    E. splint
    E. trapezium finger joint
        replacement prosthesis
    E. volar plate arthroplasty
Eaton-Lambert syndrome

Eaton-Littler
    E.-L. ligament reconstruction
    E.-L. technique
Eaton-Malerich
    E.-M. fracture-dislocation operation
    E.-M. fracture-dislocation technique
    E.-M. reduction
Eberle
    E. contracture release
    E. contracture release technique
EBGS
    electrical bone-growth stimulation
    electrical bone-growth stimulator
EBI
    electronic bone stimulation
    EBI device
    EBI external fixator
    EBI Medical OsteoGen bone
        growth stimulator
    EBI Medical Systems bone healing
        system
    EBI Medical Systems Orthofix
        fixation system
    EBI SpF-2 implantable bone
        stimulator
    EBI SpF-T implantable bone
        stimulator
ebonation
eburnate
eburnated
    e. bone
    e. bone surface
eburnation
    bony e.
    e. of cartilage
eburneum
    osteoma e.
Eby band driver
eccentric
    e. access
    e. amputation
    e. axis of ankle rotation
    e. contraction
    e. drill guide
    e. dynamic compression plate
        (EDCP)
    e. exercise
    e. function
    e. loading
    e. muscle action
    e. muscle training
    e. wear
    e. work
eccentro-osteochondrodysplasia
ecchondroma, pl. **ecchondromata**

E

ecchondrotome
ecchymosis
eccrine
    e. poroma
    e. sweat gland
ECD
    excision, curettage and drilling
echinococcosis
Echlin
    E. bone rongeur
    E. duckbill rongeur
    E. rongeur forceps
Echlin-Luer rongeur
echo
    e. time
    e. train length (ETL)
echocardiography
echography
Ecker-Lotke-Glazer
    E.-L.-G. patellar tendon repair
    E.-L.-G. tendon reconstruction
    E.-L.-G. tendon reconstruction
      technique
Eckert-Davis classification
eclipse
    e. ankle brace
    E. Gel ankle brace
    E. Gel elbow strap
    E. TENS unit
Econo
    E. 90 lumbar home traction
    E. 90 traction unit
Econo-Cerv supine cervical traction
economic self-sufficiency WHO
  Handicap Scale
economy ROM brace
EconoSoc ankle brace
Econo-Strap
E Cotton bandage
ECRB
    extensor carpi radialis brevis
    ECRB muscle
    ECRB tendon
ECRL
    extensor carpi radialis longus
    ECRL muscle
    ECRL tendon
EcstaSeat seat cushion
ECT
    European compression technique
    ECT bone screw
    ECT internal fracture fixation
    ECT internal fracture fixation
      system
ectasia
    dural e.
ectocuneiform bone

ectomesomorphic physique
ectomorph
ectomorphic physique
ectopic
    e. bone
    e. bone growth
    e. ossification
ECTR
    endoscopic carpal tunnel release
ectrodactyly
ectromelia
ECU
    extensor carpi ulnaris
    ECU muscle
    ECU tendon
ED
    elbow disarticulation
EDB
    extensor digitorum brevis
    EDB muscle
    EDB tendon
EDC
    extensor digitorum communis
EDCP
    eccentric dynamic compression plate
Eddowes
    E. disease
    E. syndrome
edema
    bone marrow e.
    constrictive e.
    dependent e.
    endoneurial e.
    goose-egg e.
    e. heat therapy
    intracompartmental e.
    leg e.
    mushy e.
    nonpitting e.
    pitting e.
    posttraumatic e.
    pretibial e.
    rheumatismal e.
    e. sock
    stump e.
    transient bone marrow e.
edematous
Eden-Hybbinette
    E.-H. arthroplasty
    E.-H. operation
    E.-H. procedure
Eden-Lange procedure
Eden test
Eder-Puestow metal olive dilator
EDF
    elongation, derotation and lateral flexion
    EDF scoliosis cast

EDG
electrodynogram
EDG system
Edgarton-Grand thumb adduction
edge
Acufex E.
E. knee brace
patellar e.
edge-detection
digital e.-d.
Edinburgh
E. method
E. Rehabilitation Status Scale
(ERSS)
Edinger-Westphal complex
Edintrak system
EDit
electric differential therapy
EDL
extensor digitorum longus
EDM
extensor digiti minimi
Edna towel clamp
EDPCS
exertional deep posterior compartment
syndrome
EDQ
extensor digiti quinti
EDS
Ehlers-Danlos syndrome
EDSS
Expanded Disability Status Scale
education
lifestyle e. (LSE)
posture e.
Edwards
E. D-L modular fixator
E. D-L modular screw rod
E. hook
E. instrumentation
E. and Lee tibiofibular diastasis
and syndesmotic injury
classification
E. modular system
E. modular system bridging sleeve
construct
E. modular system compression
construct
E. modular system construct
selection
E. modular system distraction-
lordosis construct

E. modular system dynamic
loading
E. modular system kyphoreduction
construct
E. modular system load sharing
E. modular system neutralization
construct
E. modular system rod crosslink
E. modular system rod sleeve
construct
E. modular system sacral fixation
device
E. modular system scoliosis
construct
E. modular system spinal/sacral
screw
E. modular system spinal sleeve
E. modular system spondylar
construct
E. modular system standard sleeve
construct
E. modular system Universal rod
E. polyethylene sleeve
E. procedure
E. seamless prosthesis
E. syndrome
Edwards-Levine
E.-L. hook
E.-L. rod
E.-L. sleeve
Edwin Smith papyrus
EDX, EDx
electrodiagnosis
effect
Hick e.
Ilizarov tension-stress e.
magic angle e.
neurophysiologic e.
rake-handle e.
scarring e.
spindle e.
steal e.
Steindler e.
tenodesis e.
tethering e.
efferent nerve impulse
Effler-Groves
E.-G. dissector
E.-G. hook
effleurage massage

NOTES

effort
> brief maximal e. (BME)
> e. thrombosis

effort-induced thrombosis
effusion
> ankle e.
> bloody e.
> joint e.
> knee joint e.
> shoulder joint e.

Eftekhar
> E. broken femoral stem technique
> E. concept
> E. long-stem prosthesis

Eftekhar-Charnley hip prosthesis
Egawa sign
eggcrate mattress
Eggers
> E. bone plate
> E. contact splint
> E. neurectomy
> E. operation
> E. screw
> E. tendon transfer technique
> E. tenodesis
> E. transfer

Eggsercizer
> E. CTS exerciser
> E. resistive hand exerciser

eggshell
> e. fracture
> e. procedure

eggshell-like calcification
egress of arthroscopic fluid
Egyptian foot
EHL
> extensor hallucis longus
> EHL tendon

Ehlers-Danlos
> E.-D. disease
> E.-D. syndrome (EDS)

Ehrenfeld disease
EI
> external ilium

Eichenholz stage
Eicher
> E. femoral prosthesis
> E. hip prosthesis

eighty-nine-newton test
Eilers-Armstrong unicompartmental knee prosthesis
EIP
> extensor indicis proprius
> EIP muscle
> EIP tendon

Eisenmenger complex
EJ
> elbow jerk

ejector
> Cloward dowel e.

Ekbom restless leg syndrome
Elan drill
Elan-E power drill
Elastafit tubing kit
ElastaTrac
> E. home lumbar traction system
> E. home lumbar traction unit
> E. lumbar traction

elastic
> e. ankle corset
> e. barrier
> e. cartilage
> e. compression
> e. deformation
> e. fixation
> E. Foam bandage
> e. knee cage
> e. knee cage orthosis
> e. knee cage with medial and lateral contoured knee joints
> e. knee sleeve brace
> e. limit
> e. plaster of Paris
> e. property
> e. recoil
> e. stable intramedullary nail (ESIN)
> e. stable intramedullary nailing (ESIN)
> e. stockings
> e. strain
> e. stretch
> e. traction
> e. tubing
> e. twister orthosis
> e. wristlet
> e. zone

elastic-hinge knee brace
elasticity
> modulus of e.

Elastikon
> E. dressing
> E. elastic tape

elastofibroma dorsi
Elasto-Gel
> E.-G. hot/cold wrap
> E.-G. shoulder therapy wrap

elastoidosis
Elasto-Link joint wrap
elastoma
elastomer
> conventional silicone e. (CSE)
> high performance silicone e.
> medical e. X7-2320
> polyolefin e.
> e. skin molding
> thermoplastic e. (TPE)

Elastomull
- E. dressing
- E. elastic gauze bandage
- E. splint

Elastoplast
- E. bandage
- E. dressing

elastosis

elbow
- above e. (AE)
- e. arthroplasty
- axilla, shoulder, e. (ASE)
- baseball pitcher's e.
- e. bone
- boxer's e.
- capped e.
- e. capsule
- e. cast
- compound shattered e.
- e. disarticulation (ED)
- e. dislocation
- epicondylitis of the e.
- e. extension splint
- e. extensor tendon
- fat pad of e.
- e. flexion splint
- e. flexion test
- floating e.
- e. fracture
- Frohse arcade of the e.
- golfer's e.
- e. hinge
- e. injury
- E. Injury Management Kit
- javelin thrower's e.
- e. jerk (EJ)
- e. jerk reflex test
- e. joint
- Little Leaguer's e.
- e. magnet
- milkmaid's e.
- miner's e.
- nursemaid's e.
- e. orthosis (EO)
- e. pad
- e. prosthesis
- pulled e.
- e. radiography
- e. reflex
- e. region
- e. replacement
- reverse tennis e.
- e. sleeve
- slipped e.
- Sorbie-Questor e.
- e. stability
- student's e.
- supermarket e.
- temper tantrum e.
- tennis e.
- thrower's e.
- varus-valgus stress of the e.
- Wilson procedure for extraarticular fusion of e.
- wrestler's e.

Elbow-Up Protector elbow suspension device

elbow-wrist-hand orthosis (EWHO)

elderly
- Clifton Assessment Procedures for the E. (CAPE)

electric
- e. artifact
- e. cast saw
- e. differential therapy (EDit)
- e. joint fluoroscopy
- e. wheelchair

electrical
- e. bone-growth stimulation (EBGS)
- e. bone-growth stimulator (EBGS)
- e. bone stimulation
- e. implant
- e. inactivity
- e. injury
- e. modality
- e. nerve stimulation
- e. potential
- e. silence
- e. stimulation rehabilitation
- e. stimulation therapy
- e. stimulator waveform
- e. surface stimulation
- e. surface stimulation treatment for scoliosis

Electri-Cool
- E.-C. cold therapy system
- E.-C. continuous controlled cold therapy

electroacupuncture
- Acu-Treat e.
- Electro-Acuscope e.

Electro-Acuscope
- E.-A. electroacupuncture
- E.-A. 85 stimulator

E

NOTES

electrocardiography
electrocautery
    e. apparatus
    Aspen e.
electrocoagulation
electrode
    active e.
    ArthroCare e.
    bifilar needle recording e.
    BioKnit garment e.
    bipolar needle recording e.
    bipolar stimulating e.
    coaxial needle e.
    concentric needle e.
    disk e.
    Disposatrode disposable e.
    Dupel BLUE iontophoresis e.
    Dura-Stick adhesive e.
    earth e.
    Electro-Mesh e.
    Excel Plus e.
    exploring e.
    e. glove
    e. grid
    ground e.
    indifferent e.
    LSI Easy Stims self-adhesive e.
    LSI silver self-adhesive
      disposable e.
    macro-EMG needle e.
    microcurrent e.
    monopolar needle recording e.
    multilead e.
    needle e.
    e. paste
    e. placement
    Polystim e.
    prizm Electro-Mesh Sock e.
    recording e.
    reference e.
    Silver-Thera stocking e.
    single fiber needle e.
    e. sock
    stigmatic e.
    stimulating e.
    surface e.
    Teq-Trode e.
    Ultra Stim silver e.
    unipolar needle e.
    Versa-Stim self-adhering e.
electrodesiccated bleeding point
electrodesiccation
electrodiagnosis (EDX, EDx)
    mononeuropathy e.
Electro-Diagnostic Instruments Model
  720 Bilateral Tetrapolar

electrodiagnostic medicine
electrodynogram (EDG)
electrogoniometer (elgon)
    ankle-foot e.
    parallelogram e.
    six-degrees-of-freedom e.
electrokinetic potential
Electro-Link joint wrap
electrolyte
    e. balance
    e. replacement
electromagnet
    spring-mounted e.
electromassage
electromechanical dynamometer
Electro-Mesh
    E.-M. electrode
    E.-M. sleeve
electromyocardiography
    cervical Derifield procedure e.
electromyogram (EMG)
    ulnar nerve motor/sensory e.
electromyographic activation
electromyography (EMG)
    central e.
    dynamic e.
    integrated e.
    single-fiber e. (SFEMG)
    surface e. (sEMG)
electron beam therapy
electroneuromyography (ENMG)
electroneurophysiologic
electronic
    American Medical E.'s (AME)
    e. bone stimulation (EBI)
    e. bone stimulation apparatus
    e. goniometer
Electronics electrical stimulation device
electronystagmography
electrooptical characteristic (EOC)
electrophysiologic study
electrosurgical
    e. generator
    e. instrument
    e. pencil
electrotherapeutic point stimulation
  (ETPS)
electrotherapy
    direct current e.
    Dynatron 50, 125, 525 e.
    Dynatron Mini 2000 e.
    Dynatron TX 900 e.
    Mettler e.
    PET e.
    e. system (ES)
    ultrasound e.

electrothermal arthroscopy
electrothermally assisted capsulorrhaphy
  (ETAC)
Elekta stereotactic head frame
element
    neural e.
    posterior e.
elementary fracture
elephant-ear clavicular splint
elephant-foot
    e.-f. callus
    e.-f. fracture
    e.-f. fracture nonunion
elevata
    scapula e.
elevated
    e. rim acetabular liner
    e. scapula
elevation
    e. angle
    congenital scapular e.
    e. exercise
    e. of extremity
    ice, compression, and e. (ICE)
    protection, restricted activity, ice,
      compression, e. (PRICE)
    rest, ice, compression, e. (RICE)
    scapular e.
    E.'s shoe build-up
elevator
    Adson periosteal e.
    Alexander periosteal e.
    angular e.
    Aufranc periosteal e.
    Bennett e.
    Bethune periosteal e.
    biceps e.
    Blair e.
    bone e.
    Bowen periosteal e.
    Bristow periosteal e.
    Brophy periosteal e.
    Buck periosteal e.
    Cameron-Haight periosteal e.
    Campbell periosteal e.
    Carroll-Legg periosteal e.
    Carroll periosteal e.
    Chandler bone e.
    Cheyne periosteal e.
    chisel e.
    chisel-edge e.
    Cloward osteophyte e.

Cloward periosteal e.
Cobb periosteal e.
Cohen periosteal e.
Converse periosteal e.
Coryllos-Doyen periosteal e.
Cottle-MacKenty e.
Crego periosteal e.
curved periosteal e.
Cushing-Hopkins periosteal e.
Cushing Little Joker e.
Cushing periosteal e.
Darrach periosteal e.
Davidson-Sauerbruch-Doyen
  periosteal e.
Dawson-Yuhl-Key e.
Dawson-Yuhl periosteal e.
Doyan periosteal e.
Doyen rib e.
duckbill e.
dural e.
Duval e.
Endotrac e.
extra-leverage proximal femoral e.
Farabeuf periosteal e.
Fomon periosteal e.
fracture reducing e.
Frazier e.
Freer periosteal e.
Freer septal e.
Gardner e.
hand e.
Harrington spinal e.
Henahan e.
Herczel rib e.
Hibbs chisel e.
Hoen periosteal e.
Iowa University periosteal e.
Jannetta duckbill e.
joker e.
Joseph periosteal e.
J-periosteal e.
Kahre-Williger periosteal e.
Kennerdell-Maroon e.
Key periosteal e.
Kirmission periosteal e.
Kleinert-Kutz periosteal e.
Kocher e.
Lambotte e.
lamina e.
Lane periosteal e.
Langenbeck periosteal e.
Lempert periosteal e.

E

NOTES

elevator *(continued)*
    Lewis periosteal e.
    liberator e.
    Locke e.
    Love-Adson periosteal e.
    lumbosacral fusion e.
    Malis e.
    Matson-Alexander rib e.
    Matson periosteal e.
    Matson rib e.
    McGlamry e.
    Mead periosteal e.
    modified Darrach-type e.
    Molt periosteal e.
    Moore bone e.
    e. muscle
    nasal e.
    orthopaedic shoulder e.
    OSI extremity e.
    osteophyte e.
    Penfield periosteal e.
    periosteal e.
    e. periosteotome
    Phemister e.
    posterior glenoid e.
    Presbyterian Hospital
      staphylorrhaphy e.
    Ray-Parsons-Sunday
      staphylorrhaphy e.
    Rhoton e.
    rib e.
    Roberts-Gill periosteal e.
    Rochester lamina e.
    Rochester spinal e.
    Rolyan arm e.
    Rosen e.
    round-tapped e.
    Sauerbruch rib e.
    Sayre e.
    Scott-McCracken periosteal e.
    Sebileau periosteal e.
    Sedillot periosteal e.
    Sheffield hand e.
    Sisson fracture reducing e.
    spiked Darrach-type e.
    staphylorrhaphy e.
    straight periosteal e.
    Sunday staphylorrhaphy e.
    Swanson e.
    Tegtmeier e.
    Tenzel e.
    T handle e.
    Tronzo e.
    von Langenbeck periosteal e.
    Ward periosteal e.
    Wiberg periosteal e.
    wide periosteal e.

    Willauer-Gibbon periosteal e.
    Williger periosteal e.
    Woodson e.
    Yankauer periosteal e.
    Yasargil e.
elevator-dissector
    Freer e.-d.
elevator-periosteotome
elevatus
    e. deformity
    extrinsic metatarsus primus e.
    hallux e.
    iatrogenic e.
    intrinsic metatarsus primus e.
    metatarsus primus e.
eleven-hole plate
elgon
    electrogoniometer
Eligoy metal alloy
Elite
    E. Farley retractor
    E. hip system
    E. knee brace
    E. Plus motion analyzer
    E. posterior adjustable stop
    E. posterior spring assist
    E. Power Station gym
Elithorn Maze Test
Elizabethtown osteotomy
Elliott femoral condyle blade plate
ellipsoidal articulation
ellipsoid joint
elliptical
    e. amputation
    e. incision
    e. machine
    e. overlap shadow
Ellis
    E. classification
    E. Jones peroneal tendon operation
    E. skin traction technique
    E. technique for Barton fracture
Ellis-Jones
    E.-J. peroneal tendon displacement
    E.-J. peroneal tendon technique
Ellison
    E. fixation staple
    E. iliotibial band tenodesis
    E. lateral knee reconstruction
    E. technique
Ellis-van Creveld syndrome
Elmslie
    E. peroneal tendon operation
    E. peroneal tendon procedure
    E. reconstruction
    E. triple arthrodesis
    E. weave procedure

Elmslie-Cholmely
> E.-C. foot operation
> E.-C. procedure

Elmslie-Trillat
> E.-T. osteotomy
> E.-T. patellar operation
> E.-T. patellar procedure
> E.-T. patellar realignment method
> E.-T. realignment
> E.-T. transplant

elongation
> e., derotation and lateral flexion (EDF)
> ligament e.
> peroneus brevis e.
> e. property
> repeated quick stretch from e. (RQS-E)
> tissue e.

elongation-derotation flexion
Elson middle slip test
Elvarex
> E. compression garment
> E. support garment

Ely heel-to-buttock test
emanate
Embarc bone repair material
embarrassment
> circulatory e.

emboli (*pl. of* embolus)
embolic mononeuropathy
embolism, embolus
> air e.
> arterial gas e.
> bone marrow e.
> fat e.
> pulmonary e.

embolization
embryonal rhabdomyosarcoma
EMED
> EMED gait analysis
> EMED insole

EMED-F foot-force measurement
EMED-SF
> EMED-SF pedobarograph
> EMED-SF sensor mat

emedullate
Emerald implantation system
emergency
> e. closed manipulative measure
> e. muscle

Emery-Dreifuss
> E.-D. disease
> E.-D. dystrophy

EMG
> electromyogram
> electromyography
> EMG biofeedback system
> fine wire EMG
> EMG retrainer biofeedback unit
> scanning EMG
> single-channel surface EMG
> single fiber EMG

eminence
> hypothenar e.
> medial e.
> thenar e.
> tibial e.

eminentia
emission tomography
Emmon osteotomy
empty
> e. can exercise
> e. can syndrome
> e. can test

empty-can position
empyema
empyemic scoliosis
EMS 2000 neuromuscular stimulator
en
> en bloc
> en bloc advancement
> en bloc resection

enarthrodial joint
encapsulation
encased screw
encephalitis
encephalocele
encephalopathy
> chronic traumatic e. (CTE)

encerclage
enchondral
> e. bone
> e. ossification

enchondroma
> e. of bone
> multiple e.
> solitary e.

enchondromatosis
> multiple e.

enchondromatous myxoma
encircling wire

E

NOTES

enclavement
    Regnauld e.
enclosure
    air-flow e.
encore
    E. Orthopedics
    E. Orthopedics device
encroachment
    bony e.
    cervical nerve root e.
    foraminal osteophyte e.
    osseous foraminal e.
end
    articulating bone e.
    bone e.
    bony distal e.
    e. corn
    e. cutter
    distal bone e.
    e. feel
    lateral e.
    medial e.
    e. plate
    e. play
    e. point
    e. range of motion
    e. vertebra
endarteritis obliterans
end-bearing amputation
end-biting forceps
end-cutting
    e.-c. reamer
    e.-c. reciprocating saw
endemic
    e. hypertrophy
    e. osteoarthritis
endemica
    osteoarthritis deformans e.
Ender
    E. awl
    E. femoral fracture technique
    E. flexible medullary nail
    E. nail fixation
    E. nailing
    E. pin
    E. rod
    E. rod fixation
    E. rod fixation of fracture
end-feel palpation
ending
    flower-spray e.
    nerve e.
Endius
    E. endoscopic access system
    E. spinal endoscope/camera
    E. spinal endoscopic camera
Endless Pool physical therapy pool

Endo
    E. Multi-Mode stimulator
    E. rotating knee joint prosthesis
endoabdominal fascia
EndoAvitene
EndoButton
    closed loop E.
    E. FM
endochondral
    e. bone
    e. ossification
    e. osteogenesis
endochondromatosis
endocrine fracture
EndoFix bioabsorbable interference screw
endogenous pain
Endolite
    E. prosthesis
    E. transtibial system
Endo-Model
    E.-M. hinged knee prosthesis
    E.-M. rotating knee joint prosthesis
    E.-M. sled prosthesis
endomorph
endomysial
endomysium
endoneural
    e. fibrosis
    e. tube
endoneurial edema
endoneurium degeneration
endoneurolysis
EndoPearl
    E. bioabsorbable device
    E. fixation device
endoplasmic reticulum
endoprosthesis
    acetabular e.
    Atkinson e.
    Bio-Moore e.
    femoral e.
    F.R. Thompson e.
    nonporous-coated e.
    smooth e.
    tibial e.
    TPP hip e.
    tumor-replacement e.
endoprosthetic flange
Endoprothetik
    E. CSL-Plus cemented-hip system
    E. CS-Plus cemented-hip system
end-organ
endoscope
    Agee e.
    Desormaux e.
endoscope/camera
    Endius spinal e./c.

endoscopic
> e. anterior cruciate ligament reconstruction
> e. carpal tunnel instrumentation
> e. carpal tunnel release (ECTR)
> e. carpal tunnel release system
> e. correction of scoliosis
> e. plantar fasciotomy (EPF)

endoscopy
> fiberoptic intraosseous e.
> laser-assisted spinal e. (LASE)
> lumbar epidural e.

endoskeletal
> e. alignment system (EAS)
> e. socket
> solid ankle flexible e. (SAFE)
> stationary attachment flexible e. (SAFE)

endoskeleton
endosteal
> e. hypertrophy
> e. lamella
> e. revascularization
> e. scalloping
> e. surface
> e. vessel

endosteum
endotenon
endothelial
> e. cell
> e. dysfunction

endothelium
> vascular e.

endothoracic fascia
Endotrac
> E. blade system
> E. cannula
> E. carpal tunnel release system
> E. elevator
> E. endoscopic carpal tunnel release
> E. rasp

endotracheal intubation
endovaginal lipoma
endplate
> e. activity
> e. fragmentation
> e. invagination
> e. noise
> e. ossification
> posterior e.
> e. potential (EPP)
> e. sclerosis

> e. spike
> superior e.
> vertebral body e.
> e. zone

endpoint of orthopedic test
end-stage
> e.-s. arthrosis
> e.-s. coxarthrosis
> e.-s. disruption

end-to-end
> e.-t.-e. suture
> e.-t.-e. tendon repair

end-to-side repair
endurance
> E. bone cement
> e. event
> e. exercise
> e. limit
> e. training

Enduron acetabular liner
energetics
> Apex E.

energy
> e. absorption
> e. conservation walking component
> e. expenditure
> e. intake
> kinetic e.
> e. metabolism
> muscle e.
> E. Plus shoe insert
> e. storing foot prosthesis
> strain e.

Engebretsen procedure
Engel
> E. angle
> E. plaster saw

Engelmann
> E. disease
> E. disk
> E. thigh splint

Engel-May nail
Engel-Recklinghausen disease
Engen
> E. extension orthosis
> E. palmar finger orthosis
> E. palmar wrist splint

Engh
> E. porous metal hip prosthesis
> E. total hip replacement

Engh-Glassman femoral stem

E

engine
        Acrotorque hand e.
Englehardt femoral prosthesis
English
        E. anvil nail nipper
        E. brace
        E. cane
        E. cane board
English-McNab shoulder prosthesis
engulfment abnormality
enhancer cushion
enlarged frontal horn
enlargement
        tibial tunnel e.
enlarging bur
ENMG
        electroneuromyography
Enneking
        E. classification
        E. disease stage
        E. knee arthrodesis
        E. principle
        E. question
        E. resection-arthrodesis
        E. rod
        E. staging of malignant soft tissue
        tumor
enostosis
ensheathing callus
ensiform cartilage
Ensolite padded transfer bench
Ensure-It dressing
Entegra prosthesis
entensile release
enterocutaneous fistula
enteropathic arthritis
enthesis
        Achilles tendon e.
enthesitis
enthesopathy
entocuneiform bone
entrapment
        anular ligament e.
        catheter e.
        lateral canal e.
        median nerve e.
        meniscoid e.
        nerve root e.
        e. neuropathy
        peripheral nerve e.
        peroneal nerve e.
        popliteal fossa e.
        posterior interosseous nerve e.
        posterior tibial nerve e.
        e. syndrome
        ulnar nerve e.
entrapped plantar bone

Entrex small joint arthroscopy
    instrument set
entry point
entubulation
        nerve e.
enucleate
enucleation
enucleator
        Rhoton e.
envelope
        e. arm sling
        capsuloperiosteal e.
        soft tissue e.
environmental
        e. assessment
        e. stress cracking
enzymatic debriding agent
enzyme-based lactic acid blood testing
enzyme-linked immunosorbent assay
EO
        elbow orthosis
EOC
        electrooptical characteristic
        EOC goniometer
eosinophilia-myalgia syndrome
eosinophilic
        e. granuloma
        e. granuloma of bone
epactal bone
EPB
        extensor pollicis brevis
ependymoma
EPF
        endoscopic plantar fasciotomy
epiarticular osteochondromatous
    dysplasia
EPIC
        evaluation, prediction, intervention, and
        control
        EPIC functional evaluation system
epicondylalgia
        e. externa
        radial e.
epicondylar
        e. avulsion fracture
        e. ridge
epicondyle
        femoral e.
        humeral e.
        lateral e.
        medial e.
epicondylectomy
        medial e.
epicondylitis
        e. of the elbow
        external humeral e.
        humeral e.
        lateral humeral e.

medial e.
radiohumeral e.

epicritic
    e. pain
    e. receptor
    e. sensation erythrasma
Epic wheelchair
epidermal cell tumor
epidermis, pl. epidermides
epidermodysplasia verruciformis
epidermolysis bullosa
epidermolytic acanthoma
epidermophytid reaction
epidural
    e. abscess evacuation
    e. anesthesia
    e. neurolysis
    e. space
    e. space infection
    e. steroid
    e. steroid injection (ESI)
    e. tumor evacuation
    e. venography
epidurography
epifascicular epineurotomy
Epigard dressing
epilepsy
    jacksonian e.
    myoclonic e.
    posttraumatic e.
epileptic myoclonus
Epi-Lock elbow support
epiloia
epimeric muscle
epimysiotomy
epimysium
epineural
    e. covering
    e. repair
    e. scarring
epineurectomy
    interfascicular e.
epineurial
    e. neuropathy
    e. neurorrhaphy
epineurial-perineurial neuropathy
epineurium
epineurolysis
    volar e.
epineurotomy
    anterior e.
    epifascicular e.

interfascicular e.
local e.
epiphyses (*pl. of* epiphysis)
epiphysial, epiphyseal
    e. arrest
    e. artery
    e. aseptic necrosis
    atavistic e.
    e. bar resection
    e. chondromatous giant cell tumor
    e. closure
    e. complex
    e. dysgenesis
    e. dysplasia
    e. exostosis
    e. growth plate
    e. growth plate fracture
    e. hyperplasia
    e. injury
    e. ischemic necrosis
    e. line
    e. osteochondritis
    e. osteochondroma
    e. oxygen
    e. ring
    e. slip fracture
    e. staple
    e. stapling
    e. tibial fracture
epiphysial-metaphysial osteotomy
epiphysiodesis
    Abbott-Gill e.
    Blount e.
    bone peg e.
    Heyman-Herndon e.
    medial tibial e.
    open bone graft e.
    percutaneous e.
    proximal phalangeal e.
    screw e.
    spontaneous postfracture e.
    White e.
epiphysiolysis
    femoral e.
    proximal femoral e.
epiphysiopathy
epiphysis, pl. epiphyses
    accessory e.
    capital e. (CE)
    capital femoral e.
    capitular e.
    clavicular e.

E

NOTES

epiphysis *(continued)*
    distal humeral e.
    femoral e.
    humeral e.
    iliac e.
    Morrissy percutaneous fixation of slipped e.
    Perthes e.
    pressure e.
    slipped capital femoral e. (SCFE)
    slipped under femoral e. (SUFE)
    stippled e.
    tibial e.
    traction e.
epiphysitis
    traction e.
    transient e.
Epipoint elbow support
epipteric bone
EPI Sport epicondylitis clasp
epitendineum
epitenon suture
epithelialization
epithelioid
    e. hemangioepithelioma
    e. sarcoma
epithelioma cuniculatum
epithesis
Epitrain
    E. active elbow support
    E. knitted elbow support
    E. Viscoped support
epitrochlea
epitrochlear
epitrochleoanconeus muscle
Epker osteotome
EPL
    extensor pollicis longus
eponychia
eponychium
EPP
    endplate potential
Eppright
    E. dial osteotomy
    E. Wagner shelf procedure
epsilon receptor
Epsom salts soak
Epstein
    E. bone rasp
    E. curette
    E. hip dislocation classification
    E. neurological hammer
Epstein-Thomas classification
EPTFE graft prosthesis
epX suspension sleeve
Equagesic
equalizer
    E. air walker

    E. cast brace
    E. Pro massager
    E. short leg walking cast
equation
    Bloch e.
    Jackson-Pollock skinfold e.
equilibratory ataxia
equilibrium
    e. reaction
    e. reflex
equina
    cauda e.
equine gait
equinocavovarus deformity
equinocavus foot
equinovalgus
    e. deformity
    e. foot
    pes e.
    spastic e.
    talipes e.
equinovarus
    congenital talipes e.
    e. foot
    e. hindfoot deformity
    pes e.
    e. posturing
    psychogenic e.
    talipes e. (TEV)
    Turco repair of talipes e.
equinus
    ankle e.
    anterior e.
    compensated talipes e.
    e. contracture
    e. deformity
    e. foot
    forefoot e.
    gastrocnemius e.
    gastrosoleal e.
    global metatarsus e.
    heel e.
    metatarsus primus e.
    osseous e.
    pes e.
    e. position
    residual heel e.
    residual hindfoot e.
    spastic e.
    e. step
    talipes e.
equipment
    accommodative e.
    adaptive e.
    adjustment e.
    AquaMED dry hydrotherapy e.
    Austin Medical E. (AME)
    Baltimore Therapeutic E. (BTE)

Body-Solid exercise e.
Cybex back rehabilitation e.
decompression e.
DynaDisc exercise e.
Dynamic Edge rehabilitation e.
home medical e.
insertion e.
Invertrac e.
National Operating Committee on Standards for Athletic E. (NOCSAE)
OsteoStat single-use power surgical e.
Reflex exercise and rehab e.
Response rehab and fitness e.
stainless steel e.
Vitallium e.

equivalent
human skin e.

Erb
E. atrophy
E. muscular dystrophy
E. palsy
E. point

Erb-Duchenne palsy
Erb-Landouzy disease
Erdheim-Chester disease
Erdheim syndrome
ERE
external rotation in extension

erect
e. position
e. view

erecta
dislocatio e.
luxatio e.

erector spinae
ERF
external rotation in flexion

Ergo
E. Cush back support
E. style flexion table

Ergociser
Cateye E.
E. exercise cycle

Ergoflex Premiere back support
ergogenic
ergograph
Mosso e.

ErgoLogic keyboard
ergolytic

ergometer
bicycle e.
Biodex cycle e.
Concept II rowing e.
Cybex cycle e.
cycle e.
handgrip e.
upper body e. (UBE)

ergometry
bicycle e.

ergonomic
e. assessment
e. assessment of risk and liability (EARLY)
e. factor

ergonomically
e. correct chair
e. designed transducer

ergoreceptor
ergostat
ERGOS work simulator
ergotherapy
Erichsen
E. disease
E. sign

Erich splint
Erickson-Leider-Brown technique
Eriksson
E. brachial block technique
E. cruciate ligament reconstruction
E. knee prosthesis
E. ligament technique
E. muscle biopsy cannula

ER/IR
external rotation/internal rotation
ER/IR ratio

Erlenmeyer flask deformity
Erlenmeyer-flask shape
erogenic aid
erosion
e. of articular surface
bony e.
osteoclastic e.
pedicle e.

erosive
e. arthritis
e. osteoarthritis

ERSS
Edinburgh Rehabilitation Status Scale

erythema of joint

E

NOTES

231

erythematosus
    lupus e. (LE)
    systemic lupus e. (SLE)
erythralgia
erythrasma
    epicritic sensation e.
erythrocyte sedimentation rate (ESR)
erythromelalgia
    idiopathic e.
    secondary e.
erythromycin
erythropoietin
ES
    electrotherapy system
eschar
escharotic
escharotomy
E-Series hip system
esesthopathy
    Achilles e.
ESI
    epidural steroid injection
ESIN
    elastic stable intramedullary nail
    elastic stable intramedullary nailing
ESKA modular hip system
Esmarch
    E. bandage
    E. dressing
    E. plaster knife
    E. plaster shears
    E. tourniquet
    E. tube
ESR
    erythrocyte sedimentation rate
essential
    E. Energy Cup
    E. Energy Water
    E. Energy Whole House Wand
    e. tremor
Esser skin graft
Essex-Lopresti
    E.-L. axial fixation technique
    E.-L. calcaneal fracture
      classification
    E.-L. calcaneal fracture technique
    E.-L. fixation of calcaneal fracture
    E.-L. injury
    E.-L. joint depression fracture
    E.-L. lesion
    E.-L. method
    E.-L. open reduction
    E.-L. tongue-type fracture
ESSF
    external spinal skeletal fixator
established contracture
esterified

Estersohn
    E. osteotomy
    E. osteotomy for tailor's bunion
esthesia
esthesiometry
    Semmes-Weinstein monofilament
      pressure e.
estimated blood loss
estimation
    Simple Calculated Osteoporosis
      Risk E. (SCORE)
Estok and Harris classification
Estraderm estradiol transdermal system
estrogen
ESWT
    extracorporeal shock wave therapy
ETAC
    electrothermally assisted capsulorrhaphy
ethanol
    anhydrous e.
Ethibond suture
Ethicon suture
Ethiflex suture
Ethilon suture
ethmoid forceps
Ethrone implant material
ethylene
    e. oxide
    e. oxide sterilization
    e. vinyl acetate (EVA)
etidronate
    sodium e.
etiology
    e. undetermined
    e. unknown
ETL
    echo train length
ETPS
    electrotherapeutic point stimulation
    ETPS therapy
Eucalyptamint
eukinesia
Euler
    E. angle
    E. angle of wrist motion
    E. load
eulerian angle
eumelanin
EuroCuff forearm crutch
Euroglide MKII slide board
European
    E. Chiropractic Union
    E. compression technique (ECT)
European-style screwdriver
Eurotaper 12/14 taper
Eurotech
    E. Diamond table
    E. Emerald table

E. Platinum table
E. Sapphire table

EVA
ethylene vinyl acetate
CM EVA
compression-molded ethylene vinyl acetate

evacuation
epidural abscess e.
epidural tumor e.
nail bed hematoma e.

evacuator
Hemo-Drain e.

evaluation
Balance Master rehabilitation e.
baseline capacity e.
Charcot-Marie-Tooth E.
CMT E.
Cyriax e.
Doppler pulse e.
Evans tenodesis e.
Evolution hip prosthesis e.
functional capacity e. (FCE)
Hughston knee e.
isokinetic e.
job capacity e. (JCE)
Mazur ankle e.
orthopaedic e.
physical capacity e. (PCE)
e., prediction, intervention, and control (EPIC)
preoperative e.
Smith physical capacities e. (PCE)
static e.
toddler and infant motor e. (TIME)
uniaxial balance e. (UBE)
vocational e. (VE)

evaluator
Touch-Test sensory e.

Evan
E. ankle joint instability operation
E. calcaneal lengthening osteotomy site

Evans
E. ankle reconstruction technique
E. anterior opening wedge calcaneal osteotomy
E. calcaneal lengthening
E. calcaneal reconstruction
E. fracture classification system
E. intertrochanteric fracture classification
E. lateral ankle reconstruction
E. procedure
E. tenodesis
E. tenodesis evaluation

Evans-Burkhalter
E.-B. protocol
E.-B. rehabilitation

Evazote
E. cushioning material
E. foam

event
endurance e.

eventration

Eve reconstructive procedure

Ever-Flex insole

Evershears surgical instrument device

eversion
ankle e.
heel e.
e. injury
e. osteotomy
e. stress test

eversion-external rotation deformity

evertor
e. force
e. tendon

evoked
e. compound muscle action potential
e. potential study
e. response

evolution
E. hip prosthesis
E. hip prosthesis evaluation

Ewald
E. capitellocondylar total elbow arthroplasty
E. elbow arthroplasty rating system
E. total elbow replacement
E. unconstrained elbow prosthesis

Ewald-Walker
E.-W. kinematic knee arthroplasty
E.-W. knee implant

EWHO
elbow-wrist-hand orthosis

Ewing
E. sarcoma
E. tumor

exacerbation

Exact-Fit ATH hip replacement system

E

NOTES

exaggeration reaction
EXAKT-MicroGrinding System
examination
    Apley e.
    ARM method of physical e.
    arthroscopic e.
    BB to MM e.
    belly button to medial malleolus e.
    bench e.
    Broden stress e.
    clinical e.
    comparative radiographic e.
    full spine radiographic e.
    lateral full-spine radiographic e.
    motor e.
    neurologic e.
    neurological nerve conduction
     velocity e.
    palpatory e.
    pedodynographic e.
    reflex e.
    sensory e.
    stress e.
    thermographic e.
exarticulation
Ex-Balls
excavatum
    pectus e.
Excel Plus electrode
excentric amputation
excessive
    e. joint play
    e. laxity test
    e. sweating
exchange
    isolated modular tibial insert e.
    e. nailing
excision
    e. arthroplasty
    bar e.
    Bartlett nail fold e.
    bone cyst e.
    Bose nail fold e.
    bunionette e.
    cervical disk e.
    clavicle e.
    e. and curettage
    e., curettage and drilling (ECD)
    Curtin plantar fibromatosis e.
    Das Gupta scapular e.
    disk e.
    distal clavicular e.
    Ferciot e.
    Ferciot-Thomson e.
    Flatt e.
    funicular e.
    hemivertebral e.
    e. of intervertebral disk

    intracapsular e.
    intralesional e.
    marginal e.
    McKeever-Buck fragment e.
    meniscal e.
    microlumbar disk e.
    e. of osteochondroma
    radical compartmental e.
    retropulsed bone e.
    ruptured disk e.
    split-thickness skin e. (STSE)
    Stewart distal clavicular e.
    Thompson e.
    ulnar head e.
    wide e.
    William microlumbar disk e.
excisional
    e. arthrodesis
    e. biopsy
excision-curettage technique
excitatory postsynaptic potential
exclusion clamp
excochleation
excoriation
excrescence
    bony e.
excursion
    e. amplifier sleeve
    calcaneus e.
    hindfoot e.
    insertional e.
    range of e.
    tendon e.
executive function deficit
Exerball kit
Exerband
    E. Pak bilateral tube
    E. Pak unilateral tube
ExerBand
Exerboard
    Velcro Hand E.
exercise
    active-assisted range-of-motion e.
    active-assistive e. (AAE)
    active range-of-motion e.
    aerobic e.
    anaerobic e.
    ankle-pump e.
    aquatic e.
    back e.
    Back Revolution Stick e.
    e. band
    Berger e.
    e. bone
    Buerger-Allen e.
    calf raise back e.
    Calleja e.
    e. capacity

Carpal Care e.
chain reaction e.
closed-chain e.
closed kinetic chain e. (CKCE)
closed kinetic chain progressive-
   resistance e.
co-contraction e.
Codman e.
concentric isokinetic leg press e.
contracture e.
Cooksey-Cawthorne e.
Crane shoulder e.
Daily Adjusted Progressive
   Resistance E. (DAPRE)
dead ball e.'s
DeLorme e.
dying bug e.
dynamic stump e.
eccentric e.
elevation e.
empty can e.
endurance e.
explosive e.
external rotation e.
FITT e.
flexibility e.
flexion-extension e.
forearm ischemic e.
Frenkel e.'s
gastrocnemius resistive e.
gripping e.'s
Gymnastik ball functional
   stabilization e.
hamstring-setting e.
handgrip e.
heel cord stretching e.
heel raise e.
heel rock e.
hip abductor strengthening e.
hip extension e.
hook-lying pectoral stretch e.
horizontal shoulder abduction e.
increment after e.
internal rotation e.
e. intolerance
inversion-eversion e.
e. ischemia
isokinetic e.
isometric e.
isotonic e.
kinesthetic e.
knee extension e.

knee pump e.
low-stress aerobic e.
McKenzie extension e.
muscle-setting e.
muscle-strengthening e.
e. myopathy
open-chain e.
open kinetic chain e.'s (OKCE)
orthokinetic e.
parallel squat e.
passive assistance e.
passive range-of-motion e.
passive resistive e.
passive stretch e.
pelvic floor e.
pendulum e.
peroneal strengthening e.
e. physiology
Pilates method e.
plyometric e.
pneumatic resistance e.
PNF e.
e. program
progressive-resistance e.
progressive-resistive e. (PR, PRE)
prone scapular retraction e.
proprioceptive e.
pulley e.
quadriceps-setting e.
quadriceps strengthening e.
race-pace e.
range-of-motion e.
Regen flexion e.
rehabilitation flexibility e.
remedial e.
repetitive e.
resistive e.
rotation e.
E. Sandal
e. science
seated scapular retraction e.
e. self-efficacy
E. Self-Efficacy Scale
single-row e.
six-pack hand e.
sports anemia e.
stair-climbing e.
step e.
straight leg raising e.
Super-Seven e.
supinator fossa supraclavicular fossa
   Frenkel e.'s

NOTES

exercise (continued)
    supported extension e.
    Tai Chi Chuan e.
    e. testing
    Thera-Band Max resistive e.
    therapeutic e.
    toe gripping e.
    toe raise e.
    towel e.
    unrestricted closed and open chain
      knee extension e.
    VMO e.
    volitional e.
    wall-slide e.
    Williams flexion e. (WFE)
    work hardening e.
    wrist stretch e.
exercise-associated collapse
exercise-induced
    e.-i. amenorrhea
    e.-i. anaphylaxis
    e.-i. asthma
    e.-i. breast pain
    e.-i. collapse
    e.-i. compartment syndrome
    e.-i. myokymia
    e.-i. sudden death
exerciser
    AccessTrainer e.
    animal beanbag e.
    ankle e.
    Ankle Isolator foot and ankle e.
    axial resistance e.
    bicycle e.
    Builder Grip hand e.
    Carpal Care carpal tunnel e.
    Carpal Tunnel Stretch e.
    Cat's Paw E.
    ChairCiser adjustable e.
    continuous anatomical passive e.
      (CAPE)
    Cybex II, II+ isokinetic e.
    Danniflex CPM e.
    Digi-Flex finger e.
    Digi-Flex hand e.
    DynaFlex Gyro e.
    Eggsercizer CTS e.
    Eggsercizer resistive hand e.
    Exer-Cor e.
    ExtendaFLEX e.
    finger e.
    Finger Helper hand e.
    Finger Platter hand e.
    Flextender Plus hand e.
    Grahamizer I e.
    Gripp squeeze ball hand e.
    Gyro-Flex upper extremity e.
    hand e.

    Hand Helper hand e.
    isokinetic Unex III e.
    Iso-Quadron e.
    JACE shoulder e.
    jaw e.
    Jux-A-Cisor e.
    KineTec clubfoot CPM e.
    Knead-A-Ball e.
    microcomputer upper limb e.
      (MULE)
    MiniMedBall hand e.
    Morpho E.
    Motivator FTR2000 e.
    MULE upper limb e.
    Nelson finger e.
    NordiCare Enabler e.
    NordiCare Strider e.
    NordicTrack ski e.
    NuStep e.
    Omni-Flexor wrist e.
    Oppociser hand e.
    Orthotron e.
    pedal e.
    Plyo-Sled e.
    Powerflex CMP e.
    Power Pogo stationary e.
    Power Web hand e.
    Power Web Jr. e.
    Preston Traveler CPM e.
    ProStretch e.
    Pul-Ez e.
    resistive e.
    rickshaw rehabilitation e.
    rocky boat e.
    Rotaflex e.
    Roylan ergonomic hand e.
    Seated Cable Row e.
    soft touch hand e.
    squeeze e.
    strengthening e.
    Stronghands hand e.
    Stryker CPM e.
    Stryker leg e.
    Swanson Grip-X hand e.
    Thera-Band ASSIST e.
    Thera-Band hand e.
    Thera-Band resistive e.
    Thera Cane shoulder e.
    Theraflex wrist e.
    Ther-A-Hoop e.
    Thera-Loop e.
    Thera-Putty CTS e.
    Toronto Medical CPM e.
    Tuf Nex neck e.
    Tunturi hand e.
    Versa-Trainer e.
    Walk-'n-Tone e.
    Wilco ankle e.

Wristiciser e.
Zimmer continuous anatomical
    passive e.
exercise-related headache
Exer-Cor exerciser
Exercycle
ExerFlex ball
Exer-Pedic cycle
Exerstrider walking pole
exertion
rated perceived e. (RPE)
exertional
e. anterior compartment syndrome
    (EACS)
e. deep posterior compartment
    syndrome (EDPCS)
e. hypotension
e. rhabdomyolysis
Exertools
E. Dyna-Disc
E. gymball
Exeter
E. bone lavage
E. cemented hip prosthesis
E. intramedullary bone plug
E. intramedullary bone plug device
E. stem
Exeter-Femora press fit prosthesis
EX-FI-RE
EX-FI-RE external fixation
EX-FI-RE external fixation device
EX-FI-RE external fixation system
exhaustion
postactivation e.
posttetanic e.
Exo-Bed traction unit
exoccipital bone
Exogen
E. 2000+ noninvasive ultrasound
    therapy
E. 2000 sonic accelerated fracture
    healing system
exogenous
e. fibrin clot
e. reconstruction
Exo-Overhead traction unit
Exo-Static
E.-S. cervical collar
E.-S. traction
exostectomy
lateral e.
medial e.

exostosectomy
exostosis, pl. **exostoses**
blocker's e.
bony e.
e. bursata
cuneiform-first metatarsal e.
Dupuytren e.
epiphysial e.
Haglund e.
hereditary multiple e.
hypertrophic e.
impinging e.
marginal e.
metatarsal cuneiform e.
metatarsocuneiform joint e.
multiple hereditary osteochondral e.
    (MHOCE)
osteocartilaginous e.
pump bump e.
retrocalcaneal e.
subungual e.
tackler's e.
talar neck e.
talotibial e.
traction e.
turret e.
Exotec brace
Expanded Disability Status Scale
  (EDSS)
expander
acetabular e.
Mentor tissue e.
tissue e.
expanding reamer
Expandover athletic tape
expansile
e. cyst
e. lesion
expansion
lateral extensor e.
medial extensor e.
e. screw
expansive laminaplasty
expenditure
energy e.
experimental threshold
exploration
e. and débridement
e. and revision
exploratory incision
exploring electrode

NOTES

E

explosion
  e. fracture
  front kick e.
  e. injury
explosive exercise
exposure
  Abbott-Gill epiphysial plate e.
  anterior surgical e.
  bone-tendon e.
  extrapharyngeal e.
  Henry posterior interosseous
    nerve e.
  Kocher-Langenbeck e.
  subperiosteal e.
  surgical e.
  thoracolumbar junction surgical e.
  thoracolumbar spine anterior e.
  transperitoneal e.
  upper cervical spine anterior e.
  vertebral e.
expulsion
  graft e.
exsanguinate
exsanguination tourniquet control
extend
  E. stem
  E. total hip system
ExtendaFLEX exerciser
extended
  e. activities of daily living
    (EADL)
  e. ADLs
  e. iliofemoral approach
  e. maxillotomy
  e. medial shoe counter
  e. slide trochanteric osteotomy
  e. steel shank
  e. steel-shank shoe
  e. tibial in situ bypass
extended-counter shoe
extender
  Kalish Duredge wire e.
  nail e.
  Rousek e.
  Rush e.
  Superstabilizer cemented stem e.
  Superstabilizer press-fit stem e.
  Sven-Johansson e.
Extend-It finger splint
extensibility
extensible
extensile approach
extension
  active knee e. (AKE)
  e. aid
  angle of greatest e. (AGE)
  Bardenheuer e.
  basal e.

  e. block splint
  e. block splinting method
  e. body cast
  e. bone clamp
  e. bow
  brachioradialis transfer for wrist e.
  brake lever e.
  Buck e.
  cast with dorsal toe plate e.
  cast with volar toe plate e.
  cervical rotation in e.
  Codivilla e.
  compressive e.
  e. contracture
  e. deformity
  distractive e.
  dorsal toe plate e.
  Dynasplint knee e.
  external rotation in e. (ERE)
  femoral-trunk e.
  flexion and e.
  e. gap
  headrest e.
  hip e.
  Hittenberger halo e.
  e. injury posterior atlantoaxial
    arthrodesis
  e. instability
  internal rotation in e. (IRE)
  isokinetic knee e.
  Legg-Perthes shoe e.
  lumbar e.
  e. malposition
  Maquet table e.
  e. nail
  nail e.
  NexGen offset stem e.
  e. osteotomy
  range of e.
  e. restriction
  shoe e.
  sitting knee e.
  skeletal e.
  terminal knee e.
  toe plate e.
  volitional resisted flexion and e.
extensive
  e. neoplasm
  e. posterior decompression
extensometer
  strain-gauge e.
extensor
  apparatus e.
  e. brevis arthroplasty
  e. carpi radialis brevis (ECRB)
  e. carpi radialis brevis muscle
  e. carpi radialis brevis tendon
  e. carpi radialis longus (ECRL)

e. carpi radialis longus muscle
e. carpi radialis longus tendon
e. carpi ulnaris (ECU)
e. carpi ulnaris muscle
e. carpi ulnaris tendon
e. communis muscle
e. digiti minimi (EDM)
e. digiti minimi muscle
e. digiti minimi tendon
e. digiti quinti (EDQ)
e. digiti quinti muscle
e. digiti quinti tendon
e. digitorum brevis (EDB)
e. digitorum brevis flap
e. digitorum brevis muscle
e. digitorum brevis tendon
e. digitorum communis (EDC)
e. digitorum communis muscle
e. digitorum communis tendon
e. digitorum longus (EDL)
e. digitorum longus muscle
e. digitorum longus tendon
e. digitorum transfer
e. hallucis
e. hallucis brevis muscle
e. hallucis longus (EHL)
e. hallucis longus muscle
e. hallucis longus strength
e. hallucis longus tendon
e. hallucis longus tenodesis
e. hallucis longus transfer
e. hood
e. hood mechanism
e. hood release
e. indicis proprius (EIP)
e. indicis proprius muscle
e. indicis proprius tendon
knee e.
long e.
e. mechanism dysfunction
e. pollicis brevis (EPB)
e. pollicis brevis muscle
e. pollicis brevis tendon
e. pollicis longus (EPL)
e. pollicis longus muscle
e. pollicis longus tendon
e. quinti tendon
radial wrist e.
e. retinaculum
e. substitution
e. tendon blockage
e. tendon injury

e. tendon lengthening
e. tendon repair
e. tendon transfer
e. tenotomy
e. thrust reflex
toe e.
ulnar e.
e. wad of three muscles
e. wand
wrist e.

extensus
hallux e.

exteriorization

externa
epicondylalgia e.

external
articulated e. fixator
e. band
e. elastic strap
e. fixator
e. fixator frame
e. hamstring reflex
e. humeral epicondylitis
e. ilium (EI)
e. ilium movement
e. immobilization
e. immobilizer
e. intercostal muscle
e. malleolus
e. neurolysis
e. oblique muscle
e. oblique reflex
posteroinferior e. (PIEx)
e. prehallux
e. rotation
e. rotation-abduction stress test (EAST)
e. rotation contracture
e. rotation exercise
e. rotation in extension (ERE)
e. rotation in flexion (ERF)
e. rotation/internal rotation (ER/IR)
e. rotation/internal rotation ratio
e. rotation stress test
e. rotator
e. sequential pneumatic compression boot
e. skeletal fixation apparatus
e. spinal fixation
e. spinal skeletal fixator (ESSF)
e. support
e. tibial torsion

E

NOTES

external *(continued)*
    e. traction
    e. version
external-alignment compression jig
external-coil electrical stimulation
externally
    e. powered tenodesis orthosis
    e. rotated
externum
externus
    malleolus e.
exteroceptive sensation
exteroceptor
    postural e.
extirpation
extraabdominal desmoid tumor
extraarticular
    e. ankylosis
    e. arthrodesis
    e. arthroscopy
    e. augmentation
    e. fracture
    e. graft
    e. Grice procedure
    e. hip fusion
    e. knee ligament
    e. pain syndrome
    e. pigmented villonodular synovitis
    e. pseudarthrosis
    e. reconstruction
    e. resection
    e. structure
    e. subtalar fusion
    e. subtalar joint
    e. technique
    e. tuberculosis
extrabursal approach
extracapsular
    e. ankylosis
    e. arterial ring
    e. dissection
    e. fracture
    e. ligament
    e. rupture
extracompartmental soft tissue sarcoma
extracorporeal shock wave therapy (ESWT)
extracortical chondrosarcoma
extracting forceps
extraction pliers
extractor
    Austin Moore e.
    ball e.
    Bilos pin e.
    bone e.
    bone plug e.
    break screw e.
    broach e.

    Cherry screw e.
    cloverleaf pin e.
    corkscrew femoral head e.
    femoral head e.
    femoral trial e.
    FIN e.
    Intraflex intramedullary pin e.
    Jewett e.
    Kalish Duredge wire e.
    Küntscher e.
    Mark II femoral component e.
    Mark II tibial component e.
    Massie e.
    metatarsal head e.
    Moore prosthesis e.
    Moreland femoral component e.
    e. nail drill
    Nicoll e.
    Rousek e.
    Sage e.
    Schneider e.
    Snap Lock wire/pin e.
    Southwick screw e.
    staple e.
    stem e.
    Sven-Johansson e.
    Take-Out E.
    Universal modular femoral hip component e.
    Zimmer e.
extractor-driver
    Schneider e.-d.
extractor-impactor
    Fox e.-i.
extra-depth
    e.-d. posterior acetabular retractor
    e.-d. shoe
extradural
    e. anastomosis
    e. granulation
extrafascial nerve injection
extrafusal fiber contraction
extra-large hip retractor
extra-leverage proximal femoral elevator
extramedullary
    e. alignment
    e. alignment guide
    e. fixation
    e. plasmacytoma
    e. tibial alignment jig
extraoctave fracture
extraosseous
    e. circulation
    e. factor
extraperitoneal approach
extrapharyngeal
    e. approach
    e. exposure

extrapyramidal gait
extraskeletal
    e. chondroma
    e. chondrosarcoma
    e. osteosarcoma
extra toe
extravasation
    e. extremity
    e. extrusion
    e. injury
    e. irrigation solution
extremity
    both lower e.'s (BLE)
    both upper e.'s (BUE)
    elevation of e.
    extravasation e.
    left lower e. (LLE)
    left upper e. (LUE)
    lower e. (LE)
    e. mobilization strap
    e. mobilization technique
    e. pump
    right lower e. (RLE)
    right upper e. (RUE)
    Scan-O-Gram of lower e.
    upper e. (UE)
extrinsic
    e. clubfoot
    e. entrapment test
    finger e.'s
    e. ligament
    e. metatarsus primus elevatus
    e. muscle
    e. muscle strength
    e. rearfoot post
    e. tightness test
    e. toe flexor

extruded
    e. bar polyethylene
    e. disk
extrusion
    bone graft e.
    disk e.
    extravasation e.
extubation
    postoperative e.
exuberant
    e. granulation tissue
    e. synovium
exudate
exude
Exu-Dry wound dressing
eye sign
Eyler flexorplasty
Eyre-Brook epiphysial index
EZ
    EZ Bend sponge
    EZ hand pump
    EZ Rider support chair
    EZ "T" orthopedic shirt
E-Z
    E-Z arm abduction orthosis
    E-Z Flex jaw exercising device
    E-Z Reacher
    E-Z ROC anchor
Ezeform splint
EZ-Trac orthopedic suspension device
EZ-Up inversion table
Ezy
    E. Wrap lumbosacral support
    E. Wrap shoulder immobilizer

E

NOTES

F

F latency
F wave

FA

femoral anteversion

Fabco

F. gauze bandage
F. gauze dressing

fabella syndrome
fabellofibular

f. complex
f. ligament

FABER

flexion, abduction, external rotation
FABER test

fabere

f. sign
f. test

Fabian screw
fabric

neoprene f.
Staph-Chek Synergy f.

FAC

Functional Ambulation category

facebow

Ortho-Yomy f.

facet

f. angle
f. anomaly
f. apposition
articular f.
calcaneal f.
f. capsule
f. capsule disruption
f. dislocation
f. excision technique
fibular f.
f. fracture stabilization wiring
fusion f.
f. fusion
inferior f.
f. injection
f. joint
f. joint block
f. joint disease (FJD)
f. joint dysfunction
f. joint irritation
f. joint preparation
f. joint syndrome
f. joint vacuum
lateral patellar f.
locked f.
malleolar f.
oblique wiring f.

f. plane
posterior f.
proximal fibular f.
f. replacement
f. screw system
f. subluxation
f. subluxation stabilization wiring
f. surface
f. synovial impingement
f. tropism

facetectomy

O'Donoghue f.

face validity of rehabilitation testing
facial

f. artery
F. Grading System (FGS)

facies

acromegalic f.
swan-neck f.

facilitated

f. spinal system
f. subluxation

facilitation

convergence f.
Law of F.
neuromuscular f.
f. pattern
postactivation f.
posttetanic f.
proprioceptive neuromuscular f.
(PNF)

facilitatory technique
facioauriculovertebral (FAV)
faciodigitogenital dysplasia
facioscapulohumeral (FSH)
factitious

f. injury
f. lymphedema

factor

analog neurotrophic f.
biomechanical f.
coagulation f.
f. VIII, IX deficiency
dislocation f.
ergonomic f.
extraosseous f.
high-risk f.
insulin-like growth f. (IGF)
leg protection f. (LPF)
nerve growth f.
neurotrophic f.
platelet-derived growth f. (PDGF)
RA f.
rheumatoid arthritis f.

F

factor *(continued)*
    skeletal growth f.
    transforming growth f. (TGF)
FADIR
    flexion, adduction, internal rotation
    FADIR sign
    FADIR test
fad therapy
Fahey
    F. approach
    F. pin
    F. retractor
    F. technique
Fahey-Compere pin
Fahey-O'Brien technique
failed
    f. back surgery syndrome (FBSS)
    f. back syndrome (FBS)
    f. back syndrome with documented
      pseudarthrosis
    f. femoral osteotomy
    f. implant arthroplasty
    f. joint replacement
    f. procedure
    f. surgery
    f. surgery syndrome
    f. triple arthrodesis
fail-safe mechanism
failure
    brittle bone f.
    congestive heart f.
    f. of conservative management
    differentiation f.
    fatigue f.
    Harrington rod instrumentation f.
    heart f.
    implant f.
    metal f.
    spinal implant load to f.
    stem f.
Fairbanks
    F. change
    F. sign
    F. technique
    F. technique with Sever
      modification
Fairbanks-Sever procedure
Fajersztajn crossed sciatic sign
FAL
    functional and anatomic loading
falces (*pl. of* falx)
falciform
    f. cartilage
    f. ligament
Fallat-Buckholz method
fallen arch
fallen-fragment sign
fallen-leaf sign

false
    f. acetabulum
    f. aneurysm
    f. ankylosis
    f. articulation
    f. coxa vara
    f. joint
    f. neuroma
    f. pelvis
    f. profile view
    f. rib
    f. vertebra
false-negative result
falx, pl. **falces**
    calcification of f.
    f. calcification
FAM
    functional assessment measure
familial
    f. expansile osteolysis
    f. lymphedema
    f. myoglobinuria
    f. osteoectasia
    f. periodic paralysis
    f. shape
    f. spinal muscular atrophy
family management model
fan
    Schmitt f.
    f. sign
Fanconi
    F. anemia
    F. syndrome
Fanconi-Albertini-Zellweger syndrome
Fantastic Burr nail bur
Farabeuf
    F. amputation
    F. bone-holding forceps
    F. bone rasp
    F. periosteal elevator
Farabeuf-Collin rasp
Farabeuf-Lambotte
    F.-L. bone-holding forceps
    F.-L. raspatory
far fashion
far-field potential
Farmer
    F. operation
    F. technique
far-out syndrome
Farrior wire-crimping forceps
Fartlek training
fascia, pl. **fascias, fasciae**
    Abernethy f.
    antebrachial f.
    anterior cervical f.
    Buck f.
    Camper f.

cervical f.
clavipectoral f.
Colles f.
crural f.
cuff of f.
deep f.
deltoid f.
Dupuytren f.
endoabdominal f.
endothoracic f.
gluteal f.
hypothenar f.
infraspinous f.
investing f.
f. lata
f. lata femoris
f. lata freeze-thawed graft
lumbar f.
lumbodorsal f. (LDF)
medial geniculate f.
palmar f.
plantar f.
popliteal f.
pubic f.
quadratus femoris f.
f. of quadratus lumborum muscle
retrosacral f.
Scarpa f.
f. sheath
Sibson f.
thenar f.
transversalis f.
vertebral f.
fascial
f. arthroplasty
f. band
f. compartment
f. fibromatosis
f. flap augmentation
f. graft
f. plane
f. plexus
f. release
f. sarcoma
f. septum
f. sheath covering
f. space
f. space infection
f. subcutaneous turn-down flap
f. suture
fascial-muscle interface
fasciaplasty, fascioplasty

fascias (*pl. of* fascia)
fascia-splitting incision
fascicle
anterior tibiotalar f. (ATTF)
motor f.
muscle f.
popliteomeniscal f.
sensory f.
silent f.
fascicular
f. degeneration
f. neuropathy
f. repair
fasciculation
benign f.
contraction f.
malignant f.
f. potential
proprioceptive neuromuscular f. (PNF)
fasciculus, pl. **fasciculi**
arcuate f. (AF)
fasciectomy
dermal f.
limited f.
partial f.
radical palmar f.
subtotal plantar f.
fasciitis, fascitis
diffuse f.
Dupuytren f.
iliotibial band f.
ITB f.
necrotizing f.
nodular f.
plantar f.
proliferative f.
pseudosarcomatous f.
recalcitrant plantar f.
fasciocutaneous
f. axial pattern flap
f. island flap
fasciodesis
fascio-fat graft
fasciogram
fascioplasty (*var. of* fasciaplasty)
fasciorrhaphy
fascioscapulohumeral
f. muscle atrophy disease
f. muscular atrophy
f. muscular dystrophy

NOTES

F

245

fasciotome
    intercompartment f.
    Masson f.
    Moseley f.
fasciotomy
    compartment f.
    decompression f.
    double-incision f.
    endoscopic plantar f. (EPF)
    four-compartment f.
    minimal incision plantar f.
    palmar f.
    percutaneous plantar f. (PPF)
    plantar f.
    prophylactic f.
    Rorabeck f.
    single-incision f.
    Skoog f.
    subcutaneous palmar f.
    Yount f.
fascitis (*var. of* fasciitis)
fashion
    aseptic f.
    barber-pole f.
    Bunnell zigzag f.
    cruciate f.
    far f.
    near-far f.
FASS
    foot and ankle severity scale
FAST
    Functional Assessment Staging
    FAST 1 intraosseous infusion
      system
fast
    F. Lanex rare earth screen
    f. muscle
FASTak
    F. suture anchor
    F. suture anchor system
fastener
    Intrafix ACL tibial f.
Fastex proprioceptive and agility test
FASTIN
    F. suture anchor
    F. threaded anchor
Fastlok implantable staple
FastOut device
Fas-Trac strip
fast-twitch muscle fiber
fat
    aspirated f.
    autogenous f.
    f. embolism
    f. embolism syndrome
    f. and fat-free mass (FFM)
    f. graft
    f. loading
    f. oxidation
    f. pad
    f. pad atrophy
    f. pad of elbow
    f. pad retractor
    f. pad sign
    f. pad syndrome
    f. saturation
fat-blood
    f.-b. interface (FBI)
    f.-b. interface sign
fatigue
    f. bone graft
    f. failure
    f. fracture
    implant f.
    metal f.
    f. strength
    f. stress
    f. tolerance
    volitional f.
fatty
    f. tissue
    f. tissue tumor
Faulkner curette
fault
    dynamic f.
faulty union
FAV
    facioauriculovertebral
    FAV syndrome
Fazio-Londe
    F.-L. atrophy
    F.-L. syndrome
FB
    foreign body
    FB cast cushion
FBI
    fat-blood interface
    FBI sign
FBS
    failed back syndrome
FBSS
    failed back surgery syndrome
FCE
    functional capacity evaluation
FCL
    fibular collateral ligament
FCR
    flexor carpi radialis
FCS
    full cervical spine
    FCS view
    FCS x-ray
FCU
    flexor carpi ulnaris
FDB
    flexor digitorum brevis

FDC
> flexor digitorum communis

FDICT
> frequency-difference interferential current
> therapy

FDL
> flexor digitorum longus

FDMA
> first dorsal metatarsal artery

FDP
> flexor digitorum profundus

FDQB
> flexor digitorum quinti brevis

FDS
> flexor digitorum sublimis
> flexor digitorum superficialis

Feagin shoulder dislocation test
feasibility
> vocational f.

febricitans
> pes f.

feeder
> offset suspension f.
> suspension f.
> Tumble Forms f.

feel
> end f.

feet (*pl. of* foot)
Feiss line
Feldenkrais
> F. cylinder
> F. foam roll
> F. method

Felix disease
fell on outstretched hand (FOOSH)
felon
> aseptic f.
> f. infection

felt
> f. apron Bowden cable suspension
> system
> f. brace
> f. collar splint
> f. dressing
> orthopaedic f.
> f. padding
> f. patch
> rolled f.
> F. shears

female
> f. athletic triad

> f. reamer
> f. washer

femora (*pl. of* femur)
femoral
> f. above-knee popliteal bypass
> f. aligner
> f. alignment jig
> f. antetorsion
> f. anteversion (FA)
> f. arteriography
> f. attachment
> f. bone
> f. canal restrictor
> f. circulation
> f. circumflex artery
> f. clamp
> f. component
> f. component pusher
> f. condylar defect
> f. condylar shaving
> f. condylar template
> f. condyle
> f. cortex
> f. cortical index
> f. cortical perforation
> f. cortical ring allograft
> f. cortical window
> f. cutaneous nerve
> f. derotation osteotomy
> f. diaphysial allograft
> f. diaphysis
> f. distractor
> f. drill bit
> f. endoprosthesis
> f. epicondyle
> f. epiphysiolysis
> f. epiphysis
> f. fossa
> f. fracture following total hip
> replacement classification
> f. groove
> f. guidepin
> f. guide pin
> f. head
> f. head amputation
> f. head bone removal reamer
> f. head cork screw
> f. head deformity
> f. head driver
> f. head dysplasia
> f. head extractor
> f. head line (FHL)

NOTES

F

femoral *(continued)*
 f. head and neck
 f. head/neck anteversion
 f. head vascularity
 f. impactor
 f. intramedullary guide
 f. intratrochanteric fracture
 f. medullary canal
 f. metaphysial shortening
 f. metaphysis
 f. muscle
 f. nailing
 f. neck fracture
 f. neck fracture reduction
 f. neck nail
 f. neck prosthesis
 f. neck version
 f. nerve block
 f. nerve paralysis
 f. nerve stretch test
 f. nerve traction test
 f. notch guide
 f. offset
 f. osteolysis
 f. osteomyelitis
 f. osteoporosis
 f. plate
 f. plug
 f. prosthesis broach
 f. prosthesis fixation
 f. rasp
 f. reflex
 f. region
 f. resection
 f. resector
 f. retrotorsion
 f. retroversion
 f. rollback
 f. sarcoma
 self-articulating f. (SAF)
 f. shaft
 f. shaft axis
 f. shaft fracture
 f. shaft malunion
 f. sheath
 f. supracondylar fracture
 f. torsion
 f. trial extractor
 f. tuberosity
 f. tunnel
 f. vein injury
femoral-femoral
 f.-f. bypass graft
 f.-f. crossover
femoral-trunk
 f.-t. angle
 f.-t. extension
 f.-t. flexion

femoris
 biceps f.
 fascia lata f.
 fovea capitis f.
 linea aspera f.
 profunda f.
 quadratus f. (QF)
 rectus f.
femorocrural graft
femorodistal
 f. bypass
 f. bypass procedure
femoroiliac thrombophlebitis
femoroischial transplantation
femoropatellar joint
femorotibial
 f. angle (FTA)
 f. joint (FTJ)
 f. ligament tenodesis
 f. torsion
femur, pl. **femora**
 f. button graft complex
 distal f.
 F. Finder instrument
 f. graft
 f. length (FL)
 f. length to abdominal
  circumference ratio (FL/AC)
 proximal f.
 spiral line of f.
femur-fibular-ulna complex
fence splint
fender fracture
fenestrated
 f. drape
 f. reamer
 f. stem
 f. tenotomy
fenestration
Fenlin total shoulder system
Fenton tibial bolt
Feochetti rib spreader
Ferciot
 F. excision
 F. tiptoe splint
Ferciot-Thomson excision
Ferguson
 F. bone clamp
 F. bone holder
 F. bone-holding forceps
 F. hip reduction
 F. sacral base angle
 F. scoliosis measuring method
 F. view
Ferguson-Frazier suction tube
Ferguson-Thompson-King-Moore
 osteotomy

**Ferguson-Thompson-King two-stage
osteotomy**
Fergusson
    F. forceps
    F. method for measuring scoliosis
Ferkel
    F. bipolar release
    F. C guide
    F. torticollis technique
Fernandez
    F. extensile anterior approach
    F. osteotomy
    F. point-score wrist assessment
    system
    F. scale posttraumatic wrist
    assessment system
Ferno
    F. AquaCiser underwater treadmill
    system
    F. custom therapy pool
Ferran awl
Ferrier coupler
Ferris
    F. Smith bone-biting forceps
    F. Smith-Kerrison forceps
    F. Smith-Kerrison laminectomy
    rongeur
    F. Smith rongeur
    F. Smith rongeur forceps
    F. Smith-Spurling disk rongeur
    F. Smith tissue forceps
ferromagnetic
    f. metal plate
    f. relaxation
ferumoxide injectable solution
FES
    functional electrical stimulation
    FES exercise bicycle
festinating gait
festination
fetal
    f. alcohol syndrome
    f. substantia nigra graft
fetalis
    myodystrophia f.
fever
    fracture f.
    rheumatic f.
    f. of undetermined origin (FUO)
FF
    further flexion

FFC
    fixed flexion contracture
FFI
    Foot Function Index
FFM
    fat and fat-free mass
FGS
    Facial Grading System
FHB
    flexor hallucis brevis
FHL
    femoral head line
    flexor hallucis longus
      FHL tendon transfer/augmentation
FHLD
    flexor hallucis longus dysfunction
FI
    Functional Integration
fiber
    A-delta f.
    afferent f.
    anular f.
    collagen f.
    f. density
    fast-twitch muscle f.
    intrafusal f.
    ragged-red f.
    Sharpey f.
    skeletal muscle f.
    tendinous f.
fiberglass
    f. bandage
    f. cast
    f. splint
fiber-metal peg
fiberoptic
    f. arthroscope
    f. cable
    f. intraosseous endoscopy
    f. light source
fiber-region
    anterior f.-r.
    central f.-r.
fiber-splitting incision
fibreux
    cerclage f.
fibrillar absorbable hemostat material
fibrillation
    f. potential
    synchronized f.
fibrin
    f. clot

NOTES

F

fibrin *(continued)*
    f. debris
    f. glue adhesive
fibrinoid degeneration
fibrinolysin
fibrinolysis
fibrinolytic agent
fibroadipose tissue
fibroblast
    regenerated f.
fibroblastic
    f. phase
    f. proliferation
    f. sarcoma
    f. tumor
fibrocartilage
    f. complex
    triangular f.
fibrocartilaginous
    f. disk
    f. joint
    f. pad
    f. plate
    f. tissue
fibrochondrocyte
fibroconnective tissue
fibrodysplasia ossificans progressiva
fibroelastic cartilage
fibroepithelial polyp
fibroepithelioma of Pinkus
fibroepitheliomatous
fibrofatty
    f. infiltrate
    f. tissue
fibroid tumor
fibrokeratoma
    acquired digital f.
    acral digital f.
fibrolipoma
    massive f.
fibrolipomatosis
    macrodactylia f.
fibroma
    aponeurotic f.
    calcifying aponeurotic f.
    cementing f.
    chondromyxoid f.
    desmoid f.
    desmoplastic f.
    juvenile aponeurotic f.
    Koenen periungual f.
    f. molle
    nonossifying f. (NOF)
    nonosteogenic f.
    ossifying f.
    osteogenic f.
    perineural f.
    periosteal f.

    periungual f.
    soft f.
    subungual f.
fibromatosis
    aggressive infantile f.
    f. colli
    congenital general f.
    dermal f.
    diffuse infantile f.
    Dupuytren f.
    fascial f.
    Garrod f.
    generalized f.
    infantile dermal f.
    irradiation f.
    juvenile hyaline f.
    palmar f.
    plantar f.
    pseudosarcomatous f.
    solitary f.
    sternocleidomastoid muscle f.
    subcutaneous pseudosarcomatous f.
fibromuscular disease
fibromyalgia syndrome (FMS)
fibromyalgic pain
fibromyositis
fibromyxoma
fibronectin
fibroosseous
    f. pulley
    f. ring of Lacroix
    f. sheath
    f. tunnel
fibropathic abnormality
fibroplasia
fibrosa
    myositis f.
    progressive myositis f.
fibrosarcoma
fibrosis
    anular f.
    endoneural f.
    intraneural f.
    perineural f.
    retroperitoneal f.
fibrositis
    f. ossificans progressiva
    periarticular f.
fibrosus
    anulus f.
    lacertus f.
fibrotic strut
fibrous
    f. adhesion
    f. ankylosis
    f. attachment
    f. band
    f. capsule

f. cartilage
f. cortical defect
f. dysplasia
f. dysplasia ossificans progressiva
f. hamartoma
f. histiocytoma
f. hyperplasia
f. joint
f. lesion
f. loose body
f. metaphysial defect
f. metaplasia
f. scar tissue
f. spur
f. talocalcaneal coalition
f. tissue implant
f. tumor
f. union
f. xanthoma
fibrovascular connective tissue stroma
fibroxanthoma
fibula, pl. **fibulae, fibulas**
diastasis f.
distal f.
dysplastic f.
f. protibial synostosis
proximal f.
short f.
f. shortening
fibular
f. anlage
f. bone
f. bone hook test
f. collateral ligament (FCL)
f. collateral sprain
f. compression test
f. diaphysial fracture
f. facet
f. groove
f. head
f. head resection
f. hemimelia
f. joint disruption
f. malleolus
f. margin
f. metaphysis
f. muscle
f. neck
f. onlay-inlay graft
f. ostectomy
f. osteotomy
f. peg

f. plantar marginal artery
f. pseudarthrosis
f. sesamoid
f. sesamoidal ligament
f. sesamoidectomy
f. shortening
f. strut graft
f. transfer
f. transplant
fibulas (*pl. of* fibula)
fibulectomy
partial f.
fibulocalcaneal ligament
fibulotalar
f. arthrodesis
f. ligament
fibulotalocalcaneal (FTC)
f. ligament
Ficat
F. and Arlet disease stage
F. and Arlet osteonecrosis classification
F. classification of femoral head osteonecrosis
F. femoral head osteonecrosis classification
F. procedure
F. stage of avascular necrosis classification
F. view
Ficat-Marcus grading system
Fick method
fiducial
field
F. blade
f. block
f. block anesthesia
bloodless f.
f. of dissection
f. focused nuclear magnetic resonance (FONAR)
peripheral nerve cutaneous f.
pulsating electromagnetic f.
pulsed electromagnetic f. (PEMF)
Fielding
F. femoral fracture classification
F. modification of Gallie technique
Fielding-Magliato subtrochanteric fracture classification
fifth
f. finger
f. metacarpal

NOTES

F

251

fighter's fracture
figure-eight adjustment
figure-four position
figure-of-eight
    f.-o.-e. bandage
    f.-o.-e. brace
    f.-o.-e. cast
    f.-o.-e. dressing
    f.-o.-e. harness
    f.-o.-e. suture
    f.-o.-e. taping
    f.-o.-e. test
    f.-o.-e. thoracic orthosis
    f.-o.-e. wire
    f.-o.-e. wire loop
    f.-o.-e. wiring
figure-of-four test
filarial
    f. arthritis
    f. synovitis
file
    bone f.
    orthopaedic bone f.
    orthopaedic surgical f.
filiform
fill
    fit and f.
Fillauer
    F. bar
    F. bar foot orthosis
    F. dorsiflexion assist ankle joint
    F. endoskeletal alignment system
    F. modular shuttle lock system
    F. night splint
    F. PDC ankle joint
    F. prosthesis liner
    F. Scottish Rite orthosis kit
    F. silicone suction liner
    F. silicone suspension liner
filler
    f. block
    BonePlast bone void f.
    nonosteoconductive bone-void f.
    OsteoSet bone f.
    ProOsteon implant 500 coralline
      hydroxyapatite bone void f.
    shoe f.
    Springlite toe f.
filleted graft
fillet local flap graft
film
    chiropractic x-ray f.
    lateral cervical spine f.
    scout f.
    spot f.
    stress f.
    working orthopedic surgery f.
film-screen combination

filmy adhesion
filtration system
filum
    f. spinale
    f. terminale syndrome
FIM
    functional independence measure
FIN
    flexible intramedullary nail
    FIN extractor
    FIN pin guide
    FIN system
fin
    F. & Flipper exercise log
    f. of the implant
    prosthetic stem lateral f.
finder
    angle f.
    canal f.
    Dasco Pro angle f.
    gravity-driven angle f.
    pedicle f.
finding
    bone in bone f.
    constellation of clinical f.'s
    dynamic pedodynographic f.
    thermographic f.
fine
    f. bone curette
    f. curette
    f. manipulation
    f. olive bur
    f. osteotome
    f. wire EMG
fine-angled curette
fine-tooth electric saw
finger
    adduction stress to f.
    f. agnosia
    f. angle
    f. in balloon sign
    base of f.
    baseball f.
    F. Blocking Tree
    f. bolster
    claw f.
    cloven-hoof fracture of f.
    clubbed f.
    coach's f.
    congenital trigger f.
    f. cot
    f. cot splint
    f. deformity
    f. dexterity
    distal tuberosity of f.
    drop f.
    drumstick f.
    f. exerciser

f. extension clockspring splint
f. extrinsics
fifth f.
F. Fitness Spring Ball
f. flap
f. flexion glove
f. flexion splint
f. flexor muscle
football f.
f. gauge
f. goniometer
hammer f.
F. Helper hand exerciser
hippocratic f.
f. hook
HP-100 prosthetic f.
hypoplastic f.
index f.
f. intrinsic
jammed f.
jerk f.
jersey f.
f. joint
f. joint arthroplasty
f. joint implant
f. joint implant prosthesis
f. ladder
little f.
lock f.
long f.
f. loop
lumbrical-plus f.
lumbrical syndrome f.
mallet f.
middle f.
multiple f.
f. opposition
f. pad
paradoxical lumbrical-plus f.
F. Platter hand exerciser
f. pulp
f. ray
replantation of f.
ring f.
rugby jersey f.
sausage f.
f. separator
f. sling
snap f.
spade f.
spider f.
spring f.

stuck f.
syndactylized f.
f. tourniquet
trigger f.
f. tuft
f. web
webbed f.
fingerbreadth
Finger-Hugger splint
fingernail
base of f.
beak f.
f. drill
finger-thumb reflex
fingertip
f. amputation
f. cold intolerance
f. dissection
f. guard
f. pad
fingertips-to-floor test
finger-to-finger test
finger-to-nose test
fingertrap
f. suspension
f. suture
f. traction
finish bur
finisher
Küntscher f.
Finkelstein
F. maneuver
F. sign
F. test
F. test for synovitis
Finn
F. hinged knee prosthesis
F. knee system
Finney-Flexirod prosthesis
Finney prosthesis
Finochietto
F. clamp carrier
F. rib retractor
firearm injury
Fired-Hendel procedure
firing
f. pattern
f. rate
Firm D-Ring wrist support splint
FirmFlex
F. custom orthosis
F. custom orthotic

F

NOTES

first
f. carpometacarpal joint fracture
f. cervical vertebra
f. cuneiform joint arthrodesis
f. cuneiform-navicular joint
arthrodesis
f. dorsal interosseous assist
f. dorsal metacarpal artery
f. dorsal metatarsal artery (FDMA)
f. intermetacarpal ligament
f. metacarpal
f. metatarsal-first cuneiform
arthrodesis
f. metatarsal head (FMH)
f. metatarsus rise test
f. MTP cheilectomy
f. plantar metatarsal artery (FPMA)
f. ray surgery
f. rib rasp
f. rib resection
f. web space
wrist f.

first–fifth intermetatarsal angle
first–second intermetatarsal angle
first-toe Jones repair
Fisch
F. bone drill irrigator
F. bone rongeur
F. drill

Fischer
F. pressure threshold meter
F. ring
F. tendon stripper
F. transfixing pin

fish
F. cuneiform osteotomy
F. cuneiform osteotomy technique
f. vertebra

Fisher
F. advancement flap
F. brace
F. guide
F. half pin
F. Protected Least Significant
Difference test
F. rasp

fishmouth
f. amputation
f. anastomosis
f. drain
f. end-to-end suture
f. incision

fishtail
f. deformity
f. sign

Fiskars scissors
Fisk-Fernandez volar wedge bone graft
fissure bur

fissured
f. fracture
f. nail

Fist-Palm-Side Test
Fist-Ring Test
fistula, pl. **fistulas, fistulae**
arteriovenous f. (AVF)
colocutaneous f.
enterocutaneous f.
synovial f.
vesicocutaneous f.

fistulography
FIT
Fracture Intervention Trial

fit
f. and fill
interference f.
press f.
snap f.
trial f.

Fit-Lastic
F.-L. therapy band
F.-L. therapy tubing

fitness
F. Ball
F. Safety Standards Committee

Fitnet joint testing system
Fits-All
F.-A. sling
F.-A. support

Fitstep
F. II stair climber
Universal F.

FITT
frequency, intensity, time, type
FITT exercise

fitting
immediate postsurgical f. (IPSF)
prosthetic f.
temporary prosthetic f.
Velcro f.

Fitzgerald rating
five
f. classifications of spondylolisthesis
flexor wad of f.

five-hole plate
five-incision procedure
five-in-one
f.-i.-o. knee ligament repair
f.-i.-o. knee reconstruction

five-prong rake blade retractor
Fixateur
F. Interne fixation system
F. Interne rod
F. Interne screw

fixating apparatus
fixation
abnormal f.

Ace-Colles f.
Ace-Fischer f.
Ace Unifix f.
adjunctive screw f.
Allen-Ferguson Galveston pelvic f.
AMBI f.
AMS intramedullary f.
Anderson pin f.
angled blade plate f.
anterior internal f.
anterior metallic f.
anterior plate f.
anterior screw f.
anterior spinal f.
AO external f.
AO screw f.
AO spinal internal f.
APR cement f.
Arbeitsgemeinschaft für
  Osteosynthesefragen-Association for
  the Study of Internal F. (AO-
  ASIF)
arthroscopic screw f.
Association for the Study of
  Internal F. (ASIF)
atlantoaxial rotatory f. (AARF)
Austin chevron osteotomy f.
axial f.
bar bolt f.
Barbour cervical f.
Barr open reduction and internal f.
Barr tibial fracture f.
bicortical screw f.
Biofix absorbable f.
biologic f.
blade plate f.
f. bolt
bolt f.
bone-ingrowth f.
bone suture f.
bridge plate f.
buttressing in internal f.
Calandruccio f.
Campbell screw f.
cementless f.
cerclage wire f.
cervical spine internal f.
cervical spine screw-plate f.
chevron osteotomy with rigid
  screw f.
Childress ankle f.
circular f.

circumferential wire-loop f.
cloverleaf condylar plate f.
Cole tendon f.
compression plate f.
computer-assisted percutaneous
  internal f.
condylar screw f.
coracoclavicular screw f.
coracoclavicular suture f.
cross-screw f.
DeBastiani f.
Denham external f.
dens anterior screw f.
Deverle f.
f. device
Dimon-Hughston fracture f.
f. disk
dorsal wire-loop f.
dynamic compression plate f.
dynamic condylar screw f.
dynamic external f.
f. dysfunction of the lumbar spine
ECT internal fracture f.
elastic f.
Ender nail f.
Ender rod f.
EX-FI-RE external f.
external spinal f.
extramedullary f.
femoral prosthesis f.
four-bar external f.
four-point f.
fracture f.
Gallie subtalar f.
Galveston pelvic f.
Ganz f.
Georgiade visor halo f.
Gouffon pin f.
graft f.
greenstick f.
Hackethal intramedullary bouquet f.
half-pin f.
Halifax clamp posterior cervical f.
Hammer external f.
Harrington rod f.
Herbert bone screw f.
Hex-Fix external f.
Hoffmann external f.
hook-pin f.
hook-plate f.
Hughes f.
hybrid f.

F

NOTES

fixation *(continued)*

Ikuta f.
iliac f.
Ilizarov external f.
f. imaging
ingrowth f.
Innovasive f.
interference fit f.
internal fracture f.
internal spinal f.
interosseous wire f.
intersegmental f.
Intrafix f.
intramedullary rod f.
intraosseous f.
intrapedicular f.
f. jig
Kavanaugh-Brower-Mann f.
Kempf internal screw f.
Kirschner pin f.
Kirschner wire f.
Kristiansen-Kofoed external f.
Kronner external f.
Kronner ring f.
K-wire f.
Kyle internal f.
lag screw f.
loop f.
LPPS hydroxyapatite f.
lumbar pedicle f.
lumbar spine segmental f.
lumbar spine transpedicular f.
Luque-Galveston f.
Luque loop f.
Luque rod f.
Luque segmental f.
Magerl posterior cervical screw f.
Magerl transarticular screw f.
Matta-Saucedo f.
McKeever medullary clavicle f.
medial malleolus f.
medullary nail f.
Meniscus Arrow f.
Minerva f.
minifragment plate f.
monofilament wire f.
Monticelli-Spinelli leg f.
Morrissy percutaneous slipped
  epiphysis f.
multiple-point sacral f.
Murray f.
nail plate f.
neutralization plate f.
occipitocervical f.
odontoid fracture internal f.
Olerud transpedicular f.
open reduction and internal f.
  (ORIF)

OrthoSorb pin f.
os calcis pin f.
pedicular f.
f. peg
pelvic f.
percutaneous f.
phalangeal fracture f.
Phemister acromioclavicular pin f.
pin f.
f. pin
pin-and-plaster f.
plate f.
plate-screw f.
porous ingrowth f.
posterior cervical f.
posterior screw f.
posterior segmental f.
Precision Osteolock f.
press-fit f.
prophylactic skeletal f.
provisional f.
reduction f.
ReUnite hand f.
Rezaian external f.
rigid internal f.
rod sleeve f.
Roger Anderson f.
Rogozinski spinal f.
Roy-Camille posterior screw
  plate f.
sacral fusion screw f.
sacral pedicle screw f.
sacral spine f.
sacroiliac extension f.
sacroiliac flexion f.
Sangeorzan internal f.
Schneider f.
Schuind external f.
scoliosis f.
scoliotic curve f.
screw f.
screw-and-keel f.
screw-and-plate f.
screw-and-wire f.
screw-plate f.
segmental f.
Seidel intramedullary f.
Shepherd internal screw f.
Slatis f.
SmartTack f.
Spiessel internal screw f.
spinal f.
spinopelvic transiliac f. (STIF)
spondylolisthesis reduction f.
spring f.
Stableloc II external f.
staple f.
static f.

Steinmann pin f.
strut plate f.
sublaminar f.
f. subluxation
Sukhtian-Hughes f.
suprasyndesmotic screw f.
Suretac shoulder f.
suture f.
f. technique
tension band f.
thin pin f.
three-hole suture tendon f.
TiMesh implantable hardware f.
transarticular screw f.
transarticular wire f.
transcapitellar wire f.
TransFix ACL system f.
transiliac rod f.
transpedicular f.
transsyndesmotic screw f.
transverse f.
triangular external ankle f.
True-Lok external f.
TSRH rod f.
tunnel-and-sling f.
Turvy internal screw f.
Versa-Fx femoral f.
Vidal-Adrey modified Hoffmann f.
Volkov-Oganesian external f.
VSP f.
Wagner f.
Ward-Tomasin-Vander-Griend f.
Warner-Farber ankle f.
Wasserstein f.
Webb f.
wedge f.
white f.
Wilson-Jacobs tibial f.
wire loop f.
Wisconsin wire f.
Wolvek sternal approximation f.
Zickel nail f.
Zickel subtrochanteric fracture f.

fixator

Ace-Colles external f.
Ace-Fischer external f.
Agee external f.
Agee WristJack external f.
AO internal f.
articulated external f.
biplanar f.
Block f.

cantilever external f.
carbon fiber f.
circular external f.
circular wire f.
Claiborne external f.
clamp f.
Clyburn Colles fracture f.
Clyburn external f.
Compass Hinge external f.
DeBastiani external f.
D-L internal f.
dynamic axial f. (DAF)
EBI external f.
Edwards D-L modular f.
external f.
external spinal skeletal f. (ESSF)
f. frame
Ganz anti-shock pelvic f.
half-pin external f.
Herbert screw f.
Hex-Fix monolateral external f.
hinged articulated f.
Hoffmann C-series external f.
Hoffmann Dynamic external f.
Hoffmann-Vidal external f.
HTO f.
hybrid external f.
Ilizarov circular external f.
Ilizarov external ring f.
Ilizarov hybrid f.
Jacquet f.
Kessler external f.
L-frame f.
Lima external f.
Manuflex external f.
mini-Hoffmann external f.
mini-Kessler external f.
mini-Orthofix f.
modified Hoffmann quadrilateral external f.
Monofixateur external f.
Monticelli-Spinelli f.
f. muscle
Olerud internal f.
one-bar external f.
one-plane bilateral external f.
one-plane unilateral external f.
Orthofix monolateral femoral external f.
Oxford f.
Pennig dynamic wrist f.
pin external f.

F

NOTES

fixator *(continued)*

Rezaian spinal f.
Richards Colles external f.
ring external f.
Roger Anderson external f.
spanning external f.
Stableloc Colles fracture external f.
temporary external f.
thin-wire Ilizarov f.
Thomas f.
two-plane bilateral external f.
two-plane unilateral external f.
Vermont spinal f. (VSF)
Wagner device external f.
Wagner external f.
Wiltse f.

fixator-augmented nailing

fixed

f. anatomic patellar implant
f. bearing knee implant
f. deformity
f. distraction
f. dressing
f. femoral head prosthesis
f. flexion contracture (FFC)
f. hammertoe
f. inversion
f. torticollis

fixed-angle

f.-a. AO bladeplate
f.-a. blade plate

fixed-offset guide

fixer

Wagner f.

FJD

facet joint disease

FL

femur length

FL/AC

femur length to abdominal circumference
ratio
FL/AC ratio

flaccid

f. cerebral palsy
f. flatfoot
f. gait
f. leg
f. paralysis

flaccidity

flag

f. flap
f. sign

Flagg fiberglass knee brace

flail

f. arm
f. digit
f. foot
f. implant

f. joint
f. knee
f. shoulder
f. toe

flail-elbow hinge

FLAIR

fluid attenuation inversion recovery

flake hamate fracture

flame-tip bur

Flanagan-Burem apposing hemicylindric graft

flange

endoprosthetic f.

flanged revision prosthesis

flank bone

flap

abdominal f.
abductor hallucis longus f.
adductor magnus adductor f.
adipofascial f.
advancement f.
f. amputation
anterior myocutaneous f.
anterior tibial fasciocutaneous f.
arm f.
arterial f.
Atasoy-Kleinert f.
Atasoy triangular advancement f.
Atasoy volar V-Y f.
axial pattern f.
axillary f.
biaxial f.
bilateral V-Y Kutler f.
bilobed digital neurovascular
island f.
bilobed skin f.
bipedicle dorsal f.
brachioradialis f.
buccinator myomucosal f.
bursal f.
capsular f.
capsuloperiosteal f.
Chinese f.
cocked-half f.
composite groin fascial free f.
f. congestion
cross-arm f.
cross-extremity f.
cross-finger f.
cross-leg f.
cutaneous f.
deltoid f.
deltopectoral f.
dorsal cross-finger f.
dorsalis pedis fasciocutaneous f.
Double-Z rhombic skin f.
DRAM f.
extensor digitorum brevis f.

fascial subcutaneous turn-down f.
fasciocutaneous axial pattern f.
fasciocutaneous island f.
finger f.
Fisher advancement f.
flag f.
flexor hallucis brevis f.
foot first-web f.
forearm f.
free fasciocutaneous f.
free latissimus dorsi f.
free microsurgical f.
free scapular f.
free skin f.
gastrocnemius f.
Gilbert scapular f.
gluteus maximus f.
gracilis f.
f. graft
groin f.
hemipulp f.
horseshoe-shaped f.
hypogastric f.
iliac osteocutaneous f.
iliofemoral pedicle f.
intercostal f.
inverted skin f.
island adipofascial f.
island skin f.
Kutler double lateral
  advancement f.
Kutler V-Y f.
lateral arm f.
lateral thigh f.
lateral thoracic f.
latissimus dorsi f.
lazy-V deepithelialized turn-over
  fasciocutaneous f.
Limberg f.
local f.
long posterior f.
medialis pedis f.
medial plantar fasciocutaneous f.
f. meniscal tear
microvascular free muscle f.
Moberg advancement f.
Morrison neurovascular free f.
multistaged carrier f.
muscle f.
musculocutaneous free f.
musculotendinous f.
myocutaneous f.

neurocutaneous hand f.
neurovascular free f.
nutrient f.
omental f.
f. operation
osteocutaneous free f.
osteomusculocutaneous f.
osteoperiosteal f.
palmar advancement f.
palmar cross-finger f.
parascapular f.
pectoralis major f.
pedicle groin f.
peroneal island f.
plantar artery f.
plantar V-Y advancement f.
f. plasty
posterior f.
pulp f.
radial-based f.
radial forearm f.
random pattern f.
rectus abdominis f.
rectus femoris f.
remote pedicle f.
reverse cross-finger f.
reverse-flow f.
reverse forearm island f.
rhomboid f.
rotational f.
saphenous f.
scapular f.
serratus anterior f.
single-lobed skin f.
skew f.
skin f.
sliding f.
soft tissue f.
Steichen neurovascular free f.
supramalleolar f.
sural island f.
Tait f.
temporalis fascia f.
tensor fascia femoris f.
tensor fascia lata muscle f.
thenar f.
thoracoepigastric f.
transposition f.
triangular advancement f.
turn-down tendon f.
Urbaniak neurovascular free f.
Urbaniak scapular f.

NOTES

F

flap (*continued*)
  vascularized free f.
  V-Y advancement f.
  V-Y Kutler f.
  web space f.
  wraparound neurovascular free f.
flapless amputation
flare
  f. of the condyle
  foot f.
  medial tibial f.
flared spinal rod
FlashCast
  Delta-Lite F.
flat
  f. back deformity
  f. back syndrome
  f. bone
  f. bone graft
  f. chest
  f. drill
  f. flexible foot
  F. Foot insole
  f. hand
  f. metatarsal head
  f. palpation
  f. plate
  f. plate radiography
  f. retractor
  f. splint
flat-bottomed Kerrison rongeur
flat-cut
  f.-c. arthrodesis
  f.-c. technique
flatfoot
  acquired f.
  adult acquired f.
  calcaneovalgus f.
  congenital f.
  congenital rocker-bottom f.
  f. deformity
  Durham procedure for f.
  flaccid f.
  f. gait
  hypermobile f.
  f. insole
  Kidner f.
  neonatal f.
  pediatric f.
  peroneal spastic f.
  physiologic f.
  pronated straight f.
  rigid f.
  rockerbottom f.
  spastic f.
flat-hand test
Flatt
  F. classification

F. driver
F. excision
F. finger-joint prosthesis
F. finger-thumb prosthesis
F. implant
F. recess
F. self-retaining screwdriver
F. technique
F. tendon transfer
flattening of normal lordotic curve
F&L attenuating glove
flattop talus
flatware
  Amefa F.
  Cushion Grip F.
  Melaware f.
flava (*pl. of* flavum)
flaval ligament
flavectomy
flavum, pl. **flava**
  hypertrophied ligamentum f.
Fleck
  F. fracture
  F. sign
Fleischmann bursa
flesh
  proud f.
Fletching femoral hernia implant material
flex
  f. against gravity
  F. Foam brace
  F. Foam orthosis
  F. Ranger stretch cable with pulley
Flexall gel
Flexderm wound dressing
flexed
  plantar f.
  f. position
Flex-Foam bandage
Flex-Foot Modular III prosthesis
FLEX H/A total ossicular prosthesis
flexibility
  f. conditioning program
  Cotrel-Dubousset rod f.
  f. exercise
  f. training
flexible
  f. bandage
  f. digital implant
  f. hammertoe
  f. hinge implant
  f. hinge suspension
  f. intramedullary nail (FIN)
  f. medullary nail
  f. medullary reamer
  f. orthosis

f. pes planus
f. pes valgus
f. socket
f. sound
f. talipes
Flexicair bed
Flexigrid dressing
Flexi-Grip exercise putty
Flexilite conforming elastic bandage
fleximeter
Flexinet dressing
flexing
flexion
f., abduction, external rotation
  (FABER)
f., abduction, external rotation
  contracture
active f.
f., adduction, internal rotation
  (FADIR)
f. angle
angle of greatest f. (AGF)
f. axis
back f.
f. body cast
f. body jacket
f. bumper
cervical specific rotation in f.
f. compression spine injury
  stabilization
compressive f.
f. creaking
f. distraction
distractive f.
dorsiflexion f.
elongation-derotation f.
elongation, derotation and lateral f.
  (EDF)
f. and extension
external rotation in f. (ERF)
femoral-trunk f.
forced passive full forward f.
forced plantar f.
forward f.
full fist f.
further f. (FF)
f. gap
f. glove
hip f.
f. injury posterior atlantoaxial
  arthrodesis
f. instability

internal rotation in f. (IRF)
knee f.
lateral f.
left lateral f.
lumbar lateral f.
lumbosacral f.
f. malposition
f. osteotomy
palmar f.
passive plantar f.
plantar f.
resisted active f.
f. restriction
right lateral f.
Riordan finger f.
Schober test of lumbar f.
shelf f.
sitting f.
f. spinal radiography test
spine f.
standing f.
f. teardrop fracture
toe f.
transverse axis knee f.
uninhibited f.
f. valgus deformity
volitional resisted f.
flexion-adduction
flexion-burst fracture
flexion-compression fracture
flexion-distraction
f.-d. chiropractic table
f.-d. fracture
f.-d. injury
f.-d. therapy
flexion-extension
f.-e. arc
f.-e. axis
f.-e. control cervical orthosis
f.-e. exercise
f.-e. gap
hip f.-e.
f.-e. injury
knee f.-e.
f.-e. maneuver
f.-e. MRI
f.-e. plane
f.-e. radiography
flexion-internal rotational deformity
flexion-rotation-compression maneuver
**flexion-rotation-drawer knee instability
  test**

F

NOTES

Flexirule
Flexisplint flexed arm board
FlexiSport orthotic
FlexiTherm
> F. diabetic diagnostic insole
> F. Thermographic System

FlexLite hinged knee support
Flex-Master bandage
flexometer
> Moeltgen f.

flexor
> anterior long toe f.
> f. cap
> f. carpi radialis (FCR)
> f. carpi radialis muscle
> f. carpi radialis tendon
> f. carpi ulnaris (FCU)
> f. carpi ulnaris muscle
> f. carpi ulnaris syndrome
> f. carpi ulnaris tendon
> f. digiti quinti muscle
> f. digitorum brevis (FDB)
> f. digitorum communis (FDC)
> f. digitorum communis tendon
> f. digitorum longus (FDL)
> f. digitorum longus muscle
> f. digitorum longus tendon
> f. digitorum longus tendon
> contracture
> f. digitorum longus tendon transfer
> f. digitorum profundus (FDP)
> f. digitorum profundus muscle
> f. digitorum profundus tendon
> f. digitorum quinti brevis (FDQB)
> f. digitorum slip
> f. digitorum sublimis (FDS)
> f. digitorum sublimis muscle
> f. digitorum sublimis tendon
> f. digitorum superficialis (FDS)
> f. digitorum superficialis muscle
> f. digitorum superficialis tendon
> f. to extensor tendon transfer
> extrinsic toe f.
> f. groove
> f. hallucis brevis (FHB)
> f. hallucis brevis flap
> f. hallucis brevis muscle
> f. hallucis brevis tendon
> f. hallucis longus (FHL)
> f. hallucis longus dysfunction
> (FHLD)
> f. hallucis longus muscle
> f. hallucis longus tendon
> f. hallucis longus tendon release
> f. hallucis longus tenosynovitis
> f. hallucis tendon contracture
> f. hinge orthosis
> f. hinge splint
> long toe f.

> f. mechanism
> f. origin syndrome
> f. phase
> f. plate
> f. plate release
> f. pollicis brevis (FPB)
> f. pollicis brevis muscle
> f. pollicis brevis tendon
> f. pollicis longus (FPL)
> f. pollicis longus abductor-plasty
> f. pollicis longus muscle
> f. pollicis longus tendon
> f. profundus tendon
> f. pronator slide
> f. retinaculum
> f. retinaculum of hand
> f. skin crease
> snapping thumb f.
> f. sublimis tendon
> f. tendon anastomosis
> f. tendon graft
> f. tendon laceration
> f. tendon repair
> f. tendon rupture
> f. tendon sheath
> f. tenolysis
> f. tenosynovectomy
> f. tenotomy
> toe f.
> f. wad
> f. wad of five
> f. wad of five muscles
> f. withdrawal reflex
> X-TEND-O knee f.

flexor-hinge hand-splint brace
flexorplasty
> Bunnell modification of Steindler f.
> Eyler f.
> Steindler f.

flexor-pronator
> f.-p. origin
> f.-p. origin release

flexor-to-extensor tendon transfer
FlexPosure endoscopic retractor
Flex-Sprint prosthesis
FlexStrand cable
FlexTech knee brace
Flextender Plus hand exerciser
flexural concavity
Flick-Gould technique
Flip-Flop pillow
flipped meniscus sign
flipper hand
flip test
F2L Multineck femoral stem
FLOAM ankle stirrup brace
floating
> f. arch fracture

f. cartilage
f. clavicle
f. elbow
f. gait
f. knee
f. knee fracture classification
f. ligament
f. patella
f. rib
f. thumb
f. time
f. toe
f. traction

flocculent focus of calcification
Flo-Fit Comfortseat
floor
f. of acetabulum
f. sitter
floor-reaction ankle-foot orthosis
floppy
f. infant
f. toe
flora
bacterial f.
florid
f. callus
f. reactive periostitis
f. rickets
f. synovitis
Florida
F. back brace
F. cervical brace
F. contraflexion brace
F. extension brace
F. hyperextension brace
F. J-24, J-35, J-45, J-55 brace
F. post-fusion brace
F. spinal brace
Flotan thumb
Flo-Tech prosthetic socket
Flo-Trol drinking cup
flottant
pouce f. thumb
flounce
meniscal f.
flow
blood f.
flower
F. bone
F. index
flower-spray ending

flowing hyperostosis
flow-mediated vasodilation (FMD)
flowmeter
Doppler ultrasound f.
flowmetry
laser Doppler f.
Flowtron
F. DVT
F. pneumatic compression system
BioCryo system
FLP
Functional Limitation Profile
fluctuation test
fluff dressing
FLUFTEX gauze roll
fluid
f. absorption ability
f. attenuation inversion recovery
(FLAIR)
f. balance
f. barrier boot
bursal f.
cerebrospinal f. (CSF)
f. controlled component
egress of arthroscopic f.
f. homeostasis
hypotonic f.
interstitial f.
f. overhydration
f. prosthesis
f. sign
synovial f.
FluidAir bed
Fluidotherapy sterile dry heat modality
fluorescein
f. perfusion monitoring
f. study
FluoroNav
FluoroScan
fluoroscopic table
fluoroscopy
C-arm f.
electric joint f.
intraoperative f.
portable C-arm image intensifier f.
two-plane f.
XiScan f.
flush
heparinized saline f.
peroxide f.
flute of cannulated screw

F

NOTES

fluted
- f. medullary rod
- f. reamer
- f. Sampson nail
- f. titanium nail

FLX flexible treatment coilette

Flynn
- F. femoral neck fracture reduction
- F. technique

FM
- EndoButton FM

FMD
- flow-mediated vasodilation

FMH
- first metatarsal head

fMRI
- functional magnetic resonance imaging

FMS
- fibromyalgia syndrome
- FMS Intracell stick

FO
- foot orthosis

foam
- f. casting
- f. collar
- f. cushion
- Evazote f.
- foam compression molded ethylene vinyl acetate f.
- gelatin f.
- high-density f.
- Neoplush f.
- f. pad
- Pedilen polyurethane f.
- Plastazote f.
- polyethylene f.
- prosthetic f.
- f. ring
- f. slant
- f. tape
- Temper F.
- tube f.
- f. tubing

Foamart foot impression system

focal
- f. calcification
- f. deficiency
- f. dystonia
- f. fibrocartilaginous dysplasia
- f. film distance
- f. nodular myositis
- f. pigmented villonodular synovitis
- f. scleroderma

focus, pl. foci

Foerster forceps

fold
- asymmetric skin f.
- Bartlett nail f.
- nail f.
- synovial f.

folding
- f. fracture
- f. frame wheelchair

fold-over finger splint

Folius muscle

folliculitis

fomentation therapy

Fomon
- F. chisel
- F. periosteal elevator
- F. periosteotome
- F. rasp

FONAR
- field focused nuclear magnetic resonance
- FONAR Stand-Up MRI

FOOSH
- fell on outstretched hand
- FOOSH injury

foot, pl. feet
- adolescent rigid f.
- f. alignment
- f. anesthetic
- f. angle
- f. and ankle severity scale (FASS)
- arch of f.
- f. architecture
- articulation of f.
- atavistic f.
- athlete's f.
- ball of f.
- basketball f.
- bifid f.
- broad f.
- burning f.
- calcaneocavus f.
- calcaneovalgus f.
- Carbon Copy II Light F.
- cavovarus f.
- cavus f.
- f. central compartment pressure measurement
- Charcot f.
- Cirrus composite prosthetic f.
- clavus f.
- claw f.
- cleft f.
- club f.
- f. collapse
- College Park TruStep f.
- ComfortWalk prosthetic f.
- contralateral f.
- f. cosmesis
- cosmetically acceptable f.
- C-shaped f.
- f. cushion
- dancer's f.

dangling f.
f. decompression
deconditioned f.
f. deformity
diabetic Charcot f.
digital artery of f.
ding f.
diplegic f.
f. drape
f. drop
dropped f.
Dycor prosthetic f.
f. dynamics
f. dysplasia
Egyptian f.
equinocavus f.
equinovalgus f.
equinovarus f.
equinus f.
f. first-web flap
flail f.
f. flare
flat flexible f.
Flex-Walk II prosthetic f.
forced f.
Friedreich f.
functional disability of f.
F. Function Index (FFI)
F. Function Index questionnaire
Greek f.
Hardy-Clapham classification of
  sesamoid bones of f.
F. Health Status Questionnaire
hemiplegic f.
hollow f.
hooked f.
F. Hugger foot support
hypermobile f.
hypoflexibility of f.
immersion f.
f. imprinter
inferior extensor of f.
insensate f.
f. ischemia
ischemic f.
Kingsley Steplite f.
lateral spring ligament of f.
F. Levelers custom orthotic
F. Levelers orthosis
f. lift-off
lobster-claw f.
Lo Rider prosthetic f.

low-arch f.
Madura f.
f. magnet
malodorous f.
march f.
f. model
Morand f.
Morton f.
mossy f.
multiaxis f.
neuroarthropathic f.
neuropathic f.
f. orthosis (FO)
f. orthotic management
Otto Bock 1A30 Greissinger
  Plus f.
Otto Bock 1D25 Dynamic Plus f.
paralytic f.
parrot f.
Pathfinder prosthetic f.
Persian slipper f.
f. pillow
f. placement test
planovalgus f.
plantar f.
plantigrade f.
f. plate
polydactylous cleft f.
f. progression angle (FPA)
pronated f.
pronation of the f.
f. prosthesis
f. puncture wound
Quantum f.
reel f.
Re-Flex VSP artificial f.
f. rest
rheumatoid f.
rigid f.
rockerbottom f.
f. rotation
SACH f.
SAFE f.
Seattle f.
serpentine f.
shortened f.
single-axis Syme DYCOR f.
skew f.
f. slap
f. sling
sole of f.
solid ankle, cushioned heel f.

NOTES

foot *(continued)*
    spastic flat f.
    spatula f.
    split f.
    spread f.
    S-shaped f.
    f. stabilizer
    f. stagnation
    stairclimber's f.
    f. stool
    f. strain
    superior extensor retinaculum of f.
    supination of f.
    Sure-Flex III prosthetic f.
    Syme Dycor prosthetic f.
    tabetic f.
    taut f.
    The Beachcomber prosthetic f.
    trench f.
    tripod f.
    Trow Bridge TerraRound f.
    f. type
    valgus f.
    Vari-Flex prosthetic f.
    f. volumeter
    weak f.
    Z f.
foot-ankle
    f.-a. assembly
    f.-a. brace
    f.-a. complex
football
    f. calf
    f. finger
footballer's
    f. ankle
    f. groin
    f. hernia
Footbrush
    Dr. Joseph's Original F.
footdrop
    f. brace
    f. gait
    f. night splint
Foot-Fitter
FootFlex performance stretching device
footgear
Footmaster orthotic
footpiece
    Bunker f.
    traction f.
footplate *(var. of* foot plate*)*
footprint
    f. analysis
    dynamic f.
    Harris-Beath f.
    f. index

    static f.
    tibial f.
footrest
Foot-Station 3-D foot imaging system
foot-strike
    f.-s. hemolysis
    f.-s. hemolysis anemia
foot-strike phase of gait
foot-thigh axis
footwear
    Ambulator biomechanical f.
    Ambulator conform f.
    Comfort Rite f.
forage
    f. core biopsy
    f. procedure
foramen, pl. **foramina**
    arcuate f.
    Hartigan f.
    intravertebral f. (IVF)
    ischiopubic f.
    f. magnum
    f. magnum decompression
    neural f.
    open exit f.
    sciatic f.
    f. transversarium
    Weitbrecht f.
foraminal
    f. compression test
    f. encroachment subluxation
    f. osteophyte encroachment
    f. stenosis
foraminoplasty
    laminaplasty with extended f.
foraminotomy
    neural f.
Forbes
    F. modification of Phemister graft
      technique
    F. onlay bone graft
force
    activation f.
    f. application
    contact f.
    distraction f.
    dynamic joint f.
    evertor f.
    forefoot f.
    gravity ground reaction f.
    ground reaction f.
    hamstring f.
    invertor f.
    isometric f.
    joint f.
    knee f.
    lateral compression f.
    moment of f.

Newton f.
f. nucleus
patellofemoral joint reaction f.
f. plate
f. plate foot analysis
prehension f.
reaction f.
shearing f.
subthreshold f.
tensile f.
tension f.
torque f.
f. transducer
translatory f.
weightbearing ground reaction f.

forcé

brisement f.
redressement f.

force-couple splint reduction
forced

f. adduction test
f. flexion injury
f. foot
f. passive full forward flexion
f. passive internal rotation
f. plantar flexion
f. vital capacity

forceps

Acland clamp-applying f.
Acufex curved basket f.
Acufex rotary biting basket f.
Adson clip-introducing f.
Adson drill guide f.
Adson hypophysial f.
adventitial f.
Aesculap bipolar cautery f.
alligator bone-reduction f.
alligator grasping f.
Allis tissue f.
Angell James hypophysectomy f.
angled-down f.
angled-up f.
anterior f.
AO reduction f.
Arrowsmith-Clerf pin-closing f.
arthroscopy basket f.
arthroscopy grasping f.
Asch f.
atraumatic f.
Babcock f.
baby Lane f.
Backhaus towel f.

Baer bone-cutting f.
Bane rongeur f.
Bardeleben bone-holding f.
basket f.
bearing-seating f.
Beasley-Babcock f.
Berens muscle clamp f.
biarticular bone-cutting f.
biopsy f.
bipolar f.
Bircher-Ganske cartilage f.
blunt f.
Boies f.
bone-biting f.
bone-breaking f.
bone-cutting f.
bone-grasping f.
bone-holding f.
bone punch f.
bone-splitting f.
Brand tendon-holding f.
Brand tendon-passing f.
Brown-Adson f.
Brown-Cushing f.
Brown tissue f.
bulldog clamp-applying f.
Cairns hemostatic f.
Carroll bone-holding f.
Carroll dressing f.
Carroll tendon-pulling f.
Carroll tissue f.
cartilage f.
Caspar alligator f.
cervical punch f.
Chandler spinal perforating f.
Charnley wire-holding f.
Citelli punch f.
clamp f.
Cleveland bone-cutting f.
clip-applying f.
clip-bending f.
clip-cutting f.
clip-introducing f.
coagulating f.
Crile f.
cupped grasping f.
curved basket f.
cutting f.
Dawson-Yuhl-Kerrison rongeur f.
Dawson-Yuhl-Leksell rongeur f.
Dawson-Yuhl rongeur f.
Dingman bone-holding f.

F

NOTES

forceps (*continued*)

disk f.
double-action bone-cutting f.
double-sharp f.
Dreyfus prosthesis f.
drill guide f.
eagle beak bone-cutting f.
Echlin rongeur f.
end-biting f.
ethmoid f.
extracting f.
Farabeuf bone-holding f.
Farabeuf-Lambotte bone-holding f.
Farrior wire-crimping f.
Ferguson bone-holding f.
Fergusson f.
Ferris Smith bone-biting f.
Ferris Smith-Kerrison f.
Ferris Smith rongeur f.
Ferris Smith tissue f.
Foerster f.
Friedman rongeur f.
gall duct f.
Gardner bone f.
glenoid-reaming f.
grasping f.
Greene f.
Gruppe wire prosthesis-crimping f.
Gunderson bone f.
Gunderson muscle f.
Hajek-Koffler bone punch f.
Halsted f.
Harrington clamp f.
Harrison bone-holding f.
Hartmann mosquito f.
Heermann alligator f.
hemostatic f.
Hibbs bone-cutting f.
Hinderer cartilage f.
Hirsch hypophysis punch f.
Hoen f.
Horsley bone-cutting f.
Horsley-Stille bone-cutting f.
Horsley-Stille rib shears f.
Housepan clip-applying f.
Howmedica Microfixation System f.
Hudson f.
Hurd bone-cutting f.
implant f.
Jackson broad-blade staple f.
Jackson dressing f.
Jackson tendon-seizing f.
Jacobson mosquito f.
James wound f.
Jansen monopolar f.
Jarell f.
Jarit tendon-pulling f.
jeweler's f.

Juers-Lempert rongeur f.
Kelly f.
Kern bone-holding f.
Kern-Lane bone f.
King wound f.
Kleinert-Kutz bone-cutting f.
Kleinert-Kutz rongeur f.
Kleinert-Kutz tendon f.
Knight bone-cutting f.
knotting f.
Kocher f.
Lalonde hook f.
Lambotte bone-holding f.
Landolt spreading f.
Lane screw-holding f.
Lane self-retaining bone-holding f.
Langenbeck bone-holding f.
Larsen tendon-holding f.
Leibinger Micro System plate-
   holding f.
Leksell rongeur f.
Lempert rongeur f.
LeRoy clip-applying f.
Lester muscle f.
Lewin bone-holding f.
Lewin spinal perforating f.
lion f.
lion-jaw f.
Liston bone-cutting f.
Liston-Key bone-cutting f.
Liston-Littauer bone-cutting f.
Liston-Stille bone-cutting f.
Littauer-Liston bone-cutting f.
Llorente dissecting f.
long-jaw basket f.
Lore suction tube and tip-
   holding f.
Love-Gruenwald alligator f.
Love-Kerrison rongeur f.
Lowman bone-holding f.
Luer rongeur f.
Luer-Whiting rongeur f.
Luhr Microfixation System plate-
   holding f.
Malis-Jensen microbipolar f.
Malis jeweler bipolar f.
Mantis retrograde f.
Markwalder rib f.
Martin cartilage f.
Mayfield f.
McCain TMJ f.
McGee-Priest wire f.
McGee wire-crimping f.
McIndoe rongeur f.
meniscus f.
Micro-One dissecting f.
Micro-Two f.
Mixter f.

mosquito f.
mosquito-tip grasping f.
nail-pulling f.
Nicola f.
Niro bone-cutting f.
Niro wire-twisting f.
Olivecrona clip-applying and removing f.
orthopaedic f.
Overholt clip-applying f.
perforating f.
Perman cartilage f.
pick-up f.
pin-seating f.
plain tissue f.
plate-holding f.
Poppen f.
Potts-Smith dressing f.
Preston ligamentum flavum f.
punch f.
Raimondi hemostatic f.
rat-tooth f.
reduction f.
rib f.
Riches artery f.
ring f.
Rochester-Carmalt f.
Rochester-Ochsner f.
Rochester-Pean f.
rongeur f.
rotary basket f.
Rowe disimpaction f.
Rowe glenoid-reaming f.
Rowe-Harrison bone-holding f.
Rowe modified-Harrison f.
Ruskin bone-cutting f.
Ruskin bone-splitting f.
Ruskin-Liston bone-cutting f.
Ruskin rongeur f.
Ruskin-Rowland bone-cutting f.
Russian f.
Samuels f.
Sauerbruch rib f.
Schlesinger cervical punch f.
Schlesinger rongeur f.
Schwartz clip-applying f.
Schwartz temporary clamp-applying f.
screw-holding f.
Seaber f.
seizing f.
self-centering bone-holding f.

self-retaining bone-holding f.
Selverstone rongeur f.
Semb bone f.
Semb rib f.
septal f.
sequestrum f.
Shutt Mantis retrograde f.
side-cutting basket f.
small plate f.
Smithwick clip-applying f.
smooth-tipped jeweler's f.
spatula f.
Spence rongeur f.
sponge-holding f.
spreading f.
Spurling-Kerrison rongeur f.
Steinmann tendon f.
Stevenson alligator f.
Stevenson grasping f.
Stille-Horsley bone f.
Stille-Horsley rib f.
Stille-Liston bone-cutting f.
Stille-Luer rongeur f.
Stiwer bone-holding f.
Storz Microsystems plate-holding f.
straight basket f.
Synthes Microsystems plate-holding f.
tack-and-pin f.
Takahashi f.
Take-apart f.
taper-jaw f.
tenaculum-reducing f.
tendon f.
tendon-braiding f.
tendon-holding f.
tendon-passing f.
tendon-pulling f.
tendon-retrieving f.
tendon-seizing f.
tendon-tunneling f.
Thompson hip prosthesis f.
three-edge cutting f.
thumb f.
tissue f.
titanium microsurgical bipolar f.
Toennis tumor f.
toothed tissue f.
Tudor-Edwards bone-cutting f.
tumor-grasping f.
tying f.
Ulrich bone-holding f.

F

NOTES

forceps (continued)

Ulrich-St. Gallen f.
upbiting basket f.
upcurved punch f.
Utrata f.
Van Buren sequestrum f.
vascular f.
Verbrugge bone-holding f.
Walter-Liston f.
Walton-Ruskin f.
Walton wire-pulling f.
Weller cartilage f.
Wiet cup f.
Wilde ethmoid f.
Wilde rongeur f.
wire-cutting f.
wire-extracting f.
wire-holding f.
wire prosthesis-crimping f.
wire-pulling f.
wire-tightening f.
wire-twisting f.
X-long cement f.
Zimmer-Hoen f.
Zimmer-Schlesinger f.

force-time integral (FTI)
Ford triangulation technique
forearm

f. amputation
balanced f.
carrying angle of f.
f. compartment syndrome
f. complex
f. contracture
distal f.
f. flap
f. fracture
f. ischemic exercise
f. lift assist adjustable spring-loaded device
f. lift-assist prosthesis
one-bone f.
f. splint
f. stabilizer
f. supination test
three-bone f.
f. tourniquet

forefoot

f. abduction deformity
f. abductus
f. adduction correction test
f. adductovarus
f. adductus
f. angulation
f. arthroplasty
f. block test
f. cavus
f. digital amputation

f. disruption
f. equinus
f. force
f. FPA
hooked f.
Larmon f.
narrowing of f.
f. nerve block
f. peak pressure
f. splaying
f. striker
f. valgus
f. varus

forefoot-to-rearfoot striker
foreign

f. body (FB)
f. body granuloma
f. body response
f. body screw

forequarter amputation
Forest-Hastings technique
Forestier

F. bowstring sign
F. disease

forged cobalt-chromium alloy prosthesis
fork

f. strap
f. strap prosthetic support

form

f. constancy
IKDC f.
International Knee Documentation Committee f.
Jettmobile positioning and tumble f.
Vestibulator positioning tumble f.

formal hemipelvectomy
formation

adhesion f.
beaklike osteophyte f.
bunion f.
callous f.
capsule f.
Chiari f.
cyclops f.
F. Gelfoam mattress overlay
intramembranous f.
lappet f.
new bone f.
osteomyelitic cloaca f.
osteophyte f.
periosteal new bone f.
Pfitzner theory of coalition f.
pincer nail f.
procallus f.
reactive bone f.
rouleaux f.
scar f.

spur f.
subperiosteal new bone f.
trellis f.
Formatray mandibular splint
forme, pl. **formes**
f. fruste
formes frustes neurofibromatosis
formula, pl. **formulae, formulas**
Arth-Aid Joint F.
Boyd f.
digital f.
Dreyer f.
pediatric nutritional f.
vertebral f.
Forrester
F. cervical collar brace
F. splint
Forrester-Brown
F.-B. collar
F.-B. head halter
Forte
F. harness
Fortin finger test
forward
f. bending
f. flexion
f. flexion posture
f. head posture
forward-cutting knife
Fosnaugh nail biopsy
fossa, pl. **fossae**
acetabular f.
antecubital f.
bony f.
femoral f.
glenoid f.
intercondylar f.
ischiorectal f.
Jobert f.
lower f. active, lateral knee pain, and long leg on the side ipsilateral to the weak f. (LLL)
Mohrenheim f.
olecranon f.
patellar f.
popliteal f.
sphenoidal f.
supinator f.
supraclavicular f.
upper f. active, medial knee pain, and short leg on the side ipsilateral to the weak f. (UMS)

Foster
F. bed
F. splint
F. turning frame
Foster-Kennedy maneuver
Foucher classification of epiphysial injury
foulage
foundation
Arthritis F.
level f.
Musculoskeletal Transplant F. (MTF)
Osteogenesis Imperfecta F. (OIF)
F. total knee and hip system
four-bar
f.-b. external fixation
f.-b. external fixation apparatus
f.-b. external fixation device
f.-b. linkage on knee prosthesis
f.-b. linkage prosthetic knee mechanism
f.-b. polycentric knee prosthesis
fourchée
main f.
four-compartment fasciotomy
four-corner midcarpal fusion
four-flanged nail
four-hole
f.-h. Alta straight plate
f.-h. side plate
Fourier
F. analysis
F. transform infrared spectroscopy
four-incision procedure
four-in-one
f.-i.-o. arthroplasty
f.-i.-o. cutting block
f.-i.-o. positioning block system
four-level radiculopathy
four-limb Z-plasty
Fournier test
four-part
f.-p. fracture
f.-p. variant
four-point
f.-p. fixation
f.-p. gait
f.-p. IROM brace
f.-p. IROM splint

NOTES

F

four-point (continued)
> f.-p. SuperSport functional knee brace
> f.-p. walker

four-poster
> f.-p. cervical brace
> f.-p. cervical orthosis
> f.-p. frame

four-prong finger splint
four-star exercise program
four-tap screw
fourth
> f. metatarsophalangeal joint
> f. turbinated bone

four-wire trochanter reattachment
fovea, pl. **foveae**
> f. capitis femoris
> f. centralis bone

foveal fat pad
foveate
foveated chest
foveation
Fowler
> F. central slip tenotomy
> F. knee system
> F. maneuver
> F. osteotomy
> F. position
> F. procedure
> F. spread
> F. technique
> F. tendon transfer
> F. tenodesis
> F. test

Fowler-Philip
> F.-P. angle
> F.-P. approach
> F.-P. incision

Fowles
> F. dislocation technique
> F. open reduction

fox
> F. clavicular splint
> F. extractor-impactor
> F. impactor-extractor
> F. internal fixation apparatus
> F. internal fixation device
> F. wrench

Fox-Blazina knee procedure
FP5000 pump system
FPA
> foot progression angle
> forefoot FPA
> hindfoot FPA

FPB
> flexor pollicis brevis

FPL
> flexor pollicis longus

FPMA
> first plantar metatarsal artery

F.R.
> F.R. Thompson endoprosthesis
> F.R. Thompson femoral prosthesis

fraction
> linear f.
> motor unit f.

fractional
> f. curve
> f. lengthening

fractionation
Fractomed splint
Fractura
> F. Flex bandage
> F. Flex cast

fracture
> abduction-external rotation f.
> accessory navicular f.
> accessory ossicle f.
> acetabular posterior wall f.
> acetabular rim f.
> acute avulsion f.
> adduction f.
> agenetic f.
> AIIS avulsion f.
> Aitken classification of epiphysial f.
> Allen open reduction of calcaneal f.
> alveolar bone f.
> anatomic neck f.
> Anderson-Hutchins unstable tibial shaft f.
> angulated f.
> ankle mortise f.
> anterior calcaneal process f.
> anterior column f.
> anterolateral compression f.
> AO classification of ankle f.
> apophysial f.
> arch f.
> articular mass separation f.
> articular pillar f.
> Ashhurst-Bromer ankle f. classification
> Atkin epiphysial f.
> atlas f.
> atrophic f.
> avulsion chip f.
> avulsion stress f.
> axial load teardrop f.
> backfire f.
> Bankart f.
> Barton f.
> basal neck f.
> baseball finger f.
> basilar femoral neck f.

basocervical f.
bayonet position of f.
beak f.
f. bed
bedroom f.
bending f.
Bennett basic hand f.
Bennett comminuted f.
Berndt-Hardy classification of transchondral f.
bicolumn f.
bicondylar T-shaped f.
bicondylar Y-shaped f.
bicycle spoke f.
bimalleolar ankle f.
bipartite f.
birth f.
f. blister
blow-in f.
blow-out f.
bone shaft f.
f. boot
boot-top f.
Bosworth f.
both-bone f.
both-column f.
bowing f.
f. box
boxer's f.
Boyd type II f.
f. bracing
Broberg-Morrey f.
bucket-handle f.
buckle f.
bumper f.
bunk bed f.
Burkhalter-Reyes method phalangeal f.
burst f.
butterfly f.
buttonhole f.
calcaneal avulsion f.
calcaneal displaced f.
calcaneal type I–III f.
calcaneus tongue f.
f. callus
f. callus loading
Canale-Kelly talar neck f.
capillary f.
capitellar f.
capitulum f.
carpal bone stress f.

carpal navicular f.
carpal scaphoid bone f.
carpometacarpal joint f.
cartwheel f.
Cedell f.
cemental f.
central talus f.
cephalomedullary nail f.
cervical trochanteric f.
cervical trochanteric displaced f.
chalk-stick f.
Chance vertebral f.
Chaput f.
chauffeur's f.
chip f.
chisel f.
circumferential f.
f. classification
clavicular birth f.
clay shoveler's f.
cleavage f.
closed ankle f.
closed indirect f.
closed reduction of f.
coccyx f.
Colles f.
collicular f.
Coltart f.
combined flexion-distraction injury and burst f.
combined radial-ulnar-humeral f.
comminuted bursting f.
comminuted intraarticular f.
comminuted teardrop f.
complete f.
complex f.
complicated f.
composite f.
compound comminuted f. (CCF)
compression f.
condylar compression f.
condylar femoral f.
condylar split f.
congenital f.
contrecoup f.
f. by contrecoup
controlled comminuted f.
coracoid f.
corner f.
coronal split f.
coronoid process f.
cortical f.

F

NOTES

273

fracture *(continued)*

Cotton ankle f.
cough f.
crack f.
craniofacial dysjunction f.
crush f.
crushed eggshell f.
cuboid f.
cuneiform f.
dancer's f.
Danis-Weber classification of malleolar f.
Darrach-Hughston-Milch f.
dashboard f.
f. decompression
f. deformity
Denis Browne sacral f. classification
Denis Browne spinal f. classification
Denis spinal f.
dens f.
dentate f.
depressed f.
de Quervain f.
derby hat f.
Desault f.
Descot f.
diacondylar f.
diametric pelvic f.
diaphysial f.
diastatic f.
dicondylar f.
die punch f.
direct f.
dishpan f.
f. dislocation
displaced intraarticular f.
displaced pilon f.
distal femoral epiphysial f.
distal humeral f.
distal radial f.
distraction of f.
dogleg f.
dome f.
dorsal wing f.
double f.
drill bit f.
Dupuytren f.
Duverney f.
dye-punch f.
dyscrasic f.
eggshell f.
elbow f.
elementary f.
elephant-foot f.
Ellis technique for Barton f.
f. en coin

Ender rod fixation of f.
endocrine f.
f. en rave
epicondylar avulsion f.
epiphysial growth plate f.
epiphysial slip f.
epiphysial tibial f.
Essex-Lopresti fixation of calcaneal f.
Essex-Lopresti joint depression f.
Essex-Lopresti tongue-type f.
explosion f.
extraarticular f.
extracapsular f.
extraoctave f.
fatigue f.
femoral intratrochanteric f.
femoral neck f.
femoral shaft f.
femoral supracondylar f.
fender f.
f. fever
fibular diaphysial f.
fighter's f.
first carpometacarpal joint f.
fissured f.
f. fixation
f. fixation device
flake hamate f.
Fleck f.
flexion-burst f.
flexion-compression f.
flexion-distraction f.
flexion teardrop f.
floating arch f.
folding f.
forearm f.
four-part f.
fragility f.
f. fragment
f. fragment displacement
f. fragment distraction
f. fragment nonunion
f. fragment separation
f. frame
Freiberg f.
Frykman radial f.
fulcrum f.
Gaenslen f.
Galeazzi f.
f. gap
Garden femoral neck f.
glenoid rim f.
Gosselin f.
graft f.
greater trochanteric femoral f.
greenstick f.
grenade thrower's f.

gross f.
growth plate f.
Guérin f.
gunshot f.
Gustilo-Anderson open clavicular f.
Gustilo tibial f.
Hahn-Steinthal f.
hairline f.
hamate tail f.
hangman's f.
Hawkins type I talus f.
head f.
head-splitting humeral f.
healed f.
f. healing
heat f.
hemicondylar f.
Henderson f.
Herbert scaphoid bone f.
Hermodsson f.
hickory-stick f.
high-energy f.
Hill-Sachs f.
hip avulsion f.
hockey-stick f.
Hoffa f.
Holstein-Lewis f.
hoop stress f.
horizontal f.
humeral head-splitting f.
humeral physial f.
humeral shaft f.
humeral supracondylar f.
Hutchinson f.
hyperextension teardrop f.
hyperflexion teardrop f.
ice skater's f.
idiopathic f.
impacted articular f.
impacted valgus f.
impaction f.
implant f.
impression f.
incomplete f.
indirect f.
inflammatory f.
infraction f.
infratectal transverse f.
Ingram-Bachynski hip f.
  classification
insufficiency f.
interarticular f.

intercondylar femoral f.
intercondylar humeral f.
intercondylar tibial f.
internally fixed f.
interperiosteal f.
intertrochanteric femoral f.
intertrochanteric four-part f.
F. Intervention Trial (FIT)
intraarticular calcaneal f.
intraarticular proximal tibial f.
intracapsular f.
intraoperative f.
intraperiosteal f.
inverted-Y f.
ipsilateral femoral neck f.
ipsilateral femoral shaft f.
irreducible f.
ischioacetabular f.
Jefferson cervical burst f.
Jeffery radial f. classification
joint depression f.
Jones f.
junctional f.
juvenile Tillaux f.
juxtaarticular f.
juxtacortical f.
juxtatectal transverse f.
Kapandji f.
Kilfoyle humeral medial
  condylar f. classification
knee f.
Kocher f.
Kocher-Lorenz f.
Köhler f.
laminar f.
lap seatbelt f.
lateral column calcaneal f.
lateral humeral condyle f.
laterally displaced f.
lateral malleolus f.
lateral mass f.
lateral talar process f.
lateral tibial plateau f.
lateral wedge f.
Lauge-Hansen ankle f. classification
Lauge-Hansen stage II supination-
  eversion f.
Laugier f.
lead pipe f.
Le Fort fibular f.
Le Fort II f.
Le Fort mandible f.

F

NOTES

fracture *(continued)*
Le Fort-Wagstaffe f.
lesser trochanter f.
f. line
linear f.
f. line consolidation
Lisfranc f.
Lloyd-Roberts f.
local compression f.
local decompression f.
long bone f.
longitudinal f.
long oblique f.
loose f.
Looser zone in insufficiency f.
lorry driver's f.
low-energy f.
low lumbar spine f.
low T humerus f.
lumbar spine burst f.
lumbosacral junction f.
lunate f.
Maisonneuve fibular f.
malar f.
Malgaigne pelvic f.
malleolar chip f.
mallet f.
f. malreduction
malunited calcaneus f.
malunited forearm f.
malunited radial f.
mandibular f.
march f.
marginal f.
Marmor-Lynn f.
Mason f.
Mathews olecranon f. classification
maxillary f.
medial column calcaneal f.
medial epicondyle humeral f.
medial malleolar f.
metacarpal neck f.
metaphysial tibial f.
metatarsal f.
Meyers-McKeever tibial f.
   classification
middle tibial shaft f.
midfacial f.
midfoot f.
midnight f.
midshaft f.
minimally displaced f.
mini-pilon f.
missed f.
monomalleolar ankle f.
Monteggia forearm f.
Montercaux f.
Moore f.

Mouchet f.
multangular ridge f.
multilevel f.
multipartite f.
multiple f.
multiray f.
navicular dorsal lip f.
navicular tuberosity f.
naviculocapitate f.
f. of necessity
neck f.
Neer-Horowitz classification of
   humeral f.
neoplastic f.
neurogenic f.
neuropathic f.
neurotrophic f.
Newman radial f.
nightstick f.
night-walker f.
nonarticular distal radial f.
noncontiguous f.
nondisplaced f.
nonphysial f.
nonrotational burst f.
nonunion horse-hoof f.
nonunion torsion wedge f.
nonunited f.
nutcracker f.
oblique f.
obturator avulsion f.
occipital condyle f.
occult f.
odontoid condyle f.
old f.
olecranon tip f.
one-part f.
open-book f.
open-break f.
open reduction of f.
ossification-associated f.
osteochrondral slice f.
os trigonum f.
Ovadia-Beals classification of tibial
   plafond f.
Pais f.
Palmer primary f.
Papavasiliou olecranon f.
   classification
paratrooper f.
parry f.
pars interarticularis f.
patellar sleeve f.
pathologic f.
Pauwels f.
pedicle f.
pelvic avulsion f.
pelvic rim f.

pelvic ring f.
pelvic straddle f.
penetrating f.
perforating f.
periarticular f.
periprosthetic f.
peritrochanteric f.
PER-IV f.
pertrochanteric f.
phalangeal diaphysial f.
physial plate f.
physis f.
Piedmont f.
pillow f.
pilon f.
ping-pong f.
plafond f.
plastic bowing f.
plateau f.
pond f.
Posada f.
posterior arch f.
posterior column f.
posterior element f.
posterior process f.
posterior talar process f.
posterior wall f.
postirradiation f.
postmortem f.
postoperative f.
Pott ankle f.
pressure f.
Prevent Recurrence of
  Osteoporotic F.'s (PROOF)
profundus artery f.
pronation-abduction f.
pronation-eversion f.
pronation-eversion/external
  rotation f.
proximal end tibia f.
proximal femoral f.
proximal humeral f.
proximal tibial metaphysial f.
pseudo-Jones f.
puncture f.
pyramidal f.
Quervain f.
radial head f.
radial neck f.
radial styloid f.
f. reducing elevator
reduction of f.

f. reduction
f. repair
resecting f.
retrodisplaced f.
reverse Barton f.
reverse Colles f.
reverse Monteggia f.
reverse obliquity f.
rib f.
ring f.
Rolando f.
rotational burst f.
Ruedi f.
Ruedi-Allgower tibial plafond f.
sacral f.
sacroiliac f.
Salter f.
Salter-Harris f. (type I–VI)
sandbagging long bone f.
Sanders f.
Sangeorzan navicular f.
scaphoid f.
scapular f.
secondary f.
segmental f.
Segond tibial avulsion f.
senile subcapital f.
sentinel f.
SER-IV f.
sesamoid f.
shaft f.
shear f.
Shepherd f.
short oblique f.
sideswipe elbow f.
silver-fork f.
simple f.
single-column f.
f. site
f. site nonunion Norland bone
  densitometry
skier's f.
Skillern f.
sleeve f.
small f.
Smith ankle f.
Sneppen talar f.
snowboarder's f.
spinal f.
spinous process f.
spiral oblique f.
f. splint

F

NOTES

fracture *(continued)*
 splintered f.
 split f.
 split-heel f.
 spontaneous f.
 sprain f.
 Springer f.
 sprinter's f.
 f. stabilization
 stable burst f.
 stairstep f.
 Steida f.
 stellate f.
 step-off of f.
 sternum f.
 Stieda f.
 straddle f.
 strain f.
 stress f.
 styloid f.
 subcapital f.
 subcutaneous f.
 subperiosteal f.
 subtrochanteric femoral f.
 supination-adduction f.
 supination-eversion f.
 supination-external rotation IV f.
 supracondylar humeral f.
 supracondylar Y-shaped f.
 suprasyndesmotic f.
 supratectal transverse f.
 surgical neck f.
 sustentaculum tali f.
 synchondritic f.
 T f.
 f. table
 talar avulsion f.
 talar neck f.
 talar osteochondral f.
 talus body f.
 tarsal bone f.
 T condylar f.
 teacup f.
 teardrop f.
 teardrop-shaped flexion-
  compression f.
 temporal bone f.
 tennis f.
 tension f.
 thalamic f.
 thoracic spine f.
 thoracolumbar burst f.
 three-part f.
 through-and-through f.
 thrower's f.
 Thurston-Holland f.
 tibiofibular f.
 Tillaux f.

 Tillaux-Chaput f.
 Tillaux-Kleiger f.
 toddler's f.
 tongue f.
 Torg f.
 torsional f.
 torus f.
 total talus f.
 traction f.
 transcapitate f.
 transcervical femoral f.
 transchondral f.
 transcondylar f.
 transepiphysial f.
 transhamate f.
 transiliac f.
 transsacral f.
 transscaphoid dislocation f.
 transtriquetral f.
 transverse process f.
 trapezium f.
 trimalleolar ankle f.
 triplane tibial f.
 triquetral f.
 trophic f.
 T-shaped f.
 tuberosity f.
 tuberosity avulsion f.
 tuft f.
 two-part f.
 type I, II, III, IIIA, IIIB, IIIC
  open f.
 ulnar styloid f.
 unciform f.
 uncinate process f.
 undisplaced f.
 unicondylar f.
 unstable f.
 ununited f.
 vertebral body f.
 vertebral plana f.
 vertebral stable burst f.
 vertebral wedge compression f.
 vertical f.
 vertical shear f.
 volar shear f.
 Volkmann f.
 Vostal classification of radial f.
 V-shaped f.
 wagon wheel f.
 Wagstaffe f.
 Wagstaffe-Le Fort f.
 waist f.
 Walther f.
 Watson-Jones navicular f.
 Weber B, C f.
 wedge compression f.
 wedge flexion-compression f.

wedge-shaped uncomminuted tibial plateau f.
willow f.
Wilson f.
Winquist-Hansen classification of femoral f.
f. with scoliosis
Y f.
Y-T f.
Zickel f.
ZMC f.
f. zone

fractured
f. bone mobility
f. vertebra

fracture-dislocation
atlantoaxial f.-d.
Bennett f.-d.
carpometacarpal f.-d.
Galeazzi f.-d.
intermediate cuneiform f.-d.
Lisfranc f.-d.
Monteggia f.-d.
perilunate f.-d. (PLFD)
posterior f.-d.
f.-d. reduction
tarsometatarsal f.-d.
thoracolumbar spine f.-d.
tibial plateau f.-d.
transcapitate f.-d.
transhamate f.-d.
transtriquetral f.-d.
unstable f.-d.
f.-d. with anterior ligament

fragilitas ossium congenita
fragility fracture
Fragmatome tip
fragment
alignment of fracture f.
anterolateral f.
articular f.
avascular f.
avulsion f.
bone f.
bucket-handle f.
butterfly fracture f.
capital f.
Chaput f.
chondral f.
Comet f.
corner f.
cortical f.

depression of f.
disk f.
distal f.
fracture f.
free f.
free-floating cartilaginous f.
hinged f.
hypervascular f.
intraarticular f.
loose f.
major fracture f.
osteochondral f.
retrolisthesed f.
retropulsed bony f.
step-off between bone fracture f.'s
superomedial f.
sustentacular f.
thalamic f.
Thurston-Holland f.
tuberosity f.
wedge-shaped uncomminuted f.

fragmental bone
fragmentation
endplate f.
graft f.

fraise
diamond f.

frame
Ace-Colles fracture f.
Ace-Fischer fracture f.
Ace-Fischer ring f.
Alexian Brothers overhead f.
Andrews spinal surgery f.
anterior quadrilateral triplane f.
f. application
Balkan fracture f.
bilateral f.
Böhler-Braun f.
Böhler fracture f.
Böhler reducing f.
Bradford fracture f.
Braun f.
Brooker f.
Brown-Roberts-Wells stereotactic had f.
Chalet f.
Chick CLT operating f.
CircOlectric f.
claw-type basic f.
Cole fracture f.
Cole hyperextension f.
Crawford head f.

F

NOTES

frame *(continued)*
    delta f.
    DePuy rainbow f.
    DePuy reducing f.
    double-ring f.
    Elekta stereotactic head f.
    external fixator f.
    fixator f.
    Foster turning f.
    four-poster f.
    fracture f.
    fusion f.
    GaitMaster low-profile f.
    Gardner-Wells fixation f.
    Goldthwait f.
    Granberry f.
    Hastings f.
    Heffington lumbar seat spinal f.
    Herzmark f.
    Hibbs f.
    Hitchcock stereotactic
      immobilization f.
    Hoffmann f.
    Hoffmann-Vidal double f.
    Ilizarov f.
    IV-type basic f.
    Jones abduction f.
    Jordan f.
    Kessler traction f.
    laminectomy f.
    Lex-Ton spinal f.
    Maddacrawler Crawler f.
    Malcolm-Lynn C-RXF cervical
      retractor f.
    Mayfield fixation f.
    Monticelli-Spinelli f.
    one-plane bilateral f.
    one-plane unilateral f.
    pelvic fracture f.
    phantom f.
    Pittsburgh pelvic f.
    quadrilateral f.
    rectangular f.
    Relton-Hall f.
    Risser f.
    scoliosis operating f.
    Slatis pelvic fracture f.
    sling f.
    spinal turning f.
    spine f.
    Stealth f.
    Stryker fracture f.
    Stryker turning f.
    Taylor spinal f.
    tent f.
    Thomas f.
    Thompson f.
    triangular ankle fusion f.

    triangulate triple f.
    triple f.
    two-plane bilateral f.
    two-plane unilateral f.
    Wagner f.
    Watson-Jones f.
    Weber f.
    Whitman f.
    Wilson convex f.
    Wingfield f.
    Wolfson f.
    Zimmer fracture f.
    Zimmer laminectomy f.

framer
    F. finger extension bow
    F. splint
    F. tendon passer
    F. tendon-passing needle

frank
    f. diastasis
    F. Dickson shelf procedure
    f. dislocation
    F. and Johnson modification of
      Heyman procedure
    F. Noyes function questionnaire

Fränkel
    F. neurologic deficit classification
    F. sign
    F. white line

Frankfort horizontal plane
Franz-O'Rahilly classification
frayed
    f. disk
    f. meniscus

fraying of meniscus
Frazer wrist brace
Frazier
    F. elevator
    F. suction tip

Frazier-Adson osteoplastic flap clamp
Frazier-Sachs clamp
FRD
    flexion-rotation-drawer
    FRD test

free
    f. body diagram
    f. fasciocutaneous flap
    f. fat graft
    f. flap of cartilage
    f. flap transfer
    f. fragment
    f. gracilis muscle transfer
    f. latissimus dorsi flap
    f. microsurgical flap
    f. pyridinium crosslink
    f. revascularized autograft
    f. scapular flap
    f. skin flap

f. skin graft
f. tie
f. tissue transfer
f. toe transfer
f. vascularized bone transplant
f. weight rehabilitation

Freebody
F. pin
F. stay-retractor

Freebody-Bendall-Taylor fusion technique
Freebody-Steinmann retractor
freedom
F. accommodator arch support
F. arthritis support
F. back support
degrees of f. (DOF)
F. elastic long wrist support
F. Micro Pro stimulator
f. of movement
F. neutral position splint
F. omni progressive splint
F. Palm Guard
F. Progressive Resting splint
F. sportsfit splint
F. thumbkeeper
F. thumb spica
F. thumb stabilizer
F. ultimate grip splint
F. USA wristlet

free-floating
f.-f. cartilaginous fragment
f.-f. osteotomy

Free-Flow system prosthesis
freehand
f. CT-guided biopsy
f. cut
F. prosthesis system
f. suturing technique

freely movable joint
Freeman
F. calcaneal fracture classification
F. clamp
F. modular total hip prosthesis

Freeman-high neck press fit prosthesis
Freeman-Samuelson knee prosthesis
Freeman-Sheldon syndrome
Freeman-Swanson
F.-S. knee prosthesis
F.-S. knee system

Freer
F. chisel

F. dissector
F. elevator-dissector
F. periosteal elevator
F. septal elevator

free-spinning probe
free-swinging knee gait
Free-Up massage cream
free-walking velocity
freeze-dried
f.-d. bone pin
f.-d. cancellous allograft
f.-d. graft

freeze-thawed graft
Freiberg
F. cartilage knife
F. disease
F. fracture
F. meniscectomy knife
F. traction

Freiberg-Kohler disease
Frejka
F. jacket
F. pillow
F. pillow orthosis
F. pillow splint
F. traction

fremitus
French
F. adapter
F. fracture technique
F. lateral closing-wedge osteotomy
F. rod bender
F. scale
F. supracondylar fracture operation

frenectomy
Frenkel
F. exercises
F. movement
F. track

frenulum, pl. **frenula**
frequency
f. analysis
discharge f.
f., intensity, time, type (FITT)
onset f.
recruitment f.

frequency-difference interferential current therapy (FDICT)
fresh
f. frozen allograft
f. frozen graft

freshening of bone

F

NOTES

freshen the surface
Fresnel prism
fretting corrosion
friable
Friatec manual arthroscopy instrument
fricative
friction
  f. artifact
  coefficient of f.
  cross f.
  dynamic f.
  f. lock pin
  f. massage
  patient-on-table f.
  f. rub
frictional torque
friction-reduced
  f.-r. examination table
  f.-r. segmented table
Fried-Green
  F.-G. foot operation
  F.-G. foot procedure
Fried-Hendel
  F.-H. tendon operation
  F.-H. tendon technique
Friedman
  F. bone rongeur
  F. brace
  F. rongeur forceps
  F. splint
  F. support
Friedreich
  F. ataxia
  F. disease
  F. foot
Friedrich clamp
Friedrich-Petz clamp
Fries
  F. rheumatoid arthritis score
  F. score for rheumatoid arthritis
    classification
fringe
  f. joint
  f. of osteophyte
  synovial f.
frog-leg
  f.-l. lateral view
  f.-l. position
  f.-l. splint
Fröhlich adiposogenital dystrophy
Frohse
  arcade of F.
  F. arcade of the elbow
  arch of F.
  F. ligamentous arcade
Froimson
  F. procedure

F. splint
F. technique
Froimson-Oh
  F.-O. arm procedure
  F.-O. repair
frôlement
FROM
  full range of motion
Froment
  F. paper sign
  F. ulnar nerve function test
Fromm triangle orthopedic device
frond
  synovial f.
front
  corset f.
  f. kick explosion
frontal
  f. bone
  f. bossing
  f. motion
  f. plane
  f. plane correction
  f. plane growth abnormality
  f. plane XY
  f. plane Z-plasty
  f. plate
front-entry guide
fronting of velar
frontoorbital advancement
frontside snowboard stance
frost
  F. foot operation
  F. foot procedure
  F. H-block
  F. partial matrixectomy
  F. posterior tibialis technique
  F. posterior tibialis tendon
    lengthening
  F. stitch
frostbite
  f. acroosteolysis
  f. of hand
  f. injury
frozen
  f. pelvis
  f. shoulder
  f. shoulder syndrome
Fruehevald splint
fruste
  forme f.
Frykman
  F. distal radius fracture
    classification
  F. radial fracture
F-Scan
  F-S. foot force and gait analysis
    system

F-S. foot pressure analysis
F-S. in-shoe system
F-S. pressure measurement system
FSH
facioscapulohumeral
FSI
Functional Status Index
FSQ
Functional Status Questionnaire
FSU
functional spinal unit
FT03C transducer
FTA
femorotibial angle
FTC
fibulotalocalcaneal
FTC ligament
FTI
force-time/integral
FTJ
femorotibial joint
FTSG
full-thickness skin graft
Fukuda humeral head retractor
Fukushima C-clamp
fulcrum, pl. **fulcra, fulcrums**
f. distance
f. fracture
joint f.
f. test
fulcruming
Fulford procedure
fulgurate
Fulkerson
F. functional knee score
F. oblique tibial tubercle osteotomy
full
f. cervical spine (FCS)
f. curve
f. fist flexion
f. interference pattern
f. lateral position
f. range of motion (FROM)
f. spine radiographic examination
f. thumb spica cast
f. weightbearing (FWB)
full-circle goniometer
full-curved clamp
Fuller shield dressing
full-hand splint
full-occlusal splint

full-radius
f.-r. resector
f.-r. resector knife
full-thickness
f.-t. cuff tear
f.-t. skin graft (FTSG)
fully constrained tricompartmental knee prosthesis
fulminans
purpura f.
fulminate
function
adrenergic vagal f.
ambulatory f.
bundle f.
Charnley classification of f.
cholinergic vagal f.
concentric f.
eccentric f.
intrinsic f.
Jebsen assessment of hand f.
LSUMC classification of motor
and sensory f.
motor f.
neurologic f.
perverted f.
position of f.
reflex f.
rotator cuff f.
sensory f.
splinted in position of f.
subtalar joint f. (SJF)
sudomotor f.
throwing f.
tibialis posterior f.
functional
f. activity
f. ambulation
F. Ambulation category (FAC)
f. and anatomic loading (FAL)
f. assessment measure (FAM)
F. Assessment Staging (FAST)
f. axial rotation
f. back pain
f. capacity assessment
f. capacity evaluation (FCE)
f. capacity measurement
f. disability of foot
f. electrical stimulation (FES)
f. fracture brace
f. grip pushup block
f. independence measure (FIM)

F

NOTES

functional *(continued)*
    f. instability
    F. Integration (FI)
    f. intermetatarsal angle
    f. leg length inequality
    F. Limitation Profile (FLP)
    f. loss
    f. magnetic resonance imaging
      (fMRI)
    f. neuromuscular stimulation
    f. orthotic
    f. performance
    f. phase rehabilitation
    F. Rating Score
    f. recovery
    f. refractory period
    f. restoration
    f. scoliosis
    f. short leg
    f. spinal unit (FSU)
    f. splint
    f. squats back exercise technique
    F. Status Index (FSI)
    F. Status Questionnaire (FSQ)
    f. subluxation
    f. training
functionally debilitating symptom
fungal
    f. arthritis
    f. infection
fungous synovitis
funicular excision
funiculitis
funiculus
Funk tibialis posterior tendon
   dysfunction classification syndrome
funnel
    f. breast
    f. chest
    f. technique
funnelization of metaphysis
Funsten supination splint
Funston syndrome
FUO
    fever of undetermined origin
Furacin gauze dressing
Furlong tendon stripper
Furnas bayonet osteotome
Furnas-Haq-Somers technique
Furness-Clute pin
furniture brace
furrowing
    scarring and f.
further flexion (FF)
furunculosis
fused
    f. ankle
    f. arthrodesis

    f. hip
    f. vertebra
fusiform
    f. defect
    f. periosteal new bone
fusimotor
    f. neuron
    f. system
fusion
    Adkins spinal f.
    Albee lumbar spinal f.
    Anderson ankle f.
    ankle f.
    anterior cervical f. (ACF)
    anterior cervical body f.
    anterior cervical diskectomy and f.
      (ACDF)
    anterior-inferior f.
    anterior lumbar interbody f.
    anterior lumbar vertebral
      interbody f.
    anterior and posterior f.
    anterior spinal f.
    AP f.
    atlantoaxial f.
    atlantooccipital f.
    Bailey-Badgley cervical spine f.
    BERG lumbar interbody f.
    bilateral lateral f.
    Blair ankle f.
    Bohlman triple-wire f.
    bone block f.
    Bosworth lumbar spinal f.
    Bradford f.
    Brooks cervical f.
    Brooks-Gallie cervical f.
    Brooks-Jenkins atlantoaxial f.
    Brooks-Jenkins cervical f.
    Brooks-type f.
    buried K-wire fixation in digital f.
    f. cage
    calcaneotibial f.
    cervical interbody f.
    cervical spine posterior f.
    cervicooccipital f.
    Chandler hip f.
    Charnley compression-type knee f.
    Charnley and Henderson
      extraarticular f.
    Charnley and Henderson
      intraarticular f.
    chevron f.
    Chuinard-Peterson ankle f.
    Cloward anterior spinal f.
    Cloward back f.
    CMC f.
    Coltart calcaneotibial f.
    convex f.

Copeland-Howard scapulothoracic f.
cuboid f.
Davis f.
degenerative lumbar spine f.
degenerative spondylosis
  decompression and f.
Dewar posterior cervical f.
diaphysial-epiphysial f.
DIP f.
diskectomy with Cloward f.
distal tibiofibular f.
dowel spinal f.
extraarticular hip f.
extraarticular subtalar f.
facet f.
f. facet
four-corner midcarpal f.
f. frame
Gallie atlantoaxial f.
Gallie cervical f.
Gallie subtalar ankle f.
Gallie wire f.
Gissane ankle f.
Goldstein spinal f.
f. graft
Hall facet f.
hammer toe correction with
  interphalangeal f.
Harris-Smith cervical f.
Hatcher-Smith cervical f.
Henry-Geist spinal f.
H-graft f.
Hibbs-Jones spinal f.
Hibbs spinal f.
Horwitz-Adams ankle f.
Horwitz ankle f.
hyperostotic bony f.
interbody spinal f.
interfacet wiring and f.
interphalangeal f.
interspinous process f.
intertransverse f.
intraarticular knee f.
joint f.
Kellogg-Speed lumbar spinal f.
Kennedy modification of Gallie
  ankle f.
King intraarticular hip f.
knee f.
Langenskiöld f.
lateral f.
f. limit determination

long segment spinal f.
lower cervical spine f.
lumbar spine f.
lumbar vertebral interbody f.
lumbosacral f.
lunotriquetral f.
Marcus-Balourdas-Heiple ankle f.
McKeever metatarsophalangeal f.
metatarsocuneiform joint f.
metatarsophalangeal joint f.
Müller intraarticular shoulder f.
multilevel f.
naviculocuneiform f.
f. nonunion rate
occipitoatlantoaxial f.
occipitocervical f.
pantalar f.
f. plate
posterior cervical f.
posterior lumbar interbody f.
  (PLIF)
posterior spinal f.
posterolateral interbody f. (PLIF)
posterolateral lumbosacral f.
radiolunate f.
radioscaphoid f.
Robinson anterior cervical f.
Robinson cervical spine f.
Robinson-Southwick f.
Robins-Riley spinal f.
Rowe f.
sacral spine f.
scaphocapitate f.
scapulothoracic f.
screw f.
selective thoracic spine f.
short segment spinal f.
Simmons cervical spine f.
single-level spinal f.
Smith-Petersen sacroiliac joint f.
Smith-Robinson anterior f.
Smith-Robinson cervical
  interbody f.
Soren ankle f.
spinal f.
Stamm procedure for intraarticular
  hip f.
f. stiffness
subastragalar f.
subaxial posterior cervical spinal f.
subtalar distraction bone block f.
symmetric vertebral f.

F

NOTES

fusion *(continued)*
    talar body f.
    talocalcaneal f.
    talocrural f.
    talonavicular f.
    f. technique
    thoracic facet f.
    thoracic spinal f.
    tibiocalcaneal f.
    tibiofibular f.
    tibiotalar f.
    tibiotalocalcaneal f.
    transfibular f.
    transpedal multiplanar wedge f.
    trapeziometacarpal f.
    triple tarsal f.
    triple-wire f.
    triscaphe f.
    two-stage hip f.
    upper cervical spine f.
    vertebral f.
    Watkins f.

Watson scaphotrapeziotrapezoidal f.
White posterior ankle f.
Wilson ankle f.
Wiltse bilateral lateral f.
Winter convex f.
Zielke instrumentation for scoliosis spinal f.

fustigation
Futrex body fat analyzer
Futura
    F. flexible digital implant
    F. metal hemi-toe implant
Future implant
Futuro
    F. splint
    F. wrist brace
    F. wrist support
F-wave response
FWB
    full weightbearing
FyBron dressing

G5

G5 Fleximatic massage/percussion unit

G5 Fleximatic massager/percussor massager

G5 Porta-Plus muscle stimulator

G5 Vibracare massager/percussor

G5 Vibramatic massage/percussion unit

gadopentetate-dimeglumine-enhanced magnetic resonance imaging

GADS

gas atomized dispersion strengthened

GADS technology

Gaenslen

G. fracture

G. osteomyelitis

G. sign

G. spike

G. split-heel incision

G. split-heel technique

G. test

Gaffney

G. ankle prosthesis

G. joint

gag

Dingman mouth g.

Gage

G. distal transfer

G. sign

gain

Body Oscillation Integrates Neuromuscular G. (BOING)

heat g.

GAIT

great toe arthroplasty implant technique

GAIT spacer device

gait

abductor lurch g.

G. Abnormality Rating Scale (GARS)

G. Abnormality Rating Scale Modified version (GARS-M)

adult g.

g. analysis

angle of g.

antalgic g.

apraxic g.

apropulsive g.

G., Arms, Legs, and Spine (GALS)

G., Arms, Legs, and Spine screening

arthrogenic g.

astasia-abasia g.

ataxic g.

avoidance g.

base of g.

batrachian g.

g. belt

g. biomechanics

broad-based g.

cadence of g.

calcaneal g.

cerebellar g.

Charcot g.

Charlie Chaplin g.

choreatic g.

clumsy g.

cogwheel g.

component of g.

crab g.

cross-legged g.

crouch g.

g. cycle

dancing bear g.

g. deviation

g. disorder

g. disorder, autoantibody, late-age, onset, polyneuropathy (GALOP)

g. disturbance

dorsiflexor g.

double-leg stance phase of g.

double-step g.

double-tap g.

drag-to g.

dromedary g.

drop-foot g.

drunken sailor g.

duck-waddle g.

dynamic g.

dystrophic g.

equine g.

extrapyramidal g.

festinating g.

flaccid g.

flatfoot g.

floating g.

footdrop g.

foot-strike phase of g.

four-point g.

free-swinging knee g.

gastrocnemius-soleus g.

glue-footed g.

gluteal g.

gluteus maximus g.

gluteus medius g.

heel-and-toe g.

heel contact phase of g.

heel-off phase of g.

G

gait *(continued)*
    heel-strike phase of g.
    heel-toe g.
    helicopod g.
    hemiparetic g.
    hemiplegic g.
    high-steppage g.
    hip extensor g.
    hobbling g.
    hyperextended knee g.
    hysterical g.
    instability g.
    intermittent double-step g.
    internal rotational g.
    intoeing g.
    jerky g.
    g. laboratory
    g. line
    listing g.
    g. lock splint (GLS)
    lurching g.
    marche à petits pas g.
    midstance period of g.
    g. and mobility
    myopathic g.
    narrow-base g.
    Oppenheim g.
    opposite foot strike phase of g.
    opposite toe-off phase of g.
    out-toeing g.
    painful g.
    paraparetic g.
    parkinsonian g.
    g. pathomechanics
    g. pattern
    penguin g.
    petit pas g.
    Petren g.
    pigeon-toeing g.
    g. plate
    propulsion g.
    push-off phase of g.
    reeling g.
    retropulsion of g.
    reversal of fore-aft shear phase
      of g.
    rigid g.
    scissor-leg g.
    scissors g.
    scraping toe g.
    short leg g.
    shuffling g.
    skater's g.
    slap foot g.
    slapping g.
    spastic g.
    spastic equinus g.
    stable g.
    staggering g.
    stamping g.
    stance phase of g.
    star g.
    station and g.
    g. and station
    steppage g.
    stiff g.
    stiff-knee g.
    stiff-legged g.
    stride length of g.
    strike phase of g.
    stuttering of g.
    swaying g.
    swing phase of g.
    swing-through g.
    swing-to g.
    tabetic g.
    tandem g.
    three-point g.
    tiptoe g.
    Todd g.
    toe g.
    toe-heel g.
    toeing-in g.
    toeing-out g.
    toe-off phase of g.
    toe-toe g.
    toe-walking g.
    tottering g.
    Tracto-Halter g.
    g. training
    Trendelenburg g.
    tripoding g.
    Tubersitz amputee g.
    two-point g.
    uncoordinated g.
    unsteady g.
    waddling g.
    wide-based g.

gaiter cast
GaitMaster low-profile frame
Galant
    G. sign
    G. test
Galante hip prosthesis
galaxy
    G. 900HS adjusting table
    G. McManis hylo table
Galeazzi
    G. fracture
    G. fracture-dislocation
    G. hip dislocation sign
    G. patellar operation
    G. realignment
    G. test
Galen scoliosis
Gallagher rasp

Gallannaugh plate
gall duct forceps
Gallie
  G. ankle arthrodesis
  G. approach
  G. atlantoaxial arthrodesis
  G. atlantoaxial fusion
  G. atlantoaxial fusion technique
  G. cervical fusion
  G. fusion-using cable
  G. needle
  G. procedure
  G. subtalar ankle fusion
  G. subtalar fixation
  G. wire fixation technique
  G. wire fusion
  G. wiring technique
gallium-67 scan
gallium citrate scan
Gallo traction
Gallows splint
GALOP
  gait disorder, autoantibody, late-age,
    onset, polyneuropathy
  GALOP syndrome
GALS
  Gait, Arms, Legs, and Spine
  GALS screening
Galt hand drill
galvanic
  g. bath
  g. electrode stimulator
  high-voltage pulsed g.
  g. skin response
  g. stimulation
galvanism
  high-voltage g.
Galveston
  G. fixation with TSRH crosslink
  G. metacarpal brace
  G. orientation and amnesia test
    (GOAT)
  G. pelvic fixation
  G. plate
  G. splint
  G. technique
game
  Boloxie OT Prehension G.
  Cone checkers g.
  g. knee
  g. leg

gamekeeper's
  g. injury
  g. thumb
  g. thumb dislocation
gamma
  g. camera
  g. camera imaging
  G. trochanteric locking nail
gamma-aminobutyric acid agonist
ganglion, pl. **ganglia**
  Acrel g.
  g. block
  g. cyst
  dorsal root g. (DRG)
  intraosseous g.
  metatarsophalangeal joint g.
  periosteal g.
  radiocapitellar joint g.
ganglionectomy
  dorsal root g.
ganglioneuroma
ganglionic block
ganglionostomy
gangrene
  dry g.
  gas g.
  ischemic g.
  Meleney synergistic g.
  peripheral g.
  postnatal g.
  Pott g.
  Raynaud g.
  vascular g.
  wet g.
gangrenosum
  pyoderma g.
gangrenous necrosis
Ganley
  G. and Ganley metatarsus adductus
    procedure
  G. modification of Keller
    arthroplasty
  G. splint
  G. technique
  G. tendon transfer
Gant
  G. hip arthrodesis
  G. operation
  G. osteotomy
Ganz
  G. anti-shock pelvic fixator
  G. cup

G

NOTES

289

Ganz *(continued)*
    G. fixation
    G. osteotomy
gap
    g. arthroplasty
    extension g.
    flexion g.
    flexion-extension g.
    fracture g.
    g. healing
    g. nonunion
    scapholunate g.
Garceau
    G. cheilectomy
    G. tendon technique
Garceau-Brahms arthrodesis
Garcia wrist laxity criteria
garden
    G. alignment index
    G. angle
    G. femoral neck fracture
    G. femoral neck fracture
      classification
    g. screw
    g. spade deformity
Gardner
    G. bone forceps
    G. chair
    G. elevator
    G. operation
    G. syndrome
Gardner-Diamond syndrome
Gardner-Wells
    G.-W. fixation frame
    G.-W. tongs
    G.-W. tong traction
garment
    antishock g.
    console compression g.
    Elvarex compression g.
    Elvarex support g.
    g. hook
    pneumatic g.
    pneumatic antishock g. (PASG)
Garré
    chronic sclerosing osteomyelitis
      of G.
    G. disease
    G. osteitis
    G. sclerosing osteomyelitis
Garrick test
Garrod
    G. disease
    G. fibromatosis
GARS
    Gait Abnormality Rating Scale

GARS-M
    Gait Abnormality Rating Scale Modified
      version
garter strapping
Garth view
Gartland
    G. humeral supracondylar fracture
      classification
    G. procedure
    G. Universal radial fracture
      classification
GAS
    General Adaption Syndrome
gas
    g. atomized dispersion strengthened
      (GADS)
    g. gangrene
gasless
    balloon-assisted, endoscopic,
      retroperitoneal, g. (BERG)
gas-producing streptococcal infection
gastrocnemius
    g. equinus
    g. flap
    lateral head of g.
    g. lengthening
    g. muscle
    g. recession
    g. resistive exercise
    g. rupture
    g. soleus
    g. soleus contracture
    g. tendon
    g. tendon transfer
gastrocnemius-soleus
    g.-s. complex
    g.-s. fascial strip
    g.-s. gait
    g.-s. junction
    g.-s. muscle
    g.-s. muscle group
    g.-s. recession
    g.-s. stretching
    g.-s. tendon
gastrointestinal, pl. **anastomoses**
    g. anastomosis, pl. anastomoses
      (GIA)
    g. tract
gastrosoleal equinus
Gatch bed
gate control theory of pain
Gatellier-Chastang
    G.-C. incision
    G.-C. posterolateral approach
Gates-Glidden drill
gator plastic orthosis
Gaucher disease

gauge
- acetabular g.
- aneroid g.
- B&L pinch g.
- bone screw depth g.
- bone screw ruler g.
- Charnley femoral condyle radius g.
- Charnley socket g.
- clip g.
- Cloward depth g.
- Cobb g.
- CTS g.
- depth g.
- Durkan CTS g.
- finger g.
- isometric strain g.
- Jamar hydraulic pinch g.
- measuring g.
- orthopaedic depth g.
- pain threshold g.
- Philips toe force g.
- pinch g.
- Preston pinch g.
- Rocabado posture g.
- Rosette strain g.
- screw depth g.
- socket g.
- spanner g.
- strain g.
- tourniquet g.
- uniaxial strain g.
- Vernier caliber g.

gauntlet
- g. anesthesia
- g. atrophy
- g. bandage
- g. cast
- Jobst g.
- leather lacer g.
- wrist g.

gauze
- Adaptic g.
- Cover-Roll g.
- g. dressing
- iodoform g.
- Kerlix g.
- g. packing
- petrolatum g.
- plain g.
- pledget of g.
- Safe-Wrap g.
- g. sponge

- Surgitube tubular g.
- Telfa g.
- g. wrap

Gaynor-Hart
- G.-H. position
- G.-H. x-ray position of carpal tunnel

GCT
- giant cell tumor

GDLH posterior spinal system

GD Regainer System

gear
- shoe g.

gearshift probe

gear-stick sign

GEIN
- gradual elongation intramedullary nailing

Geissling rating scale

gel
- Adcon adhesive control g.
- Adcon-L anti-adhesion barrier g.
- Aquasonic Transmission G.
- atelocollagen g.
- Carrington Dermal wound g.
- g. cast
- Ceres' Secret aloe vera g.
- Crystal polymer g.
- g. cushion
- Flexall g.
- Gel Care self-adhesive g.
- osteoinductive enhanced-graft g.
- g. pack
- silicone g.
- Silipos g.
- Silosheath g.
- g. stump sock
- g. suspension sleeve
- g. tubing
- g. warmer
- wound g.
- g. wrap

gelatin
- g. compression boot
- g. foam

gelatinous

gelatin-resorcin-formalin glue

GelBand arm band

Gel-Bank patellar strap

Gelfoam
- G. cookie
- G. pack
- G. pledget

NOTES

Gelfoam *(continued)*
    G. stamp
    thrombin-soaked G.
Gel-Foam Ultra-Wedge cushion
Geliperm dressing
Gelman
    G. foot operation
    G. foot procedure
Gelocast
    G. cast
    G. Unna boot compression dressing
    G. Unna boot compression wrap
Gelpi retractor
GELS
    gravity extension locking system
Gel-Sole shoe insert
gemellus, pl. **gemelli**
Gemini
    G. chiropractic table
    G. cup
    G. hip system prosthesis
    G. MKII mobile-bearing knee
      implant
Gem total knee system
GEN
    gradual elongation nailing
Gendron bariatric wheelchair
general
    g. ability
    G. Adaption Syndrome (GAS)
    g. adjustment
    g. capsular stretch
    g. endotracheal anesthesia
    g. thrust manipulation
generalized fibromatosis
generation
    G. II (GII)
    G. II KAFO
    G. II Unloader ADJ knee brace
    G. II Unloader Select knee brace
    Zest Anchor Advanced G. (ZAAG)
generator
    electrosurgical g.
Genesis
    G. arthroplasty hardware
    G. II foot/ankle system
    G. II foot system
    G. II mobile-bearing knee implant
    G. II total knee system
    G. knee prosthesis
    G. unicompartmental knee
genicula (*pl. of* geniculum)
genicular
    g. artery
    g. neuralgia
geniculate
    g. artery

    medial g.
    g. neuralgia
geniculum, pl. **genicula**
genital system
genitofemoral nerve
Gennari band
genotypic chondrodysplasia
gentle
    G. Threads interference screw
    g. traction
GentleStep shoe
genu
    g. recurvatum
    g. valgum
    g. valgum deformity
    g. valgus
    g. varum
    g. varum deformity
    g. varus
Genucom
    G. ACL laxity analysis system
    G. arthrometer
    G. knee flexion analysis system
Genutrain
    G. knee brace
    G. PE patellar realignment
    G. P3 knee support
GeoFlex
    G. knee
    G. knee prosthesis
geographic destruction
Geo-Matt contour cushion
Geomedic
    G. system
    G. total knee prosthesis
geometric
    g. supracondylar extension
      osteotomy
    G. total knee prosthesis
George
    G. line
    G. test
Georgiade
    G. fixation device
    G. visor cervical collar
    G. visor cervical traction
    G. visor halo fixation
    G. visor halo fixation apparatus
Geo Structure spinal implant
Gerard
    G. prosthesis
    G. resurfacing procedure
Gerbert-Mellilo method
Gerbert osteotomy
Gerdy
    G. ligament
    G. tubercle
geriatric chair trunk support

germinal matrix
germinative matrix
Gerota capsule
Gerson diet
Gerster
    G. bone clamp
    G. traction bar
Ger technique
Gertie ball
Gertzbein
    G. classification of seat-belt injury
    G. seat-belt injury classification
Gerzog bone mallet
Get-A-Grip grip
Ghajar guide
GHL
    glenohumeral ligament
Ghon-Sachs complex
Ghon tubercle
GIA
    gastrointestinal anastomosis
    GIA staple
    GIA stapler
Giannestras
    G. modification of Lapidus
      technique
    G. oblique metatarsal osteotomy
    G. step-down modified osteotomy
giant
    g. cell reaction
    g. cell reparative granuloma
    g. cell sarcoma
    g. cell tumor (GCT)
    g. cell tumor of tendon sheath
    g. motor unit action potential
    g. osteoid osteoma
    g. popliteal synovial cyst
Gianturco
    G. macrocoil
    G. prosthesis
gibbosity
gibbous
gibbus deformity of the spine
Gibney
    G. boot
    G. fixation bandage
    G. perispondylitis
    G. taping
Gibson
    G. approach
    G. bandage
    G. splint

Gibson-Piggott osteotomy
Giertz rib shears
Giertz-Shoemaker rib shears
Giertz-Stille scissors
Gifford mastoid retractor
gigantism
    hyperpituitary g.
    pituitary g.
gigas
    pes g.
Gigli
    G. saw
    G. saw blade
    G. saw guide
    G. saw osteotomy
Gigli-Strully saw
GII
    Generation II
    GII KAFO
    GII Unloader ADJ knee brace
GII
    GII EasyAnchor
    GII Snap-Pak anchor
Gilbert
    G. harvesting
    G. procedure
    G. scapular flap
Gilbert-Tamai-Weiland technique
Gilchrist
    G. splint
    G. test
Gilfillan humeral prosthesis
Giliberty
    G. acetabular prosthesis
    G. apparatus
    G. bipolar femoral head
    G. device
    G. femoral neck prosthesis
    G. hip prosthesis
Gill
    G. arthrodesis
    G. massive sliding graft
    G. modification of Campbell ankle
      procedure
    G. posterior bone block
    G. shelf procedure
    G. sliding graft technique
Gillet marching test
Gillette
    G. brace
    G. double-flexure ankle joint

NOTES

G

Gillette *(continued)*
    G. double-flexure ankle joint
      system
    G. joint orthosis
    G. joint prosthesis
    G. modification of ankle-foot
      orthosis
Gilliat-Summer nerve-damaged hand
Gillies
    G. bone graft
    G. bone hook
    G. pollicization
    G. prosthesis
Gillies-Dingman hook
Gillies-Millard
    G.-M. cocked-hat technique
    G.-M. metacarpal lengthening
Gillis suture
Gill-Manning-White
    G.-M.-W. spondylolisthesis
    G.-M.-W. spondylolisthesis
      technique
Gillquist
    G. arthroscopy
    G. procedure
    G. suction curette
    G. suction tube
Gill-Stein arthrodesis
Gilmer splint
Gil modification
Gilmore groin
Gimbel glove
gimpy
    g. knee
    g. leg
ginglymoarthrodial
ginglymoid joint
ginglymus
Girard keratoprosthesis prosthesis
girdle
    Cadenza g.
    limb g.
    pectoral g.
    pelvic g.
    shoulder g.
Girdlestone
    G. hip procedure
    G. operation
    G. pseudarthrosis
    G. resection
    G. resection arthroplasty
    G. tendon transfer
Girdlestone-Taylor procedure
Gissane
    G. angle
    G. ankle fusion
    G. arthrodesis

    crucial angle of G.
    G. spike
give-way
    g.-w. phenomenon
    g.-w. weakness
giving
    g. way
    g. way of knee
glabella
glabellar rasp
glacier
    G. ceramic 4-in-1 cutting guide
    G. ceramic knee cutting guide
    G. Pack
gladiatorum
    herpes g.
    tinea g.
gland
    eccrine sweat g.
    haversian g.
    parathyroid g.
    thyroid g.
Glasgow
    G. Coma scale
    G. screw
Glass-Bessen transfixion screw
Glasscock ear dressing
Glassman-Engh-Bobyn trochanteric slide
Gleich
    G. osteotomy
    G. osteotomy for pes valgo planus
G-lengthening of semitendinosus tendon
glenohumeral
    g. adhesive capsulitis
    g. arthrodesis
    g. dislocation repair
    g. glide
    g. joint
    g. joint cohesion
    g. joint disease
    g. joint dislocation
    g. joint stability
    g. joint subluxation
    g. ligament (GHL)
    g. pain
    g. shift
glenohumeralia
glenoid
    g. alignment peg
    g. cartilage
    g. cavitary
    g. cavity
    g. component
    g. concavity
    g. drill
    g. drill guide
    g. fixation screw
    g. fossa

g. fossa of scapula
g. implant base impactor
g. labrum
lip of g.
g. metal tray
g. neck
g. osteotomy
g. point
g. rim
g. rim fracture
g. slot
glenoid-reaming forceps
glenoplasty
posterior g.
Scott posterior g.
Gliadel implant
glide
anterior g.
anterior-inferior g.
anterior-posterior g.
cervical dorsal g.
craniocaudal g.
dorsal g.
dynamic canal g.
glenohumeral g.
g. hole for screw placement
g. hook
inferior g.
mushroom walker g.
natural apophysial g.'s (NAGS)
patellar g.
posterior g.
posterior-anterior g.
self-sustained natural
apophyseal g.'s
superior g.
sustained natural apophysial g.'s
(SNAGS)
volar g.
glider
g. cane
g. cane board
EasyStand 6000 g.
G. II patient transfer system
gliding
g. hinge joint
g. hole
g. layer
g. mechanism
g. principle
gliding-hole-first technique
glioma

gliosis
Glisson sling
global
g. cavus
G. Fx shoulder fracture system
g. metatarsus equinus
G. total shoulder arthroplasty
G. total shoulder arthroplasty
system
G. total shoulder implant
globose
glomangiosarcoma
glomus tumor
glossopharyngeal neuralgia
glove
g. anesthesia
antivibration g.
Biobrane g.
Bio-Form g.
carpal tunnel g.
compression g.
electrode g.
finger flexion g.
F&L attenuating g.
flexion g.
Gimbel g.
Handeze fingerless g.
impact g.
Isotoner g.
Jobst g.
Kevlar g.
Life Liner stick and cut-
resistant g.
Maxxus orthopedic latex surgical g.
Medak g.
Medarmor puncture-resistant g.
Necelon surgical g.
peripheral nerve g.
pressure g.
Push-Ease wheelchair g.
radial nerve g.
SoftFlex computer g.
Sorbothane antivibration g.
surgical g.
TheraKnit electrode g.
Tubigrip g.
vibration g.
weighted g.
glove-and-stocking anesthesia
GLS
gait lock splint

Norco edema glove (handwritten annotation)

NOTES

GLS (*continued*)
GLS brace
GLS suture anchor
glubionate
Gluck rib shears
glucocerebroside
glucocorticoid
gluconate
glucosteroid
glue
cyanoacrylate g.
gelatin-resorcin-formalin g.
Histoacryl g.
skin g.
Tisseel fibrin g.
glued-to-the-floor phenomenon
glue-footed gait
glutamic-oxaloacetic transaminase
glutamic-pyruvic transaminase
glutaraldehyde
gluteal
g. artery
g. bonnet
g. cleft
g. fascia
g. gait
g. lurch
g. nerve
g. reflex
g. region
g. sulcus
gluteal/hamstring raise back exercise technique
gluteus
g. maximus flap
g. maximus gait
g. maximus muscle
g. maximus tensing test
g. medius gait
g. medius muscle
g. medius paralysis
g. minimus muscle
glycation
nonenzymatic connective tissue g.
glycocalyx
glycogen sparing
glycosaminoglycan
Glynn-Neibauer technique
GMFM
Gross Motor Function Measure
gnome's calf
goal
rehabilitation g.
GOAT
Galveston orientation and amnesia test
goblet incision
Goethe bone
Gohil-Cavolo method

Golaski graft
gold
g. probe
g. salt
g. weight and wire spring implant material
Goldberg technique
golden
G. closing-wedge osteotomy
G. Comfort orthotic
G. Fitness orthotic
G. mean testing system
GoldenEye arthroscope
Goldenhar syndrome
gold-handled chuck
Goldman-Fristoe test of articulation
Goldmar opponensplasty
Goldner
G. reconstruction
G. spinal arthrodesis
Goldner-Clippinger technique
Goldner-Hayes procedure
gold-paneled chisel
GoldPoint
G. ACL functional knee brace
G. hinged knee brace
G. PCL functional knee brace
Goldstein
G. spinal fusion
G. spinal fusion technique
Goldthwait
G. brace
G. frame
G. sign
Goldthwait-Hauser procedure
golf
G. Exercise System
g. stick dissector
golfer
Thera-Band Exercise System for G.'s
golfer's
g. elbow
g. elbow test
g. wrist
Golgi
G. apparatus
G. device
G. tendon
G. tendon organ
gonadotropin
human chorionic g.
gonalgia
gonarthritis
gonarthromeningitis
gonarthrosis
gonarthrotomy
gonatagra

gonatocele
gonial angle
goniometer
    electronic g.
    EOC g.
    finger g.
    full-circle g.
    O'Brien g.
    orthopaedic g.
    Polk finger g.
    Sammons biplane g.
    Scerratti g.
    Sedan g.
    two-arm g.
    universal full-circle manual g.
    Zimmer g.
goniometric
goniometry
gonococcal
    g. arthropathy
    g. septic arthritis
gonococcic tenosynovitis
gonorrheal
    g. heel
    g. tenosynovitis
Gonstead
    G. pelvic marking system
    G. technique
gonycampsis
good
    G. Grips utensil
    G. 'N Bed wedge
    G. rasp
Goode wrap
Goodman orthopedic bed
Goodwin bone clamp
goose-egg edema
gooseneck gouge
Gordon
    G. approach
    G. joint injection technique
    G. knee phenomenon
    G. reflex
    G. reflex sign
    G. splint
    G. squeeze test
Gordon-Broström
    G.-B. single-contrast arthrogram
    G.-B. technique
Gordon-Taylor
    G.-T. hindquarter amputation
    G.-T. technique

Gore
    G. bit
    G. smoother
    G. smoother crucial tool
Gore-Tex
    G.-T. anterior cruciate ligament
    G.-T. interpositional arthroplasty
    G.-T. knee prosthesis
    G.-T. nonabsorbable suture
    G.-T. waterproof cast liner
Gorham disease
Gosselin fracture
Gotfried percutaneous compression
  plating
Gottron
    G. papule
    G. sign
Gouffon
    G. hip pin
    G. pin fixation
gouge
    Abbott g.
    Acufex g.
    Alexander g.
    Andrews g.
    Army bone g.
    arthroplasty g.
    Aufranc g.
    Bishop g.
    bone g.
    Buch-Gramcko g.
    Campbell g.
    Capener g.
    Cobb spinal g.
    curved g.
    Dawson-Yuhl g.
    Duray-Reed g.
    gooseneck g.
    Guy g.
    Hibbs g.
    Hoen g.
    Jewett g.
    Killian g.
    Lexer g.
    Lucas g.
    Metzenbaum g.
    Meyerding g.
    Moe g.
    Murphy g.
    orthopaedic g.
    oscillating g.
    Partsch g.

NOTES

G

gouge *(continued)*
  Read g.
  Rubin g.
  Sheehan g.
  Smith-Petersen curved g.
  Smith-Petersen gooseneck g.
  Smith-Petersen straight g.
  Stagnara g.
  Stille bone g.
  straight g.
  swan-neck g.
  tendon g.
  U.S. Army g.
  Watson-Jones bone g.
  West bone g.
  Zielke g.
  Zimmer g.
Gould procedure
gout
  acute g.
  articular g.
  calcium g.
  chronic tophaceous g.
  latent stage of g.
  tophaceous g.
gouty
  g. arthritis
  g. diet
  g. node
  g. pain
  g. tophaceous deposit
  g. tophus
Gowers
  G. maneuver
  G. muscular dystrophy
  G. phenomenon
  G. sign
  G. syndrome
grab
  g. bar
  g. sign
grabber
  arthroscopic g.
  disk g.
  Tab G.
  tendon g.
Graber-Duvernay procedure
grace
  G. method of ratio of metatarsal
    length
  G. plate 4-hole adapter
gracilis
  g. flap
  g. muscle
  g. muscle graft
  g. procedure
  g. syndrome

  g. tendon
  g. test
graciloplasty
  stimulated g.
grade
  g. A, B, C1, C2, D mantle
  Kellgren osteoarthritis g.
  g.'s 1–5 of mobilization
  g. I, II oscillation
  Risser g.
  Wagner g.
  Zachary sensory g.
graded
  g. Gore-Tex tape
  g. spinal anesthesia
grading
  activity g.
  g. of manipulation
  turf toe g.
gradual
  g. elongation intramedullary nailing
    (GEIN)
  g. elongation nailing (GEN)
graduated-height block
graduated tenotomy
Graf
  G. classification
  G. stabilization system
Graflex material
graft
  AAA bone g.
  acetabular augmentation g.
  ACL g.
  advancement flap g.
  Albee bone g.
  allogenic bone g.
  alloplastic g.
  antebrachial fascial g.
  anterior sliding tibial g.
  anterosuperior iliac spine g.
  autochthonous g.
  autogenous cancellous bone g.
  autogenous fibular g.
  autogenous patellar ligament g.
  autogenous semitendinosus-
    gracilis g.
  autologous cancellous bone g.
  autologous reverse g.
  autoplastic g.
  Banks bone g.
  barber-pole vein g.
  bicondylar g.
  bicortical iliac bone g.
  bicortical ilial strip g.
  bifid g.
  BioPolyMeric g.
  Blair-Brown skin g.
  bone autogenous g.

bone block g.
bone chip g.
bone marrow g.
bone peg g.
bone-tendon g.
bone-tendon-bone g.
bone-to-bone g.
Bonfiglio bone g.
bovine collagen g.
Boyd dual-onlay bone g.
BPB autologous g.
BPTB g.
Braun skin g.
bridge g.
bulk g.
cable nerve g.
cadaver bone g.
calcaneal bone g.
Calcitite g.
calvarial free bone g.
Campbell onlay bone g.
cancellous chip bone g.
cancellous insert g.
cancellous morselized bone g.
carbon fiber g.
cartilage g.
chemosterilized g.
chip g.
Chuinard autogenous bone g.
Clancy patellar tendon g.
clothespin spinal fusion g.
Codivilla bone g.
composite rib g.
composite skin g.
consolidated g.
cortical bone g.
cortical strut g.
corticocancellous bone g.
corticocancellous chip g.
cutaneous g.
cylindrical autologous dowel g.
Dacron g.
Daniel iliac bone g.
Davis muscle-pedicle g.
delayed g.
demineralized bone g.
devitalized bone g.
diamond inlay bone g.
double-looped gracilis g.
Douglas skin g.
g. dowel
dowel bone g.

Dragstedt skin g.
g. driver
dual onlay cortical bone g.
dura mater g.
Esser skin g.
g. expulsion
extraarticular g.
fascial g.
fascia lata freeze-thawed g.
fascio-fat g.
fat g.
fatigue bone g.
femoral-femoral bypass g.
femorocrural g.
femur g.
fetal substantia nigra g.
fibular onlay-inlay g.
fibular strut g.
filleted g.
fillet local flap g.
Fisk-Fernandez volar wedge
  bone g.
g. fixation
Flanagan-Burem apposing
  hemicylindric g.
flap g.
flat bone g.
flexor tendon g.
Forbes onlay bone g.
g. fracture
g. fragmentation
free fat g.
free skin g.
freeze-dried g.
freeze-thawed g.
fresh frozen g.
full-thickness skin g. (FTSG)
fusion g.
Gillies bone g.
Gill massive sliding g.
Golaski g.
gracilis muscle g.
Haldeman bone g.
hamstring g.
Harris superior acetabular g.
g. harvest
Hemashield enhanced g.
hemicondylar g.
hemicylindrical bone g.
Henderson onlay bone g.
Henry bone g.
heterodermic g.

NOTES

G

graft *(continued)*
  heterogenous g.
  Hey-Groves-Kirk bone g.
  H-graft bone g.
  Hoaglund bone g.
  homogenous g.
  homologous g.
  homoplastic g.
  H-shaped g.
  Huntington bone g.
  iliac bone g. (IBG)
  iliac crest bone g. (ICBG)
  iliac crest bone free g.
  iliac crest-inlay g.
  iliac slot g.
  iliac strut bone g.
  iliotibial band g.
  g. impingement
  Inclan bone g.
  inlay bone g.
  insert g.
  interbody g.
  intercalary g.
  interfascicular Millesi nerve g.
  interpositional tricortical g.
  interposition bone g.
  intramedullary bone g.
  ipsilateral slide g.
  irradiation sterilized g.
  island g.
  isologous g.
  Isotec patellar tendon g.
  Judet g.
  Jump g.
  keystone g.
  Krause-Wolfe skin g.
  Kutler V-Y flap g.
  LAD composite g.
  Langenskiöld bone g.
  lateral patellar autologous g.
  Lee anterosuperior iliac spine g.
  Lee bone g.
  ligamentous anterior dislocation
    composite g.
  load-bearing g.
  lyophilized bone g.
  Massie sliding g.
  massive sliding g.
  matchstick g.
  g. material alternative
  Matti-Russe bone g.
  McFarland bone g.
  McMaster bone g.
  medullary bone g.
  meniscus g.
  mesh g.
  Meyers quadratus muscle-pedicle
    bone g.

  Millesi nerve g.
  Moberg dowel g.
  morcellized bone g.
  morcellized cancellous g.
  Mueller patellar tendon g.
  multiple cancellous chip g.
  muscle pedicle bone g.
  nail bed g.
  nerve g.
  neurovascular island g.
  Nicoll cancellous bone g.
  Nicoll cancellous insert g.
  nonisometric g.
  nontubed closed distant flap g.
  nontubed open distant flap g.
  Ollier thick split free g.
  Ollier-Thiersch skin g.
  onlay bone g.
  onlay cancellous iliac g.
  OP-1 implant/bone g.
  Opteform 100HT bone g.
  osteoarticular g.
  osteocartilaginous g.
  osteochondral g.
  osteogenic protein-1 bone g.
  osteoperiosteal bone g.
  Overton dowel g.
  Papineau g.
  particulate cancellous bone g.
  patellar tendon g.
  pedicle bone g.
  pedicle fat g.
  peg bone g.
  percutaneous autogenous dowel
    bone g.
  pericardium g.
  peroneus brevis g.
  Phemister onlay bone g.
  pie-crusting skin g.
  plantaris tendon g.
  porous polyethylene g.
  posterior bone g.
  posterior cruciate ligament g.
  posterolateral bone g.
  powdered bone g.
  g. preparation
  prophylactic bone g.
  prosthetic femorodistal g.
  PTFE g.
  rectus femoris g.
  revascularization of g.
  Reverdin epidermal free g.
  rib g.
  Russe bone g.
  Ryerson bone g.
  sandwiched iliac bone g.
  scapular g.
  segmental tendon g.

semitendinosus-gracilis g.
semitendinous g.
single-condylar g.
single-onlay cortical bone g.
single-stage tendon g.
sliding bone g.
Soto-Hall bone g.
split calvarial bone g.
split-thickness skin g. (STSG)
Stark g.
g. strength
structural bone g.
g. structure
strut bone g.
subclavius tendon g.
Tait g.
Taylor-Townsend-Corlett iliac crest bone g.
temporal fascia g.
tendon g. (TG)
g. tension
tension-free Millesi nerve g.
Thiersch medium split free g.
Thiersch thin split free g.
Thomas extrapolated bar g.
tibial bone g.
tricortical iliac crest bone g.
tricortical ilial strip g.
tube flap g.
tubularization of the g.
tumbler g.
vascularized bone g.
vascularized fibular g.
vascularized osteoseptocutaneous fibular autogenous g.
vascularized rib strut g.
wedge g.
Weiland iliac crest bone g.
Whitecloud-LaRocca fibular strut g.
Wilson bone g.
Wilson-Jacobs patellar g.
Windson-Insall-Vince bone g.
Wolfe hand surgery g.
Wolfe-Kawamoto bone g.
Wolf full-thickness free g.
wraparound flap bone g.
Z-plasty local flap g.
graft-bony tunnel wall abrasion
grafting vein
Graftmaster device
Grafton
G. bone matrix/marrow combination

G. DBM putty
G. demineralized bone matrix putty material
Graham
G. ankle arthrodesis
G. muscle hook
G. nerve hook
G. traction
Grahamizer I exerciser
Gram
G. negative
G. positive
G. stain
Granberg cervical traction system
Granberry
G. frame
G. splint
G. traction
Grand Stand support stand
Grantham femur fracture classification
Grant-Small-Lehman supracondylar extension osteotomy
Grant, Surrall, and Lehman procedure
Granuflex dressing
granular
g. cell myoblastoma
g. histiocytosis
granulation
extradural g.
healing by g.
g. phase
g. tissue
granule
ProOsteon Implant 500 g.
granuloma
eosinophilic g.
foreign body g.
giant cell reparative g.
Mignon eosinophilic g.
pyogenic g.
g. pyogenicum
reparative g.
rheumatic g.
subperiosteal giant-cell reparative g.
subungual g.
swimming pool g.
tubercular g.
granulomatosis
Langerhans cell g.
Wegener g.
granulomatous
g. fungal infection

NOTES

G

granulomatous (*continued*)
    g. myositis
    g. tenosynovitis
graph
    Moseley bone age g.
    Moseley straight line g.
Graphic Rating Scale (GRS)
Grashey view
grasp
    pinch g.
    prehension g.
    thumb-pinch g.
grasper
    Acufex g.
    loose body g.
    pituitary g.
grasper-cutter
    Questus leading edge g.-c.
grasping
    g. forceps
    g. power
    g. suture
grasshopper
    g. patella
    G. positioner
Grass neurostimulator
grater reamer
Graves scapula
gravis
    myasthenia g.
    Tensilon test for myasthenia g.
gravitational
    g. insecurity
    g. line
    g. proprioception
gravity
    center of g. (CG, COG)
    g. drawer test
    g. equinus cast
    g. extension locking system
      (GELS)
    flex against g.
    g. ground reaction force
    line of g.
    g. line
    g. method of Stimson
    g. stress test
gravity-driven angle finder
gray
    G. bone drill
    g. matter
    periaqueductal g. (PAG)
    G. ramus communicans
    G. reamer
    G. revision instrument system
Grayson
    G. ligament
    G. ligament in hand

grease gun injury
great
    g. sciatic nerve
    g. toe
    g. toe amputation
    g. toe arthroplasty implant
      technique (GAIT)
    g. toe bone
    g. toe implant
    g. toe implant prosthesis
    g. toe push-off
    g. toe reflex
    g. vessel
greater
    g. multangular
    g. multangular bone
    g. multangular ridge
    g. pelvis
    g. rhomboid muscle
    g. trochanter
    g. trochanteric apophysial arrest
    g. trochanteric femoral fracture
    g. tuberosity
    g. tuberosity osteotomy
Greek foot
green
    G. arthroplasty
    G. muscle hook
    G. procedure
    G. transfer
Green-Anderson growth table
Green-Banks
    G.-B. technique
    G.-B. transfer
Greenberg clamp
Greene forceps
Greenfield
    G. osteotomy
    G. spinocerebellar ataxia
      classification
Green-Grice procedure
Green-Laird modification of the
    Reverdin osteotomy
Green-O'Brien evaluation system
Green-Reverdin osteotomy
Green-Seligson-Henry (GSH)
    G.-S.-H. nail
greenstick
    g. dorsal proximal metatarsal
      osteotomy
    g. fixation
    g. fracture
Green-Watermann osteotomy
Greifer prosthesis
Greissinger
    G. foot prosthesis
    G. Multi-Axis joint

Grelot
    image en G.
grenade
    g. thrower's arm
    g. thrower's fracture
Greulich-Pyle
    G.-P. bone age
    G.-P. technique
Greulich and Pyle skeletal maturation stage
Grice
    G. extraarticular subtalar arthrodesis
    G. incision
    G. procedure
Grice-Green
    G.-G. extraarticular subtalar arthrodesis
    G.-G. operation
    G.-G. technique
grid
    electrode g.
    g. maze board
    g. maze set
    radiographic g.
    Shar-Tek foot positioning g.
Grierson
    G. meniscal shaver
    G. tendon stripper
griffe
    main en g.
Griffith incision
grimace test
grinder
    DePuy calcar g.
grinding test
grip
    dowel g.
    Get-A-Grip g.
    key g.
    g. lock
    pencil g.
    Posey g.
    Skil-Care cushion g.
    g. strength
    g. strength test
    syringe g.
    g. tester
    ulnar side g.
Grip-Ease device
Gripp
    G. squeeze ball
    G. squeeze ball hand exerciser

Gripper acetabular cup prosthesis
gripping exercises
GripTrack Commander strength tester
Grisel
    G. disease
    G. syndrome
Gristina-Webb
    G.-W. prosthesis
    G.-W. total shoulder arthroplasty
Griswold distraction machine
grit-blasted prosthesis
Gritti
    G. amputation
    G. operation
Gritti-Stokes
    G.-S. amputation
    G.-S. distal thigh procedure
    G.-S. knee prosthesis
groin
    g. flap
    footballer's g.
    Gilmore g.
    g. pain
groin-to-ankle cast
grommet
    g. bone liner
    circumferential g.
    press-fit circumferential g.
    titanium circumferential g.
groove
    anular g.
    bicipital g.
    deltopectoral g.
    g. distal tibia
    femoral g.
    fibular g.
    flexor g.
    intercollicular g.
    intercondylar g.
    intertubercular g.
    nail g.
    parasagittal g.
    patellar g.
    patellofemoral g.
    peroneal g.
    g. of Ranvier
    spiral humeral g.
    trochlear g.
grooved
    g. director
    g. dissector

G

NOTES

grooved *(continued)*
G. Pegboard Test
g. protector
grooving
g. osteotome
g. reamer
gross
g. fracture
g. manipulation
G. Motor Function Measure (GMFM)
Grosse-Kempf
G.-K. interlocking medullary nail
G.-K. interlocking medullary nailing
G.-K. locking nail
G.-K. tibial technique
ground
g. electrode
g. lamella
purchase and press the g.
g. reaction
g. reaction force
group
activity g.
adductor muscle g.
ancillary muscle g.
AO g.
g. fascicular repair
gastrocnemius-soleus muscle g.
levator ani g.
muscle g. (MG)
PROOF g.
quadriceps muscle g.
grouped discharge
Grover
G. meniscotome
G. meniscus knife
Groves-Goldner technique
Groves opponensplasty
growing pain
growth
anchorage-dependent g.
appositional g.
g. arrest
g. arrest line
asymmetrical g.
bone g.
g. center of bone
chondroosseous g.
ectopic bone g.
g. hormone
g. hormone hypersecretion
g. hormone resistance
latitudinal g.
physial g.
g. plate
g. plate abscess
g. plate fracture

g. plate injury
g. prediction
g. retardation
g. zone
GRS
Graphic Rating Scale
Gruca
G. lower leg procedure
G. stabilization
Gruca-Weiss spring
Gruen
G. mode
G. zone
Gruppe
G. wire prosthesis
G. wire prosthesis-crimping forceps
GSB
GSB elbow prosthesis
GSB expanded version for knee prosthesis
GSH
Green-Seligson-Henry
GSH nail
G suit
GTS two-piece implant system
guard
ankle g.
Cloward cervical drill g.
drill g.
fingertip g.
Freedom Palm G.
McDavid ankle g.
McDavid hinged knee g.
Omed vented instrument g.
palm g.
pin g.
Progressive Palm G.
Ullrich drill g.
guarded osteotome
guardian
G. limb salvage system
G. Red Dot walker
guarding
muscle g.
Guardsman femoral interference screw
Gubler tumor
Gudas
G. scarf Z-plasty
G. scarf Z-plasty osteotomy
Guepar hinged knee prosthesis
Guérin fracture
Guhl
G. distraction
G. technique
guide
Accu-Cut osteotomy g.
Accu-Line g.
acetabular cup peg drill g.

Achillon instrument g.
ACL drill g.
Acufex alignment g.
Acufex tibial g.
Adapteur multifunctional drill g.
adjustable angle g.
Adson drill g.
Adson saw g.
aiming g.
alignment g.
angel wing g.
apical axis g.
Arbeitsgemeinschaft für
  Osteosynthesfragen-stopped drill g.
Arthrex femoral g.
Arthrex tibial g.
axis g.
Bailey-Gigli saw g.
Bailey saw g.
ball-tipped Küntscher g.
barrel g.
g. barrel
Blair saw g.
bone wire g.
Bow & Arrow cannulated drill g.
Bullseye femoral g.
g. bushing
calibrated pin g.
Cloward drill g.
contoured anterior spinal plate
  drill g.
Cushing-Gigli saw g.
Cushing saw g.
cutter g.
Davis saw g.
Delta Recon proximal drill g.
DePuy femoral acetabular
  overlay g.
distal femoral cutting g.
drill g.
eccentric drill g.
extramedullary alignment g.
femoral intramedullary g.
femoral notch g.
Ferkel C g.
FIN pin g.
Fisher g.
fixed-offset g.
front-entry g.
Ghajar g.
Gigli saw g.
Glacier ceramic 4-in-1 cutting g.

Glacier ceramic knee cutting g.
glenoid drill g.
handheld drill g.
Hewson cruciate g.
Hewson ligament drill g.
Hoffmann pin g.
g. hole
Howell tibial g.
humeral cutting g.
intercondylar drill g.
intramedullary g.
Lebsche saw g.
Levin drill g.
ligature g.
Lipscomb-Anderson drill g.
long axial alignment g.
long nail-mounted drill g.
MOD femoral drill g.
nail-driving g.
nail rotational g.
neutral drill g.
notch cutting g.
nut alignment g.
patellar drill g.
patellar reamer g.
patellar resection g.
PCA cutting g.
PCA medullary g.
picket fence g.
g. pin
pin g.
Poppen Gigli saw g.
ProTrac alignment g.
Puddu drill g.
Raney saw g.
reamer g.
rear-entry ACL drill g.
Reece osteotomy g.
Richards angle g.
Richards drill g.
g. rod
saw g.
scaphoid screw g.
Scott-RCE osteotomy g.
screw angle g.
Stader pin g.
stationary angle g.
Synthes wire g.
targeting drill g.
T-Bar g.
telescopic view g.
tibial cutting g.

G

NOTES

guide *(continued)*
 tibial drill g.
 tissue anchor g. (TAG)
 Todd-Wells g.
 tube g.
 tunnel drill g.
 tunnel locator g.
 Tworek screw g.
 Uslenghi drill g.
 g. wire
 wire and drill g.
 wound measuring g.
 Yasargil ligature g.
guideline
 Böhler g.
 Hartel g.
 Letournel g.
guidepin, guide pin
 AO g.
 ball g.
 ball-point g.
 ball-tip g.
 beaded reamer g.
 calibrated g.
 femoral g.
 lateral g.
 nonbeaded g.
 precurved ball-tipped g.
 Rica wire g.
 Synthes g.
 threaded g.
 tibial g.
 Watson-Jones g.
guidewire, guide wire
 beaded g.
 drill-tipped g.
Guilford cervical brace
Guilford-Wright prosthesis
Guillain-Barré syndrome
Guilland sign
guillotine
 g. amputation
 Charnley femoral inlay g.
Guldmann Overhead Trac System
Guleke bone rongeur
Guleke-Stookey approach
Gulick II tape
Guller resection
Gumboro disease
Gumley seat beat injury classification
gummatous
 g. abscess
 g. necrosis
gum rubber Martin bandage
gun
 Arthrex meniscal dart g.
 g. barrel sign
 Biofix arrow g.

 cement injection g.
 CMW cement g.
 Harris cement g.
 heat g.
 Lidge cement g.
 Reflex G.
 rivet g.
 staple g.
 Sterivap cement g.
Gunderson
 G. bone forceps
 G. muscle forceps
Gunning splint
Gunn jaw winking
gunshot
 g. fracture
 g. wound
gunstock deformity
Gunston
 G. arthroplasty
 G. polycentric knee prosthesis
Gunston-Hult knee prosthesis
Gurd
 G. procedure
 G. resection
Gustilo
 G. classification of puncture wound
 G. hip prosthesis
 G. knee prosthesis
 G. puncture wound classification
 G. tibial fracture
 G. tibial fracture classification
 G. unconstrained prosthesis
Gustilo-Anderson
 G.-A. open clavicular fracture
 G.-A. open fracture classification
 G.-A. tibial plafond fracture
  classification
Gustilo-Bias prosthesis
Gustilo-Kyle
 G.-K. cementless total hip
  arthroplasty
 G.-K. femoral component
gutter
 g. cast
 g. splint
Guttmann
 G. subtalar arthrodesis
 G. technique
guy
 G. gouge
 g. suture
Guyon
 G. amputation
 G. canal
 G. operation
 G. tunnel release
 G. tunnel syndrome

G/W Heel Lift, Inc. orthosis
gym
g. ball
Elite Power Station g.
hand g.
limb g.
Total G.
Zuni g.
gymball
Dyna-Disc g.
Exertools g.
gymnastics
Swedish g.

Gymnastik
G. ball
G. ball functional stabilization
exercise
gymnast's wrist
Gymnic
G. Plus exercise ball
Gypsona
G. cast
G. cast material
Gyro-Flex upper extremity exerciser
Gyroscan superconducting MRI

NOTES

H

H buttress support patellofemoral brace
H reflex
H region
H wave

HA

hallux abductus
hydroxyapatite
HA 65101 implant metal
HA 65101 implant metal prosthesis

Haacker sling

Haas

H. disease
H. operation
H. osteotomy
H. paralysis

Haber-Kraft osteotomy

habit scoliosis

habitual

h. control
h. dislocation

habituation

Hackethal

H. intramedullary bouquet fixation
H. nail
H. stacked nailing technique

hacking

hacksaw

HA-coated hip implant

Haddad metatarsal osteotomy

Haddad-Riordan arthrodesis

Hadfield hand board

Hadley S-curve

Hagie

H. hip pin
H. pin nail
H. sliding nail plate

HAGL

humeral avulsion of the glenohumeral ligament
HAGL lesion

Haglund

H. bump
H. disease
H. exostosis
H. foot deformity
H. syndrome

Haglund-Stille plaster spreader

Hahn

H. bone nail
cleft of H.
H. cleft
H. screw

Hahn-Steinthal

H.-S. capitellum fracture classification
H.-S. fracture
H.-S. fracture of capitellum

Haid

H. cervical plate
H. UBP system
H. Universal bone plate

Haight-Finochietto rib spreader

Haines-McDougall medial sesamoid ligament

hairline

h. crack
h. fracture

hairpin

h. knot
h. splint

Hajdu-Cheney syndrome

Hajdu staging system

Hajek

H. chisel
H. mallet

Hajek-Ballenger dissector

Hajek-Koffler bone punch forceps

Haldeman bone graft

Halder locking nail

half

h. Jimmie
h. ring
h. ring leg splint

half-and-half nail

half-circle plate

half-hitch arthroscopic knot

half-moon sign

half-pin

h.-p. external fixator
h.-p. fixation

half-shell splint

half-shoe

half-stitch arthroscopic knot

Halifax

H. clamp posterior cervical fixation
H. interlaminar clamp
H. interlaminar clamp kit

halisteresis phenomenon

hall

H. air drill
H. air-driven oscillating saw
H. bur
H. double-hole spinal stapler
H. driver
H. facet fusion
H. Kalamchi shelf procedure
H. mandibular implant system

hall (*continued*)
    H. Micro-Aire drill
    H. Micro E power instrument
    H. modular acetabular reamer system
    H. Neurairtome
    H. power drill
    H. sagittal saw
    H. screwdriver
    H. series 4 large bone instrument
    H. spinal screw
    H. stepdown drill
    H. technique
    H. Versipower drill
    H. Versipower oscillating saw
    H. Versipower reamer
    H. Versipower reciprocating saw
Hall-Dundar drill
Halle bone curette
Hall-effect strain transducer
Hallister heel cup
Hall-Pankovich medullary nail
Hallpike maneuver
hallucal sesamoid
hallucination
    stump h.
hallucis
    accessory abductor h.
    h. brevis tenodesis
    extensor h.
    hyperdynamic abductor h.
    h. longus laceration
hallux
    h. abductovalgus (HAV)
    h. abductus (HA)
    clawed h.
    h. dolorosus
    dropped h.
    h. elevatus
    h. extensus
    h. interphalangeal joint arthrodesis
    intrinsic minus h.
    h. IP joint
    h. limitus deformity
    h. malleus
    h. metatarsophalangeal interphalangeal scale (HMIS)
    h. migration
    h. nail
    rectus h.
    h. rigidus
    h. rigidus arthrodesis
    h. sesamoid
    h. valgus
    h. valgus angle (HVA)
    h. valgus deformity
    h. valgus interphalangeus angle
    h. valgus-metatarsus primus varus complex
    h. valgus night splint
    h. valgus orthosis
    h. valgus procedure
    h. varus
    h. varus correction
    h. varus deformity
Hall-Zimmer power instrument
halo
    h. body jacket
    h. brace
    BRW head ring h.
    h. cast
    h. cervical orthosis
    h. cervical traction system
    h. extension orthosis
    h. immobilization
    Lerman noninvasive h.
    h. pedestal
    pericellular h.
    Perry-Nickel cranial h.
    h. pin
    h. ring
    h. sign
    h. traction
    h. traction jacket
    h. traction orthosis
    Twin Cities Lo-Profile h.
    h. vest
    h. vest apparatus
    h. vest device
halo-cast distraction
halo-dependent traction
halo-extension traction
halo-femoral
    h.-f. distraction
    h.-f. traction
halogen lamp
halo-gravity traction device
halo-hyperextension traction
halo-Ilizarov distraction instrumentation
halo-pelvic
    h.-p. distraction
    h.-p. traction
halo-vest orthosis
halo-wheelchair traction
Halsey
    H. nail scissors
    H. needle holder
Halsted
    H. forceps
    H. maneuver
halter
    Cerva Crane h.
    DePuy h.
    Diskard head h.
    Forrester-Brown head h.

head h.
Redi head h.
Repro head h.
TMJ h.
h. traction
Upper 7 head h.
Zimfoam head h.
Zimmer head h.
hamartoma
    cartilaginous h.
    chondromatous h.
    fibrous h.
    leiomyomatous h.
    lipofibromatous h.
    neuromuscular h.
    polymorphic h.
hamartomatous lesion
Hamas
    H. technique
    H. upper limb prosthesis
hamate
    h. bone
    hook of the h.
    h. hook
    h. hook nonunion
    h. ligament
    h. tail fracture
hamate-lunate joint
hamatometacarpal ligament
Hambly procedure
Hamby twist drill
Hamilton
    H. apparatus
    H. bandage
    H. pelvic traction screw tractor
    H. Rating Scale for Depression
    H. ruler test
    H. screw
    H. traction
hammer
    Babinski percussion h.
    Berliner percussion h.
    Buck neurological h.
    Buck percussion h.
    cervical/lumbar h.
    Cloward h.
    Davis percussion h.
    Dejerine-Davis percussion h.
    Dejerine percussion h.
    h. digit syndrome
    Epstein neurological h.
    H. external fixation

    h. finger
    Küntscher h.
    orthopaedic h.
    percussion h.
    reflex h.
    slap h.
    sliding h.
    Taylor percussion h.
    h. toe
    h. toe correction with interphalangeal fusion
    h. toe deformity
    Troemner percussion h.
hammertoe, hammer toe (HT)
    dynamic h.
    fixed h.
    flexible h.
    h. repair
    h. syndrome (HTS)
Hammon
    H. foot operation
    H. foot procedure
Hammond splint
hamstring
    h. fixation technique
    h. force
    h. graft
    h. lengthening
    h. ligament augmentation
    medial h.
    h. muscle
    h. reflex
    h. release
    h. stretcher
    h. syndrome
    h. tendon
    h. tightness
hamstring-setting exercise
hamstrung knee
Hancock amputation
hand
    accoucheur h.
    all-median nerve h.
    all-ulnar nerve h.
    h. amputation
    h. anomaly
    ape h.
    apelike h.
    bear's paw h.
    h. block
    h. board
    h. brace

NOTES

311

hand (*continued*)
    h. chuck
    claw h.
    cleft h.
    club h.
    h. cock-up splint
    h. cone
    h. cuff
    Disabilities of the Arm, Shoulder, and H. (DASH)
    h. dissector
    h. dominance
    dorsal venous arch of h.
    dorsum of h.
    h. drill
    h. elevator
    h. evaluation set
    h. exercise ball
    h. exerciser
    fell on outstretched h. (FOOSH)
    flat h.
    flexor retinaculum of h.
    flipper h.
    frostbite of h.
    H. Functional Index (HFI)
    Gilliat-Summer nerve-damaged h.
    h. grasp strength
    Grayson ligament in h.
    h. grip dynamometer
    h. grip strength
    h. gym
    H. Helper
    H. Helper hand exerciser
    hemiplegic h.
    hypoplastic h.
    intrinsic minus h.
    intrinsic plus h.
    Krukenberg h.
    lobster-claw h.
    mirror h.
    mitten h.
    monkey fist h.
    Myobock artificial h.
    myopathy h.
    no man's land of h.
    oath h.
    obstetrician's h.
    opera-glass h.
    h. orthosis (HO)
    Otto Bock system electric h.
    pancake h.
    h. paralysis
    h. placement
    pretendinous band of h.
    h. prosthesis
    h. reconstruction
    h. rest
    h. saw
    skeleton h.
    spade h.
    spastic h.
    split h.
    spread h.
    tangential h.
    trident h.
    vaginal ligament of h.
    Volkmann claw h.
    h. volumeter
    web area of h.
    web border of h.
    writing h.
handbag muscle
handbreadth
HandClens ultra antiseptic spray
handcuff disease
handedness
Handeze fingerless glove
hand-foot syndrome
hand-foot-uterus syndrome
hand-glove prosthesis
handgrip
    h. ergometer
    h. exercise
handheld
    h. drill guide
    h. dynamometer (HHD)
    h. retractor
    h. weight (HHW)
hand-honed reverse cutting needle
handicap
    International Classification of Impairments, Disabilities, H.'s (ICIDH)
    Visual Analog Scale of H.
handle
    Bard-Parker h.
    Barton traction h.
    Beaver blade h.
    Charnley brace h.
    cup holder h.
    Dynagrip blade h.
    multisided blade h.
    Ortho-Grip silicone rubber h.
    stone basket screw mounted h.
    surgical knife h.
    Thera-Band h.
    Therap-Loop door h.
    T-pin h.
    traction h.
    Transfer Handle support h.
handlebar palsy
handle-type reamer
hand-operated drill
handpiece
    Coopervision irrigation/aspiration h.

Max 3 electric h.
reciprocating power h.
Hand-Schüller-Christian
H.-S.-C. disease
H.-S.-C. syndrome
handshake cast
Handy-Buck traction
Hanger ComfortFlex knee prosthesis
hanging
h. arm cast
h. cast sling
h. heel sign
h. hip
h. hip operation
h. of limb
h. toe operation
hangman's fracture
Hang Ups gravity boot
Hankin reduction
Hanna night splint
Hannover
H. classification
H. scoring system
Hansen
H. disease
H. fracture classification
H. pin
Hansen-Street
H.-S. driver-extractor
H.-S. nail
H.-S. pin
H.-S. plate
Hanslik patellar prosthesis
Hansson
Lars Ingvar H. (LIH)
Hapad
H. felt insert
H. heel pad
H. heel wedge
H. longitudinal metatarsal arch pad
H. medial arch pad
H. metatarsal arch
H. metatarsal insole
H. prefabricated wool felt pad
H. scaphoid arch
H. shoe insert
Hapset hydroxyapatite bone graft plaster
HAQ
Headache Assessment Questionnaire
HAQ Index
Hara infiltration block

hard
h. callus stage
h. collar
h. corn
h. disk
h. socket
Hardcastle
H. classification
H. classification of tarsometatarsal joint injury
hardening
work h.
Hardinge
H. expansion bolt
H. femoral approach
H. lateral approach
H. technique
H. vastus lateralis procedure
Hardt-Delima osteotome
hardware
Genesis arthroplasty h.
orthopaedic h.
h. photopenia
hardy
H. aluminum crutch
H. hypophysial curette
Hardy-Clapham
H.-C. classification of sesamoid bones of foot
H.-C. sesamoid classification
Hardy-Joyce triangle
hare
H. apparatus
H. compact traction splint
H. pin
H. splint device
H. traction
hark
H. foot operation
H. pes planus procedure
Harken prosthesis
Harloff cart
Harlow plate
Harmon
H. cervical approach
H. chisel
H. hip reconstruction
H. modified posterolateral approach
H. procedure
H. transfer
H. transfer technique

NOTES

H

Harms
   H. cage
   H. posterior cervical plate
**Harms-Moss anterior thoracic
   instrumentation**
harness
   figure-of-eight h.
   Forte h.
   Kicker Pavlik h.
   Pavlik h.
   weight-relieving Forte h.
   Wheaton Pavlik h.
   Zuni h.
Harold Crowe drill
Harpenden
   H. caliper
   H. dynamometer
Harpoon suture anchor
Harriluque
   H. sublaminar wiring modification
   H. technique
Harrington
   H. clamp forceps
   H. compression rod
   H. distraction instrumentation
   H. distraction outrigger
   H. distraction rod
   H. fixation device
   H. flat wrench
   H. hook clamp
   H. hook driver
   H. nail
   H. outrigger splint
   H. pedicle (bifid) hook
   H. rod clamp
   H. rod fixation
   H. rod and hook system
   H. rod instrumentation
   H. rod instrumentation compression
   H. rod instrumentation distraction
      outrigger device
   H. rod instrumentation failure
   H. rod instrumentation force
      application
   H. spinal elevator
   H. spreader
   H. total hip arthroplasty
Harrington-Kostuik
   H.-K. distraction device
   H.-K. instrumentation
Harris
   H. anterolateral approach
   H. bolt
   H. brace-type reamer
   H. broach
   H. cemented hip prosthesis
   H. cement gun

   H. center-cutting acetabular reamer
   H. condylocephalic nail
   H. condylocephalic nailing
   H. condylocephalic rod
   H. criteria
   H. criteria for implant loosening
   H. Design femoral prosthesis
   H. Design-2 implant
   H. femoral component removal
   H. footprint mat
   H. four-wire trochanter reattachment
   H. growth arrest line
   H. Hemi Arm Sling
   H. hip line
   H. hip nail
   H. hip scale
   H. hip score (HHS)
   H. hip status system
   H. Infant Neuromotor Test (HINT)
   H. knotter
   H. lateral approach
   H. medullary nail
   H. Micromini prosthesis
   H. plate
   H. scope
   H. splint
   H. splint sling
   H. superior acetabular graft
   H. view
   H. wire tier
Harris-Aufranc device
Harris-Beath
   H.-B. arthrodesis
   H.-B. axial calcaneus view
   H.-B. axial hindfoot x-ray
   H.-B. footprint
   H.-B. footprinting mat sign
   H.-B. footprint mat
   H.-B. operation
   H.-B. projection
Harris-Galante
   H.-G. acetabular cup
   H.-G. hip replacement acetabular
      component
   H.-G. I porous-coated acetabular
      component
   H.-G. porous hip prosthesis
   H.-G. stem
Harris-Mayo hip score
Harrison bone-holding forceps
Harrison-Nicolle polypropylene peg
Harris-Smith
   H.-S. anterior interbody drill
   H.-S. cervical fusion
Hartel guideline
Hart extension finger splint
Hartigan foramen

Hartmann
  H. bone rongeur
  H. mosquito forceps
Hartshill rectangle
harvest
  graft h.
  h. site
harvesting
  bone h.
  Gilbert h.
  Tamae h.
  Weiland h.
Harvey wire-cutting scissors
Hass
  H. osteotomy
  H. procedure
  H. type syndactyly
Hassmann-Brunn-Neer elbow technique
Hastings
  H. bipolar hemiarthroplasty
  H. frame
  H. hip prosthesis
  H. open reduction
Hatcher pin
Hatcher-Smith cervical fusion
hatchet-head
  h.-h. deformity
  h.-h. shoulder
Hatfield bone curette
Hauser
  H. Achilles lengthening procedure
  H. ambulation index
  H. bunionectomy
  H. heel cord procedure
  H. patellar operation
  H. patellar realignment technique
  H. patellar tendon procedure
  H. realignment
  H. tendo calcaneus lengthening
Hausmann
  H. Velcro-Lock mat platform
  H. weight rack
  H. Work-Well work hardening
    system
Hausted orthopedic bed
Hautant test
HAV
  hallux abductovalgus
haversian
  h. bone remodeling
  h. canal
  h. gland

  h. lamella
  h. space
  h. system
  h. vessel
Hawiva test
hawkeye
  H. suture needle
  H. suture needle for arthroscopy
Hawkins
  H. impingement sign
  H. line
  H. procedure
  H. talar fracture classification
  H. test
  H. type I talus fracture
**Hawkins-Warren athlete's shoulder
  score**
Haygarth node
Hay-Groves shelf procedure
Hay lateral approach
Haynes-Griffin mandibular splint
Haynes pin
Haynes-Stellite (HS)
  H.-S. 21 implant metal
  H.-S. implant metal prosthesis
Hays hand retractor
H-block
  Frost H.-b.
  H.-b. nail surgery
HBO
  hyperbaric oxygen
  HBO therapy
HCA
  heel cord advancement
HCl
  hydrochloride
HCMI
  Health Care Manufacturing Inc.
  HCMI Chiropractic System
HCTU
  home cervical traction unit
HD
  heloma durum
HD-2
  HD-2 cemented hip prosthesis
  HD-2 total hip prosthesis
head
  abductor hallucis oblique h.
  abductor hallucis transverse h.
  Aequalis h.
  avascular necrosis of the
    femoral h. (AVNFH)

NOTES

H

315

head *(continued)*
    BioPro ceramic TARA h.
    h. brace
    cartilaginous cap of phalangeal h.
    h. check
    cobalt-chromium h.
    collared femoral h.
    Continuum bipolar acetabular h.
    Copeland humeral resurfacing h.
    core decompression of femoral h.
    countersink screw h.
    DePuy hip prosthesis with
      Scuderi h.
    femoral h.
    fibular h.
    first metatarsal h. (FMH)
    flat metatarsal h.
    h. fracture
    Giliberty bipolar femoral h.
    h. halter
    H. hip arthroplasty
    h. holder
    humeral h.
    infrared h.
    ischemic necrosis of femoral h.
      (INFH)
    J-FX bipolar h.
    long h.
    Matroc femoral h.
    metatarsal flat h.
    Phillips screw h.
    pseudometatarsal h.
    radial h.
    screw h.
    Series-II humeral h.
    talar h.
    terminal h.
    ulnar h.
    V40 forged femoral h.
    Vitox femoral h.
    Ziramic femoral h.
    Zirconia orthopedic prosthetic h.
    Zyranox femoral h.
headache
    H. Assessment Questionnaire
      (HAQ)
    cervicogenic h.
    exercise-related h.
head-at-risk sign
headed Bio-Corkscrew
head-first slide
head-halter traction
headholder
    Aesculap h.
headlight
    Cogent LightWear h.
Headmaster collar
head-mounted display (HMD)

head-neck component
headrest
    doughnut h.
    h. extension
    Mayfield neurosurgical h.
    McConnell orthopedic h.
    pin h.
    three-prong h.
head-shaft angle
head-splitting humeral fracture
head-stem offset
healed fracture
Healey revision acetabular component
healing
    bone h.
    cartilage h.
    contact h.
    h. by first intention
    fracture h.
    gap h.
    h. by granulation
    organizational phase of tendon h.
    per primam h.
    plasmatic phase of skin h.
    h. retardation
    h. by second intention
    h. shoe
    soft tissue h.
    spiritual h.
    therapeutic ultrasound for tendon h.
Healos
    H. bone graft substitute
    H. synthetic bone grafting material
health
    H. Care Manufacturing Inc.
      (HCMI)
    H. O Meter Scale
Healthflex orthotic
Healthier seating cushion
The Healthy Back System
Heal Well night splint
heart
    athlete's h.
    h. failure
    h. rate (HR)
heart-and-hand syndrome
heart-shaped buttocks
heat
    h. allodynia
    h. application
    h. cramp
    h. cramping
    damp h.
    h. fracture
    h. gain
    h. gun
    h. injury prevention
    h. injury risk

h. loss
moist h.
H. Plus Massage lower body wrap
h. stress
h. stroke
h. syncope
h. therapy
heat-cured acrylic femoral head prosthesis
Heath mallet
heat-molded petroplastic ankle-foot orthosis
heavy
    h. cross-slot screwdriver
    h. side plate
heavy-duty
    h.-d. femur plate
    h.-d. two-tooth retractor
Heberden
    H. arthropathy
    H. disease
    H. node
    H. nodosity
    H. rheumatism
hebosteotomy
hebotomy
Hebra blade
Heck screw
Hector tendon
Hedblom rib retractor
Hedley-Hungerford hip prosthesis
Hedrocel
    H. cup
    H. proximal tibia augmentation implant
    H. tantalum metal structure
    H. titanium screw
heel
    anterior h.
    black-dot h.
    CARBONX active h.
    h. compression syndrome
    h. contact phase of gait
    h. cord
    h. cord advancement (HCA)
    h. cord lengthening
    h. cord stretch
    h. cord stretching exercise
    h. counter
    cucumber h.
    h. cup
    cushion h.

h. cushion
h. equinus
h. eversion
h. fat pad
H. Free splint
gonorrheal h.
h. height
high-prow h.
H. Hugger therapeutic heel stabilizer
h. jar
jogger's h.
h. lift
h. lock
h. pad pathology
h. pad thickening
painful h.
h. pain syndrome
policeman's h.
h. posting
h. prominence
prominent h.
h. raise exercise
reverse Thomas h.
h. rock exercise
rubber walking h.
SACH orthopedic h.
h. sleeve
h. and sole insert
solid ankle, cushioned h. (SACH)
h. spike
h. spur
h. spur/plantar fasciitis syndrome
H. Spur Special
h. spur syndrome
h. stand
h. strike
tennis h.
h. tension
Thomas h.
h. valgus
h. varus
h. varus sign
h. walk
walking h.
h. wedge
wedge adjustable cushioned h. (WACH)
heel-and-toe
    h.-a.-t. gait
    h.-a.-t. walk
    h.-a.-t. walking

NOTES

H

Heelbo decubitus heel/elbow protector
HeelCup
    Sof Gel H.
The Heeler inflatable heel protector
Heelift suspension boot
heel-off phase of gait
heel-palm test
heel-rise test
heel-strike phase of gait
heel-tap reflex
heel-tip test
heel-toe
    h.-t. gait
    h.-t. pattern
    h.-t. runner
heel-to-knee test
heel-to-shin test
heel-to-toe medial shoe wedge
Heel-Up Boot suspension boot
HeelWedge healing shoe
Heerfort syndrome
Heermann alligator forceps
Heffington lumbar seat spinal frame
Hefty-bite pin cutter
Hegge pin
Heifetz procedure
height
    heel h.
    intervertebral disk h.
Hein rongeur
Heiple arthrodesis
Heiss soft tissue retractor
Helal
    H. flap arthroplasty
    H. modification
    H. osteotomy
Helal-Gibb procedure
Helbing sign
Helenca
    H. bandage
    H. binder
Helfet test
helical computed tomography
helicopod gait
helicopodia
Heliodorus bandage
Helistat
helmet
    cranial h.
heloma
    h. durum (HD)
    h. molle (HM)
helotomy
Helparm
    Swedish H.
helper
    Hand H.

hemangiectasia
    Klippel-Trenaunay
    osteohypertrophic h.
hemangioendothelioma
hemangioendotheliosarcoma
hemangioepithelioma
    epithelioid h.
hemangioma
    capillary h.
    cavernous h.
hemangiomatosis
hemangiopericytoma
hemangiosarcoma
hemarthrosis
    acute traumatic h.
    posttraumatic h.
Hemashield enhanced graft
hematogenous
    h. infection
    h. osteomyelitis
hematoma
    iliopsoas muscle h.
    intramedullary h.
    postoperative drainage-related h.
    pulsating h.
    sciatic nerve palsy h.
    subgluteal h.
    subungual h.
hematomyelia
hematorrhachis
hematosteon
hemianopsia
    homonymous h.
hemiarthroplasty
    Austin Moore h.
    Bateman h.
    Hastings bipolar h.
    I-beam hip h.
    large humeral head h.
    Miller-Galante I h.
    Neer h.
    prosthetic h.
    Smith-Petersen h.
hemicallotasis
hemic calculus
hemicondylar
    h. fracture
    h. graft
hemicylindrical bone graft
hemidystonia
hemiepiphysiodesis
hemigigantism
hemihypertrophy
hemi-implant
    Dow Corning titanium h.-i.
hemi-interpositional implant
hemijoint arthroplasty

hemiknee
    Savastano h.
hemilaminectomy knife
hemimelia
    Achterman-Kalamachi fibular h.
    complete paraxial h.
    fibular h.
    paraxial h.
    partial h.
    radial h.
    tibial h.
hemimelic progressive osseous
  heteroplasia
hemiparetic gait
hemipelvectomy
    formal h.
    internal h.
hemipelvis
hemiphalangectomy
    Johnson h.
hemiplegia
    bilateral h.
    double h.
    spastic h.
    traumatic h.
hemiplegic
    h. amyotrophy
    h. foot
    h. gait
    h. hand
hemiprosthesis
    single-stemmed silicone h.
hemipulp flap
hemiresection interposition arthroplasty
hemisection
    triple h.
hemi/semi-laminotomy
Hemi-Silastic implant
hemispatial neglect
hemispherical
    h. pusher
    h. reamer
hemivertebra
    balanced h.
    congenital h.
    unbalanced h.
hemivertebral excision
hemochromatosis
hemodialysis-related arthropathy
Hemo-Drain evacuator
hemogenesis
hemolymphangioma

hemolysis
    foot-strike h.
    intravascular h.
hemophilic
    h. arthritis
    h. arthropathy
    h. joint
hemorrhage
    intramedullary h.
    retroperitoneal h.
    subacute subperiosteal h.
hemorrhagic
    h. bulla
    h. osteomyelitis
    h. villous synovitis
hemosiderin deposition
hemostasis
hemostat
    blunt nose h.
    h. clamp
    Crile h.
    Kelly h.
    mosquito h.
    Nu-Knit absorbable h.
    orthopaedic h.
    Surgicel fibrillar h.
    Surgicel Nu-Knit absorbable h.
hemostatic
    h. forceps
    h. thoracic clamp
hemothorax
Hemovac
    H. Hydrocoat drain
    H. suction tube
Henahan elevator
Hendel guided osteotome
Henderson
    H. arthrodesis
    H. clamp approximator
    H. classification
    H. fracture
    H. lag screw
    H. onlay bone graft
    H. posterolateral approach
    H. posteromedial approach
    H. skin incision
Henderson-Jones
    H.-J. chondromatosis
    H.-J. disease
Hendler unitunnel technique
Hendren self-retaining retractor

NOTES

H

Henle
    H. ligament
    trapezoid bone of H.
Hennessy knee brace
Henning
    H. cast spreader
    H. inside-to-outside technique
    H. instrument set
    H. mallet
    H. meniscal retractor
    H. plaster spreader
Henry
    H. acromioclavicular technique
    H. anterior strap approach
    H. anterolateral approach
    H. bone graft
    H. extensile approach
    H. incision
    H. knot
    knot of H.
    leash of H.
    ligament of H.
    master knot of H.
    H. muscle transfer
    H. paralysis
    H. posterior interosseous nerve
      approach
    H. posterior interosseous nerve
      exposure
    posterolateral approach of H.
    H. radial approach
    H. resection
Henry-Geist spinal fusion
Henschke-Mauch
    H.-M. saw
    H.-M. SNS knee prosthesis
    H.-M. SNS lower limb prosthesis
Hensen plane
heparinized
    h. Ringer lactate solution
    h. saline flush
hepatotoxicity
herbal therapy
Herbert
    H. bone screw
    H. bone screw fixation
    H. bone screw system
    H. jig
    H. knee prosthesis
    H. saw
    H. scaphoid bone fracture
    H. scaphoid bone fracture
      classification
    H. scaphoid screw
    H. screw fixator
Herbert-Fisher fracture system
    classification
Herbert-Whipple bone screw

Hercules
    H. plaster shears
    H. TM drop-adjusting table
Herczel
    H. rib elevator
    H. rib rasp
hereditaria
    myotonia h.
hereditary
    h. deforming chondrodysplasia
    h. essential myoclonus
    h. motor sensory neuropathy
      (HMSN)
    h. multiple exostosis
    h. neuropathic disease
    h. onychoosteodysplasia
    h. osteoonychodysplasia (HOOD)
    h. progressive arthroophthalmopathy
    h. sensory motor neuropathy (type
      I–III) (HSMN I–III)
    h. spinocerebellar ataxia
heredopathia atactica polyneuritiformis
Herendeen phenomenon
Heritage hip system
Herman-Gartland osteotomy
Hermes
    H. Evolution tricompartmental knee
      system
    H. total knee system
Hermodsson
    H. fracture
    H. internal rotation
    H. internal rotation technique
    H. tangential view
Hernandez-Ros bone staple
Herndon-Heyman
    H.-H. foot operation
    H.-H. foot procedure
Herndon hip classification
hernia
    footballer's h.
    muscle h.
    sportsman's h.
    synovial h.
herniated
    h. disk
    h. intervertebral disk (HID)
    h. nucleus pulposus (HNP)
herniation
    central h.
    cervical midline disk h.
    contained disk h.
    disk h.
    intervertebral disk h.
    intraspongy nuclear disk h.
    midline disk h.
    noncontained disk h.
    phalangeal h.

posterolateral h.
synovial h.
traumatic cervical disk h.
herpes
h. gladiatorum
h. simplex
herpetic whitlow
Herring lateral pillar classification
Herzenberg bolt
Herzmark frame
HESSCO 300, 500 series hydrotherapy table
Hessel-Nystrom pin
Hessing brace
heterodermic graft
heterogenesis
heterogenous graft
heterograft
heteroplasia
hemimelic progressive osseous h.
progressive osseous h.
heterotopic
h. bone
h. calcification
h. ossification
h. ossification prevention
heterotrophic ossification bridging
Heuter-Volkmann law
Hewson
H. breakaway pin
H. cruciate guide
H. drill
H. ligament button
H. ligament drill guide
H. suture passer
H. suture retriever
hex
h. handle curette
h. screw
h. wrench
hexagonal slot-cap screw
Hexalite plastic
Hexcel
H. knee prosthesis
H. total condylar knee system
H. total condylar prosthesis
Hexcelite
H. cast
H. sheet splint
Hex-Fix
H.-F. Add-A-Clamp
H.-F. external fixation

H.-F. monolateral external fixator
H.-F. Universal swivel clamp
hexhead
h. bolt
h. pin
h. screwdriver
Hey
H. amputation
H. Groves clamp
H. internal derangement
H. operation
Heyer-Schulte
H.-S. antisiphon device
H.-S. bur hole valve
H.-S. wound drain
Hey-Groves
H.-G. fascia lata technique
H.-G. ligament reconstruction technique
H.-G. procedure
Hey-Groves-Kirk
H.-G.-K. bone graft
H.-G.-K. technique
Heyman
H. hip classification
H. operation
H. panmetatarsal forefoot equinus suspension
H. procedure
H. technique
Heyman-Herndon
H.-H. clubfoot operation
H.-H. epiphysiodesis
H.-H. procedure
H.-H. release
Heyman-Herndon-Strong
H.-H.-S. capsular release
H.-H.-S. technique
HFI
Hand Functional Index
HG
HG multilock hip prosthesis
HG multilock hip stem
hGH
human growth hormone
HGO
hip guidance orthosis
H-graft
H.-g. bone graft
H.-g. fusion
HHD
handheld dynamometer

NOTES

H1209 healing shoe
H1215 healing shoe
HHS
Harris hip score
HHW
handheld weight
Hi
Hi Speed Pulse lavage
HIAD
high-impact aerobic dance
hiatal sign
hiatus
adductor h.
popliteal h.
Hibbs
H. arthrodesis
H. blade
H. bone-cutting forceps
H. chisel
H. chisel elevator
H. curette
H. curved osteotome
H. extensor tendon transfer cavus deformity
H. frame
H. gouge
H. mallet
H. metatarsocalcaneal angle
H. operation
H. procedure
H. retractor
H. spinal fusion
H. straight osteotome
H. tendosuspension
Hibbs-Jones spinal fusion
hibernoma
Hibiclens
H. scrub
H. solution
Hick effect
hickory-stick fracture
Hicks lugged plate
HID
herniated intervertebral disk
hidroacanthoma simplex
hierarchical scales of ADLs
high
h. heel shoe
h. median-high radial palsy
h. median-high ulnar palsy
h. molecular weight polyethylene (HMWPE)
h. muscular resistance bed
h. performance silicone elastomer
h. tibial osteotomy (HTO)
h. toe box
h. ulnar-high radial palsy
h. velocity low amplitude

high-air-loss bed
high-altitude
h.-a. activity
h.-a. adaptation
h.-a. maladaption
high-assimilation pelvis
high-definition video display
high-density foam
high-energy
h.-e. fracture
h.-e. trauma
highest turbinated bone
high-grade
h.-g. spondylolisthesis
h.-g. surface osteogenic sarcoma
high-impact
h.-i. activity
h.-i. aerobic dance (HIAD)
high-Knight brace
high-performance liquid chromatography (HPLC)
high-power athlete
high-pressure liquid chromatography (HPLC)
high-prow heel
high-resolution analysis
high-riding patella
high-risk factor
high-speed
h.-s. bur
h.-s. twist drill
high-steppage gait
high-tide walking brace
high-torque bur
high-voltage
h.-v. galvanism
h.-v. pulsed galvanic
h.-v. pulsed galvanic stimulation (HVPGS)
h.-v. pulsed stimulation (HVPS)
h.-v. therapy (HVT)
hila (*pl. of* hilum)
hilar
Hilgenreiner
H. angle
H. brace
H. horizontal Y line
Hilgenreiner-Pauwels line
Hilgenreiner-Perkins (H-P)
H-P line
Hill Air-Drop HA90C table
Hill-Nahai-Vasconez-Mathes technique
Hillock arch
Hill-Rom orthopedic bed
Hill-Sachs
H.-S. deformity
H.-S. fracture
H.-S. lesion

H.-S. shoulder dislocation
H.-S. sign
H.-S. view
hi-lo
h.-l. rehab bed
h.-l. table
hilum, pl. **hila**
hilus
neurovascular h.
h. of tendon
Hinderer
H. cartilage forceps
H. malar prosthesis
hindfoot
h. anatomic variation
h. arthrodesis
h. cavus
h. deformity
h. excursion
h. FPA
h. instability
h. joint complex
h. kinematic
lateral h.
h. motion
h. orthosis
h. pronation
spastic varus h.
h. supination
h. valgus
varus h.
hindfoot-midfoot collapse
hindquarter amputation
hinge
h. abduction
Adjusta-Wrist h.
AHSC-Volz h.
Arizona Health Sciences Center-
Volz h.
h. articulation
h. axis concept
Bahler h.
Camber axis h. (CAH)
Compass h.
Dee elbow h.
elbow h.
flail-elbow h.
implant h.
Kinematic rotation h.
Kudo h.
Lacey h.
medial/plantar h.

Noiles h.
offset h.
Quengel h.
Rancho swivel h.
h. rod
rotating h.
soft tissue h.
stabilizing h.
hinged
h. articulated fixator
h. constrained knee prosthesis
h. cylinder cast
h. cylinder splint
h. fragment
h. great toe replacement prosthesis
h. implant
h. implant prosthesis
h. joint
h. knee brace
h. Thomas splint
h. total knee prosthesis
hinged-distraction apparatus
hinging
hip h.
HINT
Harris Infant Neuromotor Test
HIO
hole-in-one
HIO technique
hip
h. abduction
h. abduction stress test
h. abductor strengthening exercise
anthropometric total h. (ATH)
h. arthroplasty
h. avulsion fracture
h. axis length
biologically designed h. (BDH)
h. bump
h. bursitis
h. capsule joint
h. click
h. compression screw
congenital dislocation of h. (CDH)
congenital dysplasia of h. (CDH)
cup-on-cup arthroplasty of the h.
DePuy AML h.
developmental dislocated h. (DDH)
developmental dysplasia of the h.
(DDH)
h. disarticulation prosthesis
h. disarticulation suspension

NOTES

hip *(continued)*
h. dislocation
dysplasia of h.
h. epiphysial injury
h. extension
h. extension exercise
h. extension range of motion
h. extensor gait
h. flexion
h. flexion-extension
h. flexor contracture
h. fraction compaction drill
h. fracture compaction drill bit
fused h.
h. guidance orthosis (HGO)
hanging h.
h. hemipelvectomy suspension
h. hinge back exercise technique
h. hinging
hockey player's h.
irritable h.
ischemic disease of the growing h.
  (IDGH)
h. joint angle (HJA)
h. joint aspiration under
  fluoroscopic control
h. joint syndrome
Kinamed anthropometric total h.
Link anatomical h.
Metasul metal-on-metal h.
h. mobility
observation h.
h. orthosis (HO)
pillow orthosis for h.
h. pin
h. pinning
h. pocket neuropathy
h. pointer
h. pointer contusion
Precision total h.
h. reduction
h. replacement
h. replacement prosthesis
revision of total h.
h. roll
h. rotation
Senegas approach to h.
h. skid
snapping h.
h. spica
h. spica cast
h. subluxation
tuberculosis of h.
windblown h.
windswept h.
HIPciser abduction splint
hipGRIP pelvic positioning system
hip-knee-ankle-foot orthosis (HKAFO)

Hipokrat bimodular shoulder system
Hippocrates
H. bandage
H. manipulation
hippocratic
h. finger
h. maneuver
HipSaver protective underwear
hip-to-ankle
h.-t.-a. view
h.-t.-a. x-ray
Hirayma osteotomy
Hiroshim transfer
Hirsch
H. hypophysial punch
H. hypophysis punch forceps
Hirschberg
H. reflex
H. sign
Hirschhorn
H. compression approach
H. compression technique
Hirschtick utility shoulder splint
hirudin
His-Haas
H.-H. muscle transfer
H.-H. procedure
histiocytic tumor
histiocytoma
angiomatoid malignant fibrous h.
  (AMFH)
fibrous h.
malignant fibrous h.
nevoid h.
pleomorphic fibrous h.
histiocytosis
granular h.
Langerhans cell h.
sinus h.
Histoacryl
H. glue
H. glue adhesive
histochemistry
Histofreezer
H. cryosurgical system
H. cryosurgical wart treatment kit
histogenesis
distraction h.
histologic
histomorphometry
histopathology
synovial h.
histoplasmosis
hitch
ankle h.
spinal h.
Hitchcock
H. arm procedure

H. stereotactic immobilization frame
H. tendon technique

Hi-Top
H.-T. II adjustable walker
H.-T. foot/ankle brace
H.-T. foot/ankle walker
H.-T. shoe

Hittenberger
H. halo extension
H. prosthesis

HJA
hip joint angle

HJD
Hospital for Joint Disease
HJD total hip system

HKAFO
hip-knee-ankle-foot orthosis

HLA
human leukocyte antigen
human lymphocyte antigen
HLA B27-related
spondyloarthropathy intersection
syndrome

HLT-405 instrument adjusting table

HM
heloma molle

HMD
head-mounted display

HMIS
hallux metatarsophalangeal
interphalangeal scale

HMP
hot moist pack

HMSN
hereditary motor sensory neuropathy

HMWPE
high molecular weight polyethylene

HNA
hypothalamoneurohypophysial axis

HNP
herniated nucleus pulposus

HO
hand orthosis
hip orthosis

HOA
hypertrophic osteoarthroscopy

Hoaglund bone graft

Hoaglund-States classification

hobbling gait

Hobb view

hockey
h. player's hip
h. stick dissector

hockey-stick
h.-s. fracture
h.-s. incision

Hodgen
H. hip splint
H. leg splint

Hodge plane

Hodgkinson acetabular component loosening criteria

Hodgson technique

Hodor-Dobbs procedure

Hoek-Bowen cement removal system

Hoen
H. clamp
H. forceps
H. gouge
H. periosteal elevator
H. retractor
H. rongeur
H. skull plate

Hoffa
H. disease
H. fat pad
H. fracture
H. massage
H. operation
H. sign
H. syndrome
H. tendon shortening
H. tendon-shortening method
H. test

Hoffa-Kastert disease

Hoffa-Lorenz operation

Hoffer
H. ankle procedure
H. split transfer

Hoffer-Daimler cast spreader

Hoffmann
H. apex fixation pin
H. approach
H. II compact external fixation
component
H. C-series external fixator
H. Dynamic external fixator
H. external fixation
H. external fixation system
H. frame
H. ligament clamp
H. metatarsal operation

NOTES

H

Hoffmann *(continued)*
- H. metatarsal procedure
- H. mini-lengthening fixation device
- H. muscular atrophy
- H. panmetatarsal head resection
- H. pin guide
- H. reflex
- H. sign
- H. syndrome
- H. transfixion pin

Hoffmann-Clayton procedure

Hoffmann-Vidal
- H.-V. double frame
- H.-V. external fixation apparatus
- H.-V. external fixation device
- H.-V. external fixator

Hogg chair

Hohl-Luck tibial plateau fracture classification

Hohl-Moore
- H.-M. classification
- H.-M. technique

Hohl tibial condylar fracture classification

Hohmann
- H. bone retractor
- H. bunionectomy
- H. operation
- H. osteotomy
- H. procedure

Hohmann-Thomasen metatarsal osteotomy

Hohmann-Wilson osteotomy

Hoke
- H. Achilles tendon lengthening
- H. Achilles tendon lengthening operation
- H. lumbar brace
- H. lumbar brace/corset
- H. lumbar corset
- H. osteotome
- H. procedure for tibial palsy
- H. tibial palsy procedure
- H. triple arthrodesis
- H. triple-section method

Hoke-Kite technique

Hoke-Martin traction

Hoke-Miller procedure

Hold-and-Hold positioner

Holdaway ratio

holder
- acetabular cup h.
- Alvarado knee h.
- arm h.
- arthroscopic leg h.
- Ayers needle h.
- Barraquer needle h.
- Böhler-Steinmann pin h.

- bone h.
- Castroviejo needle h.
- Charnley trochanter h.
- clamp h.
- Crile-Wood needle h.
- cup h.
- DeMartel-Wolfson clamp h.
- Donaghy angled suture needle h.
- Drummond hook h.
- Ferguson bone h.
- Halsey needle h.
- head h.
- hook h.
- hookbar h.
- Jacobson needle h.
- knee h.
- leg h.
- limb h.
- Malis needle h.
- Mayo-Hegar needle h.
- microneedle h.
- needle h.
- neonatal tracheostomy tube h.
- octopus h.
- operative leg h.
- OSI Arthroscopic Leg h.
- pin h.
- Prep-Assist leg h.
- Rhoton needle h.
- rod h.
- Ryder needle h.
- Sarot needle h.
- Schmidt rod h.
- shoulder h.
- staple h.
- Surbaugh leg h.
- thigh h.
- tibial track h.
- trochanter h.
- TSRH hook h.
- Wangensteen needle h.
- washer h.
- Watanabe pin h.
- Webster needle h.
- well-leg h.
- Yasargil needle h.

holding mitt

hold-relax
- h.-r. method
- h.-r. technique

Holdsworth spinal fracture classification

hole
- acetabular seating h.
- anchor h.
- anchoring h.
- blind anchorage h.
- bur h.
- centering h.

drill h.
gliding h.
guide h.
lag screw thread h.
offset drill h.
h. preparation method
ten-h. blade plate
hole-in-one (HIO)
h.-i.-o. technique
holism
Hollander clog
Hollingshead Index
Hollister Hot/Ice knee blanket
hollow
h. back
h. bone
h. bone trephine
h. chisel
h. foot
h. foot clawfoot deformity
h. mill Asnis cannulated screw
h. mill drill
h. mill instrumentation
h. mill reamer
Hollywood
H.-bed
H. bed extension hook set
Holmes
H. operation
H. phenomenon
Holmes-Stewart phenomenon
holmium YAG laser
holorachischisis
Holscher
H. knee retractor
H. root retractor
Holstein fracture of humerus
Holstein-Lewis fracture
Holt
H. bolt
H. nail
H. nail plate
Holter traction
Holt-Oram dysplasia
Holzheimer retractor
Homans
H. sign
H. test
home
h. assessment
h. cervical traction unit (HCTU)
h. exercise program

h. medical equipment
H. Ranger shoulder pulley
h. rehabilitation
h. spinal stabilization program
homeopathy
homeostasis
fluid h.
osseous h.
HomeStretch lumbar traction
HomeTrac
Saunders cervical H.
homogenous graft
homograft
h. implant material
h. prosthesis
homolog
meniscus h.
homologous graft
homonymous hemianopsia
homoplastic graft
homuncular organization
homunculus
HOOD
hereditary osteoonychodysplasia
hood
dorsal h.
extensor h.
retinacular h.
hoof bottom
hook
Acufex nerve h.
anatomic h.
h. approximator
APRL prosthetic h.
Austin Moore h.
Barr h.
bifid h.
h. blade
h. blocker
blunt h.
Bobechko sliding barrel h.
bone h.
Boyes-Goodfellow h.
button h.
buttressed h.
canted finger h.
Carroll skin h.
C-D h.
h. clamp
clawed pedicle h.
closed Cotrel-Dubousset h.
closed transverse process TSRH h.

NOTES

327

hook *(continued)*
    compression h.
    cranial Jacobs h.
    Culler h.
    Cushing dural h.
    h. dislodgment
    distraction h.
    h. distractor
    double-open h.
    double-pronged skin h.
    down-angle h.
    downsized circular laminar h.
    drop-entry (closed body) h.
    Drummond h.
    dura h.
    Edwards h.
    Edwards-Levine h.
    Effler-Groves h.
    finger h.
    garment h.
    Gillies bone h.
    Gillies-Dingman h.
    glide h.
    Graham muscle h.
    Graham nerve h.
    Green muscle h.
    h. of the hamate
    hamate h.
    h. of hamate bone
    Harrington pedicle (bifid) h.
    H. hemi-harness shoulder
      immobilizer
    h. holder
    Hosmer Dorrance h.
    h. impactor
    intermediate C-D h.
    Isola spinal implant system h.
    Jameson muscle h.
    Jannetta h.
    jig h.
    Joseph h.
    Keene compression h.
    Kennerdell-Maroon h.
    Kilner h.
    Kirby muscle h.
    Knodt rod and h.
    Küntscher nail-extracting h.
    Lahey Clinic dural h.
    Lambotte bone h.
    laminar C-D h.
    Leatherman h.
    lyre-shaped finger h.
    meniscus h.
    Micro-One h.
    Moe alar h.
    Moss h.
    multispan fracture h.
    nail-extracting h.

    nerve h.
    neutral h.
    O'Brien rib h.
    Oesch h.
    open C-D h.
    Osher irrigating implant h.
    PCL-oriented placement marking h.
    pediatric C-D h.
    pediatric TSRH h.
    pedicle C-D h.
    h. pin
    h. plate
    h. probe system
    prosthetic h.
    h. pusher
    ribbed h.
    right-angle h.
    Rogozinski h.
    h. rotary scissors
    Selby I, II h.
    sharp worm h.
    side-opening laminar h.
    h. site
    skin h.
    sliding barrel h.
    split-finger h.
    square-ended h.
    T-handled h.
    top-entry (open body) h.
    traction h.
    Trautman Locktite prosthetic h.
    h. trial set screw
    TSRH buttressed laminar h.
    TSRH circular laminar h.
    TSRH pedicle h.
    TSRH trial h.
    twist h.
    Tyrell h.
    UCLA CAPP TD h.
    up-angle h.
    vessel h.
    Vilex Ouchless H.
    Volkmann bone h.
    Yasargil spring h.
    Zielke bifid h.
    Zuelzer h.
hookbar holder
hooked
    h. acromion
    h. bone
    h. foot
    h. forefoot
    h. intramedullary nail
    h. knife
    h. medullary nail
hook-end intramedullary pin
hookian region
hook-lying pectoral stretch exercise

hook-nail deformity
hook-pin fixation
hook-plate fixation
hook-rod
    Cotrel-Dubousset h.-r.
    Isola h.-r.
    TSRH h.-r.
hook-to-screw L4-S1 compression
  construct
hoop stress fracture
Hoover
    H. sign
    H. test
hop
    h. index
    h. test
Hopkins plaster knife
Hoppenfeld-DeBoer
    H.-D. approach
    H.-D. technique
Hoppenfeld lateral approach
Hori technique
horizontal
    h. cleavage
    h. external rotation
    h. fracture
    h. gantry cut
    h. mattress suture
    h. meniscal tear
    h. osteotomy
    h. pedicle diameter
    h. plane
    h. position
    h. shoulder abduction exercise
hormone
    adrenocorticotropic h. (ACTH)
    growth h.
    human growth h. (hGH)
    thyrotropin-releasing h.
horn
    anterior h.
    bone graft shoe h.
    central h.
    cutaneous h.
    enlarged frontal h.
    posterior h.
    shoulder h.
horse
    charley h.
    h. foot callus
horseback rider's knee
horse-hoof fracture nonunion

horseshoe
    h. abscess
    h. appearance
    h. heel pad
    h. patellofemoral brace
    h. therapy table
horseshoe-shaped
    h.-s. felt pad
    h.-s. flap
horse-tail Achilles tendon tear
Horsley
    H. bone cutter
    H. bone-cutting forceps
    H. bone rongeur
    H. bone saw
    H. bone wax
    H. separator
Horsley-Stille
    H.-S. bone-cutting forceps
    H.-S. rib shears forceps
Horwitz
    H. ankle fusion
    H. ankle fusion approach
    H. transmalleolar arthrodesis
Horwitz-Adams
    H.-A. ankle fusion
    H.-A. arthrodesis
    H.-A. operation
HOS
    human osteogenic sarcoma
hose
    TED h.
    Venosan support h.
Hosmer
    H. above-knee rotator
    H. Dorrance hook
    H. Dorrance voluntary control four-
      bar knee mechanism
    H. single-axis friction knee
    H. single-axis locking knee
    H. VC four-bar knee orthosis
    H. WALK prosthesis
    H. weight-activated locking knee
hospital
    Imperial College, London H.
      (ICLH)
    H. for Joint Disease (HJD)
    H. for Special Surgery knee score
    H. for Special Surgery scale
    Texas Scottish Rite H. (TSRH)
    H. Trauma Index
host-allograft junction

NOTES

H

329

hot
- h. and cold contrast bath
- h. dog technique
- h. fomentation therapy
- h. joint
- h. knife
- h. moist pack (HMP)
- h. pack (HP)
- h. plate
- h. water bath
- h. weld

hot-cross-bun
- h.-c.-b. skull
- h.-c.-b. skull sign

hot/ice cold therapy cooler therapy device

Houghton-Akroyd
- H.-A. fracture technique
- H.-A. open reduction

Houle test

hourglass
- h. constriction
- h. deformity
- h. vertebra

House-Dieter malleus nipper

housemaid's knee

Housepan clip-applying forceps

House reconstruction

Houston
- H. halo cervical support
- H. halo cervical traction
- H. halo traction cervical collar
- H. operation

Hovanian
- H. latissimus dorsi muscle transfer
- H. procedure
- H. transfer technique

Howard
- H. bone block
- H. technique

Howell tibial guide

Howmedica
- H. bone anchor
- H. cement
- H. cerclage
- H. cerclage cable
- H. Duracon implant
- H. ICS screw
- H. Kinematic II knee prosthesis
- H. knee instrumentation
- H. knee system
- H. Microfixation System drill bit
- H. Microfixation System forceps
- H. Microfixation System plate cutter
- H. Microfixation System pliers
- H. monospherical implant
- H. monotube

- H. monotube external rotator
- H. PCA prosthesis
- H. total ankle system
- H. Universal compression screw
- H. Vitallium staple
- H. VSF fixation system

Howmedica-Osteonics instrument

Howorth
- H. approach
- H. procedure
- H. prosthesis

Howorth-Keillor procedure

Howse
- H. prosthesis
- H. total hip replacement

Howse-Coventry prosthesis

Howship lacuna

Hoyer
- H. lift
- H. traction

H-P
Hilgenreiner-Perkins
- H-P line

HP
hot pack

HP-100
- HP-100 prosthetic finger
- HP-100 prosthetic finger joint

HPA
hypothalamic-pituitary-adrenal

HPLC
high-performance liquid chromatography
high-pressure liquid chromatography

HPS II total hip prosthesis

HR
heart rate

H-reflex

HS
Haynes-Stellite

H-shaped
- H-s. capsular incision
- H-s. graft
- H-s. plate

HSMN I–III
hereditary sensory motor neuropathy (type I–III)

HSS
HSS knee score
HSS total condylar knee prosthesis

Hsu-Hsu percutaneous tendo calcaneus lengthening

HT
hammertoe
Hubbard tank

HTO
high tibial osteotomy
HTO fixator

HTO wedge human donor tissue allograft

HTS
hammertoe syndrome

Hubbard
H. bolt
H. physical therapy tank
H. side plate
H. tank (HT)

Hubbard-Nylok bolt
hubbed needle
Huber
H. abductor digiti quinti transfer
H. adductor digiti quinti opponensplasty
H. transfer of abductor digiti quinti

Hubscher maneuver
Huckstep nail
Hudson
H. bone bur
H. bone drill
H. brace drill
H. brace with bur
H. chuck adapter
H. forceps
H. Hydrofloat Cushion
H. TLSO brace

Hudson-Jones knee-cage brace
Hueter
H. bandage
H. line
H. sign

Hughes fixation
Hughston
H. Clinic injury classification
H. external rotation recurvatum test
H. knee evaluation
H. knee jerk test
H. knee score
H. lateral compartment reconstruction
H. plica test
H. posterolateral drawer test
H. posteromedial drawer test
H. procedure
H. realignment
H. view

Hughston-Degenhardt reconstruction
Hughston-Hauser procedure

Hughston-Jacobson
H.-J. lateral compartment reconstruction
H.-J. technique

Hughston-Losee jerk test
Hugh Young pedicle clamp
Hui-Linscheid procedure
human
h. chorionic gonadotropin
h. growth hormone (hGH)
h. leukocyte antigen (HLA)
h. lymphocyte antigen (HLA)
h. osteogenic sarcoma (HOS)
h. skin equivalent

Humby knife
humeral
h. avulsion of the glenohumeral ligament (HAGL)
h. bone
h. canal
h. chondroblastoma
h. circumflex vessel
h. component
h. condyle
h. cutting guide
h. epicondyle
h. epicondylitis
h. epiphysis
h. fracture abduction splint
h. fracture malunion
h. head
h. head retractor
h. head-splitting fracture
h. impactor
h. mechanism
h. neck
h. physial fracture
h. reamer
h. saw
h. shaft fracture
h. supracondylar fracture

humeri (*pl. of* humerus)
humeroperoneal muscular dystrophy
humeroradial articulation
humerothoracic abduction
humeroulnar
h. angle
h. articulation
h. joint

humerus, pl. **humeri**
articulatio humeri
distal h.

NOTES

H

humerus *(continued)*
    Holstein fracture of h.
    periarthrosis humeri
    proximal h.
humoral immunity
hump
    buffalo h.
    dowager's h.
humpback deformity
humpbacked spinal curvature
Humphry ligament
hunchback
Hungarian grip plate
Hungerford-Kenna PCA prosthesis
Hungerford-Krackow-Kenna knee arthroplasty
Hungerford technique
hung-up knee jerk
hunter
    H. canal
    H. open cord tendon implant
    H. Silastic prosthesis
    H. Silastic rod
    H. tendon prosthesis
Hunter-Boyes II
hunting
    h. reaction
    h. response
Huntington
    H. bone graft
    H. sign
    H. tibial technique
Hunt paradoxical phenomenon
Hunt-Thompson pantalar arthrodesis
Hurd bone-cutting forceps
Hurler
    H. disease
    H. polydystrophy
    H. syndrome
Hurler-Scheie
    H.-S. compound
    H.-S. syndrome
Husk bone rongeur
Hutchinson
    H. fracture
    melanotic Whitlow of H.
    H. teeth
HV
    HV NightSplint splint
    HV SoftSplint splint
HVA
    hallux valgus angle
HVPGS
    high-voltage pulsed galvanic stimulation
HVPS
    high-voltage pulsed stimulation
HVT
    high-voltage therapy

hyaline
    h. cartilage
    h. cartilage detritus
    h. cartilage implant
    h. necrosis
hyalinization
hyaluronate
hyaluronidase
hybrid
    h. external fixator
    h. fixation
    h. fixation of hip replacement component
    h. total hip replacement
HybridFit
    H. total hip system
    H. total knee system
hydatid resonance
Hydra-Cadence
    H.-C. gait-control unit
    H.-C. knee prosthesis
Hydragrip clamp insert
hydrarthrodial
hydrarthrosis
    intermittent h.
hydrate
hydration status
hydraulic
    h. knee unit
    h. knee unit prosthesis
    h. test system
Hydrisinol
hydro
    h. cushion
    H. Soothe recliner
hydrobromide
hydrocele
    Dupuytren h.
hydrocephalus
hydrochloride (HCl)
    propoxyphene h.
hydrocodone
hydrocollator
    CMO h.
    H. heating unit
    H. pad
    H. steam pack
hydrocolloid occlusive dressing
Hydrocol wound dressing
HydroFlex arthroscopy irrigating system
hydrofloat cushion
Hydrogel wound dressing
hydrogen
    h. peroxide
    h. washout method
hydromassage table
hydromelia
Hydron Burn Bandage

hydrops canal
Hydro-Splint II
hydrostatic pressure
hydrosyringomyelia
    communicating h.
hydrotherapy
    AquaMED dry h.
    dry h.
Hydro-Tone Bell
HydroTrack underwater treadmill system
Hydroxial hip prosthesis
hydroxyapatite (HA)
    h. adhesive
    h. bone
    h. bone replacement material
    calcium h.
    h.-coated ankle arthroplasty
    coralline h.
    h. deposition disease
    h. implant material
    LLPS h.
hydroxyapatite-coated
    h.-c. porous alumni cement
    h.-c. stem
hydroxylapatite
    PureFix h.
25-hydroxyvitamin D
hygroma
    cystic h.
Hylamer
    H. acetabular liner
    H. enhanced ultra-high molecular weight polyethylene acetabular liner
    H. orthopedic bearing polymer
Hylin rasp
hyoid bone
hypalgesia
hyperabduction
    h. maneuver
    h. syndrome test
hyperactive
    h. reflex
    h. response
hyperactivity
    physiological h.
hyperalgesia
hyperalimentation
hyperbaric
    h. oxygen (HBO)
    h. oxygen therapy

hypercalcemia
hypercortisolism
hyperdorsiflexion
hyperdynamic abductor hallucis
hyperemia
hyperemic
hyperesthesia
hyperesthetic
hyperextend
hyperextended knee gait
hyperextensibility
    joint h.
    h. of joint
hyperextension
    h. brace
    h. cast
    cruciform anterior spinal h. (CASH)
    h. deformity
    h. injury
    intraoperative neck h.
    h. orthosis
    rebound h.
    recurrent h.
    segmental h.
    h. stress
    h. teardrop fracture
    h. test
    h. trauma
hyperextension-hyperflexion injury
Hyperex thoracic orthosis
hyperflexed toe compartment syndrome
hyperflexion
    h. injury
    h. teardrop fracture
    h. trauma
hyperhidrosis, hyperidrosis
hyperintense zone
hyperkeratosis, pl. **hyperkeratoses**
    Kyrle h.
hyperkeratotic lesion
hyperkyphoscoliosis
    neuropathic h.
hyperkyphosis
hyperlordosis
hypermobile
    h. flatfoot
    h. foot
    h. joint
    h. joint syndrome
    h. pes planovalgus

NOTES

hypermobility
    compensatory h.
    joint h.
hypernephroma
hyperosteoidosis
hyperostosis
    ankylosing h.
    ankylosing spinal h.
    Caffey h.
    diffuse idiopathic skeletal h.
     (DISH)
    flowing h.
    infantile cortical h.
    Morgagni h.
    sesamoid h.
    h. syndrome
hyperostotic
    h. bony fusion
    h. spondylosis
hyperparathyroidism
    brown tumor of h.
    h. tumor
hyperpathia
hyperphalangism
hyperpituitary gigantism
hyperplantarflexion injury
hyperplasia
    epiphysial h.
    fibrous h.
hyperplastic
    h. bone
    h. chondrodysplasia
    h. osteoarthritis
hyperplastica
    synovitis h.
hyperpolarization
hyperpronation
hyperpyrexia
    malignant h.
hyperreflexia
    detrusor h.
hypersecretion
    growth hormone h.
hypersensitivity syndrome
hyperspectral near-infrared Raman
  imaging microscopy
hypertension
    calf h.
hyperthermia
    malignant h.
hyperthermic exercise-associated collapse
hypertonia
hypertonicity
hypertonus
hypertrophic
    h. arthritis
    h. cardiomyopathy
    h. chondrocyte

    h. exostosis
    h. flexor retinaculum
    h. granulation tissue
    h. interstitial neuropathy
    h. ligament
    h. osteoarthritis
    h. osteoarthroscopy (HOA)
    h. pulmonary osteoarthropathy
    h. scar
    h. spondylitis
    h. strength training
    h. synovitis
    h. vital nonunion
    h. zone
hypertrophica
    tenosynovitis h.
hypertrophied ligamentum flavum
hypertrophy
    bone h.
    cartilage h.
    cartilaginous h.
    endemic h.
    endosteal h.
    ligamentous-muscular h.
    uncinate h.
hypervascular
    h. fragment
    h. nonunion
hypesthesia, hypoesthesia
hypnoanalgesia
hypnoanesthesia
hypnopedia
hypnotic
    h. dissociation
    h. reinterpretation
    h. replacement
    h. therapy
hypoactive deep tendon reflex
hypoaldosteronism
    hyporeninemic h.
hypobaric
    H. microvalve
    H. transfemoral system
    H. transtibial system
hypochondriac region
hypochondriasis
hypochondroplasia
hypocycloidal ankle tomography
hypoechogenicity
hypoechoic intermetatarsal web space
  mass
hypoesthesia (*var. of* hypesthesia)
hypofibrinolysis
hypoflexibility of foot
hypogastric
    h. artery
    h. flap
hypoglossal nerve

hypokinetic aberration
hypokyphosis
    right thoracic curve with h.
    thoracic h.
hypolordosis
    cervical h.
hypomelia
hypomobile
hyponychium
hypophalangism
    pedal h.
hypophosphatemic bone disease
hypophysial, hypophyseal
hypophysial curette
hypoplasia
    cartilage-hair h. (CHH)
    odontoid h.
    phalangeal h.
    skeletal h.
hypoplastic
    h. disk space
    h. finger
    h. first rib
    h. hand
    h. thumb
hyporeninemic hypoaldosteronism
hypostatic abscess

hypotension
    exertional h.
    postexercise h.
hypotensive
    h. anesthesia
    h. surgery
hypothalamic-pituitary-adrenal (HPA)
    h.-p.-a. axis
hypothalamoneurohypophysial axis (HNA)
hypothenar
    h. eminence
    h. fascia
    h. hammertoe syndrome
    h. muscle
    h. reflex
hypothermia
hypothermic
hypotonia
    congenital h.
hypotonic fluid
hypotonus
hypotrophic arthritis
hysterical
    h. gait
    h. joint
    h. scoliosis

NOTES

H

IADL
    instrumental activities of daily living
iatrogenic
    i. dural tear
    i. elevatus
    i. injury
    i. lumbar kyphosis
    i. osteomyelitis
I-beam
    I-b. cement punch
    I-b. hemiarthroplasty hip prosthesis
    I-b. hip hemiarthroplasty
    I-b. hip operation
    Jergesen I-b.
IBF
    Insall-Burstein-Freeman
    IBF knee instrument
IBG
    iliac bone graft
IBM
    inclusion body myositis
IC
    intermittent claudication
ICBG
    iliac crest bone graft
ICD
    International Knee Documentation
      Committee
ICE
    ice, compression, and elevation
ice
    i. application
    i., compression, and elevation
      (ICE)
    i. immersion
    i. massage
    N'ice Stretch night splint
      suspension system with Sealed I.
    i. pack
    i. skater's fracture
    I. Wedge hot/cold therapy wrap
I.C.E. Down cold pack
Iceflex Endurance suction suspension
  sleeve
ICE-Magic pain reduction kit
Iceross Comfort Plus silicone gel liner
ICEX socket
ichnogram
ICIDH
    International Classification of
      Impairments, Disabilities, Handicaps
icing
    cutaneous i.
ICLH
    Imperial College, London Hospital

    ICLH ankle prosthesis
    ICLH double cup arthroplasty
    ICLH knee prosthesis
ICN
    inferior calcaneonavicular ligament
Icon pylon
ICRS
    Index Chemicus Registry System
      ICRS arthroscopic staging system
ICS
    inferior capsular shift
    intercostal space
ICT
    intermittent cervical traction
I&D
    incision and drainage
    irrigation and débridement
IDCN
    intermediate dorsal cutaneous nerve
Ideal spinal implant
Ideberg glenoid fracture classification
Identifit hip prosthesis
IDET
    intradiskal electrothermal therapy
      IDET procedure
IDGH
    ischemic disease of the growing hip
idiomuscular
idiopathic
    i. anterior knee pain
    i. avascular necrosis
    i. bone cavity
    i. erythromelalgia
    i. fracture
    i. genu valgum (IGV)
    i. hallux valgus
    i. hypertrophic osteoarthropathy
      (IHO)
    i. juvenile osteoporosis
    i. osteonecrosis
    i. polymyositis myopathy
    i. scoliosis
    i. skeletal
    i. skeletal hyperostosis syndrome
    i. toe-walker (ITW)
    i. toe walking
    i. transient osteoporosis
I disk
IDK
    internal derangement of the knee
IDN
    interdigital neuroma
IFC
    interferential stimulation
I-Flow nerve block infusion kit

IGF
insulin-like growth factor
IGF-binding protein
IGHL
inferior glenohumeral ligament
IGHL insertion
IGV
idiopathic genu valgum
IHO
idiopathic hypertrophic osteoarthropathy
IHW
inner heel wedge
IKDC
International Knee Documentation
Committee
IKDC form
IKDC score
Ikuta
I. clamp approximator
I. fixation
I. fixation device
I. pectoralis major transfer
ILD
ischemic limb disease
Ilfeld
I. brace
I. splint
I. splint orthosis
Ilfeld-Gustafson splint
Ilfeld-Holder deformity
iliac
i. apophysis
i. apophysis sign
i. apophysitis
i. artery
i. bone
i. bone graft (IBG)
i. buttressing procedure
i. canal
i. clamp
i. compression test
i. crest
i. crest bone block
i. crest bone free graft
i. crest bone graft (ICBG)
i. crest bone graft stabilization
i. crest bridge
i. crest dowel
i. crest-inlay graft
i. crest ossification
i. epiphysis
i. fixation
i. oblique view
i. osteocutaneous flap
i. osteotomy
i. post
i. region
i. screw

i. slot graft
i. spine
i. strut bone graft
i. tuberosity
i. vein
i. wing
i. wing resection
iliacus
i. muscle
i. syndrome
ilial
iliococcygeus muscle
iliocostalis lumborum syndrome
iliocostal muscle
iliofemoral
i. approach
i. flap artery
i. ligament
i. pedicle flap
i. thrombosis
i. triangle
iliofemoroplasty
iliohypogastric nerve
ilioinguinal
i. acetabular approach
i. nerve
i. syndrome
iliolumbar
i. artery
i. ligament
i. vein
iliometer
iliopatellar
i. band
i. ligament
iliopectineal
Bigelow i.
i. bursitis
i. line
iliopelvic
iliopsoas
i. bursitis
i. muscle
i. muscle hematoma
i. recession
i. tendon
i. test
i. transfer
iliopubic
iliosacral
i. articulation
i. and iliac fixation construct
i. implant
i. screw
iliospinal
iliotibial (IT)
i. band (ITB)
i. band fasciitis

i. band friction syndrome (ITBFS)
i. band graft
i. band graft augmentation
i. band tenodesis
i. band transfer
i. tract

iliotrochanteric ligament
ilioxiphopagus
ilium

AS i.
ASEx i.
ASIn i.
i. drainage
external i. (EI)
In-Ex i.
PIEx i.
PIIn i.
piriform sclerosis of i.
wing of i.

Ilizarov

I. ankle arthrodesis
I. ankle fusion technique
I. apparatus
I. circular external fixator
I. corticotomy
I. device
I. distractor
I. external fixation
I. external ring fixator
I. frame
I. hybrid fixator
I. limb lengthening
I. limb-lengthening system
I. limb-lengthening technique
I. method
I. ring
I. screw
I. tension-stress effect
I. wire

ILL

inequality in leg length

ill-fitting shoe
illuminator

Cogent XL i.

IM

intermetatarsal
intramedullary
intramuscular
IM joint

IMA

intermetatarsal angle

image

i. en Grelot
i. intensification
i. intensifier

Image-I analysis software
imaging

bone-forming sarcoma bone i.
cine-magnetic resonance i. (cine-MRI)
color duplex i.
contrast medium-enhanced magnetic resonance i. (CME-MRI)
delayed bone i.
diagnostic i.
dipyridamole thallium i.
dynamic magnetic resonance i.
fixation i.
functional magnetic resonance i. (fMRI)
gadopentetate-dimeglumine-enhanced magnetic resonance i.
gamma camera i.
indirect magnetic resonance arthrography nuclear bone i.
magnetic resonance i. (MRI)
magnetic source i. (MSI)
magnetization transfer magnetic resonance i. (mtMRI)
multiplanar virtual fluoroscopic i.
multiple line-scan i. (MLSI)
orthopantogram i.
orthoroentgenogram i.
radionucleotide i.
Raman spectroscopic i.
sagittal-plane i.

imbalance

isokinetic torque i.
muscle i.
rotator cuff i.

imbrication

capsular i.
MacNab line for facet i.
medial capsular i.

IMEX scleral implant
IML

intermetacarpal ligament

immature

i. bone
skeletally i.

immediate

i. amputation
i. postoperative prosthesis (IPOP)

NOTES

immediate *(continued)*
    i. postoperative stability (IPS)
    i. postsurgical fitting (IPSF)
immersion
    i. foot
    ice i.
immobilization
    cast i.
    i. degeneration
    external i.
    halo i.
    i. jacket
    joint i.
    i. method
    postoperative i.
    Rowe-Zarins shoulder i.
    sling i.
    sternal-occipital-mandibular i.
      (SOMI)
    Velcro i.
    Webril i.
immobilizer
    ankle i.
    cast i.
    Comfort wrist i.
    DonJoy Ultrasling shoulder i.
    external i.
    Ezy Wrap shoulder i.
    Hook hemi-harness shoulder i.
    joint i.
    knee i.
    Kuz-Medics disposable knee i.
    long leg i.
    OEC knee i.
    Pedi-Wrap i.
    Plastizote-Kydex cervical i.
    postoperative i.
    QuickCast wrist i.
    Raymond shoulder i.
    sateen knee i.
    shoulder abduction i.
    single-panel knee i.
    sling i.
    Slingshot shoulder i.
    sternal-occipital-mandibular i.
    sternal-occipital-manubrial i.
    Tab-Strap knee i.
    Trimline knee i.
    tri-panel knee i.
    Universal sling and swathe
      shoulder i.
    universal tri-panel knee i.
    Velcro i.
    Velpeau shoulder i.
    Watco knee i.
    Westfield acromioclavicular i.
    Y-strap knee i.

    Zimmer knee i.
    Zinco thumb-wrist i.
immobilizing bandage
immovable
    i. articulation
    i. bandage
    i. joint
immune system
immunity
    cell-mediated i.
    cellular i.
    humoral i.
immunoassay
    Alkphase-B i.
immunocompetence
immunogenicity
Immunomount
immunosuppressive therapy
IMN
    intramedullary nailing
IMP
    Innovative Medical Products
      IMP bone screw targeter
      IMP knee positioning triangle
      IMP Steri-Clamp
      IMP surgical leg pedestal
      IMP turnstile casting stand
      IMP Universal knee positioner
      IMP Universal lateral positioner
impact
    i. biomechanics
    direct vertex i.
    i. glove
    i. mitt
    I. modular porous prosthesis
    I. modular total hip system
    I. total hip prosthesis
impacted
    i. articular fracture
    i. valgus fracture
impaction
    atlantoaxial i.
    i. cancellous autografting
    digital i.
    i. fracture
impactor
    Austin Moore i.
    bone i.
    Cloward bone graft i.
    Cohort spinal i.
    Dawson-Yuhl i.
    femoral i.
    glenoid implant base i.
    hook i.
    humeral i.
    Küntscher i.
    Moe bone i.
    mushroom i.

I

orthopaedic i.
i. rod
shell i.
Smith-Petersen i.
vertebral body i.
impactor-extractor
Fox i.-e.
impact-release binding on ski
impaired competitor policy
impairment
i. assessment
BFM i.
chronotropic i.
neurovascular i.
physical i.
sensory i.
visual-spatial ability i.
IMP-Capello slimline abduction pillow
impedance
bioelectrical i.
i. plethysmography
imperfecta
dentinogenesis i.
luxatio i.
osteogenesis i. (OI)
Imperial College, London Hospital
(ICLH)
impingement
ankle i.
anterior ankle i.
anterior cord i.
anterior joint i.
anterior soft tissue i.
facet synovial i.
graft i.
lateral i.
i. lesion
i. pain
peroneal tendon i.
posterior i.
i. rod
roof i.
i. sign
i. spur
i. syndrome
i. test
tibiotalar i.
ulnocarpal i.
Impingement-Free Tibial Guide System
impinging exostosis
implant
Advanced mobile-bearing knee i.

i. alloy aluminum
AO-ASIF orthopaedic i.
i. arthroplasty
articulated chin i.
artificial joint i.
BAK/Proximity interbody fusion i.
Bannon-Klein i.
bicompartmental i.
Bicoral i.
BioAction great toe i.
bioactive i.
i. biocompatibility
BioCuff C bioresorbable spike
  washer i.
biodegradable i.
Biodel i.
Biofix biodegradable i.
biomechanical failure of i.
Biomet custom i.
BioSphere suture anchor i.
i. blank
bone i.
bovine collagen i.
Calnan-Nicolle finger i.
carbon i.
cartilage i.
Cartwright i.
ceramic i.
Charnley i.
chromium i.
chromium-cobalt-alloy i.
CKS i.
coated i.
cobalt i.
cobalt-chromium i.
i. collar
condylar i.
Continuum knee system i.
Corail HA-coated stem hip i.
COR/T i.
CT-based CAD/CAM revision
  femoral i.
curvilinear chin i.
Custodis i.
custom i.
Cutter i.
DePuy orthopedic i.
dorsal columella i.
dorsal column stimulator i.
double-stem silicone i.
DTT i.
Duracon knee i.

NOTES

implant *(continued)*
    Durallium i.
    Durapatite i.
    DynaGraft i.
    electrical i.
    Ewald-Walker knee i.
    i. failure
    i. fatigue
    fibrous tissue i.
    fin of the i.
    finger joint i.
    fixed anatomic patellar i.
    fixed bearing knee i.
    flail i.
    Flatt i.
    flexible digital i.
    flexible hinge i.
    i. forceps
    i. fracture
    Futura flexible digital i.
    Futura metal hemi-toe i.
    Future i.
    Gemini MKII mobile-bearing
      knee i.
    Genesis II mobile-bearing knee i.
    gentamicin i.
    Geo Structure spinal i.
    Gliadel i.
    Global total shoulder i.
    great toe i.
    HA-coated hip i.
    Harris Design-2 i.
    Hedrocel proximal tibia
      augmentation i.
    hemi-interpositional i.
    Hemi-Silastic i.
    i. hinge
    hinged i.
    Howmedica Duracon i.
    Howmedica monospherical i.
    Hunter open cord tendon i.
    hyaline cartilage i.
    Ideal spinal i.
    iliosacral i.
    IMEX scleral i.
    Insall-Burstein intracondylar knee i.
    Insall-Burstein total knee i.
    Interax Integrated Secure
      Asymmetric mobile-bearing
      knee i.
    Interpore i.
    joint i.
    Kalix flatfoot i.
    Kinetik great toe i. (KGTI)
    Kinetikos joint i.
    Koenig total great toe i.
    KPS bipolar vitallium-
      polyethylene i.

    LaPorta great toe i.
    Lawrence first metatarsophalangeal
      joint i.
    LCS total knee system i.
    lumbar anterior-root stimulator i.
      (LARSI)
    i. material
    McCutchen hip i.
    metacarpophalangeal i.
    i. metal
    metal-backed acetabular component
      hip i.
    metal-backed patellar i.
    metal hemi-toe i.
    metallic i.
    metal orthopedic i.
    methyl methacrylate bead i.
    Microloc knee i.
    mobile-bearing knee i.
    modular i.
    Neer II total shoulder system i.
    NeuFlex metacarpophalangeal
      joint i.
    NexGen knee i.
    Nexus i.
    Niebauer i.
    Niebauer-Cutter i.
    OP-1 TM bone i.
    orthotic attachment i.
    OsteoGen resorbable osteogenic
      bone-filling i.
    Osteonics HA femoral i.
    oxidized zirconium alloy on i.
    Partnership i.
    patellar resurfacing i.
    pectoralis muscle i.
    pedicle i.
    percutaneous dorsal column
      stimulator i.
    permanent i.
    phalangeal i.
    pin i.
    plastic ball i.
    PLLA i.
    PMMA i.
    polyglycolide i.
    polylactide i.
    polymethyl methacrylate i.
    Polypin biodegradable pin i.
    porous-coated i.
    primus i.
    processed carbon i.
    Profix mobile-bearing knee i.
    ProOsteon I. 500
    i. reaction
    i. removal
    Restore orthobiologic soft-tissue i.
    Rotaglide knee i.

rotating patellar i.
Seeburger i.
self-aligning mobile-bearing knee i.
Septacin i.
Sgarlato hammertoe i. (SHIP)
Sgarlato toe i.
Shaw-SHIP rod hammertoe i.
SHIP i.
Silastic finger i.
Silastic toe i.
silicone breast i.
silicone elastomer rubber ball i.
silicone MP i.
simple button patellar i.
single-stemmed toe i.
Sinterlock i.
Smart Screw bioabsorbable i.
spike washer i.
i. stage
STA-peg i.
i. stem
subtalar MBA i.
supraspinatus i.
Surgibone i.
Surgicel i.
i. survival rate
Sutter i.
Swanson carpal lunate i.
Swanson carpal scaphoid i.
Swanson finger joint i.
Swanson great toe i.
Swanson metacarpophalangeal i.
Swanson radial head i.
Swanson radiocarpal i.
Swanson small joint i.
Swanson trapezium i.
Swanson ulnar head i.
Swanson wrist joint i.
Swiss MP joint i.
Syed-Neblett i.
Syed template i.
synthetic bone i.
TACK i.
Techmedica i.
I. Technology LSF prosthesis
Teflon i.
TheraSeed i.
The Wedge i.
TissueTak corkscrew i.
titanium i.
titanium-alloy i.
tobramycin-impregnated PMMA i.

toe i.
total knee i.
Trac II knee i.
trial i.
tricompartmental i.
TSRH i.
UltraFix rotator cuff repair i.
unicompartmental knee i.
Unilab Surgibone surgical i.
Viladot i.
Vitallium i.
Weber hip i.
Weil i.
Weil-modified Swanson i.
Weil-type Swanson-design
  hammertoe i.
white band on degenerated i.
Wright monoblock titanium i.
Zang metatarsal cap i.
Zeichner i.
Zymderm collagen i.
implantable
  i. bone anchor
  i. bone anchor device
implantation
  autologous chondrocyte i. (ACI)
  collared press-fit femoral stem i.
  noncollared press-fit femoral
    stem i.
  periosteal i.
  screw i.
implant-cement interface
implanted bone growth stimulator
Implast
  I. adhesive
  I. bone cement
impression
  basilar i.
  i. defect
  i. fracture
imprinter
  foot i.
impulse
  afferent nerve i.
  efferent nerve i.
  i. inertial exercise trainer
  mobilization with i.
impulse-based nerve transmission
IMSC
  intramedullary supracondylar
    IMSC multihole nail

NOTES

inactivity
    i. atrophy
    electrical i.
    physical i.
InCare brace
incarial bone
Incavo wire passer
incidence
    myelopathy i.
    nonunion i.
incise drape
incised wound
incision
    anteromedial i.
    Banks-Laufman i.
    Bardenheuer i.
    battledore i.
    bifrontal i.
    Brockman i.
    Bruner i.
    Brunner modified i.
    Brunner palmar i.
    Bruser skin i.
    Burns-Haney i.
    Burwell-Scott modification of
      Watson-Jones i.
    capsular i.
    Chang-Miltner i.
    Charnley i.
    chevron i.
    Cincinnati i.
    circumscribing i.
    Colonna-Ralston i.
    Couvelaire i.
    Crawford i.
    Cubbins i.
    Curtin i.
    curved i.
    curvilinear i.
    deltoid-splitting i.
    i. dilator
    dorsal linear i.
    dorsal longitudinal i.
    dorsal transverse i.
    dorsomedial i.
    double i.
    i. and drainage (I&D)
    DuVries i.
    Dwyer i.
    elliptical i.
    exploratory i.
    fascia-splitting i.
    fiber-splitting i.
    fishmouth i.
    Fowler-Philip i.
    Gaenslen split-heel i.
    Gatellier-Chastang i.
    goblet i.

Grice i.
Griffith i.
Henderson skin i.
Henry i.
hockey-stick i.
H-shaped capsular i.
inverted-L lateral periosteal i.
inverted-Y i.
Jergesen i.
J-shaped skin i.
Kocher collar i.
Koenig-Schaefer i.
Langenbeck i.
lateral utility i.
lazy-C i.
lazy-L i.
lazy-S skin i.
L-curved i.
Loeffler-Ballard i.
longitudinal i.
L-shaped capsular i.
Ludloff i.
Mayfield i.
McLaughlin-Ryder i.
medial parapatellar i.
midaxillary line i.
muscle-splitting i.
Nicola i.
Ober i.
oblique i.
Ollier i.
palmar i.
parapatellar i.
parathenar i.
Picot i.
plantar longitudinal i.
posterior i.
posterolateral costotransversectomy i.
Pridie i.
racquet-shaped i.
relaxing i.
relieving i.
right-sided submandibular
  transverse i.
S i.
saber-cut i.
Seattle modification of Kocher i.
serpentine i.
S-flap i.
skin i.
skived i.
split i.
split-heel i.
S-shaped i.
stab i.
straight i.
subfascial i.
Sutherland-Rowe i.

tangential i.
Texas T i.
thoracoabdominal i.
transverse i.
triradiate i.
T-shaped i.
Turco oblique posteromedial i.
universal i.
upright-Y i.
U-shaped i.
volar midline oblique i.
volar zigzag finger i.
V-shaped i.
Wagner skin i.
Watson-Jones i.
webspace i.
Westin-Hall i.
Y i.
Y-shaped i.
Y-V-plasty i.
zigzag finger i.
Z-plasty i.
incisional
   i. biopsy
   i. neuroma
   i. skin-slough
incisive bone
Incisor arthroscopic blade
incisural notch
Inclan
   I. bone graft
   I. modification of Campbell ankle operation
   I. modification of Campbell ankle procedure
   I. posterior bone block
Inclan-Ober
   I.-O. arthroplasty
   I.-O. procedure
inclination
   i. angle
   angle of thoracic i.
inclinometer
   Baseline Bubble i.
inclusion
   i. body myositis (IBM)
   i. cyst
incomplete
   i. amputation
   i. coalition
   i. dislocation
   i. fracture

i. fracture of bone
i. luxation
i. paraplegia
i. reduction
i. syndactyly
i. tear
incongruency
   subtalar joint i.
incongruent articulation
incongruity
   angle of i.
incontinence
   urinary i.
incoordination
incorporation
   bone graft i.
increased
   i. carrying angle
   i. depolymerization
   i. lateral joint space
increment after exercise
incremental response
incubation period
incudomalleolar
   i. articulation
   i. joint
incurvated
incurvatum reflex
independent
   i. exercise program
   i. transfer
index, pl. indices
   acetabular i.
   acetabular head i. (AHI)
   acromial spur i. (ASI)
   ADL i.
   indices of ADLs
   alignment i.
   alpha i.
   ambulation i.
   arch i.
   arch-height i.
   Arthritis Helplessness I. (AHI)
   axial acetabular i. (AAI)
   Barthel ADL i.
   Benink tarsal i.
   beta i.
   body mass i. (BMI)
   Caregiver Strain I. (CSI)
   I. Chemicus Registry System (ICRS)
   Chippaux-Smirak arch i.

NOTES

index *(continued)*
    Convery polyarticular disability i.
    cortical i.
    cyst i.
    dynamic stability i.
    Eyre-Brook epiphysial i.
    femoral cortical i.
    i. finger
    i. finger abduction
    Flower i.
    Foot Function I. (FFI)
    footprint i.
    Functional Status I. (FSI)
    Garden alignment i.
    Hand Functional I. (HFI)
    HAQ I.
    Hauser ambulation i.
    Hollingshead I.
    hop i.
    Hospital Trauma I.
    Insall-Salvati patellar height i.
    Ishihara cervical spine curve i.
    Jette Functional Status i.
    Katz ADL i.
    Keitel i.
    Kenny ADL i.
    I. Knobber II massage tool
    laxity i.
    Lequesne Severity of
      Osteoarthritis I.
    Life Satisfaction I. (LSI)
    Lucas and Drucker Motor I.
    malleolar i.
    McDowell Impairment I. (MII)
    McMurtry kinematic i.
    i. metacarpophalangeal joint
      reconstruction
    Motricity I.
    notch width i. (NWI)
    Nottingham Extended ADL i.
    Oswestry i.
    PICA i.
    Predictive Salvage I.
    pressure excursion i.
    I. prosthesis
    Quetelet i.
    Reimers hip position migration i.
    Reimers instability i.
    Reintegration to Normal Living i.
    right and left ankle i.
    Ritchie rheumatoid arthritis i.
    Rivermead ADL i.
    Rivermead Mobility I. (RMI)
    sciatic function i. (SFI)
    Singh osteoporosis i.
    Spinal Cord Motor Index and
      Sensory Indices
    Spotorno i.
    Stahl i.
    Takakura i.
    talocalcaneal i.
    toe i.
    Waddell Chronic Back Pain
      Disability i.
    Western Ontario Instability I.
      (WOSI)
    Western Ontario and McMaster
      University osteoarthritis i.
    Western Ontario Rotator Cuff I.

index-ray amputation

Indiana
    I. conservative prosthesis
    I. reamer
    I. tome carpal tunnel syndrome
      release system

indices (*pl. of* index)

indifferent electrode

indirect
    i. fracture
    i. magnetic resonance arthrography
      nuclear bone imaging
    i. manipulation
    i. reduction
    i. triangulation

Indong Oh hip prosthesis

induction
    pain i.

inductive coupling device

indurated plantar keratoma (IPK)

induration

inelastic

inequality
    anatomic leg length i.
    functional leg length i.
    leg length i. (LLI)
    i. in leg length (ILL)

Inerpan flexible burn dressing

inertia
    moment of i.

In-Ex ilium

inextensibility

infant
    i. abduction splint
    i. clown cast shoe
    floppy i.
    Movement Assessment of I.'s
      (MAI)

infantile
    i. cortical hyperostosis
    i. dermal fibromatosis
    i. idiopathic scoliosis
    i. progressive spinal muscular
      atrophy
    i. tibia vara (ITV)
    i. trigger digit

I

infarct
> bone i.

infarction
> bone i.
> capsuloputaminal i.
> capsuloputaminocaudate i.

In-Fast bone screw system

infected
> i. bone
> i. nondraining nonunion

infection
> aerobic i.
> anaerobic i.
> aspergillosis i.
> blood-borne i.
> bone i.
> clostridial i.
> cryptococcal i.
> deep delayed i.
> deep wound i.
> epidural space i.
> fascial space i.
> felon i.
> fungal i.
> gas-producing streptococcal i.
> granulomatous fungal i.
> hematogenous i.
> Meleney i.
> musculoskeletal i.
> mycobacterial i.
> nontuberculous mycobacterial i.
> percutaneous bone marrow i.
> pin tract i.
> postoperative i.
> i. prevention
> pyogenic spinal i.
> spinal i.
> superficial i.
> suppurative joint i.
> tarsal joint i.
> web space i.

infectious
> i. arthritis
> i. bulbar necrosis
> i. tenosynovitis

inferential therapy

inferior
> i. angle
> atraumatic, multidirectional, bilateral
> rehabilitation i. (AMBRI)
> i. band cruciform ligament
> i. calcaneonavicular ligament (ICN)

> i. capsular shift (ICS)
> i. capsular split technique
> i. costal sulcus
> i. extensor of foot
> i. extensor retinaculum
> i. facet
> i. gemelli muscle
> i. glenohumeral ligament (IGHL)
> i. glenohumeral ligament insertion
> i. glide
> i. ilioischial ligament
> i. laryngeal nerve
> i. leaf
> i. movement
> i. peroneal retinaculum
> i. process
> i. radioulnar joint
> i. ramus
> i. spur
> i. spurring
> i. thyroid artery
> i. tibiofibular joint
> i. tibiofibular repair

InFerno moist heat therapy

inferoposterior acetabular capsule
retractor

infestation
> pressure ulcer-related maggot i.

INFH
> ischemic necrosis of femoral head

infiltrate
> fibrofatty i.

infiltration
> root i.

infinity
> I. femoral component
> I. hip system
> I. modular hip prosthesis

InFix interbody fusion system

inflamed synovial pouch

inflammation
> bursal i.
> i. management
> polyarticular symmetric tophaceous
> joint i.
> prepatellar bursa i.
> tendon i.

inflammatory
> i. arthropathy
> i. bowel disease associated arthritis
> i. fracture
> i. myositis

NOTES

347

inflammatory *(continued)*
    i. phase
    i. scoliosis
    i. spondyloarthropathy
    i. synovitis
    i. tenovaginitis
inflatable elbow splint
inflexion point
inflow
    i. cannula
    vascular i.
infracalcaneal bursitis
infraclavicular
    i. region
    i. triangle
infraction
    i. fracture
infracture
infraganglionic injury
infraglenoid tuberosity
infragluteal
    i. creaking
    i. crease
infraisthmal
infrapatellar
    i. bursa
    i. bursitis
    i. contracture syndrome (IPCS)
    i. fat pad
    i. ligament
    i. plica
    i. strap
    i. tendinitis
    i. tendon
    i. tendon rupture
    i. view
infrared
    i. applicator
    i. head
    i. light (IR)
    i. light-emitting diode
    i. therapy
    i. thermography
infrascapular region
infraspinatus
    i. muscle
    i. tendinitis
    i. tendon
infraspinous
    i. fascia
    i. region
infrasternal
infratectal transverse fracture
infratrochlear
Infusible pressure infusion bag
infusion-aspiration drainage

Inge
    I. retractor
    I. spreader
Ingebrightsen traction
Inglis-Cooper
    I.-C. release
    I.-C. technique
Inglis-Pellicci elbow arthroplasty rating system
Inglis-Ranawat-Straub
    I.-R.-S. elbow synovectomy
    I.-R.-S. technique
Inglis triaxial total elbow arthroplasty
Ingram
    I. bony bridge resection
    I. osteotomy
    I. procedure
Ingram-Bachynski hip fracture classification
Ingram-Canle-Beaty epiphysial-metaphysial osteotomy
Ingram-Withers-Speltz motor test
ingrowing toenail
ingrown
    i. nail
    i. toenail
ingrowth
    bone i.
    i. fixation
inguinal
    i. approach
    i. ligament
    i. ligament syndrome
    i. TEPP repair
inhalation anesthesia
inherent motion
inhibition test
inhibitive
    i. cast
    i. traction
inhibitor
    aldose reductase i.
    alpha-a_2-plasmin i.
    anion transport i.
    cholinesterase i.
    monoamine oxidase-B i.
    shoulder subluxation i. (SSI)
inhibitory postsynaptic potential
iniencephaly
inion bump
initial stance
initiation
    rhythmic i. (RI)
initiator drill
injection
    alcohol i.
    Black peroneal tendon sheath i.
    cervical nerve root i.

chymopapain i.
epidural steroid i. (ESI)
extrafascial nerve i.
facet i.
i. injury
intraarticular i.
intracranial pressure elevation
  joint i.
intramuscular i.
lumbar facet i.
lumbar nerve root i.
lumbar transforaminal epidural i.
nerve root i.
peroneal tendon sheath i.
procaine-phenol motor point i.
steroid I.
i. study
i. technique
tenosynovial i.
thecal i.
i. therapy
thoracic epidural i.
trigger point i.
zygapophysial joint i.

**injurious energy input spearing
injury**
acceleration/deceleration i.
accessory nerve i.
acquired brain i.
acromioclavicular joint i.
acute stretch i.
i. algorithm
ankle i.
anular i.
ASIA impairment scale for
  classification of spinal cord i.
athletic i.
avulsion i.
axial compression i.
axial loading i.
axillary nerve i.
axonal i.
ballistic i.
barked i.
bending toward the side of i.
bicycle i.
birth i.
bladder i.
brachial artery i.
brachial plexus i.
brachial plexus traction i. (BPTI)
Brief Test of Head I. (BTHI)

bunk bed i.
burst i.
calcaneocuboid joint nutcracker i.
Callahan extension of cervical i.
cervical nerve root i.
cervical spinal i.
cervical spine extension i.
Chopart osseous joint i.
chronic microtraumatic soft
  tissue i.
closed kinetic chain i.
closed soft tissue i.
cocking i.
cold i.
compression-plus-torque cervical i.
compressive flexion i.
compressive hyperextension i.
contrecoup i.
crush i.
cuneiform i.
Danis-Weber classification of
  ankle i.
dashboard knee i.
degloving i.
de Quervain i.
diffuse axonal i. (DAI)
discoligamentous i.
distal tibial epiphysial i.
distraction i.
Drummond and Hastings cuboid
  extrusion i.
dye punch i.
elbow i.
electrical i.
epiphysial i.
Essex-Lopresti i.
eversion i.
explosion i.
extensor tendon i.
extravasation i.
factitious i.
femoral vein i.
firearm i.
flexion-distraction i.
flexion-extension i.
FOOSH i.
forced flexion i.
Foucher classification of
  epiphysial i.
frostbite i.
gamekeeper's i.

NOTES

injury *(continued)*
    Gertzbein classification of seat-belt i.
    grease gun i.
    growth plate i.
    Hardcastle classification of tarsometatarsal joint i.
    hip epiphysial i.
    hyperextension i.
    hyperextension-hyperflexion i.
    hyperflexion i.
    hyperplantarflexion i.
    iatrogenic i.
    infraganglionic i.
    injection i.
    interosseous nerve i.
    inversion i.
    ipsilateral foot i.
    Klumpke i.
    knee ligamentous i.
    laryngeal nerve i.
    lateral compartment i.
    lateral compression i.
    lawn mower i.
    ligamentous i.
    Lisfranc i.
    long thoracic nerve i.
    low back i.
    lower plexus i.
    lumbar plexus i.
    lunate facet dye punch i.
    MacKinnon nerve i.
    mangling i.
    marching band i.
    matrix i.
    medial brachial cutaneous nerve i.
    medial compartment i.
    median nerve i.
    meniscal i.
    mesencephalic i.
    metatarsophalangeal joint i.
    midcarpal i.
    middle column i.
    missile i.
    multiple i.'s
    muscle-tendon i.
    musculocutaneous nerve i.
    nerve i.
    neural i.
    neurovascular i.
    nutcracker i.
    obturator nerve i.
    Ontario Cohort of Running-Related I.
    open-book pelvic i.
    osteochondral i.
    overuse i.
    paint gun i.

    paint thinner i.
    pelvic i.
    P-ER i.
    perihamate i.
    peripheral nerve i.
    peripisiform i.
    peritrapezial i.
    peritrapezoidal i.
    peroneal nerve i.
    physial i.
    pitching i.
    plantarflexion i.
    plantar plate i.
    pleural i.
    pneumatic tire i.
    Poland classification of physial i.
    posterior ligamentous i.
    predictor of i.
    pronation i.
    pronation-abduction i.
    pronation-eversion i.
    pronation-eversion-external rotation i.
    pseudogamekeeper's i.
    pudendal nerve i.
    Pugil stick i.
    radial artery i.
    radial nerve i.
    radioulnar joint i.
    recurrent laryngeal nerve i.
    reperfusion i.
    repetition strain i. (RSI)
    repetitive stress i.
    road burn i.
    Rockwood classification of acromioclavicular i.
    roller i.
    Rosenthal classification of nail i.
    rotator cuff i.
    running-related i.
    sacral plexus i.
    sacroiliac joint i.
    Sage-Salvatore classification of acromioclavicular joint i.
    sailboarder i.
    Salter-Harris classification of epiphysial plate i.
    Salter-Harris epiphysial i.
    Salter-Harris tibial-fibular i.
    sand toe i.
    Scales of Cognitive Ability for Traumatic Brain I. (SCATBI)
    scaphoid tuberosity i.
    scapuloclavicular i.
    sciatic nerve i.
    seat belt i.
    sesamoid i.
    I. Severity Score (ISS)

shearing i.
shotgun i.
sideswipe i.
skier's i.
snowboarding i.
softball sliding i.
soft tissue i.
spinal accessory nerve i.
spinal cord i. (SCI)
sports i.
stable cervical spine i.
steering wheel i.
sternoclavicular joint i.
straddle i.
strain-sprain i.
stress i.
stretch i.
subclavian artery i.
subclavian vein i.
subscapular artery i.
subscapular nerve i.
Sunderland first-degree nerve i.
supination i.
supination-adduction i.
supination-eversion i.
supination-external rotation i.
supination-inversion rotation i.
supination-outward rotation i.
supination-plantarflexion i.
supraganglionic i.
suprascapular nerve i.
synovial i.
talar neck class I–III i.
tarsometatarsal joint i.
thoracic duct i.
thoracic nerve i.
thoracoabdominal artery i.
thoracodorsal nerve i.
thoracolumbar spinal i.
thoracolumbar spine flexion-
  distraction i.
three-column cervical spine i.
throwing i.
tibial axial load i.
tibial nerve i.
tornado i.
tracheal i.
trampoline i.
transcutaneous crush i.
translation i.
traumatic brain i. (TBI)
traumatic burn i.

turf toe i.
two-column cervical spine i.
ulnar artery i.
ulnar collateral ligament i.
ulnar nerve i.
unstable cervical spine i.
vascular i.
vertebrobasilar i.
Weber classification of physial i.
weightbearing rotational i.
whiplash i.
wind-up i.
wringer i.
Zlotsky-Ballard classification of
  acromioclavicular i.

Inland Super Multi-Hite orthopedic bed
inlay
  i. bone graft
  Sher diabetic shoe i.
inlet view
inner
  i. heel wedge (IHW)
  I. Lip Plate
  I. Lok ankle brace
  i. malleolus
  i. table
innervation
  muscle i.
  parasympathetic i.
  reciprocal i.
  somatic i.
  sympathetic i.
Innomed
  I. arthroplasty measuring system
  I. Assistant Free surgical
    instrument
  I. bone curette
innominate
  anterior i.
  i. bone
  i. bone resection
  left i.
  i. movement
  i. osteotomy
  posterior i.
  right posterior i.
  i. vein
innovasive
  I. bone anchor
  I. device
  I. fixation

NOTES

innovation
 I. Sports bracing product
 i. Sports bracing support
innovative
 I. COR/T implant system
 I. Medical Products (IMP)
 I. Medical Products Steri-Clamp
inochondritis
inosculation phase
inotropism
Inronail finger or toenail prosthesis
INRO surgical nail
Insall
 I. anterior approach
 I. anterior cruciate ligament
  reconstruction
 I. criteria
 I. ligament reconstruction technique
 I. patella alta method
 I. patellar injury classification
 I. procedure
 I. proximal realignment
 I. ratio
Insall-Burstein
 I.-B. intracondylar knee implant
 I.-B. II modular total knee system
 I.-B. semiconstrained
  tricompartmental knee prosthesis
 I.-B. total knee implant
Insall-Burstein-Freeman (IBF)
 I.-B.-F. knee arthroplasty
Insall-Hood reconstruction technique
Insall-Salvati
 I.-S. measurement
 I.-S. patellar height index
 I.-S. ratio
insecurity
 gravitational i.
insensate foot
insert
 AliMed i.
 angled bearing i.
 articular i.
 cancellous i.
 clamp i.
 cushioned shoe i.
 custom-made i.
 Diab-A-Sheets shoe i.
 Durasul polyethylene, high wear
  resistant acetabular i.
 Energy Plus shoe i.
 Gel-Sole shoe i.
 i. graft
 Hapad felt i.
 Hapad shoe i.
 heel and sole i.
 Hydragrip clamp i.

Johnson & Johnson PFC cruciate-
 substituting i.
New York University orthotic i.
NYU orthosis i.
Orthex Relievers shoe i.
orthotic shoe i.
Osteonics Scorpio i.
Poly-Dial i.
polypropylene i.
POWERPoint orthotic shoe i.
Profix confirming tibial i.
ROHO solid seat i.
shoe i.
silicone gel socket i.
soft socket i.
sole i.
Spenco shoe i.
S-ROM Poly-Dial i.
thermomoldable i.
tibial i.
UCB shoe i.
viscoelastic heel i.
warm-and-form i.
inserter
 Buck femoral cement restrictor i.
 CDH cup i.
 cement restrictor i.
 cement spacer i.
 cerclage wire i.
 C-wire i.
 deluxe FIN pin i.
 Kirschner wire i.
 Massie i.
 Moon-Robinson prosthesis i.
 Robinson-Moon prosthesis i.
 Shaffner orthopedic i.
 spacer i.
 staple i.
 T-shaped i.
 TSRH hook i.
inserter-extractor
 compression i.-e.
insertion
 anatomic i.
 anomalous i.
 Bosworth bone peg i.
 C-D rod i.
 deltoid i.
 i. equipment
 IGHL i.
 inferior glenohumeral ligament i.
 lag screw i.
 ligamentous i.
 oblique screw i.
 pedicle screw i.
 percutaneous pin i.
 Pierrot-Murphy advancement i.
 rerouting i.

screw i.
i. tendinopathy
insertional
i. Achilles tendinosis
i. excursion
in-shoe transducer
inside-out
i.-o. Bankart shoulder instability
operation
i.-o. meniscal repair
i.-o. technique for establishing
ankle portal
inside-to-outside technique
**Insight knee positioning and alignment
system**
insole
Aliplast i.
Apex i.
Bestfoam i.
Comf-Orthotic 3/4-length i.
Comf-Orthotic sports replacement i.
Comf-Orthotic wool felt i.
Darco moldable i.
Diab-A-Foot rocker i.
Diab-A-Pad i.
Diab-A-Sole flat i.
Diab-A-Sole molded i.
Diabetic Diagnostic i.
D-Soles i.
EMED i.
Ever-Flex i.
Flat Foot i.
flatfoot i.
FlexiTherm diabetic diagnostic i.
Hapad metatarsal i.
Kinetic Wedge molded i.
molded postpartum i.
Orthex reliever i.
Plastazote i.
Plexidure i.
Poron 400 i.
PPT flat i.
PPT MXL soft molded i.
PPT Plastizote i.
PPT RX firm molded i.
ProThotics i.
PumpPals i.
Reflex Comfort i.
silicone i.
SofSole Airr i.
Sorbothane i.
Spenco i.

S-Soles i.
TechnoGel i.
viscoelastic i.
Viscoped S i.
instability
ankle i.
anterior shoulder i.
anterolateral-anteromedial rotary i.
anterolateral rotary i. (ALRI)
anterolateral rotary knee i.
anteromedial-posteromedial rotary i.
anteromedial rotary i.
articular i.
atlantoaxial i.
atraumatic multidirectional i.
axial i.
capitate-lunate i.
carpal i.
chronic functional i.
chronic lateral ankle i.
collateral ligament i.
combined i.
congenital atlantoaxial i.
distal intercalated segment i. (DISI)
dorsal intercalated segment i.
(DISI)
dorsiflexed intercalated segment i.
(DISI)
DRUJ i.
extension i.
flexion i.
functional i.
i. gait
hindfoot i.
intercalated segment i.
inversion i.
joint i.
knee i.
lateral rotatory ankle i.
lumbar spine i.
lunotriquetral i.
mechanical i.
medial column i.
membrane i.
midcarpal i. (MCI)
multidirectional i. (MDI)
one-plane i.
osseous i.
patellar i.
pelvic i.
perilunar i.
posterior shoulder i.

NOTES

instability *(continued)*
    posterolateral rotary i.
    posteromedial rotary i.
    postural i.
    progressive perilunar i.
    push-pull i.
    radiocarpal i.
    rotary ankle i.
    rotational i.
    sagittal plane i.
    scapholunate i.
    shoulder i.
    spinal i.
    straight lateral i.
    subtalar joint i.
    thumb i.
    tibiofibular joint i.
    tibiotalar i.
    traumatic anterior i.
    triquetrolunate i.
    valgus i.
    varus-valgus i.
    vertebral i.
    volar flexed intercalated segment i. (VISI)
    volar intercalary wrist i.
    wrist i.
installation procedure
install method
Insta-Nerve device
instantaneous axis of rotation
instant cold pack
Instat collagen sponge
institute
    Southern California Orthopedic I. (SCOI)
The Institute for Rehabilitation Research (TIRR)
Instron machine
instrument
    Accu-Line knee i.
    AccuSharp carpal tunnel release i.
    activating adjusting i. (AAI)
    Acufex arthroscopic i.
    Acufex MosaicPlasty i.
    American Academy of Orthopedic Surgeons Pediatrics Outcomes I.
    Arthrex arthroscopy i.
    Arthroforce III hand i.
    arthroscopic laser i.
    Atlas orthogonal percussion i.
    AxyaWeld i.
    back range-of-motion i.
    battery-powered i.
    Bone Grafter i.
    cervical range-of-motion i. (CROM)
    Collis TDR i.

    Command instrument system surgical i.
    Cotrel-Dubousset spinal i.
    Dreyfus prosthesis placement i.
    electrosurgical i.
    Femur Finder i.
    Friatec manual arthroscopy i.
    Hall Micro E power i.
    Hall series 4 large bone i.
    Hall-Zimmer power i.
    Howmedica-Osteonics i.
    IBF knee i.
    Innomed Assistant Free surgical i.
    Kirschner surgical i.
    LAM i.
    laser i.
    I. Makar biodegradable interference screw
    microsurgical i.
    Midas Rex pneumatic i.
    i. migration
    Mitek SuperAnchor i.
    Monogram total knee i.
    Nicolet Compass EMG i.
    orthopaedic cutting i.
    OrthoVise orthopedic i.
    oscilloscope i.
    paraspinal skin temperature thermocouple i.
    Partnership i.
    passivation metal i.
    Rancho external fixation i.
    reciprocal planing i.
    RingLoc i.
    Schema Assessment i. (SAI)
    ScoliTron i.
    Shea prosthesis placement i.
    single reference point i.
    i., sponge, and needle count
    SRP i.
    Steffee i.
    Sulzer Orthopaedics i.
    thermocouple i.
    Ultra-Cut i.
    WeeFIM i.
    Wiet graft-measuring i.
instrumental
    i. activities of daily living (IADL)
    i. ADLs
instrumentation
    Accu-Line knee i.
    Acufex arthroscopic i.
    anterior distraction i.
    anterior Zielke i.
    AO fixateur interne i.
    AO notched i.
    Apofix cervical i.
    Arthrotek Ellipticut hand i.

biodegradable fixation i.
bone-holding i.
cable-hook compression i.
Caspar anterior i.
C-D i.
compression Harrington i.
compression U-rod i.
Cotrel-Dubousset pedicle screw i.
distraction i.
double Zielke i.
Drummond spinal i.
Dwyer spinal i.
dynamic compression plate i.
Edwards i.
endoscopic carpal tunnel i.
halo-Ilizarov distraction i.
Harms-Moss anterior thoracic i.
Harrington distraction i.
Harrington-Kostuik i.
Harrington rod i.
hollow mill i.
Howmedica knee i.
Jacobs locking hook spinal rod i.
Kambin and Gellman lumbar
  diskectomy i.
Kaneda anterior spinal i.
Kostuik-Harrington spinal i.
locking hook i.
Louis i.
lumbar spine i.
lumbosacral spine transpedicular i.
Luque II segmental spinal i.
Luque semirigid segmental spinal i.
Mayfield i.
McElroy i.
modular i.
Moreland total hip revision i.
Moss i.
multiple hook assembly C-D i.
Passport i.
posterior cervical spinal i.
posterior distraction i.
posterior hook-rod spinal i.
Putti-Platt i.
rod-sleeve i.
sacral spine modular i.
segmental spinal i. (SSI)
Sielke i.
skin-contact i.
Smith-Richards i.
spinal i.
Steffee spinal i.

Stryker power i.
i. system
total knee i.
TSRH i.
Universal sacral spine i.
variable screw placement system i.
VSP plate i.
Wisconsin interspinous segmental
  spinal i.
Zielke pedicular i.

insufficiency
abductor i.
active i.
capsular length i.
i. fracture
ligamentous i.
mechanical i.
muscle i.
passive i.
peripheral vascular i.
posterior tibial tendon i.
PTT i.
transverse plane motion i.
vertebrobasilar i. (VBI)

insufflate

In-Tac bone-anchoring system

intact
I. dressing
neurologically i.
neurovascularly i.
i. neurovascular status
i. peripheral pulses
i. spinous lamina
i. spinous process

intake
dietary reference i. (DRI)
energy i.

integral
force-time i. (FTI)
I. hip system
I. Interlok femoral prosthesis
pressure-time i. (PTI)

integrated
I. Ankle orthotic ankle joint
i. electromyography
i. shape and imaging system
  (ISIS)

integration
body side i.
Functional I. (FI)
sensory i.

NOTES

integrity
    I. acetabular cup
    I. acetabular cup prosthesis
    I. acetabular cup screw
    i. and alignment
    biomechanical i.
    maintenance of bone plate i.
    soft tissue i.
Intelect
    I. Combo stimulator/ultrasound
    I. electric stimulator
    I. Legend stimulator
    I. 600MP microcurrent stimulator
InteliJet fluid management system
Intelligent Prosthesis Plus prosthesis
intensification
    image i.
intensifier
    C-arm image i.
    image i.
intention
    healing by first i.
    healing by second i.
    i. myoclonus
    primary i.
    i. tremor
intentional rotation
Inteq small joint suturing system
interaction
    surface shoe i.
    tibiofemoral i.
interarticular
    i. cartilage
    i. disk
    i. fracture
    i. joint
    i. ligament of head of rib
    i. sulcus
Interax
    I. Integrated Secure Asymmetric
      mobile-bearing knee implant
    I. total knee system
interbody
    i. arthrodesis
    i. graft
    i. rasp
    i. spinal fusion
intercalary
    i. allograft procedure
    i. diaphysial allograft
    i. graft
    i. resection
    i. segmental replacement
intercalated segment instability
intercarpal
    i. arthrodesis
    i. articulation
    i. joint

    i. ligament
    i. ligament capsulodesis
interchondral joint
interclavicular
    i. ligament
    i. notch
intercollicular groove
intercompartment fasciotome
intercondylar
    i. drill guide
    i. femoral fracture
    i. fossa
    i. groove
    i. humeral fracture
    i. notch
    i. process
    i. roof
    i. space
    i. tibial fracture
intercostal
    i. artery
    i. flap
    i. nerve
    i. nerve block
    i. neuralgia
    i. restriction
    i. space (ICS)
    i. vein
intercostobrachial nerve
intercritical time
intercuneiform joint
interdigital
    i. corn
    i. ligament
    i. neoplasm
    i. nerve
    i. nerve bundle
    i. neuroma (IDN)
    i. web space
interdischarge interval
interdisciplinary vocational evaluation
    program
interepicondylar axis
interface
    acetabular prosthetic i.
    bone-cement i.
    bone-implant i.
    bone-peg i.
    bony i.
    cement i.
    cement-bone i.
    cup-cement i.
    fascial-muscle i.
    fat-blood i. (FBI)
    implant-cement i.
    long-term bone-instrumentation i.
    patient-table i.
    pin-bone i.

prosthesis i.
prosthesis-cement i.
ShearBan low-friction i.
shoe-foot i.
soft tissue i.
interfacet
i. wiring
i. wiring and fusion
interfacial porosity
interfascicular
i. epineurectomy
i. epineurotomy
i. Millesi nerve graft
i. neurolysis
interference
i. fit
i. fit fixation
nerve i.
i. pattern
i. screw
i. screw technique
vertebrogenic i.
interferential
i. current
i. electrical stimulation
i. stimulation (IFC)
i. stimulator
i. therapy
InterFix
I. RP threaded spinal fusion cage
I. titanium threaded spinal fusion cage
interfragmentary
i. compression
i. lag screw
i. plate
i. wire
intergluteal cleft
interilioabdominal amputation
interinnominate asymmetry
interinnominoabdominal
i. amputation
i. cleft
interlaminar clamp
interleukin-1 beta release
interline
Lisfranc articular i.
interlocking
distal i.
i. medullary nail
i. nailing
proximal i.

intermaxillary bone
intermediary amputation
intermediate
i. amputation
i. bundle
i. callus
i. cast
i. C-D hook
i. cuneiform fracture-dislocation
i. disk
i. dorsal cutaneous nerve (IDCN)
i. interference pattern
i. lamella
i. phalangectomy
i. socket
Intermedics
I. natural hip system
I. Natural-Knee knee prosthesis
intermedius
vastus i.
intermetacarpal
i. articulation
i. joint
i. ligament (IML)
intermetatarsal (IM)
i. angle (IMA)
i. angle-reducing operation
i. angle-reducing procedure
i. artery
i. bursa
i. bursitis
i. joint
i. ligament
i. nerve
i. space
i. vein
intermetatarsophalangeal
i. bursa
i. bursitis
intermittens
dyskinesia i.
myotonia i.
myotonia congenita i.
intermittent
i. arthralgia
i. casting
i. cervical traction (ICT)
i. claudication (IC)
i. double-step gait
i. extremity pump
i. hydrarthrosis
i. impulse compression

NOTES

intermittent *(continued)*
- i. paresthesia
- i. pneumatic compression
- i. torticollis

intermuscular
- i. neuroma transposition
- i. septum

internal
- i. band
- i. carotid artery
- i. derangement
- i. derangement of the knee (IDK)
- i. femoral rotation
- i. fixation apparatus
- i. fixation, closed reduction
- i. fixation compression arthrodesis
- i. fixation compression arthrodesis of the ankle
- i. fixation plate-screw system
- i. fixation spring
- i. fracture fixation
- i. hemipelvectomy
- i. iliac artery
- i. iliac vein
- i. jugular vein
- i. malleolus
- i. movement
- i. neurolysis
- i. oblique muscle posteroinferior i. (PIIn)
- i. process
- i. rotary component of force component
- i. rotational gait
- i. rotation deformity
- i. rotation exercise
- i. rotation in extension (IRE)
- i. rotation in flexion (IRF)
- i. rotator
- i. snapping hip syndrome
- i. spinal fixation
- i. tibial torsion (ITT)
- i. tibial torsion brace
- i. tibiofibular torsion
- i. topography
- i. version

internal-external rotation
internally
- i. fixed fracture
- i. rotated

international
- I. Classification of Impairments, Disabilities, Handicaps (ICIDH)
- I. Classification for Surgery of the Hand in Tetraplegia
- I. Knee Documentation Committee (ICD, IKDC)
- I. Knee Documentation Committee form
- I. Knee Documentation Committee knee scale
- I. Knee Ligament
- I. Knee Ligament Standard Evaluation questionnaire
- I. Listing System
- I. 10-20 System

interne
- AO-ASIF fixateur i.
- AO fixateur i.
- Dick AO fixateur i.

internervous plane
intern's triangle in hip spica cast
internus
- malleolus i.
- metatarsus i.

interoceptor
- postural i.

Inter-Op
- I.-O. acetabular prosthesis
- I.-O. hip prosthesis

interossei (*pl. of* interosseus)
interosseous
- i. anastomosing channel
- i. artery
- i. branch
- i. cartilage
- i. compartment
- i. cuneocuboid ligament
- i. cuneometatarsal ligament
- i. diastasis
- i. intercuneiform ligament
- i. ligament disruption
- i. membrane (IOM)
- i. muscle
- i. nerve
- i. nerve injury
- i. nerve syndrome
- i. talocalcaneal ligament (ITCL)
- i. tendon
- i. wire fixation

interosseum
interosseus, pl. interossei
interparietal bone
interpeak interval
interpedicular distance widening joint widening
interpediculate
interpeduncular
- i. notch
- i. space

interpelviabdominal amputation
interperiosteal fracture
interphalangeal (IP)
- i. abductus
- i. amputation

i. arthrodesis
i. arthroplasty
i. articulation
i. coalition
distal i. (DIP)
i. fusion
i. joint (IPJ)
i. joint dislocation
i. joint space
i. osteoarthritis
proximal i. (PIP)
proximal interphalangeal/distal i.
   (PIP/DIP)
i. sesamoid management
i. tenodesis
interphalangealium
interphalangectomy
Interpore
I. bone
I. bone replacement material
I. implant
interposition
i. bone graft
i. membrane
soft tissue i.
interpositional
i. arthroplasty
i. tricortical graft
interpotential interval
interpubic disk
interregional displacement
Inter-Royal frame orthopedic bed
interrupted suture
intersacral canal
interscalene block
interscapular
i. amputation
i. reflex
**interscapulothoracic forequarter
   amputation**
Interseal
I. acetabular cup
I. Variant I–IV prosthesis
intersection syndrome
intersegmental
i. fixation
i. mobility
i. motion
i. movement
i. range of motion palpation
   (IRMP)

i. rotation
i. traction chiropractic table
intersesamoidal
intersesamoid ligament
interspace (IS)
atlantoodontoid i.
wedging of vertebral i.
interspinal ligament
interspinous
i. cable
i. ligament
i. process fusion
i. pseudarthrosis
i. segmental spinal instrumentation
   technique (ISSI)
i. wiring
interstice
bone i.
interstitial
i. fluid
i. lamella
i. meniscal tear
i. myofasciitis
interteardrop line
intertendinous vinculum
intertransverse
i. fusion
i. ligament
i. process arthrodesis
intertrigo
intertrochanteric
i. femoral fracture
i. four-part fracture
i. plate
i. varus osteotomy
Intertron therapy microprocessor
intertubercular
i. bursitis
i. groove
i. plane
i. sulcus
interval
acromiohumeral i. (AHI)
anterior atlantoodontoid i.
atlantoaxial i.
atlantodens i. (ADI)
atlas-dens i.
confidence i. (CI)
deltopectoral i.
interdischarge i.
interpeak i.
interpotential i.

NOTES

interval *(continued)*
    Kocher i.
    posterior atlantoodontoid i.
    recruitment i.
    response i.
    scaphocapitate i.
    Scheffé i.
    i. training
    trapeziodeltoid i.

intervening
    i. connective tissue
    i. muscle

intervention
    late i.
    prosthetic i.
    rehabilitation i.

intervertebral
    i. cartilage
    i. disk
    i. disk height
    i. disk herniation
    i. disk narrowing
    i. disk nucleus signal
    i. joint
    i. motor unit
    i. notch

intervolar plate ligament
intoe
intoeing gait
intolerance
    cold i.
    exercise i.
    fingertip cold i.

intorsion
intraacetabular
intraarticular
    i. adhesion
    i. arthrodesis
    i. calcaneal fracture
    i. cautery
    i. cautery device
    i. clavicle
    i. disk
    i. disk ligament
    i. dislocation
    i. fragment
    i. injection
    i. knee fusion
    i. loose body
    i. osteochondroma
    i. osteoid osteoma
    i. osteotomy
    i. procedure
    i. proximal tibial fracture
    i. reconstruction
    i. structure

intracapsular
    i. ankylosis
    i. excision
    i. fracture
    i. osteoid osteoma
    i. osteotomy
    i. rupture

Intracath needle
Intracell
    I. mechanical muscle device
    I. myofascial trigger-point device
    I. Sprinter stick
    I. trigger point massager

intrachondrial bone
intracompartmental
    i. edema
    i. ischemia
    i. pressure

Intracone intramedullary reamer
intracortical
    i. fibrous dysplasia
    i. osteogenic sarcoma

intracranial pressure elevation joint injection
intractable plantar keratosis (IPK)
intracuticular stitch
intradermal suture
intradiskal
    i. electrothermal therapy (IDET)
    i. pressure

intradural
    i. anastomosis
    i. dorsal spinal root rhizotomy
    i. tumor surgery

intraepiphysial osteotomy
Intrafix
    I. ACL tibial fastener
    I. fixation
    I. screw

Intraflex
    I. intramedullary pin
    I. intramedullary pin extractor

intrafocal reduction technique
intraforaminal approach
intrafusal fiber
intralesional
    i. excision
    i. resection

intramedullary (IM)
    Ace i. (AIM)
    i. alignment jig
    i. alignment rod
    i. ANK nail
    i. bar
    i. bone graft
    i. canal
    i. drill
    i. guide
    i. hematoma
    i. hemorrhage

i. lesion
i. nailing (IMN)
i. pin
i. reamer
i. rod fixation
i. saw
i. skeletal kinetic distractor (ISKD)
i. stem
i. supracondylar (IMSC)
i. supracondylar multihole nail

intramembranous
i. formation
i. ossification

intramuscular (IM)
i. injection
i. lengthening
i. nerve transposition
i. recording

intraneural
i. fibrosis
i. lipofibroma

intraoperative
i. Cell Saver
i. complication
i. dural tear
i. fluoroscopy
i. fracture
i. neck hyperextension
i. roentgenography
i. stress-relaxation
i. view
i. x-ray

intraorganically induced
intraosseous
i. abscess
i. circulation
i. fixation
i. ganglion
i. lipoma
i. lipomatosis
i. membrane
i. nerve transposition
i. osteosarcoma
i. pneumatocyst
i. probe
i. suture anchor
i. therapy
i. tibiofibular ligament
i. tophaceous gouty invasion
i. tumor
i. vascular congestion
i. venography

i. wire
i. wiring

intrapedicular fixation
intraperiosteal fracture
intraprosthetic
intrapyretic amputation
intrascaphoid angle
IntraSite dressing
intraspinous muscle
intraspongy nuclear disk herniation
intratendinous
intrathecal
i. anesthesia
i. neurolysis

intrathecally enhanced CT scan
intravascular hemolysis
intravenous
i. block anesthesia
i. pyelogram
i. regional anesthesia (IVRA)
i. therapy

intravertebral foramen (IVF)
Intrepid functional knee brace
intrinsic
i. clubfoot
i. contracture
finger i.
i. function
i. metatarsus primus elevatus
i. minus deformity
i. minus hallux
i. minus hand
i. minus position
i. muscle
i. muscle strength
i. paralysis
i. plus deformity
i. plus hand
i. restoration
i. tightness test
i. transverse connector
i. transverse connector role

introducer
Charnley i.
Dumon-Gilliard prosthesis i.
staple i.

intubation
endotracheal i.

Invacare
I. APM mattress
I. Comfort-Mate extra cushion
I. manual wheelchair

NOTES

Invacare *(continued)*
    I. padded shower chair
    I. vinyl transfer bench
invagination
    basilar i.
    endplate i.
invalid
    i. cushion
    i. ring
invasion
    intraosseous tophaceous gouty i.
    vascular i.
inventory
    Child Development I.
    Multidimensional Pain i.
    Vanderbilt Pain Management I.
    Westhaven Yale Multidimensional
      Pain I. (WHYMPI)
inversion
    i. ankle sprain
    i. ankle stress view
    fixed i.
    i. injury
    i. instability
    restricted i.
    i. stress test
inversion-eversion
    i.-e. exercise
    i.-e. rotation
InvertaChair traction device
inverted
    i. champagne bottle leg
    i. radial reflex
    i. scarf Z-osteotomy
    i. skin flap
    i. smile
inverted-L lateral periosteal incision
inverted-Y
    i.-Y Achilles tenotomy
    i.-Y fracture
    i.-Y incision
inverting knot technique
invertor force
Invertrac equipment
investing fascia
involucrum, pl. **involucra**
involuntary activity
involvement
    tumorous i.
inward rotation
Inyo nail
Ioban Vi-Drape
iodoform gauze
iodoform-impregnated plastic sheet
iodophor solution
IOM
    interosseous membrane
ion-bombarded cobalt-chromium

IonGuard orthopedic surface treatment
iontophoresis
    Dynaphor i.
ion transfer
iopamidol myelography
Iowa
    I. degenerative change
    I. hip score
    I. hip status rating system
    I. implant material
    I. internal prosthesis
    I. stem
    I. total hip prosthesis
    I. University periosteal elevator
IP
    interphalangeal
    IP joint
IPCS
    infrapatellar contracture syndrome
IPJ
    interphalangeal joint
IPK
    indurated plantar keratoma
    intractable plantar keratosis
I-plate
I-Plus
    I.-P system humeral fracture brace
    I.-P system ulnar fracture brace
Ipomax orthosis
IPOP
    immediate postoperative prosthesis
ipos
    i. arch support system
    i. heel relief orthosis
    i. heel relief shoe
    i. postoperative shoe
ipriflavone
IPS
    immediate postoperative stability
    IPS total hip system
IPSF
    immediate postsurgical fitting
ipsilateral
    i. approach
    i. femoral neck fracture
    i. femoral shaft fracture
    i. foot injury
    i. rotation
    i. side bending
    i. slide graft
    i. total elbow arthroplasty
    i. total shoulder arthroplasty
IR
    infrared light
    isotonic reversal
IRE
    internal rotation in extension

IRF
    internal rotation in flexion
iris scissors
IRMP
    intersegmental range of motion palpation
IROM
    IROM bilateral splint
    IROM Regal splint
    IROM splint with shells
iron
    Jewett bending i.
iron-deficiency anemia
Ironman Triathlon Pro-Power massager
irradiation
    i. fibromatosis
    i. sterilized graft
irreducible
    i. fracture
    i. fracture dislocation
irregular
    i. articular surface
    i. bone
    i. potential
irregularity
    tendon i.
irregular-shaped lesion
irrigating solution
irrigation
    i. bulb
    i. burn
    closed i.
    closed suction i.
    i. and débridement (I&D)
    drip-suck i.
    Pulsavac i.
    i. solution
    i. suction
    Systec i.
    i. system
    i. tube
    WaterPik i.
    wound i.
irrigator
    Arthro-Flo i.
    Baumrucker clamp i.
    Fisch bone drill i.
    jet i.
    ophthalmic i.
    pulse i.
irritability
    nerve root i.
    soft tissue i.

irritable
    i. hip
    i. joint
    i. lesion
    i. symptom
irritation
    i. callus
    facet joint i.
    nerve root i.
    sciatic nerve i.
Irvine
    I. ankle
    I. ankle arthroplasty
Irwin osteotomy
IS
    interspace
Isaacs syndrome
Isch-Dish Plus cushion
ischemia
    capillary i.
    critical limb i. (CLI)
    exercise i.
    foot i.
    intracompartmental i.
    muscle i.
    myocardial i.
    myoneural i.
    postural i.
    tourniquet i.
    vasospastic i.
    Volkmann i.
    warm i.
ischemic
    i. compression
    i. contracture
    i. disease of the growing hip (IDGH)
    i. foot
    i. forearm exercise test
    i. gangrene
    i. leg disease
    i. lesion
    i. limb
    i. limb disease (ILD)
    i. lumbago
    i. myositis
    i. necrosis
    i. necrosis of femoral head (INFH)
    i. tourniquet technique
    i. ulcer
ischia (*pl. of* ischium)

NOTES

ischial
- i. bone
- i. bursitis
- i. containment socket
- i. spine
- i. tuberosity
- i. weightbearing leg brace
- i. weightbearing orthosis
- i. weightbearing prosthesis (IWP)
- i. weightbearing ring

ischial-bearing seat
ischialgia
ischial-gluteal weightbearing socket
ischiatic scoliosis
ischiectomy
ischioacetabular fracture
ischiodynia
ischiofemoral ligament
ischiogluteal
- i. bursa
- i. bursitis

ischiohebotomy
ischionitis
ischiopubic
- i. arch
- i. foramen
- i. ramus

ischiopubiotomy
ischiorectal
- i. abscess
- i. fossa
- i. region

ischium, pl. **ischia**
Iselin disease
Isherwood projection
Ishihara cervical spine curve index
Ishizuki unconstrained elbow prosthesis
ISIS
  integrated shape and imaging system
    ISIS screening
ISKD
  intramedullary skeletal kinetic distractor
island
- i. adipofascial flap
- bone i.
- i. graft
- i. skin flap

Isobaric epidural/spinal anesthesia technique
Isobex dynamometer
isodynamic
IsoDyn knee brace
isoelastic pelvic prosthesis
isograft
  bone i.
isoinertial
isokinetic
- i. assessment

concentric bilateral i.
- i. dynamometry
- i. evaluation
- i. exercise
- i. joint apparatus
- i. knee extension
- i. movement
- i. performance
- i. resistance apparatus
- i. strength test maximal
- i. testing
- i. torque imbalance
- i. Unex III exerciser

Isola
- I. fixation system
- I. hook-rod
- I. spinal implant system accessory
- I. spinal implant system anchor
- I. spinal implant system application
- I. spinal implant system eye rod
- I. spinal implant system hook
- I. spinal implant system iliac post
- I. spinal implant system iliac screw
- I. spinal implant system plate-rod combination
- I. spinal instrumentation system
- I. vertebral screw
- I. wire

isolated
- i. avulsion
- i. dislocation
- i. modular tibial insert exchange
- i. paralysis
- i. zone

isolation drape
isolator
  Ankle I.
isologous graft
Isoloss AC material
isometer
  I. bone graft placement site detector
  CA-5000 drill-guide i.
  tension i.
isometric
- i. cervical extension strength
- i. contraction
- i. device
- i. exercise
- i. force
- i. motor testing
- i. point
- i. resistance
- i. strain gauge
- i. strength testing
- i. technique

i. traction
i. training
isometricity
isoniazid
isophendylate
Isoprene plastic splint
Iso-Quadron exerciser
Isostation B200
Isotechnologies B-200 low back machine
Isotec patellar tendon graft
Isotoner glove
isotonic
combination of i.'s (COI)
i. contraction
i. exercise
i. machine
i. motor testing
i. resistance
i. reversal (IR)
i. traction
i. training
isotope
bone mineralization i.
i. bone scan
isotropic disk
Isovue myelography
Israel
I. rasp
I. retractor
ISS
Injury Severity Score
Isseis-Aussies scoliosis operation
ISSI
interspinous segmental spinal
instrumentation technique

isthmic spondylolisthesis
isthmus, pl. **isthmi, isthmuses**
isuprel
IT
iliotibial
ITB
iliotibial band
ITB fasciitis
ITBFS
iliotibial band friction syndrome
ITCL
interosseous talocalcaneal ligament
Itrel
I. programmed transmitter-receiver
I. II, III spinal cord stimulation
system
ITT
internal tibial torsion
ITV
infantile tibia vara
ITW
idiopathic toe-walker
Ivalon prosthesis
IVF
intravertebral foramen
ivory
i. bone
i. osteoma
IVRA
intravenous regional anesthesia
IV-type basic frame
iWALKfree hands-free crutch
Iwashi clamp approximator
IWP
ischial weightbearing prosthesis

NOTES

J

J board
J disk
J pad
J septum
J sign

J-35

J-35 hyperextension brace
J-35 hyperextension orthosis

J-45

J-45 contraflexion brace
J-45 contraflexion orthosis

J-55

J-55 postfusion brace
J-55 postfusion orthosis

jab and hook punch combination
Jaboulay amputation
Jaccoud

J. arthritis
J. arthropathy
J. arthroplasty
J. syndrome

JACE

JACE hand continuous passive
   motion unit
JACE shoulder exerciser
JACE W550 CPM device

**JACE-STIM electrotherapy stimulation
unit**
jack

J. Frost hot/cold pack
Joint J.
J. test
turnbuckle j.
j. upper cut

jacket

body j.
Boston soft body j.
cervicothoracic j.
flexion body j.
Frejka j.
halo body j.
halo traction j.
immobilization j.
Kydex body j.
Lexan j.
Low Profile plastic body j.
LS⁴ custom spinal j.
Minerva cervical j.
Orfizip body j.
Orthoplast j.
plastic body j.
Prenyl j.
Royalite body j.
Sayre j.

underarm body j.
Vitrathene j.
von Lackum transection shift j.
Wilmington plastic j.

jackknife

j. position
j. test

The Jacknobber II
Jackson

ankle scoring system of Baird
   and J.
J. bone clamp
J. bone-extension clamp
J. bone-holding clamp
J. broad-blade staple forceps
J. compression test
J. dressing forceps
J. intervertebral disk rongeur
J. spinal surgery and imaging table
J. syndrome
J. tendon-seizing forceps

Jackson-Gorham syndrome
jacksonian epilepsy
Jackson-Pollock skinfold equation
Jackson-Pratt drain
Jacksonville sling
Jackson-Weiss syndrome
Jacobs

J. chuck
J. chuck adapter
J. chuck drill
J. chuck drive
J. distraction rod
J. locking hook spinal rod
J. locking hook spinal rod
   instrumentation
J. locking hook spinal rod
   instrumentation modification
J. locking hook spinal rod
   technique

Jacob shift test
Jacobson

J. bulldog clamp
J. mosquito forceps
J. needle holder
J. suture pusher
J. system

Jacoby

J. bunion splint
J. heel splint

Jacquet fixator
Jadassohn-Lewandowsky syndrome
JAFAR

Juvenile Arthritis Functional Assessment
Report

Jaffe
 J. disease
 J. press-fit prosthesis
 J. procedure
Jaffe-Capello-Averill hip prosthesis
jagged osteophyte
Jahss
 J. ankle dislocation classification
 J. classification of ankle dislocation
 J. maneuver
 J. metatarsophalangeal joint
  dislocation classification
 J. ninety-ninety method
 J. procedure
Jakob test
Jamaica Sandalthotics orthotic
Jamar
 J. grip tester
 J. hydraulic hand dynamometer
 J. hydraulic pinch gauge
 J. test
James
 J. position
 J. procedure
 J. splint
 J. wound forceps
Jameson
 J. muscle clamp
 J. muscle hook
jammed finger
Jamshidi needle
Janecki-Nelson
 J.-N. shoulder girdle resection
 J.-N. shoulder operation
**Janis tibialis posterior tendon
 dysfunction classification**
Jannetta
 J. duckbill elevator
 J. hook
Jansen
 J. bone curette
 J. disease
 J. metaphysial dysostosis
 J. monopolar forceps
 J. rasp
 J. test
Jansey
 J. procedure
 J. technique
**Jan van Breemen Function
 Questionnaire (JVBF)**
Japanese Orthopedic Association (JOA)
Japas
 J. osteotomy
 J. V-osteotomy
jar
 heel j.

Jarcho-Levin syndrome
Jarell forceps
Jarit
 J. anterior resection clamp
 J. cartilage clamp
 J. meniscal clamp
 J. pin cutter
 J. rotator
 J. small bone-holding clamp
 J. tendon-pulling forceps
Jarit-Liston bone rongeur
Jarit-Ruskin bone rongeur
JAS
 joint activated system
 JAS elbow motion device
javelin thrower's elbow
jaw
 j. claudication
 j. exerciser
 j. opening reflex (JOR)
Jay
 J. basic cushion
 J. Combi cushion
 J. J2 wheelchair
 J. Rave cushion
 J. Triad cushion
 J. Xtreme cushion
JCE
 job capacity evaluation
J-24 cervical orthosis
J2 cushion
Jeanie
 J. Rub
 J. Rub Massager
Jeanne sign
Jebsen
 J. assessment
 J. assessment of hand function
 J. hand test
Jebsen-Taylor hand function test
Jefferson cervical burst fracture
Jeffery
 J. radial fracture classification
 J. technique
Jelanko splint
Jendrassik maneuver
Jenet sign
**Jensen-Michelsen intertrochanteric hip
 fracture classification**
Jergesen
 J. I-beam
 J. I-beam plate
 J. incision
 J. tapered plate
 J. tube
jerk
 Achilles j.

J

ankle j. (AJ)
biceps j. (BJ)
elbow j. (EJ)
j. finger
hung-up knee j.
knee j. (KJ)
patellar j. (PJ)
quadriceps j.
j. sign
supinator j.
tendon j.
j. test
triceps j. (TJ)
triceps surae j.
jerky gait
jersey finger
jet
j. irrigator
j. lavage
Ortholav j.
J. Vac cement dispenser
Jet-Air splint
Jeter lag/position screw
jet-pilot position
Jette Functional Status index
Jettmobile positioning and tumble form
jeweler's
j. forceps
j. thumb
Jewett
J. bending iron
J. contraflexion brace
J. contraflexion orthosis
J. driver
J. extractor
J. gouge
J. hyperextension brace
J. hyperextension orthosis
J. nail
J. nail overlay plate
J. operation
J. pick-up screw
J. postfusion brace
J. postfusion orthosis
J. prosthesis
J. thoracolumbosacral orthosis
Jewett-Benjamin
J.-B. cervical brace
J.-B. cervical orthosis
J-59 Florida brace
J-FX bipolar head
J-GLAS prefab orthotic

J-hook deformity
JIDC
juvenile intervertebral disk calcification
jig
chamfer cut j.
Charnley tibial onlay j.
cutting j.
drilling j.
external-alignment compression j.
extramedullary tibial alignment j.
femoral alignment j.
fixation j.
Herbert j.
j. hook
intramedullary alignment j.
Miller-Galante j.
Osteonics j.
Plexiglas j.
precompression j.
spacer-tensor j.
tibial j.
Jimmie
half J.
jing
bifocal manipulative with
distraction j.
J&J
Johnson & Johnson
J&J postoperative shoe
J&J ulcer dressing
JOA
Japanese Orthopedic Association
JOA Scale
job
j. capacity evaluation (JCE)
j. redesign
j. task analysis (JTA)
Jobe-Glousman capsular shift procedure
Jobert fossa
Jobe test
Jobst
J. air band
J. appliance
J. athrombotic pump
J. boot
J. brassiere
J. gauntlet
J. glove
J. prosthesis
J. stockings
jockey cap patella
Joerns orthopedic bed

NOTES

jogger's
- j. heel
- j. toe

jogging in place test

Johannesberg staple

Johannson
- J. hip nail
- J. lag screw

Johannson-Barrington arthrodesis

Johanson-Blizzard syndrome

Johansson fracture classification

John
- J. Barnes myofascial release
- J. C. Wilson arthrodesis

Johner-Wruhs tibial fracture classification

Johns
- J. Hopkins bulldog clamp
- J. Hopkins National Low Back Pain Study

Johnson
- J. chevron osteotomy
- J. hemiphalangectomy
- J. & Johnson (J&J)
- J. & Johnson PFC cruciate-substituting insert
- J. medial meniscal suturing
- J. pelvic fracture technique
- J. procedure
- J. pronator advancement
- J. resection arthroplasty
- J. screwdriver
- J. staple technique
- J. and Strom tibialis posterior tendon dysfunction classification

Johnson-Boseker
- J.-B. scale
- J.-B. scale classification

Johnson-Elloy accord unconstrained prosthesis

Johnson-Jahss
- J.-J. classification of posterior tibial tendon tear
- J.-J. posterior tibial tendon tear classification

Johnson-Spiegl
- J.-S. hallux varus correction
- J.-S. procedure
- J.-S. tendon transfer

Johnson-Zuck-Wingate motor test

Johnston-Iowa hip prosthesis

joint
- AC j.
- acromioclavicular j.
- j. activated system (JAS)
- adjustable dynamic j. (ADJ)
- amphidiarthrodial j.
- ankle j.

anterior sternoclavicular j.
apophysial j.
j. arthrodesis
j. arthrogram
j. arthrography
j. arthrometer
j. arthropathy
j. aspiration
atlantoaxial j.
atlantooccipital j.
atlantoodontoid j.
bail-lock knee j.
ball-and-socket j.
basal j.
beaking j.
biaxial j.
bilocular j.
j. block
Budin j.
calcaneocuboid j.
calcaneonavicular j.
Cam Lock knee j.
capitate-hamate j.
capitate-lunate j.
j. capsule
j. capsule mechanoreceptor
carpal-intercarpal j.
carpometacarpal j.
carpophalangeal j.
cartilaginous j.
j. cavitation
j. cavity
CC j.
cervical j.
Charcot j.
j. chondroma
Chopart midtarsal j.
j. cinch
Clutton j.
CMC j.
coccygeal j.
composite j.
compound j.
condyloid j.
j. congruence
congruent metatarsophalangeal j.
coracoclavicular j.
costochondral j.
costotransverse j.
costovertebral j.
coxofemoral j.
cracking of j.
Cruveilhier j.
cubital j.
cubonavicular j.
cuneiform j.
cuneometatarsal j.
cuneonavicular j.

J

j. debris
j. deformity
j. degeneration
Delrin j.
j. depression fracture
diarthrodial j.
digital j.
DIP j.
j. disarticulation
j. dislocation
j. disruption
distal interphalangeal j. (DIPJ)
distal radioulnar j. (DRUJ)
distal tibiofibular j.
j. distraction
j. distraction cuff
j. distractor
double-action ankle j.
double pearl-face hip j.
double-stem silicone lesser MP j.
dry j.
j. dysfunction
j. effusion
elastic knee cage with medial and
    lateral contoured knee j.'s
elbow j.
ellipsoid j.
enarthrodial j.
erythema of j.
extraarticular subtalar j.
facet j.
false j.
femoropatellar j.
femorotibial j. (FTJ)
fibrocartilaginous j.
fibrous j.
Fillauer dorsiflexion assist ankle j.
Fillauer PDC ankle j.
finger j.
flail j.
j. force
fourth metatarsophalangeal j.
freely movable j.
fringe j.
j. fulcrum
j. fusion
Gaffney j.
Gillette double-flexure ankle j.
ginglymoid j.
glenohumeral j.
gliding hinge j.
Greissinger Multi-Axis j.

hallux IP j.
hamate-lunate j.
hemophilic j.
hinged j.
hip capsule j.
hot j.
HP-100 prosthetic finger j.
humeroulnar j.
hyperextensibility of j.
j. hyperextensibility
hypermobile j.
j. hypermobility
hysterical j.
IM j.
j. immobilization
j. immobilizer
immovable j.
j. implant
incudomalleolar j.
inferior radioulnar j.
inferior tibiofibular j.
j. instability
Integrated Ankle orthotic ankle j.
interarticular j.
intercarpal j.
interchondral j.
intercuneiform j.
intermetacarpal j.
intermetatarsal j.
j. internal derangement
interphalangeal j. (IPJ)
intervertebral j.
IP j.
irritable j.
J. Jack
knee j.
lap j.
lateral atlantoaxial j.
j. lavage
j. laxity
lesser metatarsophalangeal j.
j. leveling
limited motion metal ankle j.
j. line
j. line pain
j. line tenderness
Lisfranc j.
locking of j.
LT j.
lumbosacral j.
lunocapitate j.
Luschka j.

NOTES

joint *(continued)*
j. manipulation
j. meniscoid
metacarpocapitate j.
metacarpocarpal j.
metacarpohamate j.
metacarpophalangeal j. (MPJ)
metacarpophysial j.
metacarpotrapezoid j.
Metasul j.
metatarsal j.
metatarsal-tarsal j.
metatarsocuboid j.
metatarsocuneiform j.
metatarsophalangeal j. (MTPJ)
metatarsosesamoid j.
j. mice
midcarpal j.
middle atlantoepistrophic j.
middle carpal j.
midfoot j.
midtarsal j.
j. mobility
j. mobilization
j. model
mortise and tenon j.
movable j.
MTP j. (MTPJ)
multiaxial j.
multiple axis knee j.
naviculocuneiform j.
near-anatomic position of j.
neuropathic j.
neurotrophic j.
noncongruent metatarsophalangeal j.
nonsubluxated metatarsophalangeal j.
oblique metatarsocuneiform j.
occipital-axis j.
occipitoatlantoaxial j.
Oklahoma ankle j.
j. osteoarthritis
Otto Bock 3R65 children's
  hydraulic knee j.
Otto Bock 3R45 modular knee j.
patellofemoral j.
pisotriquetral j.
pivot j.
plane j.
plastic limited-motion j.
j. play
polyaxial j.
j. popping
j. position sense (JPS)
proximal interphalangeal j. (PIPJ)
proximal tibiofibular j.
radiocapitellar j.
radiocarpal j.
radiohumeral j.
radiolunate j.
radioscaphoid j.
radioscapholunate j.
radioulnar j.
j. reconstruction
j. release
j. replacement surgery
j. rice
3R80 modular hydraulic knee j.
rotary j.
sacrococcygeal j.
sacroiliac j.
saddle-shaped j.
scaphocapitate j.
scapholunate j.
scapuloclavicular j.
scapulothoracic j.
Scotty stainless ankle j.
Select j.
septic finger j.
sesamoidometatarsal j.
shoulder j.
SI j.
Silastic finger j.
simple j.
single-axis ankle j.
single pearl-face hip j.
single smooth-face hip j.
S-K reconstruction of distal
  radioulnar j.
slip j.
solid ankle j.
j. space
j. spacer
spheroidal j.
spiral j.
j. sprain
stable hinge j.
sternoclavicular j. (SCJ)
sternocostal j.
j. stiffness
stifle j.
STT j.
subluxated metatarsophalangeal j.
j. subluxation
subtalar j. (STJ)
superior radioulnar j.
superior tibiofibular j.
Sutter silicone
  metacarpophalangeal j.
suture pusher talofibular j.
Swanson finger j.
j. swelling
synarthrodial j.
synovial j.
talocalcaneal j.
talocalcaneonavicular j.
talocrural j.

talofibular j.
talonavicular j.
Tamarack flexure j.
tarsal j.
tarsometatarsal j.
temporomandibular j. (TMJ)
tibiofemoral j.
tibiofibular j.
tibiotalar j.
TN j.
total replacement j.
track-bound j.
transverse tarsal j.
trapeziometacarpal j.
trapeziotrapezoidal j.
triscaphe j.
trochoid j.
ulnocarpal j.
ulnohumeral j.
Ultraflex Dynamic J.
uncovertebral j.
uniaxial j.
unilocular j.
unstable j.
j. verrucous carcinoma
Virtual hip j.
von Gies j.
j. warmth
wedge-and-groove j.
weightbearing j.
j. wound
j. wrap
xiphisternal j.
zygapophysial j.

jointed
    double j.
Joint-Jack finger splint
joker
    j. dissector
    j. periosteal elevator
Jolly test
Jonas prosthesis
Jonathan Livingston Seagull patellar prosthesis
Jonell
    J. countertraction finger splint
    J. thumb splint
Jones
    J. abduction frame
    J. arm splint
    J. brace
    J. and Brackett anterior approach

J. classification of congenital tibial deficiency
J. cock-up toe operation
J. compression cast
J. compression pin
J. compression plate
J. congenital tibial deficiency classification
J. diaphysial fracture classification
J. dressing
J. fracture
J. metacarpal splint
J. position
J. resection arthroplasty
J. retinaculum reconstruction procedure
J. scissors
J. screw
J. suspension traction
J. tendosuspension
J. thoracic clamp
J. toe repair
J. towel clamp
J. traction splint
J. transfer
J. view
Jones-Barnes-Lloyd-Roberts classification
Jones-Brackett technique
Jones-Ellison ACL reconstruction
Joplin
    J. bunionectomy
    J. operation
    J. toe prosthesis
JOR
    jaw opening reflex
Jordan-Day drill
Jordan frame
Joseph
    J. hook
    J. nasal rasp
    J. osteotome
    J. periosteal elevator
    J. periosteotome
    J. splint
Jousto dropfoot splint, skid orthosis
JoyBags therapeutic heat pack
J-periosteal elevator
JPS
    joint position sense
JRA
    juvenile rheumatoid arthritis
J.R. Moore procedure

NOTES

J-shaped skin incision
JTA
    job task analysis
Judet
    J. epiphysial fracture classification
    J. graft
    J. hip status system
    J. pelvic x-ray view
    J. Press-Fit hip prosthesis
    J. quadricepsplasty
    J. radiograph
Juers-Lempert rongeur forceps
jugal
    j. bone
    j. suture
jumbo acetabular cup
jump
    J. graft
    j. sign
    squat j.
    J. Start Rehab
jumper's
    j. knee
    j. knee position
jumping leg
junction
    allograft-host j.
    atlantooccipital j.
    beaked cervicomedullary j.
    cervicothoracic j.
    gastrocnemius-soleus j.
    host-allograft j.
    lumbosacral j.
    meniscocapsular j.
    meniscosynovial j.
    metaphysial-diaphysial j.
    musculotendinous j.
    myotendinous j.
    occipitocervical j.
    tarsometatarsal j.
    thoracolumbar j.
junctional
    j. fracture
    j. kyphosis
junctura, pl. juncturae
Jüngling disease
Jung muscle
Junod boot
Jupiter and Belsky phalanx fracture
    classification
Jurgan
    J. pin
    J. pin ball
    J. pinball pin protector
    J. pin ball system

jury-rig
Juvara
    J. bunionectomy
    J. foot operation
    J. procedure
juvenile
    j. aponeurotic fibroma
    J. Arthritis Functional Assessment
    Report (JAFAR)
    j. bunion
    j. bunionectomy
    j. chronic arthritis
    j. diskitis
    j. flatfoot pathomechanics
    j. hallux valgus
    j. hinge axis concept
    j. hyaline fibromatosis
    j. idiopathic scoliosis
    j. intervertebral disk calcification
    (JIDC)
    j. kyphosis
    j. muscular atrophy
    j. muscular dystrophy
    j. plantar dermatosis
    j. polyarthritis
    j. rheumatoid arthritis (JRA)
    j. Tillaux fracture
    j. xanthogranuloma
juvenile-onset
    j.-o. ankylosing spondylitis
    j.-o. rheumatoid arthritis
juvenilis
    osteochondritis j.
    osteochondritis deformans j.
Jux-A-Cisor exerciser
juxtaarticular
    j. bone cyst
    j. fracture
    j. lesion
juxtaarticulation
juxtacortical
    j. chondroma
    j. chondrosarcoma
    j. fracture
juxtacubital reconstruction
juxtaepiphysial
juxtaspinal
juxtatectal transverse fracture
Juzo
    J. brace
    J. support
J-Vac closed drainage system
JVBF
    Jan van Breemen Function Questionnaire

K
K blade
K needle
Kaessmann
K. nail
K. screw
KAFO
knee-ankle-foot orthosis
Generation II KAFO
GII KAFO
PRAFO KAFO
Kager
K. fat pad Valleix sign
K. triangle
Kahre-Williger periosteal elevator
Kalamchi classification
Kalamchi-Dawe
K.-D. classification of congenital
tibial deficiency
K.-D. congenital tibial deficiency
classification
Kaleidoscope chair
Kalish
K. bunionectomy modification
K. Duredge wire cutter
K. Duredge wire extender
K. Duredge wire extractor
K. osteotomy
Kalix flatfoot implant
Kallassy
K. ankle support
K. brace
K. orthosis
Kaltenborn joint mobilization system
Kaltostat dressing
Kambin
K. and Gellman lumbar diskectomy
instrumentation
K. triangular working zone
Kampe corset
KAM Super Sucker
Kanavel
K. canal
K. cock-up splint
K. sign
K. triangle
Kaneda
K. anterior spinal instrumentation
K. anterior spinal/scoliosis system
(KASS)
K. distraction device
K. plate
K. rod
Kantrowitz thoracic clamp

Kapandji
K. fracture
K. fracture of radius
K. pinning technique
K. thumb opposition score
Kapandji-Sauvé
K.-S. arthrodesis
K.-S. radioulnar joint repair
Kapel
K. elbow dislocation technique
K. operation
Kaplan
K. modification of Ruiz-Mora
procedure
K. oblique line
K. open reduction
K. osteotomy
K. sign
K. technique
**Kaplan-Meier time-to-event analysis
method**
Kaposi sarcoma
kappa receptor
Kaprelian easy-access tweezers (KEAT)
Karakousis-Vezeridis
K.-V. procedure
K.-V. resection
karate
Shotokan k.
karate-inspired aerobics
Karfoil splint
Karlsson
K. and Peterson scoring scale
K. procedure
Karsch-Neugebauer syndrome
Kasdan retractor
Kashin-Bek disease
Kashiwagi
K. resection
K. technique
KASS
Kaneda anterior spinal/scoliosis system
Kast-Maffucci syndrome
Kast syndrome
KAT
Kinesthetic Ability Trainer
Kates forefoot arthroplasty
Kates-Kessel-Kay technique
Katz
K. ADL index
K. index of activities of daily
living
Kaufer tendon technique
Kaufmann technique
Kavanaugh-Brower-Mann fixation

K

Kawaii-Yamamoto procedure
Kawamura
    K. dome osteotomy
    K. pelvic osteotomy
Kay scissors
Kayser-Fleischer ring
Kazanjian splint
KB
    knee-bearing
Keane Mobility bed
Kearns-Sayre syndrome
Keasbey lesion
KEAT
    Kaprelian easy-access tweezers
Kech-Kelly osteotomy
KED
    Kendrick extrication device
keel
    All Poly Deltafit k.
    Deltafit K.
    k. of glenoid component
keeled chest
Keene
    K. compression hook
    K. obturator
Keen sign
Keesay treatment
Kehr
    K. procedure
    K. sign
Keitel index
Keithley clamp kit
Keith needle
Kelikian
    K. classification of nail deformity
    K. foot dressing
    K. modified Z bunionectomy
    K. modified Z osteotomy
    K. modified Z
      osteotomy/bunionectomy
    K. nail deformity classification
    K. procedure
    K. push-up test
Kelikian-Clayton-Loseff
    K.-C.-L. surgical syndactyly
    K.-C.-L. technique
Kelikian-McFarland procedure
Kelikian-Riashi-Gleason
    K.-R.-G. patellar tendon repair
    K.-R.-G. technique
Kellam-Waddel classification
Keller
    K. bunionectomy
    K. bunionectomy with prosthesis
    K. foot operation
    K. hallux valgus operation
    K. procedure
    K. resection arthroplasty

Keller-Blake
    K.-B. half-ring splint
    K.-B. leg splint
Keller-Brandes
    K.-B. procedure
    K.-B. resection arthroplasty
Keller-Lelièvre arthroplasty
Keller-Lelièvre-Hoffman procedure
Keller-Mann resection arthroplasty
Keller-Mayo diabetic foot arthroplasty
Keller-Regnauld arthroplasty
Kellgren
    K. degenerative disk disease
      criteria
    K. knee scale
    K. osteoarthritis grade
    K. sign
Kellgren-Lawrence grading system
Kellogg-Speed
    K.-S. fusion technique
    K.-S. lumbar spinal fusion
    K.-S. operation
Kelly
    K. clamp
    K. forceps
    K. hemostat
    K. peroneal tendon dislocation
      procedure
Kelly-Keck osteotomy
Kelly-Kelly osteotomy
keloid scar
Kelsey unloading exercise therapy
Kelvin body
Kempf-Grosse-Abalo Z-step osteotomy
Kempf internal screw fixation
Kemp test
Ken
    K. driver
    K. driver-extractor
    K. screwdriver
    K. sliding nail
Kendall A-V impulse system
Kendrick
    K. extrication device (KED)
    K. procedure
Kendrick-Sharma-Hassler-Herndon
  technique
Kenna Knee Scale
Kennedy
    K. LAD
    K. ligament augmenting device
    K. ligament technique
    K. modification of Gallie ankle
      fusion
    K. spillproof cup
Kennerdell-Maroon
    K.-M. elevator
    K.-M. hook

Kenny
- K. ADL index
- K. Self-Care Questionnaire
- K. treatment

Kenny-Caffey syndrome

Kenny-Howard
- K.-H. shoulder sling
- K.-H. splint

Keolar implant material

keratoderma blennorrhagica

keratolysis

keratolytic agent

keratoma
- indurated plantar k. (IPK)

keratome
- automated disposable k. (ADK)
- k. Beaver blade

keratosis, pl. **keratoses**
- actinic k.
- intractable plantar k. (IPK)
- plantar k.
- k. punctata
- stucco k.

Kerboull acetabular reinforcement device

Kerlix
- K. bandage
- K. cast padding
- K. dressing
- K. gauze
- K. wrap

Kern
- K. bone-holding clamp
- K. bone-holding forceps

Kernig
- K. sign
- K. test

Kern-Lane bone forceps

Kerpel bone curette

Kerr
- K. abduction splint
- K. electro-torque drill
- K. hand drill
- K. sign

Kerrison
- K. chisel
- K. curette
- K. downbiting rongeur
- K. punch

Kerr-Lagen abdominal support

Kessel-Bonney
- K.-B. extension osteotomy
- K.-B. procedure

Kessel plate

Kessler
- K. external fixator
- K. fixation device
- K. grasping suture
- K. metacarpal distractor
- K. metacarpal lengthening
- K. modified Achilles tendon repair
- K. posterior tibial tendon transfer
- K. posterior tibial tendon transfer operation
- K. prosthesis
- K. stitch
- K. suture technique
- K. traction
- K. traction frame

Kessler-Tajima suture

Ketac cement

ketamine

Kevlar glove

Kevorkian curette

key
- k. the cement
- k. grip
- K. intraarticular knee arthrodesis
- K. periosteal elevator
- k. pinch
- K. rasp
- k. release
- K. wrist brace

keyboard
- ErgoLogic k.
- Kinesis k.
- wave k.

keyboarder
- MouseMitt k.

Key-Conwell pelvic fracture classification

key-grip tenodesis

keyhole
- k. approach
- k. method
- k. punch
- k. tenodesis
- k. tenodesis technique

Key-loc wrench

Keys-Kirschner traction

keystone
- k. graft

K

NOTES

keystone (continued)
K. splint
k. structure
keyway
OEC lag screw component with k.
K-Fix Fixator system
KFS
Klippel-Feil syndrome
KGTI
Kinetik great toe implant
Khan-Lewis phonological analysis
Khodadad clip
Kickaldy-Willis arthrodesis
kick bucket
Kicker
K. Pavlik harness
K. Pavlik harness hip abduction brace
kick-point
Kid-Dee-Lite orthosis
Kidner
K. dissector
K. flatfoot
K. foot operation
K. foot procedure
K. lesion
kidney rest
Kiehn-Earle-DesPrez procedure
Kienböck
K. atrophy
K. disease
K. dislocation
K. phenomenon
Kikuchi-MacNap-Moreau approach
Kilfoyle
K. humeral medial condylar fracture classification
Kilian line
Killian gouge
Kilner hook
Kiloh-Nevin
K.-N. myopathy
K.-N. ocular form of progressive muscular dystrophy
kilopond
kilovoltage potential
Kilsyn-Evans
K.-E. principle of frontal plane correction
Kimerle anomaly
KinAir bed
Kinamed
K. anthropometric total hip
K. Exact-Fit ATH system
Kinast indirect reduction
Kin-Con
K.-C. device
K.-C. isokinetic exercise system

kinematic
K. II condylar and stabilizer total knee system
K. fully constrained tricompartmental knee prosthesis
k. gait pattern change
hindfoot k.
k. index of McMurtry
knee k.
k. linkage
K. II rotating hinge knee system
K. II rotating hinge total knee prosthesis
K. rotation hinge
k. study
Kinemax
K. modular condylar and stabilizer total knee system
K. Plus knee prosthesis
K. Plus total knee system
K. removable fixation peg
K. spacer
Kinemetric guide system
kineplastic amputation
kineplastics
kinesialgia
kinesiatrics
kinesiology
applied k. (AK)
kinesiopathologic component
kinesiopathology
kinesipathist
Kinesis keyboard
kinesitherapy
kinesthesia
kinesthesiometer
kinesthetic
K. Ability Trainer (KAT)
k. awareness
k. exercise
KineTec
K. clubfoot CPM exerciser
K. hip CPM machine
kinetic
k. cervical spine
k. chain
k. energy
k. energy theory
k. foot pain
k. gait analysis
k. rehab device (KRD)
k. splint
K. Wedge molded insole
K. Wedge orthotic
kinetics

Kinetik
K. great toe implant (KGTI)
K. great toe implant system
Kinetikos joint implant
Kinetix instrument for carpel tunnel release
Kinetron muscle strengthening apparatus
King
K. cervical brace
K. cervical traction
K. intraarticular hip fusion
K. intraarticular hip fusion procedure
K. maneuver
K. open reduction
K. scoliosis (type I–V)
K. technique
K. thoracic scoliosis classification
K. type IV curve posterior correction
K. type thoracic and lumbar curve (type I–IV)
K. wound forceps
King-Moe scoliosis
King-Richards
K.-R. dislocation technique
K.-R. operation
Kingsley Steplite foot
King-Steelquist
K.-S. hindquarter amputation
K.-S. technique
kinking
catheter k.
pedicular k.
Kinsbourne syndrome
Kirby muscle hook
Kirk
K. distal thigh amputation
K. distal thigh operation
K. orthopedic mallet
Kirkaldy-Willis
K.-W. operation
K.-W. three phases of degeneration
Kirmission periosteal elevator
Kirner deformity
Kirschenbaum
K. foot positioner
K. retractor
Kirschner
K. apparatus
K. bone drill

K. II-C shoulder system
K. device
K. integrated shoulder system
K. Medical Dimension hip replacement
K. Medical Dimension prosthesis
K. pin fixation
K. skeletal traction
K. stem
K. surgical instrument
K. tightener
K. total shoulder prosthesis
K. traction bow nut
K. wire (K-wire)
K. wire cutter
K. wire drill
K. wire driver
K. wire fixation
K. wire inserter
K. wire pin
K. wire placement
K. wire tensioner
K. wire traction bow
kissing
k. lesions
k. sequestra
k. spines
Kistler force platform
kit
Alpha suction attachment block k.
BFO K.
Bio-Dermal hydrogel k.
Canadian Academy of Sports Medicine emergency k.
carpal tunnel surgery relief k.
diabetic orthosis k.
Digital Care k.
Dr. Joseph's diabetic foot k.
DynaPak electrode k.
Elastafit tubing k.
Elbow Injury Management K.
Exerball k.
Fillauer Scottish Rite orthosis k.
Halifax interlaminar clamp k.
Histofreezer cryosurgical wart treatment k.
ICE-Magic pain reduction k.
I-Flow nerve block infusion k.
Keithley clamp k.
Leukotape P Combo Pack taping k.
MediCordz Rehabilitation K.

NOTES

kit *(continued)*
    Merit Final Flexion K.
    modular temPPTthotic k.
    nerve block infusion k.
    OsteoSet resorbable bead k.
    palmar swab k.
    parallel pin k.
    pelvic reconstruction k.
    portable diagnostic k.
    Posey bar k.
    Quick-Sil starter k.
    resistive chair exercise k.
    sensory stimulation k.
    Shoulder Therapy K.
    Skin Care k.
    Tacticon peripheral neuropathy k.
    Unna-Flex Plus venous ulcer k.
    VersaFlex tubing k.
Kitaoka clinical rating scale
Kitaoka-Leventen medial displacement metatarsal osteotomy
kite
    K. angle
    K. clubfoot cast
    K. and Lovell technique
    K. metatarsal cast
    K. slipper
KJ
    knee jerk
Kjolbe technique
Klagsbrun harvesting technique
Kleiger test
Klein
    K. drainage
    K. technique
Kleine-Levin syndrome
Kleinert
    K. modification
    K. postoperative traction brace
    K. repair
    K. splint
    K. technique of pulley reconstruction
Kleinert-Kutz
    K.-K. bone cutter
    K.-K. bone-cutting forceps
    K.-K. bone rongeur
    K.-K. clamp approximator
    K.-K. periosteal elevator
    K.-K. rasp
    K.-K. rongeur forceps
    K.-K. synovectomy rongeur
    K.-K. tendon forceps
    K.-K. tendon retriever
Kleinert-Ragdell retractor
Kleinman shear test
Klein-Vogelbach functional movement concept

Klemm nail
Klemm-Schellman nail
Klengall brace
Klenzak
    K. double-upright splint
    K. orthosis
    K. spring brace
Kline line
Kling
    K. adhesive dressing
    K. cervical brace
    K. elastic bandage
Klippel-Feil
    K.-F. malformation
    K.-F. segmentation defect
    K.-F. sign
    K.-F. syndrome (KFS)
Klippel-Trenaunay
    K.-T. osteohypertrophic hemangiectasia
    K.-T. syndrome
Klippel-Trenaunay-Weber syndrome
Klisic-Jankovic technique
Kloehn craniofacial remodeling technique
Klumpke
    K. injury
    K. palsy
    K. plexopathy
KMFTR
    Kotz modular femur and tibia resection
KMP
    KMP femoral stem
    KMP femoral stem prosthesis
knavel table
Knead-A-Ball exerciser
kneading massage
knee
    above k. (AK)
    acetabular k.
    ACL-deficient k.
    anatomic modular k. (AMK)
    anterior cruciate deficit k.
    k. arthrodesis
    k. arthroplasty
    k. arthroscopy
    Axiom total k.
    bicompartmental replacement of k.
    Biomet Ascent total k.
    k. bolster
    k. brace splint
    breaststroker's k.
    Brodie k.
    cadaveric k.
    k. cage brace
    carpenter's k.
    carpet-layer's k.
    k. complex

constant-friction k.
constrained condylar k.
Continuum P/S total k.
k. contracture
corner of k.
deficient k.
DePuy LCS mobile-bearing k.
k. disarticulation amputation
k. disarticulation suspension
dislocated k.
k. dislocation
k. extension assist
k. extension exercise
k. extension orthosis
k. extensor
flail k.
k. flexion
k. flexion during stance phase
motion gait determinant
k. flexion-extension
k. flexion reflex
k. flexion stress test
floating k.
k. force
k. fracture
k. fusion
game k.
Genesis unicompartmental k.
GeoFlex k.
gimpy k.
giving way of k.
hamstrung k.
k. holder
horseback rider's k.
Hosmer single-axis friction k.
Hosmer single-axis locking k.
Hosmer weight-activated locking k.
housemaid's k.
k. immobilizer
k. immobilizer splint
k. instability
k. instability test
internal derangement of the k.
(IDK)
k. jerk (KJ)
k. jerk reflex
k. jerk reflex test
k. joint
k. joint effusion
jumper's k.
k. kinematic
k. knob

Korn Cage k.
k. laxity test
k. ligamentous injury
k. lock
locked k.
Mauch Swing and Stance
hydraulic k.
k. MD brace
Miller-Galante k.
motorcyclist's k.
moviegoer's k.
neuropathic k.
Noiles posterior stabilized k.
Noiles rotating hinge k.
k. orthosis (KO)
Otto Bock 3R60 EBS k.
Otto Bock 3R80 modular rotary
hydraulic k.
Otto Bock Safety constant-
friction k.
PC Performer k.
K. Pillo
pneumatic four-bar linkage k.
PolymerFriction total k.
porous-coated anatomic total k.
k. positioner
k. positioning triangle
posterior cruciate ligament of k.
press-fit Condylar Total k.
ProAdvantage k.
k. prosthesis
k. pump
k. pump exercise
k. retractor
k. rotation
runner's k.
k. saver
Seattle safety k.
self-aligning k. (SAL)
septic k.
k. signature system
single-axis friction k. (SAFK)
single-axis locking k. (SALK)
k. sleeve
K. Sleeve knee support
k. sling
snowstorm k.
K. Society Score
K. Society total knee arthroplasty
roentgenography evaluation and
scoring
k. stability

NOTES

knee *(continued)*
    k. strike
    tension band of k.
    The K. Society clinical-rating scale
    total condylar k.
    Total Knee 2100 prosthetic k.
    total rotating k. (TRK)
    Translating and Congruent Mobile-
      Bearing K. (TACK)
    transverse ligament of k.
    trick k.
    USMC stance locking safety k.
    valgus k.
    varus k.
    k. varus-valgus
    voluntary control 4-bar k.
    weight-activated locking k.
      (WALK)
    windblown k.
    wrenched k.
knee-ankle-foot orthosis (KAFO)
knee-bearing (KB)
kneecap stabilizer
knee-chest
    k.-c. push
    k.-c. rocking
    k.-c. table
knee-control orthosis pad
Kneed-It kneeguard
knee-drop test
kneeGRIP
kneeguard
    Kneed-It k.
kneeling
    k. bench test
    k. position
    90-90 k. position
    k. reciprocal back exercise
      technique
KneeRanger hinged knee brace
kneeRAP wrap
Kniest syndrome
knife
    acetabular k.
    ACL graft k.
    amputation k.
    arthroscopic k.
    backward-cutting k.
    Ballenger swivel k.
    banana k.
    Bard-Parker k.
    bayonet k.
    Beaver cataract k.
    Beaver-DeBakey k.
    Bircher meniscus k.
    k. blade
    Blair k.
    Blount k.

Bovie k.
C k.
cartilage k.
cast k.
Castroviejo bladebreaker k.
Catlin amputating k.
chondroplasty k.
Collin amputating k.
Crile k.
cutting current k.
Down epiphysial k.
Downing cartilage k.
Esmarch plaster k.
forward-cutting k.
Freiberg cartilage k.
Freiberg meniscectomy k.
full-radius resector k.
Grover meniscus k.
hemilaminectomy k.
hooked k.
Hopkins plaster k.
hot k.
Humby k.
Krull acetabular k.
Langenbeck flap k.
Langenbeck resection k.
Lindvall-Stille k.
Liston amputating k.
Liston phalangeal k.
Lowe-Breck cartilage k.
Lowe-Breck meniscectomy k.
Maltz cartilage k.
McKeever cartilage k.
meniscectomy k.
meniscus k.
Midas Rex k.
Neff meniscus k.
Oretorp retractable k.
orthopaedic k.
Reiner plaster k.
retrograde-cutting hook-shaped k.
Ridlon plaster k.
rocker k.
Salenius meniscus k.
sculp k.
semilunar cartilage k.
serrated fine-cutting k.
sheathed k.
skiving k.
Smillie-Beaver k.
Smillie cartilage k.
Smillie meniscal k.
Smith cartilage k.
Stryker cartilage k.
tenotomy k.
upward-cutting triangular k.
Weck k.
Yamanda myelotomy k.

knight
 K. back brace
 K. bone-cutting forceps
Knight-Taylor
 K.-T. thoracic brace
 K.-T. thoracolumbosacral orthosis
Knight-Taylor-Williams spinal orthosis
Knirk-Jupiter elbow evaluation scale
Knit-Rite suspension sleeve
knob
 knee k.
Knobber
 Original Index K. II
Knobble massager
Knobby-Clark procedure
knocked-down shoulder
knock-knee
 k.-k. brace
 k.-k. deformity
Knodt
 K. distraction rod
 K. rod and hook
knot
 arthroscopic k.
 hairpin k.
 half-hitch arthroscopic k.
 half-stitch arthroscopic k.
 k. of Henry
 Henry k.
 lockable arthroscopic k.
 PDS k.
 k. pusher
 Revo k.
 sliding k.
 surfer's k.
 wire k.
knotter
 Harris k.
knotting forceps
Knott rod distraction device
Knowles
 K. hip pin
 K. pin nail
 K. pinning
knuckle
 k. bone
 boxer's k.
 k. pad
 k. shaped
knuckle-bender splint
Knuttsen bending view

KO
 knee orthosis
Kocher
 K. clamp
 K. classification
 K. collar incision
 K. curved L approach
 K. dissector
 K. elevator
 K. forceps
 K. fracture
 K. interval
 K. lateral J approach
 K. reduction
 K. reduction of shoulder
  dislocation
 K. retractor
Kocher-Debré-Semelaigne syndrome
Kocher-Gibson posterolateral approach
Kocher-Langenbeck
 K.-L. approach
 K.-L. exposure
 K.-L. ilioinguinal repair
Kocher-Lorenz
 K.-L. capitellum fracture
  classification
 K.-L. fracture
 K.-L. fracture of capitellum
Kocher-McFarland hip arthroplasty
Koch-Mason dressing
Kodel knee sling
Kodex drill
Koehler disease
Koenen periungual fibroma
Koenig
 K. metatarsal broach
 K. metatarsophalangeal joint
  arthroplasty
 K. MPJ prosthesis
 K. nail-splitting scissors
 K. rasp
 K. total great toe implant
Koenig-Schaefer
 K.-S. incision
 K.-S. medial approach
Kofoed
 K. Ankle Score
 K. scoring system
Köhler
 K. disease
 K. fracture

K

NOTES

Köhler *(continued)*
    K. hip protrusion grading scale
    K. line
Köhler-Pellegrini-Stieda disease
Kohs block
koilonychia
koilosternia
Kold Wrap
Kollagen dressing
Kolmogorov-Smirnov test
Kondoleon operation
König disease
Konstram angle
Kool Kit cold therapy pack
Korean hand acupuncture
Korex cork sheet
Korn
    K. Cage knee
    K. Cage knee brace
Kortzeborn
    K. hand operation
    K. procedure
Kostuik-Alexander arthrodesis
Kostuik-Errico spinal stability classification
Kostuik-Harrington
    K.-H. distraction system
    K.-H. spinal instrumentation
Kostuik screw
Kotz modular femur and tibia resection (KMFTR)
Kotz-Salzer rotationplasty
Koutsogiannis
    K. calcaneal displacement osteotomy
    K. procedure
Koutsogiannis-Fowler-Anderson osteotomy
KPS bipolar vitallium-polyethylene implant
Krackow
    K. Achilles tendon repair
    K. HTO blade staple
    K. locking loop technique
    K. locking suture technique
    K. maneuver
    K. point
    K. suture
Krackow-Cohn technique
Krackow-Thomas-Jones technique
Kramer-Craig-Noel basilar femoral neck osteotomy
Kramer modification of Hohmann osteotomy
Kraske position
Krause
    K. bone

    suture of K.
    ulnar collateral nerve of K.
Krause-Wolfe
    K.-W. prosthesis
    K.-W. skin graft
KRD
    kinetic rehab device
    KRD L2000 rehab device
Krempen-Craig-Sotelo tibial nonunion technique
Krempen-Silver-Sotelo nonunion operation
Kretschmer syndrome
Kreuscher
    K. bunionectomy
    K. operation
Kristiansen eyelet lag screw
Kristiansen-Kofoed external fixation
Kronfeld pin
Kronner
    K. external fixation
    K. external fixation apparatus
    K. external fixation device
    K. ring fixation
Krukenberg
    K. amputation
    K. hand
    K. hand operation
    K. hand reconstruction
    K. procedure
Krull acetabular knife
Kruskal-Wallis test
KS 5 ACL brace
K2 sensation prosthesis
KSO brace
KT-1000
    KT-1000 foot stabilizer
    KT-1000 joint arthrometer
    KT-1000 knee ligament arthrometer
KT-1000/Jr arthrometer
KT-1000/s surgical arthrometer
KT-2000 knee ligament arthrometer
Kudo ·
    K. hinge
    K. unconstrained elbow prosthesis
Kugelberg reconstruction
Kugelberg-Welander
    K.-W. disease
    K.-W. juvenile spinal muscle atrophy
Kuhlman
    K. cervical traction device
    K. traction
Kumar
    K. application
    K. spica cast technique
Kumar-Cowell-Ramsey technique

Kümmell
    K. disease
    K. spondylitis
Kümmell-Verneuil disease
Kümmel ulnar ray deficiency classification
Küntscher
    K. awl
    K. drill
    K. extractor
    K. finisher
    K. hammer
    K. humeral prosthesis
    K. impactor
    K. medullary nailing
    K. modified knee arthrodesis
    K. nail
    K. nail driver
    K. nail-extracting hook
    K. ossimeter
    K. pin
    K. reamer
    K. rod
    K. technique
    K. traction apparatus
    K. traction device
Küntscher-Hudson brace
Kunzel
    nerve of K.
Kurosaka interference-fit screw
Kurtzke
    K. Expanded Disability scale
    K. Functional system
    K. score
Kuschkin Ace wheelchair
Kuskokwim syndrome
Kutes arthroplasty
Kutler
    K. double lateral advancement flap
    K. V-Y flap
    K. V-Y flap graft
Kuwada Achilles tendon injury classification
Kuz-Medics disposable knee immobilizer
K-wire
    Kirschner wire
    K-wire driver
    K-wire fixation
    percutaneous K-wire
    K-wire placement
Kydex
    K. body jacket

    K. brace
    K. chairback orthosis
Kyle
    K. fracture classification
    K. fracture classification system
    K. internal fixation
Kyle-Gustilo classification
Kyle-Gustilo-Premer classification
kyllosis
kyphectomy
    Sharrard-type k.
kyphometer
    Debrunner k.
kyphoplasty
kyphorachitic pelvis
kyphoscoliorachitic pelvis
kyphoscoliosis
    neurofibromatosis k.
    k. secondary to neurofibromatosis
    severe k.
    thoracolumbar k.
kyphoscoliotic pelvis
kyphosing scoliosis
kyphosis
    acute angular k.
    adolescent k.
    anterior k.
    apprentice k.
    k. brace
    congenital k. (type I, II)
    k. correction
    k. creation
    iatrogenic lumbar k.
    junctional k.
    juvenile k.
    long-radius k.
    lumbar k.
    lumbosacral k.
    Luque rod fixation for k.
    myelodysplastic k.
    paralytic k.
    postlaminectomy k.
    postradiation k.
    posttraumatic k.
    rotational k.
    sagittal k.
    Scheuermann k.
    Scheuermann juvenile k. (SJK)
    short-radius k.
    thoracic k.
    thoracolumbar k.
kyphos resection

K

NOTES

kyphotic
- k. angle
- k. angulation
- k. curve
- k. deformity

- k. deformity pathomechanics
- k. pelvis

kyphotone
Kyrle hyperkeratosis
kyrtorrhachic

L
    L plate
    L rod
lab
    Orthopedic Casting L. (OCL)
laboratory
    Army Prosthetics Research L.
      (APRL)
    gait l.
    University of California,
      Berkeley L. (UCBL)
labral
    l. avulsion
    l. lesion
    l. tear
labrum, pl. **labra**
    acetabular l.
    anterior glenoid l.
    articular l.
    cartilaginous glenoid l.
    glenoid l.
    posterior glenoid l.
LAC
    long arm cast
lace
    no-tie stretch l.
laced blucher of shoe
lace-on brace
laceration
    boot-top l.
    burst-type l.
    chevron l.
    flexor tendon l.
    hallucis longus l.
    stellate nail bed l.
lacertus fibrosus
L.A. cervical orthosis
lace-up RocketSoc ankle brace
Lacey
    L. fully constrained
      tricompartmental knee prosthesis
    L. hinge
    L. hinged knee prosthesis
    L. rotating hinge arthroplasty
Lachman
    L. maneuver
    L. sign
    L. test
lacinate ligament
lacing ankle brace
lacrimal
    l. bone
    l. duct dilator
Lacroix
    fibroosseous ring of L.

    osseous ring of L.
    L. osseous ring
lactate
    Ringer l.
    l. threshold (LT)
lactic
    l. acidosis
    l. acidosis threshold
LactoSorb
    L. orthopedic wound material
    L. resorbable copolymer
lacuna
    bone l.
    cartilage l.
    Howship l.
    osseus l.
LAD
    ligament augmentation device
    ligamentous anterior dislocation
    LAD composite graft
    Kennedy LAD
ladder
    finger l.
    shoulder l.
    l. splint
Lafayette skinfold caliper
lag
    l. screw
    l. screw fixation
    l. screw insertion
    l. screw thread hole
**LaGrange humeral supracondylar
fracture classification**
LaGrange-Letoumel hip prosthesis
Lahey
    L. clamp
    L. Clinic dural hook
Laing
    L. concentric hip cup
    L. H-beam nail
    L. hip cup prosthesis
    L. plate
Lalonde
    L. dynamic compression bone
    clamp
    L. hook forceps
    L. oblique fracture large bone
    clamp
    L. oblique fracture medium bone
    clamp
    L. oblique metacarpal fracture bone
    clamp
    L. small bone clamp
    L. tendon approximator

L

387

LAM
    limb accurate measurement
    LAM instrument
lamb
    L. muscle transfer
    l. wool
    l. wool pad
Lambert cosine law
Lambert-Eaton myasthenic syndrome (LEMS)
Lambert-Lowman
    L.-L. bone clamp
    L.-L. chisel
Lambeth disability screening questionnaire
Lamb-Marks-Bayne technique
lamboid suture
Lambotte
    L. bone-holding clamp
    L. bone-holding forceps
    L. bone hook
    L. elevator
    L. osteotome
    L. principle
Lambrinudi
    L. drop foot operation
    L. osteotomy
    L. splint
    L. technique
    L. triple arthrodesis
lamella, pl. **lamellae**
    articular bone l.
    basic l.
    circumferential l.
    concentric l.
    endosteal l.
    ground l.
    haversian l.
    intermediate l.
    interstitial l.
    osseous l.
    periosteal l.
lamellar
    l. bone
    l. pattern
    l. separation
    l. thickening
lamellated bone
lamellation
lamina, pl. **laminae**
    l. elevator
    intact spinous l.
laminagram
laminaplasty
    expansive l.
    Tsuji l.
    l. with extended foraminoplasty

laminar
    l. bone
    l. C-D hook
    l. cortex posterior aspect
    l. fracture
    l. spreader
laminectomized spine
laminectomy
    cervical spine l.
    l. chisel
    decompressive l.
    l. frame
    multilevel l.
    osteoplastic l.
    radial l.
laminoforaminotomy
laminoplasty
    distraction l.
laminotomy and diskectomy
Lam inversion test
Lamis patellar clamp
lamp
    l. cord sign
    Derma-Wand germicidal l.
    halogen l.
Lance
    L. disease
    L. shelf procedure
Lanceford prosthesis
lancinating pain
lancing
Landeez all-terrain wheelchair
Landers-Foulks prosthesis
landmark
    anatomic l.
    bony l.
    pedicle l.
Landolt spreading forceps
Landouzy-Dejerine dystrophy
Landsmeer ligament
Lane
    L. bone-holding clamp
    L. bone lever
    L. bone screw
    L. periosteal elevator
    L. plate
    L. procedure
    L. screwdriver
    L. screw-holding forceps
    L. self-retaining bone-holding forceps
Lanex screen
Lange
    L. Achilles tendon reconstruction
    L. bone retractor
    L. hip reduction
    L. operation
    L. procedure

L. skinfold caliper
L. tendon lengthening
L. tendon-lengthening method
L. tendon lengthening and repair
Lange-Hohmann bone retractor
Langenbeck
L. amputation
L. anteromedial approach
L. bone-holding forceps
L. bone saw
L. flap knife
L. incision
L. metacarpal saw
L. operation
L. periosteal elevator
L. rasp
L. resection knife
L. retractor
L. triangle
Langenskiöld
L. bone graft
L. bony bridge resection
L. classification (stage I–VI)
L. fusion
L. grading system
L. osteotomy
L. procedure
Langer
L. axillary arch
L. axillary arch muscle
L. line
L. mesomelic dwarfism
Langerhans
L. cell granulomatosis
L. cell histiocytosis
Langoria sign
lap
l. joint
l. seatbelt fracture
laparoscopic surgeon's thumb
laparotomy
l. sheet
l. sponge
Lapidus
L. alternating air-pressure mattress
L. bed
L. bunionectomy
L. hammertoe technique
L. modified arthrodesis
L. operation
L. procedure
LAPOC prosthesis

LaPorta
L. great toe implant
L. total toe prosthesis
lappet formation
L'Aprina topical spray
laptop cushion
large
l. callus Podi-Burr
l. Cobra retractor
l. composite allograft
l. egress cannula
l. humeral head hemiarthroplasty
l. nail Podi-Burr
large-bore inflow cannula
large-head humeral component
large-nail spicule bur
Lark scooter
Larmon
L. forefoot
L. forefoot arthroplasty
L. forefoot procedure
Laron dwarfism
Larrey
L. amputation
L. operation
Larsen
L. disease
L. hip score
L. lateral ankle stabilization
   procedure
L. syndrome
L. tendon-holding forceps
Larsen-Johansson disease
LARSI
lumbar anterior-root stimulator implant
Lars Ingvar Hansson (LIH)
Larson
L. hip status system
L. ligament reconstruction
L. technique
laryngeal nerve injury
LAS
local adaptation syndrome
LASA
Lisfranc articular set angle
Laschal suture scissors
LASE
laser-assisted spinal endoscopy
   LASE probe
Lasègue
L. rebound test
L. sign

L

NOTES

laser

ArthroProbe arthroscopic l.
l. arthroscopy
Candela SPTL l.
carbon dioxide l.
cold l.
l. Doppler flowmetry
l. Doppler probe
holmium YAG l.
l. image custom arthroplasty (LICA)
l. instrument
low-energy l. (LEL)
low-power l.
l. nucleotomy
l. partial matrixectomy
red light neon l.
SilkTouch CO_2 l.
Surgilase CO_2 l.
Trimedyne Omnipulse holmium l.
VersaPulse holmium l.

laser-assisted

l.-a. capsular shift
l.-a. capsulorrhaphy
same-day microsurgical arthroscopic lateral-approach l.-a. (SMALL)
l.-a. spinal endoscopy (LASE)

Laserflo BPM
LaserPen laser therapy
lashing suture
last normal vertebra (LNV)
lata

fascia l.
tensor fascia l. (TFL)

Latarjet procedure
late

l. intervention
l. response
l. stance

latency

l. of activation
distal l.
F l.
motor l.
onset l.
peak l.
proximal l.
residual l.
sensory peak l.
terminal l.

latent

l. diastasis
l. period
l. stage of gout

lateral

l. acetabular shelf operation
l. acromial border
l. ankle sprain
l. arm flap
l. aspiration
l. atlantoaxial joint
l. atlantooccipital ligament
l. band
l. band mobilization
l. bending
l. bending view
l. bicipital sulcus
l. block test
l. bowing
l. buttress support J patellofemoral brace
l. calcaneal artery
l. canal entrapment
l. capsular release
l. capsular sign
l. cervical spine film
l. collateral ligament (LCL)
l. collateral sprain
l. column calcaneal fracture
l. column lengthening
l. column-lengthening surgery
l. column syndrome
l. compartment
l. compartment disruption
l. compartment injury
l. compartment reconstruction
l. compression (LC)
l. compression force
l. compression injury
l. condylar fracture classification
l. cord
l. cortex
l. corticospinal tract
l. curvature
l. decompression
l. decubitus position
l. deltoid splitting approach
l. deviation
l. disk protrusion
l. drainage
l. electrical surface stimulation (LESS)
l. end
l. epicondyle
l. exostectomy
l. extensor expansion
l. extensor release
l. femoral condyle
l. flexion
l. flexion dynamic visual analysis
l. flexion malposition
l. flexion restriction
l. forefoot overload
l. full-spine radiographic examination
l. fusion

l. gap sign
l. Gatellier-Chastung approach
l. guidepin
l. gutter syndrome
l. head of gastrocnemius
l. hindfoot
l. hip arthroscopy
l. hip rotation
l. humeral condyle fracture
l. humeral epicondylitis
l. hyperpressure syndrome
l. impingement
l. J approach
l. joint line
l. joint space
l. Kocher approach
l. listhesis
l. lumbar shift
l. malleolus
l. malleolus fracture
l. malleolus muscle
l. mass fracture
l. meniscectomy
l. meniscus
l. monopodal stance view
l. motion racket sport
l. oblique view
l. Ollier approach
l. parapatellar approach
l. park-bench position
l. patellar autologous graft
l. patellar compression syndrome
l. patellar facet
l. pivot shift
l. pivot shift test
l. plantar artery
l. plica
l. premalleolar bursitis
l. process
l. projection (LC)
l. quadruple complex
l. recess
l. recess stenosis (LRS)
l. retinaculum release
l. rhachotomy
l. roentgenogram
l. root pressure
l. rotary displacement
l. rotatory ankle instability
l. screw
l. sesamoid
l. sesamoidectomy

l. shear
l. shelf
l. sling procedure
l. slip
l. spring ligament of foot
l. spring-loaded lock
l. squeeze pinch
l. squeeze test
l. stability
l. step-up
l. sway
l. talar process fracture
l. talocalcaneal ligament (LTC)
l. tear
l. thigh flap
l. thoracic flap
l. tibial condyle
l. tibial plateau fracture
l. tibial tubercle
l. tilt stress ankle view
l. tilt stress ankle x-ray
l. transfer
l. transmalleolar portal
l. trap suture
l. trunk shift
l. tuberosity
l. utility incision
l. wedge
l. wedge fracture

lateralis
   malleolus l.
   vastus l. (VL)
   vastus medialis obliquus:vastus l.
    (VMO:VL)

laterality
   atlas l.

lateralization

laterally displaced fracture

lateral-to-medial thrust

lateroduction

lateropulsion

latex
   l. anaphylaxis
   l. cushion

latissimus
   l. dorsi
   l. dorsi flap
   l. dorsi muscle

latitudinal growth

latticework

Lauenstein procedure

L

NOTES

Lauge-Hansen
L.-H. ankle fracture classification
L.-H. stage II supination-eversion
fracture
Laugier
L. fracture
L. sign
Laurence-Biedl syndrome
Laurence-Moon-Biedl
L.-M.-B. law
L.-M.-B. syndrome
Laurence-Moon syndrome
Lauren view
Laurin
L. lateral patella displacement
L. lateral patellofemoral angle
lavage
bone l.
CarboJet l.
Exeter bone l.
Hi Speed Pulse l.
jet l.
joint l.
Ortholav jet l.
pulsatile jet l.
pulsatile pressure l.
Pulsavac l.
pulsed l.
Simpulse pulsing l.
Simpulse S/I l.
Lavine reduction
law
all-or-none l.
Davis l.
L. of Facilitation
Heuter-Volkmann l.
Lambert cosine l.
Laurence-Moon-Biedl l.
Ollier l.
Sherrington l.
sports medicine l.
von Schwann l.
Wolff l.
lawn mower injury
Lawrence
L. device
L. first metatarsophalangeal joint
implant
Lawrence-Seip syndrome
Lawson-Thornton plate
Lawton procedure
laxity
ankle l.
collateral ligament l.
cruciate ligament l.
l. index
joint l.
ligamentous l.

radioscaphocapitate ligament l.
subtalar l.
l. to varus stress
layer
cambium l.
capsular l.
gliding l.
Ollier l.
parietal tendon sheath l.
periosteal cambium l.
tangential l.
Lazepen-Gamidov anteromedial approach
lazy-C incision
lazy-L incision
lazy-S skin incision
lazy-V deepithelialized turn-over
fasciocutaneous flap
L-bolt
TSRH L-B.
LBP
low back pain
LBW
lean body weight
LC
lateral compression
lateral projection
LCC
long calcaneocuboid
LCC ligament
LCL
lateral collateral ligament
LCPD
Legg-Calvé-Perthes disease
LCR
ligamentous and capsular repair
LCR system
LCS
low-contact stress
LCS meniscal bearing
semiconstrained prosthesis
LCS mobile bearing knee system
LCS New Jersey knee prosthesis
LCS rotating platform
semiconstrained prosthesis
LCS substituting semiconstrained
prosthesis
LCS total knee system
LCS total knee system implant
LCS universal APG semiconstrained
prosthesis
LCT
liquid crystal thermography
L-curved incision
LDF
lumbodorsal fascia
LE
lower extremity
lupus erythematosus

Le
Le Dentu suture
Le Fort amputation
Le Fort fibular fracture
Le Fort II fracture
Le Fort mandible fracture
Le Fort I–III osteotomy
Le Fort-Wagstaffe fracture

LEA
lower extremity amputation

Leach-Igou step-cut medial osteotomy
Leach-Schepsis-Paul augmentation
lead
Axxess spinal cord stimulation l.
l. line
l. pipe fracture
l. synovitis

Leadbetter
L. hip manipulation
L. maneuver
L. technique

leader
tendon l.

leaders and trailers
lead-filled mallet
lead-line scan
leaf, pl. **leaves**
inferior l.
l. splint
superior l.

leaf-spring
AFO posterior l.-s.
l.-s. brace
plastic l.-s. (PLS)

leakage
bony slurry l.
chylous l.

Leake Dacron mandible prosthesis
lean
antalgic l.
l. body weight (LBW)

Leander
L. chiropractic table
L. motorized flexion table

leaning hop test
LEAP
Lewis expandable adjustable prosthesis

learning
spinal l.

leash of Henry
leather
l. ankle corset

l. cuff
l. lacer gauntlet
l. orthosis

Leatherman hook
leaves (*pl. of* leaf)
Lebsche
L. rongeur
L. saw guide
L. wire saw

LeCocq brace
Ledderhose disease
lederhosen disease
Ledraplastic exercise ball
Lee
L. anterosuperior iliac spine graft
L. bone graft
L. procedure
L. reconstruction
L. technique

leech
American l.
artificial l.
medicinal l.

Leeds-Keio Dacron mesh replacement
Leeds spinal procedure
Lefferts rib shears
LEFS
Lower Extremity Functional Scale

left
l. erector spinae musculature
l. innominate
l. lateral flexion
l. lower extremity (LLE)
l. lower limb (LLL)
l. lumbar convexity
l. rotation
l. thoracolumbar major curve pattern
l. upper extremity (LUE)
l. upper limb (LUL)

left-hand dominance
left-right leg displacement
left-sided
l.-s. nail
l.-s. thoracotomy

leg
anatomic short l.
l. axis
badger l.
baker's l.
bayonet l.
bowed l.

NOTES

L

leg *(continued)*
    l. brace
    champagne bottle l.
    C-Leg System artificial l.
    l. compartment release
    l. decompression
    l. drift
    l. edema
    L. Extension Power Rig
    flaccid l.
    functional short l.
    game l.
    gimpy l.
    inverted champagne bottle l.
    jumping l.
    l. length
    l. length determination
    l. length discrepancy (LLD)
    l. length inequality (LLI)
    lusty l.
    nonpreferred l.
    paretic l.
    l. positioner
    l. press
    l. protection factor (LPF)
    restless l.
    rider's l.
    scissor l.
    short l.
    l. shortening
    l. sling
    stork l.
    stovepipe l.
    table short l.
    tennis l.
    l. traction
    unilateral spastic l.
    l. walking cast

Legasus support CPM device

leg-curl
    ankle joint l.-c.

legend
    L. ACL functional knee brace
    L. Hy-Lo adjusting table
    L. PCL functional knee brace
    L. stationary adjusting table

leg-foot-toe syndrome

Legg-Calvé-Perthes
    L.-C.-P. disease (LCPD)
    L.-C.-P. syndrome

Legg-Calvé-Waldenström
    L.-C.-W. disease
    L.-C.-W. syndrome

Legg-Perthes
    L.-P. disease
    L.-P. disease orthosis
    L.-P. shoe extension
    L.-P. sling

Legg procedure

legholder, leg holder
    Alvarado l.
    Arthroplasty Products Consultants
        foot and l.
    arthroscopic l.
    Bickel l.
    Cherf l.
    LH1000 arthroscopic l.
    lithotomy l.
    Low Profile l.
    operative l.
    Prep-Assist l.
    Surbaugh l.
    SurgAssist surgical l.
    Zollinger l.

leg-holding
    l.-h. apparatus
    l.-h. device

leg-lengthening device

Lehman technique

Leibinger
    L. Micro System drill bit
    L. Micro System plate cutter
    L. Micro System plate-holding
        forceps
    L. Profyle hand system

Leibolt technique

Leica model 1600 water-cooled diamond saw

Leichtenstern sign

Leinbach
    L. device
    L. femoral prosthesis
    L. hip prosthesis
    L. olecranon screw
    L. osteotome

leiomyomatous hamartoma

Leksell
    L. adapter to Mayfield device
    L. laminectomy rongeur
    L. rongeur forceps
    L. stereotactic arc

Leksell-Stille thoracic rongeur

LEL
    low-energy laser

Lelièvre osteotomy

Lema strap

Lemmon
    L. rib contractor
    L. sternal approximator
    L. sternal spreader

Lempert
    L. bone curette
    L. bone rongeur
    L. periosteal elevator
    L. rongeur forceps

LEMS
Lambert-Eaton myasthenic syndrome
Lenart-Kullman technique
Lengemann wire
length
distal parabola toe l.
echo train l. (ETL)
femur l. (FL)
Grace method of ratio of metatarsal l.
hip axis l.
inequality in leg l. (ILL)
leg l.
limb l.
needle cord l.
pedicle screw cord l.
pedicle screw path l.
resting l.
l. of stay (LOS)
step l.
stride l.
lengthening
Achilles tendon l.
Anderson tibial l.
aponeurotic l.
Armistead ulnar l.
calcaneal neck l.
Codivilla tendon l.
Compere l.
l. contraction
DeBastiani femoral l.
distraction l.
Evans calcaneal l.
extensor tendon l.
fractional l.
Frost posterior tibialis tendon l.
gastrocnemius l.
Gillies-Millard metacarpal l.
hamstring l.
Hauser tendo calcaneus l.
heel cord l.
Hoke Achilles tendon l.
Hsu-Hsu percutaneous tendo calcaneus l.
Ilizarov limb l.
intramuscular l.
Kessler metacarpal l.
Lange tendon l.
lateral column l.
limb l.
limb-girdle l.
metacarpal l.

l. over nails procedure
percutaneous heel cord l.
percutaneous tendo Achillis l.
l. reflex
reverse undercutting l.
Silfverskiöld Achilles tendon l.
Silver-Simon l.
Spencer tendon l.
step-cut l.
Strayer l.
subscapularis-capsular l.
Tachdjian fractional l.
Tachdjian hamstring l.
Tajima metacarpal l.
tendo Achillis l. (TAL)
tendon l.
tibial l.
transiliac l.
ulnar l.
Vulpius l.
Vulpius-Compere gastrocnemius l.
Wagner femoral l.
Wagner tibial l.
Warren White Achilles tendon l.
white tendo calcaneus l.
Z-slide l.
length-tension curve
Lenox
L. bucket
L. Hill derotational knee brace
L. Hill knee orthosis
L. Hill Spectralite knee brace
lens
Nikon SMZ 2T magnifying l.
lenticular bone
lenticularis
dystonia l.
lentigo
l. maligna
l. maligna melanoma
l.'s (multiple), electrocardiographic abnormalities, ocular hypertelorism, pulmonary stenosis, abnormalities of genitalia, retardation of growth, and deafness (sensorineural) (LEOPARD)
Lentulo spiral drill
Leo Bathlifter
Leone expansion screw
LEOPARD
lentigines (multiple), electrocardiographic abnormalities, ocular hypertelorism,

NOTES

L

LEOPARD *(continued)*
    pulmonary stenosis, abnormalities of
    genitalia, retardation of growth, and
    deafness (sensorineural)
    LEOPARD syndrome
Lepird procedure
L'Episcopo hip reconstruction
L'Episcopo-Zachary procedure
leptopodia
**Lequesne Severity of Osteoarthritis
  Index**
Lere bone mill
Leri
    L. disease
    L. pleonosteosis
    L. sign
    L. syndrome
Leriche syndrome
Leri-Weill
    L.-W. disease
    L.-W. syndrome
Lerman
    L. hinge brace
    L. multiligamentous knee control
      orthosis
    L. noninvasive halo
Lerman-Minerva collar
LeRoy clip-applying forceps
lesion
    acute traumatic l.
    ALPSA l.
    articular cartilage l.
    atlantoaxial l.
    Bankart shoulder l.
    Bennett l.
    biceps interval l. (BIL)
    bone surface l.
    bony l.
    Brown-Séquard l.
    bubbly bone l.
    callosal l.
    cartilaginous l.
    chiropractic l.
    cleavage l.
    cyclops l.
    cystic bone l.
    desmoid l.
    destructive articular l.
    disk l.
    DREZ l.
    Essex-Lopresti l.
    expansile l.
    fibrous l.
    HAGL l.
    hamartomatous l.
    Hill-Sachs l.
    hyperkeratotic l.
    impingement l.

intramedullary l.
irregular-shaped l.
irritable l.
ischemic l.
juxtaarticular l.
Keasbey l.
Kidner l.
kissing l.'s
labral l.
lytic bone l.
meniscoid l.
metastatic bone l.
Monteggia equivalent l.
Morel-Lavele l.
morphea-like l.
muscular l.
nail bed l.
neoplastic l.
nerve root l.
neuromechanical l.
nonlinear l.
Nora l.
occult talar l.
Osgood-Schlatter l.
osseous l.
osteoblastic l.
osteocartilaginous l.
osteochondral l.
osteopathic l.
paraosseous l.
parosteal l.
pedal hyperpigmented l.
Perthes l.
Perthes-Bankart l.
polyostotic bone l.
posterior-superior humeral head l.
postfracture l.
pseudoneoplastic l.
retroacetabular l.
reverse Bankart l.
reverse Hill-Sachs l.
rotator cuff l.
Sinding-Larsen-Johansson l.
SLAP l.
soft tissue l.
Stener l.
striatal l.
subchondral l.
superior labrum anterior and
  posterior l.
transfer l.
transient l.
traumatic, unidirectional instability
  and Bankart l.
tuberculous l.
uncommitted metaphysial l.
upper motor neuron l.
vertebral l.

Wolin meniscoid l.
Woofry-Chandler classification of
Osgood-Schlatter l.
Wrisberg l.
Leslie-Ryan anterior axillary approach
LESS
lateral electrical surface stimulation
lesser
l. metatarsal
l. metatarsophalangeal joint
l. multangular
l. multangular bone
l. pelvis
l. rhomboid muscle
l. tarsal arthrodesis
l. tarsus cavus
l. toe
l. trochanter
l. trochanter fracture
l. tuberosity
Lester muscle forceps
Letournel
L. guideline
L. plate
Letournel-Judet
L.-J. acetabular fracture
classification
L.-J. approach
leukocyte scan
LeukoScan
Leukotape
L. P Combo Pack taping kit
L. P sportstape
Leung thumb loss classification
levator
l. ani group
l. scapulae muscle
l. scapulae syndrome
level
comfort l.
l. foundation
long and short l.
myoinositol l.
segmental l.
sorbitol l.
spinal l.
vertebral l.
leveling
joint l.
lever
l. arm
Lane bone l.

levering
Levin drill guide
Levine
L. Drennan angle
L. orthopedic outcomes
questionnaire
L. patellar tendon strap
Levis arm splint
levoscoliosis scoliosis
Levy & Rappel foot orthosis
Lewin
L. bone-holding clamp
L. bone-holding forceps
L. bunion dissector
L. collar
L. finger splint
L. punch test
L. reverse Lasègue test
L. snuff test
L. spinal perforating forceps
L. standing test
L. supine test
Lewin-Gaenslen test
Lewin-Stern
L.-S. finger splint
L.-S. thumb splint
Lewis
L. expandable adjustable prosthesis
(LEAP)
L. intercalary resection
L. nail
L. periosteal elevator
L. periosteal rasp
L. Trapezio prosthesis
Lewis-Chekofsky resection
Lewis-Prusik test
Lewit stretch technique
Lexan jacket
Lexer
L. chisel
L. gouge
L. osteotome
Lex-Ton spinal frame
Leyden-Möbius muscular dystrophy
Leyla
L. arm
L. bar
LFAC
low-frequency alternating current
LFIT
low-friction ion treatment
L-frame fixator

L

NOTES

LH1000 arthroscopic legholder
Lhermitte sign
liability
    ergonomic assessment of risk
      and l. (EARLY)
LIAD
    low-impact aerobic dance
liberator elevator
liberty
    L. CMC thumb brace
    L. One splint
    L. spinal system
LICA
    laser image custom arthroplasty
lichen
    l. nitidus
    l. planus
Lichtblau
    L. osteotomy
    L. tenotomy
Lichtman
    L. aseptic necrosis classification
    L. disease
    L. staging
    L. technique
    L. test
Lidge cement gun
Lido
    L. Active Multijoint System
    L. isokinetic dynamometer
    L. lift
    L. lift and work set
    L. Passive Multijoint System
    L. WorkSET work simulator
Lidoback isokinetic dynamometry
system
Lido-Gel
Liebolt radioulnar technique
life
    Diabetic Quality of L.
    L. Liner stick and cut-resistant
      glove
    quality of l.
    L. Satisfaction Index (LSI)
LIFEC
    lumbar intersomatic fusion expandable
      cage
LifeGait partial weightbearing therapy
device
Lifeline Wall Gym 2000 fitness system
lifestyle
    l. education (LSE)
    sedentary l.
lift
    BTE dynamic l.
    Calypso l.
    chiropractic laser nonsurgical
      face l.

    dead l.
    heel l.
    Hoyer l.
    Lido l.
    M/L l.
    shoe l.
    squat l.
    VuRyser monitor l.
LiftALERT
lift-off
    foot l.
    l. of heel in walk
    l. test
    tibial l.
    varus-valgus l.
LiftStation
Ligaclip applier
ligament
    accessory atlantoaxial l.
    accessory collateral l.
    accessory lateral collateral l.
    acromioclavicular l.
    acromiocoracoid l.
    adipose l.
    alar l.
    allograft reconstruction of fibular
      collateral l.
    ankle inferior transverse l.
    anterior collateral l.
    anterior cruciate l. (ACL)
    anterior fibular l.
    anterior-inferior tibiofibular l.
    anterior longitudinal l. (ALL)
    anterior medial ankle l.
    anterior meniscofemoral l.
    anterior oblique l. (AOL)
    anterior sacrococcygeal l.
    anterior sacroiliac l.
    anterior talofibular l. (ATFL)
    anterior talotibial l.
    anterior tibiofibular l.
    anterior tibiotalar l.
    anteroinferior glenohumeral l.
    anteromedial glenohumeral l.
    anterosuperior glenohumeral l.
    anular l.
    apical dental l.
    arcuate popliteal l.
    artificial l.
    atlantal transverse l.
    atlantoaxial l.
    atlantooccipital l.
    l. augmentation device (LAD)
    avulsed l.
    l. avulsion
    Barkow l.
    beak l.
    Bertin l.

Bichat l.
bifurcate l.
Bigelow l.
Bourgery l.
Brodie l.
Burns l.
l. button
calcaneoastragaloid l.
calcaneoclavicular l.
calcaneocuboid l.
calcaneofibular l. (CFL)
calcaneonavicular l.
calcaneotibial l.
Caldani l.
Campbell l.
capital l.
capsular l.
carpal l.
carpometacarpal l.
CC l.
cervical mover l.
CH l.
checkrein l.
Chrisman-Snook reconstruction of ankle l.
Civinini l.
l. clamp
Cleland l.
collateral fibular l.
collateral radial l.
collateral tibial l.
collateral ulnar l.
Colles l.
congenital laxity of l.
conoid l.
coracoacromial l.
coracoclavicular l.
coracohumeral l.
coronary l.
corporotransverse inferior l.
corporotransverse superior l.
costoclavicular l.
costotransverse l.
cruciate l.
Cruveilhier l.
cuboideonavicular l.
cuneonavicular l.
DATT l.
DCC l.
deltoid l.
deltotrapezius fascial l.
dentate l.

dorsoradial l. (DRL)
DPTT l.
dural l.
l. elongation
extraarticular knee l.
extracapsular l.
extrinsic l.
fabellofibular l.
falciform l.
fibular collateral l. (FCL)
fibular sesamoidal l.
fibulocalcaneal l.
fibulotalar l.
fibulotalocalcaneal l.
first intermetacarpal l.
flaval l.
floating l.
fracture-dislocation with anterior l.
FTC l.
Gerdy l.
glenohumeral l. (GHL)
Gore-Tex anterior cruciate l.
Grayson l.
Haines-McDougall medial sesamoid l.
hamate l.
hamatometacarpal l.
Henle l.
l. of Henry
humeral avulsion of the glenohumeral l. (HAGL)
Humphry l.
hypertrophic l.
iliofemoral l.
iliolumbar l.
iliopatellar l.
iliotrochanteric l.
inferior band cruciform l.
inferior calcaneonavicular l. (ICN)
inferior glenohumeral l. (IGHL)
inferior ilioischial l.
infrapatellar l.
inguinal l.
intercarpal l.
interclavicular l.
interdigital l.
intermetacarpal l. (IML)
intermetatarsal l.
International Knee L.
interosseous cuneocuboid l.
interosseous cuneometatarsal l.
interosseous intercuneiform l.

L

NOTES

ligament *(continued)*

interosseous talocalcaneal l. (ITCL)
intersesamoid l.
interspinal l.
interspinous l.
intertransverse l.
intervolar plate l.
intraarticular disk l.
intraosseous tibiofibular l.
ischiofemoral l.
lacinate l.
Landsmeer l.
lateral atlantooccipital l.
lateral collateral l. (LCL)
lateral talocalcaneal l. (LTC)
LCC l.
limited proteoglycan matrix of l.
Lisfranc l.
long calcaneocuboid l.
longitudinal l.
long plantar l. (LPL)
LRL l.
LT l.
lumbocostal l.
lunotriquetral l.
medial collateral l. (MCL)
medial patellofemoral l. (MPFL)
medial ulnar collateral l. (MUCL)
meniscofemoral l.
meniscotibial l.
metacarpal l.
metacarpoglenoidal l.
metacarpophalangeal l.
metatarsal l.
metatarsosesamoid l.
middle glenohumeral l. (MGHL)
midline l.
natatory l.
navicular cuneiform l.
naviculocuneiform l.
nuchal l.
oblique popliteal l.
oblique retinacular l.
olecranon l.
orbicular l.
ossification of the posterior
   longitudinal l. (OPLL)
patellar l.
patellofemoral l.
patellomeniscal l.
patellotibial l.
petroclinoid l.
pisiform metacarpal l.
pisohamate l.
pisometacarpal l.
popliteal l.
posterior cruciate l. (PCL)
posterior inferior tibiofibular l.

posterior longitudinal l. (PLL)
posterior oblique l. (POL)
posterior talofibular l. (PTFL)
pubocapsular l.
pubofemoral l.
quadrate l.
radial collateral l. (RCL)
radiocapitate l.
radiocarpal l.
radiolunotriquetral l.
radioscaphocapitate l.
radioscaphoid l.
radioscapholunate l.
radiotriquetral l.
rearfoot l.
l. reconstruction
l. replacement
retinacular l.
rhomboid l.
Robert l.
round l.
Rouviere l.
l. rupture sprain
sacrococcygeal l.
sacroiliac l.
sacrospinal l.
sacrospinous l.
sacrotuberal l.
sacrotuberous l.
scapholunate interosseous l.
scaphotrapezoid interosseous l.
scapular l.
scapulohumeral l.
SCC l.
sesamoid l.
sesamophalangeal l.
short calcaneocuboid l.
short plantar l. (SPL)
spinal posterior l.
spinal transverse l.
spiral oblique retinacular l.
spring l.
SRL l.
sternoclavicular l.
sternocostal l.
l. of Struthers
STT l.
subtalar interosseous l.
superior costotransverse l.
superomedial calcaneonavicular l.
supraspinous l.
syndesmotic l.
talocalcaneal l.
talofibular l.
talonavicular l.
tarsometatarsal l.
l. of tarsus
tectoral l.

tendinotrochanteric l.
tibial collateral l. (TCL)
tibial sesamoid l.
tibiocalcaneal l.
tibiofibular l.
tibionavicular l.
torn l.
trapezoid l.
traumatized l.
triangular l.
ulnar carpal collateral l.
ulnar collateral l. (UCL)
ulnocarpal l.
ulnolunate l.
ulnotriquetral l.
vaginal hand l.
vertebropelvic l.
Weitbrecht l.
l. of Wrisberg
yellow l.
Zenotech biomaterial-synthetic l.

ligament-bone
bone-patellar l.-b. (BPB)
l.-b. complex

ligamentoplasty
ligamentotaxis
multiplanar l.

ligamentous
l. ankylosis
l. anterior dislocation (LAD)
l. anterior dislocation composite graft
l. attachment
l. bouncing
l. box
l. and capsular repair (LCR)
l. complex
l. control brace
l. disruption
l. injury
l. insertion
l. instability test
l. insufficiency
l. laxity
l. luxation
l. release
l. stability
l. structure
l. support tissue
l. thickening
l. weave procedure

ligamentous-muscular hypertrophy

ligament-scar matrix
ligamentum bifurcatum
Ligamentus
L. Ankle ankle orthotic
L. Ankle orthosis

ligand adhesive
ligature
l. carrier
l. guide
l. passer
stick tie l.

light
l. cast
Cogent l.
l. conductor
l. cross-slot screwdriver
infrared l. (IR)
l. intensity training
l. microscopy
l. source
therapeutic l.
l. touch sensation
l. touch test
ultraviolet l.
L. V sign

Lightplast athletic tape
LIH
Lars Ingvar Hansson
LIH hook pin

Lilienthal rib spreader
Lima external fixator
limb
l. absence
l. accurate measurement (LAM)
artificial l.
l. ataxia
l. brace
l. bud
congenitally short l.
l. girdle
l. gym
hanging of l.
l. holder
ischemic l.
left lower l. (LLL)
left upper l. (LUL)
l. length
l. length angulation
l. length discrepancy
l. lengthening
phantom l.
plantigrade l.

L

NOTES

limb *(continued)*
    posture of l.
    l. replantation
    residual l.
    right lower l. (RLL)
    right upper l. (RUL)
    l. salvage
    seal l.
    l. synergy
    Trow Bridge TerraRound sports l.
    Utah artificial l.
Limberg flap
limb-girdle
    l.-g. lengthening
    l.-g. muscular dystrophy
limb-girdle-trunk paresis
limb-length disparity
limb-salvage
    l.-s. procedure
    l.-s. surgery
limb-sparing operation
limbus annulare
limit
    elastic l.
    endurance l.
    metal endurance l.
    motion l.
    within functional l.'s (WFL)
limitation
    motion l.
    l. of motion (LOM)
    l. of movement
limited
    l. compression-dynamic compression
      plate
    l. fasciectomy
    l. intertarsal arthrodesis
    l. joint mobility (LJM)
    l. motion metal ankle joint
    l. performance measure
    l. proteoglycan matrix of ligament
limited-contact dynamic compression
  plate
limiter
    Becker 655 motion control l.
    motion control l.
limiting condition
limitus
    bony hallux l.
    cartilaginous hallux l.
    McKeever arthrodesis for hallux l.
    Regnauld free phalangeal base
      autograft for hallux l.
    Z-slide lengthening in hallux l.
limp
    antalgic l.
    new-onset l.
    Trendelenburg l.

LINAC
    linear accelerator
    Boston LINAC
    University of Florida LINAC
Linberg syndrome
Lindell classification
Lindeman
    L. bur
    L. procedure
Lindermann bur
Linder sign
Lindgren oblique osteotomy
Lindholm
    L. Achilles lengthening procedure
    L. open surgical tendon repair
    L. technique
    L. tendo calcaneus repair
Lindseth osteotomy
Lindsjö method
Lindvall-Stille knife
line
    acetabular l.
    AC-PC l.
    action l.
    anterior axillary l. (AAL)
    anterior humeral l.
    anterior spinal l.
    antitension l.
    Beau l.
    bisector l.
    Blumensaat l.
    Bryant l.
    cement l.
    Chamberlain l.
    Chopart joint l.
    cleavage l.
    coronoid l.
    cyma l.
    l. of demarcation
    divisionary l.
    Duhot l.
    Dupuytren and Langer skin
      tension l.
    epiphysial l.
    Feiss l.
    femoral head l. (FHL)
    fracture l.
    Fränkel white l.
    gait l.
    George l.
    gravitational l.
    gravity l.
    l. of gravity
    growth arrest l.
    Harris growth arrest l.
    Harris hip l.
    Hawkins l.
    Hilgenreiner horizontal Y l.

Hilgenreiner-Pauwels l.
Hilgenreiner-Perkins l.
H-P l.
Hueter l.
iliopectineal l.
interteardrop l.
joint l.
Kaplan oblique l.
Kilian l.
Kline l.
Köhler l.
Langer l.
lateral joint l.
lead l.
Looser l.
lumbar gravitational l.
MacNab l.
Maquet l.
McGregor l.
McRae l.
Meary l.
medial joint l.
Meyer l.
Meyerding spondylolisthesis
  classification l.
midaxillary l. (MAL)
midheel l.
midmalleolar l.
midsternal l. (MSL)
Moloney l.
Moyer l.
Nélaton l.
oblique metacarpal l.
obturator/brim l.
odontoid perpendicular l.
Ogston l.
Ombredanne-Perkins l.
parajugular l.
parallel pitch l.'s
Perkins vertical l.
physial l.
plumb l.
posterior axillary l. (PAL)
posterior cervical l.
radiocapitellar l.
radiolucent l.
relaxed skin tension l.
Roser l.
Roser-Nélaton l.
sacral arcuate l.
sacral horizontal plane l. (SHPL)
sacroiliac l.

sacroiliac symphysis l.
Schoemaker l.
sclerotic l.
scurvy l.
Shenton l.
Skinner l.
spinolaminar l.
Sydney l.
teardrop l.
tibiofibular l.
trapezoid l.
trough l.
Trümmerfeld l.
Ullmann l.
Wagner l.
Wegner l.
Whitesides l.
Winberger l.
Y l.
Z l.
l. of Zahn

linea
l. aspera femoris
l. semilunaris
Lineage acetabular cup
linear
l. accelerator (LINAC)
l. amputation
l. analog pain scale
l. capsulotomy
l. fraction
l. fracture
L. hip stem
l. osteotomy
l. potentiometer
l. scar
L. total hip system
linear-variable-differential transducer
linebacker's arm
linen suture
liner
acetabular prosthetic l.
Alpha cushion l.
Alps CustomPro custom l.
bone l.
cast l.
cushion shoe l.
DePuy acetabular l.
Duraloc acetabular l.
elevated rim acetabular l.
Enduron acetabular l.
Fillauer prosthesis l.

NOTES

liner *(continued)*
    Fillauer silicone suction l.
    Fillauer silicone suspension l.
    Gore-Tex waterproof cast l.
    grommet bone l.
    Hylamer acetabular l.
    Hylamer enhanced ultra-high
      molecular weight polyethylene
      acetabular l.
    Iceross Comfort Plus silicone
      gel l.
    Medium-Plus alpha l.
    l. micromotion
    OrthoGel l.
    Plastizote shoe l.
    polyethylene l.
    Polysorb l.
    Reflection l.
    SiloLiner gel l.
    Spenco l.
    splint l.
    TEC l.
    USMC luxury l.
line-to-line reaming technique
Ling
    L. cemented hip prosthesis
    L. method
lingism
lingual
    l. artery
    l. vein
lining
    DePuy acetabular l.
    Thermold heat moldable shoe l.
link
    L. anatomical hip
    L. custom partial pelvis
      replacement system
    L. Endo-Model rotational knee
      prosthesis
    L. Endo-Model rotational knee
      system
    L. Lubinus SP II hip replacement
      system
    L. MP hip noncemented
      reconstruction prosthesis
    L. MP microporous hip stem
    musculotendinous-osseous l.
    L. Orthopaedics device
    L. Saddle Prosthesis Endo-Model
      hip replacement system
    L. Stack Split Splint
    L. toe splint
linkage
    kinematic l.
    rod l.
linked potential

lint-free drape
Linton procedure
Linvatec
    L. absorbable screw
    L. arthroscopic infusion pump
    L. bone anchor
    L. driver
    L. product
Lionberger-Bishop-Tullos anterior
   arthrodesis
lion forceps
lion-jaw forceps
lip
    l. of acetabulum
    l. of glenoid
    l. of navicular
    osteophytic bone l.
    posterior l.
    l. of taenia
    l. of tibia
lipid
    l. inclusion cyst
    l. tumor
lipoarthritis
lipoblastomatosis
lipocalcinogranulomatosis
lipochondrodystrophy
lipofibroma
    intraneural l.
lipofibromatosis
lipofibromatous hamartoma
lipohemarthrosis
lipoma
    endovaginal l.
    intraosseous l.
    pleomorphic l.
    spindle cell l.
lipomatosis
    intraosseous l.
lipomeningocele
liposarcoma
    myxoid l.
    myxoid-type l.
    pleomorphic l.
    round cell l.
    round cell-type l.
    well-differentiated myxoid l.
lipping
Lippman
    L. hip prosthesis
    L. screw
    L. test
Lipscomb
    L. metatarsophalangeal arthrodesis
    L. modified McKeever arthrodesis
    L. procedure
    L. technique

Lipscomb-Anderson
    L.-A. drill guide
    L.-A. procedure
liquid
    l. cable
    l. crystal thermography (LCT)
    l. nitrogen cryotherapy
Lisch nodule
Lisfranc
    L. amputation
    L. arthrodesis
    L. articular interline
    L. articular set angle (LASA)
    L. below-knee prosthesis
    L. disarticulation
    L. dislocation
    L. fracture
    L. fracture-dislocation
    L. injury
    L. joint
    L. joint articulation
    L. joint complex
    L. ligament
    L. operation
    L. tubercle
Lissauer zone
list
    postural l.
Lister
    L. corn
    L. technique
    L. technique of pulley
      reconstruction
    L. tubercle
listhesis
    anterior-posterior l.
    lateral l.
listing
    dynamic l.
    l. gait
    static l.
Liston
    L. amputating knife
    L. bone-cutting forceps
    L. bone rongeur
    L. operation
    L. phalangeal knife
    L. shears
    L. splint
Liston-Key bone-cutting forceps
Liston-Key-Horsley rib shears

Liston-Littauer
    L.-L. bone-cutting forceps
    L.-L. rongeur
Liston-Stille bone-cutting forceps
**LiteGait partial weight-bearing gait
  therapy device**
lithotomy
    l. legholder
    l. position
Litt
    cloth tape occlusion method of L.
Littauer-Liston bone-cutting forceps
Littauer-West rongeur
litter
    Neal-Robertson l.
Littig strut
little
    L. cargo vest
    l. finger
    L. Leaguer's elbow
    L. Leaguer's shoulder
    L. release
    L. syndrome
    L. technique
Littler
    L. operation
    L. opponensplasty
    L. pollicization
    L. technique
    wing excision of L.
Littler-Cooley
    L.-C. abductor digiti quinti transfer
    L.-C. muscle transfer
    L.-C. technique
livedo reticularis
Liverpool
    L. elbow prosthesis
    L. knee prosthesis
live splint
living
    activity of daily l. (ADL)
    center for independent l. (CIL)
    extended activities of daily l.
      (EADL)
    instrumental activities of daily l.
      (IADL)
    Katz index of activities of daily l.
Livingstone therapy
Livingston intramedullary bar
Liviscope scope
Lizzie doll

L

NOTES

LJM
limited joint mobility
LLC
long leg cast
LLD
leg length discrepancy
LLE
left lower extremity
LLI
leg length inequality
LLL
left lower limb
lower fossa active, lateral knee pain, and long leg on the side ipsilateral to the weak fossa
LLO
lower limb orthosis
Llorente dissecting forceps
Lloyd
L. adapter
L. adapter for Smith-Petersen nail
L. chiropractic table
L. nail driver
Lloyd-Roberts
L.-R. fracture
L.-R. fracture technique
Lloyd-Roberts-Catteral-Salamon classification
LLP
lower limb prosthesis
LLPS
low-load prolonged stretch
low-pressure plasma spray
LLPS hydroxyapatite
LLPS hydroxyapatite adhesive
LLS
long leg splint
LLWBC
long leg weightbearing cast
LLWC
long leg walking cast
LMB
LMB finger splint
LMB wire-foam economical resting splint
LMIS
AOFAS Lesser Metatarsophalangeal-Interphalangeal Scale
LMJA
longitudinal midtarsal joint axis
L'Nard
L. boot
L. Multi Podus orthosis
L. thoracolumbosacral orthosis
LNS
localized nodular synovitis
LNV
last normal vertebra

Lo
L. Bak spinal support
L. Rider prosthetic foot
load
applied l.
axial compression l.
l. beam
bending l.
compression l.
critical l.
Euler l.
ramp l.
rotatory l.
l. and shift test
spinal axial l.
torque l.
torsional l.
load-and-shift maneuver
load-bearing graft
load-deflection curve
load-deformation curve
load-displacement
l.-d. curve
l.-d. plot
loading
arch l.
axial l.
compression l.
concentric l.
cyclic l.
eccentric l.
Edwards modular system dynamic l.
fat l.
fracture callus l.
functional and anatomic l. (FAL)
l. mode
progressive l.
status l.
sustained l.
tension l.
l. time
vertical l.
load-sharing classification
load-to-grip displacement
Loban adhesive drape
Lobstein
L. disease
L. syndrome
lobster-claw
l.-c. deformity
l.-c. foot
l.-c. hand
lobster-type clamp
local
l. adaptation syndrome (LAS)
l. cavus

l. compression fracture
l. decompression fracture
l. epineurotomy
l. flap
l. radical resection
l. standby anesthesia
l. standby anesthesia technique
Localio-Francis-Rossano resection
Localio procedure
localization
pedicle l.
localized
l. bone destruction
l. nodular synovitis (LNS)
l. nodular tenosynovitis
localizer cast
locating pin
location
cervical sympathetic chain l.
pedicle l.
locator
Berman-Moorhead metal l.
metal l.
lock
Ball knee l.
l. finger
grip l.
heel l.
knee l.
lateral spring-loaded l.
spring-loaded knee l.
VariLock socket l.
lockable arthroscopic knot
Locke
L. bone clamp
L. elevator
locked
l. facet
l. intramedullary osteosynthesis
l. intramedullary osteosynthesis pin
l. knee
l. nailing
l. scapula
Lockhart toe splint
locking
anatomic medullary l. (AML)
l. clamp
l. disk
distal l.
l. hook instrumentation
l. horizontal mattress suture
l. of joint

l. loop
l. nail
l. nut
l. peg
l. pliers
l. prosthesis
proximal l.
sacroiliac joint l.
l. screw
locking-hook spinal rod
locking-position test
locking-suture technique
lockjaw
locknut wrench
lockout suture
locomotion
locomotor
l. ataxia
l. mechanism
l. pattern
l. system
Loeffler-Ballard incision
Lofstrand
L. brace
L. crutch
log
Fin & Flipper exercise l.
motor activity l.
Logan traction
logrolling maneuver
Lok-it screwdriver
Lok-screw double-slot screwdriver
LOM
limitation of motion
loss of motion
London unconstrained elbow prosthesis
Lone Star retractor system
long
l. alignment rod
l. arm brace
l. arm cast (LAC)
l. arm finger cast
l. arm splint
l. axial alignment guide
l. axis
l. axis of bone
l. axis ray
l. axis traction chiropractic table
L. Beach pedicle screw
l. bent-knee leg cast
l. bone deficiency
l. bone fracture

L

NOTES

long *(continued)*
- l. bone osteomyelitis
- l. calcaneocuboid (LCC)
- l. calcaneocuboid ligament
- l. coarse bur
- l. curette
- l. deltopectoral approach
- l. extensor
- l. external rotator
- l. fibular muscle
- l. finger
- l. head
- l. head biceps tendon
- l. leg cast (LLC)
- l. leg hinged brace
- l. leg immobilizer
- l. leg orthosis
- l. leg splint (LLS)
- l. leg stockings
- l. leg walking cast (LLWC)
- l. leg weightbearing cast (LLWBC)
- l. nail-mounted drill guide
- l. oblique fracture
- l. opponens orthosis
- l. plantar ligament (LPL)
- l. posterior flap
- l. radiolunate (LRL)
- l. segment spinal fusion
- l. and short level
- l. stem (LS)
- l. thoracic nerve injury
- l. thoracic nerve palsy
- l. toe flexor
- l. tract sign

Longevity V-Lign hip prosthesis
longissimus colli muscle
longitudinal
- l. axis
- l. blood supply
- l. deficiency
- l. displaced complete tear
- l. distraction
- l. epiphysial bracket
- l. fracture
- l. incision
- l. incomplete intrameniscal tear
- l. ligament
- l. ligament rupture
- l. member to anchor connector
- l. member to longitudinal member connector
- l. meniscal tear
- l. midtarsal joint axis (LMJA)
- l. plantar arch
- l. ridge
- l. spinal bar
- l. split tear

- l. tendon split
- l. traction

long-jaw basket forceps
long-latency somatosensory evoked potential
long-leg arthropathy
long-radius kyphosis
long-stemmed powered bur
long-term bone-instrumentation interface
longus
- abductor pollicis l. (APL)
- adductor hallucis l.
- l. capitis muscle
- l. cervicis (colli) muscle
- l. colli muscle
- extensor carpi radialis l. (ECRL)
- extensor digitorum l. (EDL)
- extensor hallucis l. (EHL)
- extensor pollicis l. (EPL)
- flexor digitorum l. (FDL)
- flexor hallucis l. (FHL)
- flexor pollicis l. (FPL)
- palmaris l. (PL)
- peroneus l.

loop
- Bunnell finger l.
- l. circumferential wire
- Duncan l.
- figure-of-eight wire l.
- finger l.
- l. fixation
- l. & hook strapping
- locking l.
- perineal l.
- Ransford l.
- l. scissors
- thumb l.
- toe l.
- wire l.

loop-lock cock-up splint
loop-over wrap
loose
- l. body grasper
- l. cartilage
- l. debris
- l. fracture
- l. fragment
- l. joint body
- l. knee procedure
- L. procedure
- l. shoulder

loosening
- acetabular component l.
- aseptic l.
- Harris criteria for implant l.
- screw l.
- sterile l.

looser
  L. line
  L. zone in insufficiency fracture
Looser-Milkman syndrome
Lo-Por vascular graft prosthesis
LOPS
  loss of protective sensation
Lord
  L. cup
  L. Press-Fit hip prosthesis
  L. total hip arthrodesis
Lordex lumbar spine system
lordoscoliosis
lordosis
  cervical l.
  compensatory l.
  l. creation
  dorsal l.
  lumbar spine l.
  occipitocervical l.
  l. preservation
  reversal of cervical l.
  thoracic spine l.
lordotic
  l. curve
  l. pelvis
lordoticiser
  Posture Pump l.
Lorenz
  L. brace
  L. cast
  L. hip reduction
  L. operation
  L. osteosynthesis system
  L. osteotomy
  L. procedure
  L. sign
Lorenzo screw
Lore suction tube and tip-holding forceps
lorgnette
  main en l.
lorry driver's fracture
LOS
  length of stay
Losee
  L. knee instability test
  L. modification
  L. modification of MacIntosh technique
  L. sling and reef technique

loss
  blood l.
  bone l.
  l. of correction
  estimated blood l.
  functional l.
  heat l.
  lumbar lordosis iatrogenic l.
  l. of motion (LOM)
  motor l.
  periprosthetic bone l.
  postmenopausal bone l.
  l. of protective sensation (LOPS)
  segmental bone l.
  sensory l.
Loth-Kirschner drill
lotion
  Biotone Polar l.
  Criticaid l.
  Senuva l.
Lottes
  L. nailing
  L. pin
  L. triflanged medullary nail
lotus
  l. position
  L. unicompartment prosthesis
Loughheed and White procedure
Louis
  L. instrumentation
  L. plate
Louisiana
  L. ankle wrap technique
  L. State University (LSU)
  L. State University Medical Center (LSUMC)
loupe
  binocular l.
  l. magnification
  magnifying l.
  surgical l.
love
  L. nerve root retractor
  L. splint
Love-Adson periosteal elevator
Love-Gruenwald alligator forceps
Love-Kerrison rongeur forceps
Lovell clubfoot cast
Lovett
  L. clinical scale of strength
  L. test
Lovibond angle

NOTES

loving
    L. Comfort maternity support
    L. Comfort postpartum support
Lovitt-Uhler modification of Jewett post-fusion brace
low
    l. back injury
    l. back neurosis
    l. back pain (LBP)
    L. Back Pain Symptom Checklist
    l. bone mass
    l. cervical approach
    l. impedance thermocouple
    l. lumbar spine fracture
    l. median-low ulnar palsy
    L. Profile legholder
    L. Profile plastic body jacket
    l. quarter Blucher shoe
    l. single thoracic curve
    l. T humerus fracture
    l. viscosity bone cement
low-air-loss bed
low-arch foot
low-assimilation pelvis
low-contact
    l.-c. dynamic compression plate
    l.-c. stress (LCS)
    l.-c. stress semiconstrained prosthesis
LowDye
    L. strapping
    L. taping
    L. taping technique
Lowe-Breck
    L.-B. cartilage knife
    L.-B. meniscectomy knife
Lowell
    L. reduction
    L. view
Lowe-Miller unconstrained elbow prosthesis
low-energy
    l.-e. fracture
    l.-e. laser (LEL)
Löwenstein view
lower
    l. cervical spine
    l. cervical spine fusion
    l. cervical spine posterior stabilization
    l. cervical spine procedure
    l. extremity (LE)
    l. extremity amputation (LEA)
    L. Extremity Functional Scale (LEFS)
    l. extremity noninvasive
    l. extremity prosthesis
    l. extremity surgery
    l. fossa active, lateral knee pain, and long leg on the side ipsilateral to the weak fossa (LLL)
    l. hand retractor
    l. hook trial
    l. limb dysmetria
    l. limb orthosis (LLO)
    l. limb prosthesis (LLP)
    l. lumbar spine
    l. nerve root compression
    l. plexus injury
    l. posterior lumbar spine and sacrum surgery
    l. sacral nerve root compression (LSNRC)
    l. thoracic pedicle
    l. thoracic spine
low-frequency alternating current (LFAC)
low-friction ion treatment (LFIT)
low-grade central osteogenic sarcoma
low-heeled shoe
low-impact aerobic dance (LIAD)
low-load prolonged stretch (LLPS)
Lowman
    L. balance board
    L. bone-holding clamp
    L. bone-holding forceps
    L. chisel
    L. hand retractor
    L. shelf procedure
Lowman-Gerster bone clamp
Lowman-Hoglund
    L.-H. chisel
    L.-H. clamp
low-neck femoral prosthesis
low-power laser
low-pressure
    l.-p. plasma spray (LLPS)
    l.-p. plasma-sprayed (LPPS)
low-profile
    l.-p. cup
    l.-p. dorsal plate
    l.-p. femoral prosthesis
    l.-p. halo traction
low-riding patella
low-set thumb
low-stress aerobic exercise
low-surface reactive
low-temperature plastic
low-tide walking brace
low-turnover osteoporosis
loxoscelism
loxotomy
LP
    lumbar puncture

LPF
    leg protection factor
LPL
    long plantar ligament
L-plate
        Synthes mini L-p.
LPPS
    low-pressure plasma-sprayed
    LPPS hydroxyapatite fixation
LRL
    long radiolunate
    LRL ligament
L-rod
        Luque L-r.
LRS
    lateral recess stenosis
LS
    long stem
    lumbosacral
LS⁴ custom spinal jacket
LSE
    lifestyle education
L-shaped
        L-s. capsular incision
        L-s. capsulotomy
        L-s. osteotomy
        L-s. plate
        L-s. rod
        L-s. rotator cuff tear
LSI
    Life Satisfaction Index
    LSI Easy Stims self-adhesive
        electrode
    LSI silver self-adhesive disposable
        electrode
LSNRC
    lower sacral nerve root compression
LSO
    lumbosacral orthosis
LSU
    Louisiana State University
        LSU reciprocation-gait orthosis
        LSU reciprocation-gait orthosis
        brace
        LSU reciprocator
LSUMC
    Louisiana State University Medical
        Center
        LSUMC classification of motor
        and sensory function
LT
    lactate threshold

    lunotriquetral
        LT joint
        LT ligament
LTC
    lateral talocalcaneal ligament
Lubinus
        L. acetabular component
        L. AP hip system
        L. knee prosthesis
        L. SP II anatomically adapted hip
        system
Lucae bone mallet
Lucas
        L. chisel
        L. and Drucker Motor Index
        L. gouge
Lucas-Cottrell
        L.-C. operation
        L.-C. osteotomy
Lucas-Murray knee arthrodesis
lucency
        cortical l.
        subchondral l.
        syndesmosis screw l.
lucent
luck
        L. bone drill
        L. hand procedure
        L. hip cup
        L. nail
        L. operation
Luck-Bishop bone saw
Ludington
        L. sign
        L. test
Ludloff
        L. bunionectomy
        L. incision
        L. medial approach
        L. operation
        L. osteotomy
        L. sign
        L. technique
Ludovici angle
Ludwig
        L. angle
        L. plane
LUE
    left upper extremity
Luekens wrinkle test

L

NOTES

Luer
    L. bone rongeur
    L. rongeur forceps
Luer-Friedman bone rongeur
Luer-Hartmann rongeur
Luer-Whiting rongeur forceps
Luhr
    L. fixation system
    L. Microfixation cranial plate
    L. Microfixation System drill bit
    L. Microfixation System plate
    cutter
    L. Microfixation System plate-
    holding forceps
    L. Microfixation System pliers
    L. microplate
    L. miniplate
    L. pan plate
    L. screw
LUL
    left upper limb
Lulu clamp
lumbago
    ischemic l.
lumbago-mechanical instability syndrome
lumbar
    l. abscess
    l. accessory movement technique
    l. agenesis
    l. anesthesia
    l. anterior-root stimulator implant
    (LARSI)
    l. brace
    l. canal
    l. disk
    l. diskography
    l. distraction manipulation
    l. epidural endoscopy
    l. extension
    l. extension test
    l. facet injection
    l. fascia
    l. flat back syndrome
    l. gravitational line
    l. intersomatic fusion expandable
    cage (LIFEC)
    l. kyphosis
    l. lateral flexion
    l. lateral flexion test
    l. lordosis iatrogenic loss
    l. lordosis preservation
    l. lordotic curve
    l. microtrauma
    l. nerve root injection
    l. pedicle
    l. pedicle fixation
    l. pedicle marker
    l. pedicle screw

    l. plexus injury
    l. protective mechanism test
    l. puncture (LP)
    l. range of motion
    l. reflex
    l. region
    l. roll
    l. rotation
    l. rotation test
    l. sagittal mobility
    l. scoliosis
    l. spine
    l. spine biopsy
    l. spine burst fracture
    l. spine decompression
    l. spine fusion
    l. spine instability
    l. spine instrumentation
    l. spine kyphotic deformity
    l. spine lordosis
    l. spine model
    l. spine pedicle diameter
    l. spine rotational stability
    l. spine segmental fixation
    l. spine transpedicular fixation
    l. spine trauma
    l. spine vertebral osteosynthesis
    l. spondylosis
    l. support cushion
    l. sympathectomy
    l. sympathetic block
    l. thecoperitoneal shunt syndrome
    l. traction
    l. transforaminal epidural injection
    l. tumor
    l. vein
    l. vertebra
    l. vertebral interbody fusion
lumbarization
lumbocostal ligament
lumbodorsal
    l. fascia (LDF)
    l. support corset
Lumbo 90 home care traction system
lumbopelvic
    l. complex
    l. radiograph
lumbosacral (LS)
    l. brace
    l. cartilaginous system
    l. corset
    l. dislocation
    l. flexion
    l. fusion
    l. fusion elevator
    l. joint
    l. joint angle
    l. junction

l. junction bone density
l. junction fracture
l. kyphosis
l. mechanical syndrome
l. orthosis (LSO)
l. plexus
l. radiculopathy
l. series
l. spine
l. spine transpedicular
   instrumentation
l. spondylolisthesis
l. traction
l. vertebra
Lumbotrain lumbosacral support
lumbrical
l. bar
l. intrinsic contracture
l. muscle
l. syndrome finger
l. tendon
lumbricalis muscle
lumbrical-plus
l.-p. finger
l.-p. phenomenon
Lumex
L. lightweight wheelchair
L. Tub-Guard safety rail
L. walker
lunate
l. acrylic cement wrist prosthesis
l. bone
l. dislocation
l. facet dye punch injury
l. fracture
l. sinus
lunatomalacia
lunatotriquetral coalition
Lunceford-Pilliar-Engh hip prosthesis
Lunceford total hip replacement
Lund
L. and Broden method
L. operation
L. prototype unicompartment
   prosthesis
Lundholm
L. plate
L. screw
lunocapitate
l. bone
l. joint
lunotriquetral (LT)

l. arthrodesis
l. dissociation
l. fusion
l. instability
l. ligament
l. shear test
lunula, pl. **lunulae**
Luongo hand retractor
lupus
l. anticoagulant
l. erythematosus (LE)
l. erythematosus preparation
Luque
L. cerclage wire
L. fixation device
L. II fixation system
L. instrumentation concave
   technique
L. instrumentation convex technique
L. loop fixation
L. L-rod
L. pedicle screw
L. II plate
L. rectangle
L. ring
L. rod
L. rod bender
L. rod fixation
L. rod fixation for kyphosis
L. rod migration
L. II screw
L. segmental fixation
L. II segmental spinal
   instrumentation
L. semirigid segmental spinal
   instrumentation
L. sublaminar wiring technique
L. wiring
Luque-Galveston
L.-G. fixation
L.-G. post
L.-G. rod
lurch
abductor l.
gluteal l.
Trendelenburg l.
lurching gait
Luschka
L. bursa
L. joint
L. muscle
Lusskin bone drill

NOTES

Lust phenomenon
lusty leg
luxated bone
luxatio
    l. coxae congenita
    l. erecta
    l. erecta shoulder dislocation
    l. imperfecta
luxation
    atlantoaxial l.
    incomplete l.
    ligamentous l.
    Malgaigne l.
    palmar l.
Lyden-Lehman technique
Lyden technique
Lyman-Smith
    L.-S. toe drop brace
    L.-S. traction
Lyme
    L. disease
    L. disease arthritis
lymphadenopathy
lymphangiography
lymphangioma
    cavernous l.
lymphangiosarcoma
lympha press traction
lymphatic
lymphedema
    cancer treatment-related l.
    l. complex
    congenital l.
    factitious l.
    familial l.
    l. sling
lymphocyte count

lymphoma
    angiotropic l.
lymph vessel
Lynco
    L. biomechanical orthotic system
    L. foot orthosis
Lynn
    L. Achilles lengthening procedure
    L. Achilles tendon repair technique
    L. tendo calcaneus repair
Lynx wrist, hand, finger orthosis arm positioner splint
LYOfoam
    L. C dressing
    L. wound dressing
lyophilization of bone
lyophilized bone graft
lyre-shaped finger hook
Lyser
    trapezoid bone of L.
Lysholm
    L. knee function scoring scale
    L. knee joint instability scope
    L. knee scoring questionnaire
    L. knee test
    L. score
Lysholm-Gillquist
    L.-G. knee subjective function scale
    L.-G. knee subjective function score
lysis
lysosomal absorption
Lyte Fit orthotic
lytic bone lesion
Lytle metacarpal splint

M
- M band
- M wave

3M
- 3M fiberglass cast
- 3M Maxi Driver blade
- 3M prep
- 3M skin drape
- 3M staple

M/3
- middle third

mA
- milliampere

MAC
- Miami Acute Care
- monitored anesthesia control
- MAC cervical collar

MacAusland
- M. lumbar brace
- M. operation
- M. procedure

MacCarthy procedure

maceration
- cutaneous m.

Macewen
- M. classification
- M. drill
- M. osteotomy

Macewen-Shands osteotomy

MacGregor
- M. osteotome
- M. osteotomy

Mache electromyogram setting

machine
- Accu-Tron microcurrent m.
- ankle exercise m.
- BackStrong lumbar extension m.
- Biodex isokinetic testing m.
- Bionx servohydraulic testing m.
- borazone blade cutting m.
- CamStar exercise m.
- continuous passive motion m.
- cooling m.
- CPM exerciser m.
- Cybex m.
- Duo-trac traction m.
- elliptical m.
- Griswold distraction m.
- Instron m.
- Isotechnologies B-200 low back m.
- isotonic m.
- KineTec hip CPM m.
- MB-900 AC m.
- Med-Fit Senior Circuit exercise m.
- MedX functional testing m.

MedX Mark II lumbar
- extension m.
- MedX stretch m.
- Orthion traction m.
- Paramount total body plate-
  loaded m.
- passive motion m.
- PodoFlex m.
- SAM spinal analysis m.
- Schwinn elliptical full body
  exercise m.
- m. screw
- spinal analysis m. (SAM)
- VersaClimber RX exercise m.
- Vivatek ultimate healing m.
- Wikco ankle m.

machine-gun-like pain

MacIntosh
- M. extraarticular tenodesis
- M. hip prosthesis
- M. iliotibial band tenodesis
- M. lateral pivot shift test
- M. over-the-top ACL reconstruction
- M. over-the-top repair
- M. technique
- M. tibial plateau prosthesis

MacKentry periosteal

Mackenzie amputation

Mackinnon-Dellon
- M.-D. criteria
- M.-D. staging system

MacKinnon nerve injury

Maclaren mobile buggy

MacLean-Maxwell disease

MacLeod capsular rheumatism

MacNab
- M. line
- M. line for facet imbrication
- M. operation
- M. shoulder repair

MacNab-English shoulder prosthesis

MacNichol-Voutsinas classification

macroadhesion

macrobrachia

macrocheiria

macrocnemia

macrocoil
- Gianturco m.

macrodactylia, macrodactyly
- m. fibrolipomatosis
- pedal m.
- progressive m.
- m. reduction procedure

macroelectromyography (macro-EMG)

M

415

macro-EMG
    macroelectromyography
    macro-EMG needle electrode
Macrofit hip prosthesis
macronychia
macroradiograph
macrotrauma rehabilitation program
macularis eruptive perstans
Madajet
    M. XL jet-injection anesthesia
      system
    M. XL local anesthesia
Maddacare child bath seat
Maddacrawler Crawler frame
Maddapult Asissto-Seat
Maddox rod test
Madelung
    M. deformity
    M. subluxation
Madigan-Wissinger-Donaldson proximal
  realignment
madreporic hip prosthesis
Madura foot
mafenide
    m. acetate
    m. acetate for burn
Maffucci
    M. disease
    M. syndrome
MAFO
    molded ankle-foot orthosis
    MAFO cane
Magerl
    M. hook-plate system
    M. plate-screw system
    M. posterior cervical screw fixation
    M. screw placement technique
    M. transarticular screw fixation
    M. translaminar facet screw
      fixation technique
magic
    m. angle effect
    m. angle phenomenon
    M. Wand vibrator
Magilligan measuring technique
Magna-FX cannulated screw system
MagnaPod pain relief magnet
Magnassager
    M. massager
    M. massage tool
Magnatherm
    M. SSP electromagnetic therapy
      unit
    M. SSP pulse shortwave diathermy
Magnathotic orthotic
MagneCore magnetic therapy pad

magnesium
    m. deficiency
    m. sulfate
magnet
    ankle m.
    BIOflex medical m.
    Dyonics Golden Retriever m.
    elbow m.
    foot m.
    MagnaPod pain relief m.
    m. splint
    Tectonic m.
magnetic
    m. motion transducer
    m. resonance arteriography
    m. resonance arthrography
    m. resonance imaging (MRI)
    m. resonance neurography (MRN)
    m. resonance spectroscopy
    m. resonance venography
    m. retriever
    m. source imaging (MSI)
    m. stimulation
    M. Support brace
    m. therapy
magnetization
    m. transfer
    m. transfer magnetic resonance
      imaging (mtMRI)
magnification
    loupe m.
    m. view
magnifying loupe
magnum
    M. 800 bed
    M. chisel
    M. curette
    foramen m.
    M. 101 Plus stimulator
    M. 101 Plus table
    M. 100 stimulator
magnus
    adductor m.
    nucleus raphe m. (NRM)
Magnuson
    M. abduction humeral splint
    M. débridement
    M. operation
    M. technique
    M. twist drill
    M. wire
Magnuson-Stack
    M.-S. arthroplasty
    M.-S. operation
    M.-S. procedure
    M.-S. shoulder arthrotomy
Ma-Griffith
    M.-G. end-to-end anastomosis

M.-G. percutaneous Achilles tendon repair
M.-G. ruptured Achilles tendon repair
M.-G. technique
M.-G. tendo calcaneus repair
M.-G. tendon anastomosis

Mahan procedure

MAI
Movement Assessment of Infants

Maigne test

main
m. d'accoucheur
m. en crochet
m. en griffe
m. en lorgnette
m. fourchée

maintained contraction

maintenance of bone plate integrity

Maisel suppression theory

Maisonneuve
M. amputation
M. fibular fracture
M. sign

Maitland
M. manipulation
M. technique

Majestro-Ruda-Frost
M.-R.-F. tendon operation
M.-R.-F. tendon technique

major
m. amputation
anterosuperior ilium m.
m. curve
m. fracture fragment
m. injury vector (MIV)
posteroinferior ilium m.

making
return-to-play sidelines decision m.

MAL
midaxillary line

malabsorption

maladaptation
soft tissue m.

maladaption
high-altitude m.

maladjustment

malakopathy

malalignment
dorsal m.
malicious m.
radial m.

rotational m.
varus m.

malangulation

malar
m. bone
m. fracture

Malawer
M. excision technique
M. resection

malaxation

Malcolm-Lynn
M.-L. C-RXF cervical retractor frame
M.-L. radiolucent spinal retraction system

Malcolm-Rand radiolucent headrest and retraction system

male
m. reamer
m. washer

malformation
Arnold-Chiari m.
arteriovenous m.
Chiari m.
Klippel-Feil m.
medullary venous m. (MVM)
retromedullary arteriovenous m.

Malgaigne
M. amputation
M. luxation
M. pelvic fracture

Malibu
M. cervical orthosis
M. Sandalthotics orthotic

malicious malalignment

maligna
lentigo m.

malignancy
spinal m.

malignant
m. acetabular osteolysis
m. fasciculation
m. fibrous histiocytoma
m. fibrous xanthoma
m. hyperpyrexia
m. hyperthermia
m. melanoma
m. myeloid sarcoma
m. osteopetrosis
m. schwannoma

Malis
M. CMC-II bipolar coagulator

M

NOTES

Malis *(continued)*
    M. curette
    M. elevator
    M. hinge clamp
    M. jeweler bipolar forceps
    M. ligature passer
    M. needle holder
Malis-Jensen microbipolar forceps
malleable
    m. metal finger splint
    structural aluminum m. (SAM)
    m. template
mallei (*pl. of* malleus)
malleolar
    m. chip fracture
    m. facet
    m. gel sleeve
    m. index
    m. osteotomy
    m. screw
    m. sulcus
Malleoloc
    M. anatomic ankle arthrosis
    M. ankle orthosis
    M. ankle support
malleolus, pl. malleoli
    belly button to medial m. (BB to MM)
    external m.
    m. externus
    fibular m.
    inner m.
    internal m.
    m. internus
    lateral m.
    m. lateralis
    medial m. (MM)
    m. medialis
    m. medialis tibiae
    outer m.
    posterior m.
    radial m.
    m. radialis
    m. tibiae
    tibial m.
    tip of medial m.
    ulnar m.
    m. ulnaris
malleotomy
Malleotrain ankle support
mallet
    Acufex m.
    Bergman m.
    bone m.
    boxwood m.
    cervical m.
    copper m.

    Cottle m.
    Crane m.
    Doyen bone m.
    m. finger
    m. finger deformity
    m. finger orthotic
    m. fracture
    Gerzog bone m.
    Hajek m.
    Heath m.
    Henning m.
    Hibbs m.
    Kirk orthopedic m.
    lead-filled m.
    Lucae bone m.
    Mead m.
    Meyerding m.
    Miltex m.
    Ombredanne m.
    polyethylene-faced m.
    Ralks m.
    Richards m.
    Rush m.
    slotted m.
    Steinbach m.
    Surgical No Bounce m.
    Swanson m.
    m. thumb
    m. toe
    m. toe deformity
    Williger bone m.
    Wolfe-Böhler m.
malleus, pl. mallei
    chirurgicum mallei
    hallux m.
malleus-incus prosthesis
Mallory
    M. prosthesis
    M. technique
Mallory-Head
    M.-H. femoral stem
    M.-H. modular calcar system
    M.-H. porous primary femoral prosthesis
    M.-H. I, II prosthesis
    M.-H. rasp
    M.-H. revision operation
    M.-H. total hip prosthesis
    M.-H. total hip revision
malnutrition
    protein m.
malodorous foot
mal perforans ulcer
malposed vertebra
malposition
    extension m.
    flexion m.

lateral flexion m.
rotational m.
malreduction
fracture m.
malrotation
Malteno tube implant material
maltracking patella
Maltz
M. cartilage knife
M. rasp
malum
m. coxae senilis
m. deformans
malunion
angulatory m.
calcaneal m.
femoral shaft m.
humeral fracture m.
talar m.
varus m.
malunited
m. acetabulum
m. calcaneus fracture
m. forearm fracture
m. radial fracture
mamillary process
management
biologic fracture m.
conservative m.
failure of conservative m.
foot orthotic m.
inflammation m.
interphalangeal sesamoid m.
neuromechanical spinal
chiropractic m.
nonoperative orthopedic m.
nonsurgical m.
preoperative m.
pressure ulcer m.
reflex tracheostomy m.
Mancini plate
**Mandelbaum-Nartolozzi-Carney patellar
tendon repair**
mandible ossification
mandibular
m. angle
m. fracture
m. nerve
m. osteotomy
m. spine
maneuver
Adson m.

Allen m.
Allis m.
Apley m.
Bárány-Nylen m.
Barlow m.
Bigelow m.
Bouvier m.
Christiani m.
circumduction m.
closed manipulative m.
costoclavicular m.
Credé m.
cross-leg Patrick m.
Dandy m.
Dix-Hallpike m.
Finkelstein m.
flexion-extension m.
flexion-rotation-compression m.
Foster-Kennedy m.
Fowler m.
Gowers m.
Hallpike m.
Halsted m.
hippocratic m.
Hubscher m.
hyperabduction m.
Jahss m.
Jendrassik m.
King m.
Krackow m.
Lachman m.
Leadbetter m.
load-and-shift m.
logrolling m.
McElvenny m.
McKenzie extension m.
McMurray circumduction m.
Mendelsohn m.
Meyn-Quigley m.
military brace m.
milking m.
Ortolani m.
osteoclasis m.
Parvin m.
Patrick cross-leg m.
Phalen m.
postural fixation back m.
Queckenstedt m.
relative response attributable to
the m. (RRAM)
reverse Bigelow m.
rotation-compression m.

M

NOTES

maneuver (*continued*)
 scalene m.
 Schreiber m.
 shear m.
 Slocum m.
 Smith m.
 Soto-Hall m.
 Spurling m.
 Steel m.
 Stimson m.
 Valsalva m.
 Walton m.
 Watson m.
 Wellmerling m.
 Whitman m.
 Wright m.
Mangled Extremity Severity Score (MESS)
mangling injury
manipulation
 m. of articulation
 back m.
 m. board
 chiropractic joint m.
 chiropractic manual m.
 contact m.
 diversified m.
 fine m.
 general thrust m.
 grading of m.
 gross m.
 Hippocrates m.
 indirect m.
 joint m.
 Leadbetter hip m.
 lumbar distraction m.
 Maitland m.
 medical m.
 myofascial m.
 noncontact m.
 opening wedge m.
 osteopathic m.
 passive joint m.
 rotational m.
 soft tissue m.
 specific thrust m.
 spinal m.
 thrust m.
 m. with distraction
manipulative
 m. procedure
 m. technique
 m. therapy
Mankin
 M. resection
 M. technique

Manktelow
 M. pectoralis major transfer
 M. transfer procedure
Mann
 M. bunionectomy
 M. modified McKeever arthrodesis
 M. procedure
 M. protocol
 M. resection arthroplasty
 M. technique
Mann-Coughlin
 M.-C. arthrodesis
 M.-C. procedure
Mann-Coughlin-DuVries cheilectomy
Mann-DuVries arthroplasty
Mann-Thompson-Coughlin arthrodesis
Manske-McCarroll opponensplasty
Manske-McCarroll-Swanson centralization
Manske technique
Mantis retrograde forceps
mantle
 cement m.
 grade A, B, C1, C2, D m.
manual
 m. adjustment
 m. cavitation
 m. contact
 m. fracture reduction
 m. locking knee prosthesis
 m. medicine
 m. muscle test
 m. muscle testing (MMT)
 m. pressure
 m. push-pull technique
 m. reflex neurotherapy
 m. resistance
 m. talar tilt
 m. therapy
 m. traction
 m. treatment
 m. wheelchair
 m. work
manubriosternal angle
manubrium, pl. **manubria**
Manuflex external fixator
manus
 m. plana
 m. valga
 m. vara
Manutrain active wrist support
MAP
 Multiaxial Assessment of Pain
Maple Leaf hip orthosis
mapping
 behavioral m.
 m. the defect
 dermatome m.

MSI m.

paraspinal m.

Maquet

    M. advancement

    M. anteromedial osteoplasty

    M. dome

    M. dome osteotomy

    M. line

    M. procedure

    M. table extension

    M. technique

Maramed

    M. Miami fracture brace system

    M. ThermoFlex

marathon

marathoner's toe

marble

    m. bone

    m. bone pin

march

    m. foot

    m. fracture

marche à petits pas gait

marching band injury

Marcove-Lewis-Huvos shoulder girdle resection

Marcus-Balourdas-Heiple

    M.-B.-H. ankle fusion

    M.-B.-H. ankle fusion technique

    M.-B.-H. transmalleolar arthrodesis

Marfan syndrome

margin

    anterior tibial m.

    fibular m.

marginal

    m. excision

    m. exostosis

    m. fracture

    m. osteophyte

    m. resection

margo, pl. **margines**

Marie-Bamberger disease

Marie-Charcot-Tooth disease

Marie-Foix sign

Marie-Strümpell

    M.-S. arthritis

    M.-S. disease

    M.-S. spondylitis

Marion screw

Mark

    M. II Chandler total knee retractor

    M. II concave total knee retractor

    M. II distal femur distractor

    M. II femoral component extractor

    M. III halo system

    M. II Kodros radiolucent awl

    M. II lateral collateral ligament retractor

    M. II modular weight retractor

    M. II Sorrells hip arthroplasty

    M. II Sorrells hip arthroplasty retractor system

    M. II S total knee retractor

    M. II Stubbs short prong collateral ligament retractor

    M. II Stulberg hip positioner

    M. II Stulberg leg positioner

    M. II tibial component extractor

    M. II wide PCL knee retractor

    M. II Wixson hip positioner

    M. II Z knee retractor

Markell

    M. brace boot

    M. Mobility Health Clogs

    M. Mobility Shoes

    M. open-toe boot

    M. open-toe shoe

    M. tarso medius straight shoe

    M. tarso pronator outflare shoe

marker

    biochemical m.

    lumbar pedicle m.

    pedicle m.

    retroreflective m.

    skin m.

    tantalum-ball m.

    thoracic pedicle m.

    X-Act podiatric m.

Markham-Meyerding retractor

Markley retention pin

Marks-Bayne technique for thumb duplication

Markwalder

    M. bone rongeur

    M. rib forceps

Markwort ankle support

Marlex

    M. mesh

    M. methyl methacrylate prosthesis

Marlin

    M. cervical collar

    M. cervical orthosis

M

NOTES

Marmor
    M. modular knee prosthesis
    M. replacement
Marmor-Lynn fracture
maroon spoon
Maroteaux
    spondyloepiphysial dysplasia of M.
Maroteaux-Lamy
    M.-L. disease
    M.-L. syndrome
Marquardt
    M. angulation osteotomy
    M. bone rongeur
Marquet fracture table
marrow
    bone m.
    m. canal
    m. cavity
    m. disease
    m. nailing
    red m.
    m. stimulation
    yellow m.
MARS
    Modular Acetabular Revision System
    MARS revision acetabular
      component
Marshall
    M. knee score
    M. ligament repair
    M. ligament repair technique
    M. patelloquadriceps tendon
      substitution
Marshall-McIntosh technique
Martel sign
martensitic stainless steel
Martin
    M. cartilage chisel
    M. cartilage clamp
    M. cartilage forceps
    M. cartilage scissors
    M. diamond wire cutter
    M. disease
    M. loop circumferential wire
    M. meniscal clamp
    M. muscular clamp
    M. osteotomy
    M. patellar wiring technique
    M. screw
    M. sheet rubber bandage
Martin-Gruber
    M.-G. anastomosis
    M.-G. connection
Martini bone curette
Marx osteoradionecrosis protocol
Mary
    angle of M.

Maryland
    M. Foot Score
    M. Foot Score Profile
MAS
    milliamperage x seconds
Mason
    M. fracture
    M. fracture classification system
    M. radial head fracture
      classification
    M. splint
Mason-Allen
    M.-A. suture
    M.-A. Universal hand splint
mass
    bony m.
    cellular periosteal
      osteocartilaginous m.
    center of m.
    fat and fat-free m. (FFM)
    hypoechoic intermetatarsal web
      space m.
    low bone m.
    osteocartilaginous m.
    plantar-hindfoot-midfoot bony m.
    pre-Achilles m.
    m.'s sign
    soft tissue m.
massage
    aqua PT water m.
    m. ball
    callus m.
    connective tissue m. (CTM)
    cross-friction m.
    deep friction m.
    deep stroking and kneading m.
    effleurage m.
    friction m.
    Hoffa m.
    ice m.
    kneading m.
    Shiatsu therapeutic m.
    Silhouette therapeutic m.
    soft tissue m.
    stimulating m.
    Swedish m.
    Teledyne Water Pik misting m.
    m. therapy
    M. Time Pro hydromassage table
    transverse friction m.
    vibratory m.
massager
    AcuVibe m.
    Body Sticks m.
    Cryocup ice m.
    Equalizer Pro m.
    G5 Fleximatic
      massager/percussor m.

Intracell trigger point m.
Ironman Triathlon Pro-Power m.
Jeanie Rub M.
Knobble m.
Magnassager m.
Medisana M.
Morfam Quality Jeanie Rub m.
Omni Roller m.
Original Backknobber muscle m.
Original Index Knobber II m.
Power Pillow cervical m.
Reach Easy m.
Saso Variable Speed M.
Scrip Muscle Master m.
T-Bar trigger-point m.
Thera Cane m.

massager/percussor
G5 Vibracare m.

masseur
masseuse
Massie
M. driver
M. extractor
M. inserter
M. II nail
M. nail assembly
M. plate
M. screwdriver
M. sliding graft
M. sliding nail

massive
m. fibrolipoma
m. herniated disk
m. osteolysis
m. osteoplysis
m. sliding graft

Masson fasciotome
massotherapy
MAST
military antishock trousers

master
Balance M.
Body M.
m. cement
Cobra M.
m. knot of Henry
NeuroCom balance m.
PRO Balance M.
M. screwdriver
SMART Balance M.
M. step foot prosthesis

Masterson
M. curved clamp
M. pelvic clamp
M. straight clamp

Master-Stim interferential stimulator
Mastin muscular clamp
mastocytosis
mastoid
m. curette
m. process
m. rongeur

Mast-Spieghel-Pappas classification
mat
Airex m.
air flow m.
AliMed sensor floor m.
children's m.
Easyslide sliding m.
EMED-SF sensor m.
Harris-Beath footprint m.
Harris footprint m.
Minislide sliding m.
Scoot-Gard m.
sting m.
m. table

Matchett-Brown
M.-B. cemented hip prosthesis
M.-B. hip arthroplasty
M.-B. internal prosthesis

matchstick
m. graft
m. test

mater
dura m.

material
acrylic implant m.
Alisoft splinting m.
allogenic lyophilized bone graft
implant m.
AlloGro bone graft m.
alloplastic m.
alpha-BSM bone repair m.
alpha-BSM bone substitute m.
aluminum oxide arthroplasty m.
American Society for Testing
and M.'s (ASTM)
amorphous eosinophilic m.
Aquaplast splinting m.
bioabsorbable m.
bioceramic implant m.
bone implant m.
Bone Plast bone replacement m.

M

NOTES

material *(continued)*
    bone-tendon graft m.
    Bonfiglio bone replacement m.
    Calcitite graft m.
    Carboplast II sheet orthotic m.
    cellular response to implant m.
    celluloid implant m.
    CHAG bone graft substitute m.
    composite m.
    copolymer orthotic m.
    corundum ceramic implant m.
    Dacron synthetic ligament m.
    Durapatite bone replacement m.
    Duraval Hook & Loop strap m.
    DYNAfabric m.
    Embarc bone repair m.
    Ethrone implant m.
    Evazote cushioning m.
    m. failure break point
    fibrillar absorbable hemostat m.
    Fletching femoral hernia
      implant m.
    gold weight and wire spring
      implant m.
    Graflex m.
    Grafton demineralized bone matrix
      putty m.
    Gypsona cast m.
    Healos synthetic bone grafting m.
    homograft implant m.
    hydroxyapatite bone replacement m.
    hydroxyapatite implant m.
    implant m.
    Interpore bone replacement m.
    Iowa implant m.
    Isoloss AC m.
    Keolar implant m.
    LactoSorb orthopedic wound m.
    Malteno tube implant m.
    methyl methacrylate implant m.
    Nicoll bone replacement m.
    Omega splinting m.
    Ommaya reservoir implant m.
    Opteform bone graft m.
    OrthoDyn bone substitute m.
    Ortho-Glass synthetic m.
    Ortho-Jel impression m.
    Osteogenics BoneSource synthetic
      bone replacement m.
    paraffin implant m.
    Pe Lite thermoplastic crepe m.
    PerioGlas bone graft m.
    Plasti-Pore prosthetic m.
    polyether implant m.
    polyethylene implant m.
    polyurethane implant m.
    polyvinyl alcohol splinting m.
    polyvinyl implant m.

    Porocoat prosthetic m.
    porous prosthetic m.
    ProOsteon bone graft m.
    Proplast I, II porous implant m.
    Proplast prosthetic m.
    purulent m.
    Pyrost bone graft m.
    Schepens hollow silicone
      hemisphere implant m.
    Scutan temporary splint m.
    Shearing posterior chamber
      implant m.
    shell implant m.
    silicone m.
    Silon silicone thermoplastic
      splinting m.
    solid buckling implant m.
    solid silicone exoplant implant m.
    Spitz-Holter valve implant m.
    splinting m.
    Stimoceiver implant m.
    Synergy flexible splinting m.
    synthetic m.
    thermomoldable m.
    ThermoSKY orthotic m.
    tissue mandrel implant m.
    titanium implant m.
    Unilab Surgibone bone
      replacement m.
    Virtullene brace m.
    viscoelastic m.
    Vitallium implant m.
    Vitox alumina ceramic m.
    zirconium oxide arthroplasty m.
    Zorbacel shock-absorbing m.
Matev sign
Mathews
    M. drill point
    M. hand drill
    M. load drill
    M. olecranon fracture classification
Mathew scale
Mathieu rasp
Mathys prosthesis
matricectomy *(var. of* matrixectomy)
matrix, pl. **matrices**
    bone m.
    Collagraft bone graft m.
    demineralized bone m. (DBM)
    germinal m.
    germinative m.
    m. Grafton putty
    m. injury
    ligament-scar m.
    nail m.
    m. seating system
    sterile m.

matrix-bone marrow slurry
matrixectomy, matricectomy
    chemical m.
    Frost partial m.
    laser partial m.
    partial m.
    phenol m.
    phenol-alcohol m.
    Steindler m.
    total m.
    Winograd partial m.
    Zadik total m.
Matroc femoral head
Matrol femoral head prosthesis
Matson
    M. periosteal elevator
    M. procedure
    M. rib elevator
Matson-Alexander rib elevator
Matta-Saucedo fixation
matter
    gray m.
    white m.
Matthew cross-leg clamp
Matthews-Green pin
matting
    Dycem roll m.
Matti-Russe
    M.-R. bone graft
    M.-R. technique
mattress
    Akros extended care m.
    Akros pressure m.
    AkroTech m.
    antidecubitus m.
    chiropractic m.
    Clinisert m.
    DeCube m.
    eggcrate m.
    Invacare APM m.
    Lapidus alternating air-pressure m.
    Nirvana m.
    OptiMax Supreme pressure
      reduction m.
    overlay m.
    PressureGuard m.
    Q Star Voyager pressure
      reduction m.
    RIK fluid m.
    Sofflex m.
    Sof Matt pressure relieving m.
    m. suture

    Tempur-Pedic pressure relieving
      Swedish m.
    T-Foam m.
    Tri-Float pressure reduction m.
Mattrix spinal cord stimulation system
maturation
    accelerated bone m.
    bone m.
    delayed bone m.
    m. phase
    skeletal m.
    m. zone
maturity
    bone m.
    Oxford method for scoring
      skeletal m.
    skeletal m.
Mau
    M. and Ludloff procedure
    M. osteotomy
Mauch
    M. S'n'S
    M. Swing and Stance hydraulic
      knee
Mauck
    M. knee procedure
    M. operation
Mauclaire disease
max
    M. 3 electric handpiece
    Thera-Band M.
MaxCast
    M. cast
    M. casting tape
Maxi-Driver driver
MaxiFloat wheelchair cushion
maxillary
    m. fracture
    m. process
    m. spine
maxillectomy
    Cocke m.
    subtotal m.
maxillofacial bone screw
maxillotomy
    extended m.
Maxima II transcutaneous electrical
  nerve stimulator
maximal
    isokinetic strength test m.
    m. oxygen uptake

M

NOTES

maximal *(continued)*
    m. stimulus
    m. voluntary contraction (MVC)
Maxim Modular Knee System
maximum
    m. conduction velocity
    m. control (MC)
    m. eversion velocity
    m. inversion velocity
    one-repetition m. (1-RM)
    m. oxygen uptake
    m. pressure picture (MPP)
    m. radial bow
    repetition m. (RM)
Maxon suture
Maxwell body
Maxwell-Brancheau
    M.-B. arthroereisis (MBA)
    M.-B. procedure
Maxxus orthopedic latex surgical glove
May anatomical bone plate
Mayer
    M. orthotic
    M. reflex
    M. splint
    M. transfer operation
Mayfield
    M. adapter
    M. fixation frame
    M. forceps
    M. head rest
    M. incision
    M. instrumentation
    M. miniature clip applier
    M. neurosurgical headrest
    M. temporary aneurysm clip
      applier
Mayo
    M. ankle arthroplasty
    M. approach
    M. block anesthesia
    M. bunionectomy
    M. carpal instability classification
    M. clamp
    M. Clinic congruent elbow plate
    M. Clinic forefoot score
    M. Clinic hip scoring system
    M. elbow distraction device
    M. elbow fracture classification
    M. elbow performance score
    M. hallux valgus modified
      operation
    M. metatarsal head resection
    M. nerve block
    M. resection arthroplasty
    M. rigid cervical collar
    M. scissors

    M. semiconstrained elbow
      prosthesis
    M. total ankle prosthesis
    M. total elbow arthroplasty
Mayo-Collins retractor
Mayo-Hegar needle holder
Mayo-Stone-Valenti hallux limitus/rigidus
    arthroplasty
Mayo-Thomas collar
Mazas totally constrained elbow
    prosthesis
Mazet
    M. knee disarticulation
    M. technique
Mazur
    M. ankle elevation classification
    M. ankle evaluation
    M. ankle rating
    M. operation
MB-900 AC machine
MBA
    Maxwell-Brancheau arthroereisis
M-Brace knee brace
MBS
    Multi Balance System
      MBS snap-on orthotic
MC
    maximum control
    metacarpal
      MC walker brace
MCA
    motorcycle accident
McAfee approach
McArdle
    M. disease
    M. syndrome
McAtee compression screw device
McAtee-Tharias-Blazina arthroplasty
McBride
    M. bunionectomy
    M. bunion hallux valgus
    M. bunion hallux valgus operation
    M. femoral prosthesis
    M. hallux abductovalgus reduction
    M. hallux valgus reduction
    M. pin
    M. plate
    M. procedure
    M. tripod
    M. tripod pin traction
McBride-Moore prosthesis
McCabe-Farrior rasp
McCain
    M. TMJ arthroscopic system
    M. TMJ cannula
    M. TMJ curette
    M. TMJ forceps
McCarroll-Baker procedure

McCarty hip procedure
McCash
 M. hand procedure
 M. hand surgery
McCauley foot procedure
McClintoch brace
McCollough internal tibial torsion brace
McConnell
 M. extensile approach
 M. median and ulnar nerve
  approach
 M. orthopedic headrest
 M. patellofemoral treatment plan
 M. shoulder positioner
 M. taping technique method
 M. technique
McCormick-Blount procedure
McCullough retractor
McCune-Albright syndrome
McCutchen hip implant
McDavid
 M. ankle guard
 M. hinged knee guard
 M. knee brace
McDermott radiological classification
McDonald dissector
McDowell Impairment Index (MII)
McElfresh-Dobyns-O'Brien technique
McElroy
 M. curette
 M. instrumentation
McElvenny
 M. foot procedure
 M. maneuver
 M. technique
McElvenny-Caldwell procedure
McFarland bone graft
McFarland-Osborne
 M.-O. lateral approach
 M.-O. technique
McFarlane technique
McGee
 M. prosthesis needle
 M. splint
 M. wire-crimping forceps
McGee-Priest wire forceps
McGehee elbow prosthesis
McGill
 M. pain checklist
 M. Pain Questionnaire
 M. pain scale

McGlamry
 M. elevator
 M. and Feldman modification
 M. procedure
McGlamry-Downey procedure
McGregor line
McGuire
 M. pelvic positioner
 M. rating
 M. score
MCI
 midcarpal instability
McIndoe
 M. bone rongeur
 M. rongeur forceps
 M. scissors
McIntire splint
McIvor ENT retractor
McKay
 M. hip procedure
 M. osteotomy
McKay-Simons
 M.-S. clubfoot operation
 M.-S. CSR
 M.-S. CSR operation
McKee
 M. brace
 M. femoral prosthesis
 M. totally constrained elbow
  prosthesis
 M. tri-fin nail
McKee-Farrar
 M.-F. acetabular cup
 M.-F. total hip arthroplasty
 M.-F. total hip prosthesis
McKeever
 M. arthrodesis for hallux limitus
 M. bunionectomy
 M. cartilage knife
 M. medullary clavicle fixation
 M. metatarsophalangeal arthrodesis
 M. metatarsophalangeal fusion
 M. open reduction
 M. operation
 M. patellar cap prosthesis
 M. patellar resurfacing device
 M. procedure
 M. Vitallium knee prosthesis
McKeever-Buck
 M.-B. elbow operation
 M.-B. elbow technique
 M.-B. fragment excision

M

NOTES

McKeever-Collison long-stem prosthesis
McKeever-MacIntosh tibial plateau prosthesis
McKenzie
    M. bone drill
    M. cervical roll
    M. enlarging bur
    M. extension exercise
    M. extension maneuver
    M. lumbar roll
    M. method
    M. night roll
    M. perforating twist drill
    M. Repex table
McKittrick transmetatarsal amputation
McKusick-type metaphysial chondrodysplasia
MCL
    medial collateral ligament
    MCL brace
McLain-Weinstein spinal tumor classification
McLaughlin
    M. acromioplasty
    M. approach
    M. arthroplasty
    M. carpal scaphoid screw
    M. modification of Bunnell pull-out suture
    M. nail
    M. operation
    M. osteosynthesis apparatus
    M. osteosynthesis device
    M. plate
    M. procedure
    M. subscapularis transfer
McLaughlin-Hay technique
McLaughlin-Ryder incision
McLeod padded clavicular splint
McLight PCL brace
McMaster bone graft
McMaster-Toronto arthritis patient preference disability questionnaire
McMurray
    M. circumduction maneuver
    M. osteotomy
    M. sign
    M. test
McMurtry
    kinematic index of M.
    M. kinematic index
McNaught prosthesis
MCP
    metacarpophalangeal
    MCP finger joint prosthesis
MCR
    midcarpal radial
    MCR portal

McRae line
McReynolds
    M. driver
    M. driver-extractor
    M. method
    M. open fracture reduction technique
    M. open reduction
McShane-Leinberry-Fenlin acromioplasty
MCU
    midcarpal ulnar
    MCU portal
McWhorter posterior shoulder approach
MD
    muscular dystrophy
    MD brace
MDCN
    medial dorsal cutaneous nerve
MDI
    multidirectional instability
MDS microdebrider
Mead
    M. bone rongeur
    M. mallet
    M. periosteal elevator
meal
    bone m.
mean
    m. flow velocity
    m. value
Mears-Rubash approach
Mears sacroiliac plate
Meary
    M. line
    M. metatarsotalar angle
measure
    Canadian Occupational Performance M.
    emergency closed manipulative m.
    functional assessment m. (FAM)
    functional independence m. (FIM)
    Gross Motor Function M. (GMFM)
    limited performance m.
    outcome m.
    parallel goniometric m.
    reconstructive m.
    standard goniometric m.
measured stress
measurement
    Agliette m.
    alignment m.
    anthropometric m.
    appendicular bone mass m.
    arthrometer m.
    arthrometric knee laxity m.
    Blackburn-Peel m.
    calcaneal compartment pressure m.
    clear space m.

curve m.
EMED-F foot-force m.
foot central compartment
  pressure m.
functional capacity m.
Insall-Salvati m.
limb accurate m. (LAM)
Mehta rib angle m.
motion m.
pain m.
pedodynographic m.
range-of-motion m.
roof arc m.
Schober m.
skinfold m.
spasticity m.
tibiofibular overlap m.
tissue pressure m.
Zwipp subtalar joint instability m.
measurer
  Bunnell digital exertion m.
measuring
  m. gauge
  precise lesion m. (PLM)
mechanical
  m. agent
  m. axis
  combined m. (CM)
  m. dermatome
  m. dysfunction
  m. instability
  m. insufficiency
  m. low back pain syndrome
  m. modality
  m. pain threshold (MPTh)
mechanic pin vice
mechanics
  altered intervertebral m.
  altered regional m.
  body m.
  walking m.
mechanism
  abductor m.
  adhesion/cohesion m.
  Adjustable Leg and Ankle
   Repositioning M. (ALARM)
  capsuloligamentous m.
  central extensor m. (CEM)
  clamping m.
  Cook-Gordon m.
  m. of correction

cranial-sacral respiratory m.
 (CRSM)
digital extensor m.
extensor hood m.
fail-safe m.
flexor m.
four-bar linkage prosthetic knee m.
gliding m.
Hosmer Dorrance voluntary control
 four-bar knee m.
humeral m.
locomotor m.
MicroStable liner locking m.
neurotraumatic m.
Noiles rotating hinge knee m.
physiological venous pump m.
post-and-cam m.
primary cranial sacral
 respiratory m.
quadriceps m.
screw-home m.
slider crank m.
tendo Achillis m.
terminal extensor m. (TEM)
UHR locking ring m.
Windlass m.
mechanoreceptor
  m. activity
  m. Golgi tendon organ
  joint capsule m.
  pacinian m.
  Ruffini m.
Meckel cavity
Mecring acetabluar prosthesis
Medak glove
Medarmor puncture-resistant glove
Med-Fit
  M.-F. cranial-sacral table
  M.-F. Senior Circuit exercise
   machine
medial
  m. aspect
  m. aspiration
  m. bicipital sulcus
  m. bicortical screw
  m. border
  m. brachial cutaneous nerve injury
  m. brachial nerve
  m. capsular imbrication
  m. capsulorrhaphy
  m. clear space
  m. collateral ligament (MCL)

NOTES

medial *(continued)*
m. collateral sprain
m. column calcaneal fracture
m. column instability
m. compartment
m. compartment disruption
m. compartment injury
m. cortical overlap technique
m. crossover toe
m. deviation of the second toe
m. disk protrusion
m. displacement
m. dorsal cutaneous nerve (MDCN)
m. drainage
m. eminence
m. eminence resection
m. end
m. epicondylar apophysis
m. epicondyle
m. epicondylectomy
m. epicondyle humeral fracture
m. epicondylitis
m. exostectomy
m. extensor expansion
m. femoral condyle
m. gastrocnemius bursitis
m. geniculate
m. geniculate artery
m. geniculate fascia
m. hamstring
m. head of the gastrocnemius
  rupture
m. head-stem offset
m. heel-and-sole wedge
m. heel skive technique
m. heel wedge (MHW)
m. heel wedge orthosis
m. hip rotation
m. humeral condyle
m. joint line
m. longitudinal arch
m. malleolar fracture
m. malleolar/small bone fragment
  clamp
m. malleolus (MM)
m. malleolus cast
m. malleolus fixation
m. malleolus resection
m. malleolus of tibia
m. meniscectomy
m. meniscus
m. metacarpal bone
m. movement
m. neurovascular bundle
m. oblique (MO)
m. parapatellar arthrotomy
m. parapatellar capsular approach
m. parapatellar incision

m. patellar plica
m. patellofemoral ligament (MPFL)
m. plantar artery
m. plantar fasciocutaneous flap
m. portal
m. proximal tibial angle
m. quadruple complex
m. ray adduction deformity
m. release
m. repair
m. rollover
m. rotation procedure
m. sesamoid
m. shelf
m. shelf/medial plica
m. sole wedge
m. sole wedge orthosis
m. sole-wedge shoe modification
m. stem pivot
m. sural cutaneous nerve
m. swivel dislocation
m. talocalcaneal bar
m. talonavicular capsule
m. tennis elbow tendinosis
m. tibial epiphysiodesis
m. tibial flare
m. tibial stress syndrome (MTSS)
m. tibial syndrome (MTS)
m. torsion
m. T-strap
m. tubercle
m. ulnar collateral ligament
  (MUCL)
m. unicortical screw
m. V-Y capsulotomy
m. wall
medialis
malleolus m.
m. pedis flap
vastus m.
medialization ratio
medial/lateral
m. femoral condyle
m. meniscus
medial/plantar hinge
median
m. nerve
m. nerve block
m. nerve compression
m. nerve entrapment
m. nerve injury
m. nerve palsy
m. raphe
m. sagittal plane
Medi-Band bandage
medical
m. adhesive
M. Design brace

m. elastomer X7-2320
M. Examination and Diagnostic Coding System (MEDICS)
m. manipulation
M. Research Council (MRC)
M. Research Council system
m. subcutaneous reflection

medication
antiinflammatory m.
nonsteroidal antiinflammatory m.

medicinal leech

medicine
allopathic m.
alternative m.
American College of Sports M. (ACSM)
m. ball
Chinese m.
complimentary alternative m. (CAM)
dance m.
electrodiagnostic m.
manual m.
Native American m.
occupational and environmental m. (OEM)
osteopathic m.
physical m. (PM)
podiatric m.
sports m.
vertebral m.

MediCordz Rehabilitation Kit

MEDICS
Medical Examination and Diagnostic Coding System

Medicus bed

Mediflow
M. waterbase pillow
M. Waterpillow

Mediloy
M. implant metal
M. implant metal prosthesis

mediolateral (M/L)
m. position
m. radiocarpal angle
m. stress
m. tilt

mediotarsal amputation

Medipedic Multicentric knee brace

Mediplast

MEDI Plus compression stockings

Medipore H surgical tape

Medi-Rip dressing

MediRule II measuring device

Medisana Massager

Mediskin hemostatic sponge

Medi-Stim stimulator

medium
Amipaque contrast m.
m. callus Podi-Burr
m. carbide cone bur
m. fine bur
Microfil contrast m.
m. nail Podi-Burr
m. profile femoral prosthesis

Medium-Plus alpha liner

medius
digitus m.

Medmetric
M. knee ligament arthrometer
M. KT-1000 knee laxity arthrometer

Medoff
M. axial compression screw
M. sliding plate

Meds eye protector

Medtronic spinal cord stimulation system

medulla, pl. **medullae**

medullary
m. bone graft
m. callus
m. canal
m. canal reamer
m. cavity
m. nail
m. nail fixation
m. nailing
m. paraganglioma
m. pin
m. prosthesis
m. saw
m. venous malformation (MVM)
m. vent tubing

medullectomy

medullization

medulloarthritis

medullostomy
tarsal m.

MedX
M. functional testing machine
M. Mark II lumbar extension machine
M. stretch machine

M

NOTES

Meek
M. clavicular strap
M. pelvic traction belt
Mega-Air bed
megahorn meniscus
megalodactyly
megaprosthesis
Mega Tilt and Turn bed
Mehn-Quigley technique
Mehta rib angle measurement
Meige syndrome
melagra
melalgia
melamine resin
melanoma
acral lentiginous m.
Breslow classification of m.
Clark classification of m.
lentigo maligna m.
malignant m.
metastatic m.
nodular m.
plantar malignant m.
melanosis circumscripta preblastomatosis of Dubreuilh
melanotic
m. panaris
m. Whitlow of Hutchinson
Melaware flatware
Meleney
M. infection
M. synergistic gangrene
melioidosis
musculoskeletal m.
melioidotic
Melone distal radius fracture classification
melon-seed body
melorheostosis
melosalgia
Melzack Pain Questionnaire
membrane
anterior atlantooccipital m.
atlantooccipital anterior m.
basement m.
cricothyroid m.
m. instability
interosseous m. (IOM)
interposition m.
intraosseous m.
mucous m.
periprosthetic m.
Preclude spinal m.
suprasyndesmotic m.
synovial m.
m. tack
thickened synovial m.
trauma-induced m.

membranous
m. bone
m. ossification
m. osteogenesis
Memford-Gurd arthroplasty
memory
m. board
m. splint
Mendel-Bekhterev
M.-B. reflex
M.-B. sign
Mendelsohn
M. maneuver
M. modification of matrixectomy suture technique
Menelaus triceps transfer
meningeal syndrome
meningioma
meningism
meningismus
meningitis
meningocele
meningococcal purpura
meningoencephalomyelitis
meningomyelitis
meningomyelocele
meniscal
m. aponeurosis
m. arrow
m. autograft transplantation
m. clamp
m. curette
m. cyst
m. excision
m. flounce
m. injury
m. lateral tear
m. mirror
m. radial tear
m. repair
m. repair needle
m. scissors
m. spoon
m. staple
m. transverse tear
meniscectomy
arthroscopic m.
m. knife
lateral m.
medial m.
partial m.
Patel medial m.
m. scissors
subtotal lateral m.
total m.
menisci (*pl. of* meniscus)
meniscitis

meniscocapsular
m. junction
m. tear
meniscofemoral
m. capsule
m. ligament
meniscoid
m. entrapment
joint m.
m. lesion
meniscopexy
meniscoplasty
meniscorrhaphy
meniscosynovial junction
meniscotibial
m. capsule
m. ligament
meniscotome
Bircher m.
Bowen-Grover m.
curved m.
Grover m.
Storz m.
meniscotomy chisel
meniscus, pl. menisci
M. Arrow fixation
bridge of m.
clefting of m.
degenerative m.
discoid lateral m.
m. forceps
frayed m.
fraying of m.
m. graft
m. homolog
m. hook
m. knife
lateral m.
medial m.
medial/lateral m.
megahorn m.
M. Mender II system
resection of m.
m. retractor
m. scissors
torn m.
trapped m.
Mennell
M. sign
M. test

MENS
microamperage electrical nerve
stimulation
MENS unit
Mensor-Scheck
M.-S. hanging-hip operation
M.-S. technique
mental torticollis
Mentor
M. Self-Cath soft catheter
M. tissue expander
Mephisto Mobils professional shoe
MEPP
miniature end-plate potential
MERAC
Musculoskeletal Evaluation,
Rehabilitation and Conditioning
meralgia
merchant
M. congruence angle
M. and Dietz ankle score
M. radiograph
M. view
mercury
millimeters of m. (mmHg)
meridian
M. Intersegmental table
M. ST femoral implant component
m. therapy
Merit Final Flexion Kit
Merland perimedullary arteriovenous fistula classification
Merle
M. d'Aubigné hip score
M. d'Aubigné and Postel hip
rating scale
Merlin arthroscopy blade
Merocel pack
merry
M. Walker
M. Walker ambulation device
Mersilene
M. Kessler stitch
M. sling
M. suture
M. tape
Meryon sign
mesencephalic injury
mesenchymal
m. cell
m. chondrosarcoma
m. tumor

M

NOTES

mesenchyme
mesenchymoma
    pluripotential m.
mesenteric vasculitis
mesh
    chromium-cobalt m.
    m. graft
    Marlex m.
    metal m.
    sintered titanium m.
    stainless steel m.
    tantalum m.
mesher
    Zimmer skin graft m.
mesiodistal plane
mesocuneiform bone
mesotendineum
mesotendon
mesothenar muscle
MESS
    Mangled Extremity Severity Score
MET
    metabolic equivalent of task
metabolic
    m. bone disease
    m. equivalent of task (MET)
    m. syndrome (MS)
    m. variable
metabolism
    energy m.
metacarpal (MC)
    m. amputation
    m. base
    m. beak
    m. block
    m. bone
    duplicated m.
    fifth m.
    first m.
    m. lengthening
    m. ligament
    m. neck
    m. neck fracture
    m. osteotomy
    thumb m.
metacarpectomy
metacarpocapitate joint
metacarpocarpal joint
metacarpoglenoidal ligament
metacarpohamate joint
metacarpophalangeal (MCP, MP)
    m. arthroscopy
    m. articulation
    m. dislocation
    m. implant
    m. joint (MPJ)
    m. joint arthroplasty
    m. ligament

metacarpophysial
    m. joint
    m. joint extension contracture
metacarpotrapezoid joint
metacarpus
metachromatic mucoid substance
metaepiphysis
metal
    Alivium implant m.
    Biophase implant m.
    Biotex implant m.
    m. clamp
    Coballoy implant m.
    Co-Cr-Mo alloy implant m.
    Co-Cr-W-Ni alloy implant m.
    m. endurance limit
    m. failure
    m. fatigue
    m. femoral head prosthesis
    m. foot plate
    HA 65101 implant m.
    Haynes-Stellite 21 implant m.
    m. hemi-toe implant
    m. hybrid orthosis
    implant m.
    m. implant corrosion
    m. locator
    m. measuring triangle
    Mediloy implant m.
    m. mesh
    Orthochrome implant m.
    m. orthopedic implant
    m. pin
    porous m.
    Protasul implant m.
    m. pusher
    m. pylon
    Sinterlock implant m.
    m. splint
    Tivanium implant m.
    Vinertia implant m.
    Vitallium implant m.
    Zimaloy implant m.
metal-backed
    m.-b. acetabular component
    m.-b. acetabular component hip
      implant
    m.-b. acetabular cup
    m.-b. patellar implant
    m.-b. plastic-on-metal prosthesis
    m.-b. socket
metallic
    m. bead
    m. debris
    m. implant
metalloproteinase
    tissue inhibitor of m. (TIMP)
metallosis

metal-on-metal articulating intervertebral disk prosthesis

metaphyses (*pl. of* metaphysis)

metaphysial
- m. abscess
- m. aclasis
- m. artery
- m. chondrodysplasia
- m. to diaphysial width ratio
- m. fibrous cortical defect
- m. fibrous defect
- m. head resection with prosthesis
- m. osteotomy
- m. shortening
- m. spike
- m. stapler
- m. tibial fracture
- m. tuberculosis
- m. wedge

metaphysial-articular nonunion

metaphysial-diaphysial
- m.-d. angle
- m.-d. junction

metaphysial-epiphysial angle

metaphysis, pl. **metaphyses**
- distal m.
- femoral m.
- fibular m.
- funnelization of m.
- tibial m.

metaphysitis

metaplasia
- cartilaginous m.
- fibrous m.
- osteocartilaginous m.

metaplastic ossification

metastasis, pl. **metastases**
- bony m.
- osteoblastic m.
- Picker Magnascanner for bone m.
- spinal m.

metastatic
- m. bone lesion
- m. bone survey
- m. disease
- m. melanoma
- m. spinal tumor

Metasul
- M. hip joint component
- M. joint
- M. metal-on-metal hip

- M. metal-on-metal hip prosthesis system

metatarsal (MT)
- m. artery
- m. axis
- m. bar shoe modification
- m. block
- m. bone
- m. callosity
- m. cookie
- m. cuneiform exostosis
- dorsiflexed m.
- m. flatfoot bar
- m. flat head
- m. fracture
- m. head extractor
- m. head osteotomy
- m. head resection
- m. joint
- lesser m.
- m. ligament
- m. neck
- m. neck osteotomy
- m. oblique osteotomy
- m. ossification
- osteochondrosis of m.
- m. osteology
- m. overload syndrome
- m. pad
- m. parabola
- m. phalangeal fifth angle
- m. proximal dome osteotomy
- m. ray
- m. Reverdin osteotomy
- m. shaft
- m. traction
- m. V-shaped osteotomy

metatarsalgia
- Morton m.
- secondary m.
- transfer m.

metatarsal-tarsal joint

metatarsectomy

metatarsi (*pl. of* metatarsus)

metatarsocalcaneal angle

metatarsocuboid joint

metatarsocuneiform (MTC)
- m. angle
- m. arthrodesis
- m. articulation
- m. joint

M

NOTES

metatarsocuneiform *(continued)*
    m. joint exostosis
    m. joint fusion
metatarsophalangeal (MT, MTP)
    m. arthroplasty
    m. capsulotomy
    m. creaking
    m. crease
    m. joint (MTPJ)
    m. joint arthrodesis
    m. joint capsule
    m. joint disarticulation
    m. joint dislocation
    m. joint fusion
    m. joint ganglion
    m. joint injury
    m. joint synovitis
    m. subluxation
metatarsophalangeal-interphalangeal scale
metatarsophalangealium
metatarsosesamoid
    m. joint
    m. ligament
metatarsotalar angle
metatarsus, pl. **metatarsi**
    m. abductus
    m. adductocavus
    m. adductovarus
    m. adductus (MTA)
    m. adductus angle
    m. adductus deformity
    m. cavus
    m. internus
    m. primus adductus (MPA)
    m. primus atavicus
    m. primus declination angle
    m. primus elevatus
    m. primus equinus
    m. primus osteotomy
    m. primus varus (MPV)
    m. primus varus deformity
    m. rectus
    m. valgus
    m. varus (MTV)
    m. varus deformity
metatropic dwarfism
metazonal region
Met Bar shoe modification
Metcalf spring drop brace
meter
    Fischer pressure threshold m.
    pinch m.
methacrylate
    antibiotic-impregnated
      polymethyl m.
    centrifuged methyl m.
    methyl m.

    polymethyl m. (PMMA)
    m. resin
methemoglobin
method
    Abbott m.
    antegrade m.
    anthropometric m.
    biofeedback-assisted m.
    Bleck m.
    Borggreve m.
    Buck m.
    Budin-Chandler m.
    bundle-nailing m.
    cable cerclage m.
    Callahan m.
    Carrel m.
    Caton m.
    Chaput m.
    Cobb m.
    computer-assisted design-controlled
      alignment m. (CAD/CAM)
    contoured adduction trochanteric-
      controlled alignment m. (CAT-
      CAM)
    cup and cone m.
    Delore m.
    depth caliper-meter stick m.
    disk diffusion m.
    dynamic traction m.
    Edinburgh m.
    Elmslie-Trillat patellar
      realignment m.
    Essex-Lopresti m.
    extension block splinting m.
    Fallat-Buckholz m.
    Feldenkrais m.
    Ferguson scoliosis measuring m.
    Fick m.
    Gerbert-Mellilo m.
    Gohil-Cavolo m.
    Hoffa tendon-shortening m.
    Hoke triple-section m.
    hold-relax m.
    hole preparation m.
    hydrogen washout m.
    Ilizarov m.
    immobilization m.
    Insall patella alta m.
    install m.
    Jahss ninety-ninety m.
    Kaplan-Meier time-to-event
      analysis m.
    keyhole m.
    Lange tendon-lengthening m.
    Lindsjö m.
    Ling m.
    Lund and Broden m.
    McConnell taping technique m.

McKenzie m.
McReynolds m.
Mose m.
Mosley anterior shoulder repair m.
nail length gauge m.
Neufeld dynamic m.
ninety-ninety m.
Oil-Red-O m.
one-inclinometer m.
OnTrack treatment m.
Oxford m.
Palmer m.
pedicle m.
m. of perpendiculars
Pilates exercise m.
pin-and-plaster m.
Ponseti clubfoot treatment m.
Ranawat-Dorr-Inglis m.
receptor-tonus m.
retrograde m.
Risser m.
Russe-Gerhardt m.
Schede m.
Schober m.
Stamm m.
Stimson gravity m.
Stulberg m.
Tajima m.
total mesenteric apron m.
Trager m.
two-inclinometer m.
Wagner limb lengthening m.
Zwipp m.
methotrexate toxicity
methyl
　m. methacrylate
　m. methacrylate adhesive
　m. methacrylate bead
　m. methacrylate bead implant
　m. methacrylate cement
　m. methacrylate implant material
methylcellulose
methylene
　m. blue
　m. blue dye
methylprednisolone
　m. acetate
　m. sodium succinate
methylxanthine
Metrecom
　M. digitizer
　M. spinal analyzer

Mettler
　M. electrotherapy
　M. Trio neuromuscular electrical
　　stimulator
Metzenbaum
　M. chisel
　M. gouge
　M. scissors
Meuli arthroplasty
Meurig Williams plate
Meyer
　M. cervical orthosis
　M. dysplasia
　M. line
Meyer-Betz
　M.-B. disease
　M.-B. syndrome
Meyer-Burgdorff osteotomy
Meyerding
　M. bone skid
　M. chisel
　M. curved osteotome
　M. gouge
　M. mallet
　M. retractor
　M. spondylolisthesis classification
　　line
　M. straight osteotome
Meyerding-Van Demark technique
Meyers-McKeever
　M.-M. tibial fracture classification
Meyers quadratus muscle-pedicle bone graft
Meyhoeffer bone curette
Meynet node
Meyn-Quigley maneuver
Meyn reduction of elbow dislocation
MFA
　Musculoskeletal Function Assessment
　　MFA questionnaire
M-F heel protector
MG
　muscle group
　MG II knee prosthesis
　MG II total knee system
MGHL
　middle glenohumeral ligament
　MGHL cord
MGH osteotome
MHOCE
　multiple hereditary osteochondral
　exostosis

M

NOTES

MHW
    medial heel wedge
Miami
    M. Acute Care (MAC)
    M. Acute cervical collar
    M. Acute collar cervical traction
    M. fracture brace
    M. J cervical collar
    M. J collar cervical traction
    M. TLSO scoliosis brace
Mibelli
    porokeratosis of M.
MICA 3x sleeve
mice (*pl. of* mouse)
Michaelis rhomboid
Michael Reese articulated prosthesis
Michal deformity
Michel clip
Michele
    M. long-stem prosthesis
    M. vertebral biopsy
    M. vertebral trephine
Michelson-Sequoia air drill
Michigan
    M. Bone Health Study
    M. Hand Outcomes
    M. Hand Outcomes Questionnaire
micro
    M. QuickAnchor
    M. Series wire driver
    m. waveform
Micro-Aire
    M.-A. débridement of bone surface
    M.-A. drill
    M.-A. oscillating saw
    M.-A. osteotome
    M.-A. reamer
microamperage
    m. electrical nerve stimulation
      (MENS)
    m. neural stimulation (MNS)
microanastomosis
microavulsion
microcirculation
microcoil
microcomputer upper limb exerciser
    (MULE)
microcrystalline collagen
microcurrent
    m. electrode
    m. therapy
microdebrider
    MDS m.
microdiskectomy
    arthroscopic m. (AMD)
    uniportal arthroscopic m.

MicroFET2
    M. muscle tester
    M. muscle testing device
Microfil contrast medium
Microfoam dressing
microfracture
microgeodic syndrome
micrographia
microinterlock
microirrigating cannula
microirrigator
MicroLite suture anchor
Microloc
    M. knee implant
    M. knee prosthesis
    M. knee system
microlumbar
    m. diskectomy (MLD)
    m. disk excision
    m. diskography
micromelic dwarfism
micrometric screw
Micro-Mill knee instrument system
MicroMite anchor suture
micromotion
    liner m.
microneedle holder
microneurography midlatency SEP
microneurosurgical technique
Micro-One
    M.-O. dissecting forceps
    M.-O. hook
microoscillating saw
microparticulated protein product
MicroPhor iontophoretic drug delivery
    system
micropin
    Pischel m.
microplate
    Luhr m.
micropodia
microprocessor
    Intertron therapy m.
microsagittal saw
microsaw
    Zimmer m.
microscissors
microscope
    double binocular operating m.
    operating m.
microscopy
    confocal m.
    hyperspectral near-infrared Raman
     imaging m.
    light m.
    transmission electron m.

Microsect
    M. curette
    M. shaver
MicroStable liner locking mechanism
microstaple
    Barouk m.
microsurgical
    m. diskectomy (MSD)
    m. instrument
    m. thoracoscopic vertebrectomy
microtiter protein kinase assay
microtrauma
    cervical m.
    lumbar m.
    repetitive m.
    thoracic m.
Micro-Two forceps
microvalve
    Hypobaric m.
microvascular
    m. clamp
    m. free muscle flap
    m. osseous transfer
    m. surgical anastomosis
microvasculature
Microvel prosthesis
microwave diathermy (MWD)
Micro-Z neuromuscular stimulator
Midas
    M. Rex acorn
    M. Rex bone cutter
    M. Rex bur
    M. Rex drill
    M. Rex instrumentation system
    M. Rex knife
    M. Rex pneumatic instrument
midaxillary
    m. line (MAL)
    m. line incision
midbody of vertebra
midcalf
midcarpal
    m. arthrodesis
    m. arthroscopy
    m. injury
    m. instability (MCI)
    m. joint
    m. portal
    m. radial (MCR)
    m. ulnar (MCU)

Middeldorpf
    M. splint
    M. triangle
mid-diaphysial axis
middle
    m. atlantoepistrophic joint
    m. carpal joint
    m. column injury
    m. finger
    m. finger amputation
    m. glenohumeral ligament (MGHL)
    m. sacral artery
    m. sacral vein
    m. third (M/3)
    m. third of shaft
    m. thyroid vein
    m. tibial shaft fracture
middle-ear barotrauma
middle-finger test
midfacial fracture
midfemur
midfoot
    m. abductus
    m. adductus
    m. arthritis
    m. arthrodesis
    m. arthropathy
    m. cavus
    m. fracture
    m. joint
    m. scale
midheel line
Midland
    M. multifunctional mat platform
    M. tilt table
midlateral
    m. approach
    m. capsule
    m. portal
midline
    m. disk herniation
    M. Hi-Lo Mat Platform
    m. ligament
    m. medial approach
midmalleolar line
midmedial capsule
midnight fracture
midpalmar
    m. abscess
    m. space

M

NOTES

midpatellar
    m. portal
    m. tendon
midsagittal plane
midshaft
    m. fracture
    m. metatarsal osteotomy
midstance period of gait
midsternal line (MSL)
midsubstance tear
midtarsal
    m. dome osteotomy
    m. joint
    m. osteoarthritis
    m. V-osteotomy
midtarsus
midthigh amputation
Midwest Regional Spinal Cord Injury Center
Mignon eosinophilic granuloma
migration
    m. of acetabular cup
    brace m.
    hallux m.
    instrument m.
    Luque rod m.
    m. of prosthesis
    rod m.
    staple m.
    trochanteric m.
migratory
    m. arthralgia
    m. arthritis
MII
    McDowell Impairment Index
Mikasa subacromial bursography
Mikhail bone block
Mikulicz
    M. angle
    M. operation
    M. pad
    M. procedure
    M. sponge
Mikulicz-Vladimiroff amputation
Milch
    M. condylar fracture classification
    M. cuff resection
    M. cuff resection of ulna technique
    M. elbow fracture classification
    M. elbow operation
    M. elbow technique
    M. fracture classification syndrome
    M. plate
    M. radioulnar joint repair
Miles bone chisel
milestone
    motor m.

Milewski driver
Milford mallet finger technique
military
    m. antishock trousers (MAST)
    m. brace maneuver
    m. brace position
    m. posture test
    m. tuck position
milk-alkali disease
milking
    m. maneuver
    m. of vessel
milkmaid's
    m. elbow
    m. elbow dislocation
milkman's
    m. pseudofracture
    m. syndrome
milk test
mill
    bone m.
    Lere bone m.
    OrthoBlend powered bone m.
mille
    m. pattes screw
    m. pattes technique
Millender arthroplasty
Millender-Nalebuff wrist arthrodesis
Miller
    M. flatfoot operation
    M. foot procedure
    M. rasp
Miller-Galante
    M.-G. I condylar total knee system
    M.-G. I hemiarthroplasty
    M.-G. hip prosthesis
    M.-G. jig
    M.-G. knee
    M.-G. knee arthroplasty
    M.-G. II knee prosthesis
    M.-G. revision knee system
    M.-G. total knee system
Millesi
    M. modified technique
    M. nerve graft
milliamperage x seconds (MAS)
milliampere (mA)
millimeter (mm)
millimeters of mercury (mmHg)
millimetric rule
milliner's needle
milling cutter
Mills
    M. dressing
    M. test
Miltex
    M. bone saw
    M. mallet

M. nail nipper
M. wire twister
Miltner-Wan calcaneus resection
Milwaukee
M. cervicothoracolumbosacral
orthosis
M. scoliosis brace
M. scoliosis orthosis
M. shoulder syndrome
mimocausalgia
Minaar
M. classification of coalition
M. classification system
M. coalition classification
mind-body therapy
MindSet toe splint
mineralization
Miner osteotome
miner's elbow
Minerva
M. cast
M. cervical brace
M. cervical jacket
M. fixation
M. orthosis
M. vest
mini
m. AO screw
m. applier
M. Bio-Phase suture anchor
M. GLS anchor
m. lag screw system (MLS)
**Mini-Acutrak small bone fixation
system**
miniature
m. end-plate potential (MEPP)
m. multipurpose clamp
mini-C-arm
XiScan m.-C-a.
mini-core disease
minifixator
articulate m.
Mini-Flap drain system
minifragment
m. plate fixation
m. screw
mini-Hoffmann external fixator
mini-Hohmann podiatric retractor
mini-Kessler external fixator
mini-Lambotte osteotome
mini-Lexer osteotome
minimal incision plantar fasciotomy

minimally displaced fracture
minima patella
MiniMedBall hand exerciser
mini-meniscus blade
minimi
abductor digiti m. (ADM)
extensor digiti m. (EDM)
opponens digiti m. (ODM)
minimum incision surgery (MIS)
minimus
digitus m.
mini-open rotator cuff repair
mini-Orthofix fixator
mini-pilon fracture
miniplate
Luhr m.
Mini-Revo Screws suture anchor
Mini-ROC anchor
Minislide sliding mat
ministaple
Bio-R-Sorb resorbable poly-L-lactic
acid m.
ministem shaft
mini-Stryker power drill
mini-Ullrich bone clamp
**Minkoff-Jaffe-Menendez posterior
approach**
Minkoff-Nicholas procedure
Minneapolis hip prosthesis
Minnesota
M. Manual Dexterity Test
M. Rate of Manipulation test
M. Spatial Relations Test
minor
m. amputation
m. curve
M. sign
Minos air drill
Mira
M. cautery
M. drill
M. reamer
Mirage Spinal System
mirror
Apfelbaum m.
dental m.
m. hand
meniscal m.
Mirua-Komada release
MIS
minimum incision surgery
misalignment

NOTES

M

miserable misalignment syndrome
missed fracture
misshapen
missile injury
Mital
    M. elbow release
    M. elbow release operation
    M. elbow release technique
Mitchel-Adam multipurpose clamp
Mitchell
    M. bunionectomy
    M. distal osteotomy
    M. hallux valgus procedure
    M. operation
    M. osteotome
    M. osteotomy/bunionectomy
    M. posterior displacement
      osteotomy
    M. step-down osteotomy
Mitek
    M. absorbable anchor
    M. anchor system
    M. bone anchor
    M. FASTIN threaded anchor
    M. GII easy anchor
    M. GII Snap-Pak
    M. GII suture anchor system
    M. GL anchor
    M. knotless anchor
    M. ligament anchor
    M. micro anchor
    M. Micro QuickAnchor
    M. Mini GLS anchor
    M. Mini QuickAnchor
    M. Panalok RC anchor
    M. rotator cuff anchor
    M. SuperAnchor instrument
    M. Tacit threaded anchor
    M. vapor
    M. VAPR tissue removal system
mitella
miter technique
mitochondrial myopathy
mitochondrion, pl. mitochondria
mitt
    holding m.
    impact m.
    motion control m.
    paraffin m.
    wash m.
mitten hand
Mittlemeir
    M. broach
    M. ceramic hip prosthesis
    M. noncemented femoral prosthesis
Mitutoyo digital caliper
MIV
  major injury vector

mixed
    m. amputation
    m. connective tissue disease
    m. connective tissue disorder
    m. cord syndrome
mixer
    MixEvac bone cement m.
MixEvac bone cement mixer
Mixter
    M. forceps
    M. ligature-carrier clamp
    M. right-angle clamp
Miyakawa
    M. knee operation
    M. knee procedure
Mize-Bucholz-Grogen approach
Mizuno-Hirohata-Kashiwagi technique
Mizuno technique
MKG knee support
MKS II knee brace
M/L
  mediolateral
  M/L lift
MLD
  microlumbar diskectomy
MLS
  mini lag screw system
MLSI
  multiple line-scan imaging
MM
  medial malleolus
mm
  millimeter
mmHg
  millimeters of mercury
MMT
  manual muscle testing
MNCV
  motor nerve conduction velocity
MNS
  microamperage neural stimulation
MO
  medial oblique
Moberg
    M. advancement flap
    M. arthrodesis
    M. deltoid muscle transfer
    M. deltoid-to-triceps transfer
    M. dowel graft
    M. key-grip tenodesis
    M. key-pinch procedure
    M. osteotome
    M. Picking Up Test
    M. screw
    M. splint
mobile-bearing
    m.-b. knee arthroplasty
    m.-b. knee implant

mobile wad
Mobilimb CPM device
mobility
    active m.
    m. aid
    coordinated m.
    fractured bone m.
    gait and m.
    hip m.
    intersegmental m.
    joint m.
    limited joint m. (LJM)
    lumbar sagittal m.
    muscle tissue m.
    passive m.
    rotation m.
    sacral m.
    sacroiliac joint m.
    sagittal m.
    segmental m.
    side-bending m.
    symphysial m.
    m. testing
    translation m.
    unisegmental m.
    vertical symphysial m.
    m. WHO Handicap Scale
mobilization
    ASTM augmented soft tissue m.
    augmented soft tissue m. (ASTM)
    Duran passive m.
    grades 1–5 of m.
    joint m.
    lateral band m.
    nonthrust m.
    soft tissue m.
    spinal joint m.
    m. with impulse
MOD
    MOD femoral drill guide
    MOD unicompartmental knee
      system
modality
    deep heat m.
    electrical m.
    Fluidotherapy sterile dry heat m.
    mechanical m.
    nonthermal m.
    passive treatment m.
    superficial heat m.
    thermal m.

mode
    Gruen m.
    loading m.
model
    M. 810 axial closed-loop hydraulic
      mechanical testing
    Bennett pain m.
    corpectomy m.
    Currey m.
    Denis Browne three-column m.
    family management m.
    foot m.
    joint m.
    lumbar spine m.
    Tanner developmental m.
modeling
    cortical bone m.
modification
    Bloom-Raney m.
    Bonfiglio m.
    C-D screw m.
    Clark-Southwick-Odgen m.
    dietary m.
    Duncan-Lovell m.
    Fairbanks technique with Sever m.
    Gil m.
    Harriluque sublaminar wiring m.
    Helal m.
    Jacobs locking hook spinal rod
      instrumentation m.
    Kalish bunionectomy m.
    Kleinert m.
    Losee m.
    McGlamry and Feldman m.
    medial sole-wedge shoe m.
    metatarsal bar shoe m.
    Met Bar shoe m.
    Neer m.
    Seddon m.
    Sequeira-Khanuja m.
    shoe m.
    Stauffer m.
    Strickland m.
    Youngwhich m.
modified
    M. American Shoulder and Elbow
      Surgeons Shoulder Patient Self-
      Evaluation Form patient
      questionnaire
    m. Boyd amputation
    m. Boyd amputation of ankle and
      distal tibial physis

M

NOTES

modified *(continued)*
m. Boyd ankle arthrodesis
m. Broström-Evans procedure
m. Broström procedure
m. Chrisman-Snook ankle reconstruction
m. Cocklin toe operation
m. Cotrel cast
m. Crawford Campbell inlaid bone-grafting technique
m. Darrach-type elevator
m. Frankel classification
m. Fukuda-type retractor
m. Gait Abnormality Rating Scale
m. Grace plate
m. Harris hip score
m. Hoffmann quadrilateral external fixator
m. Hohmann bunionectomy
m. Hoke-Miller flatfoot procedure
m. Keller resection arthroplasty
m. Kessler suture
m. Kessler-Tajima suture
m. Kienböck disease
m. Lapidus arthrodesis
m. Lapidus procedure
m. Mau bunionectomy
m. Mau osteotomy
m. McBride bunionectomy
m. mold and surface replacement arthroplasty
m. Moore hip locking prosthesis
m. Oppenheimer splint
M. Rankin scale
m. Robert Jones dressing
m. Rowe shoulder score
m. Sillence classification
m. tonsillar prong
m. two-portal endoscopic carpal tunnel release
m. Wagner classification system
m. Watson-Jones ankle tenodesis
m. Wilson osteotomy
m. Zarins and Rowe

Modny
M. drill
M. pin

modular
M. Acetabular Revision System (MARS)
m. Austin Moore hip prosthesis
m. implant
m. instrumentation
m. Iowa Precoat total hip prosthesis
m. large-head component
m. Lenbach hip system
m. Moniflex hip stem

3R80 m. hydraulic knee joint
m. socket
m. S-ROM total hip system
m. temPPTthotic kit
m. total hip prosthesis
m. unicompartmental knee prosthesis

module
Allen Diagnostic M.
Peak gait m.

modulus
m. of elasticity
Young m.

Moe
M. alar hook
M. bone curette
M. bone impactor
M. gouge
M. intertrochanteric plate
M. modified Cotrel cast
M. modified Harrington rod
M. osteotome
M. scoliosis operation
M. scoliosis technique
M. square-end rod
M. system

Moe-Kettleson distribution of curves in scoliosis
Moeller-Barlow disease
Moeltgen flexometer
Mogensen procedure
Mohrenheim fossa
Mohr finger splint
Mohs technique
Moire topographic scoliosis assessment
moist
m. heat
m. heat therapy
Restore Clean 'N M.
Molander-Olerud shoulder score
mold
m. acetabular arthroplasty
Aufranc concentric hip m.
Biothotic orthotic m.
caudad anterior m.
cephalad anterior m.
molded
AFO m.
m. ankle-foot orthosis (MAFO)
m. lumbosacral orthosis
m. posterior plaster splint
m. postpartum insole
m. Thomas collar
molding
compression m.
elastomer skin m.
polyethylene compression m.
m. sock

Mold-In-Place back support
moleskin
    m. padding
    m. strip dressing
    m. traction tape
Molestick padding
Molesworth-Campbell elbow approach
  operation
Molesworth osteotomy
molle
    fibroma m.
    heloma m. (HM)
Moloney line
Molt periosteal elevator
molybdenum
    stainless steel and m. (SMO)
moment
    anterior bending m.
    m. arm
    m. of force
    m. of inertia
    posterior bending m.
    three-point bending m.
momentum
    angular m.
Momma-Too Maternity Support
MOM tractograph
Monarch knee brace
Monark
    M. bicycle
    M. Rehab Trainer
monarthric
monarthritis
    viral m.
monarticular synovitis
Mönckeberg sclerosis
Mondini dysplasia
Moniflex hip stem
monitor
    blood pressure m. (BPM)
    M. Master M. support
    MyoTrac EMG biofeedback m.
    NervePace nerve conduction m.
    Polar Vantage XL heart m.
    Polar wrist m.
    TABS Elite mobility m.
    Vantage Performance m. (VPM)
monitored anesthesia control (MAC)
monitoring
    blood pressure m.
    fluorescein perfusion m.
    screw position perioperative m.

    somatosensory evoked potential m.
    spinal cord function
      intraoperative m.
MonitorMate monitor arm
monkey fist hand
monkey-paw
Monk hip prosthesis
monoamine oxidase-B inhibitor
monoarthritis
monoarticular septic arthritis
monoblock
    m. femoral component
    m. femoral stem prosthesis
monocane
monoclonal gammopathy
monodactyly
Monodos orthosis
monofilament
    calibrated m.
    nylon m.
    m. pressure test
    Semmes-Weinstein m.
    Softip m.
    m. suture
    m. wire
    m. wire fixation
Monofixateur external fixator
Monogram total knee instrument
monolithic
    m. A1203 cup
    m. A1203 cup prosthesis
monomalleolar ankle fracture
mononeuritis multiplex
mononeuropathy
    diabetic femoral m.
    m. electrodiagnosis
    embolic m.
    m. multiplex
monophasic
    m. action potential
    m. endplate activity
    m. waveform
monoplace hyperbaric chamber
monoplegia
    monostotic m.
monopolar
    m. cautery
    m. needle recording electrode
monosodium urate crystal
monospherical total shoulder
  arthroplasty

M

NOTES

monostotic
    m. fibrous dysplasia
    m. monoplegia
monosynaptic reflex arc stereotactic arc
monotube
    M. external fixator system
    Howmedica m.
Monro bursa
Monteggia
    M. dislocation
    M. equivalent lesion
    M. forearm fracture
    M. fracture-dislocation
    M. fracture-dislocation of ulna
Montenovesi rongeur
Montercaux fracture
Monticelli-Spinelli
    M.-S. circular external fixation
      system
    M.-S. distraction
    M.-S. distraction technique
    M.-S. distractor
    M.-S. fixator
    M.-S. frame
    M.-S. leg fixation
Montreal hip positioner
moon
    M. boot
    M. Boot brace
    M. Boot shoe
    M. Walker
Mooney
    M. brace
    M. cast
Moon-Robinson
    M.-R. prosthesis inserter
    M.-R. stapes prosthesis
Moore
    M. bone drill
    M. bone elevator
    M. bone reamer
    M. driver
    M. femoral neck prosthesis
    M. fixation pin
    M. fracture
    M. hip endoprosthesis system
    M. hip prosthesis
    M. nail
    M. osteotomy
    M. osteotomy-osteoclasis
    M. posterior approach
    M. prosthesis extractor
    M. prosthesis-mortising chisel
    M. sliding nail plate
    M. stem
    M. technique
    M. template

    M. tibial plateau fracture
      classification
Moore-Blount
    M.-B. driver
    M.-B. screwdriver
Moore-Southern approach
mooring
mop-end
    m.-e. Achilles tendon tear
    m.-e. appearance
    m.-e. mid-substance tear
Morand foot
morcellate
morcellation
    Robinson m.
    Robinson-Chung-Farahvar
      clavicular m.
morcellize
morcellized
    m. bone
    m. bone graft
    m. cancellous graft
Moreira
    M. bolt
    M. plate
Moreland
    M. femoral component extractor
    M. osteotome
    M. total hip revision
      instrumentation
Moreland-Marder-Anspach femoral stem
    removal
Morel-Lavele lesion
Morel syndrome
Moretz prosthesis
Morfam Quality Jeanie Rub massager
Morgagni hyperostosis
Morgan-Casscells
    M.-C. meniscus suturing
    M.-C. meniscus suturing technique
morphea-like lesion
morphine pump
Morpho Exerciser
morphogenesis
morphogenetic protein
morphologically
morphometry
    pedicle m.
Morquio
    M. disease
    M. sign
    M. syndrome
Morquio-Brailsford syndrome
Morquio-Ullrich
    M.-U. disease
    M.-U. syndrome
Morrey-Bryan total elbow arthroplasty

Morrey elbow arthroplasty rating system

Morris

    M. biphase screw

    M. retractor

Morris-Hand-Dunn anterior arthrodesis

Morrison

    M. neurovascular free flap

    M. technique

Morrissy

    M. percutaneous fixation of slipped epiphysis

    M. percutaneous slipped epiphysis fixation

Morscher cervical plate

Morse

    M. taper

    M. tapered prosthetic post

    M. taper lock of modular hip implant component

mortise

    ankle m.

    bone m.

    cuneiform m.

    m. and tenon joint

    tibial m.

    m. view

mortising chisel

Morton

    M. disease

    M. foot

    M. interdigital neuroma

    M. metatarsalgia

    M. neuralgia

    M. neurectomy

    M. neuroma neurolysis

    M. neuromata

    M. sign

    M. syndrome

    M. test

    M. toe

    M. toe support

Morton-Horwitz nerve cross-over sign

mosaic

    m. arthroplasty

    m. plantar verruca

    m. wart

mosaicplasty

    arthroscopic m.

    m. technique

MosaicPlasty system

Mose

    M. concentric rings

    M. method

Moseley

    M. bone age graph

    M. fasciotome

    M. glenoid rim prosthesis

    M. straight line graph

Mosley anterior shoulder repair method

mosquito

    m. clamp

    m. forceps

    m. hemostat

mosquito-tip grasping forceps

Moss

    M. cage

    M. fixation system

    M. hook

    M. instrumentation

    M. rod

    M. screw

Mosso ergograph

mossy foot

moth-eaten destruction

Mother Jones dressing

Mother-To-Be

    M.-T.-B. abdominal support

    M.-T.-B. Support Maternity Support

motion

    accessory m.

    active ankle joint complex range of m. (AAROM)

    active-assisted range of m. (AAROM)

    active integral range of m. (AIROM)

    active and passive range of m.

    active range of m. (AROM)

    m. activity

    alternating range of m. (ARM)

    angular m.

    angulation m.

    ankle dorsiflexion range of m. (ADROM)

    ankle inversion-eversion range of m.

    AP translatory m.

    arc of m.

    axis of rib m.

    back range of m. (BROM)

    m. barrier

    bucket-handle rib m.

M

NOTES

motion *(continued)*
    constant massive m.
    continuous passive m. (CPM)
    m. control
    controlled ankle m. (CAM)
    m. control limiter
    m. control mitt
    m. control procedure
    coupled m.
    degrees-of-freedom joint m.
    m. demand
    distractive m.
    double-flexion knee m.
    end range of m.
    Euler angle of wrist m.
    frontal m.
    full range of m. (FROM)
    hindfoot m.
    hip extension range of m.
    inherent m.
    intersegmental m.
    m. limit
    m. limitation
    limitation of m. (LOM)
    loss of m. (LOM)
    lumbar range of m.
    m. measurement
    osteokinematic m.
    m. palpation
    passive intervertebral m. (PIVM)
    passive range of m. (PROM)
    pattern of m.
    m. performance
    physiologic m.
    pistoning m.
    plantarflexory m.
    protective limitation of range
      of m.
    pump-handle rib m.
    m. quality
    range of m. (ROM)
    rectilinear m.
    m. response
    restricted range of m.
    restriction of m.
    rotary m.
    sacroiliac joint m.
    sagittal m.
    scapulothoracic m.
    m. segment
    shoulder range of m.
    m. slack
    sling suspension range of m.
    stable to m.
    subtalar m.
    synergistic finger m.
    synergistic wrist m.
    m. testing
    m. therapy
    toe range of m.
    total active m. (TAM)
    total eversion range of m.
    total passive m. (TPM)
    total range of m. (TROM)
    translation m.
    translatory m.
    trial range of m.
    triaxial m.
    triplane m.
    uninhibited ankle m.
    valgus knee m.
    m. velocity
    winging m.
motion-preserving procedure
Motivator FTR2000 exerciser
motoneuron *(var. of* motor neuron)
motor
    m. activity
    m. activity log
    m. branch
    m. conduction velocity
    m. deficit
    m. development
    m. dysfunction
    m. examination
    m. fascicle
    m. function
    m. function assessment
    m. function deficit
    m. latency
    m. loss
    m. milestone
    m. neglect testing
    m. nerve conduction velocity
      (MNCV)
    m. neurolysis
    m. neuron
    m. neuronal pool
    m. neuron disease
    m. neuropathy
    m. point
    m. point block
    m. recovery
    m. reflex
    m. response
    m. restlessness
    m. and sensory neuropathy, type
      I–II
    m. speech disorder
    m. strength
    m. unit
    m. unit action potential (MUAP)
    m. unit fraction
    m. unit potential (MUP)

m. vehicle accident (MVA)
m. weakness
motorcycle accident (MCA)
motorcyclist's knee
motorized
m. bur
m. meniscal cutter
m. meniscal shaver
m. reamer
m. shaving system
m. suction shaver
m. trimmer
motor neuron, motoneuron
Motricity Index
mottled
mottling
Mouchet
M. disease
M. fracture
Mould arthroplasty
Moule screw pin
Mouradian
M. humeral fixation system
M. rod
M. screw
mouse, pl. **mice**
joint mice
M. Nest mouse rest
MouseMitt keyboarder's
movable joint
move
push-pull m.
movement
active hip m.
adventitious m.
anterior-inferior m.
anterior-posterior m.
anterosuperior external ilium m. (ASEx)
anterosuperior internal ilium m. (ASIn)
arcuate m.
m. artifact
M. Assessment of Infants (MAI)
assistive m.
atlas-axis m.
caliper rib m.
compensatory m.
m. disorder
dissociation m.
dynamic m.
external ilium m.

freedom of m.
Frenkel m.
inferior m.
innominate m.
internal m.
intersegmental m.
isokinetic m.
limitation of m.
medial m.
passive m.
posteroinferior external m.
posteroinferior internal m.
primary or intentional m.
primary rotation m.
quasi-independent Y-axis m.
resistive m.
sagittal m.
m. science
Swedish m.
total body m.
trick m.
unilateral posterior-anterior m.
universal coronal m.
mover
prime m.
moviegoer's knee
movie sign
moxa heat therapy
moxibustion heat therapy
Moyer line
Moynihan towel clamp
MP
metacarpophalangeal
MP35N implant metal prosthesis
MPA
metatarsus primus adductus
M-Pact
M-P. cast cutter
M-P. cast spreader
M-P. cast vacuum
M-P. flexible orthotic
MPF
myofascial pain syndrome
MPFL
medial patellofemoral ligament
MPJ
metacarpophalangeal joint
MPM bandage
MPP
maximum pressure picture
MPTh
mechanical pain threshold

M

NOTES

MPV
    metatarsus primus varus
MRC
    Medical Research Council
        MRC muscle function classification
MRI
    magnetic resonance imaging
        dynamic MRI
        flexion-extension MRI
        FONAR Stand-Up MRI
        Gyroscan superconducting MRI
        MRI testing
MRI-compatible plate and screw system
MRI-directed surgery
MRN
    magnetic resonance neurography
MS
    metabolic syndrome
    multiple sclerosis
MS322 muscle stimulator
MSC cold pack
MSD
    microsurgical diskectomy
MSI
    magnetic source imaging
        MSI mapping
MSL
    midsternal line
MST-6A1-4V implant metal prosthesis
MT
    metatarsal
    metatarsophalangeal
    muscle testing
        MT bar
MTA
    metatarsus adductus
        MTA brace
MTC
    metatarsocuneiform
MTE allograft
MTF
    Musculoskeletal Transplant Foundation
mtMRI
    magnetization transfer magnetic
    resonance imaging
MTP
    metatarsophalangeal
        MTP joint (MTPJ)
MTPJ
    metatarsophalangeal joint
    MTP joint
MTS
    medial tibial syndrome
MTSS
    medial tibial stress syndrome
MTV
    metatarsus varus

MUAP
    motor unit action potential
Mubarak-Hargens
    M.-H. decompression
    M.-H. decompression technique
mucate
MUCL
    medial ulnar collateral ligament
mucoid degeneration
mucopolysaccharide
    sulfated m.
mucopolysaccharidosis,
    pl. **mucopolysaccharidoses**
mucous
    m. cyst
    m. membrane
mucus
Mudder sign
mud pack bath
Mueli wrist prosthesis
Mueller
    M. anterolateral femorotibial
      ligament tenodesis
    M. arthrodesis
    M. ATF ankle brace
    M. compression apparatus
    M. compression blade plate
    M. cup
    M. distractor
    M. dual-lock hip prosthesis
    M. femoral supracondylar fracture
      classification
    M. fixation device
    M. hinged knee brace
    M. hip arthroplasty
    M. humerus fracture classification
    M. intertochanteric varus osteotomy
    M. knee operation
    M. knee procedure
    M. lateral compartment
    M. Lite ankle brace
    M. orthopedic shoulder brace
    M. patellar tendon graft
    M. retractor
    M. technique
    M. template
    M. tibial fracture classification
    M. total hip replacement prosthesis
    M. transposition osteotomy
    M. Ultralite brace
    M. Weiss syndrome
    M. wrap-around knee brace
    M. wrench
Mueller-Charnley hip prosthesis
Mulder
    M. click
    M. sign

MULE
    microcomputer upper limb exerciser
    MULE upper limb exerciser
Mulholland and Gunn criteria
Müller
    M. intraarticular shoulder fusion
    M. osteotomy
    M. plate
    M. saw
Muller prosthesis
Mulligan Silastic prosthesis
multangular
    m. bone
    greater m.
    lesser m.
    m. ridge fracture
multi
    M. Axis Ankle
    M. Balance System (MBS)
    M. Podus boot
    M. Podus boot system
    M. Podus foot system
multiaction pin cutter
multiarticular
multiaxial
    M. Assessment of Pain (MAP)
    m. joint
    m. screw
multiaxis
    m. foot
    m. prosthesis
MultiBoot orthosis
multicentric
    m. osteogenic sarcoma
    m. reticulohistiocytosis
Multidex chronic wound treatment system
Multidimensional Pain inventory
multidirectional instability (MDI)
multidisciplinary
multielectrode
multifidus
    m. muscle
    m. syndrome
Multiflex foot prosthesis
multifocal osteomyelitis
multilead electrode
Multileaf Collimator
multilevel
    m. fracture
    m. fusion
    m. laminectomy

Multi-Lig knee brace
Multi-Lock
    M.-L. hand operating table
    M.-L. hip prosthesis
    M.-L. knee brace
multipack
    Ortho-ice m.
multipartite
    m. fracture
    m. patella
multipennate muscle
multiplace hyperbaric chamber
multiplanar
    m. computed tomography scan
    m. CT scan
    m. deformity
    m. ligamentotaxis
    m. virtual fluoroscopic imaging
multiplane echo probe
multiple
    m. action cutter
    m. axis knee joint
    m. cancellous chip graft
    m. digits
    m. discharge
    m. enchondroma
    m. enchondromatosis
    m. epiphysial dysplasia
    m. finger
    m. flexible medullary nail
    m. fracture
    m. hereditary osteochondral exostosis (MHOCE)
    m. hook assembly
    m. hook assembly C-D instrumentation
    m. injuries
    m. line-scan imaging (MLSI)
    m. myeloma
    m. neurofibroma
    m. osteochondromatosis
    m. pinhole occluder
    m. pterygium syndrome
    m. ray
    m. ray amputation
    m. sclerosis (MS)
    m. synostoses syndrome
    m. tarsal coalitions
    m. trauma
multiple-point sacral fixation
multiplex
    mononeuritis m.

M

NOTES

multiplex *(continued)*
    mononeuropathy m.
    myoclonus m.
    paramyoclonus m.
multipolar bipolar cup
Multipulse 1000 compression pump
multipurpose
    m. angled clamp
    m. curved clamp
multiradius unconstrained prosthesis
multiray fracture
multisegmental
    m. spinal distortion
    m. spinal stenosis
multisided blade handle
multisized reamer
multispan fracture hook
multistaged carrier flap
Multitak
    M. SS system
    M. suture snap system
Mumford
    M. procedure
    M. resection
Mumford-Gurd
    M.-G. arthroplasty
    M.-G. operation
mummification necrosis
Munchmeyer disease
Munster cast
MUP
    motor unit potential
Murphy
    M. Achilles tendon advancement
    M. brace
    M. gouge
    M. heel cord advancement
    M. lateral approach
    M. nail
    M. osteotome
    M. punch test
    M. skid
    M. sling
    M. splint
Murphy-Lane bone skid
Murray
    M. fixation
    M. knee prosthesis
    M. and Welch-BDH prosthesis
Murray-Jones arm splint
Murray-Thomas arm splint
muscle
    abdominal m.
    abductor digiti minimi m.
    abductor digiti quinti m.
    abductor hallucis m.
    abductor pollicis brevis m.
    abductor pollicis longus m.

accessory soleus m.
adductor hallucis m.
adductor pollicis m.
Aeby m.
agonist m.
agonistic m.
Albinus m.
m. analysis
anconeus m.
antagonistic m.
appendicular skeletal m. (ASM)
BBC m.'s
m. belly
biceps brachii m.
biceps femoris m.
bicipital m.
m. biopsy clamp
Bowman m.
brachialis m.
brachioradialis m.
buccinator m.
casserian m.
Casser perforated m.
Chassaignac axillary m.
m. contractility
m. contracture
m. contusion
coracobrachial m.
m. cramp
cricopharyngeal sphincter m.
cucullaris m.
deepithelialized rectus abdominis m.
  (DRAM)
deltoid m.
digastric m.
m. disorder
dorsal interosseous m.
Dupré m.
ECRB m.
ECRL m.
ECU m.
EDB m.
EIP m.
elevator m.
emergency m.
m. energy
m. energy technique
epimeric m.
epitrochleoanconeus m.
extensor carpi radialis brevis m.
extensor carpi radialis longus m.
extensor carpi ulnaris m.
extensor communis m.
extensor digiti minimi m.
extensor digiti quinti m.
extensor digitorum brevis m.
extensor digitorum communis m.
extensor digitorum longus m.

extensor hallucis brevis m.
extensor hallucis longus m.
extensor indicis proprius m.
extensor pollicis brevis m.
extensor pollicis longus m.
extensor wad of three m.'s
external intercostal m.
external oblique m.
extrinsic m.
fascia of quadratus lumborum m.
m. fascicle
fast m.
femoral m.
m. fiber action potential
m. fiber conduction velocity
fibular m.
finger flexor m.
fixator m.
m. flap
flexor carpi radialis m.
flexor carpi ulnaris m.
flexor digiti quinti m.
flexor digitorum longus m.
flexor digitorum profundus m.
flexor digitorum sublimis m.
flexor digitorum superficialis m.
flexor hallucis brevis m.
flexor hallucis longus m.
flexor pollicis brevis m.
flexor pollicis longus m.
flexor wad of five m.'s
Folius m.
gastrocnemius m.
gastrocnemius-soleus m.
gluteus maximus m.
gluteus medius m.
gluteus minimus m.
gracilis m.
greater rhomboid m.
m. group (MG)
m. guarding
hamstring m.
handbag m.
m. hernia
hypothenar m.
iliacus m.
iliococcygeus m.
iliocostal m.
iliopsoas m.
m. imbalance
inferior gemelli m.
infraspinatus m.

m. innervation
m. insufficiency
internal oblique m.
interosseous m.
intervening m.
intraspinous m.
intrinsic m.
m. ischemia
Jung m.
Langer axillary arch m.
lateral malleolus m.
latissimus dorsi m.
lesser rhomboid m.
levator scapulae m.
long fibular m.
longissimus colli m.
longus capitis m.
longus cervicis (colli) m.
longus colli m.
lumbrical m.
lumbricalis m.
Luschka m.
mesothenar m.
multifidus m.
multipennate m.
m. and neurological stimulation
  electrotherapy device
nonstriated m.
oblique m.
obturator externus m.
obturator internus m.
omohyoid m.
opponens digiti quinti m.
opponens pollicis m. (OP)
palmar interosseous m.
palmaris digitorum superficialis m.
palmaris longus m.
paraspinal m.
paravertebral m.
m. patterning sequence
pectineus m.
pectoralis major m.
pectoralis minor m.
m. pedicle bone graft
peroneal m.
peroneus brevis m.
peroneus longus m.
peroneus quartus m.
peroneus tertius m.
Phillips m.
piriform m.
plantaris m.

M

NOTES

muscle *(continued)*
platysma m.
m. play
pollicis longus m.
popliteal m.
postaxial m.
posterior deltoid m.
postural m.
preaxial m.
profundus m.
pronator quadratus m.
pronator teres m.
m. protein synthesis
psoas m.
quadrate m.
quadratus femoris m.
quadratus lumborum m.
quadratus plantae m.
quadriceps femoris m.
rectus abdominis m.
rectus femoris m.
red m.
m. relaxant
released ulnar intrinsic m.
m. repositioning
rhomboid m.
rider's m.
Riolan m.
rotator m.
sacrococcygeal m.
sacrospinal m.
sartorius m.
scalene m.
scapulohumeral m.
scapulothoracic m.
semimembranosus m.
semispinal m.
semitendinosus m.
serratus anterior m.
m. sheath
short fibular m.
shunt m.
Sibson m.
skeletal m.
m. slide
m. sliding operation
slow m.
smooth m.
soleus m.
somatic m.
m. spasm
sphincter m.
m. spindle
spurt m.
sternocleidomastoid m.
sternohyoid m.
sternomastoid m.
sternothyroid m.

m. strain
strap m.
m. stretch reflex
striated m.
striped m.
subclavius m.
subcostal m.
suboccipital m.
subscapularis m.
subvertebral m.
supinator m.
supraspinatus m.
supraspinous m.
synergistic m.
teres major m.
teres minor m.
m. testing (MT)
thenar m.
third fibular m.
tibial m.
tibialis anterior m.
tibialis posterior m.
m. tissue mobility
toe extensor m.
toe flexor m.
m. tone
tonic m.
trachelomastoid m.
m. transfer
transversus abdominis m.
trapezius m.
triangular m.
triceps surae m.
tricipital m.
twitch m.
unipennate m.
unstriated m.
vastus intermedius m.
vastus lateralis m.
vastus medialis m.
vestigial m.
voluntary m.
white m.
Wilson m.
yoked m.
muscle-balancing procedure
muscle-plasty
Speed V-Y m.-p.
muscle-setting exercise
muscle-splitting incision
muscle-strengthening exercise
muscle-tendon
m.-t. attachment
m.-t. injury
m.-t. transplantation
muscle-to-bone suture
muscular
m. atrophy

m. attachment
m. clamp
m. contraction
m. coordination
m. cramp
m. dystrophy (MD)
m. lesion
m. neurofibromatosis
m. reeducation
m. reflex
m. rehabilitation
m. tissue
m. torticollis
m. trophoneurosis
muscularity
musculature
axial m.
left erector spinae m.
paraspinal m.
paravertebral m.
peroneal m.
right erector spinae m.
musculoaponeurotic
musculocutaneous
m. amputation
m. free flap
m. nerve
m. nerve block
m. nerve injury
m. nerve paralysis
musculoelastic
musculofascial
musculointestinal
musculoligamentous
musculomembranous
musculophrenic
musculorum
dystonia m.
musculoskeletal
M. Evaluation, Rehabilitation and Conditioning (MERAC)
M. Function Assessment (MFA)
m. infection
m. melioidosis
M. Transplant Foundation (MTF)
m. trauma
M. Tumor Society
musculospiral paralysis
musculotendinous
m. cuff
m. flap
m. junction

m. system
m. unit
musculotendinous-osseous link
Musgrave
M. footprint pedobarograph
M. Footprint System
mushroom
m. impactor
m. walker glide
mushy edema
musician's plight
muslin sling
Mustard iliopsoas transfer
mutilans
arthritis m.
m. rheumatoid arthritis
mutilation
amniotic deformity, adhesion, m. (ADAM)
MV1, MV2 receptor
MVA
motor vehicle accident
MVC
maximal voluntary contraction
MVM
medullary venous malformation
MVP
Biodex Multi-Joint System 3 MVP
MWD
microwave diathermy
M3-X fixation system
myalgia
myasthenia
m. angiosclerotica
m. gravis
myatonia
myatrophy
mycetoma
Carter m.
recurrent m.
mycobacterial
m. arthritis
m. infection
Mycocide
mycotic club nail
myectomy
myectopy
myelalgia
myelapoplexy
myelasthenia
myelatelia
myelatrophy
myelauxe

M

NOTES

myelencephalitis
myelinated
myelinopathy
myelinosis
myelitis
    acute transverse m.
myeloblastoma
myelocele
myelocystocele
myelocystomeningocele
myelodiastasis
myelodysplasia
myelodysplastic kyphosis
myeloencephalitis
myelofibrosis
myelogenous callus
myelogram
myelographic
myelography
    air m.
    computer-assisted m. (CAM)
    iopamidol m.
    Isovue m.
    opaque m.
    oxygen m.
myelolipoma
myeloma
    multiple m.
    solitary m.
myelomalacia
myelomeningitis
myelomeningocele
myelomere
myeloneuritis
myeloparalysis
myelopathy
    cervical spondylotic m.
    m. incidence
    noncompressive m.
    progressive subacute m.
    radiation-related m.
    spinal stenotic m.
    transverse m.
    vacuolar m.
myelophthisis
myeloplegia
myeloproliferative disorder
myeloradiculitis
myeloradiculopathy
myelorrhagia
myelorrhaphy
    commissural m.
myelosclerosis
myelosyphilis
myelotomy
    Bischof m.
Myers knee retractor
mylohyoid

myoasthenia
myoblast
myoblastoma
    granular cell m.
Myobock
    M. artificial hand
    M. system
myobradia
myocardial
    m. bridging
    m. ischemia
myocele
myocelialgia
myocelitis
myocellulitis
myocerosis
myocervical collar
myoclasis
myoclonia
myoclonic epilepsy
myoclonus
    action m.
    epileptic m.
    hereditary essential m.
    intention m.
    m. multiplex
    nocturnal m.
    palatal m.
    spinal m.
myocoele
myocrismus
myocutaneous flap
myocytoma
myodegeneration
myodemia
myodesis
myodiastasis
myodynamic
myodynamics
myodynia
myodysneuria
myodystonia
myodystrophia fetalis
myodystrophy
myoedema
myoelastic
myoelectrical
myoelectrically silent
myoelectric control prosthesis
myoencephalopathy
myofascia
myofascial
    m. closure
    m. manipulation
    m. pain
    m. pain syndrome (MPF)
    m. release
    m. tenderness

m. trigger point
m. unit
myofasciitis
interstitial m.
myofibril
myofibroblast
myofibroma
myofibrosis
myofibrositis
MyoForce test
myofusio-periostitis
myogelosis
myogenic
m. paralysis
m. tonus
m. torticollis
myoglobinuria
familial m.
myography
acoustic m.
myohypertrophia
myoinositol level
myoischemia
myokerosis
myokinesis
myokymia
exercise-induced m.
myokymic discharge
myolipoma
myologia
myology
myolysis
myoma
myomalacia
myomatosis
myomectomy, myomatectomy
myomelanosis
myonecrosis
clostridial m.
myoneuralgia
myoneural ischemia
myoneurasthenia
myoneurectomy
myoneuroma
myoneurosis
myonosus
myopachynsis
myopalmus
myoparalysis
myoparesis
myopathic
m. arthrogryposis

m. atrophy
m. gait
m. motor unit potential
m. paralysis
m. recruitment
m. scoliosis
myopathophysiology
myopathy
acquired m.
benign congenital m.
carcinomatous m.
centronuclear m.
exercise m.
m. hand
idiopathic polymyositis m.
Kiloh-Nevin m.
mitochondrial m.
myotubular m.
nemaline rod-body m.
polymyositis m.
postinfectious m.
rheumatoid arthritis m.
sarcotubular m.
steroid m.
structural congenital m.
Welander distal m.
zebra body m.
zidovudine-induced m.
myophagism
myoplastic muscle stabilization
myoplasty
myopsychopathy
myorrhaphy
myorrhexis
myosarcoma
Myoscan sensor
myoschwannoma
myosclerosis
myositis
acute progressive m.
cervical tension m. (CTM)
clostridial m.
m. fibrosa
focal nodular m.
granulomatous m.
inclusion body m. (IBM)
inflammatory m.
ischemic m.
m. ossificans
m. ossificans progressiva
proliferative m.
rheumatoid m.

M

NOTES

myositis *(continued)*
    m. serosa
    streptococcal m.
    suppurative m.
    tension m.
    viral m.
myospasm
myostasis
myosteoma
myosthenic
myosthenometer
myosuture
myosynizesis
myotasis
myotatic
    m. reflex
    m. unit
myotendinous junction
myotenontoplasty
myotenositis
myotenotomy
myotomal pain
myotome
myotomy
myotonia
    m. acquisita
    m. atrophica
    chondroplastic m.
    m. congenita
    m. congenita intermittens
    congenital m.
    drug-induced m.

    m. dystrophica
    m. hereditaria
    m. intermittens
    Schwartz-Jampel m.
myotonic
    m. discharge
    m. muscular dystrophy
    m. potential
myotonoid
myotonometer
myotonus
MyoTrac
    M. device
    M. EMG biofeedback monitor
    M. single-channel
myotrophic
myotrophy
myotube
myotubular myopathy
myovascular
mytenositis
myxedema
myxofibroma
myxoid
    m. chondrosarcoma
    m. cyst
    m. liposarcoma
myxoid-type liposarcoma
myxoma
    enchondromatous m.
    soft tissue m.
myxosarcoma

NA
neuropathic arthropathy
NAAP
National Arthritis Action Plan
Nada-Chair Back-Up portable back sling
Naden-Rieth prosthesis
NADPH
nicotinamide-adenine dinucleotide phosphate
Naffziger
N. sign
N. syndrome
N. test
Nägele pelvis
NAGS
natural apophysial glides
reverse NAGS

nail
adjustable n.
Ainsworth modification of Massie n.
Alta tibial n.
antegrade femoral n.
antegrade/retrograde compression n.
anteroposterior n.
AO slotted medullary n.
AP n.
n. assembly
Augustine boat n.
n. avulsion
Bailey-Dubow n.
Barr bolt n.
beak n.
n. bed
n. bed graft
n. bed hematoma evacuation
n. bed lesion
bent n.
Bickel intramedullary n.
Biomet ankle arthrodesis n.
blind medullary n.
boat n.
Böhler n.
brittle n.
Brooker double-locking unreamed tibial n.
Brooker femoral n.
Brooker-Wills n.
Calandruccio n.
cannulated n.
centromedullary n.
Chandler unreamed interlocking tibial n.
Chick n.

Christensen interlocking n.
closed Küntscher n.
closed unlocked n.
cloverleaf Küntscher n.
clubbed n.
condylocephalic n.
crutch and belt femoral closed n.
Curry hip n.
Delitala T-nail n.
delta femoral n.
Delta Recon n.
delta tibial n.
Derby n.
Diamond n.
diamond-shaped medullary n.
digital n.
double-ended n.
double-hollow n.
n. drill
n. driver
n. dust
dynamic locking n.
dystrophic n.
elastic stable intramedullary n. (ESIN)
Ender flexible medullary n.
Engel-May n.
n. extender
n. extension
extension n.
femoral neck n.
fissured n.
flexible intramedullary n. (FIN)
flexible medullary n.
fluted Sampson n.
fluted titanium n.
n. fold
n. fold removal
four-flanged n.
Gamma trochanteric locking n.
Green-Seligson-Henry n.
n. groove
Grosse-Kempf interlocking medullary n.
Grosse-Kempf locking n.
GSH n.
Hackethal n.
Hagie pin n.
Hahn bone n.
Halder locking n.
half-and-half n.
Hall-Pankovich medullary n.
hallux n.
Hansen-Street n.
Harrington n.

N

nail *(continued)*
Harris condylocephalic n.
Harris hip n.
Harris medullary n.
Holt n.
hooked intramedullary n.
hooked medullary n.
Huckstep n.
IMSC multihole n.
ingrown n.
INRO surgical n.
interlocking medullary n.
intramedullary ANK n.
intramedullary supracondylar
 multihole n.
Inyo n.
Jewett n.
Johannson hip n.
Kaessmann n.
Ken sliding n.
Klemm n.
Klemm-Schellman n.
Knowles pin n.
Küntscher n.
Laing H-beam n.
left-sided n.
n. length gauge method
Lewis n.
Lloyd adapter for Smith-Petersen n.
locking n.
Lottes triflanged medullary n.
Luck n.
Massie II n.
Massie sliding n.
n. matrix
n. matrix phenolization (NMP)
McKee tri-fin n.
McLaughlin n.
medullary n.
Moore n.
multiple flexible medullary n.
Murphy n.
mycotic club n.
nested n.
Neufeld n.
No-Lok self-locking n.
noncannulated n.
nonreamed n.
Nylok self-locking n.
onychocryptosis n.
open n.
open-section n.
Orthofix intramedullary n.
OrthoSorb pin n.
Palmer bone n.
PGP n.
Pidcock n.
pincer n.

Pitcock n.
n. plate
n. plate apparatus
n. plate device
n. plate fixation
n. plate removal
prebent n.
Pugh sliding n.
reamed n.
Recon n.
retrograde intramedullary n.
ReVision n.
Richards reconstruction n.
right-sided n.
n. root
n. rotational guide
Rush flexible medullary n.
Rush pin n.
Russell-Taylor delta tibial n.
Russell-Taylor interlocking
 medullary n.
Rydell n.
Sage forearm n.
Sage radial n.
Sage triangular n.
Sampson medullary n.
Sarmiento n.
Schneider medullary n.
Seidel humeral locking n.
self-broaching n.
self-locking n.
n. set
sliding n.
Slocum n.
slotted n.
Smillie n.
Smith-Petersen femoral neck n.
Smith-Petersen transarticular n.
specialized n.
spring-loaded n.
standard medullary n.
n. starter
static locking n.
Steinmann extension n.
Street forearm n.
striated n.
supracondylar medullary n.
n. suture
Sven-Johansson femoral neck n.
telescoping n.
Temple University n.
Terry n.
Thatcher n.
Thompson n.
Thornton n.
Tiemann n.
titanium n.
triangular medullary n.

triflanged Lottes n.
triflanged medullary n.
True/Flex intramedullary n.
turtle neck n.
Uniflex humeral n.
Uniflex intramedullary n.
Universal n.
Venable-Stuck n.
Vesely-Street split n.
Vitallium Küntscher n.
V-medullary n.
watch crystal n.
Watson-Jones n.
Webb bolt n.
Williams n.
Winograd technique for ingrown n.
Z fixation n.
Zickel subcondylar n.
Zickel subtrochanteric n.
Zickel supracondylar medullary n.
Zimmer telescoping n.

nail-bending device
nail-driving guide
nail-extracting hook
nailing

antegrade n.
blind medullary n.
bundle nailing
centromedullary n.
closed Küntscher n.
closed medullary n.
condylocephalic n.
crutch and belt femoral closed n.
elastic stable intramedullary n.
  (ESIN)
Ender n.
exchange n.
femoral n.
fixator-augmented n.
gradual elongation n. (GEN)
gradual elongation intramedullary n.
  (GEIN)
Grosse-Kempf interlocking
  medullary n.
Harris condylocephalic n.
interlocking n.
intramedullary n. (IMN)
Küntscher medullary n.
locked n.
Lottes n.
marrow n.
medullary n.

open medullary n.
retrograde n.
static lock n.
tibiocalcaneal medullary n.
Vertstreken closed medullary n.
Zickel n.

nail-patella syndrome
nail-pulling forceps
nail-screw sideplate assembly
Nakamura brace
Nakayama staple
Nalebuff arthrodesis
Nalebuff-Millender lateral band
  mobilization technique
Namaqualand hip dysplasia
nana

pelvis n.

NAP

nerve action potential

napkin

n. ring calcar allograft
n. ring compression

Napoleon hat sign
naprapathy
Nara arthroplasty
Naraghi-DeCoster reduction clamp
narrow

n. AO dynamic compression plate
n. toebox shoe

narrow-base gait
narrow-blade retractor
narrowed joint space
narrowing

arthritic ankle joint n.
n. of forefoot
intervertebral disk n.
n. of spinal canal

narrow-neck mini-Hohmann retractor
nasal

n. elevator
n. spine

nascent motor unit potential
natatory

n. cord
n. ligament

Nathan-Trung modification of
  Krukenberg hand reconstruction
national

N. Arthritis Action Plan (NAAP)
N. Arthritis Data Workgroup
N. Association of Medical
  Equipment Suppliers

N

NOTES

national *(continued)*

N. Collegiate Athletic Association drug testing policy

N. Collegiate Athletic Association prohibited drug

N. Collegiate Athletic Association spine injury prevention rule

N. Football Head and Neck Injury Registry

N. Institute of Arthritis and Musculoskeletal and Skin Diseases (NIAMS)

N. Operating Committee on Standards for Athletic Equipment (NOCSAE)

Native American medicine

natural apophysial glides (NAGS)

Natural-Hip

N.-H. prosthesis

N.-H. system

N.-H. titanium hip stem

Natural-Knee

N.-K. II system

N.-K. unconstrained prosthesis

Natural-Lok acetabular cup prosthesis

naturopathy

Naughton-Dunn triple arthrodesis

Nauth

N. traction apparatus

N. traction device

navicular

accessory n.

n. arthritis

bifurcate n.

n. body

n. bone

cartilaginous n.

n. cookie in shoe

cornuate n.

n. cuneiform ligament

divided n.

n. dorsal lip fracture

n. drop test

n. to first metatarsal angle

lip of n.

n. osteonecrosis

n. prominence

protrusion of the n.

n. screw

n. shoe cookie

n. shoe pad

tarsal n.

n. tuberosity

n. tuberosity fracture

n. wedging

naviculectomy

naviculocapitate

n. fracture

n. fracture syndrome

naviculocuneiform

n. breach

n. coalition

n. fusion

n. joint

n. joint arthrodesis

n. ligament

Navigator power wheelchair

Navitrack computer-assisted surgery system

NC

neurogenic claudication

NCS

nerve conduction study

NCT

nerve compression test

NCV

nerve conduction velocity

Neal-Robertson litter

near-anatomic position of joint

near-constant frequency trains

near-far fashion

near-field potential

nearthrosis

NEB

New England Baptist

NEB acetabular cup

NEB arthroplasty

NEB total hip prosthesis

Necelon surgical glove

necessity

fracture of n.

neck

basal n.

n. brace

congenital wry n.

crick in the n.

n. diameter

femoral head and n.

fibular n.

n. fracture

glenoid n.

humeral n.

metacarpal n.

metatarsal n.

n. pain syndrome

phalangeal n.

radial n.

n. reflex

n. roll

n. shaft

skeletal wry n.

supple n.

surgical n.

talar n.

n. wrap
wry n.
Neckcare pillow
Neck-Hugger cervical support pillow
neck-righting reflex
Neck-Roll aromatherapy hot/cold pack
neck-shaft angle (NSA)
Necktrac
N. traction
N. traction device
necrosis
aseptic n.
atraumatic n.
avascular n. (AVN)
bone n.
central n.
coagulation n.
coagulative n.
corticosteroid-induced avascular n.
dry n.
epiphysial aseptic n.
epiphysial ischemic n.
gangrenous n.
gummatous n.
hyaline n.
idiopathic avascular n.
infectious bulbar n.
ischemic n.
mummification n.
Paget quiet n.
pressure n.
radiographic avascular n.
Ratliff avascular n. classification
septic n.
skin n.
steroid-induced avascular n.
superficial n.
total n.
n. ustilaginea
Zenker n.
necrotic
n. bone
n. tissue
necroticans
osteochondritis n.
necrotizing fasciitis
necrotomy
osteoplastic n.
NEECHAM Confusion Scale
needle
Astralac n.
atraumatic n.

Beath n.
Bergstrom n.
Bier lumbar puncture n.
n. biopsy
bone biopsy n.
bore n.
bougie n.
Bunnell tendon n.
conventional cutting n.
n. cord length
cutting n.
Deschamps n.
diamond point n.
diskogram n.
n. electrode
Framer tendon-passing n.
Gallie n.
hand-honed reverse cutting n.
Hawkeye suture n.
n. holder
hubbed n.
Intracath n.
Jamshidi n.
K n.
Keith n.
McGee prosthesis n.
meniscal repair n.
milliner's n.
osteodysplasty of Melnick and N.'s
n. placement
Plum-Blossom acupuncture n.
Quincke n.
retrobulbar prosthesis n.
reverse cutting n.
ribbed n.
Seirin acupuncture n.
Sklar ligature n.
spinal n.
Stimuplex block n.
swaged n.
taper cut n.
tendon n.
The Painless One acupuncture n.
Thomas n.
Tuohy lumbar puncture n.
Verbrugge n.
Veress n.
Wangensteen n.
Webster n.
needle-nose
n.-n. rongeur
n.-n. vise-grip pliers

N

NOTES

needlescope

Neer

   N. acromioplasty
   N. acromioplasty for rotator cuff tear
   N. capsular shift procedure
   N. femur fracture classification
   N. hemiarthroplasty
   N. II humeral component
   N. humeral replacement prosthesis
   N. humerus fracture classification
   N. impingement sign
   N. impingement test
   N. lateral view
   N. modification
   N. open reduction
   N. posterior shoulder reconstruction
   N. ring
   N. shoulder fracture classification
   N. shoulder prosthesis (I, II)
   N. II shoulder system
   N. II total knee system
   N. II total shoulder system implant
   N. transscapular view
   N. umbrella prosthesis
   N. unconstrained shoulder arthroplasty

Neer-Horowitz

   N.-H. classification of humeral fracture
   N.-H. humerus fracture classification

Neer-Vitallium humeral prosthesis

Neff

   N. femorotibial nail system
   N. meniscus knife

negative

   n. afterpotential
   n. casting
   n. congruence angle
   n. impression cast
   n. ulnar variance (NUV)
   n. work

neglect

   hemispatial n.
   traumatic brain injury-related n.
   visual n.

neglected rupture

Neibauer-Cutter prosthesis

Neiguan point acupressure

Neil-Moore perforator drill

Neivert osteotome

Nélaton

   N. ankle dislocation
   N. line
   N. operation
   N. rubber tube drain

Nelson

   N. finger exerciser
   N. rib retractor
   N. rib spreader
   N. scissors
   N. sign

nemaline rod-body myopathy

neoadjuvant chemotherapy

neocortex

neoformation

   nodular n.

neolimbus

neonatal

   n. flatfoot
   n. sandbag
   n. septic arthritis
   n. tracheostomy tube holder

neoplasm

   bone n.
   extensive n.
   interdigital n.

neoplastic

   n. fracture
   n. lesion

Neoplush foam

neoprene

   n. ankle support
   n. back support
   n. dressing
   n. elbow sleeve
   n. fabric
   n. knee sleeve
   n. shoe
   n. wrist brace
   n. wrist orthosis
   n. wrist strap

Ne-Osteo bone morphogenic protein

neotendon

neovascularization

nerve

   abductor digiti minimi n.
   accessory n.
   n. action potential (NAP)
   antebrachial cutaneous n.
   anterior thoracic n.
   anterior tibial n.
   Arnold n.
   articular n.
   axillary n.
   n. block infusion kit
   Bock n.
   calcaneal n.
   n. cap
   cluneal n.
   common digital n.
   common peroneal n.
   n. compression test (NCT)
   n. conduction study (NCS)

n. conduction velocity (NCV)
n. conduction velocity test
n. crossing
cubital n.
cutaneous n.
deep peroneal n.
digital branch of plantar n.
dorsal cutaneous n.
dorsal scapular n.
dorsomedial cutaneous n.
n. ending
n. entrapment site
n. entrapment syndrome
n. entubulation
femoral cutaneous n.
n. fiber action potential
genitofemoral n.
gluteal n.
n. graft
great sciatic n.
n. growth factor
n. hook
hypoglossal n.
iliohypogastric n.
ilioinguinal n.
inferior laryngeal n.
n. injury
intercostal n.
intercostobrachial n.
interdigital n.
n. interference
intermediate dorsal cutaneous n.
  (IDCN)
intermetatarsal n.
interosseous n.
n. involvement testing
n. of Kunzel
mandibular n.
medial brachial n.
medial dorsal cutaneous n.
  (MDCN)
medial sural cutaneous n.
median n.
musculocutaneous n.
obturator n.
n. palsy
pectoral n.
peripheral n.
peroneal n.
phrenic n.
plantar n.
popliteal n.

posterior tibial n. (PTN)
radial digital n.
radial sensory n.
recurrent laryngeal n.
recurrent meningeal n.
regeneration of n.
n. root
n. root block
n. root compression
n. root decompression
n. root entrapment
n. root injection
n. root irritability
n. root irritation
n. root lesion
n. rootlet ablation
sacral n.
saphenous n.
scapular n.
sciatic n.
sensorimotor n.
sensory n.
n. separator
n. sheath tumor
sinuvertebral n.
somatic n.
spinal accessory n.
n. stretching
superficial peroneal n.
superficial radial n. (SRN)
superior laryngeal n.
suprascapular n.
sural n.
sympathetic n.
thoracic n.
thoracodorsal n.
tibial n.
n. tracing
n. transmission
n. trunk action potential
ulnar n. (UN)
vagus n.
vertebral n.
n. wrapping
NervePace nerve conduction monitor
Nervoscope
nested
n. nail
n. step stool
netting
splint pan n.

N

NOTES

network
  achilleocalcaneal vascular n.
Neubeiser adjustable forearm splint
Neufeld
  N. apparatus
  N. cast
  N. device
  N. driver
  N. dynamic method
  N. nail
  N. pin
  N. plate
  N. roller traction
  N. screw
NeuFlex metacarpophalangeal joint implant
Neumann syndrome
Neurain drill
Neurairtome
  N. drill
  Hall N.
neural
  n. arch resection technique
  n. crest
  n. element
  n. foramen
  n. foraminal stenosis (NFS)
  n. foraminotomy
  n. injury
  n. strength training
  n. tension
  n. tissue
  n. tube defect
  n. tube defect-related anomaly of vertebra
  n. tumor
neuralgia
  adhesive n.
  brachial n.
  genicular n.
  geniculate n.
  glossopharyngeal n.
  intercostal n.
  Morton n.
  occipital n.
  sciatic n.
  stump n.
  tension n.
  traumatic prepatellar n.
  trigeminal n.
  vagoglossopharyngeal n.
  vidian n.
neuralgic amyotrophy
neurapraxia
  cervical cord n. (CCN)
  Seddon n.
  traction n.
  transient n.

neurasthenia
neuraxial compression
neurectomy
  adductor tenotomy and obturator n. (ATON)
  Eggers n.
  Morton n.
  obturator n.
  Phelps n.
  ulnar motor n.
neurilemoma
neuritic amyotrophy
neuritis
  axial n.
  brachial n.
  obturator nerve n.
  peripheral n.
  pudendal n.
  radicular n.
  sciatic n.
  suprascapular n.
  sural n.
  wallet n.
neuroablative
Neuro-Aide testing device
neuroanastomosis
neuroarthropathic foot
neuroarthropathy
  atrophic n.
  Charcot n.
neuroarticular
  n. dysfunction
  n. subluxation
  n. syndrome
neuroblastoma
neurocentral synchondrosis
neurocirculation
NeuroCom balance master
neurocutaneous hand flap
neurodevelopmental
  n. approach
  n. training
  n. treatment
NeuroDrape surgical drape
neurodystrophic
neuroectodermal tumor
neurofibroma
  multiple n.
  nonplexiform cutaneous n.
  plexiform n.
neurofibromatosis
  formes frustes n.
  n. kyphoscoliosis
  kyphoscoliosis secondary to n.
  muscular n.
neurofibrosarcoma
neurofibrositis
neurofunctional subluxation

neurogenic
    n. arthrogryposis
    n. atrophy
    n. bladder
    n. bowel
    n. claudication (NC)
    n. disease
    n. disorder
    n. fracture
    n. motor evoked potential (NMEP)
    n. shock
    n. syndrome
    n. torticollis
neurography
    magnetic resonance n. (MRN)
neuroleptanalgesia
neuroleptic
neurologic
    n. assessment
    n. complication
    n. deficit
    n. disorder
    n. examination
    n. function
    n. pain
neurological
    n. nerve conduction velocity
      examination
    n. testing
neurologically intact
neurolysis
    alcohol n.
    chemical n.
    distal n.
    epidural n.
    external n.
    interfascicular n.
    internal n.
    intrathecal n.
    Morton neuroma n.
    motor n.
    phenol n.
neurolytic block
neuroma, pl. **neuromata**
    amputation stump n.
    bulb n.
    n. in continuity
    cutaneous n.
    dorsal n.
    false n.
    incisional n.
    interdigital n. (IDN)

    Morton neuromata
    Morton interdigital n.
    posttraumatic n.
    refractory n.
    n. sign
    spindle n.
    sural n.
    traumatic n.
neuromatosis
neuromatous
neuromechanical
    n. correction
    n. lesion
    n. spinal chiropractic management
neuromeningeal pathway
neuromuscular
    n. block
    n. component
    n. disease
    n. electrical stimulation (NMES)
    n. electrical stimulation therapy
    n. facilitation
    n. gait pattern change
    n. hamartoma
    n. junction disorder
    n. proprioceptive process
    n. reflex treatment
    n. scoliosis
    n. scoliosis orthotic treatment
    n. III stimulator
    n. transfer
neuromusculoskeletal
neuromyotonia
neuromyotonic discharge
neuron
    fusimotor n.
    motor n.
    serotonergic n.
neuronitis
    Parsonage-Turner n.
neuropathic
    n. ankle
    n. arthritis
    n. arthropathy (NA)
    n. collapse
    n. foot
    n. foot deformity
    n. forefoot ulceration
    n. fracture
    n. hyperkyphoscoliosis
    n. joint
    n. joint disease

NOTES

N

neuropathic *(continued)*
    n. joint dislocation
    n. knee
    n. motor unit potential
    n. osteoarthropathy
    n. recruitment
    n. spinal arthropathy
    n. ulcer
neuropathogenic
neuropathophysiology
    normalization of n.
neuropathy
    alcoholic n.
    amyloid n.
    brachial plexus n.
    chemotherapy-related n.
    compressive n.
    diabetic n.
    entrapment n.
    epineurial n.
    epineurial-perineurial n.
    fascicular n.
    hereditary motor sensory n. (HMSN)
    hereditary sensory motor n. (type I–III) (HSMN I–III)
    hip pocket n.
    hypertrophic interstitial n.
    motor n.
    motor and sensory n., type I–II
    periepineurial n.
    peripheral n.
    peroneal n.
    porphyritic n.
    radiation-related n.
    spontaneous median n.
    sural n.
    ulnar n.
neurophysiologic effect
neurophysiology
neuroplasty
neuroprosthesis
neuropsychological screening
neuroreflexive
neurorrhaphy
    epineurial n.
    perineurial n.
neurosis, *pl.* **neuroses**
    low back n.
    torsion n.
neuroskeletal
neurostimulator
    Biotens n.
    Grass n.
    Staodyne EMS+2 n.
neurosuture
neurosyphilis
neurotendinous

neurotherapy
    manual reflex n.
neurothlipsis
neurotization
neurotmesis
    Seddon n.
neurotomy
neurotraumatic mechanism
neurotripsy
neurotrophic
    n. atrophy
    n. factor
    n. food ulcer
    n. fracture
    n. joint
    n. ulceration
Neurotube bioabsorbable nerve conduit
neurovascular (NV)
    n. anatomy
    n. bundle
    n. complication
    n. corn
    n. free flap
    n. hilus
    n. impairment
    n. injury
    n. island graft
    n. status
    n. structure
neurovascularly intact
neutral
    n. angle
    n. anteversion
    n. drill guide
    n. hip position
    n. hook
    n. position splint
    n. rotation
    n. triangle
    n. wrist curl
    n. zone (NZ)
neutralization
    anterior n.
    n. plate
    n. plate fixation
neutron radiography
nevi (*pl. of* nevus)
Neviaser
    N. acromioclavicular technique
    N. arthroplasty
    N. classification of frozen shoulder
    N. frozen shoulder classification
    N. operation
    N. test
    N. theory
Neviaser-Wilson-Gardner
    N.-W.-G. procedure

N.-W.-G. technique
N.-W.-G. transfer
Nevin ankle brace
nevoid histiocytoma
nevus, pl. **nevi**
new
   n. bone formation
   N. England Baptist (NEB)
   N. England Baptist acetabular cup
   N. England Baptist hip arthroplasty
   N. England scoliosis brace
   n. happy bur
   N. Jersey ankle
   N. Jersey hemiarthroplasty
     prosthesis
   N. Jersey LCS shoulder prosthesis
   N. Jersey LCS total knee
     prosthesis
   N. Mind Set toe splint
   N. Schwinn 900 bicycle
   N. Schwinn elliptical bicycle
   N. Versaback gym ball
   N. York diagnostic criteria
   N. York diagnostic criteria
     classification
   N. York diagnostic criteria for
     rheumatoid arthritis
   N. York Orthopedic front-opening
     orthosis
   N. York University (NYU)
   N. York University orthotic insert
newer-generation device
Newington
   N. brace
   N. orthosis
newly woven bone
Newman
   N. plate
   N. radial fracture
   N. radial neck and head fracture
     classification
Newman-Keuls procedure
new-onset limp
Newport
   N. hip system
   N. MC hip orthosis
   N. MC hip orthosis brace
Newton
   N. ankle prosthesis
   N. force
newtonian body

newton-meter
   concentric plantar flexion peak
     torque n.-m.
Nexerciser Plus
NexGen
   N. complete knee system
   N. component
   N. knee implant
   N. offset stem extension
Nextep knee brace
Nexus
   N. hip prosthesis
   N. implant
   N. wheelchair seating system
NFS
   neural foraminal stenosis
NIAMS
   National Institute of Arthritis and
     Musculoskeletal and Skin Diseases
N'ice
   N. Stretch night splint
   N. Stretch night splint suspension
     system with Sealed Ice
Nicholas
   N. five-in-one reconstruction
   N. five-in-one reconstruction
     technique
   N. ligament technique
   N. manual muscle tester
Nickelplast blank
Nicola
   N. arthroplasty
   N. forceps
   N. incision
   N. rasp
   N. scissors
   N. shoulder operation
   N. shoulder procedure
Nicoladoni suture
Nicolet Compass EMG instrument
Nicoll
   N. bone
   N. bone replacement material
   N. cancellous bone graft
   N. cancellous insert graft
   N. classification
   N. extractor
   N. fracture operation
   N. fracture repair procedure
   N. plate
   N. rasp
   N. tendon prosthesis

N

NOTES

nicotinamide-adenine dinucleotide
  phosphate (NADPH)
nidus
    radiolucent n.
Niebauer
    N. finger-joint replacement
     prosthesis
    N. implant
    N. metacarpophalangeal joint
     Silastic prosthesis
    N. trapeziometacarpal arthroplasty
    N. trapezium replacement prosthesis
Niebauer-Cutter implant
Niebauer-King technique
Nievergelt-Pearlman syndrome
night
    n. brace
    n. splint
    n. splinting
    N. Splint support
Nightimer carpal tunnel support
nightstick fracture
night-walker fracture
nigricans
    acanthosis n.
Nikon SMZ 2T magnifying lens
Nilsson lateral ankle stabilization
  procedure
Nimmo receptor-tonus technique
ninety-ninety
    n.-n. intraosseous wire Nitinol
     flexible wire
    n.-n. method
    n.-n. traction
nipper
    English anvil nail n.
    House-Dieter malleus n.
    Miltex nail n.
    n.'s nail drill
Niro
    N. bone-cutting forceps
    N. wire-twisting forceps
Nirschl
    N. operation
    N. technique
Nirvana mattress
Nitalloy
2-nite
nitidus
    lichen n.
nitinol
nitrofurazone
nitrogen
    n. balance
    urinary n.
nitroglycerin
nitroprusside
Nitro wheelchair

NMEP
    neurogenic motor evoked potential
NMES
    neuromuscular electrical stimulation
     NMES therapy
NMP
    nail matrix phenolization
NMR
    nuclear magnetic resonance
no
    no man's land of hand
    no touch rule
Nobel test
nociception
nociceptive
    n. receptor
    n. transmission
nociceptor
    n. agent
    angry backfiring C n.
    bombardment by n.
NOCSAE
    National Operating Committee on
     Standards for Athletic Equipment
nocturnal myoclonus
node
    Bouchard n.
    gouty n.
    Haygarth n.
    Heberden n.
    Meynet n.
    Osler n.
    Parrot n.
    Schmorl n.
nodosa
    arthritis n.
    panarteritis n.
    polyarteritis n.
nodose rheumatism
nodosity
    Heberden n.
nodular
    n. fasciitis
    n. melanoma
    n. neoformation
    n. tenosynovitis
nodularity
    tendon n.
nodulation
nodule
    Bouchard n.
    Lisch n.
    rheumatoid n.
    Schmorl n.
    synovial n.
    tendon n.
NOF
    nonossifying fibroma

NoHands Mouse-Foot-Operated
  Computer Mouse System
Noiles
    N. fully constrained
      tricompartmental knee prosthesis
    N. hinge
    N. posterior stabilized knee
    N. rotating hinge knee
    N. rotating hinge knee mechanism
noise
    endplate n.
Nolan system collimator mounted
  contact shield
No-Lok
    N.-L. bolt
    N.-L. screw
    N.-L. self-locking nail
nomenclature
    dynamic listing n.
    static listing n.
nomogram
nonabsorbable suture
nonadherent gauze dressing
nonambulation
no-name, no-fame bursa
nonarticular
    n. arthritis
    n. distal radial fracture
nonaugmented repair
nonbeaded guidepin
nonbeveled
nonbipedal
noncannulated nail
noncemented total hip arthroplasty
noncollared press-fit femoral stem
  implantation
noncompliance
noncompressive myelopathy
noncongruent metatarsophalangeal joint
noncontact manipulation
noncontained
    n. disk
    n. disk herniation
noncontiguous fracture
noncontractile
nondermatomal pattern
nondisplaced fracture
nondissociative
    carpal instability n. (CIND)
nonenzymatic connective tissue glycation
nonfenestrated stem

nonfluency
nonfused arthrodesis
nonglabrous skin
nonhinged
    n. knee prosthesis
    n. linked prosthesis
nonimpulsed base nerve transmission
noninvasive
    lower extremity n.
    n. technique
nonisometric graft
nonlamellar bone
nonlamellated bone
nonlinear lesion
nonnarcotic analgesic
nonoperative
    n. orthopedic management
    n. treatment
nonosseous
    n. tarsal coalition
    n. tissue trauma
nonossified tarsal navicular cartilage
nonossifying fibroma (NOF)
nonosteoconductive bone-void filler
nonosteogenic fibroma
nonphysial fracture
nonpitting edema
nonplexiform cutaneous neurofibroma
nonporous-coated endoprosthesis
nonpreferred leg
nonradicular pattern
nonreamed nail
nonreconstructable
nonreplantable amputation
nonrotational burst fracture
non-self-tapping screw
nonspasmodic torticollis
nonspecific
    n. arthralgia
    n. cardiomyopathy
nonstanding lateral oblique view
nonsteroidal
    n. antiinflammatory drug (NSAID)
    n. antiinflammatory medication
nonstriated muscle
nonstructural curve
nonsubluxated metatarsophalangeal joint
nonsubperiosteal cortical defect
nonsuppurative osteomyelitis
nonsurgical management
nonthermal modality

NOTES

nonthreaded
    n. pin
    n. wire
nonthrust mobilization
nontotal-contact disorder
nontraumatic
    n. idiopathic osteonecrosis
    n. synovitis
nontubed
    n. closed distant flap graft
    n. open distant flap graft
nontuberculous mycobacterial infection
nonunion
    atrophic n.
    avascular n.
    bayonet n.
    bioelectrical repair of delayed
      union or n.
    defect n.
    draining infected n.
    dry infected n.
    elephant-foot fracture n.
    fracture fragment n.
    n. of fracture site
    n. fracture trauma
    gap n.
    hamate hook n.
    n. horse-hoof fracture
    horse-hoof fracture n.
    hypertrophic vital n.
    hypervascular n.
    n. incidence
    infected nondraining n.
    metaphysial-articular n.
    oligotrophic fracture n.
    n. osteomyelitis
    n. rate
    scaphoid n.
    supracondylar n.
    synovial n.
    talar body n.
    n. torsion wedge fracture
    torsion wedge fracture n.
    vascular n.
    wedge n.
nonunited fracture
nonwalking cast
nonweightbearing (NWB)
    n. brace
    n. crutch walk
    n. crutch walking
    n. view
    n. x-ray
Nora lesion
NordiCare
    N. Back Therapy System
    N. Enabler exerciser
    N. Strider exerciser

NordicTrack
    N. Motion Analyzer
    N. ski exerciser
no-reflow phenomenon
Norian SRS cement
normal
    n. anatomic position
    n. last shoe
    n. lordotic curve
    upper limits of n.
normalization of neuropathophysiology
Normalize Press-Fit hip prosthesis
Norman
    N. tibial bolt
    N. tibial pin
normoxia
Norm testing and rehabilitation system
North
    N. American blastomycosis
    N. American Malignant
      Hyperthermia protocol
Northville brace
Northwick Park Index of Independence in ADL
Norton ball reamer
Norton-Brown orthosis
Norwich press fit prosthesis
Norwood iliotibial band tenodesis
nose
    anteater n.
no-stretch RocketSoc brace
notariorum
    paralysis n.
notch
    acetabular n.
    A-frame n.
    clavicular n.
    coracoid n.
    costal n.
    cotyloid n.
    cuboid n.
    n. cut
    n. cutting guide
    incisural n.
    interclavicular n.
    intercondylar n.
    interpeduncular n.
    intervertebral n.
    radial sigmoid n.
    scapular n.
    sciatic n.
    semilunar n.
    sigmoid n.
    spinoglenoid n.
    suprasternal n.
    trochlear n.
    ulnar n.
    vertebral n.

n. view
n. width index (NWI)
notcher device
notchplasty
n. blade
n. procedure
Nothnagel acroparesthesia
no-tie stretch lace
notochord
persistent n.
no-touch technique
Nottingham Extended ADL index
nourished
well developed, well n. (WD, WN)
Novagel gel sheet
Novus
N. LC threaded interbody fusion cage
N. LT titanium threaded interbody fusion cage
Noyes flexion rotation drawer test
nozzle
suction n.
NRM
nucleus raphe magnus
NRS
numeric rating scale
NSA
neck-shaft angle
NSAID
nonsteroidal antiinflammatory drug
N-telopeptide (NTx)
N-Terface dressing
NTx
N-telopeptide
Nu
Nu Gauze bandage
Nu Gauze dressing
Nu Gauze packing
nubbin
nuchal
n. ligament
n. region
n. rigidity
nuclear
n. arthrogram
n. magnetic resonance (NMR)
n. magnetic resonance scan
nuclei (*pl. of* nucleus)
Nucleotome
N. probe
N. system

nucleotomy
laser n.
nucleus, pl. **nuclei**
force n.
periaqueductal gray n.
prosthetic disk n. (PDN)
n. pulposus
pulpy n.
n. raphe magnus (NRM)
nudge control on prosthesis
Nu-Knit absorbable hemostat
NuKO knee orthosis
numeric rating scale (NRS)
Nurick
N. classification of spondylosis
N. spondylosis classification
Nurolon suture
nursemaid's elbow
Nussbaum bracelet
NuStep
N. exerciser
N. total body recumbent stepper
nut
n. alignment guide
Close Encounter n.
Kirschner traction bow n.
locking n.
nylon n.
traction bow n.
VDS hex n.
nutation
counter n.
nutcracker
n. fracture
n. injury
n. sign
NutraFill hydrophilic dressing
NutraStat wound dressing
nutrient
n. artery
n. flap
NUTRI-SPEC testing
nutrition
parenteral n.
tissue n.
total parenteral n. (TPN)
nutritional osteomalacia
NUV
negative ulnar variance
Nuwave transcutaneous electrical nerve stimulator

N

NOTES

NV
neurovascular
NWB
nonweightbearing
NWI
notch width index
Nylatex
N. strap
N. wrap
Nylok self-locking nail
nylon
n. monofilament

n. nut
n. suture
n. teaspoon
Nystroem nail driver
Nystroem-Stille driver
NYU
New York University
NYU orthosis insert
NYU-Hosmer electric elbow and prehension actuator
NZ
neutral zone

OA
osteoarthritis
OA knee brace
OAdjuster knee brace
OAP
osteoarthropathy
OAR
Ottawa Ankle Rule
oarsman's wrist
OAS
Oral Analogue Scale
OASIS
osteotomy analysis simulation software
OASIS wound dressing
OAsys knee brace
oath hand
OATS
osteochondral autograft transfer system
OATS technique
OAV
oculoauriculovertebral
OAWO
opening abductory wedge osteotomy
Ober
O. anterior transfer
O. incision
O. operation
O. posterior drainage
O. release
O. tendon technique
O. test
Ober-Barr
O.-B. procedure for brachioradialis transfer
O.-B. transfer technique
obese
o. bed
o. knee osteoarthritis
o. support
o. walker
objective sign
OBLA
onset of blood lactate accumulation
obligate translation
oblique
o. amputation
o. bandage
o. closing wedge osteotomy (OCWO)
o. displacement
o. facet wiring
o. fracture
o. incision
medial o. (MO)
o. meniscal tear

o. metacarpal line
o. metatarsocuneiform joint
o. midtarsal joint axis (OMJA)
o. muscle
o. osteotomy for tibial deformity
o. osteotomy with derotation
o. popliteal ligament
o. retinacular ligament
o. retinacular ligament tightness test
o. screw insertion
o. slide osteotomy
o. view
o. wire
o. wiring facet
obliquity
pelvic o.
obliquus
vastus medialis obliquus (VMO)
obliterans
arteriosclerosis o.
endarteritis o.
oblong polyethylene acetabular cup
O₂Boot
O'Brien
O. capsular shift procedure
O. goniometer
O. pelvic halo operation
O. radial fracture classification
O. rib hook
O. staple
observation hip
obstetrician's hand
obturator
o. artery
o. avulsion fracture
blunt o.
conical o.
core biopsy o.
o. externus muscle
o. internus muscle
o. internus tendon
Keene o.
o. nerve
o. nerve injury
o. nerve neuritis
o. neurectomy
o. oblique view
o. sign
o. sleeve
o. sulcus
obturator/brim line
OBUS back support
Obwegeser
O. sagittal mandibular osteotomy

O

Obwegeser *(continued)*
   O. sagittal mandibular osteotomy
     technique
occipital
   o. bone
   o. condyle
   o. condyle fracture
   o. neuralgia
   o. region
occipital-axis joint
occipital-fiber analysis
occipitoatlantal dislocation
occipitoatlantoaxial
   o. fusion
   o. joint
   o. joint complex
occipitocervical
   o. angle
   o. arthrodesis
   o. articulation
   o. fixation
   o. fusion
   o. junction
   o. lordosis
   o. plate
   o. stabilization
occluder
   multiple pinhole o.
occlusal splint
occlusive dressing
occult
   o. fracture
   o. primary malignant tumor
   o. talar lesion
occulta
   spina bifida o. (SBO)
occupation
   sedentary o.
occupational
   o. behavior
   o. and environmental medicine
     (OEM)
   o. rating
   o. risk
   o. role
   o. science
   o. stress syndrome (OSS)
   o. therapy (OT)
OCD
   osteochondritis dissecans
ochronosis
ochronotic
   o. arthritis
   o. arthropathy
OCL
   Orthopedic Casting Lab
   OCL volar splint

O'Connor
   O. finger dexterity test
   O. operating arthroscope
   O. tweezer dexterity test
octagon roll
OCT compound
octopus holder
ocular
   o. prosthesis
   o. scoliosis
   o. sign
oculoauriculovertebral (OAV)
   o. dysplasia
oculoplethysmography (OPG)
OCWO
   oblique closing wedge osteotomy
OD
   osteochondritis dissecans
Oden peroneal tendon subluxation
   classification
Odland ankle prosthesis
ODM
   opponens digiti minimi
O'Donoghue
   O. ACL reconstruction
   O. cotton cast
   O. dressing
   O. facetectomy
   O. knee splint
   O. procedure
   O. stirrup splint
   O. test
   triad of O.
   unhappy triad of O.
odontoid
   o. agenesis
   o. condyle
   o. condyle fracture
   o. fracture internal fixation
   o. fracture stabilization
   o. hypoplasia
   o. perpendicular line
   o. process
   o. process osteosynthesis
   o. x-ray view
odontoid-axial area
odontoidectomy
ODQ
   opponens digiti quinti
OEC
   OEC knee immobilizer
   OEC lag screw component with
     keyway
   OEC Mini 6600 imaging system
   OEC popliteal pad
   OEC splint
   OEC wrist/forearm support
Oehler symptom

OEM
occupational and environmental medicine
Oesch hook
offloading knee brace
offset
o. cane
o. drill hole
femoral o.
head-stem o.
o. hinge
medial head-stem o.
o. suspension feeder
o. V-osteotomy
offset-V procedure
Ogata technique
Ogden
O. Anchor soft tissue device
O. bone anchor
O. epiphysial fracture classification
O. fracture classification
O. fracture classification system
O. knee dislocation classification
O. plate
O. plate system
O. tissue reattachment mini system
Ogee acetabular component
Ogston
O. line
O. operation
Oh
Oh cemented hip prosthesis
Oh Press-Fit hip prosthesis
Oh-Spectron prosthesis
OI
osteogenesis imperfecta
OIC
osteogenesis imperfecta congenita
OIF
Osteogenesis Imperfecta Foundation
oil
Decubitene oxygenated o.
Oil-Red-O method
OIT
osteogenesis imperfecta tarda
OKCE
open kinetic chain exercises
Oklahoma
O. ankle joint
O. ankle joint orthosis
O. ankle prosthesis
O. cable system

OKQ
Osteoporosis Knowledge Questionnaire
old
o. fracture
o. man's back
o. smoothie bur
o. unreduced dislocation
Olds pin
olecranarthritis
olecranarthrocace
olecranarthropathy
olecranization
olecranoid
olecranon
o. bursa
o. bursitis
o. fossa
o. ligament
o. osteochondritis
o. process
o. region
o. tip fracture
oleoma
Olerud
O. internal fixator
O. and Molander fracture classification
O. pedicle fixation system
O. PSF fixation system
O. PSF rod
O. PSF screw
O. transpedicular fixation
oligoarthritis
undifferentiated o.
oligoarticular
o. arthritis
o. disease
oligodendroglioma
oligotrophic fracture nonunion
olisthesis
olisthetic vertebra
olisthy
Olivecrona
O. clip-applying and removing forceps
O. rasp
olive-shaped bur
olive wire
Ollier
O. arthrodesis approach
O. disease
O. dyschondroplasia

O

NOTES

Ollier *(continued)*
    O. incision
    O. lateral approach
    O. law
    O. layer
    O. operation
    O. osteochondromatosis
    O. rake retractor
    O. syndrome
    O. technique
    O. thick split free graft
Ollier-Thiersch skin graft
O'Malley jaw fracture splint
Ombredanne mallet
Ombredanne-Perkins line
Omed vented instrument guard
Omega
    O. compression hip screw system
    O. Plus compression hip system
    O. splinting material
omental flap
Omer-Capen
    O.-C. carpectomy
    O.-C. technique
OMJA
    oblique midtarsal joint axis
Ommaya
    O. reservoir device
    O. reservoir implant material
Omni
    O. knee brace
    O. Roller massager
Omniace RT3200N electromyographic amplifier
Omniderm dressing
Omnifit
    O. dual geometry microstructured prosthesis
    O. HA hip stem prosthesis
    O. HA hip stent
    O. knee prosthesis
    O. Plus hip system
    O. PSL microstructured prosthesis
    O. total knee system
Omnifit-C
    Osteonics O.-C
OmniFlex
    O. hip prosthesis
    O. knee orthosis
Omni-Flexor
    O.-F. device
    O.-F. wrist exerciser
OMNI pretibial buttress
Omnitron exercise testing
omoclavicular
omodynia
omohyoid muscle
omosternum

Omotrain active shoulder support
omovertebral bone
OMT
    osteomanipulative therapy
    osteopathic manipulative therapy
one
    o. and one-half spica cast
    o. wound-one scar concept
one-bar external fixator
one-bone forearm
one-half
    o.-h. patellar tendon transplant
    o.-h. spica cast
one-handed kitchen tool
one-inclinometer method
one-leg
    o.-l. hop for distance test
    o.-l. stance test
one-part fracture
one-plane
    o.-p. bilateral external fixator
    o.-p. bilateral frame
    o.-p. deformity
    o.-p. instability
    o.-p. unilateral external fixator
    o.-p. unilateral frame
one-repetition maximum (1-RM)
one-sided dog-ear repair
one-stage amputation
one-time sharp débridement tray
onlay
    o. bone graft
    o. bone graft cast
    o. cancellous iliac graft
onset
    o. of blood lactate accumulation (OBLA)
    delayed o.
    o. frequency
    o. latency
Ontario Cohort of Running-Related Injury
OnTrack treatment method
onychauxis
onychectomy
onychoclavus
onychocryptosis nail
onychodystrophy
onychogryphosis
onycholysis
onychomadesis
onychomycosis
    proximal subungual o. (PSO)
    subungual o.
    superficial white o. (SWO)
onychomycotic toenail
onychoosteodysplasia
    hereditary o.

onychophosis
onychotomy
Ony-Clear
onyxis
OP
    opponens pollicis muscle
OP-1
    osteogenic protein-1
        OP-1 implant/bone graft
        OP-1 TM bone implant
opaque
    o. arthrography
    o. myelography
    o. synovium
open
    o. amputation
    o. base wedge osteotomy
    o. base wedge
      osteotomy/bunionectomy
    o. biopsy
    o. bone graft epiphysiodesis
    o. C-D hook
    o. disk surgery
    o. dislocation
    o. double-decked hook cervical
      system
    o. drainage
    o. exit foramen
    o. fracture wound drain
    o. kinetic chain exercises (OKCE)
    o. medullary nailing
    o. nail
    o. palm technique
    o. pinning
    o. reduction
    o. reduction of fracture
    o. reduction and internal fixation
      (ORIF)
    o. tenotomy
    o. wedge (OW)
    o. wound
open-air splint
open-book
    o.-b. fracture
    o.-b. pelvic injury
open-bowl cement technique
open-break fracture
open-chain exercise
open-end wrench
opening
    o. abductory wedge osteotomy
      (OAWO)

Sierra 2-load voluntary o.
voluntary o. (VO)
o. wedge manipulation
o. wedge manipulation and
    reapplication of plaster
o. wedge osteotomy
open-section nail
open-staple capsulorrhaphy
open-toe shoe
opera-glass hand
operating
    o. microscope
    o. room
    o. time
operation
    Abbe o.
    Abbott o.
    Abbott-Lucas shoulder o.
    Adams hip o.
    Adelmann o.
    Akin o.
    Albee o.
    Albee-Delbert o.
    Albert knee o.
    Alouette o.
    Amstutz resurfacing o.
    Anderson o.
    Anderson-Hutchins o.
    Annandale o.
    anterior ankle shift o.
    Armistead ulnar lengthening o.
    ASIF screw fixation o.
    Aufranc-Turner o.
    Auto-Implant o.
    Avila o.
    Axer o.
    Badgley o.
    Baker patellar advancement o.
    Baker translocation o.
    Baldwin Bowers radioulnar joint o.
    Bankart o.
    Bankart-Putti-Platt o.
    Barker o.
    Barr tendon transfer o.
    Barsky o.
    Barwell o.
    Bateman shoulder o.
    Bauer-Tondra-Trusler o.
    Baumgard-Schwartz tennis elbow o.
    Bennett quadriceps plastic o.
    Bent o.
    Berger o.

O

NOTES

operation *(continued)*

Bier o.
Blundell-Jones o.
Bora o.
Bosworth shelf o.
Boyd o.
Brackett-Osgood-Putti-Abbott o.
Brahms foot o.
bridle posterior tibial tendon
   transfer o.
Bristow o.
Brittain o.
Brockman foot o.
Brooks cervical fusion o.
Brooks-Gallie cervical o.
Brooks-Jenkins cervical o.
Broström-Gould ankle instability o.
Brown knee approach o.
Buck o.
Bunnell posterior tibial tendon
   transfer o.
Butler fifth toe o.
Caldwell-Coleman flatfoot o.
Caldwell-Durham tendon o.
Campbell ankle o.
Carmody-Batson o.
Carnesale hip approach o.
Cave o.
Cave-Rowe shoulder dislocation o.
centralization of radius o.
Chopart o.
Cloward o.
Cocklin toe o.
Codivilla o.
Cole o.
Colonna shelf o.
Compere o.
Conn o.
Contour DF-80 total hip o.
Copeland-Howard shoulder o.
Cotrel-Dubousset derotation o.
Cracchiolo-Sculco implant o.
Credo o.
Crutchfield o.
Cubbins o.
Davies-Colley o.
Diamond-Gould syndactyly o.
Dickson o.
Dickson-Diveley foot o.
Dieffenbach o.
Dunn hip o.
Dupuytren o.
Durham flatfoot o.
DuVries modified McBride hallux
   valgus o.
Dwyer clawfoot o.
Eaton-Malerich fracture-
   dislocation o.

Eden-Hybbinette o.
Eggers o.
Ellis Jones peroneal tendon o.
Elmslie-Cholmely foot o.
Elmslie peroneal tendon o.
Elmslie-Trillat patellar o.
Evan ankle joint instability o.
Farmer o.
flap o.
French supracondylar fracture o.
Fried-Green foot o.
Fried-Hendel tendon o.
Frost foot o.
Galeazzi patellar o.
Gant o.
Gardner o.
Gelman foot o.
Girdlestone o.
Grice-Green o.
Gritti o.
Guyon o.
Haas o.
Hammon foot o.
hanging hip o.
hanging toe o.
Hark foot o.
Harris-Beath o.
Hauser patellar o.
Herndon-Heyman foot o.
Hey o.
Heyman o.
Heyman-Herndon clubfoot o.
Hibbs o.
Hoffa o.
Hoffa-Lorenz o.
Hoffmann metatarsal o.
Hohmann o.
Hoke Achilles tendon
   lengthening o.
Holmes o.
Horwitz-Adams o.
Houston o.
I-beam hip o.
Inclan modification of Campbell
   ankle o.
inside-out Bankart shoulder
   instability o.
intermetatarsal angle-reducing o.
Isseis-Aussies scoliosis o.
Janecki-Nelson shoulder o.
Jewett o.
Jones cock-up toe o.
Joplin o.
Juvara foot o.
Kapel o.
Keller foot o.
Keller hallux valgus o.
Kellogg-Speed o.

Kessler posterior tibial tendon transfer o.
Kidner foot o.
King-Richards o.
Kirkaldy-Willis o.
Kirk distal thigh o.
Kondoleon o.
Kortzeborn hand o.
Krempen-Silver-Sotelo nonunion o.
Kreuscher o.
Krukenberg hand o.
Lambrinudi drop foot o.
Lange o.
Langenbeck o.
Lapidus o.
Larrey o.
lateral acetabular shelf o.
limb-sparing o.
Lisfranc o.
Liston o.
Littler o.
Lorenz o.
Lucas-Cottrell o.
Luck o.
Ludloff o.
Lund o.
MacAusland o.
MacNab o.
Magnuson o.
Magnuson-Stack o.
Majestro-Ruda-Frost tendon o.
Mallory-Head revision o.
Mauck o.
Mayer transfer o.
Mayo hallux valgus modified o.
Mazur o.
McBride bunion hallux valgus o.
McKay-Simons clubfoot o.
McKay-Simons CSR o.
McKeever o.
McKeever-Buck elbow o.
McLaughlin o.
Mensor-Scheck hanging-hip o.
Mikulicz o.
Milch elbow o.
Miller flatfoot o.
Mital elbow release o.
Mitchell o.
Miyakawa knee o.
modified Cocklin toe o.
Moe scoliosis o.

Molesworth-Campbell elbow approach o.
Mueller knee o.
Mumford-Gurd o.
muscle sliding o.
Nélaton o.
Neviaser o.
Nicola shoulder o.
Nicoll fracture o.
Nirschl o.
Ober o.
O'Brien pelvic halo o.
Ogston o.
Ollier o.
Osborne-Cotterill elbow dislocation o.
Osgood o.
Overholt o.
over-the-top knee o.
Paci o.
Paddu knee o.
Palmer-Widen o.
Pauwels o.
Pheasant elbow o.
Phelps o.
Phemister o.
Putti-Platt o.
resurfacing o.
reverse Mauck knee o.
revision total hip o.
Ridlon o.
Rose foot o.
Roux-Goldthwait o.
Sargent knee o.
Sayre o.
Schanz o.
screw fixation o.
Selig hip o.
Smith-Robinson o.
Sofield femoral deficiency o.
Souter hip o.
Stener-Gunterberg hip o.
Stewart arm o.
subcutaneous o.
Suppan foot o.
Sutherland hip o.
Syme o.
Tharies hip replacement o.
T-plasty modification of Bankart shoulder o.
Vulpius equinus deformity o.
Weaver-Dunn acromioclavicular o.

NOTES

O

operation *(continued)*
    West and Soto-Hall patella o.
    Zadik foot o.
    Zickel subtrochanteric fracture o.
operative
    o. ankylosis
    o. arthroscopy
    o. arthrotomy
    o. leg holder
    o. legholder
    o. roentgenogram
    o. site
OPG
    oculoplethysmography
O'Phelan technique
ophthalmic
    o. irrigator
    o. scoliosis
opiate receptor antagonist
Opiela brace
opioid
    o. antagonist
    o. receptor
opisthenar
opisthotonic position
OPLL
    ossification of the posterior longitudinal
    ligament
Opmi microscopic drape
Oppenheim
    O. amyotonia
    O. brace
    O. disease
    O. gait
    O. reflex
    O. sign
    O. stroke test
    O. syndrome
Oppenheimer
    O. spring wire
    O. spring-wire splint
    O. with reverse knuckle-bender
    splint
Oppociser
    O. exercise device
    O. hand exerciser
opponens
    o. bar
    o. digiti minimi (ODM)
    o. digiti quinti (ODQ)
    o. digiti quinti muscle
    o. orthosis
    o. pollicis muscle (OP)
    o. pollicus
    o. splint
    o. transfer
opponensplasty
    abductor digiti minimi o.

abductor digiti quinti o.
    Bunnell o.
    Camitz o.
    Goldmar o.
    Groves o.
    Huber adductor digiti quinti o.
    Littler o.
    Manske-McCarroll o.
    Phalen-Miller o.
    ring sublimis o.
    Riordan finger o.
opposite
    o. foot strike phase of gait
    o. toe-off phase of gait
opposition
    o. contracture
    finger o.
    o. test
    thumb o.
Opraflex
    O. drape
    O. dressing
OpSite wound dressing
opsonic activity
Opteform
    O. bone graft material
    O. 100HT bone graft
Optetrak
    O. comprehensive knee system
    O. total knee replacement system
optical
    o. stereophotogrammetry
    o. trapping
Opti-Curve therapeutic pillow
Opti-Fix
    O.-F. II acetabular cup
    O.-F. femoral prosthesis
    O.-F. hip stem
    O.-F. I, II prosthesis
    O.-F. total hip system
optimal alignment
OptiMax Supreme pressure reduction
    mattress
optimizing motion palpation
option
    O. hip system
    O. Orthotic Series
optoelectric
    o. measuring apparatus
    o. measuring system
    o. signal detection apparatus
Optotrak motion measurement system
OPTP
    Orthopaedic Physical Therapy Products
    OPTP Slant
O'Rahilly limb deficiency classification

oral
- O. Analogue Scale (OAS)
- o. nutritional supplement

Oratec
- O. chisel
- O. device
- O. thermal shrinking probe

orbicular
- o. ligament
- o. zone

orbit
- angular process of o.

Orbital shoulder stabilizer brace
orbitosphenoidal bone
order of activation
ordinal classification
Oregon Poly II ankle prosthesis
Oretorp retractable knife
Orfit splint
Orfizip
- O. body jacket
- O. knee cast
- O. wrist cast

organ
- Golgi tendon o.
- mechanoreceptor Golgi tendon o.

organization
- homuncular o.

organizational phase of tendon healing
orientation
- phalangeal articular o.
- visual o.
- o. WHO Handicap Scale

ORIF
- open reduction and internal fixation

origin
- adductor o.
- deltoid o.
- fever of undetermined o. (FUO)
- flexor-pronator o.
- tripartite muscle o.

original
- O. Backknobber muscle massager
- O. Backnobber massage tool
- O. Index Knobber II
- O. Index Knobber II massager
- O. Index Knobber II massage tool
- O. Jacknobber II muscle-massage device

Oris pin
Orlando hip-knee-ankle-foot orthosis

ORLAU
- Orthotic Research and Locomotor Assessment Unit
  - ORLAU swivel walker
  - ORLAU swivel walker orthosis

Orlon with Lycra stump sock
Ormandy screw
Ormco pin
ORN
- osteoradionecrosis

oropharyngeal approach
Orozco plate
Orr-Buck traction
Orthairtome
- O. II drill
- O. wire driver

Orthawear antiembolism stockings
orthesis
orthetics
Orth-evac autotransfusion system
Orthex
- O. cannulated bone screw
- O. reliever insole
- O. Relievers shoe insert

Orthion traction machine
Ortho
- O. DX electromedical stimulator
- O. Dx stimulator for knee rehabilitation

Ortho-Arch II orthotic
Ortho-Biotic recliner
OrthoBlast
- O. osteoinductive bioimplant
- O. paste

OrthoBlend powered bone mill
OrthoBone pillow
Ortho-Cel pad
Orthochrome
- O. implant metal
- O. implant metal prosthesis

Orthocomp cement
orthodigita
Orthodoc presurgical planning system
orthodox procedure
orthodromic velocity
OrthoDyn bone substitute material
Orthodyne Enhancer unit
Ortho-evac postoperative transfusion system
Orthofit 9000, 9001 orthotic
Orthofix
- O. apparatus

O

NOTES

Orthofix *(continued)*
    O. Cervical-Stim bone growth stimulator
    O. external fixation device
    O. intramedullary nail
    O. ISKD device
    O. M-100 distractor
    O. monolateral femoral external fixator
    O. Ogden anchor
    O. pin
    O. prosthesis
    O. screw
Orthoflex
    O. dressing
    O. elastic plaster bandage
Ortho-Foam
    O.-F. elbow/heel pad
    O.-F. protector
Orthofuse implantable growth stimulator
OrthoGel liner
OrthoGen bone growth stimulator
Ortho-Glass
    O.-G. splint
    O.-G. synthetic material
Ortho-Grip silicone rubber handle
Ortho-ice multipack
Ortho-Jel impression material
orthokinetic exercise
orthokinetics
    Orthokinetics travel chair
    orthopaedic o.
Ortho-last splint
Ortholav
    O. irrigation and suction device
    O. jet
    O. jet lavage
Ortholen sheet
Ortholign spinal orthosis
Ortholoc
    O. Advantim revision knee system
    O. Advantim total knee system
    O. implant metal prosthesis
    O. II unconstrained prosthesis
OrthoLogic
    O. 1000 bone growth stimulation
    O. 1000 bone growth stimulator
orthomechanical
orthomechanotherapy
Orthomedics
    O. brace
    O. Stretch and Heel splint
    O. Ultra-Guard hip orthosis
orthomelic
Orthomerica
    O. TC AFO system
    O. UFO
Ortho-mesh

Orthomet
    O. Axiom total knee system
    O. Perfecta total hip system
Orthomite II adhesive
Ortho-Mold
    O.-M. lumbar body
    O.-M. spinal brace
    O.-M. splint
orthomolecular medicine/megavitamin therapy
orthonormal diameter
orthopaedic, orthopedic
    Advanta O.'s
    o. bed
    o. bone file
    o. broach
    o. bur
    O.'s Casting Lab (OCL)
    o. cement
    o. chisel
    o. curette
    o. cutting instrument
    o. depth gauge
    o. dynamometer
    Encore O.'s
    o. evaluation
    o. felt
    o. forceps
    o. goniometer
    o. gouge
    o. hammer
    o. hardware
    o. hemostat
    o. impactor
    o. knife
    o. orthokinetics
    o. osteotome
    o. oxford shoe
    O. Physical Therapy Products (OPTP)
    O.'s Positioning Seat
    o. propeller
    o. prosthesis
    o. rasp
    o. reamer
    o. rehabilitation
    o. retractor
    o. rongeur
    o. scissors
    o. shoulder elevator
    o. stockinette
    o. strap clavicular splint
    Sulzer O.'s
    o. surgery
    o. surgical file
    o. surgical pliers
    o. surgical stripper
    O. Systems Inc. (OSI)

o. table
O. Trauma Association
classification
orthopaedist, orthopedist
OrthoPak
O. II bone growth stimulator
O. bone growth stimulator system
Ortho-Pal body support
orthopantogram imaging
orthopedic (*var. of* orthopaedic)
orthopedist (*var. of* orthopaedist)
orthopercussion
Orthoplast
O. dressing
O. fracture brace
O. isoprene splint
O. jacket
O. plastic
O. slipper cast
orthoPLUG
orthopod
orthopraxis
orthopraxy spurious spinous process
orthoRaps postsurgical wound wrap
orthoroentgenogram imaging
orthoroentgenography
Orthoset radiopaque bone cement
orthosis, pl. **orthoses**
abduction hip o.
accommodative o.
Adjustable Advanced Reciprocating
Gait O. (ARGO)
A-frame o.
airplane splint o.
AliCork Foot O.
Aliplast custom-molded foot o.
ambulation training o.
Amfit custom o.
ankle o. (AO)
ankle contracture o.
ankle-foot o. (AFO)
ankle-foot plastic o.
ankle stabilizing o. (ASO)
anteroposterior control o.
Anti-Shox o.
Atlanta brace o.
Atlanta-Scottish Rite abduction o.
bail-lock knee joint o.
balanced forearm o. (BFO)
balance padding o.
bar-and-shoe o.
Bauerfeind Malleolic Ankle O.

Beaufort seating o.
Bebax o.
Bennett o.
BFO O.
BioCast wrist/hand o.
Biothotic foot o.
Boston brace thoracolumbosacral o.
Boston postoperative hip o.
cable-twister o.
calcaneal spur cookie o.
Caligamed ankle o.
caliper o.
Canadian Knee O.
CASH thoracolumbosacral o.
C-bar o.
cervical o. (CO)
cervical thoracic o.
cervicothoracic o. (CTO)
cervicothoracolumbosacral o.
(CTLSO)
chairback lumbosacral o.
clavicle o.
cock-up splint o.
Comfy Elbow O.
Comfy Knee O.
Controller shoulder o.
copolymer ankle-foot o.
corrective o.
Craig-Scott o.
cruciform anterior spinal
hyperextension o.
CTLSO o.
Daytona cervical o.
DDH o.
Denis Browne bar foot o.
developmental dislocated hip o.
Diabetic D-Sole foot o.
dial-lock o.
dorsiflexion assist ankle joint
ankle-foot o.
o. drop-lock ring
dual-photon electrospinal o.
DuraBoot o.
Dynamic elbow o.
Dynamic knee o.
Dynamic wrist o.
elastic knee cage o.
elastic twister o.
elbow o. (EO)
elbow-wrist-hand o. (EWHO)
Engen extension o.
Engen palmar finger o.

O

orthosis *(continued)*
externally powered tenodesis o.
E-Z arm abduction o.
figure-of-eight thoracic o.
Fillauer bar foot o.
FirmFlex custom o.
Flex Foam o.
flexible o.
flexion-extension control cervical o.
flexor hinge o.
floor-reaction ankle-foot o.
foot o. (FO)
Foot Levelers o.
four-poster cervical o.
Frejka pillow o.
gator plastic o.
Gillette joint o.
Gillette modification of ankle-
    foot o.
G/W Heel Lift, Inc. o.
hallux valgus o.
halo cervical o.
halo extension o.
halo traction o.
halo-vest o.
hand o. (HO)
heat-molded petroplastic ankle-
    foot o.
hindfoot o.
hip o. (HO)
hip guidance o. (HGO)
hip-knee-ankle-foot o. (HKAFO)
Hosmer VC four-bar knee o.
hyperextension o.
Hyperex thoracic o.
Ilfeld splint o.
Ipomax o.
ipos heel relief o.
ischial weightbearing o.
J-24 cervical o.
J-45 contraflexion o.
Jewett-Benjamin cervical o.
Jewett contraflexion o.
Jewett hyperextension o.
Jewett postfusion o.
Jewett thoracolumbosacral o.
J-35 hyperextension o.
Jousto dropfoot splint, skid o.
J-55 postfusion o.
Kallassy o.
Kid-Dee-Lite o.
Klenzak o.
knee o. (KO)
knee-ankle-foot o. (KAFO)
knee extension o.
Knight-Taylor thoracolumbosacral o.
Knight-Taylor-Williams spinal o.
Kydex chairback o.

L.A. cervical o.
leather o.
Legg-Perthes disease o.
Lenox Hill knee o.
Lerman multiligamentous knee
    control o.
Levy & Rappel foot o.
Ligamentus Ankle o.
L'Nard Multi Podus o.
L'Nard thoracolumbosacral o.
long leg o.
long opponens o.
lower limb o. (LLO)
LSU reciprocation-gait o.
lumbosacral o. (LSO)
Lynco foot o.
Malibu cervical o.
Malleoloc ankle o.
Maple Leaf hip o.
Marlin cervical o.
medial heel wedge o.
medial sole wedge o.
metal hybrid o.
Meyer cervical o.
Milwaukee
    cervicothoracolumbosacral o.
Milwaukee scoliosis o.
Minerva o.
molded ankle-foot o. (MAFO)
molded lumbosacral o.
Monodos o.
MultiBoot o.
neoprene wrist o.
Newington o.
Newport MC hip o.
New York Orthopedic front-
    opening o.
Norton-Brown o.
NuKO knee o.
Oklahoma ankle joint o.
OmniFlex knee o.
opponens o.
Orlando hip-knee-ankle-foot o.
ORLAU swivel walker o.
Ortholign spinal o.
Orthomedics Ultra-Guard hip o.
o. overlapped uprights
overlapped uprights in o.
parapodium o.
passive prehension o. (PPO)
patellar tendon-bearing o. (PTBO)
patellar tendon weightbearing
    brace o.
patellar tracking o.
patellofemoral o.
pediatric pressure relief ankle
    foot o.
Phelps o.

pillow o.
plantar arch support o.
plantar fasciitis o. (PFO)
plastic ankle-foot o.
plastic floor reaction ankle-foot o.
Plastizote cervical collar o.
pneumatic o.
polypropylene ankle-foot o.
polypropylene glycol-ankle-foot o.
  (PPG-AFO)
polypropylene glycol-
  thoracolumbosacral o. (PPG-TLSO)
poster o.
posterior leaf-spring ankle-foot o.
postoperative lumbosacral o.
prehension o.
pressure-relieving o.
Profile Sitting O.
Pro-glide o.
Progressive ankle o.
prosthesis and o. (P&O)
PTB ankle-foot o.
PTB plastic o.
Pucci pediatrics hand o.
Pucci rehab knee o.
reciprocal finger prehension o.
reciprocation gait o. (RGO)
resting o.
rib belt o.
rigid o.
Rochester hip-knee-ankle-foot o.
SACH o.
sacroiliac o. (SIO)
safety pin o.
Sawa shoulder o.
Scottish Rite hip o.
Seattle o.
Select joint o.
semirigid polypropylene ankle-
  foot o.
serial stretch orthoses
Shaeffer rigid o.
short leg o.
short opponens o.
shoulder o. (SO)
shoulder-elbow-wrist-hand o.
  (SEWHO)
single-photon electrospinal o.
skull-occiput-mandibular
  immobilization o.
Slim Option shoe o.
soft collar cervical o.

SOLEutions custom o.
SOMI o.
spinal o. (SO)
Sport-Stirrup o.
spring-loaded lock o.
spring-wire ankle-foot o.
standard shell ankle-foot o.
standing frame o.
static o.
steel sole plate o.
sternal-occipital-mandibular
  immobilizer o.
sternooccipital mandibular
  immobilizer o.
supramalleolar o. (SMO)
Swede-O-Universal o.
Swedish knee cage o.
Tachdjian o.
Taylor thoracolumbosacral o.
tenodesis o.
themoplastic ankle-foot o.
therapeutic o.
Thera-Pos elbow o.
Therapy Carrot Finger O. (TCFO)
Theratotic firm foot o.
Theratotic soft foot o.
Thomas collar cervical o.
Thomas heel o.
thoracic o. (TO)
thoracic spine o.
thoracolumbar o.
thoracolumbosacral o. (TLSO)
Tib-Transformer o.
TIRR foot-ankle o.
ToeOFF o.
tone-reducing ankle-foot o.
  (TRAFO)
Toronto parapodium o.
total contact o. (TCO)
total contact bivalve ankle-foot o.
total hip stabilization o.
TPE ankle-foot o.
TPE biomechanical foot o.
TRAFO o.
Transpire wrist o.
trilateral knee-ankle-foot o.
trunk-hip-knee-ankle-foot o.
  (THKAFO)
turnbuckle wrist o.
two-poster cervical o.
UCB foot o.
UCBL o.

O

NOTES

orthosis *(continued)*
UCOlite o.
Ultrabrace knee o.
underarm o.
University of California Berkeley
  Laboratory o.
upper limb o. (ULO)
VAPC dorsiflexion assist o.
Vari-Duct hip and knee o.
Viscoheel K, N o.
Viscoheel SofSpot o.
Viscolas o.
von Rosen splint hip o.
weight-relieving o.
Williams o.
wrist-driven flexor hinge o.
wrist-driven lateral prehension o.
wrist-driven wrist-hand o.
wrist-hand o. (WHO)
XPE foot o.
Zinco ankle o.
Orthosleep Pillow
OrthoSorb
O. absorbable pin
O. pin fixation
O. pin nail
O. rod
orthostatic
Orthotech Controller knee brace
Orthotec pressurized fluid irrigation
  system
orthotic
Aerodyn o.
Alden CDI o.
Alznner o.
Amfit o.
Anti-Shox sports o.
o. attachment implant
BIOflex o.
Biofoot o.
BioSole GEL o.
Biothotic o.
Blanke inverted tibialis posterior
  tendon o.
Blue Line o.
o. coiled spring twister
DesignLine o.
o. device
Diab-A-Thotics o.
DressFlex o.
DSIS o.
D-Soles o.
Duraleve custom molded foot o.
FirmFlex custom o.
FlexiSport o.
Foot Levelers custom o.
Footmaster o.
functional o.

Golden Comfort o.
Golden Fitness o.
Healthflex o.
Jamaica Sandalthotics o.
J-GLAS prefab o.
Kinetic Wedge o.
Ligamentus Ankle ankle o.
Lyte Fit o.
Magnathotic o.
Malibu Sandalthotics o.
mallet finger o.
Mayer o.
MBS snap-on o.
M-Pact flexible o.
Ortho-Arch II o.
Orthofit 9000, 9001 o.
ParFlex o.
o. plate
Polydor Preforms o.
PRAFO adjustable o.
PreCustom O.
pressure-relief ankle-foot o.
  (PRAFO)
ProLite Plus runner's o.
prosthetic and o. (P&O)
Pro Support Systems o.
Pucci Air o.
QuikFormables o.
Rediform o.
O. Research and Locomotor
  Assessment Unit (ORLAU)
Rohadur-Polydor o.
Rohadur-Schaefer o.
Rohadur-Whitman o.
SACH o.
SAFE o.
Sandalthotics postural support o.
shoe o.
o. shoe insert
Slimthetics o.
Sof Sole motion control o.
Soft Super Sport o.
Soft Support Preforms o.
SOLEutions soft plus o.
SOLEutions sport shell o.
solid ankle, cushioned heel o.
Sporthotics o.
Sport Preforms o.
stationary attachment flexible
  endoskeletal o.
Stratos o.
Superfeet Custom Pre-Fabricated O.
Superform Contours o.
Super Jock n' Jill store
  Superfeet o.
Supralen cradle o.
Supralen Schaefer o.
Swiss Balance o.

Thermo HK/Rohadur o.
Thermo HK/Tepefom o.
Thinline uncovered o.
total contact shell ankle-foot o.
UCOheal o.
UltraStep o.
Universal plantar fasciitis o. (UFO)
Wire-Foam O.
XO-soft-sole o.
orthotist
orthotome resector
Ortho-Trac
O.-T. adhesive skin traction
bandage
O.-T. pneumatic vest
orthotripsy
Orthotron exerciser
Ortho-Turn transfer aid
Ortho-Vent
O.-V. bandage
O.-V. traction
OrthoVise orthopedic instrument
OrthoWedge healing shoe
Ortho-Yomy facebow
Ortolani
O. click
O. maneuver
O. sign
os
os acromiale
os calcis pin fixation
os trigonum fracture
OS-5/Plus 2 knee brace
Osada
O. portable handpiece system
O. saw
Osborne
O. plate
O. posterior approach
O. punch
Osborne-Cotterill
O.-C. elbow dislocation
O.-C. elbow dislocation operation
O.-C. elbow technique
O.-C. procedure
**OSCAR ultrasonic bone cement
removal system**
oscillating
o. gouge
o. saw
oscillation
grade I, II o.

oscillator
oscilloscope instrument
Osebold-Remondini syndrome
Osgood
O. modified technique
O. operation
O. rotational osteotomy
Osgood-Schlatter
O.-S. disease
O.-S. knee brace
O.-S. lesion
O.-S. syndrome
Osher irrigating implant hook
OSI
Orthopaedic Systems Inc.
OSI Arthroscopic Leg holder
OSI extremity elevator
OSI laxity tester
OSI modular table system
OSI Well Leg Support
OSI-Schlein shoulder positioner
Osler node
OsmoCyte Island wound-care dressing
Osmond-Clarke
O.-C. foot procedure
O.-C. technique
osphyomyelitis
osphyotomy
OSS
occupational stress syndrome
ossa tarsi
OssaTron
O. noninvasive extracorporeal shock
wave therapy device
O. shock wave
osseoaponeurotic
osseocartilaginous thoracic cage
Osseodent surgical drill
osseofibrous
osseointegrated prosthesis
osseointegration
osseomucoid
osseous
o. adjustment
o. attachment
o. bridge
o. bridge prevention
o. coalition
o. defect
o. drift
o. dystrophy
o. equinus

NOTES

O

osseous *(continued)*
    o. foraminal encroachment
    o. homeostasis
    o. instability
    o. lamella
    o. lesion
    o. patella outgrowth
    o. pin
    o. prominence
    o. ring of Lacroix
    o. structure
    o. tissue
    o. tunnel
osseus lacuna
ossicle
    accessory o.
ossicular chain replacement prosthesis
ossiferous
ossific
ossificans
    myositis o.
    osteitis o.
    pelvospondylitis o.
    periostitis o.
ossification
    bilateral heterotopic o.
    bipartite o.
    Brooker classification of
      heterotopic o. I–IV
    cartilaginous o.
    ectopic o.
    enchondral o.
    endochondral o.
    endplate o.
    heterotopic o.
    iliac crest o.
    intramembranous o.
    mandible o.
    membranous o.
    metaplastic o.
    metatarsal o.
    paraarticular heterotopic o.
    periarticular heterotopic o.
    perichondral o.
    periosteal o.
    pisiform o.
    o. of the posterior longitudinal
      ligament (OPLL)
    o. primary center
    o. secondary center
    trapezium o.
    trapezoid o.
    triquetrum o.
ossification-associated fracture
ossifluent abscess
ossiform
ossify
ossifying fibroma

ossimeter
    Küntscher o.
Ossotome bur
ostealgia
ostealgic
osteal resonance
ostectomy
    fibular o.
    partial o.
osteitis
    alveolar o.
    condensing o.
    o. deformans
    o. distal phalanx
    Garré o.
    o. necroticans pubis
    o. ossificans
    pagetoid o.
    o. pubis
    rarefying o.
    sclerosing nonsuppurative o.
    suppurative o.
ostemia
ostempyesis
osteoanagenesis
OsteoAnalyzer device
osteoanesthesia
osteoaneurysm
OsteoArthritic knee brace
osteoarthritis (OA)
    ankle o.
    o. deformans
    o. deformans endemica
    degenerative o.
    endemic o.
    erosive o.
    o. grading classification
    hyperplastic o.
    hypertrophic o.
    interphalangeal o.
    joint o.
    midtarsal o.
    obese knee o.
    o. padded night sleeve brace
    posttraumatic o.
    primary degenerative o.
    tarsometatarsal o.
    traumatic o.
osteoarthropathy (OAP)
    hypertrophic pulmonary o.
    idiopathic hypertrophic o. (IHO)
    neuropathic o.
    pneumogenic o.
    pulmonary o.
    pustulotic o.
    tabetic o.
osteoarthroscopy
    hypertrophic o. (HOA)

osteoarthrosis
osteoarthrotomy
osteoarticular
    o. allograft
    o. allograft transplantation
    o. defect
    o. graft
    o. tuberculosis
osteoblastic
    o. bone regeneration
    o. lesion
    o. metastasis
    o. osteogenic sarcoma
osteoblastoma
    spinal o.
osteoblast proliferation fluorometric assay
Osteobond copolymer bone cement
osteobunionectomy
osteocachexia
osteocampsia
OsteoCap hip prosthesis
osteocartilaginous
    o. exostosis
    o. graft
    o. lesion
    o. loose body
    o. mass
    o. metaplasia
osteochondral
    o. allograft
    o. autograft transfer system (OATS)
    o. contusion
    o. defect
    o. fracture arthrography
    o. fracture of the dome of the talus
    o. fragment
    o. graft
    o. injury
    o. lesion
    o. prominence
    o. ridge
osteochondritis
    capitellar o.
    crushing o.
    o. deformans juvenilis
    o. deformans juvenilis dorsi
    o. dissecans (OCD, OD)
    epiphysial o.
    o. juvenilis

    o. necroticans
    olecranon o.
    puncture wound o.
    syphilitic o.
osteochondroarthropathy
osteochondrodesmodysplasia
osteochondrodysplasia
osteochondrodystrophia deformans
osteochondrodystrophy
osteochondrofibroma
osteochondrolysis
osteochondroma
    congenital o.
    epiphysial o.
    excision of o.
    intraarticular o.
    pedunculated o.
    sessile-type o.
osteochondromatosis
    multiple o.
    Ollier o.
    synovial o.
osteochondromyxoma
osteochondropathy
osteochondrophyte
osteochondrosarcoma
osteochondrosis
    o. deformans tibiae
    o. of metatarsal
osteochondrotic loose body
osteochrondral slice fracture
Osteo-Clage Cable System
osteoclasis
    Blount technique for o.
    o. maneuver
osteoclast
    Collin o.
    Rizzoli o.
    o. tension staple
osteoclastic
    o. erosion
    o. giant cell
    o. resorption
osteoclast-mediated
    o.-m. bone
    o.-m. osteoporosis
osteoclastoma
osteoconduction
osteocutaneous free flap
osteocystoma
osteocyte
osteodesmosis

NOTES

osteodiastasis
osteodistractor
    Ace/Normed o.
osteodynia
osteodysplasty of Melnick and Needles
osteodystrophy
    Albright hereditary o.
    azotemic o.
    parathyroid o.
    pulmonary o.
    renal o.
osteoectasia
    familial o.
osteoectomy
osteoenchondroma
osteoepiphysis
osteofascial compartment
osteofibrochondrosarcoma
osteofibroma
osteofibromatosis
osteofibrosis
osteofibrous dysplasia
Osteofil allograft paste
OsteoGen
    O. bone growth stimulation
    O. implantable bone growth
      stimulator
    O. resorbable osteogenic bone-
      filling implant
osteogenesis
    distraction o.
    endochondral o.
    o. imperfecta (OI)
    o. imperfecta congenita (OIC)
    O. Imperfecta Foundation (OIF)
    o. imperfecta tarda (OIT)
    membranous o.
    periosteal o.
osteogenic
    o. cell
    o. fibroma
    o. osteomalacia
    o. protein-1 (OP-1)
    o. protein-1 bone graft
    o. sarcoma
Osteogenics BoneSource synthetic bone
  replacement material
OsteoGram bone density test
Osteoguide
osteohalisteresis
osteohydatidosis
osteoid
    calcified o.
    o. osteoma
    o. seam
    unmineralized o.
osteoinduction
osteoinductive enhanced-graft gel

osteokinematic motion
osteokinematics
osteolipochondroma
osteolipoma
Osteolock
    O. acetabular component
    O. HA femoral component
    O. hip prosthesis
    Precision O.
osteology
    metatarsal o.
osteolysis
    acetabular o.
    debris-incited o.
    debris-induced o.
    familial expansile o.
    femoral o.
    malignant acetabular o.
    massive o.
    posttraumatic o.
    pubic o.
osteolytic sarcoma
osteoma
    cavalryman's o.
    compact o.
    o. durum
    o. eburneum
    giant osteoid o.
    intraarticular osteoid o.
    intracapsular osteoid o.
    ivory o.
    osteoid o.
    parosteal o.
    solitary o.
    o. spongiosum
    subperiosteal-paraarticular–type
      osteoid o.
osteomalacia
    nutritional o.
    osteogenic o.
    renal tubular o.
    senile o.
osteomalacic pelvis
osteomanipulative therapy (OMT)
Osteomark bone-loss urine test
osteomatoid
osteomatosis
Osteomed screw
osteomesopyknosis
osteometry
osteomusculocutaneous flap
osteomyelitic
    o. cloaca formation
    o. sinus
osteomyelitis
    Ackerman criteria for o.
    acute hematogenous o. (AHO)
    anaerobic o.

ankle o.
blastomycotic o.
chloramphenicol o.
cystic o.
femoral o.
Gaenslen o.
Garré sclerosing o.
hematogenous o.
hemorrhagic o.
iatrogenic o.
long bone o.
multifocal o.
nonsuppurative o.
nonunion o.
pedal o.
pin-tract o.
postfracture o.
posttraumatic chronic o.
primary subacute o.
probe test for o.
pyogenic vertebral o.
sclerosing nonsuppurative o.
secondary hematogenous o.
spinal o.
subacute hematogenous o.
suppurative o.
synovitis-acne-pustulosis-
hyperostosis o. (SAPHO)
tuberculous spinal o.
tuberculous vertebral o.
typhoid o.
vertebral o.
osteomyelodysplasia
osteon
osteonal
o. bone union
o. lamellar bone
Osteone air drill
osteonecrosis
dysbaric o.
Ficat classification of femoral
head o.
idiopathic o.
navicular o.
nontraumatic idiopathic o.
posttraumatic o.
steroid-induced o.
osteoneuralgia
Osteonics
O. acetabular cup
O. acetabular dome hole plug
O. HA femoral implant

O. hip prosthesis
O. jig
O. Omnifit-C
O. Omnifit-HA component
O. Omnifit-HA hip stem
O. Scorpio insert
O. Scorpio posterior cruciate
retaining total knee system
Stryker Howmedica O.
osteoonychodysplasia
hereditary o. (HOOD)
Osteopatch bone density test
osteopathia striata
osteopathic
o. lesion
o. manipulation
o. manipulative therapy (OMT)
o. manipulative treatment
o. medicine
o. scoliosis
osteopathology
osteopathy
alimentary o.
osteopenia
transient o.
osteopenic
o. bone
o. bone stock
osteoperiosteal
o. bone graft
o. flap
osteoperiostitis
osteopetrorickets
osteopetrosis
malignant o.
osteophlebitis
osteophore
osteophyte
apophysial joint o.
bony o.
bridging o.
o. elevator
o. formation
fringe of o.
jagged o.
marginal o.
posterior o.
osteophytic
o. bone lip
o. spur
osteophytosis
osteoplaque

O

NOTES

osteoplastic
    o. amputation
    o. flap clamp
    o. laminectomy
    o. necrotomy
    o. reconstruction
osteoplasty
    Maquet anteromedial o.
osteoplysis
    massive o.
osteopoikilosis
osteopoikilotic
osteoporosis
    disuse o.
    dual photon densitometry test
      for o.
    femoral o.
    idiopathic juvenile o.
    idiopathic transient o.
    O. Knowledge Questionnaire (OKQ)
    low-turnover o.
    osteoclast-mediated o.
    posttraumatic o.
    o. pseudoglioma syndrome
    regional migratory o.
    senile o.
    Singh index of o.
    transient o.
osteoporotic
    o. bone
    o. spine
Osteopower modular handpiece system
osteoprogenitor cell
osteoprotegerin
osteoradionecrosis (ORN)
osteorrhagia
osteorrhaphy
osteosarcoma
    conventional o.
    extraskeletal o.
    intraosseous o.
    parosteal o.
    periosteal o.
    recurrent parosteal o.
    secondary o.
    spinal o.
    telangiectatic o.
OsteoSet
    O. bone filler
    O. bone graft substitute
    O. resorbable bead kit
OsteoSet-T medicated bone graft substitute
osteosis
osteospongioma
OsteoStat
    O. disposable power tool

    O. single-use power surgical
      equipment
Osteo-Stim
    O.-S. implantable bone growth
      stimulation
    O.-S. implantable bone growth
      stimulator
osteosuture
osteosynovitis
osteosynthesefragen
osteosynthesis
    anterior column o.
    locked intramedullary o.
    lumbar spine vertebral o.
    odontoid process o.
    plate-screw o.
    posterior column o.
    thoracic spine vertebral o.
    thoracolumbar spine vertebral o.
    vertebral o.
    Wagner multiple K-wire o.
osteotabes
osteotelangiectasia
osteothrombophlebitis
osteothrombosis
OsteoTite bone screw
osteotome
    AcuDriver o.
    Acufex o.
    air compression o.
    Albee o.
    Alexander costal o.
    Anderson-Neivert o.
    Andrews o.
    Army o.
    arthroscopic o.
    Aufranc o.
    backcutting o.
    bayonet o.
    Blount o.
    Bowen o.
    box o.
    Campbell o.
    Carroll-Legg o.
    Carroll-Smith-Petersen o.
    Cavin o.
    Cebotome o.
    Cherry o.
    Cinelli o.
    Clayton o.
    Cloward spinal fusion o.
    Cobb o.
    Compere o.
    Cottle o.
    Crane o.
    curved o.
    Dautrey o.
    Dawson-Yuhl o.

Dingman o.
disposable one-piece o.
Epker o.
fine o.
Furnas bayonet o.
grooving o.
guarded o.
Hardt-Delima o.
Hendel guided o.
Hibbs curved o.
Hibbs straight o.
Hoke o.
Joseph o.
Lambotte o.
Leinbach o.
Lexer o.
MacGregor o.
Meyerding curved o.
Meyerding straight o.
MGH o.
Micro-Aire o.
Miner o.
mini-Lambotte o.
mini-Lexer o.
Mitchell o.
Moberg o.
Moe o.
Moreland o.
Murphy o.
Neivert o.
orthopaedic o.
Padgett o.
Parkes o.
Peck o.
Rhoton o.
Rish o.
rotary o.
Sheehan o.
Silver o.
Simmons o.
Smith-Petersen curved o.
Smith-Petersen straight o.
Stille o.
straight o.
Swanson o.
Swiss pattern o.
thin o.
unguarded o.
U.S. Army o.
Weck o.
West o.

osteotomize

osteotomy
Abbott-Gill o.
abduction o.
abductory midfoot o.
abductory wedge o.
acetabular shelf o.
adduction o.
Agliette supracondylar o.
Akin proximal phalangeal o.
Akron midtarsal o.
Amspacher-Messenbaugh closing
  wedge o.
Amstutz-Wilson o.
o. analysis simulation software
  (OASIS)
Anderson-Fowler calcaneal
  displacement o.
angulation o.
anterior calcaneal o.
arcuate o.
Austin o.
Axer lateral opening wedge o.
Axer varus derotational o.
Bailey-Dubow o.
Baker-Hill o.
Balacescu closing wedge o.
ball-and-socket trochanteric o.
Barouk microscrew with
  shortening o.
barrel-stave o.
basal chevron o.
basal closing wedge o.
base o.
base-of-the-neck o.
base wedge o.
basilar closing wedge metatarsal o.
basilar crescentic o.
basilar plantarflexory metatarsal o.
Bellemore-Barrett closing wedge o.
Berens o.
Berman-Gartland metatarsal o.
Bernese periacetabular o.
bicorrectional Austin o.
bifurcation o.
biplane Dwyer o.
biplane trochanteric o.
biplaning of o.
block o.
Blount displacement o.
Blundell-Jones hip o.
Blundell-Jones varus o.

O

NOTES

osteotomy *(continued)*
 Bonney-Kessel dorsiflexionary tilt-up o.
 Booth wire o.
 Borden-Spencer-Herman o.
 Brackett o.
 Brett o.
 Brett-Campbell tibial o.
 o. bunionectomy
 calcaneal L o.
 calcaneal sliding corrective o.
 Campbell tibial o.
 Canale o.
 canal innominate o.
 capital crescentic shelf o.
 Carstan reverse wedge o.
 Cartam-Treander reverse wedge o.
 Chambers o.
 chevron-Akin double o.
 chevron modification of the Mitchell o.
 Chiari innominate o.
 Chiari-Salter-Steel pelvic o.
 closed base wedge o. (CBWO)
 closed intramedullary o.
 closing abductory-wedge o. (CAWO)
 closing base-wedge o.
 closing wedge greenstick dorsal proximal metatarsal o.
 Cole o.
 compensatory basilar o.
 compromise o.
 controlled rotational o.
 corrective lengthening o.
 countersinking o.
 Coventry distal femoral o.
 Coventry proximal tibial o.
 Coventry vagal o.
 Crawford L-shaped o.
 Crego femoral o.
 crescentic base wedge o.
 crescentic basilar first metatarsal o.
 crescentic calcaneal o.
 crescentic shelf o. (CSO)
 crescent-shaped o.
 cuboid-calcaneal o.
 cuboid wedge o.
 cuneiform o.
 cup-and-ball o.
 curved o.
 cylindrical o.
 decompressive o.
 Dega pelvic o.
 delayed femoral o.
 DeRosa-Graziano step-cut o.
 derotational o.
 dial pelvic o.

 dial periacetabular o.
 diaphysial o.
 Dickinson-Coutts-Woodward-Handler o.
 Dickson geometric o.
 Dillwyn-Evans o.
 Dimon o.
 Dimon-Hughston intertrochanteric o.
 displacement anterior cavus V o.
 distal L o.
 distal oblique sliding o.
 dome proximal tibial o.
 dome-shaped o.
 dorsal-V o.
 dorsiflexion metatarsal o.
 dorsiflexory wedge o.
 double o.
 Dunn o.
 Dunn-Hess trochanteric o.
 Dwyer calcaneal o.
 Elizabethtown o.
 Elmslie-Trillat o.
 Emmon o.
 epiphysial-metaphysial o.
 Eppright dial o.
 Estersohn o.
 Evans anterior opening wedge calcaneal o.
 eversion o.
 extended slide trochanteric o.
 extension o.
 failed femoral o.
 femoral derotation o.
 Ferguson-Thompson-King-Moore o.
 Ferguson-Thompson-King two-stage o.
 Fernandez o.
 fibular o.
 Fish cuneiform o.
 flexion o.
 Fowler o.
 free-floating o.
 French lateral closing-wedge o.
 Fulkerson oblique tibial tubercle o.
 Gant o.
 Ganz o.
 geometric supracondylar extension o.
 Gerbert o.
 Giannestras oblique metatarsal o.
 Giannestras step-down modified o.
 Gibson-Piggott o.
 Gigli saw o.
 Gleich o.
 glenoid o.
 Golden closing-wedge o.
 Grant-Small-Lehman supracondylar extension o.

greater tuberosity o.
Greenfield o.
Green-Laird modification of the
  Reverdin o.
Green-Reverdin o.
greenstick dorsal proximal
  metatarsal o.
Green-Watermann o.
Gudas scarf Z-plasty o.
Haas o.
Haber-Kraft o.
Haddad metatarsal o.
Hass o.
Helal o.
Herman-Gartland o.
high tibial o. (HTO)
Hirayma o.
Hohmann o.
Hohmann-Thomasen metatarsal o.
Hohmann-Wilson o.
horizontal o.
iliac o.
Ingram o.
Ingram-Canle-Beaty epiphysial-
  metaphysial o.
innominate o.
intertrochanteric varus o.
intraarticular o.
intracapsular o.
intraepiphysial o.
Irwin o.
Japas o.
Johnson chevron o.
Kalish o.
Kaplan o.
Kawamura dome o.
Kawamura pelvic o.
Kech-Kelly o.
Kelikian modified Z o.
Kelly-Keck o.
Kelly-Kelly o.
Kempf-Grosse-Abalo Z-step o.
Kessel-Bonney extension o.
Kitaoka-Leventen medial
  displacement metatarsal o.
Koutsogiannis calcaneal
  displacement o.
Koutsogiannis-Fowler-Anderson o.
Kramer-Craig-Noel basilar femoral
  neck o.
Kramer modification of
  Hohmann o.

Lambrinudi o.
Langenskiöld o.
Leach-Igou step-cut medial o.
Le Fort I–III o.
Lelièvre o.
Lichtblau o.
Lindgren oblique o.
Lindseth o.
linear o.
Lorenz o.
L-shaped o.
Lucas-Cottrell o.
Ludloff o.
Macewen o.
Macewen-Shands o.
MacGregor o.
malleolar o.
mandibular o.
Maquet dome o.
Marquardt angulation o.
Martin o.
Mau o.
McKay o.
McMurray o.
metacarpal o.
metaphysial o.
metatarsal head o.
metatarsal neck o.
metatarsal oblique o.
metatarsal proximal dome o.
metatarsal Reverdin o.
metatarsal V-shaped o.
metatarsus primus o.
Meyer-Burgdorff o.
midshaft metatarsal o.
midtarsal dome o.
Mitchell distal o.
Mitchell posterior displacement o.
Mitchell step-down o.
modified Mau o.
modified Wilson o.
Molesworth o.
Moore o.
Mueller intertochanteric varus o.
Mueller transposition o.
Müller o.
oblique closing wedge o. (OCWO)
oblique slide o.
Obwegeser sagittal mandibular o.
open base wedge o.
opening abductory wedge o.
  (OAWO)

O

NOTES

osteotomy *(continued)*
opening wedge o.
Osgood rotational o.
Pauwels proximal o.
Pauwels valgus o.
Pauwels Y o.
peg-in-hole o.
Peimer reduction o.
pelvic o.
Pemberton pericapsular o.
percutaneous o.
pericapsular o.
phalangeal o.
Phemister o.
o. pin
plantar flexor proximal
  metatarsal o.
Platou o.
posterior iliac o.
posterior spinal wedge o.
Potts eversion o.
Potts tibial o.
radial recession o.
radial wedge o.
Ranawat-DeFiore-Straub o.
Rappaport o.
reduction o.
Regnauld o.
Reverdin o.
Reverdin-Green o.
Reverdin-Laird o.
reverse Austin o.
reverse closing base wedge o.
reverse Dillwyn-Evans calcaneal o.
Root-Siegal varus derotational o.
rotational scarf o.
Roux o.
sagittal split o.
sagittal-Z o.
Sakoff o.
Salter innominate o.
Salter pelvic o.
Samilson crescentic calcaneal o.
sandwich o.
Sarmiento intertrochanteric o.
Scanz o.
scarf Z o.
Schanz angulation o.
Schanz femoral o.
Schede hip o.
Schwartz dorsiflexory o.
segmental alveolar o.
shortening o.
Siffert intraepiphysial o.
Siffert-Storen intraepiphysial o.
Simmonds-Menelaus metatarsal o.
Simmonds-Menelaus proximal
  phalangeal o.

Simmons o.
Smith-Petersen o.
Sofield o.
Southwick biplane trochanteric o.
Speed o.
spike o.
spinal o.
Sponsel oblique o.
Stamm metatarsal o.
Steel triple innominate o.
Steel triradiate o.
step o.
step-cut o.
step-down o.
Stren intraepiphyseal o.
subcapital o.
subcondylar o.
subtraction o.
subtrochanteric o.
Sugioka transtrochanteric
  rotational o.
supracondylar femoral
  derotational o.
supracondylar varus o.
supramalleolar derotational o.
supramalleolar varus derotation o.
supratubercular wedge o.
Sutherland-Greenfield o.
Swanson o.
talar neck o.
talocalcaneal o.
tarsal wedge o.
Thompson telescoping V o.
through-and-through V-shaped
  horizontal o.
tibial tuberosity o.
total maxillary o.
translational o.
transpedal multiplanar wedge o.
transtrochanteric rotational o.
transtrochanteric valgus o. (TVO)
trapezoidal resection o.
Trethowan metatarsal o.
Trillat o.
triplane o.
triple innominate o.
trochanteric o.
tubercle o.
U o.
unplanned valgus o.
V o.
Vanore o.
varus rotational o. (VRO)
varus rotation shortening o.
vertical sagittal split o. (VSO)
visor o.
visor/sandwich o.
V-shaped o.

Wagdy double-V o.
Waterman o.
Weber humeral o.
Weber subcapital o.
wedge o.
Weil o.
Whitman o.
Wilson double oblique o.
Wilson oblique displacement o.
Wiltse ankle o.
Wiltse varus supramalleolar o.
Y o.
Yancey o.
Yu o.
osteotomy/bunionectomy
base wedge o./b.
closed wedge o./b.
crescentic base wedge o./b.
Kelikian modified Z o./b.
Mitchell o./b.
open base wedge o./b.
rotational scarf o./b.
scarf Z o./b.
supertubercular wedge o./b.
osteotomy-osteoclasis
Moore o.-o.
osteotribe
osteotripsy
osteotrite
Osteotron stimulator for bone union
osteotylus
OsteoView
O. 2000 imaging system
O. x-ray device
ostium, pl. **ostia**
ostraceous
ostracosis
Ostrum-Furst syndrome
Ostrup harvesting technique
Oswestry
O. Disability Score
O. index
O. Low Back Pain Disability
Oswestry-O'Brien spinal stapler
OT
occupational therapy
Ottawa Ankle Rule (OAR)
Otto
O. Bock 1A30 Greissinger Plus foot
O. Bock 1D25 Dynamic Plus foot
O. Bock dynamic prosthesis

O. Bock 3R65 children's hydraulic knee joint
O. Bock 3R60 EBS knee
O. Bock 3R45 modular knee joint
O. Bock 3R80 modular rotary hydraulic knee
O. Bock Safety constant-friction knee
O. Bock system electric hand
O. disease
O. pelvis
O. pelvis dislocation
Oudard procedure
out
draped o.
step out, turn o. (SOTO)
toeing o.
outcome
o. measure
Michigan Hand O.'s
Outerbridge
O. classification
O. degenerative arthritis staging
O. ridge
O. scale
Outerbridge-Kashiwagi procedure
outer malleolus
outflow cannula
outgrowth
osseous patella o.
outlet
cervical o.
supraspinatus o.
o. view
out-of-cast ankle brace
outpatient
o. physical therapy
o. rehabilitation
output
cardiac o.
urinary o.
outrigger
o. arm
o. cast
dorsal wrist splint with o.
Harrington distraction o.
o. splint
O. wire
outside-in technique
outside-the-boot brace
outside-to-outside arthroscopy technique
outsole

NOTES

O

out-toeing
    o.-t. gait
outward rotation
Ovadia-Beals
    O.-B. classification of tibial
      plafond fracture
    O.-B. tibial plafond fracture
      classification
oval
    o. amputation
    o. curved-cup curette
    o. washer
over-bed table
overcorrection
overdistraction
Overdyke hip prosthesis
overextension
overflexion
overgrowth
    bony o.
    terminal o.
overhead
    o. exercise test
    o. olecranon traction
overhinge
    variable flexion o. (VFO)
Overholt
    O. clip-applying forceps
    O. operation
overhydration
    fluid o.
overlap
    tibiofibular o.
overlapped uprights in orthosis
overlapping fifth toe
overlay
    Bodyline sleeper mattress o.
    o. drafting
    Formation Gelfoam mattress o.
    o. mattress
    o. plate
    Stimulite honeycomb mattress o.
    x-ray o.
overload
    compression o.
    lateral forefoot o.
    torsional o.
overmotivation
overpull
overreaching
overriding fifth toe

oversewn
oversize tennis shoe
over-straight toe
overstrain
overstretch weakness
over-the-door traction unit
over-the-top
    o.-t.-t. knee operation
    o.-t.-t. knee procedure
    o.-t.-t. position
Overton dowel graft
overtraining syndrome
over-tying wire
overuse
    o. injury
    o. injury assessment
    o. syndrome
OW
    open wedge
Owen gauze dressing
Owens silk
Oxford
    O. fixator
    O. meniscal unicompartment
      prosthesis
    O. method
    O. method for scoring skeletal
      maturity
    O. uncompartmental device
oxidation
    carbohydrate o.
    fat o.
oxide
    ethylene o.
oxidized
    o. zirconium
    o. zirconium alloy on implant
oximeter
    pulse o.
Oxycel oxidized cellulose
oxygen
    dysbaric o.
    epiphysial o.
    hyperbaric o. (HBO)
    o. myelography
    o. seizure
    o. tension
    o. therapy
    transcutaneous o.
oyster-shell brace

P
    passive
P/3
    proximal third
PA
    posteroanterior
Paas disease
pachydactylia
pachydactylous
pachydactyly
pachyonychia congenita
pachyperiostitis
pachypodous
pacinian mechanoreceptor
Paci operation
pack
    Adaptic p.
    Arctic Blaze hot/cold p.
    Avitene p.
    Back-Ease aromatherapy hot/cold p.
    Baxter personal Von-Loc ice p.
    BodyIce cold p.
    cold p.
    Coldhot p.
    Colpacs p.
    cool p.
    CP2 inflatable cold p.
    DynaHeat hot p.
    gel p.
    Gelfoam p.
    Glacier P.
    hot p. (HP)
    hot moist p. (HMP)
    Hydrocollator steam p.
    ice p.
    I.C.E. Down cold p.
    instant cold p.
    Jack Frost hot/cold p.
    JoyBags therapeutic heat p.
    Kool Kit cold therapy p.
    Merocel p.
    MSC cold p.
    Neck-Roll aromatherapy hot/cold p.
    Polar P.
    Softouch Cold/Hot P.
    P. technique
    TheraBeads microwaveable moist
      heat p.
    Thera-Med cold p.
    Thermal P.
    ThermalSoft hot & cold p.'s
    Thermophore hot p.
    Ultimate Cold N' Hot P.
    vaginal p.
    Whitehall Glacier P.

Pack-Ehrlich deep iliac dissection
packing
    Adaptic p.
    gauze p.
    Nu Gauze p.
    wound p.
Pacs
    Boo-Boo P.
PACU
    postanesthesia care unit
pad
    ABD p.
    abdominal lap p.
    Achilles heel p.
    Airex balance p.
    AirLITE support p.
    Aliplast p.
    alternating pressure p.
    antidecubitus p.
    aperture p.
    Aquaflex gel p.
    Aquatech cast p.
    Aquatherm bed p.
    Arthropor cup p.
    artificial fat p.
    balance p.
    Bauerfeind silicone heel p.
    buttocks p.
    buttress p.
    calcaneal fat p.
    Charnley foam suture p.
    cloverleaf met foot p.
    cold p.
    crest buttress p.
    dancer's p.
    digital p.
    distal star p.
    elbow p.
    fat p.
    fibrocartilaginous p.
    finger p.
    fingertip p.
    foam p.
    foveal fat p.
    Hapad heel p.
    Hapad longitudinal metatarsal
      arch p.
    Hapad medial arch p.
    Hapad prefabricated wool felt p.
    heel fat p.
    Hoffa fat p.
    horseshoe heel p.
    horseshoe-shaped felt p.
    Hydrocollator p.

P

pad *(continued)*
    infrapatellar fat p.
    J p.
    knee-control orthosis p.
    knuckle p.
    lamb's wool p.
    MagneCore magnetic therapy p.
    metatarsal p.
    Mikulicz p.
    navicular shoe p.
    OEC popliteal p.
    Ortho-Cel p.
    Ortho-Foam elbow/heel p.
    painful heel p.
    patellar fat p.
    patellar orthosis p.
    Pedi-Cushions p.
    Pedifix crest p.
    Pedifix hammertoe p.
    Pelite p.
    Pen/Alps distal p.
    plantar fat p.
    pre-Achilles fat p.
    prefabricated wool felt p.
    premalleolar fat p.
    pubic p.
    Redigrip knee p.
    reticulated polyurethane p.
    retropatellar fat p.
    ROHO heel p.
    scalene fat p.
    scaphoid shoe p.
    Scholl p.
    second skin p.
    sensor p.
    shock-absorbent heel p.
    shoe heel p.
    silicone p.
    Silipos digital p.
    Sof-Rol cast p.
    Sof Sole Sof Gel heel p.
    Sorbothane recoil p.
    S'port Max stabilization p.
    spur p.
    Staph-Chek p.
    Sure Sport p.
    T-Foam bed p.
    Thermapad p.
    Thermophore moist heat p.
    thickness of heel p.
    Vac-Pac p.
    valgus knee control p.
    varus knee control p.
    Zimfoam p.

padded
    p. aluminum splint
    p. board splint
    p. bolster

    p. button
    p. clamp
    p. plywood splint
    p. tongue blade splint

padding
    cast p.
    contoured felt p.
    cotton cast p.
    Delta-Rol cast p.
    felt p.
    Kerlix cast p.
    moleskin p.
    Molestick p.
    pressure relief p.
    Protouch synthetic orthopedic p.
    QuickStick p.
    Reston p.
    Sifoam p.
    splint p.
    Therafoam p.
    Thero-Skin gel p.
    Webril cotton p.

Paddu knee operation
Padgett
    P. electric dermatome
    P. osteotome
    P. prosthesis

pad/protector
    Decubinex p./p.

PAG
    periaqueductal gray

Pagddu procedure
Paget
    P. disease
    P. juvenile syndrome
    P. osteitis deformans
    P. quiet necrosis
    P. test

Paget-associated osteogenic sarcoma
pagetoid
    p. bone
    p. osteitis

Paget-Schrötter syndrome
pain
    aches and p.'s
    Achilles tendon p.
    aching p.
    acute p.
    adolescent back p.
    AHCPR guidelines for treatment of
      acute low back p.
    amputation-related bone p.
    p. at rest
    back p.
    bandlike p.
    Behavioral Assessment of P. (BAP)
    boring p.
    burning p.

causalgic p.
cervical myofascial p.
chronic low back p. (CLBP)
chronic subtalar joint p.
contralateral p.
p. control infusion pump
cross leg p.
deafferentation p.
dermatomal p.
diskogenic neck p.
p. drawing
dull aching p.
p. dysfunction syndrome
endogenous p.
epicritic p.
exercise-induced breast p.
fibromyalgic p.
functional back p.
gate control theory of p.
glenohumeral p.
gouty p.
groin p.
growing p.
idiopathic anterior knee p.
impingement p.
p. induction
joint line p.
kinetic foot p.
lancinating p.
low back p. (LBP)
machine-gun-like p.
p. measurement
Multiaxial Assessment of P. (MAP)
myofascial p.
myotomal p.
neurologic p.
patellofemoral p. (PFP)
perimalleolar p.
periscapulitis shoulder p.
persistent p.
phantom limb p.
pillar p.
plantar p.
postherpetic p.
postoperative p.
posttraumatic p.
prickling p.
Pronex pneumatic device for cervical p.
p. provocation test
radicular p.

recalcitrant p.
referred neuritic p.
referred trigger point p.
rest p. (RP)
Roland index of low back p.
scapulothoracic p.
sclerotomal p.
searing p.
shooting p.
splint-like p.
static foot p.
sympathetically mediated p.
p. threshold gauge
ticlike p.
vise-like p.
volley of p.
p. with weightbearing
pain-all-over syndrome
PainFree pump
painful
  p. arc
  p. arc sign
  p. arc syndrome
  p. femoral head prosthesis
  p. gait
  p. heel
  p. heel pad
  p. minor intervertebral dysfunction (PMID)
  p. spur
  p. stump
  p. toe
The Painless One acupuncture needle
pain-related sleep disturbance
paint
  p. gun injury
  p. thinner injury
paired
  p. discharge
  p. response
  p. scintigraphy
  p. stimulus
Pais fracture
Pak
  Apollo hot/cold P.
PAL
  posterior axillary line
Palacos
  P. cement adhesive
  P. radiopaque bone cement
Paladon

NOTES

P

palatal myoclonus
palatine bone
Palex expansion screw
Paley classification
palindromic
    p. arthropathy
    p. rheumatism
palliative care
pallor
palm
    p. guard
    p. space
palmar
    p. advancement flap
    p. aponeurosis
    p. approach
    p. arch
    p. clip
    p. cock-up splint
    p. creaking
    p. crease
    p. cross-finger flap
    p. fascia
    p. fasciotomy
    p. fibromatosis
    p. flexion
    p. grasp reflex
    p. incision
    p. interosseous muscle
    p. luxation
    p. pinch
    p. plate
    p. swab kit
    p. synovectomy
    p. tilt
    p. wrist
    p. wrist splint
palmaris
    p. digitorum superficialis muscle
    p. longus (PL)
    p. longus muscle
    p. longus tendon
palmature
Palmer
    P. bone nail
    P. method
    P. primary fracture
    P. screw
    P. technique
    P. transscaphoid perilunar
      dislocation
    P. triangular fibrocartilage complex
      lesion classification
Palmer-Dobyns-Linscheid ligament repair
Palmer-Gonstead-Firth listing system
Palmer-Widen
    P.-W. operation
    P.-W. shoulder technique

palm-to-axilla dressing
palm-up test
palpable band
palpation
    p. of anterior superior iliac spine
    digital p.
    end-feel p.
    flat p.
    p. of iliac crest
    intersegmental range of motion p.
      (IRMP)
    motion p.
    optimizing motion p.
    pincer p.
    p. of posterior superior iliac spine
    screening p.
    static p.
    p. testing
palpatory
    p. diagnosis
    p. examination
    p. skill
PALS
    Pediatric Advanced Life Support
palsy
    ataxic cerebral p.
    athetoid cerebral p.
    backpack p.
    Bell p.
    brachial plexus p.
    cerebral p. (CP)
    combined nerve p.
    crutch p.
    drummer-boy p.
    Duchenne-Erb p.
    dyskinetic cerebral p.
    Erb p.
    Erb-Duchenne p.
    flaccid cerebral p.
    handlebar p.
    high median-high radial p.
    high median-high ulnar p.
    high ulnar-high radial p.
    Hoke procedure for tibial p.
    Klumpke p.
    long thoracic nerve p.
    low median-low ulnar p.
    median nerve p.
    nerve p.
    peripheral nerve p.
    peroneal nerve p.
    posterior interosseous nerve p.
    postnatal cerebral p.
    prisoner's p.
    progressive supranuclear p.
    radial nerve p.
    Saturday night p.
    sciatic p.

spastic cerebral p.
tardy ulnar p.
thenar p.
thoracic nerve p.
tourniquet p.
ulnar nerve p.

Paltrinieri-Trentani
P.-T. prosthesis
P.-T. resurfacing
P.-T. resurfacing procedure

Palumbo
P. ankle stabilizer
P. dynamic patellar brace
P. knee support
P. patella tracker
P. stabilizing brace

Panacryl suture
Panalok absorbable anchor
panaris
melanotic p.
panarteritis nodosa
panarthritis
panastragaloid arthrodesis
pancake hand
panclavicular dislocation
pancreatic enzyme therapy
pandemic
Panje voice button prosthesis
panmetatarsal
p. head resection
p. tendon suspension
Panner disease
panniculus adiposus
pannus
p. deformity
p. of synovium
Panogauze Hydrogel wound dressing
panosteitis
Panoview
P. arthroscope
P. arthroscopic system
panplexopathy
pan splint
pant
prophylactic abduction p.
pantalar
p. arthrodesis
p. fusion
pantalocrural
p. arthritic destruction
p. arthritis

pantaloon
p. brace
p. spica cast
p. walking cast
Pantopaque
pantrapezial arthritis
pants-over-vest
p.-o.-v. capsulorrhaphy
p.-o.-v. technique
panty
Cadenza p.
PAOD
peripheral arterial occlusive disease
Papavasiliou
P. olecranon fracture classification
papaverine
papillary adenoma
Papineau
P. graft
P. technique
papule
Gottron p.
papyrus
Edwin Smith p.
PAR
postanesthesia recovery
paraarticular
p. arthrodesis
p. calcification
p. heterotopic ossification
Parabath paraffin heat treatment
parabola
metatarsal p.
Para-Care paraffin therapy bath
paracervical
parachute
Corkscrew P.
p. jumper's dislocation
p. reflex
P. technique
p. test
p. therapy
Parachutist ankle brace
paradoxical
p. lumbrical-plus finger
paraffin
p. bath (PB)
p. heat therapy
p. implant material
p. mitt
p. treatment
p. wax therapeutic application

NOTES

P

paraganglioma
    medullary p.
paraglenoid sulcus
parajugular line
parallel
    p. goniometric measure
    p. pin kit
    p. pitch lines
    p. squat exercise
parallelism
parallelogram electrogoniometer
paralysis, pl. **paralyses**
    adductor pollicis p.
    p. agitans
    atrophic muscular p.
    backpack p.
    brachial plexus p.
    Chaves-Rapp p.
    common peroneal nerve p.
    compression p.
    cruciate p.
    crutch p.
    Cruveilhier p.
    Dewar-Harris p.
    Dickson p.
    familial periodic p.
    femoral nerve p.
    flaccid p.
    gluteus medius p.
    Haas p.
    hand p.
    Henry p.
    intrinsic p.
    isolated p.
    musculocutaneous nerve p.
    musculospiral p.
    myogenic p.
    myopathic p.
    p. notariorum
    peripheral p.
    peroneal p.
    Pott p.
    pressure p.
    Remak p.
    rucksack p.
    serratus anterior p.
    spastic p.
    spinomuscular p.
    tourniquet p.
    ulnar nerve p.
    Vastamäki p.
    Volkmann ischemic p.
    Whitman p.
    writer's p.
paralytic
    p. chest
    p. contracture
    p. foot

    p. kyphosis
    p. scoliosis
paramalleolar artery
ParaMax
    P. ACL guide system
    P. angled driver
paramedian
    p. approach
    p. sagittal plane
parameniscus
paramount
    P. total body plate-loaded machine
    P. 3-Way Press Bench
paramyoclonus multiplex
paramyotonia congenita
paraosseous lesion
paraparesis
paraparetic gait
parapatellar
    p. arthrotomy
    p. incision
    p. plica
    p. synovitis
paraphysiologic zone
paraplegia
    incomplete p.
    postoperative p.
    Pott p.
    spastic p.
    traumatic p.
parapodium orthosis
pararectus approach
parasacral block
parasagittal
    p. groove
    p. scar
parascapular flap
paraspinal
    p. abscess
    p. approach
    p. mapping
    p. muscle
    p. muscle spasm
    p. musculature
    p. rod application
    p. skin temperature thermocouple
      instrument
paraspinous muscular spasm
parasympathetic
    p. innervation
    p. nervous system (PNS)
parasympatholytic
paratendinitis
    Achilles p.
paratenon
paratenonitis
parathenar incision

parathyroid
    p. gland
    p. osteodystrophy
paratonia
paratrooper fracture
paravertebral
    p. abscess
    p. block
    p. muscle
    p. muscle spasm
    p. musculature
    p. sympathetic chain
paraxial hemimelia
Pare elbow dislocation reduction
parenteral nutrition
paresis
    limb-girdle-trunk p.
paresthesia, pl. **paresthesias**
    Berger p.
    intermittent p.
paresthetica
    cheiralgia p.
paretic leg
ParFlex orthotic
Parham
    P. band
    P. support
Parham-Martin
    P.-M. band
    P.-M. bone-holding clamp
    P.-M. fracture apparatus
    P.-M. fracture device
parietal
    p. bone
    p. pleura
    p. tendon sheath layer
    p. tuberosity
Paris
    elastic plaster of P.
    P. manual therapy table
    plaster of P. (POP)
park
    P. aneurysm
    transverse line of P.
Parkes osteotome
Parkinson disease
parkinsonian gait
Parona space
paronychia bur
parosteal
    p. chondrosarcoma
    p. lesion

    p. osteogenic sarcoma
    p. osteoma
    p. osteosarcoma
parosteitis
parosteosis
paroxysmal burning
PAR-Q
    Physical Activity Readiness
    Questionnaire
parquetry set
Parrish-Mann hammertoe technique
Parrish procedure
parrot
    p. foot
    P. node
    P. pseudoparalysis
parrot-beak tear
parry fracture
pars
    p. defect
    p. interarticularis fracture
Parsonage-Aldren-Turner syndrome
Parsonage-Turner
    P.-T. neuronitis
    P.-T. syndrome
partial
    p. adactyly
    p. ankylosis
    p. aphalangia
    p. diskectomy
    p. dislocation
    p. fasciectomy
    p. fibulectomy
    p. hand amputation
    p. hemimelia
    p. matrixectomy
    p. meniscectomy
    p. ossicular
    reconstruction/replacement
    prosthesis
    p. ossicular replacement prosthesis
    (PORP)
    p. ostectomy
    p. patellectomy
    p. sit-ups back exercise technique
    p. thromboplastin time (PTT)
    p. weightbearing (PWB)
partially
    p. necrotic osseous trabecula
    p. threaded pin
participation
    sports p.

NOTES

P

particle of bone
particulate
    p. cancellous bone graft
    p. synovitis
    p. wear debris
partnership
    P. implant
    P. instrument
    P. system
partridge
    P. band
    P. strap
Partsch
    P. chisel
    P. gouge
Parvin
    P. gravity technique
    P. maneuver
    P. reduction
PASA
    proximal articular set angle
PASG
    pneumatic antishock garment
passage
    adiabatic fast p.
    wire p.
passer
    Batzdorf cervical wire p.
    Brand tendon p.
    Bunnell tendon p.
    Charnley wire p.
    Concept two-pin p.
    curved p.
    DeMayo suture p.
    Framer tendon p.
    Hewson suture p.
    Incavo wire p.
    ligature p.
    Malis ligature p.
    Shuttle-Relay suture p.
    suture p.
    tendon p.
    Wedeen wire p.
    wire p.
passing suture
passivation metal instrument
passive (P)
    p. accessory motion test
    p. assistance exercise
    p. dorsiflexion
    p. gliding technique
    p. insufficiency
    p. intervertebral motion (PIVM)
    p. joint manipulation
    p. mobility
    p. mobility testing
    p. motion device
    p. motion machine

    p. movement
    p. night stretch splint
    p. patellar glide test
    p. patellar tilt test
    p. physiological test
    p. plantar flexion
    p. positioning device
    p. prehension orthosis (PPO)
    p. range of motion (PROM)
    p. range-of-motion exercise
    p. resistive exercise
    p. restraint
    p. spacer
    p. straight leg raising
    p. stretch
    p. stretch exercise
    p. traction table
    p. treatment modality
Passow chisel
Passport instrumentation
paste
    absorbable collagen p. (ACP)
    bone p.
    Coe-pak p.
    electrode p.
    OrthoBlast p.
    Osteofil allograft p.
    Regenafil allograft p.
    Unna p.
PAT
    Physical Ability Test
Patau syndrome
patch
    Carrel p.
    p. dressing
    felt p.
patella, pl. patellae
    absent p.
    p. alta
    apex patellae
    apex of head of p.
    p. baja
    p. ballottement
    p. bipartita
    bipartite p.
    p. bone saw
    chondromalacia patellae
    p. cubiti
    p. cup
    débridement p.
    dislocated p.
    floating p.
    grasshopper p.
    high-riding p.
    jockey cap p.
    low-riding p.
    maltracking p.
    minima p.

multipartite p.
plastic p.
prosthetic p.
P. Pusher
skyline x-ray view of p.
slipping p.
squinting p.
subluxing p.
superior pole of p.
p. tracker
p. turndown approach
undersurface of p.
patellalgia
patellapexy
patellaplasty
patellar
p. advancement
p. affection
p. aligner
p. alignment
p. apprehension sign
p. apprehension test
p. band
P. Band knee protector
p. bar
p. bone-tendon-bone autograft
p. bursa
p. bursitis
p. button
p. cement clamp
p. chondromalacia
p. clonus
p. clunk syndrome
p. contour
p. dislocation cast
p. drill guide
p. edge
p. fat pad
p. fossa
p. glide
p. glide test
p. groove
p. inhibition test probe-to-bone test
p. instability
p. intraarticular dislocation
p. jerk (PJ)
p. ligament
p. ligament-patellar ratio
p. malalignment syndrome
p. orthosis pad
p. pair syndrome
p. plug

p. portal
p. realignment
p. reamer guide
p. reamer shaft
p. reduction clamp
p. reflex
p. region
p. resection guide
p. resurfacing
p. resurfacing implant
p. retinacula release
p. retinaculum
p. retraction test
p. rotation
p. shelf
p. skyline view
p. sleeve fracture
p. stabilizer
p. stabilizing brace (PSB)
p. subluxation
p. taping
p. tap test
p. tendinitis
p. tendon
p. tendon-bearing (PTB)
p. tendon-bearing below-knee
  prosthesis
p. tendon-bearing brace
p. tendon-bearing orthosis (PTBO)
p. tendon-bearing–supracondylar
p. tendon-bearing–supracondylar-
  suprapatellar (PTB-SC-SP)
p. tendon-bearing suspension
  (PTBS)
p. tendon bone block
p. tendon graft
p. tendon repair
p. tendon socket (PTS)
p. tendon stabilization (PTS)
p. tendon substitution
p. tendon transfer (PTT)
p. tendon weightbearing brace
  orthosis
p. tendon weightbearing cast
p. tracking
p. tracking orthosis
p. transplant
p. tuberosity
patellectomy
partial p.
total p.
West-Soto-Hall p.

NOTES

patelloadductor reflex
patellofemoral
    p. alignment
    p. arthritis
    p. articulation
    p. brace
    p. compartment
    p. congruence
    p. crepitation
    p. disorder
    p. dysarthrosis
    p. dysfunction (PFD)
    p. dysplasia
    p. groove
    p. groove cartilage
    p. joint
    p. joint radiography
    p. joint reaction force
    p. ligament
    p. orthosis
    p. pain (PFP)
    p. pain syndrome (PPS)
    p. realignment
    p. stress syndrome
patellomeniscal ligament
patelloquadriceps
    p. tendon
    p. tendon substitution
patellotibial ligament
Patel medial meniscectomy
Paterson
    P. procedure
    P. technique
Pathfinder prosthetic foot
pathogenesis
pathognomonic sign
pathokinesiologic
pathologic
    p. amputation
    p. barrier
    p. dislocation
    p. fracture
    p. reflex
    p. spondylolisthesis
pathological plica
pathology
    bone p.
    heel pad p.
pathomechanical state
pathomechanics
    gait p.
    juvenile flatfoot p.
    kyphotic deformity p.
    spinal fusion p.
pathomechanism
pathway
    neuromeningeal p.

patient-controlled
    p.-c. analgesia (PCA)
    p.-c. anesthesia (PCA)
patient-on-table friction
patient positioning
patient-resisted internal rotation
patient-table interface
Patrick
    P. cross-leg maneuver
    P. drill
    P. sign
    P. test
    P. trigger area
Patrick/fabere test
Patten-Bottom-Perthes brace
pattern
    AO fracture p.
    calcaneal gait p.
    cloverleaf p.
    Collimator plugging p.
    compression p.
    curve p.
    dermatomal p.
    DISI collapse p.
    double major curve p.
    facilitation p.
    firing p.
    full interference p.
    gait p.
    heel-toe p.
    interference p.
    intermediate interference p.
    lamellar p.
    left thoracolumbar major curve p.
    locomotor p.
    p. of motion
    nondermatomal p.
    nonradicular p.
    plantar pressure p.
    PNF p.
    posterior depression p.
    primitive locomotor p.
    recruitment p.
    reduced interference p.
    right thoracic, left lumbar curve p.
    right thoracic, left thoracolumbar
      curve p.
    right thoracic minor curve p.
    single-unit p.
    storiform p.
    stretch p.
    p. of thrust
    two-point step-to gait p.
    type II curve p.
    whorled p.
patterning
    Aston p.
PattStrap knee support

patty
    cement p.
    cottonoid p.
pauciarticular arthritis
Paufique blade
Paulos ligament technique
Paulson knee retractor
Paulus plate
Pauly point
Pauwels
    P. angle
    P. femoral neck fracture
    classification
    P. fracture
    P. operation
    P. proximal osteotomy
    P. technique
    P. valgus osteotomy
    P. Y osteotomy
Pauzat disease
Pavlik
    P. bandage
    P. harness
    P. harness splint
    P. sling
Pavlov ratio
paw
Payr sign
PB
    paraffin bath
    peroneus brevis
PBS
    peroneus brevis split
PC
    PC Performer knee
    PC Performer knee prosthesis
PCA
    patient-controlled analgesia
    patient-controlled anesthesia
    porous-coated anatomic
    PCA cutting guide
    PCA hip stem
    PCA medullary guide
    PCA Original prosthesis
    PCA primary total knee system
    PCA Standard prosthesis
    PCA total hip replacement
    PCA unconstrained tricompartmental
    prosthesis
    PCA unicompartmental knee
    prosthesis

    PCA Universal total knee
    instrument system
PCB
    proximal communicating branch
PCE
    physical capacity evaluation
    Smith physical capacities evaluation
PCL
    posterior cruciate ligament
    PCL Pro
PCL-oriented
    PCL-o. placement (POP)
    PCL-o. placement marking hook
PDA
    plantar digital artery
PDGF
    platelet-derived growth factor
PDLS
    physical daily living skills
PDN
    prosthetic disk nucleus
    PDN device
PDS
    polydioxanone suture
    PDS band
    PDS knot
    PDS suture
pDXA
    peripheral dual-energy x-ray
    absorptiometry
Peabody
    P. and Munro procedure
    P. splint
Peacock
    P. transposing index ray
    P. transposing technique
peak
    P. anterior compression plate
    system
    P. Fixation System
    P. gait module
    p. height velocity (PHV)
    p. latency
    P. Motus Motion Measurement
    System
    p. pressure
    p. torque
    p. torque test
peak-pressure analysis
Pean clamp
pear bur

NOTES

P

pear-shaped
    p.-s. body
    p.-s. vertebra
Pearson
    P. attachment to Thomas splint
    P. intramedullary saw
    P. splint attachment
Pease bone drill
Pease-Thomson traction
Pebax
    P. counter unit
    P. fastening strap
PEC
    PEC modular total knee system
    PEC total hip system
Pec-Dec
Peck osteotome
pectineus muscle
pectoral
    p. girdle
    p. nerve
    p. reflex
pectoralis
    p. major flap
    p. major muscle
    p. minor muscle
    p. muscle implant
pectus
    p. carinatum
    p. excavatum
    p. recurvatum
pedal
    p. disability benefit
    p. exerciser
    p. hyperpigmented lesion
    p. hypophalangism
    p. macrodactylia
    p. osteomyelitis
Pedar
    P. pressure insole system
    P. pressure measurement system
Pedar-in-shoe measurement system
PED block
pedestal
    cast equipped with rubber p.
    halo p.
    IMP surgical leg p.
    shelf p.
    p. sign
    surgical leg p.
pedestaled
pedestrian accident
pediatric
    P. Advanced Life Support (PALS)
    p. blade plate
    p. C-D hook
    p. Cotrel-Dubousset rod
    p. flatfoot

    p. nutritional formula
    p. PRAFO brace
    p. pressure relief ankle foot orthosis
    p. system
    p. TSRH hook
    P. Ultrasound Bone Analyzer
pedicle
    adjoining p.
    p. anatomy
    p. axis angle
    p. bone graft
    p. C-D hook
    p. clamp
    p. connector
    contralateral hypoplastic/agenetic p.
    p. cortex disruption
    p. diameter
    p. entrance point
    p. erosion
    p. fat graft
    p. finder
    p. fracture
    p. groin flap
    p. implant
    p. landmark
    p. localization
    p. location
    lower thoracic p.
    lumbar p.
    p. marker
    p. method
    p. morphometry
    p. plate
    p. screw
    p. screw breakage
    p. screw construct
    p. screw cord length
    p. screw hardware prominence
    p. screw insertion
    p. screw path length
    p. screw plating
    p. screw pull-out strength
    p. screw system
    p. sounder
    p. sounding probe
    thoracic p.
pedicled
    p. fibular transfer
    p. transplant
Pedic sponge
pedicular
    p. fixation
    p. kinking
pediculosis
pedicure
Pedi-Cushions pad

Pedifix
  P. crest pad
  P. forefoot compression sleeve
  P. hammertoe pad
Pedilen polyurethane foam
Pediplast cushion
pedis
  calcar p.
  pollex p.
  tinea p.
pedistal
  Body P.
Pedi-Wrap immobilizer
pedobarogram
pedobarograph
  Biokinetics p.
  EMED-SF p.
  Musgrave footprint p.
pedobarographic analysis
pedobarography
  dynamic p. (DPB)
pedodynamometer
pedodynograph
pedodynographic
  p. examination
  p. measurement
pedogram
pedograph
pedography
pedometer
Pedors orthopedic shoe
pedorthics
pedorthist peritenon
pedorthotic
pedorthotist
pedoscope
Pedrialle template
pedunculated
  p. loose body
  p. osteochondroma
PEER
  pronation-eversion-external rotation
Peet Z-plasty
peg
  anchoring p.
  p. base plate
  Beath bone intramedullary p.
  bone p.
  p. bone graft
  p. device
  fiber-metal p.
  fibular p.

fixation p.
glenoid alignment p.
Harrison-Nicolle polypropylene p.
Kinemax removable fixation p.
locking p.
polyethylene p.
Smith subtalar joint arthroereisis p.
  (STA-peg)
stringing p.
peg-and-socket technique
pegboard
  p. lateral positioning device
  Purdue p.
pegged tibial prosthesis
pegging
  bone p.
peg-in-hole
  p.-i.-h. arthroereisis
  p.-i.-h. osteotomy
Peimer reduction osteotomy
Pelite pad
Pe Lite thermoplastic crepe material
Pelken sign
Pellegrini disease
Pellegrini-Stieda disease
pelves (*pl. of* pelvis)
pelvic
  p. abscess
  p. angle
  p. avulsion fracture
  p. band
  p. bench
  p. block
  p. brace
  p. brim
  p. C-clamp
  p. circumference
  p. discontinuity
  p. drainage
  p. fixation
  p. flexion contracture (PFC)
  p. floor exercise
  p. fracture frame
  p. girdle
  p. hyperextension traction
  p. injury
  p. instability
  p. kinematic chain
  p. lateral shift
  p. lateral tilt
  p. obliquity
  p. osteotomy

NOTES

P

pelvic *(continued)*
p. pain and organic dysfunction
p. plane
p. reconstruction kit
p. region bursitis
p. region contusion
p. rim fracture
p. ring
p. ring fracture
p. rock (PR)
p. rock test
p. rotation
p. rotation motion gait determinant
p. shift motion gait determinant
p. side-shift
p. sling
p. splint
p. splinting
p. straddle fracture
p. tilt motion gait determinant
p. traction belt
p. unleveling
pelvic-femoral angle
pelvis, pl. **pelves**
achondroplastic p.
assimilation p.
beaked p.
bony p.
caoutchouc p.
cordate p.
cordiform p.
coxalgic p.
dual drop p. (DDP)
dwarf p.
false p.
frozen p.
greater p.
high-assimilation p.
kyphorachitic p.
kyphoscoliorachitic p.
kyphoscoliotic p.
kyphotic p.
lesser p.
lordotic p.
low-assimilation p.
Nägele p.
p. nana
osteomalacic p.
Otto p.
Prague p.
pseudoosteomalacic p.
rachitic p.
Rokitansky p.
rostrate p.
rubber p.
scoliotic p.
split p.
spondylolisthetic p.

p. spuria
stove-in p.
pelvofemoral muscular dystrophy
pelvospondylitis ossificans
Pemberton
P. acetabuloplasty
P. pericapsular osteotomy
P. spur-crushing clamp
PEMF
pulsed electromagnetic field
PEMF bone growth stimulation
pen
STA-Pen writer p.
weighted p.
Pen/Alps distal pad
pencil
p. and cup deformity
electrosurgical p.
p. grip
skin p.
sterile p.
penciling of ribs on x-ray
pencil-tip drill
Penco Walker Sleds
pendulum exercise
penetrating
p. drill
p. fracture
penetration
anterior cortex p.
Penfield
P. 4 dissector
P. periosteal elevator
penguin gait
Pennal classification
Penn finger drill
Pennig dynamic wrist fixator
Pennsylvania bimanual work sample
Penrose drain
Pentothal Sodium
pentoxifylline
peptic ulcer
peptido-leukotriene
P-ER
pronation-external rotation
P-ER injury
perception
constant-touch p.
p. deficit
visual p.
PercScope percutaneous diskectomy
percussion
p. hammer
p. sign
p. tenderness
Trömner p.
Percuss-O-Matic jackhammer device

percutaneous
p. Achilles tendon repair
p. autogenous dowel bone graft
p. bone marrow infection
p. core bone biopsy
p. corticotomy
p. dorsal column stimulator implant
p. epiphysiodesis
p. fixation
p. heel cord lengthening
p. K-wire
p. lumbar diskectomy
p. needle placement
p. osteotomy
p. pin
p. pin insertion
p. pinning
p. plantar fasciotomy (PPF)
p. reduction
p. stapling
p. tendo Achillis lengthening
p. tenotomy
p. transmalleolar drilling

Percy
P. amputating saw
P. amputation retractor
P. plate

Perez postoperative pain scale
Perfecta
P. femoral stem
P. hip prosthesis
P. Interseal total hip system
P. I, II prosthesis

PerFixation
P. screw
P. system

perforating
p. artery
p. bur
p. forceps
p. fracture
p. twist drill

perforation
attritional p.
cortical p.
femoral cortical p.

perforator
Boyd p.
Dodd p.
p. drill

performance
p. area

p. component
p. context
functional p.
isokinetic p.
P. knee prosthesis
P. modular total knee system
motion p.
safety p.
Test of Infant Motor P. (TIMP)
P. unicompartmental knee system
P. Wrap knee support

performance-enhancing steroid
performer ultralight knee brace
perfusion
digital blood p.
pulsatile hypothermic p.

perianal
p. sensation
p. skin

periaqueductal
p. gray (PAG)
p. gray nucleus

periarthritis
periarthrosis humeri
periarticular
p. abscess
p. calcification
p. fibrositis
p. fracture
p. heterotopic ossification
p. tissue

pericapsular osteotomy
pericapsulitis
pericardium graft
pericellular halo
perichondral
p. circulation
p. ossification
p. ring

perichondrium
PERI-COMFORT cushion
pericyte
Zimmerman p.

periepineurial neuropathy
perihamate injury
perilesional bone
Peri-Loc prosthesis
perilunar
p. instability
p. transscaphoid dislocation

NOTES

515

perilunate
    p. carpal dislocation
    p. fracture-dislocation (PLFD)
perimalleolar pain
perimysial
perimysiitis
perimysium
perinea (*pl. of* perineum)
perineal
    p. loop
    p. post
    p. sensation
perineometer
    Peritron p.
perineum, pl. **perinea**
perineural
    p. block
    p. fibroma
    p. fibrosis
    p. tissue
perineurial neurorrhaphy
perineurium, pl. **perineuria**
period
    absolute refractory p.
    functional refractory p.
    incubation p.
    latent p.
    postinjury p.
    refractory p.
    relative refractory p.
    silent p.
periodic arthralgia
periodization of training
PerioGlas bone graft material
perionychium
perioperative
    p. antibiotic therapy
    p. reduction
periostalgia
    chronic p.
periostea (*pl. of* periosteum)
periosteal
    p. arthritis
    p. band
    p. bone collar
    p. button
    p. cambium layer
    p. chondroma
    p. chondrosarcoma
    p. desmoid
    p. elevator
    p. fibroma
    p. ganglion
    p. implantation
    p. lamella
    MacKentry p.
    p. new bone
    p. new bone formation

    p. ossification
    p. osteogenesis
    p. osteosarcoma
    p. reaction
    round-tapped p.
    p. sarcoma
    p. sleeve
    p. tissue
    p. vessel
periosteopathy
periosteoplastic amputation
periosteotome
    Alexander costal p.
    Alexander-Farabeuf p.
    Ballenger p.
    Brown p.
    costal p.
    elevator p.
    Fomon p.
    Joseph p.
periosteotomy
periosteum, pl. **periostea**
periostitis
    florid reactive p.
    p. ossificans
    suppurative p.
periostotome
periostotomy
peripatellar
    p. retinacular support
    p. tendinitis
peripheral
    p. arterial occlusive disease
    (PAOD)
    p. arteriography
    p. artery
    p. chemical sympathectomy
    p. dual-energy x-ray absorptiometry
    (pDXA)
    p. gangrene
    p. nerve
    p. nerve block
    p. nerve block anesthesia
    p. nerve cutaneous field
    p. nerve entrapment
    p. nerve glove
    p. nerve injury
    p. nerve palsy
    p. nerve tumor classification
    p. nervous system (PNS)
    p. neuritis
    p. neurocompressive disorder
    p. neuropathy
    p. paralysis
    p. polyneuritis
    p. vascular disease (PVD)
    p. vascular insufficiency
    p. vascular obstructive disease

p. vascular surgery (PVS)
p. vascular system (PVS)
peripisiform injury
peripolar zone
periprosthetic
p. bone loss
p. bone resorption
p. fracture
p. membrane
periscapulitis shoulder pain
perispondylitis
Gibney p.
peritendinitis
Achilles p.
p. crepitans
p. serosa
peritendinous scar
peritendon
peritenon
pedorthist p.
peritoneum
peritrapezial
p. arthritis
p. injury
peritrapezoidal injury
peritrochanteric fracture
Peritron perineometer
periungual fibroma
PER-IV fracture
Perkins
P. test
P. traction
P. vertical line
Perlstein brace
Perma-Hand silk suture
Permalock
Weber P.
Perman cartilage forceps
permanent
p. callus
p. disability
p. implant
p. partial disability (PPD)
p. partial disability rating
p. and total disability (PTD)
peroneal
p. artery
p. compartment syndrome
p. dislocation
p. groove
p. island flap
p. muscle

p. muscle spasm
p. muscular atrophy
p. musculature
p. nerve
p. nerve entrapment
p. nerve injury
p. nerve palsy
p. neuropathy
p. paralysis
p. retinaculum
p. sign
p. sinus
p. spastic flatfoot
p. strengthening exercise
p. tendinitis
p. tendon
p. tendon displacement
p. tendon impingement
p. tendon procedure
p. tendon sheath injection
p. tendon subluxation
p. tenolysis
p. tenosynovitis
p. tunnel
p. tunnel compression test
p. vein
peronealis
trochlea p.
peroneum
peroneus
p. brevis (PB)
p. brevis elongation
p. brevis graft
p. brevis to longus anastomosis
p. brevis muscle
p. brevis split (PBS)
p. brevis tendon
p. brevis transfer
p. longus
p. longus muscle
p. longus tendinopathy (PLT)
p. longus tendon
p. quartus muscle
p. tertius muscle
p. tertius tendon
peroxide
p. flush
hydrogen p.
perpendicular
method of p.'s
p. strumming
per primam healing

NOTES

P

Perrin-Ferraton disease
Perry
    P. extensile anterior approach
    P. sensor
    P. technique
Perry-Nickel
    P.-N. cranial halo
    P.-N. technique
Perry-O'Brien-Hodgson
    P.-O.-H. technique
    P.-O.-H. triple tenodesis
Perry-Robinson cervical technique
Persian slipper foot
persistent
    p. clonus
    p. notochord
    p. occiput/atlas disrelationship
    p. pain
    p. sciatic artery
perstans
    macularis eruptive p.
Perthes
    P. disease
    P. epiphysis
    P. lesion
    P. procedure
    P. reamer
    P. tourniquet test
Perthes-Bankart lesion
pertrochanteric fracture
perverted function
pes
    p. anserine bursitis
    p. anserinus
    p. anserinus syndrome
    p. anserinus transplant
    p. arcuatus
    p. arcuatus clawfoot deformity
    p. calcaneus
    p. cavovalgus
    p. cavovarus
    p. cavus
    p. cavus clawfoot deformity
    p. equinovalgus
    p. equinovarus
    p. equinovarus adductus
    p. equinus
    p. febricitans
    p. gigas
    p. plano valgus
    p. planovalgus
    p. planovalgus abductus
    p. planovalgus deformity
    p. plantigrade planus
    p. planus deformity
    p. pronatus
    p. valgo planus
    p. valgo planus deformity

    p. valgus planus
    p. varus
PET
    positron emission tomography
    PET electrotherapy
petaling the cast
petechia, pl. **petechiae**
Peterson
    P. syndrome
    P. traction
PET/Eurotech Generation 2000 table
petit
    p. pas gait
    P. triangle
Petren gait
Petrie spica cast
pétrissage
petroclinoid ligament
petrolatum gauze
petrosal bone
petrous temporal bone
Pettibon chiropractic procedure
PFA
    proximal reference axis
PFC
    pelvic flexion contracture
    PFC curved unconstrained
        prosthesis
    PFC femoral prosthesis
    PFC hip stem
    PFC modular total knee system
    PFC offset tibial tray
    PFC Sigma knee system
    PFC TC3 modular knee system
    PFC total hip replacement system
PFD
    patellofemoral dysfunction
    polyurethane foam dressing
Pfeiffer syndrome
PFFD
    proximal focal femoral deficiency
Pfitzner theory of coalition formation
PF Night Splint II splint
PFO
    plantar fasciitis orthosis
    PFO night splint
PFP
    patellofemoral pain
PFT
    postoperative flexor tendon
    PFT traction brace
PGA-PLA
    polyglycolic acid-polylactic acid
    PGA-PLA biomaterial
PGP
    P. flexible nail system
    P. nail
PGS-3000 pulsed galvanic stimulator

phagocytosis
phalangeal
    p. articular orientation
    p. articulation
    p. bone
    p. clamp
    p. condylectomy
    p. degloving
    p. diaphysial fracture
    p. dislocation
    p. fracture fixation
    p. herniation
    p. hypoplasia
    p. implant
    p. malunion correction
    p. microgeodic syndrome
    p. neck
    p. osteotomy
    p. polydactyly
    p. synostosis
phalangectomy
    intermediate p.
phalanges (*pl. of* phalanx)
phalangization
phalangophalangeal amputation
phalanx, pl. **phalanges**
    accessory p.
    delta p.
    distal p. (DP)
    osteitis distal p.
    proximal p. (PP)
    tufted p.
    waist of the p.
Phalen
    P. maneuver
    P. position
    P. wrist flexion test
Phalen-Miller opponensplasty
phantom
    p. frame
    p. limb
    p. limb pain
    p. limb syndrome
    p. pain phenomenon
    p. sensation
phantosmia
pharmacodynamic
pharmacokinetic
pharyngeal tissue
phase
    blood pool p.
    p. 2 elbow program

    fibroblastic p.
    flexor p.
    granulation p.
    inflammatory p.
    inosculation p.
    maturation p.
    propulsive p.
    remodeling p.
    reparative p.
    stance p.
    swing p.
Pheasant
    P. diskotome
    P. elbow operation
    P. elbow technique
Phelps
    P. brace
    P. neurectomy
    P. operation
    P. orthosis
    P. partial resection
    P. scapulectomy
    P. splint
Phemister
    P. acromioclavicular pin fixation
    P. biopsy trephine
    P. elevator
    P. medial approach to tibia
    P. onlay bone graft
    P. onlay bone graft technique
    P. operation
    P. osteotomy
    P. posteromedial approach
    P. rasp
Phemister-Bonfiglio technique
phenol
    p. cauterization
    p. chemosurgery
    p. matrixectomy
    p. neurolysis
phenol-alcohol matrixectomy
phenolization
    nail matrix p. (NMP)
phenomenon, pl. **phenomena**
    bioelectric p.
    brake p.
    Burner p.
    combined flexion p.
    crankshaft p.
    give-way p.
    glued-to-the-floor p.
    Gordon knee p.

NOTES

P

phenomenon *(continued)*
Gowers p.
halisteresis p.
Herendeen p.
Holmes p.
Holmes-Stewart p.
Hunt paradoxical p.
Kienböck p.
lumbrical-plus p.
Lust p.
magic angle p.
no-reflow p.
phantom pain p.
pivot-shift p.
pronation p.
Queckenstedt p.
radial p.
Raynaud p.
referred anatomic p.
referred trigger point p.
relaxation p.
release p.
Rust p.
staircase p.
temporary cavity p.
tibial p.
toe p.
Valleix p.
vertebral steal p.
Westphal p.
wind-up p.
phenylephrine
phenyltoloxamine
Philadelphia
P. cervical collar
P. collar cervical support
P. collar cervical traction
P. Plastizote cervical brace
P. rigid collar
Philips
P. Angiodiagnostics 96 apparatus
P. linear accelerator
P. toe force gauge
Phillips
P. head screw
P. head screwdriver
P. muscle
P. recessed-head screw
P. screw head
P. splint
phlebography
phlebolith
phlebothrombosis
phlogistic agent
phocomelia
complete p.
distal p.
proximal p.

phocomelic dwarfism
Phoenix
P. foot system
P. Outrigger splint
P. total hip prosthesis
phonophoresis
hydrocortisone p.
p. plantarflexion
ultrasound p.
Phoresor
P. II iontophoretic drug delivery
system
P. PM900 iontophoresis system
phosphatase
alkaline p.
bone-specific alkaline p. (BSAP)
tartrate resistant acid p. (TRAP)
phosphate
calcium p.
nicotinamide-adenine dinucleotide p.
(NADPH)
technetium-99m p.
tetracalcium p.
tricalcium p.
phospholipid
photogrammetry
x-ray p.
photon densitometry
photopenia
hardware p.
photoplethysmography (PPG)
digital p.
phrenic nerve
phthinoid chest
PHV
peak height velocity
phycomycosis
physes (*pl. of* physis)
physial, physeal
p. angle
p. bar
p. bridge
p. cartilage
p. closure
p. damage
p. disruption
p. distraction
p. growth
p. injury
p. line
p. mamillary process
p. plate fracture
p. region
p. scar
p. stapling
physiatric
physiatrics
physiatrist

physiatry
physical
    P. Ability Test (PAT)
    p. activity
    P. Activity Readiness Questionnaire (PAR-Q)
    p. agent
    p. capacity evaluation (PCE)
    p. daily living skills (PDLS)
    p. impairment
    p. inactivity
    p. independence WHO Handicap Scale
    p. medicine (PM)
    p. medicine and rehabilitation (PMR)
    p. therapy (PT)
    p. therapy table
    p. training (PT)
    p. work
    p. work capacity (PWC)
physiognomy
PhysioGymnic exercise ball
physiologic
    p. barrier
    p. flatfoot
    p. lock of the motion segment
    p. motion
    p. response
    p. saline
    p. valgus
physiological
    p. hyperactivity
    p. venous pump mechanism
physiology
    exercise p.
physiolysis
    central p.
Physio-Roll-R-Cise
Physio-Roll VisuaLiser exercise ball
Physio-Stim
    P.-S. bone growth stimulator
    P.-S. Lite bone growth stimulator
physiotherapist
physiotherapy
    aqua PT dry p.
physique
    ectomesomorphic p.
    ectomorphic p.
physis, pl. **physes**
    distal tibial p.
    p. fracture

    modified Boyd amputation of ankle and distal tibial p.
phytonutrient
PI
    posteroinferior
piano key sign
piano-wire dorsiflexion brace
PICA
    posterior inferior cerebellar artery
    PICA index
pick
    P. chisel
    dental p.
Picker Magnascanner for bone metastasis
picket
    p. fence guide
    P. Fence leg positioner
pick-up
    p.-u. forceps
    p.-u. test
Picot incision
picture
    maximum pressure p. (MPP)
Pidcock
    P. nail
    P. pin
piecemeal
pie-crusting skin graft
Piedmont fracture
Pierrot-Murphy
    P.-M. advancement insertion
    P.-M. tendon technique
PIEx
    posteroinferior external
    PIEx ilium
    PIEx subluxation
piezoelectric
    p. accelerometer
    p. potential
Piezo electro-needleless stimulator
piezogenic
Piffard curette
pigeon
    p. breast
    p. chest
pigeon-toeing gait
pigmented
    p. nodular synovitis of tendon sheath
    p. villonodular bursitis
    p. villonodular synovitis (PVS)

NOTES

P

pigtail tendon stripper
PIIn
posteroinferior internal
PIIn ilium
PIIn subluxation
Pilates
P. exercise method
P. method exercise
pillar
articular p.
p. pain
p. tenderness
Pillet hand prosthesis
Pilliar
P. prosthesis
P. total hip replacement
Pillo
Knee P.
Pillo-Pedic cervical traction pillow
pillow
abduction p.
antibacterial p.
Bio-Gel decubitus p.
Bodynapper Comfort P.
Capello slim-line abduction p.
Carter elevation p.
Carter foam p.
cervical sleep p.
p. collar
Comfort Club tub p.
Comfort-U total body p.
Crescent Complete Sleeper p.
Crescent memory p.
Crescent-Pillo p.
D-Core support p.
Dream P.
Flip-Flop p.
foot p.
p. fracture
Frejka p.
IMP-Capello slimline abduction p.
Mediflow waterbase p.
Neckcare p.
Neck-Hugger cervical support p.
Opti-Curve therapeutic p.
OrthoBone p.
p. orthosis
p. orthosis for hip
Orthosleep P.
Pillo-Pedic cervical traction p.
Pillo-Wedge p.
Pron p.
shoulder abduction p.
Silicore foot p.
snooze p.
Softeze water p.
p. splint

Tempur-Pedic pressure relieving
Swedish p.
T-Foam p.
Theracloud p.
Therapeutica Sleeping P.
Therasleep Cervical P.
Tri-Core cervical support p.
Wal-Pil-O neck p.
Pillo-Wedge pillow
pill rolling tremor
pilomotor
p. dysfunction
p. response
pilon
p. fracture
p. fracture classification
pilonidal dimple
Pil-O-Splint wrist splint
pilot
p. bur
p. drill
P. point screw

pin
A p.
absorbable polymeric p.
absorbable polyparadioxanone p.
Ace p.
Acufex distractor p.
alignment p.
Allofix freeze-dried cortical
bone p.
Apex p.
Arthrex zebra p.
arum fixation p.
ASIF screw p.
Asnis p.
Austin Moore p.
p. ball system
Barr p.
beaded hip p.
Beath p.
Belos compression p.
bevel-point Rush p.
Bilos p.
Biofix system p.
bioresorbable p.
Böhler p.
Böhler-Knowles hip p.
Böhler-Steinmann p.
Bohlman p.
breakaway p.
Breck p.
calcaneal p.
calibrated p.
Canakis beaded hip p.
cancellous p.
Charnley p.
p. chuck

p. clamp
clavicle p.
cloverleaf p.
Co-Cr-Mo p.
collapsible p.
Compere threaded p.
Compton clavicle p.
Conley p.
cortical p.
Craig p.
Crawford-Adams p.
Crego-McCarroll p.
p. crimper
Crowe pilot point on Steinmann p.
Crowe tip p.
Crutchfield p.
p. cutter
Davis p.
Day fixation p.
DCS p.
deluxe FIN p.
Denham p.
DePuy p.
derotational p.
Deyerle II p.
distraction p.
drill p.
Ender p.
p. external fixator
Fahey p.
Fahey-Compere p.
femoral guide p.
Fischer transfixing p.
Fisher half p.
p. fixation
fixation p.
Freebody p.
freeze-dried bone p.
friction lock p.
Furness-Clute p.
Gouffon hip p.
p. guard
p. guide
Hagie hip p.
halo p.
Hansen p.
Hansen-Street p.
Hare p.
Hatcher p.
Haynes p.
p. headrest
Hegge p.

Hessel-Nystrom p.
Hewson breakaway p.
hexhead p.
hip p.
Hoffmann apex fixation p.
Hoffmann transfixion p.
p. holder
hook p.
hook-end intramedullary p.
p. implant
Intraflex intramedullary p.
intramedullary p.
Jones compression p.
Jurgan p.
Kirschner wire p.
Knowles hip p.
Kronfeld p.
Küntscher p.
LIH hook p.
locating p.
locked intramedullary
  osteosynthesis p.
Lottes p.
marble bone p.
Markley retention p.
Matthews-Green p.
McBride p.
medullary p.
metal p.
Modny p.
Moore fixation p.
Moule screw p.
Neufeld p.
nonthreaded p.
Norman tibial p.
Olds p.
Oris p.
Ormco p.
Orthofix p.
OrthoSorb absorbable p.
osseous p.
osteotomy p.
partially threaded p.
percutaneous p.
Pidcock p.
Pritchard Mark II p.
Pugh hip p.
rasp p.
resorbable polydioxanon p.
restorative p.
p. retractor
ReUnite orthopedic p.

NOTES

P

523

pin *(continued)*
Rhinelander p.
Riordan p.
Risser p.
Rissler-Stille p.
Roger Anderson p.
Rush intramedullary fixation p.
Safir p.
Sage p.
Scand p.
Schanz p.
Schneider p.
Schweitzer p.
self-broaching p.
self-tapering p.
Serrato forearm p.
Shriners p.
p. site
skeletal p.
p. sleeve
Smart P.
Smillie p.
Smith-Petersen fracture p.
SMO Moore p.
smooth Steinmann p.
Snap fixation p.
socket p.
spring p.
Stader p.
Steinmann fixation p.
Street medullary p.
strut-type p.
p. suture
Tachdjian p.
tapered p.
threaded Steinmann p.
tibial p.
titanium half p.
p. track
p. tract infection
traction p.
transarticular p.
transcapitellar p.
transfixing p.
trochanteric p.
Turner p.
Tutofix cortical p.
union broach retention p.
Varney p.
Venable-Stuck fracture p.
p. vise
von Saal medullary p.
Walker hollow quill p.
Watanabe p.
Webb p.
p. wheel
wrench p.
Z p.

Zimfoam p.
Zimmer p.
pin-and-plaster
p.-a.-p. fixation
p.-a.-p. method
pin-bone interface
pincement
pincer
p. nail
p. nail formation
p. palpation
p. testing
pinch
p. callus
p. gauge
P. Gauge and Jackson Strength Evaluation System
p. grasp
key p.
lateral squeeze p.
p. meter
palmar p.
p. power
p. restoration
p. strength
p. tree
pinchometer
Prestop p.
ping-pong
p.-p. bone
p.-p. fracture
Pinkus
fibroepithelioma of P.
Pinnacle acetabular cup system
Pinn-ACL guide system
Pinn anterior cruciate ligament guide system
pinning
Asnis p.
closed p.
hip p.
Knowles p.
open p.
percutaneous p.
Sherk-Probst percutaneous p.
Sofield p.
Wagner closed p.
pinprick
p. hyperalgesia test
p. sensation
pin-seating forceps
pin-to-bar clamp
Pinto distractor
pin-tract osteomyelitis
pinwheel
Cleanwheel disposable neurological p.

Safe-T-Wheel p.
Wartenberg p.
Pinwheel System
Piotrowski sign
PIP
proximal interphalangeal
PIP articulation
PIP flexion creaking
PIP/DIP
proximal interphalangeal/distal
interphalangeal
PIP/DIP strap
piperacillin/tazobactam therapy
pipe tree
PIPJ
proximal interphalangeal joint
Pipkin
P. fracture classification system
P. posterior hip dislocation
classification
P. subclassification of Epstein-
Thomas classification
pi-plate dorsal distal radius plate
Pirie
P. bone
talonavicular ossicle of P.
piriform
p. muscle
p. sclerosis of ilium
piriformis
p. sign
p. syndrome
Pirogoff amputation
Pischel micropin
pisiform
p. bone
p. bursa
p. metacarpal ligament
p. ossification
pisohamate ligament
pisometacarpal ligament
pisotriquetral
p. arthritis
p. joint
pistol-grip hand drill
piston
cannulated expulsion p.
p. prosthesis
p. sign
pistoning motion
pitch
calcaneal p.

pitching injury
Pitcock nail
pitted cartilage
pitting edema
Pittsburgh pelvic frame
pituitary
p. gigantism
p. grasper
p. rongeur
PIVM
passive intervertebral motion
PIVM testing
pivot
Accu-Line dual p.
calcar p.
p. of calcar
p. joint
medial stem p.
P. Pole walking device
pivoting
p. and cutting activity
p. sports
pivot-shift
p.-s. phenomenon
p.-s. sign
p.-s. test
pivot-sport activity
PJ
patellar jerk
PL
palmaris longus
placement
bone graft p.
electrode p.
glide hole for screw p.
hand p.
Kirschner wire p.
K-wire p.
needle p.
PCL-oriented p. (POP)
percutaneous needle p.
plate p.
portal p.
posterolateral bone graft p.
p. reflex
rod p.
sacral screw p.
variable screw p. (VSP)
placing reflex
plafond
p. fracture

NOTES

P

plafond (*continued*)
tibial p.
varus p.

plain
p. gauze
p. pattern plate
p. rotary scissors
p. screwdriver
p. tissue forceps

Plak-Vac oral suction brush

plan
McConnell patellofemoral
treatment p.
National Arthritis Action P.
(NAAP)
preoperative p.

plana
coxa p.
manus p.
vertebra p.

plane
AC-PC p.
anatomic p.
axial p.
coronal p.
facet p.
fascial p.
flexion-extension p.
Frankfort horizontal p.
frontal p.
Hensen p.
Hodge p.
horizontal p.
internervous p.
intertubercular p.
p. joint
Ludwig p.
median sagittal p.
mesiodistal p.
midsagittal p.
paramedian sagittal p.
pelvic p.
primary movement p.
sagittal p.
spinous p.
sternoxiphoid p.
subcostal p.
suprasternal p.
thigh-shank p.
thoracic p.
transverse p.
varus-valgus p.
vertical p.

planer
calcar p.
Rubin bone p.
Rubin cartilage p.

plane-type acromioclavicular articulation

planning
preoperative p.
rehabilitation p.

Planostretch stockings

planovalgus
p. deformity
p. foot
hypermobile pes p.
pes p.
talipes p.

plantalgia

plantar
p. angulation
p. aponeurosis
p. approach
p. arch support orthosis
p. arterial arch
p. artery
p. artery flap
p. axial view
p. Babinski response
p. bony prominence
p. bromidrosis
p. buckling
p. calcaneal spur
p. calcaneonavicular ligament-tibialis
posterior tendon advancement
p. callosity
p. capsular release
p. capsule
p. capsuloligamentous complex
p. compartment
p. condylectomy
p. corn
p. digital artery (PDA)
p. ecchymosis sign
p. fascia
p. fascial release
p. fasciitis
p. fasciitis night splint
p. fasciitis orthosis (PFO)
p. fasciitis syndrome
p. fasciitis taping
p. fasciotomy
p. fat pad
p. fibromatosis
p. flexed
p. flexed stress radiograph
p. flexion
p. flexion-inversion deformity
p. flexor proximal metatarsal
osteotomy
p. foot
p. keratosis
p. lateral base
p. longitudinal incision
p. malignant melanoma
p. metatarsal angle

p. metatarsal artery
p. nerve
p. pain
p. plate
p. plate injury
p. plate release
p. pressure
p. pressure pattern
p. reflex
p. shift
p. stress ankle x-ray
p. sweating
p. tendopathy
p. toe pulp
p. transposition
p. vault
p. V infiltration block
p. V-Y advancement flap
p. wart (PW)

plantar-dorsiflexion
plantarflex
plantarflexing
plantarflexion
p. injury
phonophoresis p.
p. stress view
plantarflexion-inversion test
plantarflexory motion
plantar-hindfoot-midfoot bony mass
plantaris
p. muscle
p. tendon
p. tendon graft
plantar-lateral release
plantar-medial release
plantarward
plantigrade
p. foot
p. limb
p. platform
planus
Anderson-Fowler anterior calcaneal osteotomy pes p.
collapsing pes valgo p.
flexible pes p.
Gleich osteotomy for pes valgo p.
lichen p.
pes plantigrade p.
pes valgo p.
pes valgus p.
rigid pes p.

Selakovich procedure for pes valgo p.
talipes p.
plasma
p. beta-endorphin
p. cell dyscrasia
coagulated p.
p. volume shift
plasmacytoma
aggressive solitary p.
extramedullary p.
Plasmanate
plasma-sprayed
low-pressure p.-s. (LPPS)
p.-s. titanium
plasmatic phase of skin healing
plasmin
plast
Putti bone p.
Plastalume
P. bulb-ended splint
P. straight splint
Plastazote
P. blank
P. foam
P. insole
plaster
Batchelor p.
p. cast application burn
closing wedge manipulation and reapplication of p.
Hapset hydroxyapatite bone graft p.
opening wedge manipulation and reapplication of p.
p. of Paris (POP)
p. of Paris bandage
p. of Paris cast
p. of Paris splint
p. saw
p. slab splint
p. sole
p. sore
p. toe cap
Velpeau p.
x-ray in p. (XIP)
x-ray out of p. (XOP)
Zoroc p.
plastic
p. achillotenotomy
p. ankle-foot orthosis
p. ball implant
p. body jacket

NOTES

P

plastic *(continued)*
- p. bowing fracture
- p. cast
- p. collar
- p. deformation
- p. end cap
- p. femoral plug
- p. floor reaction ankle-foot orthosis
- p. heel cup
- Hexalite p.
- p. leaf-spring (PLS)
- p. limited-motion joint
- low-temperature p.
- p. marrow canal restrictor
- Orthoplast p.
- p. patella
- p. repair
- p. strain
- thermolabile p.
- unitary p.

PlastiCast adjustable joint cast system
plasticity
- connective tissue p.
- cortical p.

Plasticor prosthesis
Plasti-Pore
- P.-P. ossicular replacement prosthesis
- P.-P. prosthetic material

Plastiport
- P. TORP
- P. TORP prosthesis

Plastizote
- P. arch support
- P. cervical collar
- P. cervical collar orthosis
- P. foot bed
- P. orthotic device
- P. shoe liner

Plastizote-Kydex cervical immobilizer
PLAST-O-FIT thermoplastic bandage
plasty
- Bosworth-type reverse p.
- Coleman p.
- Durham p.
- flap p.
- rotation p.
- side-swing p.
- skin p.
- trans-bone p.
- V-Y p.
- Y-V p.

plate
- 90-90 p.
- acetabular reconstruction p.
- AcroMed VSP p.
- adolescent condylar blade p.
- alar p.

Alta condylar buttress p.
Alta distal fracture p.
anchor p.
anterior cervical p. (ACP)
anterior sacroiliac joint p.
antiglide p.
AO-ASIF compression p.
AO condylar blade p.
AO contoured T p.
AO dynamic compression p.
AO hook p.
AO reconstruction p.
AO semitubular p.
AO small fragment p.
AO spoon p.
Arbeitsgemeinschaft für Osteosynthesfragen-Morscher p.
Armstrong p.
ASIF broad dynamic compression bone p.
ASIF right-angle blade p.
ASIF T-p.
athletic shoe carbon fiber p.
autocompression p.
avulsion of nail p.
axial p.
Badgley p.
Bagby angled compression p.
barrel p.
Batchelor p.
p. bender
biodegradable p.
blade p.
Blair talar body fusion blade p.
Blair tibiotalar arthrodesis blade p.
Blanchard traction device blade p.
Blount blade p.
bone flap fixation p.
Bosworth spine p.
Boyd side p.
bridge p.
broad AO dynamic compression p.
Burns p.
butterfly-shaped monoblock vertebral p.
buttress pie p.
buttress-type p.
Calandruccio side p.
calcaneal Y p.
cap-and-anchor p.
carbon fiber-reinforced p.
cartilaginous growth p.
Caspar cervical p.
cervical p.
cloverleaf p.
coaptation p.
cobra-head p.
Collison p.

compression p.
Concise side p.
condylar p.
connecting p.
Continuum total knee base p.
contoured anterior spinal p. (CASP)
contoured T-plate p.
cortical p.
craniocervical p.
crosslink p.
cruciform tibial base p.
C-shaped p.
3D p.
deck p.
DePuy p.
Deyerle p.
double Cobra p.
double-H p.
Driessen hinged p.
p. driver
dual p.
Dwyer-Hall p.
dynamic compression p. (DCP)
eccentric dynamic compression p. (EDCP)
Eggers bone p.
eleven-hole p.
Elliott femoral condyle blade p.
end p.
epiphysial growth p.
femoral p.
ferromagnetic metal p.
fibrocartilaginous p.
five-hole p.
p. fixation
fixed-angle blade p.
flat p.
flexor p.
foot p., footplate
force p.
four-hole Alta straight p.
four-hole side p.
frontal p.
fusion p.
gait p.
Gallannaugh p.
Galveston p.
growth p.
Hagie sliding nail p.
Haid cervical p.
Haid Universal bone p.

half-circle p.
Hansen-Street p.
Harlow p.
Harms posterior cervical p.
Harris p.
heavy-duty femur p.
heavy side p.
Hicks lugged p.
Hoen skull p.
Holt nail p.
hook p.
hot p.
H-shaped p.
Hubbard side p.
Hungarian grip p.
Inner Lip P.
interfragmentary p.
intertrochanteric p.
Jergesen I-beam p.
Jergesen tapered p.
Jewett nail overlay p.
Jones compression p.
Kaneda p.
Kessel p.
L p.
Laing p.
Lane p.
Lawson-Thornton p.
Letournel p.
limited compression-dynamic compression p.
limited-contact dynamic compression p.
Louis p.
low-contact dynamic compression p.
low-profile dorsal p.
L-shaped p.
Luhr Microfixation cranial p.
Luhr pan p.
Lundholm p.
Luque II p.
Mancini p.
Massie p.
May anatomical bone p.
Mayo Clinic congruent elbow p.
McBride p.
McLaughlin p.
Mears sacroiliac p.
Medoff sliding p.
metal foot p.
Meurig Williams p.
Milch p.

NOTES

P

plate *(continued)*
modified Grace p.
Moe intertrochanteric p.
Moore sliding nail p.
Moreira p.
Morscher cervical p.
Mueller compression blade p.
Müller p.
nail p.
narrow AO dynamic
  compression p.
Neufeld p.
neutralization p.
Newman p.
Nicoll p.
occipitocervical p.
Ogden p.
Orozco p.
orthotic p.
Osborne p.
overlay p.
palmar p.
Paulus p.
pediatric blade p.
pedicle p.
peg base p.
Percy p.
pi-plate dorsal distal radius p.
p. placement
plain pattern p.
plantar p.
Polytechnic foot-pressure
  measuring p.
precurved p.
pressure p.
protection p.
pterygoid p.
Pugh p.
pylon attachment p.
quadrangular positioning p.
reconstruction p.
resorbable p.
Richards-Hirschhorn p.
Rohadur gait p.
roof p.
round-hole compression p.
Roy-Camille p.
Schweitzer spring p.
semitubular blade p.
semitubular compression p.
Senn p.
serpentine p.
seven-hole p.
seventeen-hole p.
Sherman bone p.
side p.
Simmons p.
six-hole p.

slide p.
slotted femur p.
Smith-Petersen intertrochanteric p.
SMO p.
p. spacer washer
spinous process p.
spoon p.
spring p.
stabilization p.
stainless steel p.
static compression p.
Steffee pedicle p.
Steffee screw p.
stem base p.
subchondral p.
supracondylar p.
symmetrical thoracic vertebral p.
symmetric sacral p.
Synthes dorsal distal radius p.
Synthes pie p.
Syracuse anterior I p.
Tacoma sacral p.
tarsal p.
T buttress p.
tectal p.
Temple University p.
tendon p.
tension band p.
thoracolumbosacral p.
Thornton nail p.
three-hole p.
tibial base p.
titanium hollow screw
  osseointegrating reconstruction p.
  (THORP)
titanium mandibular p.
toe p.
Townley tibial plateau p.
Townsend-Gilfillan p.
trial base p.
T-shaped AO p.
TSRH p.
tubular bone p.
Tupman p.
twisted p.
two-hole p.
UCBL foot p.
universal bone p. (UBP)
Uslenghi p.
variable screw p. (VSP)
V blade p.
Venable p.
vertebral end p.
Vitallium Luhr p.
V nail p.
volar p.
VSP p.
Wainwright p.

Weber antiglide p.
Wenger p.
Whitman p.
Wilson p.
wing p.
Wright p.
Wurzburg p.
X p.
X-shaped p.
Y bone p.
Y-shaped p.
Zimmer femoral condyle blade p.
Zimmer side p.
Zimmer Y p.
Z-shaped p.
Zuelzer hook p.

plateau
bicondylar tibial p.
p. fracture
proximal tibial p.
tibial p.

plate-holding forceps
platelet
p. concentrate
p. count

platelet-derived growth factor (PDGF)
plate-like atelectasis
plate-screw
p.-s. fixation
p.-s. osteosynthesis
p.-s. system

platform
p. crutch
Hausmann Velcro-Lock mat p.
Kistler force p.
Midland multifunctional mat p.
Midline Hi-Lo Mat P.
plantigrade p.

plating
compression p.
diaphysial p.
Gotfried percutaneous
compression p.
pedicle screw p.
posterior spinal p.
variable spinal p. (VSP)

Platinum stationary table
Platou osteotomy
platybasia
platysma muscle
platyspondylia, platyspondylisis

play
end p.
excessive joint p.
joint p.
muscle p.
return to p. (RTP)

Playmaker
P. functional knee brace
P. support

PlayTuf knee brace
PLB
primary lymphoma of bone

pledget
Betadine-soaked p.
p. dressing
p. of gauze
Gelfoam p.

pleomorphic
p. fibrous histiocytoma
p. lipoma
p. liposarcoma
p. rhabdomyosarcoma

pleonosteosis
Leri p.

plethysmography
digital p.
impedance p.

pleura, pl. **pleurae**
parietal p.

pleural injury
Plexidure insole
plexiform
p. fibrohistiocytic tumor
p. neurofibroma

Plexiglas
P. jig
P. spacer

PlexiPulse
P. DVT prophylaxis system
P. intermittent pneumatic
compression device

plexopathy
brachial p.
congenital p.
Klumpke p.

plexus
p. block
brachial p.
cervical p.
fascial p.
lumbosacral p.

NOTES

P

plexus *(continued)*
    sacral p.
    subdermal p.
PLFD
    perilunate fracture-dislocation
plica, pl. **plicae**
    bucket-handle p.
    infrapatellar p.
    lateral p.
    medial patellar p.
    medial shelf/medial p.
    parapatellar p.
    pathological p.
    suprapatellar p.
    symptomatic synovial p.
    p. syndrome
    synovial p.
    tendon p.
    p. test
plication
    capsular p.
    disk p.
    soft tissue p.
plicectomy
pliers
    Compaction p.
    extraction p.
    Howmedica Microfixation
      System p.
    locking p.
    Luhr Microfixation System p.
    needle-nose vise-grip p.
    orthopaedic surgical p.
    Power-Grip p.
    slip-joint p.
    Sontec p.
    square-end p.
    Storz Microsystems p.
    Synthes Microsystems p.
    wire bending p.
PLIF
    posterior lumbar interbody fusion
    posterolateral interbody fusion
plight
    musician's p.
plinth
PLL
    posterior longitudinal ligament
PLM
    precise lesion measuring
    PLM device
plombage
    bone p.
plot
    load-displacement p.
plotter
    X-Y p.

PLS
    plastic leaf-spring
PLT
    peroneus longus tendinopathy
plug
    bone femoral p.
    bone-graft p.
    Buck p.
    cement p.
    p. cutter
    Exeter intramedullary bone p.
    femoral p.
    Osteonics acetabular dome hole p.
    patellar p.
    plastic femoral p.
    polyethylene femoral buck p.
plumbism
plumb line
plumb-line analysis
Plum-Blossom acupuncture needle
plunger
    dome p.
plunger-type femoral pressurizer
pluripotential
    p. mesenchymal tumor
    p. mesenchymoma
plus
    Nexerciser P.
    Steri-Cuff P.
Plyoback
    P. II
    P. Rebounder
Plyoball
plyometric
    p. exercise
    p. resistance
plyometrics
Plyo-Sled exerciser
Plystan prosthesis
PM
    physical medicine
PMA
    progressive muscular atrophy
PMD
    progressive muscular dystrophy
PMID
    painful minor intervertebral dysfunction
PMMA
    polymethyl methacrylate
    PMMA bone cement
    PMMA centralizer
    PMMA implant
PMR
    physical medicine and rehabilitation
    polymyalgia rheumatica
    posteromedial release

PMT
    PMT halo system
    PMT halo system brace
Pneu Knee brace
pneumarthrosis
pneumatic
    p. ankle tourniquet
    p. antishock garment (PASG)
    p. compression boot
    p. compression sleeve
    p. compression stockings
    p. compression therapy
    p. drill accessory
    p. external compression device
    p. four-bar linkage knee
    p. garment
    p. orthosis
    p. pedal compression
    p. resistance exercise
    p. splint
    p. tire injury
    p. tourniquet cuff
pneumatocyst
    intraosseous p.
pneumoarthrogram
pneumoarthrography
pneumogenic osteoarthropathy
pneumonitis
pneumothermomassage
pneumothorax
Pneu-trac
    P.-t. cervical collar
    P.-t. neck brace
PNF
    proprioceptive neuromuscular facilitation
    proprioceptive neuromuscular fasciculation
    PNF exercise
    PNF pattern
    PNF technique
PNS
    parasympathetic nervous system
    peripheral nervous system
P&O
    prosthesis and orthosis
    prosthetic and orthotic
podalgia
podarthritis
podedema
podiatric medicine
podiatrist

podiatry
    doctor of p.
    P. Institute procedures for ankle arthrodesis
    P. Institute rasp
Podi-Burr
    large callus P.-B.
    large nail P.-B.
    medium callus P.-B.
    medium nail P.-B.
    P.-B. nail bur
podismus
poditis
pododynamometer
pododynia
PodoFlex
    P. machine
    P. reflexology device
podogeriatrics
podogram
podograph
podologist
podology
podomechanotherapy
podometer
podopediatrics
podospasm
Podospray
    Darco P.
    P. nail drill system
    P. podiatry drill
Pogon chair
Pogrund lateral approach
point
    anchoring p.
    associated myofascial trigger p.
    Back Shu paraspinal p.
    bleeding p.
    break p.
    cannulated drill p.
    carbon steel drill p.
    contact p.
    Crowe pilot p.
    Crutchfield drill p.
    dorsal p.
    drill p.
    electrodesiccated bleeding p.
    end p.
    entry p.
    Erb p.
    glenoid p.
    inflexion p.

NOTES

P

point (*continued*)
    isometric p.
    Krackow p.
    material failure break p.
    Mathews drill p.
    motor p.
    myofascial trigger p.
    Pauly p.
    pedicle entrance p.
    pressure p.
    primary myofascial trigger p.
    Raney-Crutchfield drill p.
    referred p.
    satellite myofascial trigger p.
    secondary myofascial trigger p.
    single reference p. (SRP)
    Steinmann pin with Crowe pilot p.
    tender p. (TeP)
    p. tenderness
    trigger p.
    Trousseau p.
    twist drill p.
    Universal drill p.
    vector p.
pointed
    p. awl
    p. toe shoe
pointer
    hip p.
    shoulder p.
Pointer-Plus
pointillage
point-of-reduction clamp
Poirier
    space of P.
Poisson ratio
poker
    p. back
    p. spine
POL
    posterior oblique ligament
Poland
    P. anomaly
    P. classification of physial injury
    P. epiphysial fracture classification
    P. syndrome
polar
    P. Care 500 cryotherapy device
    P. Pack
    P. Vantage XL heart monitor
    P. Wrap cold therapy
    P. wrist monitor
    p. zone
Polaris knee rehab brace
polarization
Polar-Mate coagulator
Polarus
    P. humeral rod

    P. Plus humeral fixation system
    P. positional humeral fixation
      system
pole
    Exerstrider walking p.
    walking p.
policeman's heel
policy
    impaired competitor p.
    National Collegiate Athletic
      Association drug testing p.
    P. and Review Committee for
      Human Research
polio
poliomyelitis treatment
Polk finger goniometer
pollex
    p. abductus
    p. pedis
pollicis
    adductor p.
    p. longus muscle
    opponens p.
pollicization
    Buck-Gramcko p.
    Gillies p.
    Littler p.
    Riordan p.
pollicized ray
Pollock sign
polyacetal resin
polyarteritis nodosa
polyarthric
polyarthritis
    juvenile p.
    vertebral p.
polyarthropathy
polyarticular
    p. juvenile rheumatoid arthritis
    p. symmetric tophaceous joint
      inflammation
polyaxial
    p. cervical screw
    p. joint
polybutester suture
polybutilate-coated polyester
Polycel bone composite prosthesis
polycentric
    p. knee prosthesis
    p. rotation
    p. unconstrained prosthesis
    P. and Wide-Track knee system
polydactylous cleft foot
polydactyly
    central p.
    phalangeal p.
    postaxial p.
    preaxial p.

short rib p.
thumb p.
Wassel classification of thumb p.
Polydek suture
Polyderm hydrophilic polyurethane foam dressing
Poly-Dial
P.-D. insert
P.-D. prosthesis
P.-D. socket
polydioxanone suture (PDS)
Polydor Preforms orthotic
polydystrophy
Hurler p.
polyester
Dacron p.
polybutilate-coated p.
p. suture
polyether implant material
polyethylene
ArCom processed p.
p. button
carbon fiber-reinforced p.
p. compression molding
p. debris
p. drain
Durasul p.
extruded bar p.
p. femoral buck plug
p. femoral buck plug procedure
p. foam
high molecular weight p. (HMWPE)
p. implant material
p. liner
p. liner implant component
p. patellar implant prosthesis
p. peg
porous p.
p. proximal brim in quadrilateral contour
p. sleeve
p. socket
p. suture
p. talar prosthesis
ultrahigh molecular weight p. (UHMWPE)
polyethylene-faced
p.-f. driver
p.-f. mallet
Polyform splint
polygalactic acid suture

polyglactin suture
polyglycolic acid suture
polyglycolide implant
polyglyconate suture
polylactide
p. absorbable screw
p. implant
Poly-Lock bonding
PolyMem wound care dressing
polymer
biodegradable synthetic p.
cold-curing p.
Hylamer orthopedic bearing p.
self-curing p.
viscoelastic p.
PolymerFriction total knee
polymeric
p. debris
p. dressing
polymerization of bone cement
polymetatarsalia
polymethyl
p. methacrylate (PMMA)
p. methacrylate bone cement
p. methacrylate implant
polymethylmethacrylate biomaterial
polymorphic hamartoma
polymyalgia rheumatica (PMR)
polymyositis myopathy
polyneuritiformis
heredopathia atactica p.
polyneuritis
peripheral p.
polyneuropathy
gait disorder, autoantibody, late-age, onset, p. (GALOP)
sensory p.
polyolefin elastomer
polyostotic
p. bone lesion
p. fibrous dysplasia
polyp
fibroepithelial p.
polyphasic action potential
Polypin biodegradable pin implant
polypropylene
p. ankle-foot orthosis
p. glycol-ankle-foot orthosis (PPG-AFO)
p. glycol-thoracolumbosacral orthosis (PPG-TLSO)
p. insert

NOTES

P

535

polypropylene *(continued)*
    p. prosthesis
    p. suture
polyradiculoneuropathy
    acute inflammatory demyelinating p. (AIDP)
polyradiculopathy
    acute inflammatory p.
    diabetic p.
polyserositis
Polyskin dressing
Polysorb
    P. heel cup
    P. liner
    P. suture
Polystim electrode
Polytechnic foot-pressure measuring plate
polytetrafluoroethylene (PTFE)
polytomography
polyurethane
    p. bandage
    p. cast
    p. foam dressing (PFD)
    p. implant material
polyvinyl
    p. alcohol splint
    p. alcohol splinting material
    p. chloride (PVC)
    p. implant material
PolyWic dressing
pommel cushion
Poncet
    P. disease
    P. rheumatism
poncho restraint
pond
    P. adjustable splint
    p. fracture
Ponseti
    P. clubfoot treatment method
    P. splint
    P. technique
Pontenza arthrodesis
pontine micturition center
pontoon spica cast
pool
    Aquaciser p.
    AquaMotion p.
    aquatic therapy p.
    Endless Pool physical therapy p.
    Ferno custom therapy p.
    motor neuronal p.
    SwimEx p.
    p. therapy
poor
    p. alignment

    p. bone stock
    p. cosmesis
POP
    PCL-oriented placement
    plaster of Paris
    POP cast
Popeye arm
popliteal
    p. angle
    p. artery
    p. crease
    p. entrapment syndrome
    p. fascia
    p. flexion creaking
    p. fossa
    p. fossa entrapment
    p. fossa neural blockade
    p. hiatus
    p. ligament
    p. muscle
    p. nerve
    p. pressure sign
    p. pterygium syndrome
    p. recess
    p. region
    p. sciatic nerve block
    p. space
    p. tendon
    p. vein
    p. vessel
popliteomeniscal fascicle
popliteus
    p. bypass
    p. tendinitis
    p. tendon
popoff suture
Poppen
    P. forceps
    P. Gigli saw guide
    P. ridge sensitometer
popping
    joint p.
pop rivet
porcine prosthesis
PORD
    posterior reduction device
porencephalic cyst
Porocoat
    P. AML noncemented prosthesis
    P. porous coating
    P. prosthetic material
    Tri-Lock total hip prosthesis with P.
Poro-in-between sole
porokeratoma
porokeratosis, pl. **porokeratoses**
    p. of Mibelli

poroma
    eccrine p.
Porometal noncemented femoral
  prosthesis
Poron
    P. cellular urethane
    P. 400 insole
poroplastic splint
porosity
    interfacial p.
porotic bone
porous
    p. cementless component
    p. coating
    p. ingrowth fixation
    p. metal
    p. polyethylene
    p. polyethylene graft
    p. prosthetic material
    p. surfaced prosthesis
porous-coated
    p.-c. acetabular cup
    p.-c. anatomic (PCA)
    p.-c. anatomic prosthesis
    p.-c. anatomic total hip
      replacement
    p.-c. anatomic total knee
    p.-c. component
    p.-c. femur prosthesis
    p.-c. hip prosthesis
    p.-c. implant
PORP
    partial ossicular replacement prosthesis
    Richards hydroxyapatite PORP
porphyria
porphyritic neuropathy
portable
    p. C-arm image intensifier
      fluoroscopy
    p. diagnostic kit
    P. Topical Hyperbaric Oxygen
      Extremity Chamber
portal
    1–2 p.
    3–4 p.
    4–5 p.
    p. accessory
    anterior p.
    anterocentral arthroscopic p.
    anteroinferior p.
    anterolateral p.
    anteromedial p.

    arthroscopic entry p.
    Caspari arthroscopic p.
    central transpatellar tendon p.
    desktop therapy p.
    direct lateral p.
    inside-out technique for establishing
      ankle p.
    lateral transmalleolar p.
    MCR p.
    MCU p.
    medial p.
    midcarpal p.
    midlateral p.
    midpatellar p.
    patellar p.
    p. placement
    Portal Pro 2 treatment chair
    posterior p.
    posteroinferior p.
    posterolateral p.
    posteromedial p.
    proximal midpatellar medial and
      lateral p.'s
    radiocarpal p.
    stab wound arthroscopy entry p.
    straight posterior p.
    subacromial p.
    superior p.
    superolateral p.
    superomedial p.
    suprapatellar p.
    Swedish p.
    transmalleolar p.
    transpatellar tendon p.
    transtendocalcaneus p.
    6U p.
    Wilmington arthroscopic p.
Porter-Richardson-Vainio
    P.-R.-V. synovectomy
    P.-R.-V. technique
portion
    accessory p.
    cord p.
    devitalized p.
    proximal p.
Portmann drill
portmanteau procedure
Portola Valley Scale
port-wine stain
Porzett splint
Posada fracture

NOTES

P

537

Posey
- P. bar kit
- P. bed cradle
- P. belt
- P. drop seat
- P. grip
- P. Palm Cone
- P. sling

Positex knee wedge

position
- angular p.
- antiembolic p.
- arch and slouch p.
- barber chair p.
- bayonet fracture p.
- beach chair p.
- Bonner p.
- Brickner p.
- cottonloader p.
- decubitus p.
- de Kleyn p.
- dorsal lithotomy p.
- dorsal recumbent p.
- dorsiflexion-plantar flexion p.
- empty-can p.
- equinus p.
- erect p.
- figure-four p.
- flexed p.
- Fowler p.
- frog-leg p.
- full lateral p.
- p. of function
- Gaynor-Hart p.
- horizontal p.
- intrinsic minus p.
- jackknife p.
- James p.
- jet-pilot p.
- Jones p.
- jumper's knee p.
- kneeling p.
- 90-90 kneeling p.
- Kraske p.
- lateral decubitus p.
- lateral park-bench p.
- lithotomy p.
- lotus p.
- mediolateral p.
- military brace p.
- military tuck p.
- neutral hip p.
- normal anatomic p.
- opisthotonic p.
- over-the-top p.
- Phalen p.
- prayer p.
- prone p.

- proximal bow p.
- quasistatic stressed p.
- rectus p.
- recumbent p.
- resting calcaneal stance p. (RCSP)
- reverse Trendelenburg p.
- scissor-leg p.
- semi-Fowler p.
- semisitting p.
- p. sense
- side-lying p.
- side-posture p.
- Sims p.
- sitting p.
- sniffer's p.
- p. in space
- spinal fusion p.
- subtalar joint neutral p. (STNP)
- supine p.
- three-quarters prone p.
- tibial sesamoid p. (TSP)
- translational p.
- Trendelenburg p.

positional
- p. dyskinesia
- p. release therapy

positioner
- acetabular cup p.
- Allen arthroscopic elbow p.
- Allen arthroscopic knee p.
- Allen arthroscopic wrist p.
- arm p.
- Assistant Free Stulberg leg p.
- Bareskin knee p.
- Biomet Second Assistant knee p.
- cup p.
- De Mayo hip p.
- Grasshopper p.
- Hold-and-Hold p.
- IMP Universal knee p.
- IMP Universal lateral p.
- Kirschenbaum foot p.
- knee p.
- leg p.
- Mark II Stulberg hip p.
- Mark II Stulberg leg p.
- Mark II Wixson hip p.
- McConnell shoulder p.
- McGuire pelvic p.
- Montreal hip p.
- OSI-Schlein shoulder p.
- Picket Fence leg p.
- Prep-Assist p.
- Profex arthroscopic leg p.
- Schlein shoulder p.
- shoulder abduction p.
- Stulberg hip p.

Stulberg Mark II leg p.
SurgAssist leg p.
Ther-A-Shapes p.
Universal knee p.
Universal lateral p.
Vac-Pac p.
Wixson hip p.

positioning
patient p.
proper neck p.

positive
p. ability
p. afterpotential
p. impingement sign
p. rim sign
p. sharp wave
p. supporting reflex
p. ulnar variance (PUV)

positron
p. emission tomographic scan
p. emission tomography (PET)

post
extrinsic rearfoot p.
iliac p.
Isola spinal implant system iliac p.
Luque-Galveston p.
Morse tapered prosthetic p.
perineal p.
status p.
thumb p.
P. total shoulder arthroplasty

postactivation
p. depression
p. exhaustion
p. facilitation
p. potentiation

postacute sprain
Postalume finger splint
post-and-cam mechanism
postanesthesia
p. care unit (PACU)
p. recovery (PAR)

postaxial
p. muscle
p. polydactyly

postcalcaneal bursitis
postcast compression reflex
postcasting syndrome
postcompetition rehabilitation
postconcussive syndrome
Postel hip status system

posterior
anterior and p. (AP)
p. apprehension test
p. arch
p. arch fracture
p. atlantoaxial arthrodesis
p. atlantoodontoid interval
p. axillary line (PAL)
p. bending moment
p. bone block
p. bone graft
p. bow
p. capsule
p. capsulorrhaphy
p. capsulotomy
p. cervical fixation
p. cervical fusion
p. cervical line
p. cervical spinal instrumentation
p. colliculus
p. column fracture
p. column osteosynthesis
p. column sign
p. compartment
p. component
p. construct
p. cord syndrome
p. costotransversectomy approach
p. cruciate
p. cruciate condylar knee system
p. cruciate ligament (PCL)
p. cruciate ligament graft
p. cruciate ligament of knee
p. cruciate ligament tear
p. cruciate sprain
p. curvature
p. deltoid muscle
p. deltoid-to-triceps transfer
p. depression pattern
p. distraction instrumentation
p. drainage
p. drawer sign
p. drawer test
p. element
p. element fracture
p. endplate
p. facet
p. facet dislocation
p. facet displacement
p. fixation system biomechanics
p. flap
p. flap technique

NOTES

P

539

posterior *(continued)*
   p. fracture-dislocation
   p. glenoid elevator
   p. glenoid labrum
   p. glenoplasty
   p. glide
   p. hiatal sign
   p. hip dislocation
   p. hook-rod spinal instrumentation
   p. horn
   p. horn meniscal tear
   p. iliac osteotomy
   p. iliofemoral technique
   p. impingement
   p. incision
   p. inferior cerebellar artery (PICA)
   p. inferior tibiofibular ligament
   p. innominate
   p. innominate rotation
   p. interosseous branch
   p. interosseous nerve compression
    syndrome
   p. interosseous nerve entrapment
   p. interosseous nerve palsy
   p. interspinous wiring
   p. inverted U approach
   p. joint syndrome
   p. knee pull syndrome
   p. leaf-spring ankle-foot orthosis
   p. ligamentous injury
   p. lip
   p. longitudinal fiber region
   p. longitudinal ligament (PLL)
   p. lower cervical spine stabilization
   p. lower cervical spine surgery
   p. lumbar interbody fusion (PLIF)
   p. lumbar interbody fusion surgery
   p. lumbar spine and sacrum
    surgery
   p. malleolus
   p. midline approach
   p. mold splint
   p. nerve decompression
   p. oblique fiber region
   p. oblique ligament (POL)
   p. oblique meniscal tear
   p. oblique sprain
   p. occipitocervical approach
   p. osteophyte
   p. pelvic tilt
   p. pharyngeal abscess
   p. portal
   p. process fracture
   p. radial collateral artery
   p. reduction device (PORD)
   p. release
   p. rhizotomy
   p. rod system

   p. rotation on the left side
   p. rotation on the right side
   p. sacroiliac spine (PSIS)
   p. sag sign
   p. screw fixation
   p. segmental fixation
   p. shoulder dislocation
   p. shoulder instability
   p. spinal fusion
   p. spinal plating
   p. spinal wedge osteotomy
   p. spur
   p. stability
   p. stress test
   p. superior humeral head defect
   p. superior iliac spine (PSIS)
   superior labrum anterior and p.
    (SLAP)
   p. talar process fracture
   p. talofibular ligament (PTFL)
   p. thigh bar
   p. tibial artery
   p. tibial nerve (PTN)
   p. tibial nerve entrapment
   p. tibial pulse (PTP)
   p. tibial spine
   p. tibial tendinitis (PTT)
   p. tibial tendon (PTT)
   p. tibial tendon dysfunction
    (PTTD)
   p. tibial tendon insufficiency
   p. tibial tendon transfer
   p. translation
   p. transolecranon approach
   p. triangle
   p. tuberosity
   p. upper cervical spine surgery
   p. wall fracture
posterior-anterior
   p.-a. glide
   p.-a. pressure
   p.-a. screw
posterior-inferior
   p.-i. capsular shift procedure
   p.-i. spine
posteriorly
posterior-superior
   p.-s. humeral head lesion
   p.-s. oblique projection
posteroanterior (PA)
posterodistal
posteroinferior (PI)
   p. external (PIEx)
   p. external movement
   p. ilium major
   p. internal (PIIn)
   p. internal movement
   p. portal

posterolateral
    p. approach
    p. approach of Henry
    p. aspect
    p. bone graft
    p. bone graft placement
    p. bundle
    p. capsule
    p. compartment
    p. costotransversectomy incision
    p. costotransversectomy technique
    p. decompression
    p. drainage
    p. drawer sign
    p. drawer test
    p. herniation
    p. interbody fusion (PLIF)
    p. lumbosacral fusion
    p. portal
    p. release
    p. rotary instability
    p. structure

posteromedial
    p. approach
    p. bow
    p. capsule
    p. compartment
    p. corner
    p. dislocation
    p. drainage
    p. drawer sign
    p. pivot-shift test
    p. portal
    p. region
    p. release (PMR)
    p. rotary instability

posteroproximal
poster orthosis
postexercise hypotension
postfracture
    p. cyst
    p. lesion
    p. osteomyelitis
    p. swelling
    p. syndrome

postganglionic technique
postherpetic pain
postinfectious
    p. arthritis
    p. myopathy

posting
    heel p.

    strip p.
    wedge p.

postinjury period
postirradiation
    p. fracture
    p. osteogenic sarcoma

postisometric
    p. relaxation
    p. relaxation traction technique
    p. stretch technique

postlaminectomy
    p. kyphosis
    p. two-level spondylolisthesis

postmenopausal
    p. arthritis
    p. bone loss

postmortem fracture
postnatal
    p. cerebral palsy
    p. gangrene

postoperative
    p. bracing
    p. casting
    p. complication
    p. corticosteroid
    p. drainage-related hematoma
    p. extubation
    p. flexor tendon (PFT)
    p. fracture
    p. immobilization
    p. immobilizer
    p. infection
    p. lumbosacral orthosis
    p. pain
    p. paraplegia
    p. regimen
    p. synovitis
    p. therapy
    p. wound care

postphlebitis syndrome
postpoliomyelitic contracture
postpolio syndrome
postpyelomyelitis syndrome
postradiation kyphosis
postreduction x-ray
poststatic dyskinesia (PSDK)
posttetanic
    p. exhaustion
    p. facilitation
    p. potentiation

posttraumatic
    p. algodystrophic syndrome

NOTES

P

posttraumatic *(continued)*
    p. angulation
    p. apoplexy
    p. arthritis
    p. arthrosis
    p. cavus
    p. chronic cord syndrome
    p. chronic osteomyelitis
    p. degenerative disease Lance
     acetabuloplasty
    p. dystrophy
    p. edema
    p. epilepsy
    p. hemarthrosis
    p. kyphosis
    p. neuroma
    p. osteoarthritis
    p. osteolysis
    p. osteonecrosis
    p. osteoporosis
    p. pain
    p. sacroiliac dysfunction
    p. spinal deformity
    p. syringomyelia
postulnar bone
postural
    p. analysis
    p. balance
    p. complex
    p. component
    p. control
    p. development
    p. exteroceptor
    p. fixation back maneuver
    p. instability
    p. interoceptor
    p. ischemia
    p. list
    p. muscle
    p. receptor
    p. reflex
    p. strain
    p. sway
    p. syndrome
    p. tremor
    p. variation
posture
    batrachian p.
    benediction p.
    cavus p.
    P. Curve lumbar cushion
    decerebrate p.
    decorticate p.
    p. education
    forward flexion p.
    forward head p.
    p. of limb
    P. Pump lordoticiser

    P. Pump Spine Trainer
    recumbent p.
    P. S'port
    P. Wedge seat cushion
Posture-Rite lap desk
posturing
    equinovarus p.
posturography
    computerized dynamic p. (CDP)
potassium-40 count
potential
    action p. (AP)
    auditory evoked p. (AEP)
    bioelectric p.
    biphasic action p.
    bizarre repetitive p.
    brainstem auditory evoked p.
     (BAEP)
    brief, small, abundant p. (BSAP)
    brief, small, abundant,
     polyphasic p. (BSAPP)
    complex motor unit action p.
    compound mixed nerve action p.
    compound motor nerve action p.
    compound muscle action p.
     (CMAP)
    compound muscle-motor action p.
     (CMAP)
    compound sensory nerve action p.
    denervation p.
    dermatosensory evoked p.
    electrical p.
    electrokinetic p.
    endplate p. (EPP)
    evoked compound muscle action p.
    excitatory postsynaptic p.
    far-field p.
    fasciculation p.
    fibrillation p.
    giant motor unit action p.
    inhibitory postsynaptic p.
    irregular p.
    kilovoltage p.
    linked p.
    long-latency somatosensory
     evoked p.
    miniature end-plate p. (MEPP)
    monophasic action p.
    motor unit p. (MUP)
    motor unit action p. (MUAP)
    muscle fiber action p.
    myopathic motor unit p.
    myotonic p.
    nascent motor unit p.
    near-field p.
    nerve action p. (NAP)
    nerve fiber action p.
    nerve trunk action p.

neurogenic motor evoked p. (NMEP)
neuropathic motor unit p.
piezoelectric p.
polyphasic action p.
pseudopolyphasic action p.
regeneration motor unit p.
resting membrane p.
satellite p.
sensory evoked p.
sensory nerve action p. (SNAP)
serrated action p.
short-latency somatosensory evoked p.
somatosensory evoked p. (SEP, SSEP)
spinal evoked p.
streaming p.
tetraphasic action p.
triphasic action p.
visual evoked p.

potentiation
postactivation p.
posttetanic p.

potentiometer
linear p.

Pott
P. abscess
P. ankle fracture
P. disease
P. dwarfism
P. gangrene
P. paralysis
P. paraplegia
P. puffy tumor
P. spinal curvature

Potter arthrodesis
Potts
P. eversion osteotomy
P. splint
P. tibial osteotomy

Potts-Smith dressing forceps
pouce flottant thumb
pouch
antibiotic bead p.
bead p.
inflamed synovial p.
suprapatellar p.

pouch-type sling
Poulet disease
poundal
pounds of traction

Pouteau syndrome
powder
p. board
thrombin p.

powdered bone graft
power
P. Anthro Shoe
p. bur
p. drill
grasping p.
p. oscillating saw
P. Pillow cervical massager
pinch p.
P. Play knee brace
P. Pogo stationary exerciser
p. rasp
p. reamer
thumb pinch p.
P. Trainer cycle
P. Web hand exerciser
P. Web Jr. exerciser
p. wheelchair

Powerbelt exercise system
PowerCut drill blade
power-driven
p.-d. reamer
p.-d. saw

powered metaphysial stapler
Powerflex
P. CMP exerciser
P. tape

Power-Grip pliers
Powermatic table
POWERPoint orthotic shoe insert
PowerStar bipolar scissors
Powerstep foot support
PP
proximal phalanx

PPD
permanent partial disability
PPD rating

PPF
percutaneous plantar fasciotomy

PPG
photoplethysmography

PPG-AFO
polypropylene glycol-ankle-foot orthosis
PPG-AFO brace

PPG-TLSO
polypropylene glycol-thoracolumbosacral orthosis
PPG-TLSO brace

NOTES

P

PPO
> passive prehension orthosis

PPS
> patellofemoral pain syndrome

PPT
>> PPT flat insole
>> PPT insole system
>> PPT MXL soft molded insole
>> PPT orthotic device
>> PPT Plastizote insole
>> PPT RX firm molded insole
>> PPT sheet
>> PPT soft tissue orthotic system

PQ
> pronator quadratus
>> PQ Premium heel cup

PR
> pelvic rock
> progressive-resistive exercise

PRAFO
> pressure-relief ankle-foot orthotic
>> PRAFO adjustable orthotic
>> PRAFO KAFO
>> PRAFO PKA KAFO attachment

Prague pelvis

Pratt
>> P. open reduction
>> P. symptom
>> P. T-clamp
>> P. technique

prayer
>> p. position
>> p. view

PRE
> progressive-resistive exercise

pre-Achilles
>> p.-A. bursa
>> p.-A. bursitis
>> p.-A. fat pad
>> p.-A. mass

preassembled metal-backed socket

preaxial
>> p. muscle
>> p. polydactyly

prebent nail

precaution
>> cardiac p.'s
>> universal p.'s

precise lesion measuring (PLM)

Precision
>> P. hip stem
>> P. Osteolock
>> P. Osteolock femoral component system
>> P. Osteolock femoral prosthesis
>> P. Osteolock fixation
>> P. Osteolock hip prosthesis

>> P. Strata hip system
>> P. total hip

Preclude spinal membrane

precoat
>> P. hip prosthesis
>> P. Plus femoral prosthesis

precompression jig

precontoured unit rod

precurved
>> p. ball-tipped guidepin
>> p. plate

PreCustom Orthotic

prediction
>> Anderson-Green growth p.
>> growth p.

Predictive Salvage Index

predictor of injury

predislocation syndrome

predisposition
>> congenital p.

preemptive blockade technique

prefabricated wool felt pad

preganglionic
>> p. sympathectomy
>> p. technique

prehallux
>> external p.
>> p. osseous prominence

prehension
>> p. force
>> p. grasp
>> p. orthosis

preinterparietal bone

Preiser disease

preload

premalleolar fat pad

premanipulative testing

premature
>> p. closure
>> p. consolidation

Premier press fit prosthesis

prenatal dislocation

Prenyl jacket

preoperative
>> p. drawing
>> p. evaluation
>> p. management
>> p. plan
>> p. planning
>> p. roentgenography
>> p. tomography

prep
>> 3M p.

preparation
>> bone-patellar tendon-bone p.
>> facet joint p.
>> graft p.
>> lupus erythematosus p.

rod contour p.
skin p.
Spälteholz p.
wire contour p.

Prep-Assist
P.-A. leg holder
P.-A. legholder
P.-A. positioner

prepatellar
p. bursa
p. bursa inflammation
p. bursitis

Prep-IM
presacral block
Presbyterian
P. Hospital staphylorrhaphy elevator
P. Hospital T-clamp

prescription
ACSM Guidelines for Exercise
Testing and P.

preservation
lordosis p.
lumbar lordosis p.

prespondylolisthesis
press
CamStar power leg p.
p. fit
leg p.
Shuttle MVP leg p.
supine chest p.
p. up

press-fit
p.-f. acetabular implant insertion
technique
p.-f. circumferential grommet
p.-f. condylar knee arthroplasty
p.-f. Condylar Total knee
p.-f. condylar total knee prosthesis
p.-f. cup
p.-f. femoral component
p.-f. fixation
p.-f. stem
p.-f. total condylar knee system

pressure
ankle systolic p.
blood p.
bone marrow p. (BMP)
central posterior-anterior p.
compartmental p.
p. cushion
disk p.
Doppler ankle systolic p.

p. epiphysis
p. excursion index
forefoot peak p.
p. fracture
p. glove
hydrostatic p.
intracompartmental p.
intradiskal p.
lateral root p.
manual p.
p. necrosis
p. paralysis
peak p.
plantar p.
p. plate
p. point
posterior-anterior p.
p. relief padding
p. relief shoe
rolfing p.
P. Sentinel reamer
sequential p.
p. sore
systolic blood p.
p. therapy
p. threshold
tissue p.
toe p.
p. tolerance
tourniquet p.
p. transducer
p. transducer-monitor system
p. ulcer
p. ulcer assessment
p. ulcer classification
p. ulcer cleansing
p. ulcer dressing
p. ulcer management
p. ulcer prevention
p. ulcer-related maggot infestation
ultraviolet light p.

PressureGuard mattress
pressure-relief
p.-r. ankle-foot orthotic (PRAFO)
p.-r. cushion

pressure-relieving orthosis
pressure-sensitive
p.-s. area
p.-s. tissue

Pressure-Specified Sensory Device
pressure-time integral (PTI)
pressure-tolerant tissue

NOTES

P

pressurized cement
pressurizer
    acetabular p.
    plunger-type femoral p.
Preston
    P. ligamentum flavum forceps
    P. overhead pulley
    P. pinch gauge
    P. screw
    P. Traveler CPM exerciser
Prestop pinchometer
pretarget filtration system
pretendinous
    p. band
    p. band of hand
    p. cord
pretibial
    p. bearing (PTB)
    p. buttress (PTB)
    p. edema
prevention
    heat injury p.
    heterotopic ossification p.
    infection p.
    osseous bridge p.
    pressure ulcer p.
    rod rotation p.
Prevent Recurrence of Osteoporotic Fractures (PROOF)
prevertebral space
PRICE
    protection, restricted activity, ice, compression, elevation
Price muscular biopsy clamp
prickling pain
Pridie
    P. ankle arthrodesis
    P. incision
Pridie-Koutsogiannis procedure
Primaderm dressing
Primapore wound dressing
primary
    p. amputation
    p. arthroplasty
    p. bone union
    p. closure
    p. cranial sacral respiratory mechanism
    p. curve
    p. cystic arthrosis
    p. degenerative arthritis
    p. degenerative osteoarthritis
    p. intention
    p. or intentional movement
    p. lymphoma of bone (PLB)
    p. movement plane
    p. myofascial trigger point
    p. peroneus longus tendinopathy

    p. progressive amyotrophy
    p. repair
    p. rotation movement
    p. sequestrum
    p. spongiosa
    p. stem (PS)
    p. subacute osteomyelitis
    p. subtalar arthrodesis
    p. tumor
    p. x-ray beam
prime mover
Primer modified Unna boot
primitive
    p. bone
    p. dislocation
    p. locomotor pattern
    p. reflex
primus
    digitus p.
    P. flexible great toe
    p. implant
princeps pollicis artery
principal stress
principle
    anatomic fracture reduction p.
    axial compression p.
    biomechanical p.
    Enneking p.
    gliding p.
    Lambotte p.
    SAID p.
    spherical gliding p.
prism
    Fresnel p.
prisoner's palsy
Pritchard
    P. II elbow prosthesis
    P. Mark II pin
    P. total elbow prosthesis
Pritchard-Walker
    P.-W. semiconstrained elbow prosthesis
    P.-W. total elbow prosthesis
Pritchett-Mallin-Matthews arthrodesis
Pritsch talar osteochondroma classification
prizm
    p. Electro-Mesh Sock electrode
    p. Electro-Mesh Z-Stim-II stimulator
Pro
    P. Osteon 500 bone graft substitute
    PCL P.
    P. Support Systems orthotic
Pro-8 ankle brace
ProAdvantage knee

probability
    bone cyst fracture p.
PRO Balance Master
probe
    Acufex p.
    angled p.
    arthroscopic p.
    Bipolar Circumactive P. (BICAP)
    blunt-tip p.
    Bunnell dissecting p.
    Bunnell forwarding p.
    calibrated p.
    dissecting p.
    free-spinning p.
    gearshift p.
    gold p.
    intraosseous p.
    LASE p.
    laser Doppler p.
    multiplane echo p.
    Nucleotome p.
    Oratec thermal shrinking p.
    pedicle sounding p.
    reverse-cutting meniscal p.
    skin temperature monitoring p.
    spinning p.
    p. test for osteomyelitis
    ultrasonic p.
    Woodson p.
procaine-phenol motor point injection
procallus formation
Procase Ankle-Lock brace
procedure
    Adams p.
    Akin p.
    Albee shelf p.
    AMBRI p.
    anchovy p.
    Anderson-Fowler p.
    antenna p.
    anterior stabilization p.
    AO p.
    Arbeitsgemeinschaft für
      osteosynthesefragen p.
    arthroscopic transglenoid suture
      stabilization p.
    articulatory p.
    Auto-Implant p.
    Axer-Clark p.
    Badgley combination p.
    Baker Achilles tendon
      lengthening p.

    Bankart p.
    Barsky p.
    Bartlett p.
    Basic I, II cranial adjusting p.
    Baxter-D'Astous p.
    beefburger p.
    Bell-Tawse p.
    Bennett quadriceps plastic p.
    Bentson p.
    Berman-Gartland p.
    B.H. Moore p.
    Bickel-Moe p.
    Bilhaut-Cloquet p.
    Blair p.
    Blatt p.
    Blatt-Ashworth p.
    bone block p.
    bony p.
    Bose p.
    Bosworth shelf p.
    Boyd-Bosworth p.
    Boyd-McLeod p.
    Boyd-Sisk p.
    Boytchev p.
    Brahms p.
    Brantigan-Voshell p.
    Braun p.
    Bridle p.
    Bristow p.
    Bristow-Helfet p.
    Bristow-Latarjet p.
    Bristow-May p.
    Brockman p.
    Broström p.
    Bryan p.
    Bunnell-Williams p.
    Calandriello p.
    callus distraction p.
    Campbell-Akbarnia p.
    Campbell ankle p.
    Campbell-Goldthwait p.
    capsular imbrication p.
    capsular shift p.
    Castle p.
    Chambers p.
    Chandler p.
    Charnley ankle fusion p.
    checkrein p.
    chevron p.
    Chiari shelf p.
    chiropractic adjustment p.

NOTES

P

procedure *(continued)*

Chrisman-Snook weave p.
Clayton p.
Cobb tibialis posterior tendon dysfunction p.
Cole p.
Connolly p.
Conrad-Frost Achilles tenotomy p.
Copeland-Howard shoulder p.
core drilling p.
Cotting ingrown nail p.
Cotton p.
Cracchiolo p.
Cummins p.
Darrach p.
Das Gupta p.
debulking p.
degloving p.
denervation p.
DePalma staple p.
Dewar posterior cervical fixation p.
Dickson-Diveley p.
Dorrance p.
Downey-McGlamery p.
Downey-Rubin overlapping toe repair p.
DREZ p.
DuVries p.
Dwyer p.
Eden-Hybbinette p.
Eden-Lange p.
Edwards p.
eggshell p.
Elmslie-Cholmely p.
Elmslie peroneal tendon p.
Elmslie-Trillat patellar p.
Elmslie weave p.
Engebretsen p.
Eppright Wagner shelf p.
Evans p.
Eve reconstructive p.
extraarticular Grice p.
failed p.
Fairbanks-Sever p.
femorodistal bypass p.
Ficat p.
Fired-Hendel p.
five-incision p.
forage p.
four-incision p.
Fowler p.
Fox-Blazina knee p.
Frank Dickson shelf p.
Frank and Johnson modification of Heyman p.
Fried-Green foot p.
Froimson p.
Froimson-Oh arm p.

Frost foot p.
Fulford p.
Gallie p.
Ganley and Ganley metatarsus adductus p.
Gartland p.
Gelman foot p.
Gerard resurfacing p.
Gilbert p.
Gill modification of Campbell ankle p.
Gillquist p.
Gill shelf p.
Girdlestone hip p.
Girdlestone-Taylor p.
Goldner-Hayes p.
Goldthwait-Hauser p.
Gould p.
Graber-Duvernay p.
gracilis p.
Grant, Surrall, and Lehman p.
Green p.
Green-Grice p.
Grice p.
Gritti-Stokes distal thigh p.
Gruca lower leg p.
Gurd p.
Hall Kalamchi shelf p.
hallux valgus p.
Hambly p.
Hammon foot p.
Hardinge vastus lateralis p.
Hark pes planus p.
Harmon p.
Hass p.
Hauser Achilles lengthening p.
Hauser heel cord p.
Hauser patellar tendon p.
Hawkins p.
Hay-Groves shelf p.
Heifetz p.
Helal-Gibb p.
Herndon-Heyman foot p.
Hey-Groves p.
Heyman p.
Heyman-Herndon p.
Hibbs p.
His-Haas p.
Hitchcock arm p.
Hodor-Dobbs p.
Hoffer ankle p.
Hoffmann-Clayton p.
Hoffmann metatarsal p.
Hohmann p.
Hoke-Miller p.
Hoke tibial palsy p.
Hovanian p.
Howorth p.

Howorth-Keillor p.
Hughston p.
Hughston-Hauser p.
Hui-Linscheid p.
IDET p.
iliac buttressing p.
Inclan modification of Campbell
  ankle p.
Inclan-Ober p.
Ingram p.
Insall p.
installation p.
intercalary allograft p.
intermetatarsal angle-reducing p.
intraarticular p.
Jaffe p.
Jahss p.
James p.
Jansey p.
Jobe-Glousman capsular shift p.
Johnson p.
Johnson-Spiegl p.
Jones retinaculum reconstruction p.
J.R. Moore p.
Juvara p.
Kaplan modification of Ruiz-
  Mora p.
Karakousis-Vezeridis p.
Karlsson p.
Kawaii-Yamamoto p.
Kehr p.
Kelikian p.
Kelikian-McFarland p.
Keller p.
Keller-Brandes p.
Keller-Lelièvre-Hoffman p.
Kelly peroneal tendon
  dislocation p.
Kendrick p.
Kessel-Bonney p.
Kidner foot p.
Kiehn-Earle-DesPrez p.
King intraarticular hip fusion p.
Knobby-Clark p.
Kortzeborn p.
Koutsogiannis p.
Krukenberg p.
Lance shelf p.
Lane p.
Lange p.
Langenskiöld p.
Lapidus p.

Larmon forefoot p.
Larsen lateral ankle stabilization p.
Latarjet p.
lateral sling p.
Lauenstein p.
Lawton p.
Lee p.
Leeds spinal p.
Legg p.
lengthening over nails p.
Lepird p.
L'Episcopo-Zachary p.
ligamentous weave p.
limb-salvage p.
Lindeman p.
Lindholm Achilles lengthening p.
Linton p.
Lipscomb p.
Lipscomb-Anderson p.
Localio p.
Loose p.
loose knee p.
Lorenz p.
Loughheed and White p.
lower cervical spine p.
Lowman shelf p.
Luck hand p.
Lynn Achilles lengthening p.
MacAusland p.
MacCarthy p.
macrodactalia reduction p.
Magnuson-Stack p.
Mahan p.
manipulative p.
Manktelow transfer p.
Mann p.
Mann-Coughlin p.
Maquet p.
Matson p.
Mauck knee p.
Mau and Ludloff p.
Maxwell-Brancheau p.
McBride p.
McCarroll-Baker p.
McCarty hip p.
McCash hand p.
McCauley foot p.
McCormick-Blount p.
McElvenny-Caldwell p.
McElvenny foot p.
McGlamry p.
McGlamry-Downey p.

NOTES

P

procedure (*continued*)
    McKay hip p.
    McKeever p.
    McLaughlin p.
    medial rotation p.
    Mikulicz p.
    Miller foot p.
    Minkoff-Nicholas p.
    Mitchell hallux valgus p.
    Miyakawa knee p.
    Moberg key-pinch p.
    modified Broström p.
    modified Broström-Evans p.
    modified Hoke-Miller flatfoot p.
    modified Lapidus p.
    Mogensen p.
    motion control p.
    motion-preserving p.
    Mueller knee p.
    Mumford p.
    muscle-balancing p.
    Neer capsular shift p.
    Neviaser-Wilson-Gardner p.
    Newman-Keuls p.
    Nicola shoulder p.
    Nicoll fracture repair p.
    Nilsson lateral ankle stabilization p.
    notchplasty p.
    O'Brien capsular shift p.
    O'Donoghue p.
    offset-V p.
    orthodox p.
    Osborne-Cotterill p.
    Osmond-Clarke foot p.
    Oudard p.
    Outerbridge-Kashiwagi p.
    over-the-top knee p.
    Pagddu p.
    Paltrinieri-Trentani resurfacing p.
    Parrish p.
    Paterson p.
    Peabody and Munro p.
    peroneal tendon p.
    Perthes p.
    Pettibon chiropractic p.
    polyethylene femoral buck plug p.
    portmanteau p.
    posterior-inferior capsular shift p.
    Pridie-Koutsogiannis p.
    Proxiderm p.
    Putti-Platt shoulder p.
    realignment p.
    reefing p.
    Regnauld p.
    Reichenheim-King p.
    resurfacing p.
    Reverdin-Green foot p.
    Reverdin-Green-Laird p.
    reverse Jones p.
    reverse Mauck knee p.
    reverse Putti-Platt p.
    revision p.
    Ridlon p.
    Roaf, Kirkaldy-Willis, and
     Cattero p.
    Rockwood p.
    Rockwood-Matsen capsular shift p.
    Root p.
    Rose foot p.
    Roux-Goldthwait p.
    Ruiz-Mora p.
    Ryerson p.
    sacroiliac buttressing p.
    Saha p.
    salvage p.
    Samilson p.
    sartorial slide p.
    Sauvé-Kapandji p.
    Schrock p.
    Scuderi p.
    Selakovich p.
    semitendinosus p.
    Sgarlato p.
    Sgarlato hammertoe implant p.
    Sham p.
    shelf p.
    short lever specific contact p.
    Silfverskiöld p.
    Silver p.
    sling p.
    Slocum knee p.
    Somerville p.
    Souter hip p.
    Southwick slide p.
    spinal locking p.
    Spira p.
    Spittler p.
    SPLATT p.
    split anterior tibial tendon p.
    stabilization of the chevron p.
    Stack shoulder p.
    Staheli shelf p.
    Stamm and Wilson overlapping toe
     management p.
    STA-peg p.
    Steindler p.
    Steytler-Van Der Walt p.
    Stone p.
    Strayer Achilles lengthening p.
    Stromeyer Achilles tenotomy p.
    Sutherland hip p.
    Syme p.
    Tachdjian p.
    Taylor p.
    tendon checkrein p.
    terminal Syme p.

Thomas p.
Thomas-Thompson p.
Tikhoff-Linberg radical arm p.
p. time
Trillat p.
triple-wire p.
Tsai-Stillwell p.
TUBS p.
upper cervical spine p.
Valenti p.
Van Ness p.
Verebelyi-Ogston decancellation p.
Vulpius p.
Vulpius-Stoffel p.
wafer p.
Wallenberg p.
Watson-Cheyne-Burghard p.
Watson-Jones p.
Weaver-Dunn p.
Webb p.
Weber p.
Weston shelf p.
White slide p.
Whitman talectomy p.
Whitman-Thompson p.
Williams p.
Woodward p.
Yoke transposition p.
Young p.
Youngswick-Austin p.
Yount p.
Zadik foot p.
Zancolli clawhand deformity p.
Zancolli-Lasso p.
Zancolli static lock p.
Zaricznyj p.
Zarins-Rowe p.

process

abnormal posterior talar p.
absent spinous p.
acromion p.
articular p.
bifid spinous p.
bone destructive p.
capitular p.
Civinini p.
cleft spinous p.
condyloid p.
conoid p.
coracoacromial p.
coracoid p.
coronoid p.

cubital p.
deficient spinous p.
dislocation of articular p.
inferior p.
intact spinous p.
intercondylar p.
internal p.
lateral p.
mamillary p.
mastoid p.
maxillary p.
neuromuscular proprioceptive p.
odontoid p.
olecranon p.
orthopraxy spurious spinous p.
physial mamillary p.
sacralized transverse p.
spinous p.
spurious articular p.
Steida bony p.
Stieda p.
styloid p.
superior p.
supracondylar p.
talar p.
talus lateral posterior p.
transverse p.
unciform p.
ungual p.
xiphoid p.
Zimmer PMMA precoat p.

processed carbon implant
ProCol bovine bioprosthesis tendon
procurvatum deformity
ProCyte transparent dressing
Proderm topical spray
product

Body Glove orthopaedic p.
cyclooxygenase p.
Innovation Sports bracing p.
Innovative Medical P.'s (IMP)
Linvatec p.
microparticulated protein p.
Orthopaedic Physical Therapy P.'s (OPTP)
resistive exercise p.'s (REP)

production

bone p.
torque p.

Profex

P. arthroscopic leg positioner
P. arthroscopic tourniquet

NOTES

P

proficiency
    Bruininks-Oseretsky Test of
      Motor P.
profile
    acromial p.
    Functional Limitation P. (FLP)
    P. hip prosthesis
    P. hip stem
    Maryland Foot Score P.
    reduced p. (RP)
    risk factor p.
    P. Sitting Orthosis
    Staheli rotational p.
    P. total hip system
    wrist speed p.
Profix
    P. confirming tibial insert
    P. metaphysial tibial stem
    P. mobile-bearing knee implant
    P. nonporous tibial base
    P. porous femoral component
    P. total knee replacement system
ProFlex wrist support
ProFlo vascular compression therapy
Profore
    P. Four-Layer bandage system
    P. wound dressing
ProForma prosthesis
profunda
    p. brachii artery
    p. femoris
profundus
    p. advancement
    p. artery fracture
    flexor digitorum p. (FDP)
    p. muscle
    p. tendon
Pro-glide
    P.-g. orthosis
    P.-g. splint
program
    ABAQUS modeling p.
    aquatic exercise p.
    aquatic stabilization p.
    Camp Diversity arthritis p.
    Carpal Care rehabilitative p.
    exercise p.
    flexibility conditioning p.
    four-star exercise p.
    home exercise p.
    home spinal stabilization p.
    independent exercise p.
    interdisciplinary vocational
      evaluation p.
    macrotrauma rehabilitation p.
    phase 2 elbow p.
    rehabilitation therapeutic p.
    Rothman Institute total hip p.

    stretching p.
    TotalGym Exercise P.
    trunk stabilization rehabilitation p.
    Ultimate Hand Helper
      strengthening p.
    walking p.
    weight-training p.
    Westcott Pyramid P.
    Williams exercise p.
    work hardening p.
programmable VariGrip II prosthetic control system
progression
    curve p.
    p. to full weightbearing
    p. of training
    p. walking component
progressiva
    dysbasia lordotica p.
    fibrodysplasia ossificans p.
    fibrositis ossificans p.
    fibrous dysplasia ossificans p.
    myositis ossificans p.
progressive
    P. Ambulation Scale
    P. ankle orthosis
    p. diaphysial dysplasia
    p. loading
    p. lumbar extension rehabilitation
    p. macrodactylia
    p. muscle relaxation
    p. muscular atrophy (PMA)
    p. muscular dystrophy (PMD)
    p. myositis fibrosa
    p. neurologic disorder
    p. nuclear amyotrophy
    p. osseous heteroplasia
    P. Palm Guard
    p. perilunar instability
    p. resistance brace
    p. spinal amyotrophy
    p. subacute myelopathy
    p. supranuclear palsy
    p. systemic sclerosis
    p. weight
    p. weightbearing
progressively larger reamer
progressive-resistance exercise
progressive-resistive exercise (PR, PRE)
Progress splint
proinflammatory state
projection
    axial calcaneal p.
    axial sesamoid p.
    bursal p.
    cephaloscapular p.
    convergence p.
    dorsoplantar p.

Harris-Beath p.
Isherwood p.
lateral p. (LC)
posterior-superior oblique p.
stress dorsiflexion p.

prolapse
disk p.

Prolene suture
proliferating zone
proliferation
angiofibroblastic p.
bizarre parosteal
osteochondromatous p. (BPOP)
fibroblastic p.
reactive periosteal p.
p. therapy
villous lipomatous p.

proliferative
p. arthritis
p. fasciitis
p. myositis
p. synovitis

Proline Stomatex shoulder brace
ProLite Plus runner's orthotic
prolotherapy
PROM
passive range of motion

prominence
heel p.
navicular p.
osseous p.
osteochondral p.
pedicle screw hardware p.
plantar bony p.
prehallux osseous p.
rotational p.
tibial tubercle p.

prominent
p. heel
p. spur

promontory, promontorium
sacral p.

pronate
pronated
p. foot
p. pes cavus
p. straight flatfoot

pronation
p. contracture
p. control
p. of the foot
hindfoot p.

p. injury
p. phenomenon
p. sign
p. spring-control device
subtalar p.
p. and supination

pronation-abduction
p.-a. fracture
p.-a. injury

pronation-eversion
p.-e. fracture
p.-e. injury

pronation-eversion-external
p.-e.-e. rotation (PEER)
p.-e.-e. rotation injury

pronation-eversion/external rotation fracture
pronation-external rotation (P-ER)
pronation/spring control (PSC)
pronation-supination
pronator
p. drift
p. drill
p. quadratus (PQ)
p. quadratus muscle
p. reflex
p. teres (PT)
p. teres muscle
p. teres release
p. teres syndrome
p. teres tendon

pronatory gait
pronatus
pes p.

prone
p. blocking technique
p. extension test
p. external rotation test
p. knee-bend test
p. knee flexion test
p. position
p. rectus test
p. reduction
p. sacral push
p. scapular retraction exercise

Pronex
P. home traction
P. patient controlled pneumatic traction device
P. pneumatic cervical traction
P. pneumatic device for cervical pain

NOTES

P

prong
    modified tonsillar p.
pronometer
Pron pillow
Pronto cement
PROOF
    Prevent Recurrence of Osteoporotic
       Fractures
    PROOF group
ProOsteon
    P. bone graft material
    P. Implant 500
    P. implant 500 coralline
       hydroxyapatite bone void filler
    P. Implant 500 granule
Propac
    Champ Insulated P. II
propagation velocity
Propel cannulated interference screw
propeller
    orthopaedic p.
proper
    p. digital nerve branch
    p. neck positioning
properitoneal space
properly seated
property
    elastic p.
    elongation p.
prophylactic
    p. abduction pants
    p. antibiotic therapy
    p. anticoagulation
    p. bone graft
    p. fasciotomy
    p. operative stabilization
    p. resection
    p. skeletal fixation
    p. taping
prophylaxis, pl. prophylaxes
    deep venous thrombosis p.
    dextran p.
    DVT p.
Proplast
    P. HA
    P. I, II porous implant material
    P. prosthesis
    P. prosthetic material
proportionate dwarfism
proprioception
    gravitational p.
proprioceptive
    p. deficit
    p. exercise
    p. neuromuscular facilitation (PNF)
    p. neuromuscular facilitation
      approach

    p. neuromuscular fasciculation
      (PNF)
    p. rehabilitation
    p. training
proprioceptor
propriosensory training
proprius
    extensor indicis p. (EIP)
    p. tendon
Prop'r Toes hammertoe cushion
propulsion
    p. biomechanics
    p. gait
propulsive phase
prostaglandin
PROSTALAC
    prosthetic antibiotic-loaded acrylic
      cement
    PROSTALAC total hip prosthesis
    PROSTALAC total joint prosthesis
prosternation
prosthesis, pl. prostheses
    above-knee p., AK p.
    acetabular p.
    acrylic bar p.
    ACS Gemini p.
    ACS Profile p.
    ACS Star p.
    AcuMatch M Series modular
      femoral hip p.
    advanced mobile-bearing p.
    Advance PS total knee p.
    Advantim total knee p.
    Advantim unconstrained p.
    Aequalis humeral p.
    Aequalis shoulder p.
    Aesculap-PM noncemented
      femoral p.
    AFI total hip replacement p.
    AGC femoral p.
    AGC knee p.
    AGC tibial p.
    AHP digital p.
    AHSC elbow p.
    AHSC-Volz elbow p.
    Airlite p.
    Airprene hinged knee p.
    AK p. (*var. of* above-knee p.)
    Alivium implant metal p.
    Allen-Brown p.
    Allurion foot p.
    alumina-alumina total hip
      replacement p.
    alumina cemented total hip p.
    alumina-on-alumina p.
    AMC total wrist p.
    American Heyer-Schulte chin p.

American Heyer-Schulte-Hinderer
malar p.
American Heyer-Schulte Radovan
tissue expander p.
AMK unconstrained p.
AML Plus p.
AML Tang femoral p.
AML total hip p.
Amstutz cemented hip p.
Anametric total knee p.
Anatomic Precoat hip p.
anatomic surface p.
Anderson acetabular p.
ankle p.
Apollo hip p.
APR acetabular p.
APR femoral p.
APR II p.
APRL hand p.
Arafiles elbow p.
Arizona Health Science Center-Volz
elbow p.
Arthropor cup p.
Arthropor II acetabular p.
Atlas modular humeral p.
Attenborough total knee p.
Aufranc cobra hip p.
Aufranc-Turner cemented hip p.
Austin Moore femoral head p.
Autophor ceramic total hip p.
Autophor femoral p.
Avanta MCP joint implant
finger p.
Avanta metacarpophalangeal
implant p.
Averett hip p.
Averill press fit p.
Balance hip p.
ball-and-socket ankle p.
Bankart shoulder p.
Bantam CDH p.
Bateman femoral neck p.
Bateman finger p.
Bateman UPF p.
Bateman UPF II bipolar p.
Bateman UPF II shoulder p.
BDH p.
Beachcomber waterproof p.
bead-blasted p.
Bechtol hip p.
Bechtol shoulder p.
Bechtol system p.

Becker hand p.
Beck-Steffee total ankle p.
below-elbow p.
below-knee p.
Bi-Angular shoulder p.
Biaxial Weave composite p.
bicentric p.
bicompartmental knee implant p.
bicondylar ankle p.
bicondylar knee p.
Bi-Metric hip p.
Bi-Metric Interlok femoral p.
Bi-Metric porous primary
femoral p.
Bio-Chromatic hand p.
Bioclad with pegs reinforced
acetabular p.
BioFit Press-Fit acetabular p.
Bioglass p.
Bio-Groove acetabular p.
Bio-Groove Macrobond HA
femoral p.
Biomet AGC knee p.
Biomet hip p.
Biometric p.
Biomet total toe p.
Bio-Modular shoulder p.
Biophase implant metal p.
Biotex implant metal p.
bipolar femoral head p.
bipolar hip replacement p.
Björk p.
BK p.
Blauth knee p.
Blazina p.
Bock knee p.
Bograb Universal offset
ossicular p.
Bombelli-Mathys-Morscher hip p.
bone p.
bovine collagen material p.
Brigham p.
Bryan total knee implant p.
Buchholz p.
Buechel-Pappas total ankle p.
Byars mandibular p.
CAD/CAM p.
CAD femoral stem p.
Caffinière trapeziometacarpal p.
Calandruccio cemented hip p.
calcar replacement femoral p.
Callender technique hip p.

NOTES

P

prosthesis *(continued)*
Calnan-Nicolle finger p.
Calnan-Nicolle
metatarsophalangeal p.
Calnan-Nicolle synthetic joint p.
camouflage p.
Canadian hip disarticulation p.
Capello press-fit p.
capitellocondylar unconstrained
elbow p.
Carbon Copy high performance
foot p.
Carbon Copy HP foot p.
Carbon Copy II Foot p.
Carbon Copy II Light p.
Cardona keratoprosthesis p.
carpal lunate implant p.
carpal scaphoid implant p.
Cathcart Orthocentric hip p.
CDH Precoat Plus hip p.
cementless p.
Centralign precoat hip p.
ceramic femoral head p.
ceramic ossicular p.
Ceramion p.
CFS hip p.
Charnley acetabular cup p.
Charnley cemented p.
Charnley-Hastings p.
Charnley low-friction hip p.
Charnley-Müller hip p.
Charnley total hip p.
Chatzidakis hinged Vitallium
implant p.
CHD p.
Chopart partial foot p.
Choyce MK II keratoprosthesis p.
Christiansen hip p.
Cinch instant suction B.K. p.
Cintor knee p.
Cirrus foot p.
clamshell p.
Clayton p.
Cloutier unconstrained knee p.
CML p.
Coballoy implant metal p.
cobalt-chromium-alloy p.
Co-Cr-Mo alloy p.
Co-Cr-W-Ni alloy p.
Cofield shoulder p.
cold-mold p.
cold-weld femoral p.
collar-calcar support femoral p.
College Park TruStep foot p.
Compartmental II knee p.
p. component
p. component subsidence
compression-molded p.

computer-assisted design/computer-
assisted manufacturing p.
Conaxial ankle p.
conoidal ankle p.
constrained hinged knee p.
constrained nonhinged knee p.
Continuum unconstrained p.
Contour internal p.
conventional single-axis knee p.
Coonrad hinged p.
Coonrad-Morrey elbow p.
Coonrad semiconstrained elbow p.
Corail press-fit p.
C-2 OsteoCap hip p.
CPT p.
crimped Dacron p.
cruciate condylar unconstrained p.
cruciate-retaining p.
cruciate-sacrificing p.
CSF p.
p. cup
custom p.
custom-threaded p.
DANA shoulder p.
D'Aubigne femoral p.
Deane unconstrained knee p.
DeBakey p.
debonded femoral stem p.
Dee totally constrained elbow p.
p. dehiscence
de La Caffinière
trapeziometacarpal p.
DeLaura knee p.
DeLaura-Verner knee p.
DePalma hip p.
DePuy AML Porocoat stem p.
Deune knee p.
digital p.
Dimension-C femoral stem p.
Dimension hip p.
direct-impact p.
distal radioulnar joint p.
doffing p.
donning p.
Dorrance hand p.
Dow Corning Wright finger
joint p.
p. driver
DRUJ p.
dual-lock total hip p.
Duocondylar knee p.
Duo-Lock hip p.
duopatellar unconstrained p.
Dupaco knee p.
Duracon p.
Duraloc p.
Dycor Geriatric ADL single axis
foot p.

Dynaplex knee p.
Eaton trapezium finger joint replacement p.
Edwards seamless p.
E-2 foot p.
Eftekhar-Charnley hip p.
Eftekhar long-stem p.
Eicher femoral p.
Eicher hip p.
Eilers-Armstrong unicompartmental knee p.
elbow p.
Endolite p.
Endo-Model hinged knee p.
Endo-Model rotating knee joint p.
Endo-Model sled p.
Endo rotating knee joint p.
energy storing foot p.
Engh porous metal hip p.
Englehardt femoral p.
English-McNab shoulder p.
Entegra p.
EPTFE graft p.
Eriksson knee p.
Evolution hip p.
Ewald unconstrained elbow p.
Exeter cemented hip p.
Exeter-Femora press fit p.
femoral neck p.
finger joint implant p.
Finney p.
Finney-Flexirod p.
Finn hinged knee p.
fixed femoral head p.
flanged revision p.
Flatt finger-joint p.
Flatt finger-thumb p.
Flex-Foot Modular III p.
FLEX H/A total ossicular p.
Flex-Sprint p.
Flex-Walk p.
Flex-Walk II p.
fluid p.
foot p.
forearm lift-assist p.
forged cobalt-chromium alloy p.
four-bar linkage on knee p.
four-bar polycentric knee p.
Free-Flow system p.
Freeman-high neck press fit p.
Freeman modular total hip p.
Freeman-Samuelson knee p.

Freeman-Swanson knee p.
F.R. Thompson femoral p.
fully constrained tricompartmental knee p.
Gaffney ankle p.
Galante hip p.
Gemini hip system p.
Genesis knee p.
GeoFlex knee p.
Geomedic total knee p.
Geometric total knee p.
Gerard p.
Gianturco p.
Gilfillan humeral p.
Giliberty acetabular p.
Giliberty femoral neck p.
Giliberty hip p.
Gillette joint p.
Gillies p.
Girard keratoprosthesis p.
Gore-Tex knee p.
great toe implant p.
Greifer p.
Greissinger foot p.
Gripper acetabular cup p.
Gristina-Webb p.
grit-blasted p.
Gritti-Stokes knee p.
Gruppe wire p.
GSB elbow p.
GSB expanded version for knee p.
Guepar hinged knee p.
Guilford-Wright p.
Gunston-Hult knee p.
Gunston polycentric knee p.
Gustilo-Bias p.
Gustilo hip p.
Gustilo knee p.
Gustilo unconstrained p.
HA 65101 implant metal p.
Hamas upper limb p.
hand p.
hand-glove p.
Hanger ComfortFlex knee p.
Hanslik patellar p.
Harken p.
Harris cemented hip p.
Harris Design femoral p.
Harris-Galante porous hip p.
Harris Micromini p.
Hastings hip p.
Haynes-Stellite implant metal p.

NOTES

P

prosthesis *(continued)*
HD-2 cemented hip p.
HD-2 total hip p.
heat-cured acrylic femoral head p.
Hedley-Hungerford hip p.
Henschke-Mauch SNS knee p.
Henschke-Mauch SNS lower
 limb p.
Herbert knee p.
Hexcel knee p.
Hexcel total condylar p.
HG multilock hip p.
Hinderer malar p.
hinged constrained knee p.
hinged great toe replacement p.
hinged implant p.
hinged total knee p.
hip disarticulation p.
hip replacement p.
Hittenberger p.
homograft p.
Hosmer WALK p.
Howmedica Kinematic II knee p.
Howmedica PCA p.
Howorth p.
Howse p.
Howse-Coventry p.
HPS II total hip p.
HSS total condylar knee p.
Hungerford-Kenna PCA p.
Hunter Silastic p.
Hunter tendon p.
Hydra-Cadence knee p.
hydraulic knee unit p.
Hydroxial hip p.
I-beam hemiarthroplasty hip p.
ICLH ankle p.
ICLH knee p.
Identifit hip p.
immediate postoperative p. (IPOP)
Impact modular porous p.
Impact total hip p.
Implant Technology LSF p.
Index p.
Indiana conservative p.
Indong Oh hip p.
Infinity modular hip p.
Inronail finger or toenail p.
Insall-Burstein semiconstrained
 tricompartmental knee p.
Integral Interlok femoral p.
Integrity acetabular cup p.
Intelligent Prosthesis Plus p.
p. interface
Intermedics Natural-Knee knee p.
Inter-Op acetabular p.
Inter-Op hip p.
Interseal Variant I–IV p.

Iowa internal p.
Iowa total hip p.
ischial weightbearing p. (IWP)
Ishizuki unconstrained elbow p.
isoelastic pelvic p.
Ivalon p.
Jaffe-Capello-Averill hip p.
Jaffe press-fit p.
Jewett p.
Jobst p.
Johnson-Elloy accord
 unconstrained p.
Johnston-Iowa hip p.
Jonas p.
Jonathan Livingston Seagull
 patellar p.
Joplin toe p.
Judet Press-Fit hip p.
Keller bunionectomy with p.
Kessler p.
Kinematic fully constrained
 tricompartmental knee p.
Kinematic II rotating hinge total
 knee p.
Kinemax Plus knee p.
Kirschner Medical Dimension p.
Kirschner total shoulder p.
KMP femoral stem p.
knee p.
Koenig MPJ p.
Krause-Wolfe p.
K2 sensation p.
Kudo unconstrained elbow p.
Küntscher humeral p.
Lacey fully constrained
 tricompartmental knee p.
Lacey hinged knee p.
LaGrange-Letoumel hip p.
Laing hip cup p.
Lanceford p.
Landers-Foulks p.
LAPOC p.
LaPorta total toe p.
LCS meniscal bearing
 semiconstrained p.
LCS New Jersey knee p.
LCS rotating platform
 semiconstrained p.
LCS substituting semiconstrained p.
LCS universal APG
 semiconstrained p.
Leake Dacron mandible p.
Leinbach femoral p.
Leinbach hip p.
Lewis expandable adjustable p.
 (LEAP)
Lewis Trapezio p.
Ling cemented hip p.

Link Endo-Model rotational
knee p.
Link MP hip noncemented
reconstruction p.
Lippman hip p.
Lisfranc below-knee p.
Liverpool elbow p.
Liverpool knee p.
locking p.
London unconstrained elbow p.
Longevity V-Lign hip p.
Lo-Por vascular graft p.
Lord Press-Fit hip p.
Lotus unicompartment p.
low-contact stress
semiconstrained p.
Lowe-Miller unconstrained elbow p.
lower extremity p.
lower limb p. (LLP)
low-neck femoral p.
low-profile femoral p.
Lubinus knee p.
lunate acrylic cement wrist p.
Lunceford-Pilliar-Engh hip p.
Lund prototype unicompartment p.
MacIntosh hip p.
MacIntosh tibial plateau p.
MacNab-English shoulder p.
Macrofit hip p.
madreporic hip p.
malleus-incus p.
Mallory p.
Mallory-Head I, II p.
Mallory-Head porous primary
femoral p.
Mallory-Head total hip p.
manual locking knee p.
Marlex methyl methacrylate p.
Marmor modular knee p.
Master step foot p.
Matchett-Brown cemented hip p.
Matchett-Brown internal p.
Mathys p.
Matrol femoral head p.
Mayo semiconstrained elbow p.
Mayo total ankle p.
Mazas totally constrained elbow p.
McBride femoral p.
McBride-Moore p.
McGehee elbow p.
McKee-Farrar total hip p.
McKee femoral p.

McKee totally constrained elbow p.
McKeever-Collison long-stem p.
McKeever-MacIntosh tibial
plateau p.
McKeever patellar cap p.
McKeever Vitallium knee p.
McNaught p.
MCP finger joint p.
Mecring acetabluar p.
Mediloy implant metal p.
medium profile femoral p.
medullary p.
metal-backed plastic-on-metal p.
metal femoral head p.
metal-on-metal articulating
intervertebral disk p.
metaphysial head resection with p.
MG II knee p.
Michael Reese articulated p.
Michele long-stem p.
Microloc knee p.
Microvel p.
migration of p.
Miller-Galante hip p.
Miller-Galante II knee p.
Minneapolis hip p.
Mittlemeir ceramic hip p.
Mittlemeir noncemented femoral p.
modified Moore hip locking p.
modular Austin Moore hip p.
modular Iowa Precoat total hip p.
modular total hip p.
modular unicompartmental knee p.
Monk hip p.
monoblock femoral stem p.
monolithic A1203 cup p.
Moon-Robinson stapes p.
Moore femoral neck p.
Moore hip p.
Moretz p.
Moseley glenoid rim p.
MP35N implant metal p.
MST-6A1-4V implant metal p.
Mueli wrist p.
Mueller-Charnley hip p.
Mueller dual-lock hip p.
Mueller total hip replacement p.
Muller p.
Mulligan Silastic p.
multiaxis p.
Multiflex foot p.

NOTES

P

prosthesis *(continued)*
Multi-Lock hip p.
multiradius unconstrained p.
Murray knee p.
Murray and Welch-BDH p.
myoelectric control p.
Naden-Rieth p.
Natural-Hip p.
Natural-Knee unconstrained p.
Natural-Lok acetabular cup p.
NEB total hip p.
Neer humeral replacement p.
Neer shoulder p. (I, II)
Neer umbrella p.
Neer-Vitallium humeral p.
Neibauer-Cutter p.
New Jersey hemiarthroplasty p.
New Jersey LCS shoulder p.
New Jersey LCS total knee p.
Newton ankle p.
Nexus hip p.
Nicoll tendon p.
Niebauer finger-joint replacement p.
Niebauer metacarpophalangeal joint
  Silastic p.
Niebauer trapezium replacement p.
Noiles fully constrained
  tricompartmental knee p.
nonhinged knee p.
nonhinged linked p.
Normalize Press-Fit hip p.
Norwich press fit p.
nudge control on p.
ocular p.
Odland ankle p.
Oh cemented hip p.
Oh Press-Fit hip p.
Oh-Spectron p.
Oklahoma ankle p.
Omnifit dual geometry
  microstructured p.
Omnifit HA hip stem p.
Omnifit knee p.
Omnifit PSL microstructured p.
OmniFlex hip p.
Opti-Fix femoral p.
Opti-Fix I, II p.
Oregon Poly II ankle p.
Orthochrome implant metal p.
Orthofix p.
Ortholoc implant metal p.
Ortholoc II unconstrained p.
orthopaedic p.
p. and orthosis (P&O)
osseointegrated p.
ossicular chain replacement p.
OsteoCap hip p.
Osteolock hip p.

Osteonics hip p.
Otto Bock dynamic p.
Overdyke hip p.
Oxford meniscal unicompartment p.
Padgett p.
painful femoral head p.
Paladon p.
Paltrinieri-Trentani p.
Panje voice button p.
partial ossicular
  reconstruction/replacement p.
partial ossicular replacement p.
  (PORP)
patellar tendon-bearing below-
  knee p.
PCA Original p.
PCA Standard p.
PCA unconstrained
  tricompartmental p.
PCA unicompartmental knee p.
PC Performer knee p.
pegged tibial p.
Perfecta hip p.
Perfecta I, II p.
Performance knee p.
Peri-Loc p.
PFC curved unconstrained p.
PFC femoral p.
Phoenix total hip p.
Pillet hand p.
Pilliar p.
piston p.
Plasticor p.
Plasti-Pore ossicular replacement p.
Plastiport TORP p.
Plystan p.
Polycel bone composite p.
polycentric knee p.
polycentric unconstrained p.
Poly-Dial p.
polyethylene patellar implant p.
polyethylene talar p.
polypropylene p.
porcine p.
Porocoat AML noncemented p.
Porometal noncemented femoral p.
porous-coated anatomic p.
porous-coated femur p.
porous-coated hip p.
porous surfaced p.
Precision Osteolock femoral p.
Precision Osteolock hip p.
precoat hip p.
Precoat Plus femoral p.
Premier press fit p.
press-fit condylar total knee p.
Pritchard II elbow p.
Pritchard total elbow p.

Pritchard-Walker semiconstrained
  elbow p.
Pritchard-Walker total elbow p.
Profile hip p.
ProForma p.
Proplast p.
PROSTALAC total hip p.
PROSTALAC total joint p.
prosthetic antibiotic-loaded acrylic
  cement total joint p.
Protasul femoral p.
Protasul-10 noncemented femoral p.
Protasul-64 WF Zweymuller
  femoral p.
Protek p.
provisional p.
proximal humeral p.
proximal third femoral p.
PTB-SC-SP p.
PTB supracondylar p.
PTB suprapatellar p.
PTS soft wedge p.
Quantum Foot p.
radial head implant p.
Radovan tissue expander p.
Ranawat-Burstein hip p.
Randelli shoulder p.
Rastelli p.
Reflection I p.
Reflection Interfit p.
Reflection V p.
Re-Flex VSP p.
retaining knee p.
Reverdin p.
Richards hip p.
Richards maximum contact cruciate-
  sparing p.
Richard Smith p.
Richards Spectron metal-backed
  acetabular p.
Richards Zirconia femoral head p.
Ring knee p.
Ring total hip p.
Ring UPM press-fit p.
RMC p.
RM isoelastic hip p.
Robert Brigham semiconstrained p.
Robert Brigham total knee p.
Rock-Mulligan p.
Roper-Day p.
Rosenfeld hip p.
rotating femoral head p.

rotating hinge knee p.
Rothman Institute femoral p.
Roy-Camile p.
SACH foot p.
sacrificing knee p.
saddle p.
SAF p.
SAFE II p.
Salzer p.
Sampson p.
Sarmiento STH-2 hip p.
Sauerbruch p.
Savastano Hemi-Knee p.
Savastano unconstrained p.
Savastano unicompartment p.
Sbarbaro hip p.
Sbarbaro tibial plateau p.
Scarborough p.
Schlein semiconstrained elbow p.
Schlein total elbow p.
Schlein trisurface ankle p.
Schuknecht Gelfoam wire p.
Schuknecht Teflon wire piston p.
seating of p.
Seattle Foot p.
Secur-Fit HA PSL X'tra p.
Select ankle p.
Select modular shoulder p.
self-bearing ceramic hip p.
self-centering Universal hip p.
semiconstrained tricompartmental
  knee p.
Sense-of-Feel p.
SensorHand p.
Sharrard-Trentani p.
Shaw-Sgarlato hammertoe
  implant p.
Sheehan knee p.
Sherfee p.
Shier knee p.
shoulder disarticulation p.
Silastic ball spacer p.
Silastic radial head p.
Silastic standard elastometer p.
Silastic thumb p.
Silflex intramedullary p.
silicone trapezium p.
single-axis ankle p.
sintered implant p.
Sinterlock implant metal p.
Sivash hip p.
SMA p.

NOTES

prosthesis *(continued)*

Smith ankle p.
Smith-Brown long-stem p.
Smith-Petersen hip cup p.
SMO p.
solid ankle, cushioned heel p.
Solution p.
Souter-Strathclyde elbow p.
Souter unconstrained elbow p.
Spectron hip p.
Speed radius cap p.
spherocentric fully constrained
  tricompartmental knee p.
Spotorno hip p.
Springlite lower limb p.
S-ROM Arthropor I–III p.
S-ROM Arthropor oblong p.
S-ROM femoral stem p.
S-ROM hip p.
S-ROM super cup p.
S-ROM ZZT I, II p.
stainless steel implant metal p.
Stanmore shoulder p.
Stanmore totally constrained
  elbow p.
stemmed tibial p.
Stenzel rod p.
Stevens-Street elbow p.
St. Georg-Buchholz ankle p.
St. Georg fully constrained p.
St. Georg sledge
  unicompartment p.
STH-2 hip p.
St. Jude p.
Street-Stevens humeral p.
substituting knee p.
suction suspension p.
Sulzer p.
SuperCup acetabular cup p.
Sure-Flex p.
surgical p.
Surgitek p.
Sutter double-stem silicone
  implant p.
Sutter MCP finger joint p.
Swanson finger joint p.
Swanson flexible hallux valgus p.
Swanson great toe p.
Swanson metacarpal p.
Swanson metatarsal p.
Swanson Silastic elbow p.
Swanson T-shaped great toe
  Silastic p.
Swanson wrist p.
Syme amputation p.
Syme foot p.
Synatomic total knee p.
synthetic p.

Taperloc femoral p.
TARA total hip p.
Target p.
Tavernetti-Tennant knee p.
TCCK unconstrained knee p.
Teflon tri-leaflet p.
p. template
tendon p.
Thackray hip p.
Tharies hip replacement p.
thermomechanical implant metal p.
T28 hip p.
Thompson femoral neck p.
Thompson hemiarthroplasty hip p.
Thompson-Parkridge-Richards
  ankle p.
threaded titanium acetabular p.
  (TTAP)
thrust plate p. (TPP)
Ti-Bac II hip p.
tibial plateau p.
Ti/CoCr hip p.
Ti-Con p.
Tilastin hip p.
Tillman p.
Titan cemented hip p.
titanium hip p.
titanium implant p.
Ti-Thread p.
Titian hip p.
Tivanium hip p.
Tivanium implant metal p.
TMA p.
toe p.
TORP p.
total articular replacement
  arthroplasty p.
Total Concept ankle/foot p.
total condylar p. III (TCP-III)
total condylar III fully
  constrained p.
total condylar knee p.
total condylar semiconstrained
  tricompartmental p.
total hip replacement p.
total joint replacement p.
Total Knee p.
total knee replacement p.
total ossicular replacement p.
  (TORP)
Total Shock p.
Townley-horizontal platform p.
Townley TARA p.
Townley total knee p.
TPR ankle p.
Trac II knee p.
transtibial immediate
  postoperative p.

trapezial p.
trapeziometacarpal joint
  replacement p.
trapezium implant p.
Trapezoidal-28 hip p.
Trapezoidal-28 internal p.
TR-28 hip p.
Triad p.
trial p.
Tri-Axial p.
triaxial semiconstrained elbow p.
tricompartmental knee p.
Tricon-M cruciate-sparing p.
Tricon-M patellar p.
trileaflet p.
Tri-Lock press-fit p.
Trilogy p.
Tronzo p.
Trow Bridge Terra-Round all-
  terrain p.
trunnion-bearing hip p.
TruStep foot p.
TTAP p.
TTAP-ST acetabular p.
TT Pylon p.
Turner p.
two-prong stem finger p.
UCI ankle p.
UCI unconstrained p.
UHMWPE p.
ulnar head implant p.
Ultimate knee p.
unconstrained tricompartmental
  knee p.
unicompartmental knee p.
unicondylar p.
Universal I, II p.
Universal femoral head p.
Universal hip p.
upper extremity myoelectric p.
upper limb p. (ULP)
Valls hip p.
Vanghetti limb p.
Varikopf hip p.
VerSys p.
Viladot p.
Vinertia implant metal p.
Vitallium humeral replacement p.
Vitallium-W implant metal p.
Volz wrist p.
Wadsworth unconstrained elbow p.
Wagner p.

Walldius Vitallium mechanical
  knee p.
Warsaw hip p.
Waugh knee p.
Waugh total ankle replacement p.
Wayfarer modifiable foot p.
Weller total hip joint p.
well-seated p.
Whitesides Ortholoc II condylar
  femoral p.
Whitesides total knee p.
William Harris hip p.
Wilson-Burstein hip internal p.
Wright knee p.
Wright titanium p.
wrist joint implant p.
Xenophor femoral p.
Young hinged knee p.
Young-Vitallium hinged p.
Zimaloy femoral head p.
Zimaloy implant metal p.
Zimmer Centralign Precoat hip p.
Zimmer hip p.
Zimmer shoulder p.
Zimmer tibial p.
Zirconia femoral head p.
Zirconia orthopedic p.
zirconium oxide ceramic p.
Z-stent p.
ZTT I, II acetabular cup p.
Zweymuller cementless hip p.
prosthesis-cement interface
prosthetic
  p. ambulation
  American Board of Certification of
    Orthotics and P.'s
  American Hand P.'s (AHP)
  p. antibiotic-loaded acrylic cement
    (PROSTALAC)
  p. antibiotic-loaded acrylic cement
    total joint prosthesis
  p. arthroplasty
  Cirrus foot p.
  p. cone
  p. disk nucleus (PDN)
  p. disk nucleus device
  p. femorodistal graft
  p. fitting
  p. foam
  p. gait training
  p. hemiarthroplasty
  p. hook

NOTES

P

prosthetic *(continued)*
    p. intervention
    p. and orthotic (P&O)
    p. patella
    P. Problem Inventory Scale
    P. Problem Inventory Scale
      classification
    p. replacement
    p. socket
    p. spacer
    p. speech aid
    p. stance phase shock
    p. stem lateral fin
    p. support
    p. training
Flex-Walk
    F.-W. II prosthesis
    F.-W. prosthesis
    F.-W. II prosthetic foot
prosthetics
prosthetist
prosthetist/orthotist
ProStretch exerciser
Protasul
    P. femoral prosthesis
    P. implant metal
**Protasul-10 noncemented femoral
prosthesis**
**Protasul-64 WF Zweymuller femoral
prosthesis**
Pro-Tec patellar tendon strap
protection
    digital artery p.
    p. plate
    p., restricted activity, ice,
      compression, elevation (PRICE)
protective
    p. extension reaction
    p. limitation of range of motion
    p. shield
    p. weightbearing
protector
    Alvarado collateral ligament p.
    ankle ligament p. (ALP)
    Bandage Gard cast p.
    Cast Gard cast p.
    grooved p.
    Heelbo decubitus heel/elbow p.
    Jurgan pinball pin p.
    Meds eye p.
    P. meniscus suturing system
    M-F heel p.
    Ortho-Foam p.
    Patellar Band knee p.
    ROHO heel p.
    Seal-Tight cast p.
    ShowerSafe waterproof cast and
      bandage p.

    The Heeler inflatable heel p.
    tissue p.
Protecto splint
Protege manual flexion distraction table
protein
    bone morphogenetic p. (BMP)
    cartilage oligomeric matrix p.
      (COMP)
    C-reactive p.
    dietary p.
    IGF-binding p.
    p. malnutrition
    morphogenetic p.
    Ne-Osteo bone morphogenic p.
protein-1
    osteogenic p.-1 (OP-1)
protein-based bone graft substitute
Protek prosthesis
proteoglycan synthesis
prothelen set
ProThotics insole
prothrombin time (PT)
prothrombotic state
protocol
    Bruce p.
    Duran-Houser p.
    Evans-Burkhalter p.
    Mann p.
    Marx osteoradionecrosis p.
    North American Malignant
      Hyperthermia p.
    p. of Walsh
proton density
Protoplast cement
Protouch synthetic orthopedic padding
ProTrac
    P. alignment guide
    P. cruciate reconstruction system
    P. measurement device
    P. system for knee surgery
protraction
protractor
    arthrodial p.
    Demariniff p.
    triplanar p.
    Zimmer p.
protruding disk
protrusio
    p. acetabuli
    p. cage
    p. deformity
    p. ring
    p. shell
protrusion
    central disk p.

disk p.
p. distance
lateral disk p.
medial disk p.
p. of the navicular
protuberans
dermatofibrosarcoma p.
proud flesh
Providence Scoliosis System
provisional
p. amputation
p. calcification
p. callus
p. fixation
P. Fixation TC-100 plating system
p. prosthesis
p. stabilization
Proxiderm
P. procedure
P. wound closure system
proximal
p. annular pulley of the thumb
p. articular facet angle
p. articular set angle (PASA)
p. bow position
p. carpal row
p. cement spacer
p. communicating branch (PCB)
p. compression test
p. and distal realignment
p. drill-guide assembly
p. end tibia fracture
p. femoral epiphysiolysis
p. femoral focal deficiency
p. femoral fracture
p. femoral metaphysial shortening
p. femoral resection
p. femur
p. fibula
p. fibular facet
p. focal femoral deficiency (PFFD)
p. humeral fracture
p. humeral prosthesis
p. humerus
p. interlocking
p. interphalangeal (PIP)
p. interphalangeal/distal
  interphalangeal (PIP/DIP)
p. interphalangeal joint (PIPJ)
p. interphalangeal joint approach
p. intrinsic release
p. latency

p. locking
p. medial brim
p. metatarsal approach
p. midpatellar medial and lateral
  portals
p. nerve release
p. phalangeal epiphysiodesis
p. phalanx (PP)
p. phocomelia
p. portion
p. radioulnar articulation
p. radius
p. reference axis (PFA)
p. row carpectomy
p. set angle deviation
p. subungual onychomycosis (PSO)
p. tendon rupture
p. thigh band
p. third (P/3)
p. third femoral prosthesis
p. third of shaft
p. tibia
p. tibial metaphysial fracture
p. tibial plateau
p. tibiofibular joint
p. tibiofibular joint dislocation
p. tibiofibular subluxation
p. tibiofibular synostosis
p. ulna
p. Wagner metaphysial shortening
proximal-to-distal
p.-t.-d. dissection technique
p.-t.-d. ring
proximoataxia
proximolateral
prune-belly syndrome
PS
primary stem
PSB
patellar stabilizing brace
PSC
pronation/spring control
PSDK
poststatic dyskinesia
pseudankylosis
pseudarthrosis, pseudoarthrosis
ball-and-socket giant p.
closed p.
congenital tibial p.
documented p.
extraarticular p.

NOTES

P

pseudarthrosis *(continued)*
    failed back syndrome with
      documented p.
    fibular p.
    Girdlestone p.
    interspinous p.
    radial p.
    p. rate
    p. repair
    synovial p.
    tibial p.
pseudoacetabulum
pseudoachondroplasia
pseudoanemia
    athlete's p.
    dilutional p.
pseudoaneurysm
pseudoarthritis
    ball-and-socket giant p.
    congenital p.
pseudoarthrosis *(var. of* pseudarthrosis)
pseudoarticulation
pseudo-Babinski sign
pseudoboutonnière deformity
pseudocapsule chondrosarcoma
pseudoclaudication
pseudoclawing
pseudocortex
pseudocoxalgia
pseudocyst
    calcaneal p.
pseudodislocation
pseudoepiphysis
pseudoexostosis
pseudofacilitation
pseudofracture
    milkman's p.
pseudogamekeeper's injury
pseudogout
pseudohead
pseudo-Hurler deformity
pseudohypertrophic dystrophy
pseudohypertrophy
pseudohypoparathyroidism
pseudo-Jones fracture
pseudometatarsal head
pseudomyotonic discharge
pseudoneoplastic lesion
pseudoneuroma
pseudoosteomalacic pelvis
pseudoosteomyelitis
pseudoparalysis
    congenital atonic p.
    Parrot p.
pseudoperiosteal reaction
pseudopodium
pseudopolyphasic action potential
pseudo-Pott disease

pseudoradicular syndrome
pseudosarcomatous
    p. fasciitis
    p. fibromatosis
    p. reaction
pseudostability test
pseudosubluxation
pseudotendon
pseudothrombophlebitis (PTP)
pseudotumorous mucin deposition
pseudovarus
    cubitus p.
PSIS
    posterior sacroiliac spine
    posterior superior iliac spine
PSO
    proximal subungual onychomycosis
psoas
    p. abscess
    p. muscle
    p. tendon syndrome
psoriasis
    arthritis-associated p.
psoriatic arthritis
psychogenic equinovarus
psychological adjustment
psychomotor
psychosomatic
PT
    physical therapy
    physical training
    pronator teres
    prothrombin time
      PT tilt table
PTB
    patellar tendon-bearing
    pretibial bearing
    pretibial buttress
      PTB ankle-foot orthosis
      PTB brace
      PTB cast
      PTB plastic orthosis
      PTB supracondylar prosthesis
      PTB suprapatellar prosthesis
PTBO
    patellar tendon-bearing orthosis
PTBS
    patellar tendon-bearing suspension
PTB-SC-SP
    patellar tendon-bearing–supracondylar-
      suprapatellar
      PTB-SC-SP prosthesis
PTD
    permanent and total disability
pterygium colli
pterygoid
    p. bone

p. chest
p. plate

PTFE
polytetrafluoroethylene
PTFE graft

PTFL
posterior talofibular ligament

PTI
pressure-time integral

PTN
posterior tibial nerve

PTP
posterior tibial pulse
pseudothrombophlebitis

PTS
patellar tendon socket
patellar tendon stabilization
PTS knee brace
PTS soft wedge prosthesis

PTT
partial thromboplastin time
patellar tendon transfer
posterior tibial tendinitis
posterior tibial tendon
PTT insufficiency

PTTD
posterior tibial tendon dysfunction

pubalgia

pubic
p. bone
p. diastasis
p. fascia
p. osteolysis
p. pad
p. ramus
p. symphysis

pubiotomy

pubis
osteitis p.
osteitis necroticans p.
symphysis p.

pubocapsular ligament
pubococcygeus
pubofemoral ligament
puboischial area
puborectalis
Pucci
P. Air orthotic
P. pediatrics hand orthosis
P. rehab knee orthosis
P. splint

pucker sign

Puddu
P. drill guide
P. tendon technique

pudendal
p. artery
p. block
p. nerve injury
p. neuritis

Pudenz flushing chamber
puerperal synovitis
Pugh
P. driver
P. hip pin
P. plate
P. sliding nail
P. traction

Pugil stick injury
Puka chisel
Pul-Ez
P.-E. exerciser
P.-E. shoulder pulley

pull
p. screw
spinous p.

pulled elbow
puller
Ultra-Drive plug p.

pulley
A1–A4 anular p.
C1–C3 cruciate p.
p. exercise
fibroosseous p.
Flex Ranger stretch cable with p.
Home Ranger shoulder p.
Preston overhead p.
Pul-Ez shoulder p.
Range-Master p.
p. reconstruction
SABA p.
shoulder p.
weights and p.'s

pull-out
p.-o. button
p.-o. strength
p.-o. suture

pulmonary
p. atelectasis
p. barotrauma
p. complication
p. embolism
p. osteoarthropathy
p. osteodystrophy

NOTES

P

pulp
    p. amputation
    p. approach
    finger p.
    p. flap
    plantar toe p.
    p. traction
pulposus
    herniated nucleus p. (HNP)
    nucleus p.
pulpy nucleus
pulsatile
    p. hypothermic perfusion
    p. jet lavage
    p. pneumatic plantar-compression
      device
    p. pressure lavage
pulsating
    p. electromagnetic field
    p. hematoma
Pulsavac
    P. irrigation
    P. lavage
    P. III wound débridement system
pulse
    blood volume p. (BVP)
    dorsalis pedis p.
    dorsal pedal p.
    intact peripheral p.'s
    p. irrigator
    p. oximeter
    posterior tibial p. (PTP)
    p. status-pull test
    p. volume recorder (PVR)
pulsed
    p. diathermy
    p. electric magnetic field bone
      growth stimulation
    p. electromagnetic field (PEMF)
    p. galvanic stimulator
    p. lavage
    p. short-wave therapy
    p. ultrasound
pulselessness
Pulvertaft
    P. end-to-end suture
    P. fish-mouth stitch
    P. interweave suture
    P. weave tendon repair technique
pulvinar
    p. fibrofatty debris
    p. region
pumice stone
pump
    ALZET continuous infusion
      osmotic p.
    ankle rehab p.
    arthroscopic p.

    A-V Impulse foot p.
    p. bump
    p. bump area
    p. bump deformity
    p. bump exostosis
    cement p.
    continuous wave arthroscopy p.
    extremity p.
    EZ hand p.
    intermittent extremity p.
    P. It Up pneumatic socket volume
      management system
    Jobst athrombotic p.
    knee p.
    Linvatec arthroscopic infusion p.
    morphine p.
    Multipulse 1000 compression p.
    pain control infusion p.
    PainFree p.
    sequential extremity p.
    Vacumix vacuum p.
    venous foot p.
pump-handle rib motion
PumpPals insole
punch
    Acufex rotary p.
    arthroscopic p.
    p. biopsy
    bone graft p.
    bone hole p.
    boxer's p.
    Caspari suture p.
    Casselberry suture p.
    cervical laminectomy p.
    Charnley femoral prosthesis
      neck p.
    cruciate p.
    Deyerle p.
    p. drunk syndrome
    p. forceps
    Hirsch hypophysial p.
    I-beam cement p.
    Kerrison p.
    keyhole p.
    Osborne p.
    Rowe glenoid p.
    Schlesinger p.
    suction p.
    tibial p.
    tubular p.
punctata
    chondrodysplasia p.
    keratosis p.
puncture
    p. fracture
    lumbar p. (LP)
    spinal p.

p. wound
p. wound osteochondritis
Puno-Winter-Byrd (PWB)
P.-W.-B. system
purchase
bony p.
p. and press the ground
socket p.
toe-ground p.
Purdue pegboard
pure
p. limb apraxia limb asymmetry
p. syndactyly
PureFix hydroxylapatite
purposeful activity
purpura
p. fulminans
meningococcal p.
pursestring suture
purulent
p. material
p. synovitis
push
p. cuff
knee-chest p.
P. medical brace
prone sacral p.
spinous p.
Push-Ease
P.-E. Quad Cuff
P.-E. wheelchair glove
pusher
Charnley femoral prosthesis p.
femoral component p.
hemispherical p.
hook p.
Jacobson suture p.
knot p.
metal p.
Patella P.
Revo loop handle knot p.
push-off
great toe p.-o.
p.-o. by great toe
p.-o. phase of gait
p.-o. velocity
push-pull
p.-p. activity
p.-p. ankle stress view
p.-p. hip view
p.-p. instability

p.-p. move
p.-p. test
push-up
p.-u. block
p.-u. test
pustulotic osteoarthropathy
putative segmental instantaneous axis of rotation
Puth abduction splint
Putti
P. bone plast
P. bone rasp
P. knee arthrodesis
P. posterior approach
P. posterior bone block
scapular sign of P.
P. sign
P. splint
Putti-Platt
P.-P. arthroplasty
P.-P. instrumentation
P.-P. operation
P.-P. shoulder procedure
putty
AliMed p.
AlloMatrix bone graft p.
AlloMatrix injectable p.
BeOK hand exercise p.
Blue Brand Therapy P.
color-coded therapy p.
Flexi-Grip exercise p.
Grafton DBM p.
matrix Grafton p.
Thera-Plast p.
Therapy P.
PUV
positive ulnar variance
PVC
polyvinyl chloride
PVC drain
PVC tubing
PVD
peripheral vascular disease
PVD dressing
PVR
pulse volume recorder
PVS
peripheral vascular surgery
peripheral vascular system
pigmented villonodular synovitis
PW
plantar wart

NOTES

P

PWB
partial weightbearing
Puno-Winter-Byrd
    PWB transpedicular spine fixation
    system
PWC
physical work capacity
pyarthrosis
pycnodysostosis
PYD
pyridinium collagen crosslink
pyridinoline collagen crosslink
pyelogram
intravenous p.
pyknodysostosis
Pyle
bone age according to Greulich
    and P.
P. disease
pylon
AirStance p.
p. attachment plate
Icon p.
P. intramedullary nail system
metal p.
Stratus impact-reducing p.
vertical shock p.

pyocyanin
pyoderma gangrenosum
pyogenic
p. arthritis
p. bursitis
p. granuloma
p. spinal infection
p. vertebral osteomyelitis
pyogenicum
granuloma p.
pyomyositis
staphylococcal p.
Pyramesh cage
pyramid
p. attachment
suction p.
pyramidal
p. fracture
p. tract
pyridinium collagen crosslink (PYD)
pyridinoline collagen crosslink (PYD)
Pyrilinks-D urine assay
pyrolytic
p. carbon
p. carbon device
Pyrost bone graft material

Q
- Q angle
- Q disk
- Q Star Voyager pressure reduction mattress

Q angle
QCT
- quantitative computed tomography

QF
- quadratus femoris

qigong
Qingyangshen (QYS)
QNA
- quadriceps neutral angle

Q-Ray bracelet
QSAC
- quadrant sparing acetabular component

QSART
- quantitative sudomotor axon reflex test

QST
- quantitative sensory testing

quad
- q. bar
- q. board
- q. cane

quadpolar IF waveform
quadrangular
- q. cartilage
- q. positioning plate

quadrant
- Q. advanced shoulder brace
- q. of death
- q. sparing acetabular component (QSAC)
- q. test

quadrate
- q. ligament
- q. ligament of Denuce
- q. muscle

quadratus
- q. femoris (QF)
- q. femoris fascia
- q. femoris muscle
- q. lumborum muscle
- q. lumborum syndrome
- q. plantae muscle
- pronator q. (PQ)

quadriceps
- q. active test
- q. angle
- q. aponeurosis
- q. apron
- q. atrophy
- q. contraction test
- q. contracture
- q. contusion
- q. De Lorme boot
- q. femoris muscle
- q. femoris muscle cast
- q. jerk
- q. mechanism
- q. muscle group
- q. neutral angle (QNA)
- q. reflex
- q. strengthening exercise
- q. tendon
- q. wasting

quadricepsplasty
- Coonse-Adams q.
- Judet q.
- Thompson q.
- V-Y q.

quadriceps-setting exercise
Quadriflex
quadrilateral
- q. brim
- q. frame
- q. ischial weight-bearing socket
- q. space syndrome

quadriparesis
quadripartite bone
quadriplegia
- spastic q.
- transient q.

quadriplegic
quadruped back exercise technique
quadruple
- q. amputation
- q. complex

Quadtro
- Q. cushion
- Q. cushion with Isoflap valve

QualCare knee brace
QualCraft
- Q. ankle support
- Q. short elastic wrist support
- Q. splint
- Q. strap

quality
- Agency for Healthcare Research and Q. (AHCPR)
- q. of life
- motion q.
- Q. of Well-Being Scale

quantitative
- q. computed tomography (QCT)
- q. mechanical pain testing
- q. sensory testing (QST)

quantitative *(continued)*
q. sudomotor axon reflex test
(QSART)
q. ultrasound (QUS)
quantity
scalar q.
vector q.
Quantum
Q. foot
Q. Foot prosthesis
Q. 400 traction
Quartzo device
quasi-independent Y-axis movement
quasistatic stressed position
Quebec Back Pain Disability Scale
Queckenstedt
Q. maneuver
Q. phenomenon
Q. sign
Q. test
Queckenstedt-Stookey test
Quengel
Q. apparatus
Q. cast
Q. device
Q. hinge
Quénu-Küss tarsometatarsal injury
classification
Quénu nail plate removal technique
Quervain
Q. disease
Q. fracture
question
Enneking q.
questionnaire
American Academy of Orthopaedic
Surgeons/Hip Society q.
Behavioral Assessment of Pain Q.
Children's Comprehensive Pain Q.
(CCPQ)
Cincinnati knee scoring q.
Clinical Analysis Q. (CAQ)
Community Integration Q. (CIQ)
Coping Strategies Q. (CSQ)
Disabilities of Arm, Shoulder and
Hand q.
Foot Function Index q.
Foot Health Status Q.
Frank Noyes function q.
Functional Status Q. (FSQ)
Headache Assessment Q. (HAQ)
International Knee Ligament
Standard Evaluation q.
Jan van Breemen Function Q.
(JVBF)
Kenny Self-Care Q.
Lambeth disability screening q.
Levine orthopedic outcomes q.

Lysholm knee scoring q.
McGill Pain Q.
McMaster-Toronto arthritis patient
preference disability q.
Melzack Pain Q.
MFA q.
Michigan Hand Outcomes Q.
Modified American Shoulder and
Elbow Surgeons Shoulder Patient
Self-Evaluation Form patient q.
Osteoporosis Knowledge Q. (OKQ)
Physical Activity Readiness Q.
(PAR-Q)
Roland-Morris Q. (RMQ)
Short Musculoskeletal Function
Assessment q.
Shoulder Pain and Disability Index
patient q.
Shoulder Severity Index patient q.
Simple Shoulder Test patient q.
Subjective Shoulder Rating Scale
patient q.
Varni-Thompson Pediatric Pain Q.
Questus leading edge grasper-cutter
Quetelet index
QuickAnchor
Micro Q.
Mitek Micro Q.
Mitek Mini Q.
Quickbox container
QuickCast
Q. splint
Q. wrist immobilizer
Quickie
Q. Carbon wheelchair
Q. EX wheelchair
Q. GPS wheelchair
Q. GP Swing-Away wheelchair
Q. GPV wheelchair
Q. Kidz wheelchair
Q. Recliner wheelchair
Q. Ti wheelchair
Quick-Sil
Q.-S. silicone system
Q.-S. starter kit
QuickStick padding
quick stretch
QuickTack
Q. device
Q. periosteal fixation system
quiescence
quiet hip disease
Quigley traction
QuikFormables orthotic
Quik splint
Quinby pelvic fracture classification
Quincke needle

quinti
    abductor digiti q. (ADQ)
    extensor digiti q. (EDQ)
    Huber transfer of abductor
      digiti q.
    opponens digiti q. (ODQ)

quotient
    acetabular head q.
QUS
    quantitative ultrasound

NOTES

RA
> rheumatoid arthritis
>> RA factor
>> RA test

rabbeting
race-pace exercise
rachialgia
rachicentesis, rachiocentesis
rachilysis
rachiochysis
rachiodynia
rachiokyphosis
rachiomyelitis
rachioparalysis
rachiopathy
rachioplegia
rachioscoliosis
rachiotome
rachiotomy, rachitomy
rachisagra
rachischisis
rachitic
> r. cat-back
> r. pelvis
> r. rosary sign
> r. scoliosis

rachitomy (*var. of* rachiotomy)
rack
> Hausmann weight r.

racket amputation
racquetball
racquet-shaped incision
RADAR
> Rapid Assessment of Disease Activity in Rheumatology

radial
> r. agenesis
> r. antebrachial region
> r. artery
> r. artery injury
> r. bearing
> r. bone
> r. bursa
> r. clubhand
> r. collateral ligament (RCL)
> r. column
> r. deficiency
> r. deviation
> r. digital nerve
> r. drift
> r. epicondylalgia
> r. forearm flap
> r. fracture reduction
> r. head
> r. head anlage

> r. head dislocation
> r. head fracture
> r. head implant prosthesis
> r. head subluxation
> r. hemimelia
> r. laminectomy
> r. malalignment
> r. malleolus
> r. meniscal tear
> midcarpal r. (MCR)
> r. neck
> r. neck fracture
> r. nerve glove
> r. nerve injury
> r. nerve palsy
> r. phenomenon
> r. pseudarthrosis
> r. ray defect
> r. recession osteotomy
> r. reflex
> r. sensory nerve
> r. sensory nerve entrapment syndrome
> r. shaft
> r. sigmoid notch
> r. slab splint
> r. styloid fracture
> r. sulcus
> r. trial
> r. tuberosity
> r. tunnel
> r. tunnel syndrome
> r. wedge osteotomy
> r. wrist extensor
> r. wrist extensor tendinitis

radial-based flap
radialis
> flexor carpi r. (FCR)
> malleolus r.
> r. sign

radialized
radian
radiate ligament of head of rib
radiation-related
> r.-r. myelopathy
> r.-r. neuropathy

radiation therapy
radiatum
radical
> r. compartmental excision
> r. flexor release
> r. nail bed ablation
> r. palmar fasciectomy
> r. resection

radicotomy

radicular
    r. artery
    r. neuritis
    r. pain
radiculectomy
radiculitis
    acute brachial r.
    cervical r.
radiculomyelopathy
radiculoneuritis
radiculopathy
    cervical r.
    four-level r.
    lumbosacral r.
radicurogram
radii (*pl. of* radius)
radioactive
radiocapitate ligament
radiocapitellar
    r. articulation
    r. joint
    r. joint ganglion
    r. line
    r. subluxation
radiocarpal
    r. angle
    r. arthritis
    r. arthrodesis
    r. arthroscopy
    r. articulation
    r. dislocation
    r. instability
    r. joint
    r. ligament
    r. portal
radiodiagnostic study
radiogram
radiograph
    anterior drawer stress r.
    cross-table lateral r.
    Judet r.
    lumbopelvic r.
    Merchant r.
    plantar flexed stress r.
    skyline r.
    spot r.
    stress r.
    tangential standing r.
    Velpeau axillary r.
    weightbearing tangential r.
    West Point axillary lateral r.
radiographic
    r. avascular necrosis
    r. grid
radiography
    biplanar r.
    Broden stress r.
    carpometacarpal joint r.

    elbow r.
    flat plate r.
    flexion-extension r.
    neutron r.
    patellofemoral joint r.
    scanogram r.
    serendipity view in shoulder r.
    shoulder r.
    stress r.
    upright skeletal r.
radiohumeral
    r. articulation
    r. bursa
    r. bursitis
    r. epicondylitis
    r. joint
radioisotope
    r. clearance assay
    r. gallium scan
    r. indium-labeled white blood cell scan
    r. technetium scan
    r. thallium
radiolucency
radiolucent
    r. line
    r. nidus
    r. roll
    r. sound
    r. splint
    r. wrist fixation system
radiolunate
    r. fusion
    r. joint
    long r. (LRL)
    short r. (SRL)
radiolunotriquetral ligament
radionucleotide imaging
radionuclide bone scan
radiopaque bone cement
radioscaphocapitate (RSC)
    r. ligament
    r. ligament laxity
radioscaphoid
    r. articulation
    r. fusion
    r. joint
    r. ligament
radioscapholunate
    r. joint
    r. ligament
radiotherapy
    coxa vara deformity pelvic r.
radiotranslucent rod
radiotriquetral ligament
radioulnar
    r. articulation
    r. dislocation

r. dissociation
r. joint
r. joint injury
r. subluxation
r. surface
r. synostosis (type I, II)
radius, pl. **radii**
absent r.
r. of angulation
anular ligament of r.
distal r.
Kapandji fracture of r.
proximal r.
thrombocytopenia-absent r. (TAR)
Radley-Liebig-Brown
R.-L.-B. approach
R.-L.-B. resection
Radovan tissue expander prosthesis
ragged-red fiber
Ragnell retractor
rail
Bed-Bar support r.
Lumex Tub-Guard safety r.
Raimiste sign
Raimondi hemostatic forceps
Rainbow cast sandal
raise
single-leg toe r.
raising
contralateral straight leg r.
crossed straight leg r. (CSLR)
diurnal variation in straight leg r.
passive straight leg r.
straight leg r. (SLR)
well-leg r.
rake-handle effect
rake retractor
rales and rhonchi
Ralks
R. bone drill
R. fingernail drill
R. mallet
Ralston-Thompson pseudarthrosis technique
Raman spectroscopic imaging
ramp load
ramus
dorsal r.'s
inferior r.
ischiopubic r.
pubic r.

Ranawat-Burstein
R.-B. hip prosthesis
R.-B. porous stem
Ranawat classification
Ranawat-DeFiore-Straub
R.-D.-S. osteotomy
R.-D.-S. technique
Ranawat-Dorr-Inglis method
Rancho
R. ankle foot control device
R. anklet foot control apparatus
R. Cube System
R. external fixation instrument
R. swivel hinge
Ranchos Los Amigos Scale
Rand
R. Functional Limitations Battery
R. Physical Capacities Battery
Randelli shoulder prosthesis
random pattern flap
Raney
R. bone drill
R. flexion jacket brace
R. perforator drill
R. saw guide
Raney-Crutchfield
R.-C. drill point
R.-C. tongs
R.-C. tong traction
range
r. of excursion
r. of extension
r. of motion (ROM)
r. of motion brace
r. of motion rehabilitation
r. of motion therapeutic stretching
r. of motion therapy
Range-Master pulley
range-of-motion
r.-o.-m. exercise
r.-o.-m. measurement
r.-o.-m. restriction
r.-o.-m. testing
Ranke complex
Ransford loop
Ranvier
groove of R.
zone of R.
raphe
anterolateral r.
median r.

NOTES

Rapid Assessment of Disease Activity
  in Rheumatology (RADAR)
RAP-n-roll
Rappaport osteotomy
rarefaction
rarefying osteitis
rasp, raspatory
  Acufex convex r.
  Alexander r.
  Alexander-Farabeuf r.
  angled r.
  Arthrofile orthopaedic r.
  Aufricht glabellar r.
  Austin Moore r.
  Bacon r.
  Bardeleben r.
  Beaver-tail r.
  bell r.
  Black r.
  Bristow r.
  Brown r.
  carbon-tungsten r.
  Charnley r.
  convex r.
  Coryllos r.
  Cottle r.
  Cottle-MacKenty r.
  custom r.
  DePuy r.
  diamond r.
  Doyen costal r.
  Doyen rib r.
  Endotrac r.
  Epstein bone r.
  Farabeuf bone r.
  Farabeuf-Collin r.
  femoral r.
  first rib r.
  Fisher r.
  Fomon r.
  Gallagher r.
  glabellar r.
  Good r.
  Herczel rib r.
  Hylin r.
  interbody r.
  Israel r.
  Jansen r.
  Joseph nasal r.
  Key r.
  Kleinert-Kutz r.
  Koenig r.
  Langenbeck r.
  Lewis periosteal r.
  Mallory-Head r.
  Maltz r.
  Mathieu r.
  McCabe-Farrior r.

  Miller r.
  Nicola r.
  Nicoll r.
  Olivecrona r.
  orthopaedic r.
  Phemister r.
  r. pin
  Podiatry Institute r.
  power r.
  Putti bone r.
  rib r.
  Rubin r.
  Schneider r.
  Schneider-Sauerbruch r.
  Seawell r.
  Thompson r.
  triangular r.
  ulnar r.
  Yasargil micro r.
  Zollner r.
raspatory
  Farabeuf-Lambotte r.
Rastelli prosthesis
ratchet
  r. clamp
  r. flexor tenodesis splint
ratcheting T-handle
ratchet-type brace
ratchety weakness
rate
  basal metabolic r. (BMR)
  erythrocyte sedimentation r. (ESR)
  firing r.
  fusion nonunion r.
  heart r. (HR)
  implant survival r.
  nonunion r.
  pseudarthrosis r.
  resting heart r. (RHR)
  sedimentation r.
  steady state heart r. (SSHR)
  strontium-85 resorption r.
  vertebral osteosynthesis fusion r.
  Westergren sedimentation r.
rated perceived exertion (RPE)
Rath treatment table
rating
  American Shoulder and Elbow
    Surgeons r.
  Fitzgerald r.
  Mazur ankle r.
  McGuire r.
  occupational r.
  permanent partial disability r.
  PPD r.
ratio
  AB/AD r.
  abductor/adductor r.

ankle-brachial pressure r.
arch-height r.
Blackburne r.
Blackburn-Peel r.
bone age r.
Brattström condylar height r.
canal-to-calcar isthmus r.
carpal height r.
Dorr r.
ER/IR r.
external rotation/internal rotation r.
femur length to abdominal
   circumference r. (FL/AC)
FL/AC r.
Holdaway r.
Insall r.
Insall-Salvati r.
medialization r.
metaphysial to diaphysial width r.
patellar ligament-patellar r.
Pavlov r.
Poisson r.
respiratory exchange r.
r. scale in rehabilitation testing
VMO:VL EMG r.
waist-to-hip r.

Ratliff avascular necrosis classification
rat-tooth forceps
Rauchfuss
   R. sling
   R. triangle
rave
   fracture en r.
raw bone
ray
   r. amputation
   r. axis
   border r.
   central r.
   finger r.
   long axis r.
   metatarsal r.
   multiple r.
   Peacock transposing index r.
   plantarflexed
   pollicized r.
   r. resection
   R. screw
   stiff r.
   R. TFC threaded fusion cage
   transposing index r.

Ray-Clancy-Lemon technique
Rayhack technique
Raymond shoulder immobilizer
Raynaud
   R. disease
   R. gangrene
   R. phenomenon
   R. syndrome
Ray-Parsons-Sunday staphylorrhaphy
   elevator
Rayport muscular biopsy clamp
Ray-Tec sponge
RB1 suture
RC
   rehabilitation counseling
   rotator cuff
RCB
   rotator cuff buttress
RCL
   radial collateral ligament
RCSP
   resting calcaneal stance position
reabsorption
   bony r.
Reach Easy massager
reacher
   Double Duty cane r.
   E-Z R.
reaction
   compensation r.
   epidermophytid r.
   equilibrium r.
   exaggeration r.
   r. force
   giant cell r.
   ground r.
   hunting r.
   implant r.
   periosteal r.
   protective extension r.
   pseudoperiosteal r.
   pseudosarcomatous r.
   r. time
   vagal r.
reactive
   r. arthritis
   r. bone formation
   low-surface r.
   r. periosteal proliferation
   r. synovitis
Read gouge

R

NOTES

Real-EaSE neck and shoulder relaxer
realignment
    distal r.
    Elmslie-Trillat r.
    Galeazzi r.
    Genutrain PE patellar r.
    Hauser r.
    Hughston r.
    Insall proximal r.
    Madigan-Wissinger-Donaldson
      proximal r.
    patellar r.
    patellofemoral r.
    r. procedure
    proximal and distal r.
    Roux-Goldthwait r.
Reality Orientation Chart
reamed
    r. nail
    sequentially r.
reamer
    acetabular r.
    acorn r.
    Aequalis r.
    Anspach r.
    Arthrex coring r.
    Aufranc r.
    Austin Moore r.
    ball r.
    blunt tapered T-handled r.
    bone r.
    r. brace
    brace-type r.
    calcar r.
    Campbell r.
    cannulated Henderson r.
    chamfer r.
    Charnley deepening r.
    Charnley expanding r.
    Charnley taper r.
    Charnley trochanter r.
    cheese-grater hemispherical r.
    Christmas tree r.
    r. clamp
    concave-surface r.
    congruous cup-shaped r.
    conical r.
    corrugated r.
    cup r.
    debris-retaining r.
    deepening r.
    DePuy r.
    end-cutting r.
    expanding r.
    female r.
    femoral head bone removal r.
    fenestrated r.
    flexible medullary r.

    fluted r.
    grater r.
    Gray r.
    grooving r.
    r. guide
    Hall Versipower r.
    handle-type r.
    Harris brace-type r.
    Harris center-cutting acetabular r.
    hemispherical r.
    hollow mill r.
    humeral r.
    Indiana r.
    Intracone intramedullary r.
    intramedullary r.
    Küntscher r.
    male r.
    medullary canal r.
    Micro-Aire r.
    Mira r.
    Moore bone r.
    motorized r.
    multisized r.
    Norton ball r.
    orthopaedic r.
    Perthes r.
    power r.
    power-driven r.
    Pressure Sentinel r.
    progressively larger r.
    Richards r.
    rigid r.
    Rush rod awl r.
    Smith-Petersen r.
    spherical r.
    spiral cortical r.
    spiral trochanteric r.
    spot-face r.
    step-cut r.
    straight power r.
    Swanson r.
    tapered r.
    tapered hand r.
    T-handled r.
    triangular bone r.
    triple r.
    trochanteric r.
    Wagner acetabular r.
reaming awl
reamputation
reanastomosis of blood supply
rear-entry ACL drill guide
rearfoot
    r. deformity
    r. ligament
    r. stability system (RSS)
    r. valgus
    r. varus

re-arthroscoped
reassessment
reattachment
    Amstutz r.
    Doll trochanteric r.
    four-wire trochanter r.
    Harris four-wire trochanter r.
    Volz-Turner r.
REB band
Rebel knee brace
rebound
    r. hyperextension
    r. tenderness
rebounder
    Plyoback R.
recalcitrant
    r. neuropathic ulcer
    r. pain
    r. plantar fasciitis
receiver operating characteristic
recent dislocation
receptor
    delta r.
    epicritic r.
    epsilon r.
    kappa r.
    MV1, MV2 r.
    nociceptive r.
    opioid r.
    postural r.
    sigma r.
    stretch r.
receptor-tonus method
recess
    acetabular r.
    anular periradial r.
    Flatt r.
    lateral r.
    popliteal r.
    ulnar synovial r.
recession
    Bleck iliopsoas r.
    gastrocnemius r.
    gastrocnemius-soleus r.
    iliopsoas r.
    Strayer gastrocnemius r.
    Strayer gastrocnemius-soleus r.
    tongue-in-groove r.
    ulnar r.
recipient
    r. site
    r. team

reciprocal
    r. arm raise back exercise
      technique
    r. finger prehension orthosis
    r. innervation
    r. isokinetic testing
    r. planing instrument
    r. relaxation
reciprocating
    r. motor saw
    r. power handpiece
reciprocation gait orthosis (RGO)
reciprocator
    LSU r.
Recklinghausen
    R. canal
    R. disease
recliner
    Hydro Soothe r.
    Ortho-Biotic r.
reclining frame wheelchair
recoil
    elastic r.
Recon
    R. nail
    R. proximal drill guide bolt
reconstruction
    ACL r.
    Allman modification of Evans
      ankle r.
    Andrews iliotibial band r.
    ankle r.
    anterior capsulolabral r. (ACLR)
    arthroscopically assisted anterior
      cruciate ligament r.
    arthroscopic transhumeral r.
    augmented r.
    autogenous patellar tendon r.
    Bankart r.
    bifurcated vein graft for
      vascular r.
    Bristow shoulder r.
    Broström ligament r.
    Brown knee joint r.
    Bunnell technique of pulley r.
    capsular-shift r.
    Cho anterior cruciate ligament r.
    Chrisman-Snook r.
    Clancy-Andrews r.
    Clancy cruciate ligament r.
    complex acetabular r.
    cruciate ligament r.

R

NOTES

reconstruction *(continued)*
D'Aubigne femoral r.
D'Aubigne resection r.
Eaton-Littler ligament r.
Ecker-Lotke-Glazer tendon r.
Ellison lateral knee r.
Elmslie r.
endoscopic anterior cruciate
   ligament r.
Eriksson cruciate ligament r.
Evans calcaneal r.
Evans lateral ankle r.
exogenous r.
extraarticular r.
five-in-one knee r.
Goldner r.
hand r.
Harmon hip r.
House r.
Hughston-Degenhardt r.
Hughston-Jacobson lateral
   compartment r.
Hughston lateral compartment r.
index metacarpophalangeal joint r.
Insall anterior cruciate ligament r.
intraarticular r.
joint r.
Jones-Ellison ACL r.
juxtacubital r.
Kleinert technique of pulley r.
Krukenberg hand r.
Kugelberg r.
Lange Achilles tendon r.
Larson ligament r.
lateral compartment r.
Lee r.
L'Episcopo hip r.
ligament r.
Lister technique of pulley r.
MacIntosh over-the-top ACL r.
modified Chrisman-Snook ankle r.
Nathan-Trung modification of
   Krukenberg hand r.
Neer posterior shoulder r.
Nicholas five-in-one r.
O'Donoghue ACL r.
osteoplastic r.
r. plate
pulley r.
Rosenberg endoscopic anterior
   cruciate ligament r.
Silfverskiöld Achilles tendon r.
sternoclavicular joint r.
sural island flap for foot and
   ankle r.
Swanson r.
tenoplastic r.
thumb r.

Torg knee r.
two-stage tendon graft r.
Verdan osteoplastic thumb r.
Vulpius Achilles tendon r.
Watson-Jones r.
Whitman femoral neck r.
Zancolli r.
reconstructive measure
recorder
pulse volume r. (PVR)
recording
r. electrode
intramuscular r.
recovery
fluid attenuation inversion r.
   (FLAIR)
functional r.
motor r.
r. phase rehabilitation
postanesthesia r. (PAR)
r. room (RR)
recreational therapy (RT)
recrudescence
recruitment
r. frequency
r. interval
myopathic r.
neuropathic r.
r. pattern
rectangle
Hartshill r.
Luque r.
rectangular
r. amputation
r. awl
r. frame
rectilinear
r. bone scan
r. motion
rectus
r. abdominis flap
r. abdominis muscle
r. adductor syndrome
r. femoris
r. femoris contracture
r. femoris flap
r. femoris graft
r. femoris muscle
r. femoris tendon
r. foot type
r. hallux
metatarsus r.
r. position
r. sheath
recumbency
recumbent
r. bicycle
r. cycle

r. position
r. posture
recurrent
r. disorder
r. hyperextension
r. laryngeal nerve
r. laryngeal nerve injury
r. median nerve block
r. meningeal nerve
r. mycetoma
r. parosteal osteosarcoma
r. patellar dislocation
r. synovitis
recurvatum
r. angulation deformity
cubitus r.
genu r.
pectus r.
r. test
red
R. Cross freeze-dried allograft
r. light neon laser
r. marrow
r. muscle
r. response
Reddihough scale
redesign
job r.
Redi-Around finger splint
Rediform orthotic
Redigrip
R. knee pad
R. pressure bandage
Redi head halter
Redi-Trac
R.-T. traction apparatus
R.-T. traction device
Redi-Vac cast cutter
redressement forcé
redresser
dual pin r.
redressment
reduced
r. interference pattern
r. profile (RP)
reducible
reduction
Ace bandage r.
Agee force-couple splint r.
Allen r.
anatomic r.
Aston cartilage r.

Barsky macrodactyly r.
Becton open r.
Bell-Tawse open r.
Boitzy open r.
Burwell-Charnley classification of fracture r.
Calandriello hip r.
calcaneal fracture r.
closed r. (CR)
concentric r.
congruent r.
Cooper r.
Crego hip r.
Crosby r.
Cubbins open r.
r. deformity
delayed open r.
Dias-Giegerich open r.
Eaton closed r.
Eaton-Malerich r.
Essex-Lopresti open r.
femoral neck fracture r.
Ferguson hip r.
r. fixation
Flynn femoral neck fracture r.
force-couple splint r.
r. forceps
Fowles open r.
fracture r.
r. of fracture
fracture-dislocation r.
Hankin r.
Hastings open r.
hip r.
Houghton-Akroyd open r.
incomplete r.
indirect r.
internal fixation, closed r.
Kaplan open r.
Kinast indirect r.
King open r.
Kocher r.
Lange hip r.
Lavine r.
Lorenz hip r.
Lowell r.
manual fracture r.
McBride hallux abductovalgus r.
McBride hallux valgus r.
McKeever open r.
McReynolds open r.
Neer open r.

NOTES

reduction *(continued)*
  open r.
  r. osteotomy
  Parvin r.
  percutaneous r.
  perioperative r.
  Pratt open r.
  prone r.
  radial fracture r.
  Ridlon hip r.
  r. ring
  shoulder r.
  side posture r.
  Speed-Boyd open r.
  Speed open r.
  spondylolisthesis r.
  stable r.
  sternoclavicular joint r.
  Stimson r.
  surgical r.
  swan-neck deformity r.
  r. syndactyly
  r. technique
  tibiofibular joint r.
  trial r.
  Wayne County r.
  Weber-Brunner-Freuler open r.
Reebok
  R. shoe
  R. Slide System
  R. Step System
Reece
  R. orthopedic shoe
  R. osteotomy guide
Reed cast belt
reeducation
  muscular r.
reefing
  capsular r.
  r. procedure
reel foot
reeling gait
Reese
  R. dermatome
  R. osteotomy guide system
reevaluate
reexploration
reference
  biomechanical frame of r.
  r. electrode
referred
  r. anatomic phenomenon
  r. neuritic pain
  r. point
  r. trigger point pain
  r. trigger point phenomenon
refill
  capillary r.

reflection
  R. I, V, and FSO acetabular cup
  Campbell triceps r.
  R. Interfit prosthesis
  R. liner
  medical subcutaneous r.
  R. I prosthesis
  R. V prosthesis
  vertebral neural r.
Re-Flex
  R.-F. VSP artificial foot
  R.-F. VSP prosthesis
reflex
  absent r.
  accommodation r.
  Achilles tendon r.
  adductor r.
  anal r.
  ankle jerk r.
  antagonistic r.
  aponeurotic r.
  r. arc
  asymmetric incurvatum r.
  asymmetric tonic neck r. (ATNR)
  automatic neonatal walking r.
  axon r.
  Babinski r.
  Bekhterev deep r.
  Bekhterev-Mendel r.
  biceps r.
  blink r.
  body righting r.
  brachioradialis r.
  Brain r.
  Brudzinski r.
  bulbocavernosus r.
  Chaddock r.
  R. Comfort insole
  cremasteric r.
  crossed adductor r.
  crossed extensor r.
  crossed flexor r.
  cry r.
  cutaneous axon r.
  deep tendon r. (DTR)
  delayed r.
  deltoid r.
  depressed r.
  derotational r.
  r. development
  digital r.
  dorsal r.
  elbow r.
  equilibrium r.
  r. examination
  R. exercise and rehab equipment
  extensor thrust r.
  external hamstring r.

external oblique r.
femoral r.
finger-thumb r.
flexor withdrawal r.
r. function
gluteal r.
Gordon r.
great toe r.
R. Gun
H r.
r. hammer
hamstring r.
heel-tap r.
Hirschberg r.
Hoffmann r.
hyperactive r.
hypoactive deep tendon r.
hypothenar r.
incurvatum r.
interscapular r.
inverted radial r.
jaw opening r. (JOR)
knee flexion r.
knee jerk r.
lengthening r.
lumbar r.
Mayer r.
Mendel-Bekhterev r.
motor r.
muscle stretch r.
muscular r.
r. muscular contraction
myotatic r.
neck r.
neck-righting r.
r. neurovascular dystrophy
Oppenheim r.
palmar grasp r.
parachute r.
patellar r.
patelloadductor r.
pathologic r.
pectoral r.
placement r.
placing r.
plantar r.
positive supporting r.
postcast compression r.
postural r.
primitive r.
pronator r.
quadriceps r.

radial r.
r. rebound component of whiplash
Remak r.
righting r.
Romberg r.
scapular r.
scapulohumeral r.
slow stretch r.
sole r.
sole-tap r.
somatosomatic r.
Stookey r.
stretch r.
sudomotor startle r.
supinator jerk r.
supinator longus r.
suprapatellar r.
r. sympathetic dystrophy (RSD)
tarsophalangeal r.
tendon r.
r. therapy
r. threshold
tibioadductor r.
tilting r.
toe r.
tonic neck r.
r. tracheostomy management
triceps surae r.
ulnar r.
vertebra prominens r.
vertical suspension r.
vestibulospinal r.
viscerosomatic r.
von Bekhterev r.
wrist flexion r.
ReFlexion first MPJ implant system
reflexogenic
reflexology
refractory
r. neuroma
r. period
refracture
Refsum syndrome
refusion
Regal Acrylic/Stretch prosthetic sock
Regenafil allograft paste
regenerated fibroblast
regeneration
r. motor unit potential
r. of nerve
osteoblastic bone r.

NOTES

regeneration *(continued)*
    tibial bone defect r.
    r. torus
Regen flexion exercise
regimen
    postoperative r.
region
    axillary r.
    basilar r.
    calcaneal r.
    cervical r.
    deltoid r.
    elbow r.
    femoral r.
    gluteal r.
    H r.
    hookian r.
    hypochondriac r.
    iliac r.
    infraclavicular r.
    infrascapular r.
    infraspinous r.
    ischiorectal r.
    lumbar r.
    metazonal r.
    nuchal r.
    occipital r.
    olecranon r.
    patellar r.
    physial r.
    popliteal r.
    posterior longitudinal fiber r.
    posterior oblique fiber r.
    posteromedial r.
    pulvinar r.
    radial antebrachial r.
    superomedial r.
    true acetabular r.
    ulnar antebrachial r.
    volar antebrachial r.
regional
    r. anesthesia
    r. block
    r. migratory osteoporosis
registration
    sensory r.
registry
    National Football Head and Neck
      Injury R.
Regnauld
    R. enclavement
    R. free phalangeal base autograft
      for hallux limitus
    R. hallux rigidus classification
    R. modification of Keller
      arthroplasty
    R. osteotomy
    R. procedure

Regnauld-type great toe degeneration
regular stem
Rehab
    2+2 R. Collar
    Jump Start R.
    R. TROM brace
rehabilitation
    acute phase r.
    aquatic r.
    r. assessment
    r. care
    community r.
    r. counseling (RC)
    cryotherapy r.
    day treatment r.
    electrical stimulation r.
    Evans-Burkhalter r.
    r. flexibility exercise
    free weight r.
    functional phase r.
    r. goal
    home r.
    r. intervention
    r. muscle strengthening
    muscular r.
    Ortho Dx stimulator for knee r.
    orthopaedic r.
    outpatient r.
    physical medicine and r. (PMR)
    r. planning
    postcompetition r.
    progressive lumbar extension r.
    proprioceptive r.
    range of motion r.
    recovery phase r.
    remote locomotor r.
    Stage model of industrial r.
    Synergy joint r.
    r. therapeutic program
    r. treatment
    vocational r. (VR)
rehabilitator
    Ankle Isolator ankle r.
Reichenheim-King procedure
Reichenheim technique
Reichert-Mundinger stereotactic device
Reimers
    R. hip position migration index
    R. instability index
reimplantation
Reiner
    R. bone rongeur
    R. plaster knife
Reinert acetabular extensile approach
reinforcement
    Bragard r.
    r. ring
reinnervation

Reintegration to Normal Living index
reinterpretation
    hypnotic r.
Reiter
    R. disease
    R. syndrome
ReJuveness scar treatment
rekindling test
relapsing ankle sprain
relation to subadjacent segment
relative
    r. refractory period
    r. response attributable to the
       maneuver (RRAM)
    r. risk (RR)
Relax-A-Bac posture support
relaxant
    muscle r.
    skeletal muscle r.
relaxation
    ferromagnetic r.
    r. phenomenon
    postisometric r.
    progressive muscle r.
    reciprocal r.
    r. response
    r. training
relaxed skin tension line
relaxer
    Real-EaSE neck and shoulder r.
relaxing incision
Re-Lax-O chiropractic table
release
    adductor tendon and lateral
       capsular r.
    anterior hip r.
    anterior shoulder r.
    anterolateral r.
    Baxter nerve r.
    Beaty lateral r.
    bipolar r.
    brevis r.
    Brown two-portal carpal tunnel r.
    capsular r.
    carpal tunnel r. (CTR)
    Chow endoscopic carpal tunnel r.
    circumferential r.
    clubfoot r.
    complete subtalar r. (CSR)
    distal intrinsic r.
    distal soft tissue r. (DSTR)
    Dupuytren contracture r.

    Eberle contracture r.
    endoscopic carpal tunnel r. (ECTR)
    Endotrac endoscopic carpal
       tunnel r.
    entensile r.
    extensor hood r.
    fascial r.
    Ferkel bipolar r.
    flexor hallucis longus tendon r.
    flexor plate r.
    flexor-pronator origin r.
    Guyon tunnel r.
    hamstring r.
    Heyman-Herndon r.
    Heyman-Herndon-Strong capsular r.
    Inglis-Cooper r.
    interleukin-1 beta r.
    John Barnes myofascial r.
    joint r.
    key r.
    Kinetix instrument for carpel
       tunnel r.
    lateral capsular r.
    lateral extensor r.
    lateral retinaculum r.
    leg compartment r.
    ligamentous r.
    Little r.
    medial r.
    Mirua-Komada r.
    Mital elbow r.
    modified two-portal endoscopic
       carpal tunnel r.
    myofascial r.
    Ober r.
    patellar retinacula r.
    r. phenomenon
    plantar capsular r.
    plantar fascial r.
    plantar-lateral r.
    plantar-medial r.
    plantar plate r.
    posterior r.
    posterolateral r.
    posteromedial r. (PMR)
    pronator teres r.
    proximal intrinsic r.
    proximal nerve r.
    radical flexor r.
    retinacular r.
    retrogeniculate hamstring r.
    Sengupta quadriceps r.

NOTES

release *(continued)*
> Siegel hip r.
> Snow-Littler r.
> soft tissue r.
> spinal fascial r.
> tarsal tunnel r. (TTR)
> tendon r.
> triceps surae r.
> trigger finger r.
> trigger thumb r.
> Turco clubfoot r.
> Turco posteromedial r.
> Ueba r.
> ulnar nerve r.
> unipolar r.
> Williams-Haddad r.
> Z-plasty r.

released ulnar intrinsic muscle
Reliance CM femoral implant component
relieving incision
relocation test
Relton-Hall frame
Remak
> R. paralysis
> R. reflex

remedial exercise
remediation
> biokinetic r.

remobilization
remodeling
> bone r.
> cortical bone r.
> haversian bone r.
> r. phase

remote
> r. locomotor rehabilitation
> r. pedicle flap

removable cast
removal
> Cameron femoral component r.
> cast r.
> cement r.
> Collis-Dubrul femoral stem r.
> r. of excess cement
> Harris femoral component r.
> implant r.
> Moreland-Marder-Anspach femoral stem r.
> nail fold r.
> nail plate r.
> stem r.
> Winograd nail plate r.

remover
> Biomet Ultra-Drive cement r.
> Craig pin r.

renal
> r. osteodystrophy
> r. tubular osteomalacia

Renaut body
Renee creak sign
Renolux convertible car seat
reoperation
REP
> resistive exercise products
> REP Bands exercise band

repair
> Abraham-Pankovich tendo calcaneus r.
> Achilles tendon r. (ATR)
> ACL r.
> acromioclavicular joint r.
> all-inside r.
> arthroscopic Bankart r.
> Atasoy-type flap for nail injury r.
> augmented r.
> Baldwin Bowers radioulnar joint r.
> Bankart shoulder r.
> Becker tendon r.
> bioabsorbable tack r.
> Black r.
> bone graft r.
> Bosworth tendo calcaneus r.
> Boyd-Anderson biceps tendon r.
> brachial plexus r.
> Broström lateral ankle ligament r.
> Bunnell tendon r.
> capsule r.
> Caspari r.
> delayed primary r.
> dog-ear r.
> dural r.
> DuVries hammertoe r.
> dynamic r.
> Ecker-Lotke-Glazer patellar tendon r.
> end-to-end tendon r.
> end-to-side r.
> epineural r.
> extensor tendon r.
> fascicular r.
> first-toe Jones r.
> five-in-one knee ligament r.
> flexor tendon r.
> fracture r.
> Froimson-Oh r.
> glenohumeral dislocation r.
> group fascicular r.
> hammertoe r.
> inferior tibiofibular r.
> inguinal TEPP r.
> inside-out meniscal r.
> Jones toe r.
> Kapandji-Sauvé radioulnar joint r.

Kelikian-Riashi-Gleason patellar tendon r.
Kessler modified Achilles tendon r.
Kleinert r.
Kocher-Langenbeck ilioinguinal r.
Krackow Achilles tendon r.
Lange tendon lengthening and r.
ligamentous and capsular r. (LCR)
Lindholm open surgical tendon r.
Lindholm tendo calcaneus r.
Lynn tendo calcaneus r.
MacIntosh over-the-top r.
MacNab shoulder r.
Ma-Griffith percutaneous Achilles tendon r.
Ma-Griffith ruptured Achilles tendon r.
Ma-Griffith tendo calcaneus r.
Mandelbaum-Nartolozzi-Carney patellar tendon r.
Marshall ligament r.
medial r.
meniscal r.
Milch radioulnar joint r.
mini-open rotator cuff r.
nonaugmented r.
one-sided dog-ear r.
Palmer-Dobyns-Linscheid ligament r.
patellar tendon r.
percutaneous Achilles tendon r.
plastic r.
primary r.
pseudarthrosis r.
rod fracture r.
rotator cuff r.
Scuder r.
semitendinosus augmentation of patellar tendon r.
Sever-L'Episcopo shoulder r.
shoulder r.
Speed sternoclavicular r.
Staples r.
Staples-Black-Broström ligament r.
Strickland tendon r.
suture anchor shoulder r.
Talesnick scapholunate r.
tendon r.
Teuffer tendo calcaneus r.
tissue r.
transacromial coracoacromial ligament r.
transglenoid suture r.
triad knee r.
triple ligamentous r.
Tsuge tendon r.
Turco-Spinella tendo calcaneus r.
vertical loop suture technique for meniscus r.
volar plate r.
Watson-Jones fracture r.
Zone Specific II meniscal r.

reparative
r. granuloma
r. phase

repeated
r. quick stretch (RQS)
r. quick stretch from elongation (RQS-E)
r. quick stretch superimposed upon an existing contraction (RQS-SEC)

reperfusion injury
repetition
r. maximum (RM)
r. strain injury (RSI)
r. time (TR)

repetitive
r. discharge
r. exercise
r. microtrauma
r. nerve stimulation
r. strain disorder
r. stress disorder
r. stress injury
r. stress syndrome (RSS)
r. trauma
r. trauma disorder (RTD)

replacement
allograft ligament r.
alumina bioceramic joint r.
Amstutz total hip r.
anatomic porous r. (APR)
Ascension MCP total joint r.
Ascension PIP total joint r.
Averill total hip r.
r. bone
Buechel-Pappas total ankle r.
calcar r.
Capello total hip r.
cementless total hip r.
Charnley total hip r.
dynamic double tendon r.
elbow r.
electrolyte r.

NOTES

replacement *(continued)*
    Engh total hip r.
    Ewald total elbow r.
    facet r.
    failed joint r.
    hip r.
    Howse total hip r.
    hybrid total hip r.
    hypnotic r.
    intercalary segmental r.
    Kirschner Medical Dimension
     hip r.
    Leeds-Keio Dacron mesh r.
    ligament r.
    Lunceford total hip r.
    Marmor r.
    PCA total hip r.
    Pilliar total hip r.
    porous-coated anatomic total hip r.
    prosthetic r.
    Ring UPM total hip r.
    Ring UPM total knee r.
    SAF hip r.
    Scandinavian total ankle r. (STAR)
    Scarborough total hip r.
    self-articulating femoral hip r.
    self-bearing ceramic total hip r.
    Stanmore knee r.
    Stanmore total hip r.
    surface r.
    Tharies hip r.
    tile plate facet r.
    total ankle r. (TAR)
    total hip r. (THR)
    total joint r. (TJR)
    total knee r. (TKR)
    TR-28 total hip r.
replantable amputation
replantation
    r. of amputated digit
    autogenous meniscal cartilage r.
    r. bandage
    r. of finger
    limb r.
RepliCare wound dressing
Replica total hip replacement system
repolarization
report
    Juvenile Arthritis Functional
     Assessment R. (JAFAR)
repositioner
    Wilson-Cook prosthesis r.
repositioning
    muscle r.
reproducibility
reproducible
Repro head halter
rerouted tendon

rerouting
    Blair-Omer r.
    r. insertion
    Zancolli biceps tendon r.
research
    Alvarado Orthopedic R.
    The Institute for Rehabilitation R.
     (TIRR)
    Vioxx Gastrointestinal Outcomes R.
     (VIGOR)
resectable
resecting fracture
resection
    anterior tarsal r.
    r. arthrodesis
    r. arthroplasty
    Badgley iliac wing r.
    bar r.
    bone r.
    bony bridge r.
    calcaneal r.
    calcaneonavicular bar r.
    Carrell r.
    caudal lamina r.
    Clayton procedure with
     panmetatarsal head r.
    cuff r.
    Darrach r.
    r. dermodesis
    Dillwyn-Evans r.
    distal femoral r.
    en bloc r.
    epiphysial bar r.
    extraarticular r.
    femoral r.
    fibular head r.
    first rib r.
    Girdlestone r.
    Guller r.
    Gurd r.
    Henry r.
    Hoffmann panmetatarsal head r.
    iliac wing r.
    Ingram bony bridge r.
    innominate bone r.
    intercalary r.
    intralesional r.
    Janecki-Nelson shoulder girdle r.
    Karakousis-Vezeridis r.
    Kashiwagi r.
    Kotz modular femur and tibia r.
     (KMFTR)
    kyphos r.
    Langenskiöld bony bridge r.
    Lewis-Chekofsky r.
    Lewis intercalary r.
    Localio-Francis-Rossano r.
    local radical r.

R

Malawer r.
Mankin r.
Marcove-Lewis-Huvos shoulder
    girdle r.
marginal r.
Mayo metatarsal head r.
medial eminence r.
medial malleolus r.
r. of meniscus
metatarsal head r.
Milch cuff r.
Miltner-Wan calcaneus r.
Mumford r.
panmetatarsal head r.
Phelps partial r.
prophylactic r.
proximal femoral r.
radical r.
Radley-Liebig-Brown r.
ray r.
Rockwood r.
Stener-Gunterberg r.
Thompson r.
Tikhoff-Linberg shoulder girdle r.
transoral odontoid r.
tumor r.
vertebral body stapling wedge r.
wafer distal ulna r.
Weaver-Dunn r.
wedge r.
wedge matrix r. (WMR)

resection-arthrodesis
Enneking r.-a.

resection-realignment

resector
Accu-Line femoral r.
Accu-Line tibial r.
r. blade
femoral r.
full-radius r.
orthotome r.
synovial r.
tibial r.

residence ridge

residual
r. cement
r. heel equinus
r. hindfoot equinus
r. latency
r. limb
r. tension

residuum, pl. **residua**

resilience

resin
melamine r.
methacrylate r.
polyacetal r.

Resist-A-Band exercise band

resistance
growth hormone r.
isometric r.
isotonic r.
manual r.
plyometric r.
strength against r.
Thera-Band System of
    Progressive R.
r. training

resistant clubfoot

Resist-A-Tube exercise band

resisted
r. active flexion
r. dorsiflexion
r. external rotation

resistive
r. chair exercise kit
r. exercise
r. exercise products (REP)
r. exerciser
r. exercise table
r. movement

resonance
field focused nuclear magnetic r.
    (FONAR)
hydatid r.
nuclear magnetic r. (NMR)
osteal r.

resorbable
r. ceramic
r. plate
r. polydioxanon pin

resorption
bone r.
osteoclastic r.
periprosthetic bone r.
tuftal r.

respiratory exchange ratio

Respond II muscle stimulator

response
average evoked r.
axon r.
blink r.
brainstem auditory evoked r.
    (BAER)

NOTES

response *(continued)*
    decremental r.
    delayed r.
    evoked r.
    foreign body r.
    F-wave r.
    galvanic skin r.
    hunting r.
    hyperactive r.
    incremental r.
    r. interval
    late r.
    motion r.
    motor r.
    paired r.
    physiologic r.
    pilomotor r.
    plantar Babinski r.
    red r.
    R. rehab and fitness equipment
    relaxation r.
    sensory r.
    visual evoked r.

rest
    bed r.
    Core Hibak R.
    Core Lobak R.
    Core Sitback R.
    foot r.
    hand r.
    r., ice, compression, elevation
      (RICE)
    kidney r.
    Mayfield head r.
    Mouse Nest mouse r.
    r. pain (RP)
    pain at r.

Restcue bed
resting
    r. calcaneal stance position (RCSP)
    r. foot sling
    r. forefoot supination angle
    r. heart rate (RHR)
    r. length
    r. membrane potential
    r. orthosis
    r. pan splint
    r. shear stiffness
    r. tremor
    r. zone

restless leg
restlessness
    motor r.

Reston
    R. dressing
    R. padding

restoration
    R. acetabular system

    functional r.
    R. GAP acetabular cup
    intrinsic r.
    pinch r.
    R. Secur-Fit X'tra acetabular shell

Restoration-HA hip system
restorative pin
restore
    R. ACL guide system
    R. CalciCare dressing
    R. Clean 'N Moist
    R. orthobiologic soft-tissue implant

restraint
    active r.
    passive r.
    poncho r.
    universal canvas body r.

restricted
    r. inversion
    r. range of motion

restriction
    extension r.
    flexion r.
    intercostal r.
    lateral flexion r.
    r. of motion
    range-of-motion r.
    rotational r.
    skin r.
    soft tissue r.

restrictive bandage
restrictor
    BioStop G bone cement r.
    cement r.
    femoral canal r.
    plastic marrow canal r.

result
    false-negative r.

resurfacing
    Achilles tendon r.
    Amstutz r.
    bone r.
    r. operation
    Paltrinieri-Trentani r.
    patellar r.
    r. procedure
    Salzer r.

resurrection bone
retainer
    Thermoskin heat r.

retaining knee prosthesis
retardation
    deafness, onychoosteodystrophy,
      mental r. (DOOR)
    growth r.
    healing r.

retention
r. drill
r. suture
reticula (*pl. of* reticulum)
reticular
r. bone bruise
r. cell sarcoma
reticularis
livedo r.
reticulated polyurethane pad
reticulin stain
reticulocytosis
cerebroside r.
reticuloendothelial system
reticuloendotheliosis
reticulohistiocytosis
multicentric r.
reticulum, pl. **reticula**
endoplasmic r.
sarcoplasmic r.
retinacular
r. artery
r. hood
r. ligament
r. release
retinaculum, pl. **retinacula**
caudal r.
extensor r.
flexor r.
hypertrophic flexor r.
inferior extensor r.
inferior peroneal r.
patellar r.
peroneal r.
superior peroneal r. (SPR)
Weitbrecht r.
retraction
Schink metatarsal r.
retractor
Adson cerebellar r.
Adson hemilaminectomy r.
Allport r.
Alm wound r.
amputation r.
appendiceal r.
Army-Navy r.
Assistant Free long prong collateral
ligament r.
Assistant Free Shubbs short prong
collateral ligament r.
Assistant Free wide PCL r.
Aufranc cobra r.

Badgley laminectomy r.
Balfour self-retaining r.
Ballantine hemilaminectomy r.
Bankart r.
Beckman r.
Bennett bone r.
Bennett tibial r.
Bertin hip r.
blade-point r.
blade-spike r.
Blount anvil r.
Blount knee r.
Bodnar r.
Boyle-Davis r.
Busenkell posterior hip r.
Campbell nerve root r.
Carroll-Bennett r.
Carroll hand r.
Caspar r.
cerebellar r.
Chandler knee r.
Charnley horizontal r.
Charnley initial incision r.
Charnley knee r.
Charnley pin r.
Charnley self-retaining r.
Cloward blade r.
cobra r.
Collis r.
Collis-Taylor r.
Cooley rib r.
crank frame r.
Crego r.
curved r.
Cushing r.
Darrach r.
Deaver r.
deep r.
D'Errico r.
digital self-retaining r.
Doane knee r.
double bent Hohmann acetabular r.
double-ended right-angle r.
double-hook Lovejoy r.
Downey hemilaminectomy r.
Dozier radiolucent Bennett r.
dual nerve root suction r.
East-West r.
Elite Farley r.
extra-depth posterior acetabular r.
extra-large hip r.
Fahey r.

R

NOTES

retractor *(continued)*
    fat pad r.
    Finochietto rib r.
    five-prong rake blade r.
    flat r.
    FlexPosure endoscopic r.
    Freebody-Steinmann r.
    Fukuda humeral head r.
    Gelpi r.
    Gifford mastoid r.
    handheld r.
    Hays hand r.
    heavy-duty two-tooth r.
    Hedblom rib r.
    Heiss soft tissue r.
    Hendren self-retaining r.
    Henning meniscal r.
    Hibbs r.
    Hoen r.
    Hohmann bone r.
    Holscher knee r.
    Holscher root r.
    Holzheimer r.
    humeral head r.
    inferoposterior acetabular capsule r.
    Inge r.
    Israel r.
    Kasdan r.
    Kirschenbaum r.
    Kleinert-Ragdell r.
    knee r.
    Kocher r.
    Lange bone r.
    Lange-Hohmann bone r.
    Langenbeck r.
    large Cobra r.
    Love nerve root r.
    lower hand r.
    Lowman hand r.
    Luongo hand r.
    Markham-Meyerding r.
    Mark II Chandler total knee r.
    Mark II concave total knee r.
    Mark II lateral collateral
      ligament r.
    Mark II modular weight r.
    Mark II S total knee r.
    Mark II Stubbs short prong
      collateral ligament r.
    Mark II wide PCL knee r.
    Mark II Z knee r.
    Mayo-Collins r.
    McCullough r.
    McIvor ENT r.
    meniscus r.
    Meyerding r.
    mini-Hohmann podiatric r.
    modified Fukuda-type r.

Morris r.
Mueller r.
Myers knee r.
narrow-blade r.
narrow-neck mini-Hohmann r.
Nelson rib r.
Ollier rake r.
orthopaedic r.
Paulson knee r.
Percy amputation r.
pin r.
Ragnell r.
rake r.
rib r.
ribbon r.
Richardson r.
ring r.
Rosenberg r.
Rowe humeral head r.
Sauerbruch r.
Scholten sternal r.
Scoville r.
Seeburger r.
self-retaining r.
Senn r.
sharp r.
Sherwin knee r.
Sims r.
single-prong broad acetabular r.
skid humeral head r.
Smillie knee r.
Sofield r.
soft tissue blade r.
Southwick two-tined r.
standard 2-inch blade r.
standard 4-inch blade r.
stiff ribbon r.
Tang r.
Taylor r.
thin glenoid r.
three-prong rake blade r.
three-two Weitlaner self-retaining r.
tibial r.
Tupper hand-holder and r.
two-prong rake r.
upper hand r.
U-shaped r.
Verbrugge-Hohmann bone r.
Volkmann rake r.
Wagner r.
Watanabe r.
Weit-Arner r.
Weitlaner r.
Wichman r.
Williams self-retaining r.
Wilson gonad r.
Wink r.
Z r.

retraining
    VMO r.
retriever
    Carroll tendon r.
    Hewson suture r.
    Kleinert-Kutz tendon r.
    magnetic r.
retroacetabular lesion
retro-Achilles bursa
retrobulbar prosthesis needle
retrocalcaneal
    r. bursa
    r. bursitis
    r. disorder
    r. exostosis
    r. spur
retrocalcaneobursitis
retrodisplaced fracture
retroflexion
    tibial r.
retrogeniculate hamstring release
retrograde
    r. Beaver blade
    r. degeneration
    r. drilling
    r. intramedullary nail
    r. meniscal blade
    r. method
    r. nailing
retrograde-cutting hook-shaped knife
retrolisthesed fragment
retrolisthesis positional dyskinesia
retromedullary arteriovenous
  malformation
retropatellar
    r. fat pad
    r. fat pad contracture
retroperitoneal
    r. approach
    r. decompression
    r. fibrosis
    r. hemorrhage
    r. space
retropharyngeal
    r. abscess
    r. approach
    r. fascial cleft
    r. space
retropulsed
    r. bone excision
    r. bony fragment
retropulsion of gait

retroreflective marker
retrosacral fascia
retrospondylolisthesis
retrosternal
    r. abscess
    r. dislocation
retrotorsion
    femoral r.
    tibial r.
retrovascular cord
retroversion
    r. of acetabular cup
    angle of r.
    femoral r.
    tibial r.
Rett syndrome
return
    r. to play (RTP)
    r. of sensation
return-to-play
    r.-t.-p. consideration
    r.-t.-p. injury assessment
    r.-t.-p. musculoskeletal assessment
    r.-t.-p. sidelines decision making
ReUnite
    R. hand fixation
    R. orthopedic pin
    R. orthopedic screw
    R. resorbable orthopedic fixation
    system
revascularization
    endosteal r.
    r. of graft
revascularized tissue
Revelation hip system
Reverdin
    R. bunionectomy
    R. epidermal free graft
    R. osteotomy
    R. prosthesis
Reverdin-Green
    R.-G. bunionectomy
    R.-G. foot procedure
    R.-G. osteotomy
Reverdin-Green-Laird procedure
Reverdin-Laird
    R.-L. bunionectomy
    R.-L. osteotomy
Reverdin-McBride bunionectomy
reversal
    r. of antagonist (ROA)
    r. of cervical lordosis

R

NOTES

reversal *(continued)*
r. of fore-aft shear phase of gait
isotonic r. (IR)
stabilizing r. (SR)

reverse
r. Austin osteotomy
r. Bankart lesion
r. Barton fracture
r. Bigelow maneuver
r. buckling
r. closing base wedge osteotomy
r. Colles fracture
r. cross-finger flap
r. cutting needle
r. Dillwyn-Evans calcaneal
osteotomy
r. forearm island flap
r. Hill-Sachs defect
r. Hill-Sachs lesion
r. Hill-Sachs sign
r. Jones procedure
r. knuckle-bender splint
r. Lasègue test
r. last shoe
r. lunge back exercise technique
r. Mauck knee operation
r. Mauck knee procedure
r. Monteggia fracture
r. NAGS
r. obliquity fracture
r. pivot shift
r. pivot shift test
r. Putti-Platt procedure
r. tennis elbow
r. Thomas heel
r. Trendelenburg position
r. undercutting lengthening
r. wedge technique
r. windlass
r. wrist curl

reverse-cutting meniscal probe
reverse-flow flap
reverse-threaded screw
**reversible ischemic neurologic disability
(RIND)**
revised
Symptoms Checklist 90 R. (SCL-90R)

revision
exploration and r.
r. hip arthroplasty
R. hip stem
Mallory-Head total hip r.
r. procedure
stump r.
r. of total hip
r. total hip operation

ReVision nail

Revo
R. knot
R. loop handle knot pusher
R. retrievable cancellous screw
R. rotator cuff repair system
R. suture anchor

Rezaian
R. external fixation
R. external fixation apparatus
R. external fixation device
R. interbody device
R. spinal fixator

RGO
reciprocation gait orthosis

R-HAB
Rincoe human action bionic
R-HAB lighter weight ankle

rhabdomyolysis
exertional r.

rhabdomyoma
rhabdomyosarcoma
alveolar r.
embryonal r.
pleomorphic r.

rhachotomy
Capener lateral r.
decompression r.
lateral r.

rHead implant system
rheobase
rheostosis
rheumatic
r. fever
r. granuloma
r. scoliosis

rheumatica
polymyalgia r. (PMR)

rheumatism
Besnier r.
chronic r.
Heberden r.
MacLeod capsular r.
nodose r.
palindromic r.
Poncet r.
tuberculous r.
World Health
Organization/International League
Against R. (WHO/LAR)

rheumatismal edema
rheumatoid
r. arthritis (RA)
r. arthritis factor
r. arthritis myopathy
r. arthritis synovitis
r. cyst
r. deformity
r. disease

r. disorder
r. foot
r. myositis
r. nodule
r. spondylitis
r. vasculitis
rheumatologic disorder
rheumatologist
rheumatology
American College of R. (ACR)
Rapid Assessment of Disease
Activity in R. (RADAR)
Rhinelander pin
**Rhino Triangle polypropylene hip
abduction brace**
rhizomelic spondylosis
rhizomelic-type chondrodysplasia
rhizomesomelic bone dysplasia
rhizotomy
intradural dorsal spinal root r.
posterior r.
selective posterior r. (SPR)
RHOCS
right-handed orthogonal coordinate
system
rhomboid
r. flap
r. ligament
Michaelis r.
r. muscle
rhonchus, pl. **rhonchi**
rales and rhonchi
Rhoton
R. elevator
R. enucleator
R. needle holder
R. osteotome
RHR
resting heart rate
rhythm
scapulohumeral r.
rhythmic
r. handgrip work
r. initiation (RI)
r. initiation technique
r. stabilization
RI
rhythmic initiation
rib
r. approximator
bed of r.
r. belt

r. belt orthosis
bicipital r.
bucket-handle r.
r. cage
cervical r.
r. contractor
r. contusion
costochondral junction of r.'s
r. cutter
r. drill
r. elevator
false r.
floating r.
r. forceps
r. fracture
r. graft
hypoplastic first r.
interarticular ligament of head
of r.
radiate ligament of head of r.
r. rasp
r. retractor
rudimentary r.
slipping r.
spurious r.
sternal r.
Stiller r.
true r.
vertebral r.
vertebrocostal r.
vertebrosternal r.
ribbed
r. hook
r. needle
ribbed-sole shoe
Ribble bandage
ribbon
r. retractor
r. sign
ribonucleoprotein (RNP)
rib-vertebral angle
Rica
R. bone drill
R. wire guidepin
Ricard amputation
RICE
rest, ice, compression, elevation
rice
r. body
joint r.
Richards
R. angle guide

R

NOTES

Richards *(continued)*
    R. arthrodesis
    R. bone clamp
    R. classic compression hip screw
    R. Colles external fixator
    R. drill guide
    R. fixation staple
    R. fixator system
    R. hip endoprosthesis system
    R. hip prosthesis
    R. hydroxyapatite PORP
    R. lag screw
    R. lag screw device
    R. locking rod
    R. Lovejoy bone drill
    R. mallet
    R. maximum contact cruciate-sparing prosthesis
    R. modular hip system
    R. modular stem
    R. Phillips screwdriver
    R. pistol-grip drill
    R. reamer
    R. reconstruction nail
    R. sideplate
    R. Solcotrans orthopedic drainage-reinfusion system
    R. Spectron metal-backed acetabular prosthesis
    R. Zirconia femoral head prosthesis
Richards-Hirschhorn plate
Richard Smith prosthesis
Richardson
    R. retractor
    R. rod
    R. subtalar arthrodesis
Riche-Cannieu
    R.-C. anastomosis
    R.-C. connection
Riches artery forceps
Richet
    R. bandage
    R. tibial-astragalocalcaneal canal
Richie brace
Richmond
    R. bolt
    R. subarachnoid screw
    R. subarachnoid screw sensor
    R. subarachnoid twist drill
Richter
    R. bone drill
    R. bone screwdriver
rickets
    adult r.
    florid r.
    vitamin D-dependent r. (VDDR)
    vitamin D-resistant r. (VDRR)
rickshaw rehabilitation exerciser

Rideau technique
rider's
    r. bone
    r. bursa
    r. leg
    r. muscle
    r. sprain
    r. tendon
ridge
    dorsal r.
    epicondylar r.
    greater multangular r.
    longitudinal r.
    osteochondral r.
    Outerbridge r.
    residence r.
    talar r.
    trapezial r.
    vastus lateralis r.
Ridlon
    R. hip reduction
    R. operation
    R. plaster knife
    R. procedure
Riecken PQ premium heel cup
rig
    Leg Extension Power R.
right
    r. erector spinae musculature
    r. lateral flexion
    r. and left ankle index
    r. lower extremity (RLE)
    r. lower limb (RLL)
    r. posterior innominate
    r. rotation
    r. thoracic curve
    r. thoracic curve with hypokyphosis
    r. thoracic, left lumbar curve pattern
    r. thoracic, left thoracolumbar curve pattern
    r. thoracic minor curve pattern
    r. upper extremity (RUE)
    r. upper limb (RUL)
    r. ventricular cardiomyopathy
right-angle
    r.-a. dental drill
    r.-a. hook
right-ankle bur
right-hand dominance
right-handed orthogonal coordinate system (RHOCS)
righting
    r. reflex
    trunk r.
right/left
    r./l. discrimination
    r./l. timing

right-sided
r.-s. nail
r.-s. submandibular transverse
   incision
r.-s. thoracotomy

rigid
r. bar
r. below-the-knee cast
r. body
r. collar
r. curve
r. curve scoliosis
r. dressing
r. equinovarus deformity
r. flatfoot
r. flatfoot deformity
r. foot
r. foot cavus
r. frame wheelchair
r. gait
r. internal fixation
r. metal pelvic band
r. orthosis
r. pedicle screw
r. pes planus
r. postoperative brace
r. reamer
r. rockerbottom (RRB)
r. round back
r. sound

rigidity
C-D instrumentation r.
cogwheel r.
Cotrel pedicle screw r.
nuchal r.
spinal fixation r.

rigidus
hallux r.

RIK
RIK fluid mattress
RIK FootHugger fluid heel boot

Riley-Day syndrome

rim
acetabular r.
alar r.
glenoid r.
sclerotic marginal r.
r. sign
tibial r.

Rincoe
R. human action bionic (R-HAB)
R. human action bionic ankle

RIND
reversible ischemic neurologic disability

ring
Ace-Colles half r.
arterial r.
r. block anesthesia
carbon fiber half r.
cartilaginous r.
Charnley centering r.
congenital r.
constriction r.
cricoid r.
r. curette
r. cushion
doughnut r.
drop-lock r.
epiphysial r.
r. external fixator
extracapsular arterial r.
r. finger
r. finger–small finger syndactyly
Fischer r.
foam r.
r. forceps
r. fracture
half r.
halo r.
Ilizarov r.
invalid r.
ischial weightbearing r.
Kayser-Fleischer r.
R. knee prosthesis
Lacroix osseous r.
Luque r.
r. man shoulder
Mose concentric r.'s
Neer r.
orthosis drop-lock r.
pelvic r.
perichondral r.
protrusio r.
proximal-to-distal r.
reduction r.
reinforcement r.
r. retractor
r. sign
r. structure
r. sublimis opponensplasty
r. syndrome
R. total hip prosthesis
R. UPM press-fit prosthesis
R. UPM total hip replacement

NOTES

ring *(continued)*
    R. UPM total knee replacement
    V1 halo r.
ringer
    R. arthroscopy
    R. lactate
RingLoc
    R. acetabular series
    R. instrument
Riolan
    R. bone
    R. muscle
Riordan
    R. club hand classification
    R. finger flexion
    R. finger opponensplasty
    R. pin
    R. pollicization
    R. sign
    R. tendon transfer technique
rise
    single heel r.
    r. time
Riseborough-Radin
    R.-R. fracture classification system
    R.-R. intercondylar fracture
      classification
riser
    stress r.
Rish osteotome
risk
    r. factor profile
    heat injury r.
    occupational r.
    relative r. (RR)
Risser
    R. frame
    R. grade
    R. localizer scoliosis cast
    R. method
    R. pin
    R. sign
    R. stage
    R. technique
    R. turnbuckle cast
Rissler-Stille pin
Ritchie rheumatoid arthritis index
Rivermead
    R. ADL index
    R. Mobility Index (RMI)
    R. Motor Assessment
rivet
    r. gun
    pop r.
Rizzoli osteoclast
RLE
    right lower extremity

RLL
    right lower limb
RM
    repetition maximum
      RM isoelastic hip prosthesis
1-RM
    one-repetition maximum
RMC
    RMC knee replacement device
    RMC prosthesis
RMI
    Rivermead Mobility Index
RMQ
    Roland-Morris Questionnaire
R/O
    rule out
ROA
    reversal of antagonist
road burn injury
Roaf, Kirkaldy-Willis, and Cattero procedure
Robert
    R. Brigham semiconstrained
      prosthesis
    R. Brigham total knee prosthesis
    R. Jones bandage
    R. Jones dressing
    R. Jones splint
    R. ligament
    R. view
Roberts
    R. approach
    R. technique
Roberts-Gill periosteal elevator
Robinson
    R. anterior cervical diskectomy
    R. anterior cervical fusion
    R. arthrometer
    R. arthroplasty
    R. cervical spine fusion
    R. morcellation
    R. spinal arthrodesis
Robinson-Chung-Farahvar clavicular morcellation
Robinson-Moon prosthesis inserter
Robinson-Riley cervical arthrodesis
Robinson-Smith spinal arthrodesis
Robinson-Southwick
    R.-S. fusion
    R.-S. fusion technique
Robins-Riley spinal fusion
Robodoc robot
robot
    Robodoc r.
robotic
robust rheumatoid arthritis

ROC

ROC anchor
ROC anchoring device

Rocabado posture gauge

Rochester

R. bone trephine device
R. compression system
R. harvest bone cutter
R. hip-knee-ankle-foot orthosis
R. lamina elevator
R. recipient bone cutter
R. spinal elevator

Rochester-Carmalt forceps

Rochester-Ochsner forceps

Rochester-Pean forceps

rock

R. ankle exercise board
pelvic r. (PR)
R. & Roller exercise board

rocker

r. balance square
r. bar
r. board
r. boot
r. bottom sole
Carolina r.
r. knife
Uniplane r.

rockerbottom

r. flatfoot
r. flatfoot deformity
r. foot
rigid r. (RRB)
r. shoe

RocketSoc ankle brace

rocking

knee-chest r.

Rock-Mulligan prosthesis

Rockwood

R. anterior acromioplasty
R. classification
R. classification of
acromioclavicular injury
R. posterior capsulorrhaphy
R. procedure
R. resection
R. shoulder screw

Rockwood-Green technique

Rockwood-Matsen capsular shift procedure

rocky boat exerciser

rod

alignment guide r.
Alta advance tibial/humeral r.
Alta CFX reconstruction r.
Alta tibial-humeral r.
aluminum master r.
Amset R-F r.
auto-reinforced polyglycolide r.
Bailey-Dubow r.
r. bender
r. bending
Bickel intramedullary r.
centralizing r.
r. clamp
cold rolled r.
compression r.
concave r.
r. contour preparation
convex r.
Cotrel-Dubousset r.
Dacron-impregnated silicone r.
degradable polyglycolide r.
delta r.
distraction r.
r. distraction device
double-L spinal r.
dual square-ended Harrington r.
Edwards D-L modular screw r.
Edwards-Levine r.
Edwards modular system
Universal r.
Ender r.
Enneking r.
Fixateur Interne r.
flared spinal r.
fluted medullary r.
r. fracture repair
guide r.
Harrington compression r.
Harrington distraction r.
Harris condylocephalic r.
hinge r.
r. holder
Hunter Silastic r.
impactor r.
impingement r.
intramedullary alignment r.
Isola spinal implant system eye r.
Jacobs distraction r.
Jacobs locking hook spinal r.
Kaneda r.
Knodt distraction r.

NOTES

rod *(continued)*
Küntscher r.
L r.
r. linkage
locking-hook spinal r.
long alignment r.
L-shaped r.
Luque r.
Luque-Galveston r.
r. migration
Moe modified Harrington r.
Moe square-end r.
Moss r.
Mouradian r.
Olerud PSF r.
OrthoSorb r.
pediatric Cotrel-Dubousset r.
PGA r.
r. placement
Polarus humeral r.
precontoured unit r.
radiotranslucent r.
Richards locking r.
Richardson r.
r. rotation prevention
round-ended distraction r.
Rush r.
Russell-Taylor delta r.
Sage r.
Sampson r.
Schneider r.
screw alignment r.
Selby I, II r.
Serrato forearm r.
Shaw-SHIP r.
Sheffield r.
silicone-dacron tendon r.
r. sleeve fixation
spinal fixation r.
square-ended distraction r.
Stenzel r.
straight threaded r.
surgical r.
R. TAG suture anchor system
telescoping medullary r.
r. template
tendon r.
threaded r.
U Luque vertebral r.
unit spinal r.
V-A alignment r.
VDS compression r.
VSF r.
Williams r.
Wiltse system aluminum master r.
Wiltse system spinal r.
Wissinger r.

Zickel r.
Zielke r.
rod-hook construct
rod-mounted
r.-m. targeting apparatus
r.-m. targeting device
rod-sleeve instrumentation
Roeder manipulative aptitude test device
roentgen
r. stereophotogrammetric analysis (RSA)
r. stereophotogrammetry
roentgenogram
biplane r.
lateral r.
operative r.
templating r.
two-plane r.
roentgenography
intraoperative r.
preoperative r.
stress r.
roentgenometrics
roentgen-stereophotogrammatic study
Roger
R. Anderson compression device
R. Anderson external fixation apparatus
R. Anderson external fixation device
R. Anderson external fixator
R. Anderson fixation
R. Anderson pin
R. Anderson splint
R. Anderson stabilization device
R. Anderson system
R. Anderson table
R. Anderson traction
Rogers cervical fusion technique
Rogozinski
R. hook
R. screw system
R. spinal fixation
R. spinal fixation system
R. spinal rod system
Rohadur gait plate
Rohadur-Polydor orthotic
Rohadur-Schaefer orthotic
Rohadur-Whitman orthotic
ROHO
ROHO bed
ROHO heel pad
ROHO heel protector
ROHO Pack-It cushion
ROHO pediatric seating system
ROHO solid seat insert
Rokitansky pelvis

Roland index of low back pain
Roland-Morris Questionnaire (RMQ)
Rolando fracture
role
    intrinsic transverse connector r.
    occupational r.
rolfing
    r. therapy
    r. treatment
Rolimeter
    Aircast R.
roll
    cervical r.
    chest r.
    r. control bolster
    cotton r.
    Dutchman's r.
    Feldenkrais foam r.
    FLUFTEX gauze r.
    hip r.
    lumbar r.
    McKenzie cervical r.
    McKenzie lumbar r.
    McKenzie night r.
    neck r.
    octagon r.
    radiolucent r.
    Skillbuilder half r.
    r. stitch
    towel r.
    Tumble Forms r.
Roll-A-Bout
Rollator Nova walker
rollback
    femoral r.
rolled felt
roller
    r. bandage
    r. injury
    Sorbothane rice sheller r.
RollerBack self-massage device
rolling
    skin r.
Rollocane
rollover
    medial r.
Rolyan
    R. AquaForm wrist and thumb
      spica splint
    R. arm elevator
    R. foot support
    R. Gel Shell spica splint

    R. Reach N Range Pulley System
    R. TakeOff Sprint brace
    R. tibial fracture brace
Rolz device
ROM
    range of motion
    ROM knee brace
    ROM therapy
    ROM walker brace
Roman arch
Romano curved drilling system
Romberg
    R. reflex
    R. sign
    R. test
Rome criteria
rongeur
    Adson r.
    angled jaw r.
    angled pituitary r.
    angular bone r.
    Bacon bone r.
    Baer bone r.
    Bane bone r.
    Bane-Hartmann bone r.
    basket r.
    bayonet r.
    Beyer r.
    Beyer-Stille bone r.
    Blumenthal bone r.
    bone-nibbling r.
    bone punch r.
    Bruening-Citelli r.
    Campbell r.
    cervical r.
    Cherry-Kerrison laminectomy r.
    Cicherelli bone r.
    Cintor bone r.
    Cleveland bone r.
    Cloward disk r.
    Cloward-English laminectomy r.
    Cloward-Harper laminectomy r.
    Cloward intervertebral disk r.
    Codman-Harper laminectomy r.
    Codman-Kerrison laminectomy r.
    Codman-Leksell laminectomy r.
    Codman-Schlesinger cervical
      laminectomy r.
    Cohen r.
    Colclough laminectomy r.
    Corbett bone r.
    curved bone r.

NOTES

rongeur *(continued)*
    Cushing disk r.
    Dale first rib r.
    Dean bone r.
    Decker r.
    Defourmentel bone r.
    disk r.
    double-action r.
    downbiting r.
    duckbill r.
    Echlin bone r.
    Echlin duckbill r.
    Echlin-Luer r.
    Ferris Smith r.
    Ferris Smith-Kerrison laminectomy r.
    Ferris Smith-Spurling disk r.
    Fisch bone r.
    flat-bottomed Kerrison r.
    r. forceps
    Friedman bone r.
    Guleke bone r.
    Hartmann bone r.
    Hein r.
    Hoen r.
    Horsley bone r.
    Husk bone r.
    Jackson intervertebral disk r.
    Jarit-Liston bone r.
    Jarit-Ruskin bone r.
    Kerrison downbiting r.
    Kleinert-Kutz bone r.
    Kleinert-Kutz synovectomy r.
    Lebsche r.
    Leksell laminectomy r.
    Leksell-Stille thoracic r.
    Lempert bone r.
    Liston bone r.
    Liston-Littauer r.
    Littauer-West r.
    Luer bone r.
    Luer-Friedman bone r.
    Luer-Hartmann r.
    Markwalder bone r.
    Marquardt bone r.
    mastoid r.
    McIndoe bone r.
    Mead bone r.
    Montenovesi r.
    needle-nose r.
    orthopaedic r.
    pituitary r.
    Reiner bone r.
    Ruskin r.
    Ruskin-Jansen bone r.
    Ruskin-Liston bone r.
    Ruskin-Rowland bone r.
    Schell bone r.
    Schlesinger cervical r.
    Schlesinger intervertebral disk r.
    Semb bone r.
    Semb-Stille bone r.
    Shearer r.
    single-action r.
    Smith-Petersen r.
    Spurling r.
    Spurling-Kerrison upbiting and downbiting r.
    Stille r.
    Stille-Horsley bone r.
    Stille-Liston bone r.
    Stille-Luer bone r.
    Stille-Luer duckbill r.
    Stille-Luer-Echlin r.
    Stille-Ruskin bone r.
    straight bone r.
    straight pituitary r.
    Super Cut laminectomy r.
    synovial r.
    upbiting r.
    upcut r.
    Walton-Liston bone r.
    Walton-Ruskin bone r.
    Watson-Williams intervertebral disk r.
    Weil-Blakesley intervertebral disk r.
    Wilde intervertebral disk r.

rongeured

Rood technique

roof
    acetabular r.
    r. arc measurement
    r. impingement
    intercondylar r.
    r. plate
    r. wedge

roofplasty

roof-reinforcement ring hip arthroplasty component

room
    Allender vertical laminar flow r.
    Charnley laminar flow r.
    operating r.
    recovery r. (RR)
    surgical dressing r. (SDR)
    training r.

Roos
    R. approach
    R. overhead exercise test
    R. rib cutter

root
    r. anomaly
    r. canal broach
    cervical r.
    r. infiltration
    nail r.

nerve r.
R. procedure
r. tension sign
Root-Siegal varus derotational osteotomy
rope
r. stretching device
The R. stretch-and-traction device
The R. stretching device
Roper-Day prosthesis
ropey
ropiness
Rorabeck fasciotomy
rose
R. foot operation
R. foot procedure
Rosen
R. bur
R. elevator
R. splint
Rosenberg
R. endoscopic anterior cruciate
ligament reconstruction
R. retractor
R. view
Rosenfeld hip prosthesis
Rosenthal classification of nail injury
Roser line
Roser-Nélaton line
rosette
r. Beaver blade
R. strain gauge
rostrate pelvis
Rotablator rotating bur
Rotaflex exerciser
Rotaglide
R. knee implant
R. total knee system
rotary
r. ankle instability
r. basket
r. basket forceps
r. bur
r. control
r. deviation
r. displacement
r. drawer test
r. instability test
r. joint
r. motion
r. osteotome
r. stability

rotated
externally r.
internally r.
rotating
r. femoral head prosthesis
r. hinge
r. hinge knee prosthesis
r. patellar implant
r. turner
rotation
abduction-external r. (AER)
abnormal instantaneous axis of r.
anterior innominate r.
axial r.
axis of r.
r. axis
Borggreve limb r.
center of axial r.
cervical general r.
r. device
r. drawer test
eccentric axis of ankle r.
r. exercise
external r.
external rotation/internal r. (ER/IR)
flexion, abduction, external r.
(FABER)
flexion, adduction, internal r.
(FADIR)
foot r.
forced passive internal r.
functional axial r.
Hermodsson internal r.
hip r.
horizontal external r.
instantaneous axis of r.
intentional r.
internal-external r.
internal femoral r.
intersegmental r.
inversion-eversion r.
inward r.
ipsilateral r.
knee r.
lateral hip r.
left r.
lumbar r.
medial hip r.
r. mobility
neutral r.
outward r.
patellar r.

R

NOTES

rotation *(continued)*
    patient-resisted internal r.
    pelvic r.
    r. plasty
    polycentric r.
    posterior innominate r.
    pronation-eversion-external r.
      (PEER)
    pronation-external r. (P-ER)
    putative segmental instantaneous
      axis of r.
    r. recurvatum test
    resisted external r.
    right r.
    sagittal r.
    spine r.
    supination-external r. (SER)
    supination-external r. IV (SER-IV)
    synchronous scapuloclavicular r.
    r. testing
    thoracolumbosacral orthosis—flexion,
      extension, lateral bending, and
      transverse r. (TLSO-FELR)
    tibiofibular r.
    vertebral r.
rotational
    r. alignment
    r. burst fracture
    r. contracture
    r. correction
    r. deformity
    r. flap
    r. instability
    r. kyphosis
    r. malalignment
    r. malposition
    r. manipulation
    r. prominence
    r. restriction
    r. scarf osteotomy
    r. scarf osteotomy/bunionectomy
    r. scoliosis
rotation-compression maneuver
rotationplasty
    Kotz-Salzer r.
    tibial hindfoot
      osteomusculocutaneous r.
    Van Ness r.
    Winkelmann r.
rotator
    r. cuff (RC)
    r. cuff buttress (RCB)
    r. cuff calcific tendinitis
    r. cuff calcified deposit
    r. cuff contusion
    r. cuff degeneration
    r. cuff function
    r. cuff imbalance

    r. cuff impingement syndrome
    r. cuff injury
    r. cuff lesion
    r. cuff repair
    r. cuff tear
    r. cuff tear arthroplasty
    r. cuff tendinopathy
    r. cuff tendon
    external r.
    Hosmer above-knee r.
    Howmedica monotube external r.
    internal r.
    Jarit r.
    long external r.
    r. muscle
    short external r.
    r. unit
rotatores syndrome
rotatory
    r. atlantoaxial subluxation
    r. load
    r. torque
rotatory-variable-differential transducer
Rotes joint mobility scale
Rothman
    R. Institute femoral prosthesis
    R. Institute total hip program
Roto-Rest bed
RotorloC absorbable rotator cuff suture
    anchor
rotoscoliosis
rototome
Rotter-Erb syndrome
roughened cartilage
roughening
roughen the surface
rouleaux formation
round
    r. bur
    r. cell liposarcoma
    r. cell-type liposarcoma
    r. ligament
    r. shoulder
    r. shoulder deformity
roundback stem
round-ended distraction rod
round-hole compression plate
round-tapped
    r.-t. elevator
    r.-t. periosteal
Rousek
    R. extender
    R. extraction set
    R. extractor
Roussy-Lévy
    R.-L. disease
    R.-L. syndrome
Rouviere ligament

R

Roux
    R. osteotomy
    R. sign
Roux-duToit staple capsulorrhaphy
Roux-Goldthwait
    R.-G. operation
    R.-G. procedure
    R.-G. realignment
row
    carpal r.
    proximal carpal r.
Rowe
    R. blanket
    R. calcaneal fracture classification
    R. disimpaction forceps
    R. fusion
    R. glenoid punch
    R. glenoid-reaming forceps
    R. humeral head retractor
    R. modified-Harrison forceps
    modified Zarins and R.
    R. posterior shoulder approach
Rowe-Harrison bone-holding forceps
Rowe-Lowell
    R.-L. fracture-dislocation
      classification
    R.-L. hip dislocation classification
Rowe-Zarins shoulder immobilization
rowing and sculling
Rowland-Hughes splint
Royalite body jacket
Roy-Camile prosthesis
Roy-Camille
    R.-C. plate
    R.-C. posterior screw plate fixation
Roylan ergonomic hand exerciser
Royle-Thompson transfer technique
RP
    reduced profile
    rest pain
RPE
    rated perceived exertion
RQS
    repeated quick stretch
RQS-E
    repeated quick stretch from elongation
RQS-SEC
    repeated quick stretch superimposed upon
      an existing contraction
RR
    recovery room
    relative risk

RRAM
    relative response attributable to the
      maneuver
RRB
    rigid rockerbottom
RSA
    roentgen stereophotogrammetric analysis
RSC
    radioscaphocapitate
RSD
    reflex sympathetic dystrophy
RSI
    repetition strain injury
RSS
    rearfoot stability system
    repetitive stress syndrome
RT
    recreational therapy
RTD
    repetitive trauma disorder
RTP
    return to play
rub
    friction r.
    Jeanie R.
rubber
    r. band traction
    r. bolster
    r. drain
    r. pelvis
    r. shod
    r. shod clamp
    r. sling
    r. sole cast walker
    r. spacer
    r. walking heel
    r. wedge walker
Rubbermaid adjustable bath/shower seat
Rubin
    R. bone planer
    R. cartilage planer
    R. gouge
    R. rasp
Rubinstein-Taybi syndrome
Rubix-Cube
rubor
rucksack paralysis
rudimentary
    r. bone
    r. rib
RUE
    right upper extremity

NOTES

Ruedi-Allgower
    R.-A. classification
    R.-A. tibial plafond fracture
Ruedi fracture
Ruffini mechanoreceptor
rugby jersey finger
rugger
    r. jersey sign
    r. jersey spine
Ruiz-Mora
    R.-M. correction
    R.-M. procedure
RUL
    right upper limb
rule
    millimetric r.
    National Collegiate Athletic
      Association spine injury
      prevention r.
    no touch r.
    Ottawa Ankle R. (OAR)
    r. out (R/O)
ruler
    Berndt hip r.
    ulnar r.
Rumel
    R. aluminum bridge splint
    R. myocardial clamp
    R. rubber clamp
    R. thoracic clamp
runner
    r. bump
    heel-toe r.
    r. knee
    Sprint R.
    r. toe
running
    r. suture
    treadmill r.
running-related injury
rupture
    Achilles tendon r. (ATR)
    adductor longus muscle r.
    anterior talofibular ligament r.
    buttonhole r.
    closed r.
    collateral ligament r.
    crescentic r.
    cruciate ligament r.
    distal biceps brachii tendon r.
    extracapsular r.
    flexor tendon r.
    gastrocnemius r.
    infrapatellar tendon r.
    intracapsular r.
    longitudinal ligament r.
    medial head of the
      gastrocnemius r.

    neglected r.
    proximal tendon r.
    spontaneous r.
    stress r.
    subscapularis r.
    syndesmosis r.
    tendon r.
    transverse ligament r.
    ulnar collateral ligament r.
ruptured
    r. disk
    r. disk excision
rush
    R. bender
    R. bone clamp
    R. driver
    R. driver-bender-extractor
    R. extender
    R. flexible medullary nail
    R. intramedullary fixation pin
    R. mallet
    R. pin nail
    R. pin reamer awl
    R. rod
    R. rod awl reamer
Ruskin
    R. bone-cutting forceps
    R. bone-splitting forceps
    R. rongeur
    R. rongeur forceps
Ruskin-Jansen bone rongeur
Ruskin-Liston
    R.-L. bone-cutting forceps
    R.-L. bone rongeur
Ruskin-Rowland
    R.-R. bone-cutting forceps
    R.-R. bone rongeur
Russe
    R. bone graft
    R. classification
    R. technique
Russe-Gerhardt method
Russell
    R. fibular head autograft
    R. skeletal traction
    R. splint
Russell-Silver dwarfism
Russell-Taylor
    R.-T. classification
    R.-T. delta rod
    R.-T. delta tibial nail
    R.-T. femoral interlocking nail
      system
    R.-T. interlocking medullary nail
    R.-T. screw
Russian
    R. forceps
    R. waveform

rust
 R. amputation saw
 R. disease
 R. phenomenon
 R. sign
 r. syndrome
Rüter classification
R-Value exercise ball

Rx Comfort sock
Rydell nail
Ryder needle holder
Ryerson
 R. bone graft
 R. procedure
 R. technique
 R. triple arthrodesis

NOTES

R

SA

skeletal age

SAARD

slow-acting antirheumatic drug

SABA pulley

Sabel cast walker

saber

s. shin

s. shin deformity

s. tibia

saber-cut

s.-c. approach

s.-c. incision

Sabolich above-knee socket system

SAC

short arm cast

sideline assessment of concussion

space available for the cord

sac

bursal s.

common dural s.

thecal s.

SACH

solid ankle, cushioned heel

SACH foot

SACH foot adapter

SACH foot prosthesis

SACH orthopedic heel

SACH orthosis

SACH orthotic

Sach nerve separator

saclike cavity

sacra (*pl. of* sacrum)

sacral

s. agenesis

s. ala

s. alar screw

s. approach

s. arcuate line

s. artery

s. bar technique

s. base angle

s. base distortion

s. block

s. bone

s. bone tip

s. bursa

s. canal

s. cyst

s. dermatome

s. fracture

s. fusion screw fixation

s. horizontal plane line (SHPL)

s. mobility

s. nerve

s. nerve root sparing

s. pedicle screw

s. pedicle screw fixation

s. plexus

s. plexus injury

s. promontory

s. screw placement

s. segment

s. spine

s. spine decompression

s. spine fixation

s. spine fusion

s. spine modular instrumentation

s. spine stabilization

s. support

s. tilt

s. triangle

s. tuberosity

s. vertebra

sacralgia

sacralization

sacralized transverse process

sacrectomy

sacrificing knee prosthesis

sacrococcygeal

s. abscess

s. articulation

s. chordoma

s. joint

s. ligament

s. muscle

sacrodynia

Sacro-Eze lumbar support

sacrofemoral angle

sacrohorizontal angle

sacroiliac (SI)

s. approach

s. articulation

s. belt

s. binder

s. block

s. buttressing procedure

s. disarticulation

s. dislocation

s. extension fixation

s. flexion fixation

s. fracture

s. hypermobility syndrome

s. joint

s. joint arthropathy

s. joint inflammatory
  spondyloarthropathy

s. joint injury

s. joint locking

s. joint mobility

S

sacroiliac *(continued)*
  s. joint motion
  s. joint syndrome
  s. ligament
  s. line
  s. orthosis (SIO)
  s. subluxation
  s. symphysis line
sacroiliitis
sacrooccipital technique (SOT)
sacrospinal
  s. ligament
  s. muscle
sacrospinalum
sacrospinous ligament
sacrotomy
sacrotuberal ligament
sacrotuberous ligament
sacrovertebral angle
sacrum, pl. sacra
  transverse process of s.
saddle
  s. back
  basal block cervical s.
  s. block anesthesia
  cervical s.
  s. clamp
  Cloward surgical s.
  s. cushion
  s. prosthesis
saddlebag
  Seidel s.
saddle-shaped joint
SAF
  self-articulating femoral
  SAF hip replacement
  SAF prosthesis
SAFE
  solid ankle flexible endoskeletal
  stationary attachment flexible
    endoskeletal
  SAFE foot
  SAFE orthotic
  SAFE II prosthesis
Safe-T mate anti-rollback device
Safe-T-Wheel pinwheel
safety
  s. performance
  s. pin orthosis
  s. pin splint
safety-bolt suture
Safe-Wrap gauze
SAFHS
  sonic-accelerated fracture-healing system
  SAFHS ultrasound device
Safir pin
SAFK
  single-axis friction knee

sag
  sling seat s.
sage
  S. cheilectomy
  S. driver
  S. driver-extractor
  S. extractor
  S. forearm nail
  S. pin
  S. radial nail
  S. rod
  S. triangular nail
Sage-Clark
  S.-C. cheilectomy
  S.-C. technique
Sager traction splint
Sage-Salvatore
  S.-S. acromioclavicular joint injury
    classification
  S.-S. classification of
    acromioclavicular joint injury
sagittal
  s. band
  s. deformity
  s. kyphosis
  s. mobility
  s. motion
  s. movement
  s. pedicle angle
  s. pedicle diameter
  s. plane
  s. plane instability
  s. roll spondylolisthesis
  s. rotation
  s. spinal canal diameter
  s. split osteotomy
  s. stress test
  s. stress x-ray
  s. surgical saw
sagittal-plane imaging
sagittal-Z osteotomy
Saha
  S. procedure
  S. shoulder muscle classification
  S. transfer technique
Sahara clinical bone sonometer
SAI
  Schema Assessment instrument
SAID
  specific adaptation to imposed demand
  SAID principle
sailboarder injury
Sakellarides calcaneal fracture
  classification
Sakellarides-Deweese technique
Sakoff osteotomy
SAL
  self-aligning knee

Salenius meniscus knife
Saleto-400
Saleto-600
Saleto-800
salient angle
saline
    s. acceptance test
    physiologic s.
    s. solution
saline-enhanced MR arthrogram
SALK
    single-axis locking knee
salt
    gold s.
Salter
    S. criteria
    S. epiphysial fracture classification
    S. fracture
    S. innominate osteotomy
    S. pelvic osteotomy
    S. sling
    S. technique
Salter-Harris
    S.-H. classification of epiphysial
       plate injury
    S.-H. epiphysial injury
    S.-H. fracture (type I–VI)
    S.-H. tibial-fibular injury
    S.-H. tibial-fibular injury
       classification
Salter-Harris-Rang epiphysial fracture
    classification
Salter-Thompson classification
Saltiel brace
salvage
    s. arthrodesis
    limb s.
    s. procedure
Salzer
    S. prosthesis
    S. resurfacing
SAM
    spinal analysis machine
    structural aluminum malleable
       SAM spinal analysis machine
       SAM splint
Sam
    S. Jr. posture analyzer
    S. splint
same-day microsurgical arthroscopic
    lateral-approach laser-assisted
    (SMALL)

Samilson
    S. crescentic calcaneal osteotomy
    S. procedure
    sliding plane osteotomy of S.
Sammarco-DiRaimondo modification of
    Elmslie technique
Sammons biplane goniometer
sample
    Pennsylvania bimanual work s.
Sampson
    S. medullary nail
    S. prosthesis
    S. rod
Samuels forceps
SANC
    short arm navicular cast
sandal
    Benefoot & Birkenstock orthotic s.
    Exercise S.
    Rainbow cast s.
Sandalthotics postural support orthotic
sandbag
    neonatal s.
sandbagging long bone fracture
Sanders
    S. CT Classification
    S. fracture
    S. intraarticular calcaneal fracture
       classification
    S. type
Sandimmune
sand toe injury
sandwiched iliac bone graft
sandwich osteotomy
Sanfilippo syndrome
Sangeorzan
    S. internal fixation
    S. navicular fracture
sanguineous
Sani-Grinder
sanitizer
Sani Vac
Santa Casa distractor
saphenous
    s. artery
    s. flap
    s. nerve
    s. vein
SAPHO
    synovitis-acne-pustulosis-hyperostosis
       osteomyelitis
       SAPHO syndrome

S

NOTES

sapphire
    S. table
    S. View arthroscope
Saratoga cycle
Sarbo sign
sarcoid
    s. arthritis
    Boeck s.
sarcoidosis
sarcoma
    alveolar soft-part s.
    bicompartmental soft tissue s.
    botryoid s.
    chondroblastic s.
    clear cell s.
    deep intracompartmental soft
      tissue s.
    epithelioid s.
    Ewing s.
    extracompartmental soft tissue s.
    fascial s.
    femoral s.
    fibroblastic s.
    giant cell s.
    high-grade surface osteogenic s.
    human osteogenic s. (HOS)
    intracortical osteogenic s.
    Kaposi s.
    low-grade central osteogenic s.
    malignant myeloid s.
    multicentric osteogenic s.
    osteoblastic osteogenic s.
    osteogenic s.
    osteolytic s.
    Paget-associated osteogenic s.
    parosteal osteogenic s.
    periosteal s.
    postirradiation osteogenic s.
    reticular cell s.
    sclerosa osteoblastic osteogenic s.
    small cell osteogenic s.
    soft tissue s.
    subcutaneous intracompartmental
      soft tissue s.
    subcutaneous soft tissue s.
    synovial cell s.
sarcomatous change
sarcopenia
sarcoplasmic reticulum
sarcotubular myopathy
Sargent knee operation
Sarmiento
    S. fracture brace
    S. intertrochanteric osteotomy
    S. nail
    S. short leg patellar tendon-bearing
      cast

    S. STH-2 hip prosthesis
    S. trochanteric fracture technique
Sarot needle holder
sartorial slide procedure
sartorius
    s. muscle
    s. tendon
SAS
    short arm splint
    shoulder arm system
    SAS II brace
    SAS shoe
Saso Variable Speed Massager
Sat-A-Lite contoured wedge seat
    cushion
sateen knee immobilizer
satellite
    s. myofascial trigger point
    s. potential
Saticon tube camera
Satterlee
    S. amputating saw
    S. bone saw
saturation
    arterial oxygen s.
    fat s.
Saturday night palsy
Saturn carpal tunnel splint
saucerization
Saucony shoe
Sauerbruch
    S. prosthesis
    S. retractor
    S. rib elevator
    S. rib forceps
    S. rib shears
Saunders
    S. cervical HomeTrac
    S. mobilization wedge
    S. traction
sausage
    s. digit
    s. finger
    s. toe
Sauvé-Kapandji
    S.-K. arthroplasty
    S.-K. procedure
Savastano
    S. hemiknee
    S. Hemi-Knee prosthesis
    S. Hemi-Knee system
    S. unconstrained prosthesis
    S. unicompartment prosthesis
saver
    intraoperative Cell S.
    knee s.
saw
    Adams s.

Adson wire s.
Aesculap s.
air-driven oscillating s.
amputation s.
Bailey wire s.
bayonet s.
Beaver s.
Bier amputation s.
Bishop s.
bone s.
Charriere amputation s.
Charriere bone s.
circular s.
Cottle s.
counter rotating s.
crescentic s.
crosscut s.
Delrin-handle bone s.
DeMartel wire s.
electric cast s.
end-cutting reciprocating s.
Engel plaster s.
fine-tooth electric s.
Gigli s.
Gigli-Strully s.
s. guide
Hall air-driven oscillating s.
Hall sagittal s.
Hall Versipower oscillating s.
Hall Versipower reciprocating s.
hand s.
Henschke-Mauch s.
Herbert s.
Horsley bone s.
humeral s.
intramedullary s.
Langenbeck bone s.
Langenbeck metacarpal s.
Lebsche wire s.
Leica model 1600 water-cooled diamond s.
Luck-Bishop bone s.
medullary s.
Micro-Aire oscillating s.
microoscillating s.
microsagittal s.
Miltex bone s.
Müller s.
Osada s.
oscillating s.
patella bone s.
Pearson intramedullary s.

Percy amputating s.
plaster s.
power-driven s.
power oscillating s.
reciprocating motor s.
Rust amputation s.
sagittal surgical s.
Satterlee amputating s.
Satterlee bone s.
single-blade s.
single-sided bone s.
Skil s.
Sklar bone s.
Stryker s.
Tuke s.
twin-blade oscillating s.
Weiss amputation s.
Zimmer oscillating s.

Sawa
S. shoulder brace
S. shoulder orthosis

sawblade
Stablecut s.

sawcut

Sayre
S. bandage
S. elevator
S. jacket
S. operation
S. splint
S. suspension apparatus
S. suspension traction

Sbarbaro
S. hip prosthesis
S. spica cast
S. tibial plateau prosthesis

SBO
spina bifida occulta

SB+ testing and treatment

SB− testing and treatment

SC
sternoclavicular
supracondylar
SC suspension

scaffold
collagen s.

Scaglietti
S. closed reduction technique
S. procedure scale

scalar
s. classification
s. quantity

NOTES

scale

Abbreviated Injury S. (AIS)
Abnormal Involuntary Movement S. (AIMS)
Adelaar-Williams-Gould ten-point s.
Adolescent and Pediatric Pain Tool S.
Alberta Infant Motor S. (AIMS)
American Musculoskeletal Tumor Society rating s.
American Orthopaedic Foot and Ankle Society Ankle-Hindfoot S.
American Shoulder and Elbow Surgeons s.
American Spinal Injury Association impairment s.
Angus-Cowell s.
ankle-hindfoot s.
AOFAS Lesser Metatarsophalangeal-Interphalangeal S. (LMIS)
Arthritis Impact Measurement S. (AIMS)
Arthritis Quality of Life S.
Ashworth s.
ASIA impairment s.
balance beam s.
Borg s.
Boyd Modification of the Tardieu spastic measurement s.
Broberg-Morrey elbow function s.
Charnley-Merle D'Aubigné disability grading s.
Charnley pain and function grading s.
Clyde Mood s.
S.'s of Cognitive Ability for Traumatic Brain Injury (SCATBI)
Crowe hip s.
DASH s.
Disabilities of the Arm, Shoulder, and Hand s.
disability s.
economic self-sufficiency WHO Handicap S.
Edinburgh Rehabilitation Status S. (ERSS)
Exercise Self-Efficacy S.
Expanded Disability Status S. (EDSS)
foot and ankle severity s. (FASS)
French s.
Gait Abnormality Rating S. (GARS)
Geissling rating s.
Glasgow Coma s.
Graphic Rating S. (GRS)
hallux metatarsophalangeal interphalangeal s. (HMIS)
Harris hip s.
Health O Meter S.
Hospital for Special Surgery s.
International Knee Documentation Committee knee s.
JOA S.
Johnson-Boseker s.
Karlsson and Peterson scoring s.
Kellgren knee s.
Kenna Knee S.
Kitaoka clinical rating s.
Knirk-Jupiter elbow evaluation s.
Köhler hip protrusion grading s.
Kurtzke Expanded Disability s.
linear analog pain s.
Lower Extremity Functional S. (LEFS)
Lysholm-Gillquist knee subjective function s.
Lysholm knee function scoring s.
Mathew s.
McGill pain s.
Merle d'Aubigné and Postel hip rating s.
metatarsophalangeal-interphalangeal s.
midfoot s.
mobility WHO Handicap S.
modified Gait Abnormality Rating S.
Modified Rankin s.
NEECHAM Confusion S.
numeric rating s. (NRS)
Oral Analogue S. (OAS)
orientation WHO Handicap S.
Outerbridge s.
Perez postoperative pain s.
physical independence WHO Handicap S.
Portola Valley S.
Progressive Ambulation S.
Prosthetic Problem Inventory S.
Quality of Well-Being S.
Quebec Back Pain Disability S.
Ranchos Los Amigos S.
Reddihough s.
Rotes joint mobility s.
Scaglietti procedure s.
Severin hip dysplasia s.
social integration World Health Organization Handicap S.
Sports Activity S.
Stanford Hypnotic Clinical S.
Steinberg rating s.
Symptoms and Sports Participation Rating S.
Tardieu spasticity measurement s.
Tegner activity rating s.

The Knee Society clinical-rating s.
UCLA Shoulder Rating s.
visual analog s.
Volpicelli functional ambulation s.
Wechsler Adult Intelligence s.
Wechsler Memory s.

scalene
s. block
s. fat pad
s. maneuver
s. muscle

scalenotomy
scalenus anterior syndrome
scalloping
endosteal s.
s. of vertebra
vertebral s.

scalpel
Bard-Parker s.

scalprum
scan
adenosine thallium s.
bone s.
CT s.
DEXA s.
DXA s.
gallium-67 s.
gallium citrate s.
intrathecally enhanced CT s.
isotope bone s.
lead-line s.
leukocyte s.
multiplanar computed tomography s.
multiplanar CT s.
nuclear magnetic resonance s.
positron emission tomographic s.
radioisotope gallium s.
radioisotope indium-labeled white
  blood cell s.
radioisotope technetium s.
radionuclide bone s.
rectilinear bone s.
technetium-99m diphosphonate s.
technetium-99m pyrophosphate s.
technetium-99m sulfur colloid s.
thallium s.
three-phase bone s.
triple-phase bone s.
triple-phase isotope bone s.
white blood cell s.

Scandinavian total ankle replacement (STAR)

Scand pin
scanner
Acoma s.
All-Tronics s.
thermographic s.

scanning
s. densitometry
s. EMG

Scan-O-Gram of lower extremity
scanogram radiography
scanography
Scanz osteotomy
scaphocapitate
s. fusion
s. interval
s. joint
s. syndrome

scaphocapitolunate arthrodesis (SCL)
scaphoid
bipartite s.
s. bone
carpal s.
s. cookie in shoe
s. fracture
s. humpback deformity
s. lift test
s. nonunion
s. scapula
s. screw guide
s. shift test
s. shoe cookie
s. shoe pad
s. tuberosity injury
waist of s.

scaphoiditis
scaphoid-lunate
Scaphoid-Microstaple system
scapholunate (SL)
s. advanced collapse (SLAC)
s. angle
s. arthritis collapse (SLAC)
s. dissociation
s. gap
s. instability
s. interosseous ligament
s. joint

scaphotrapeziotrapezoid arthrodesis
scaphotrapezoid interosseous ligament
scaphotrapezoid-trapezial (STT)
scapula, pl. scapulae
alar s.
s. alata

NOTES

scapula *(continued)*
  body of s.
  s. elevata
  elevated s.
  glenoid fossa of s.
  Graves s.
  locked s.
  scaphoid s.
  snapping s.
  winging of s.
scapulalgia
scapular
  s. approximation test
  s. border
  s. dysfunction
  s. elevation
  s. flap
  s. fracture
  s. graft
  s. ligament
  s. nerve
  s. notch
  s. peroneal atrophy
  s. reflex
  s. sign of Putti
  s. winging
scapulary
scapulectomy
  Das Gupta s.
  Phelps s.
scapuloclavicular
  s. articulation
  s. injury
  s. joint
scapulocostal syndrome
scapulodynia
scapulohumeral
  s. atrophy
  s. bursa
  s. ligament
  s. muscle
  s. reflex
  s. rhythm
scapulolateral view
scapuloperoneal syndrome
scapulopexy
scapulothoracic
  s. arthrodesis
  s. bursitis
  s. dissociation
  s. fusion
  s. joint
  s. motion
  s. muscle
  s. pain
scapulovertebral border
scar
  area s.

s. band
s. formation
hypertrophic s.
keloid s.
linear s.
parasagittal s.
peritendinous s.
physial s.
s. tissue
Scarborough
  S. prosthesis
  S. total hip replacement
scarf
  s. bandage
  s. Z osteotomy
  s. Z osteotomy/bunionectomy
  s. Z-plasty
scarlatinal synovitis
Scarpa fascia
scarring
  s. cosmesis
  s. effect
  epineural s.
  s. and furrowing
SCATBI
  Scales of Cognitive Ability for Traumatic
  Brain Injury
  SCATBI Assessment
SCC
  short calcaneocuboid
  SCC ligament
SCD
  sequential compression device
  SCD stockings
Scerratti goniometer
SCFE
  slipped capital femoral epiphysis
Schaberg-Harper-Allen technique
Schaffer squeeze
Schanz
  S. angulation osteotomy
  S. collar
  S. collar brace
  S. disease
  S. dressing
  S. femoral osteotomy
  S. operation
  S. pin
  S. screw
  S. syndrome
Schatzker tibial plateau fracture
  classification
Schauwecker
  S. patellar tension band wire
  S. patellar wiring
  S. patellar wiring technique
Schede
  S. bone curette

S. hip osteotomy
S. method
Scheffé
S. interval
S. test
Scheie syndrome
Schell bone rongeur
Schema Assessment instrument (SAI)
Schepens hollow silicone hemisphere implant material
Schepsis-Leach technique
Scherisorb dressing
Scher nail biopsy
Scheuermann
S. disease
S. dystrophic spondylosis
S. juvenile kyphosis (SJK)
S. kyphosis
S. syndrome
Schiek Belt
Schink metatarsal retraction
Schlatter disease
Schlatter-Osgood disease
Schlein
S. clamp
S. elbow arthroplasty
S. semiconstrained elbow prosthesis
S. shoulder positioner
S. total elbow prosthesis
S. trisurface ankle prosthesis
Schlesinger
S. cervical punch forceps
S. cervical rongeur
S. intervertebral disk rongeur
S. punch
S. rongeur forceps
S. sign
Schmeisser
S. spica
S. spica cast
Schmid
S. disease
S. metaphysial dysostosis
Schmidt rod holder
Schmitt fan
Schmorl
S. disease
S. node
S. nodule
Schneider
S. driver-extractor
S. extractor

S. extractor-driver
S. fixation
S. hip arthrodesis
S. medullary nail
S. nail driver
S. pin
S. rasp
S. rod
Schneider-Sauerbruch rasp
Schnute wedge resection technique
Schober
S. measurement
S. method
S. technique
S. test
S. test of lumbar flexion
Schoemaker line
Scholl pad
Scholten sternal retractor
Schreiber maneuver
Schrock
S. arthroplasty
S. procedure
Schuind external fixation
Schuknecht
S. Gelfoam wire prosthesis
S. Teflon wire piston prosthesis
Schultze acroparesthesia
Schutte shovelnose basket
Schwann
S. cell
S. tumor
schwannoma
cellular s.
collagenous s.
malignant s.
Schwartz
S. clip-applying forceps
S. dorsiflexory osteotomy
S. syndrome
S. temporary clamp-applying forceps
Schwartz-Blajwas-Marcinko irrigation system
Schwartze chisel
Schwartz-Jampel
S.-J. myotonia
S.-J. syndrome
Schwarz finger extension bow
Schweitzer
S. pin
S. spring plate

NOTES

Schwinn
S. Air-Dyne bicycle
S. bi-directional Windjammer upper
body cycle
S. elliptical full body exercise
machine
S. Fitness Advisor
S. Spinner bicycle
S. 900 stationary bicycle
SCI
spinal cord injury
sciatic
s. foramen
s. function index (SFI)
s. leg block
s. nerve
s. nerve injury
s. nerve irritation
s. nerve palsy hematoma
s. neuralgia
s. neuritis
s. notch
s. palsy
s. scoliosis
s. tension sign
sciatica
science
exercise s.
movement s.
occupational s.
scintigraphy
bone s.
combined s.
indium-111 s.
paired s.
triphase technetium s.
scissor-leg
s.-l. gait
s.-l. position
scissor leg
scissors
Acufex s.
adventitial s.
arthroscopic s.
Aslan endoscopic s.
Babcock wire-cutting s.
Bantam wire-cutting s.
Beebe wire-cutting s.
Bellucci alligator s.
blunt-tip iris s.
cartilage s.
collar and crown s.
Crafoord thoracic s.
crown and collar s.
curved Mayo s.
Dean s.
dissecting s.
Fiskars s.

s. gait
Giertz-Stille s.
Halsey nail s.
Harvey wire-cutting s.
hook rotary s.
iris s.
Jones s.
Kay s.
Koenig nail-splitting s.
Laschal suture s.
loop s.
Martin cartilage s.
Mayo s.
McIndoe s.
meniscal s.
meniscectomy s.
meniscus s.
Metzenbaum s.
s. nail drill
Nelson s.
Nicola s.
orthopaedic s.
plain rotary s.
PowerStar bipolar s.
serrated s.
Sistron s.
Sistrunk s.
Slip-N-Snip s.
Smillie meniscal s.
Smith s.
Stephen s.
straight s.
suture s.
tissue s.
Walton s.
Webster meniscectomy s.
Weck microsuture cutting s.
Weller cartilage s.
wire-cutting s.
SCIWORA
spinal cord injury without radiographic
abnormality
SCJ
sternoclavicular joint
SCL
scaphocapitolunate arthrodesis
scleroderma
focal s.
sclerosa osteoblastic osteogenic sarcoma
sclerosing
s. nonsuppurative osteitis
s. nonsuppurative osteomyelitis
sclerosis, pl. scleroses
amyotrophic lateral s. (ALS)
anterolateral s. (ALS)
Baló s.
bone s.
diaphysial s.

endplate s.
Mönckeberg s.
multiple s. (MS)
progressive systemic s.
subchondral s.
systemic s.
zonal s.

sclerotic
s. bone
s. line
s. marginal rim
s. segment
sclerotomal pain
sclerotome pain chart
SCL-90R
Symptoms Checklist 90 Revised
SCOI
Southern California Orthopedic Institute
SCOI arthroscopic tenodesis
SCOI shoulder brace
scoliokyphosis
scoliometer
scoliosis
adolescent s.
adolescent idiopathic s. (AIS)
adult s.
Aussies-Isseis unstable s.
bregmatic bone Brissaud s.
Brissaud s.
s. cast
cicatricial s.
Cobb method for measuring s.
compensatory s.
congenital s.
s. correction
s. correction with Dwyer cable
Cotrel s.
coxitic s.
curve progression in s.
degenerative lumbar s.
dextrorotary s.
dextroscoliosis s.
double major curve s.
double thoracic curve s.
Dwyer correction of s.
electrical surface stimulation
   treatment for s.
empyemic s.
endoscopic correction of s.
Fergusson method for measuring s.
s. fixation
fracture with s.

functional s.
Galen s.
habit s.
hysterical s.
idiopathic s.
infantile idiopathic s.
inflammatory s.
ischiatic s.
juvenile idiopathic s.
King-Moe s.
King s. (type I–V)
kyphosing s.
levoscoliosis s.
lumbar s.
Moe-Kettleson distribution of
   curves in s.
myopathic s.
neuromuscular s.
ocular s.
s. operating frame
ophthalmic s.
osteopathic s.
s. overlap brace
paralytic s.
rachitic s.
S. Research Society Hughston knee
   scope
rheumatic s.
rigid curve s.
rotational s.
sciatic s.
static s.
structural s.
s. surgery
thoracic curve s.
thoracolumbar idiopathic s.
thoracolumbar spine s.
uncompensated rotary s.
Winter-King-Moe s.
scoliotic
s. curve
s. curve fixation
s. pelvis
scoliotone
ScoliTron instrument
scooter
Lark s.
Scoot-Gard mat
scope
Doppler s.
Harris s.
Liviscope s.

NOTES

scope *(continued)*
Lysholm knee joint instability s.
Scoliosis Research Society
Hughston knee s.

SCORE
Simple Calculated Osteoporosis Risk
Estimation

score
AAOS Knee Society Clinical
Rating S.
American Knee Society s.
AOFAS s.
ASES shoulder s.
Bandi patellofemoral s.
Carter-Rowe shoulder s.
Catterall hip s.
Champion Trauma S. (CTS)
Charnley hip s.
composite knee s.
D'Aubigne-Postel postoperative
function s.
duPont Bunion Rating S.
Fries rheumatoid arthritis s.
Fulkerson functional knee s.
Functional Rating S.
Harris hip s. (HHS)
Harris-Mayo hip s.
Hawkins-Warren athlete's
shoulder s.
Hospital for Special Surgery
knee s.
HSS knee s.
Hughston knee s.
IKDC s.
Injury Severity S. (ISS)
Iowa hip s.
Kapandji thumb opposition s.
Knee Society S.
Kofoed Ankle S.
Kurtzke s.
Larsen hip s.
Lysholm s.
Lysholm-Gillquist knee subjective
function s.
Mangled Extremity Severity S.
(MESS)
Marshall knee s.
Maryland Foot S.
Mayo Clinic forefoot s.
Mayo elbow performance s.
McGuire s.
Merchant and Dietz ankle s.
Merle d'Aubigné hip s.
modified Harris hip s.
modified Rowe shoulder s.
Molander-Olerud shoulder s.
Oswestry Disability S.
Sherman s.

skeletal injury s.
Tegner knee reconstruction
activity s.
trauma s.

scored cartilage
scoring
Knee Society total knee
arthroplasty roentgenography
evaluation and s.
Scorpio total knee system
Scotchcast
S. 2 cast tape
S. length splinting system
scotoma, pl. **scotomata**
absolute s.
Scott
S. ankle splint
S. arthroplasty
S. double-strap ankle support
S. elastic ankle strap
S. glenoplasty technique
S. hinged knee support
S. humeral splint
S. posterior glenoplasty
S. Uniform tennis elbow splint
S. wrist wrap
Scottish
S. Rite brace
S. Rite hip orthosis
S. Rite splint
Scott-McCracken periosteal elevator
Scott-RCE osteotomy guide
scotty
s. dog sign
S. stainless ankle joint
scout film
Scoville
S. curette
S. retractor
Scranton transmalleolar arthrodesis
scraper
Bradley femoral canal
preparation s.
scraping toe gait
screen
Fast Lanex rare earth s.
Lanex s.
split s.
screening
Gait, Arms, Legs, and Spine s.
GALS s.
ISIS s.
neuropsychological s.
s. palpation
screw
Absolute absorbable s.
Ace s.
AcroMed s.

alar s.
s. alignment bar
s. alignment rod
Alta cancellous s.
Alta cortical s.
Alta cross-locking s.
Alta lag s.
Alta supracondylar s.
Alta transverse s.
AMBI hip s.
Amset R-F s.
anchor s.
s. angle guide
s. angulation
AO-ASIF s.
AO cancellous s.
AO cortex s.
AO lag s.
AO spongiosa s.
Arthrex sheathed interference s.
arthrodesis s.
ASIF cancellous s.
ASIF cortical s.
ASIF malleolar s.
Asnis III cannulated s.
Aten olecranon s.
Autogenesis automator for
  Ilizarov s.
axial compression s.
s. backout
Barouk cannulated bone s.
Basile hip s.
Bechtol s.
bicortical s.
Bio-Absorbable interference s.
BioCuff C bioresorbable
  cannulated s.
Bio-Interference tibial s.
Biologically Quiet interference s.
Bionx absorbable cannulated s.
Bionx self-reinforced PLLA
  smart s.
BioRCI s.
BioScrew absorbable interference s.
BioSorbFX SR self-reinforced plate
  and s.
Bold compression s.
bone mulch s.
Bosworth coracoclavicular s.
s. breakage
buttress thread s.
Campbell cannulated s.

cancellous bone s.
cannulated cancellous lag s.
cannulated hip s.
CAPIS s.
carpal scaphoid s.
Carrell-Girard s.
Caspar cervical s.
chrome cobalt s.
Clearfix s.
Cohort bone s.
Collison s.
compression hip s.
compression lag s.
s. compressor
Concise compression hip s.
cortex s.
cortical bone s.
cortical cancellous s.
Cotrel pedicle s.
Coventry s.
crown drill s.
cruciate head bone s.
cruciform head bone s.
Cubbins s.
DeMuth hip s.
s. depth calibrator
s. depth gauge
DePuy interference s.
Deyerle interlocking s.
distal locking s.
distraction s.
double-threaded Herbert s.
Duo-Drive s.
Dwyer spinal s.
Dynamic condylar s. (DCS)
dynamic hip s. (DHS)
ECT bone s.
Edwards modular system
  spinal/sacral s.
Eggers s.
encased s.
EndoFix bioabsorbable
  interference s.
s. epiphysiodesis
expansion s.
Fabian s.
femoral head cork s.
Fixateur Interne s.
s. fixation
s. fixation operation
flute of cannulated s.
foreign body s.

NOTES

screw *(continued)*
four-tap s.
s. fusion
Garden s.
Gentle Threads interference s.
Glasgow s.
Glass-Bessen transfixion s.
glenoid fixation s.
Guardsman femoral interference s.
Hahn s.
Hall spinal s.
Hamilton s.
s. head
Heck s.
Hedrocel titanium s.
Henderson lag s.
Herbert bone s.
Herbert scaphoid s.
Herbert-Whipple bone s.
hex s.
hexagonal slot-cap s.
hip compression s.
hollow mill Asnis cannulated s.
hook trial set s.
Howmedica ICS s.
Howmedica Universal
  compression s.
iliac s.
iliosacral s.
Ilizarov s.
s. implantation
s. insertion
s. insertion technique
Instrument Makar biodegradable
  interference s.
Integrity acetabular cup s.
interference s.
interfragmentary lag s.
Intrafix s.
Isola spinal implant system iliac s.
Isola vertebral s.
Jeter lag/position s.
Jewett pick-up s.
Johannson lag s.
Jones s.
Kaessmann s.
Kostuik s.
Kristiansen eyelet lag s.
Kurosaka interference-fit s.
lag s.
Lane bone s.
lateral s.
Leinbach olecranon s.
Leone expansion s.
Linvatec absorbable s.
Lippman s.
locking s.
Long Beach pedicle s.

s. loosening
Lorenzo s.
Luhr s.
lumbar pedicle s.
Lundholm s.
Luque II s.
Luque pedicle s.
machine s.
malleolar s.
Marion s.
Martin s.
maxillofacial bone s.
McLaughlin carpal scaphoid s.
medial bicortical s.
medial unicortical s.
Medoff axial compression s.
micrometric s.
mille pattes s.
mini AO s.
minifragment s.
Moberg s.
Morris biphase s.
Moss s.
Mouradian s.
multiaxial s.
navicular s.
Neufeld s.
No-Lok s.
non-self-tapping s.
Olerud PSF s.
Ormandy s.
Orthex cannulated bone s.
Orthofix s.
Osteomed s.
OsteoTite bone s.
Palex expansion s.
Palmer s.
pedicle s.
PerFixation s.
PGA s.
Phillips head s.
Phillips recessed-head s.
Pilot point s.
s. placement C-guide
polyaxial cervical s.
polylactide absorbable s.
s. position perioperative monitoring
posterior-anterior s.
Preston s.
Propel cannulated interference s.
pull s.
Ray s.
ReUnite orthopedic s.
reverse-threaded s.
Revo retrievable cancellous s.
Richards classic compression hip s.
Richards lag s.
Richmond subarachnoid s.

rigid pedicle s.
Rockwood shoulder s.
Russell-Taylor s.
sacral alar s.
sacral pedicle s.
Schanz s.
Scuderi s.
Selby I, II s.
self-tapping bone s.
SemiFix s.
set s.
Shanz s.
Sharpey s.
Shelton bone s.
Sherman bone s.
Simmons double-hole spinal s.
Simmons-Martin s.
sliding compression hip s.
small fragment s.
small-headed s.
spherical-headed s.
spongiosa s.
s. stabilization
stainless steel s.
Steffee plate and s.
step s.
Storz s.
s. stripout
Stryker lag s.
subarticular s.
superior thoracic pedicle s.
Swiss cancellous s.
syndesmotic s.
Synthes compression hip s.
s. tap
Thatcher s.
thoracolumbar pedicle s.
Thornton s.
threaded cancellous s.
thumb s.
tibial head s.
s. tip
titanium s.
Tivanium cancellous bone s.
s. toggle
s. torque
Townley bone graft s.
Townsend-Gilfillan s.
traction tongs s.
transarticular s.
transfixion s.
transpedicular s.

transverse s.
triangulated pedicle s.
TSRH pedicle s.
tulip pedicle s.
Tunneloc bone mulch s.
unicortical s.
Universal fixation s.
Uppsala s.
Vari-Angle s.
varus-valgus adjustment s.
VDS s.
Venable s.
Venable-Stuck s.
Virgin hip s.
Vitallium s.
VLC compression s.
VSF s.
Wagner-Schanz s.
Weise jack s.
Wiltse pedicle s.
wood s.
Woodruff s.
Wurzburg s.
Yuan s.
Zimmer compression hip s.
Zuelzer s.

screw-and-keel fixation
screw-and-plate fixation
screw-and-wire fixation
screwdriver
Allen head s.
automatic s.
Becker s.
Bio-Interference s.
Bosworth s.
cannulated s.
CAPIS s.
Children's Hospital s.
Collison s.
cross-slot s.
cruciform s.
Cubbins bone s.
DePuy s.
Dorsey screw-holding s.
European-style s.
Flatt self-retaining s.
Hall s.
heavy cross-slot s.
hexhead s.
Johnson s.
Ken s.
Lane s.

NOTES

screwdriver *(continued)*
    light cross-slot s.
    Lok-it s.
    Lok-screw double-slot s.
    Massie s.
    Master s.
    Moore-Blount s.
    Phillips head s.
    plain s.
    Richards Phillips s.
    Richter bone s.
    self-retaining s.
    Shallcross s.
    Sherman s.
    Sherman-Pierce s.
    single cross-slot s.
    single-slot s.
    skull plate s.
    straight hex s.
    Stryker s.
    torque s.
    Trinkle s.
    Universal hex s.
    VDS s.
    White s.
    Williams s.
    Woodruff s.
    Zimmer s.
screw-holding forceps
screw-home mechanism
screw-in ceramic acetabular cup
Screw-Lok tap
screw-plate
    s.-p. approach
    Calandruccio impaction s.-p.
    s.-p. fixation
    Zimmer impaction s.-p.
screw-rod
    Wiltse s.-r.
screw-to-screw compression construct
Scrip Muscle Master massager
scroll bone
scrub
    Hibiclens s.
SCS
    spinal canal stenosis
SCSP, SC-SP
    supracondylar-suprapatellar
Scuderi
    S. procedure
    S. screw
    S. technique
Scuder repair
sculling
    rowing and s.
Scully
    S. Hip S'port
    S. Hip S'port hip device

sculp
    Concise cementing s.
    s. knife
Scultetus
    S. bandage
    S. binder
scurvy line
Scutan temporary splint material
S-cutting block
SD
    shoulder disarticulation
    SD sorb staple
SDD
    sterile dry dressing
SDR
    surgical dressing room
Seaber forceps
seal-fin deformity
seal limb
Seal-Tight cast protector
seam
    osteoid s.
searching big toe
searing pain
seat
    antithrust s.
    Backjoy s.
    s. belt
    s. belt injury
    Carrie car s.
    Comfy toilet lift s.
    Dream Ride car s.
    ischial-bearing s.
    Maddacare child bath s.
    Orthopedic Positioning S.
    Posey drop s.
    Renolux convertible car s.
    Rubbermaid adjustable
      bath/shower s.
    Snug s.
    Special S.
    Spelcast car s.
    Tall-ette toilet s.
    Tubsider Kneeling S.
seated
    S. Cable Row exerciser
    s. hamstring curl
    properly s.
    s. root test
    s. scapular retraction exercise
seating
    s. chisel
    s. of prosthesis
    trial s.
    s. wedge
Seattle
    S. foot
    S. Foot prosthesis

S. LightFoot 2
S. modification of Kocher incision
S. orthosis
S. safety knee
S. splint
Seawell rasp
Sebileau periosteal elevator
second
  s. cervical vertebra
  cycle per s. (cps, c/sec)
  s. impact syndrome
  s. metatarsal artery
  milliamperage x s.'s (MAS)
  s. skin pad
secondary
  s. amputation
  s. bone union
  s. closure
  s. disability
  s. erythromelalgia
  s. fracture
  s. hematogenous osteomyelitis
  s. hip-spine syndrome
  s. metatarsalgia
  s. myofascial trigger point
  s. osteosarcoma
  s. posttraumatic syringomyelia
  s. stabilizer
second-generation cementing technique
second-look arthroscopy
section
  bar s.
  calcaneonavicular bar s.
sectioning
  sequential s.
**Secure Yet Gentle surgical dressing
system**
Secur-Fit HA PSL X'tra prosthesis
Sedan goniometer
sedation therapy
Seddon
  S. classification
  S. coin test
  S. dorsal spine costotransversectomy
  S. modification
  S. neurapraxia
  S. neurotmesis
  S. technique
sedentary
  s. lifestyle
  s. occupation
  s. work

Sedillot periosteal elevator
sedimentation rate
Seeburger
  S. implant
  S. retractor
segment
  apical s.
  central s.
  motion s.
  physiologic lock of the motion s.
  relation to subadjacent s.
  sacral s.
  sclerotic s.
  spinal s.
  vertebral motion s.
segmental
  s. alveolar osteotomy
  s. bone defect
  s. bone loss
  s. compression construct
  s. deficiency
  s. dysfunction
  s. fixation
  s. fracture
  s. hyperextension
  s. level
  s. mobility
  s. mobility testing
  s. spinal correction system (SSCS)
  s. spinal instrumentation (SSI)
  s. tendon graft
  s. vertebral
    cellulotenoperiosteomyalgic
    syndrome (SVCPMS)
**segmentally demineralized bone
technology**
segmentation
  s. defect
  supernumerary lumbar s.
**segmented orthopedic system total hip
and knee system**
Segond tibial avulsion fracture
Seidel
  S. bone-holding clamp
  S. humeral locking nail
  S. intramedullary fixation
  S. saddlebag
**Seinsheimer femoral fracture
classification**
Seirin acupuncture needle
seismotherapy
seizing forceps

S

NOTES

seizure
    acute repetitive s. (ARS)
    oxygen s.
Selakovich
    S. procedure
    S. procedure for pes valgo planus
Selby
    S. I, II fixation system
    S. I, II hook
    S. I, II rod
    S. I, II screw
select
    S. ankle prosthesis
    S. joint
    S. joint orthosis
    S. modular shoulder prosthesis
    S. shoulder system
selection
    bone plate s.
    Edwards modular system
      construct s.
selective
    s. posterior rhizotomy (SPR)
    Theraform S.'s
    s. thoracic spine fusion
Selectively Lockable knee brace
self-adhering varus/valgus wedge
self-aligning
    s.-a. knee (SAL)
    s.-a. mobile-bearing knee implant
self-articulating
    s.-a. femoral (SAF)
    s.-a. femoral hip replacement
self-bearing
    s.-b. ceramic hip prosthesis
    s.-b. ceramic total hip replacement
self-broaching
    s.-b. nail
    s.-b. pin
self-care
self-centering
    s.-c. bone-holding forceps
    s.-c. Universal hip prosthesis
self-curing polymer
self-efficacy
    exercise s.-e.
self-help ability
self-locking nail
self-mutilation
self-propelling wheelchair
self-reinforcing polylevolactic acid (SR-PLLA)
self-retaining
    s.-r. bone-holding forceps
    s.-r. clamp
    s.-r. retractor
    s.-r. screwdriver
self-sealing cannula

self-sustained natural apophyseal glides
self-tapering pin
self-tapping bone screw
Selig hip operation
Sell-Frank-Johnson
    S.-F.-J. extensor shift
    S.-F.-J. extensor shift technique
Sellors rib contractor
Selverstone rongeur forceps
Semb
    S. bone forceps
    S. bone-holding clamp
    S. bone rongeur
    S. rib forceps
Semb-Stille bone rongeur
sEMG
    surface electromyography
semicanal of humerus sulcus
semicircular flap amputation
semiconstrained
    s. total elbow arthroplasty
    s. tricompartmental knee prosthesis
SemiFix screw
semiflexion
semi-Fowler position
semilunar
    s. bone
    s. cartilage
    s. cartilage knife
    s. notch
    s. sulcus
semilunaris
    linea s.
semiluxation
semimembranosus
    s. bursitis
    s. complex
    s. muscle
    s. tendinitis
    s. tendon
semiopen sliding tenotomy
semirigid
    s. ankle brace
    s. fiberglass cast (SRF)
    s. polypropylene ankle-foot orthosis
    s. postoperative dressing
    s. shell
semisitting position
semispinal muscle
semi suture-loop technique
semitendinosus
    s. augmentation of patellar tendon
      repair
    s. muscle
    s. procedure
    s. technique
    s. tendon

s. tendon transfer
s. tenodesis
semitendinosus-gracilis graft
semitendinous graft
semitubular
s. blade plate
s. compression plate
Semmes-Weinstein
S.-W. monofilament
S.-W. monofilament pressure
esthesiometry
S.-W. monofilament pressure test
Senegas
S. approach to hip
S. hip approach
senescence
Sengupta quadriceps release
senile
s. hallux valgus
s. hip disease
s. osteomalacia
s. osteoporosis
s. subcapital fracture
senilis
coxa s.
malum coxae s.
Senn
S. plate
S. retractor
senna
sensation
altered s.
catching s.
diminished s.
exteroceptive s.
light touch s.
loss of protective s. (LOPS)
perianal s.
perineal s.
phantom s.
pinprick s.
return of s.
sharp s.
shocklike s.
touch s.
vibration s.
sense
joint position s. (JPS)
position s.
vibration s.
Sense-of-Feel prosthesis
sensibility recovery sequence

sensitivity
vibration s.
sensitometer
Poppen ridge s.
sensor
capacitive s.
DermaTemp infrared
thermographic s.
Myoscan s.
s. pad
Perry s.
Richmond subarachnoid screw s.
Servo Pro force s.
SensorHand prosthesis
sensorimotor, sensory motor
s. deficit
s. nerve
s. stimulation approach
sensorineural, sensory/neural
s. abnormality
sensory
s. awareness
s. component
s. deficit
s. delay
s. evoked potential
s. examination
s. fascicle
s. function
s. impairment
s. integration
s. loss
s. motor
s. nerve
s. nerve action potential (SNAP)
s. nerve conduction velocity
s. peak latency
s. polyneuropathy
s. registration
s. response
s. stimulation kit
sensory-motor training
sensory/neural (*var. of* sensorineural)
sentinel fracture
Senuva lotion
Seoffert triple arthrodesis
SEP
somatosensory evoked potential
microneurography midlatency SEP
separation
AC joint s.
acromioclavicular s.

NOTES

separation *(continued)*
   articular mass s.
   atlantoaxial s.
   degree of s.
   fracture fragment s.
   lamellar s.
   shoulder s.
   sternoclavicular joint s.
   transepiphysial s.
separator
   abduction knee s.
   finger s.
   Horsley s.
   nerve s.
   Sach nerve s.
   toe s.
sepsis
septa (*pl. of* septum)
Septacin implant
septal forceps
septic
   s. arthritis
   s. bursitis
   s. finger joint
   s. knee
   s. necrosis
Septobal bead
septum, pl. **septa**
   Bigelow s.
   fascial s.
   intermuscular s.
   J s.
Sequeira-Khanuja modification
sequela, pl. **sequelae**
sequence
   Carr-Purcell s.
   Carr-Purcell-Meiboom-Gill s.
   muscle patterning s.
   sensibility recovery s.
sequencing bead patterns set
sequential
   s. compression device (SCD)
   s. extremity pump
   s. pneumatic compression boot
   s. pneumatic pump traction
   s. pressure
   s. sectioning
sequentially reamed
sequestered disk
sequestra (*pl. of* sequestrum)
sequestral
sequestrated disk
sequestration
sequestrectomy
sequestrotomy
sequestrum, pl. **sequestra**
   avascular s.
   bone s.

   bony s.
   button s.
   s. forceps
   kissing sequestra
   primary s.
   tuberculous s.
SER
   supination-external rotation
Serafin technique
serendipity
   s. view
   s. view in shoulder radiography
serial
   s. casting
   s. stretch orthoses
   s. wedge cast
series
   Davis s.
   lumbosacral s.
   Option Orthotic S.
   RingLoc acetabular s.
   Valpar component work sample s.
Series-II humeral head
SER-IV
   supination-external rotation IV
   SER-IV fracture
Serola sacroiliac belt
seroma
seronegative
   s. arthropathy
   s. enthesopathy and arthropathy syndrome
   s. rheumatoid arthritis
seropositive rheumatoid arthritis
serosa
   myositis s.
   peritendinitis s.
serosanguineous
serotonergic neuron
serous
   s. abscess
   s. synovitis
serpentine
   s. foam collar
   s. foot
   s. incision
   s. plate
serrated
   s. action potential
   s. fine-cutting knife
   s. scissors
serration
Serrato
   S. forearm pin
   S. forearm rod
serratus
   s. anterior flap

s. anterior muscle
s. anterior paralysis

serum calcium

service

Carticel cartilage-cell culturing s.

Servo Pro force sensor

Servox device

sesamoid

accessory s.
bipartite tibial s.
s. bone
s. clamp
s. disruption
fibular s.
s. fracture
hallucal s.
hallux s.
s. hyperostosis
s. injury
lateral s.
s. ligament
medial s.
tibial s.
tibial hallux s.

sesamoidectomy

s. dissector
fibular s.
lateral s.

sesamoiditis

sesamoidometatarsal joint

sesamophalangeal ligament

sessile

sessile-type osteochondroma

set

acetabular trial s.
ACL guide s.
aluminum contouring template s.
s. angle
s. angle of toe
AO minifragment s.
Bankart shoulder repair s.
bone drill s.
Brown-Mueller T-fastener s.
Craig vertebral biopsy s.
Entrex small joint arthroscopy instrument s.
grid maze s.
hand evaluation s.
Henning instrument s.
Hollywood bed extension hook s.
Lido lift and work s.
nail s.

parquetry s.
prothelen s.
Rousek extraction s.
s. screw
sequencing bead patterns s.
SmartPin instrument s.
Stille bone drill s.
Stille-pattern trephine and bone drill s.
vari-balance board s.
volumeter s.

set-hold adjustment

Seton hip brace

Setopress dressing

setter

bone plug s.

setting

bone s.
Mache electromyogram s.

Seutin plaster shears

seven-hole plate

seventeen-hole plate

Sever

S. disease
S. modification of Fairbank technique

severance

severe s.

severe

s. kyphoscoliosis
s. rigid thoracic curve
s. severance

Severin

anatomical classification system of S.
S. classification
S. hip criteria
S. hip dysplasia scale

Sever-L'Episcopo

S.-L. repair of shoulder
S.-L. shoulder repair

SEWHO

shoulder-elbow-wrist-hand orthosis

sex-linked muscular dystrophy

SFA

superficial femoral artery

SFEMG

single-fiber electromyography

SFI

sciatic function index

S-flap incision

NOTES

S

Sgarlato
> S. device
> S. hammertoe implant (SHIP)
> S. hammertoe implant procedure
> S. procedure
> S. toe implant

shadow
> elliptical overlap s.
> s. shield

Shadow-Line ACF spine retractor system
Shaeffer rigid orthosis
Shaffner orthopedic inserter
shaft
> bone s.
> Cloward drill s.
> distal third of s.
> femoral s.
> s. fracture
> metatarsal s.
> middle third of s.
> ministem s.
> neck s.
> patellar reamer s.
> proximal third of s.
> radial s.

Shallcross screwdriver
Sham procedure
shank
> s. bone
> extended steel s.
> steel s.
> Zimmer-Hudson s.

Shannon 44 bur
Shanz screw
shape
> Erlenmeyer-flask s.
> familial s.

Shapiro
> S. classification
> S. classification of mechanisms of growth arrest

Sharbaro driver
sharing
> Edwards modular system load s.

Shark pediatric wheelchair
sharp
> acetabular angle of S.
> S. acetabular angle
> s. dissection
> s. retractor
> s. sensation
> s. trocar
> s. worm hook

sharp/dull discrimination
Sharpey
> S. fiber
> S. screw

sharp-pointed wire
Sharp-Purser Test
SharpShooter
> S. tissue repair system
> S. tissue repair technique

Sharrard
> S. posterior transfer
> S. transfer technique

Sharrard-Trentani prosthesis
Sharrard-type kyphectomy
Shar-Tek foot positioning grid
shaver
> arthroscopic s.
> automated s.
> Cuda s.
> cutting s.
> Dyonics s.
> Grierson meniscal s.
> Microsect s.
> motorized meniscal s.
> motorized suction s.
> sucker s.
> synovial s.

shaving
> arthroscopic s.
> femoral condylar s.
> s. system

Shaw-Sgarlato hammertoe implant prosthesis
Shaw-SHIP
> S.-S. rod
> S.-S. rod hammertoe implant

Shea
> S. drill
> S. prosthesis placement instrument

shear
> airplane s.'s
> anterior s.
> Baer rib s.'s
> Bethune-Coryllos rib s.
> Bethune rib s.'s
> biarticular bone s.'s
> Brunner rib s.'s
> Brunn plaster s.'s
> Collins rib s.'s
> Cooley rib s.'s
> Esmarch plaster s.'s
> Felt s.'s
> s. fracture
> Giertz rib s.'s
> Giertz-Shoemaker rib s.'s
> Gluck rib s.'s
> Hercules plaster s.'s
> lateral s.
> Lefferts rib s.'s
> Liston s.'s
> Liston-Key-Horsley rib s.'s
> s. maneuver

Sauerbruch rib s.'s
Seutin plaster s.'s
s. stiffness
Stille plaster s.'s
s. strain
s. stress
s. test
s. testing
vertical s. (VS)

ShearBan low-friction interface
Shearer rongeur
shearing
s. callosity
s. callus
s. force
s. injury
S. posterior chamber implant
material

shear-off device
sheath
arthroscopic s.
carotid s.
digital flexor tendon s.
fascia s.
femoral s.
fibroosseous s.
flexor tendon s.
giant cell tumor of tendon s.
muscle s.
pigmented nodular synovitis of
tendon s.
rectus s.
synovial s.
tendinous s.
tendon s.
tenosynovial s.
visceral tendon s.

sheathed knife
sheath/liner
Silipos Distal Dip prosthetic s./l.

Sheehan
S. chisel
S. gouge
S. knee prosthesis
S. osteotome

sheepskin
sheet
Alpha flat s.
Antishear gel s.
Barrier lower extremity s.
s. cork
iodoform-impregnated plastic s.

Korex cork s.
laparotomy s.
Novagel gel s.
Ortholen s.
PPT s.
sterile s.

sheeting
Carboplast II s.
Silastic s.
sterile s.

Sheffield
S. hand elevator
S. rod
S. support

shelf
s. acetabuloplasty
Blumer s.
s. flexion
lateral s.
medial s.
patellar s.
s. pedestal
s. procedure

shell
AFO standard s.
s. allograft
calf s.
s. impactor
s. implant material
IROM splint with s.'s
protrusio s.
Restoration Secur-Fit X'tra
acetabular s.
semirigid s.
S-ROM contained s.
thigh s.
total hip articular replacement by
internal eccentric s.'s (THARIES)
Unna paste s.

shelling off of cartilage
Shelton
S. bone screw
S. femoral fracture classification

shelving
Shenton line
Shepherd
S. fracture
S. internal screw fixation

shepherd's crook deformity
Sher diabetic shoe inlay
Sherfee prosthesis

NOTES

Sherk-Probst
    S.-P. percutaneous pinning
    S.-P. technique
Sherlock threaded suture anchor
Sherman
    S. block test
    S. bone plate
    S. bone screw
    S. remote podiatric vacuum system
    S. score
    S. screwdriver
Sherman-Pierce screwdriver
Sherman-Stille drill
Sherrington law
Sherwin knee retractor
ShiatsuBACK back support
Shiatsu therapeutic massage
shield
    AME pin site s.
    arthroscopic s.
    bunion s.
    contact s.
    Nolan system collimator mounted
      contact s.
    protective s.
    shadow s.
    Sof-Gel palm s.
    Sportelli system collimator mounted
      contact s.
shielding
    stress s.
Shier knee prosthesis
Shifrin wire twister
shift
    anterior talus s.
    atraumatic, multidirectional, bilateral
      rehabilitation inferior (capsular s.)
    capsular s.
    glenohumeral s.
    inferior capsular s. (ICS)
    laser-assisted capsular s.
    lateral lumbar s.
    lateral pivot s.
    lateral trunk s.
    pelvic lateral s.
    plantar s.
    plasma volume s.
    reverse pivot s.
    Sell-Frank-Johnson extensor s.
    s. sign
    talar s.
    s. test
    trochanteric s.
    trunk s.
shifter
    AliMed Conductive Patient S.
shifting
    vessel s.

shin
    s. bone
    saber s.
    s. splint
shingling
SHIP
    Sgarlato hammertoe implant
    SHIP implant
Shirley drain
shirt
    EZ "T" orthopedic s.
shish kebab technique
shock
    s. absorption
    s. artifact
    neurogenic s.
    prosthetic stance phase s.
    spinal s.
    s. treatment
    vasogenic s.
shock-absorbent
    s.-a. heel pad
    s.-a. sole
shocklike sensation
Shockmaster heel cushion
shock-wave therapy (SWT)
shod
    rubber s.
shoe
    accommodative s.
    AccuTread s.
    Acor Quikform I, II s.
    Ambulator H1200 healing s.
    Ambulatory s.
    Apex Ambulator s.
    Ariat s.
    arthritic s.
    Asics GEL-MC s.
    balmoral laced s.
    Bebax s.
    Bevin s.
    Birkenstock s.
    Blucher laced s.
    broad-toed s.
    Brooks s.
    calcaneal spur pad in s.
    Canfield s.
    cast s.
    Comed postoperative s.
    s. cookie
    corrective s.
    custom-made s.
    custom-molded s.
    cut-out s.
    Dansko s.
    Darco surgical s.
    Darco Wedge s.
    depth inlay s.

Depth orthopedic s.
s. dermatitis
diabetic pressure relief s.
extended-counter s.
extended steel-shank s.
s. extension
extra-depth s.
s. filler
s. gear
GentleStep s.
healing s.
s. heel pad
HeelWedge healing s.
H1209 healing s.
H1215 healing s.
high heel s.
Hi-Top s.
ill-fitting s.
infant clown cast s.
s. insert
ipos heel relief s.
ipos postoperative s.
J&J postoperative s.
laced blucher of s.
s. lift
low-heeled s.
low quarter Blucher s.
Markell Mobility S.'s
Markell open-toe s.
Markell tarso medius straight s.
Markell tarso pronator outflare s.
Mephisto Mobils professional s.
s. modification
Moon Boot s.
narrow toebox s.
navicular cookie in s.
neoprene s.
normal last s.
open-toe s.
orthopaedic oxford s.
s. orthotic
OrthoWedge healing s.
oversize tennis s.
Pedors orthopedic s.
pointed toe s.
Power Anthro S.
pressure relief s.
Reebok s.
Reece orthopedic s.
reverse last s.
ribbed-sole s.
rockerbottom s.

SAS s.
Saucony s.
scaphoid cookie in s.
Softie s.
soft-vamp s.
s. sole
space s.
stiff-soled s.
straight last s.
s. stretcher
tarsal pronator s.
Terrmocork diabetic s.
Thera-Medic s.
therapeutic s.
torque heel s.
Tru-Fit custom molded s.
Tru-Mold s.
Urban Walkers s.
vamp of s.
Vibram rockerbottom s.
Viking postoperative s.
Viva s.
WACH orthopedic s.
s. wear
Weaver rockerbottom s.
s. wedge
wedge adjustable cushioned heel s.
wedged s.
wide toebox s.
wooden s.
wooden-soled s.
Xsensibles s.
Xtra Depth s.
Zimmer postoperative s.
Zohar s.

shoe-foot interface
Shoemaker lateral approach
shooting pain
short

s. arm brace
s. arm cast (SAC)
s. arm fiberglass cast
s. arm gauntlet cast
s. arm navicular cast (SANC)
s. arm splint (SAS)
s. arm sugar-tong splint
s. bone
s. calcaneocuboid (SCC)
s. calcaneocuboid ligament
s. coarse bur
s. curette
s. external rotator

NOTES

short *(continued)*
 s. fibula
 s. fibular muscle
 s. fine bur
 s. leg
 s. leg caliper brace
 s. leg cast (SLC)
 s. leg double-upright brace
 s. leg gait
 s. leg orthosis
 s. leg plaster cast
 s. leg splint
 s. leg syndrome
 s. leg walker
 s. leg walking brace
 s. leg walking cast (SLWC)
 s. lever accessory movement
  technique
 s. lever specific contact procedure
 S. Musculoskeletal Function
  Assessment (SMFA)
 S. Musculoskeletal Function
  Assessment questionnaire
 s. oblique fracture
 s. opponens orthosis
 s. plantar ligament (SPL)
 s. radiolunate (SRL)
 s. rib polydactyly
 s. segment spinal fusion
 s. stature
 s. thumb
 s. walking cast
 s. Z bunionectomy
short-acting block anesthesia
shortened foot
shortening
 Achilles tendon s.
 Broughton-Olney-Menelaus tibial
  diaphysial s.
 closed femoral diaphysial s.
 s. collectomy
 s. contraction
 digital s.
 distal Wagner femoral
  metaphysial s.
 femoral metaphysial s.
 fibula s.
 fibular s.
 Hoffa tendon s.
 leg s.
 metaphysial s.
 s. osteotomy
 proximal femoral metaphysial s.
 proximal Wagner metaphysial s.
 skeleton s.
 tibial diaphysial s.
 Wagner femoral metaphysial s.

 Winquist-Hansen-Pearson closed
  femoral diaphysial s.
short-latency somatosensory evoked
 potential
short-limb dwarfism
short-radius kyphosis
shortwave diathermy (SWD)
shotgun injury
Shotokan karate
shot wadding
shoulder
 s. abduction immobilizer
 s. abduction pillow
 s. abduction positioner
 s. abduction test
 s. amputation
 s. ankylosis
 apprehension s.
 s. apprehension sign
 archer's s.
 s. arm system (SAS)
 s. arthrodesis
 s. arthroplasty
 baseball s.
 Bigliani/Flatow complete s.
 s. blade
 s. bone
 bull's eye s.
 s. clock
 s. complex
 s. contracture
 s. controller
 s. cuff
 s. depression test
 s. disarticulation (SD)
 s. disarticulation prosthesis
 s. dislocation
 s. dome
 double contrast arthrotomography
  of s.
 drop s.
 s. dystopia
 S. Ease abduction support
 flail s.
 frozen s.
 s. girdle
 hatchet-head s.
 s. holder
 s. horn
 s. impingement sign
 s. instability
 s. joint
 s. joint effusion
 knocked-down s.
 s. ladder
 Little Leaguer's s.
 loose s.
 Neviaser classification of frozen s.

s. orthosis (SO)
S. Pain and Disability Index patient questionnaire
s. pointer
s. pulley
s. radiography
s. range of motion
s. reduction
s. repair
ring man s.
s. ROM arc
round s.
s. saddle sling
s. separation
S. Severity Index patient questionnaire
Sever-L'Episcopo repair of s.
s. spica cast
s. spica splint
stubbed s.
s. subluxation
s. subluxation inhibitor (SSI)
s. subluxation inhibitor brace
swimmer's s.
tennis s.
terrible triad of the s.
S. Therapy Kit
weightlifter's s.
s. wheel
shoulder-elbow-wrist-hand orthosis (SEWHO)
shoulder-girdle syndrome
shoulder-hand-finger syndrome
shoulder-hand syndrome
shoulderRAP wrap
shoulder-to-head check
ShowerSafe
S. waterproof cast and bandage cover
S. waterproof cast and bandage protector
Show'rbag
SHPL
sacral horizontal plane line
Shriners pin
shrinker
stump s.
Shriver-Johnson interphalangeal arthrodesis
shucking
shuck test
shuffling gait

shunt
s. muscle
Sundt s.
ventriculoperitoneal s.
Shur-Band self-closure elastic bandage
shuttle
S. Balance trainer
S. cardiomuscular conditioner
Caspari s.
S. MiniClinic resistance system
S. MVP leg press
Shuttle-Relay suture passer
Shutt Mantis retrograde forceps
Shwachman syndrome
SI
sacroiliac
SI belt
SI joint
sialoprotein
bone s.
sibilant
Sibson
S. fascia
S. muscle
sicca
caries s.
synovitis s.
sickle-cell anemia
sickle-shape Beaver blade
side
s. bending
crest sign s.
s. cutter
dollar sign s.
S. Kick I, II table
s. lunge back exercise technique
s. plate
posterior rotation on the left s.
posterior rotation on the right s.
s. posture reduction
side-bending
s.-b. barrier
s.-b. mobility
side-cut pin cutter
side-cutting
s.-c. basket forceps
s.-c. blade
s.-c. bur
s.-c. Swanson bar
side-glide test
side-jump test

NOTES

Sidekick foot support
sideline assessment of concussion (SAC)
sidelines triage
side-lying
 s.-l. back exercise technique
 s.-l. hip abductor
 s.-l. iliac compression test
 s.-l. position
side-opening laminar hook
sideplate
 s. barrel
 barreled s.
 compression s.
 Richards s.
 sliding compression screw with s.
side-posture position
side-shift
 pelvic s.-s.
side-swing plasty
sideswipe
 s. elbow fracture
 s. injury
Siegel hip release
Sielke instrumentation
Sieman table
Siemens linear accelerator
Sierra 2-load voluntary opening
Siffert-Forster-Nachamie arthrodesis
Siffert intraepiphysial osteotomy
Siffert-Storen intraepiphysial osteotomy
Sifoam padding
sigma receptor
sigmoid notch
sign
 abduction s.
 Achilles bulge s.
 Adam s.
 adduction s.
 Adson s.
 alien hand s.
 Allen s.
 Allis s.
 Amoss s.
 André Thomas s.
 Anghelescu s.
 antecedent s.
 anterior drawer s.
 anterior foot draw s.
 anterior hiatal s.
 anterior tibial s.
 anvil s.
 apprehension s.
 arterial occlusion s.
 Ashhurst s.
 Babinski s.
 Bancroft s.
 Barlow s.
 Bassett s.

Battle s.
bayonet s.
Beevor s.
benediction attitude s.
bite s.
Bloomberg s.
bone bruise s.
bottle s.
Bouchard s.
bowstring s.
bow-tie s.
Bragard s.
Brudzinski s.
Bryant s.
Burton s.
C s.
camelback s.
Carman meniscus s.
cement-wedge s.
Chaddock s.
Chinese red line s.
choppy sea s.
Clark s.
clawhand s.
Cleeman s.
click s.
cockade s.
Codman s.
cogwheel s.
Collier s.
comma s.
commemorative s.
Comolli s.
contralateral s.
Coopernail s.
crescent s.
crest s.
cupid's bow contour s.
David Letterman s.
Dawbarn s.
deep lateral femoral notch s.
Dejerine s.
Demianoff s.
Desault s.
Destot s.
dimple s.
divot s.
dollar s.
doll's eye s.
double-arc s.
double camelback s.
drawer s.
drivethrough s.
drop-arm s.
Dupuytren s.
Earle s.
Egawa s.
Erichsen s.

eye s.
fabere s.
FADIR s.
Fairbanks s.
Fajersztajn crossed sciatic s.
fallen-fragment s.
fallen-leaf s.
fan s.
fat-blood interface s.
fat pad s.
FBI s.
finger in balloon s.
Finkelstein s.
fishtail s.
flag s.
Fleck s.
flipped meniscus s.
fluid s.
Forestier bowstring s.
Fränkel s.
Froment paper s.
Gaenslen s.
Gage s.
Galant s.
Galeazzi hip dislocation s.
gear-stick s.
Goldthwait s.
Gordon reflex s.
Gottron s.
Gowers s.
grab s.
Guilland s.
gun barrel s.
half-moon s.
halo s.
hanging heel s.
Harris-Beath footprinting mat s.
Hawkins impingement s.
head-at-risk s.
heel varus s.
Helbing s.
hiatal s.
Hill-Sachs s.
Hirschberg s.
Hoffa s.
Hoffmann s.
Homans s.
Hoover s.
hot-cross-bun skull s.
Hueter s.
Huntington s.
iliac apophysis s.

impingement s.
J s.
Jeanne s.
Jenet s.
jerk s.
jump s.
Kager fat pad Valleix s.
Kanavel s.
Kaplan s.
Keen s.
Kehr s.
Kellgren s.
Kernig s.
Kerr s.
Klippel-Feil s.
Lachman s.
lamp cord s.
Langoria s.
Lasègue s.
lateral capsular s.
lateral gap s.
Laugier s.
Leichtenstern s.
Leri s.
Lhermitte s.
Light V s.
Linder s.
long tract s.
Lorenz s.
Ludington s.
Ludloff s.
Maisonneuve s.
Marie-Foix s.
Martel s.
masses s.
Matev s.
McMurray s.
Mendel-Bekhterev s.
Mennell s.
Meryon s.
Minor s.
Morquio s.
Morton s.
Morton-Horwitz nerve cross-over s.
movie s.
Mudder s.
Mulder s.
Naffziger s.
Napoleon hat s.
Neer impingement s.
Nelson s.
neuroma s.

S

NOTES

639

sign *(continued)*
    nutcracker s.
    objective s.
    obturator s.
    ocular s.
    Oppenheim s.
    Ortolani s.
    painful arc s.
    patellar apprehension s.
    pathognomonic s.
    Patrick s.
    Payr s.
    pedestal s.
    Pelken s.
    percussion s.
    peroneal s.
    piano key s.
    Piotrowski s.
    piriformis s.
    piston s.
    pivot-shift s.
    plantar ecchymosis s.
    Pollock s.
    popliteal pressure s.
    positive impingement s.
    positive rim s.
    posterior column s.
    posterior drawer s.
    posterior hiatal s.
    posterior sag s.
    posterolateral drawer s.
    posteromedial drawer s.
    pronation s.
    pseudo-Babinski s.
    pucker s.
    Putti s.
    Queckenstedt s.
    rachitic rosary s.
    radialis s.
    Raimiste s.
    Renee creak s.
    reverse Hill-Sachs s.
    ribbon s.
    rim s.
    ring s.
    Riordan s.
    Risser s.
    Romberg s.
    root tension s.
    Roux s.
    rugger jersey s.
    Rust s.
    Sarbo s.
    Schlesinger s.
    sciatic tension s.
    scotty dog s.
    shift s.
    shoulder apprehension s.

    shoulder impingement s.
    somatic s.
    Soto-Hall s.
    Speed s.
    spilled cup s.
    spilled teacup s.
    spine s.
    spur s.
    stair s.
    stepladder s.
    Strümpell s.
    Strunsky s.
    suction s.
    sulcus s.
    supinator fat pad s.
    swallow-tail s.
    terminal J s.
    Terry Thomas s.
    theater s.
    thermoregulatory s.
    thick patella s.
    Thomas s.
    Thompson s.
    thorn s.
    Thurston-Holland flag s.
    tibialis s.
    Tinel s.
    Tinel-Hoffmann s.
    toe spread s.
    toggle s.
    too-many-toes s.
    Trendelenburg s.
    tripod s.
    trough s.
    tuck s.
    Turyn s.
    Uhthoff s.
    V s.
    vacant glenoid s.
    Valleix s.
    Vanzetti s.
    Voshell s.
    Waddell s.
    Waldenström s.
    Walker-Murdoch wrist s.
    Wartenberg s.
    Werenskiold s.
    wet leather s.
    Wilson s.
    Wimberger s.
    windshield wiper s.
    wink s.
    winking owl s.
    Yergason s.
SignaDRESS hydrocolloid dressing
signal
    intervertebral disk nucleus s.
    s. void

Sigvaris stockings
Silapap
Silastic
  S. ball
  S. ball spacer prosthesis
  S. ball therapy
  S. button
  S. drain
  S. finger implant
  S. finger joint
  S. gel dressing
  S. lunate arthroplasty
  S. radial head prosthesis
  S. sheeting
  S. standard elastometer prosthesis
  S. thumb prosthesis
  S. toe implant
silence
  electrical s.
silent
  s. fascicle
  s. hip stage
  myoelectrically s.
  s. period
  s. thrombosis
Silesian
  S. bandage
  S. bandage prosthetic support
  S. belt
Silflex intramedullary prosthesis
Silfverskiöld
  S. Achilles tendon lengthening
  S. Achilles tendon reconstruction
  S. disease
  S. procedure
  S. technique
  S. test
silhouette
  s. capsulectomy
  s. spinal system
  S. therapeutic massage
silicone
  s. arthritis
  s. breast implant
  s. elastomer rubber ball implant
  s. gel
  s. gel socket insert
  s. implant arthroplasty
  s. insole
  s. material
  s. MP implant
  s. pad

  s. rubber arthroplasty
  s. rubber sphere
  s. spacer
  s. synovitis
  s. thermoplastic splinting (STS)
  s. trapezium prosthesis
  Wonderflex s.
  s. wrist arthroplasty
silicone-dacron tendon rod
silicone-only suspension (SOS)
Silicore foot pillow
Silipos
  S. digital pad
  S. Distal Dip prosthetic sheath/liner
  S. gel
  S. mesh cap
  S. mesh tubing
  S. Silicone Wonder Cup
  S. suspension sleeve
silk
  s. mesh gauze dressing
  Owens s.
  s. suture
SilkTouch CO_2 laser
Sillence osteogenesis imperfecta classification
SiloLiner gel liner
Silon silicone thermoplastic splinting material
Silopad
  S. body sleeve
  S. toe sleeve
Silosheath
  S. gel
  S. sock
silver
  S. bunionectomy
  s. dollar technique
  S. osteotome
  S. procedure
  s. sulfadiazine
silver-fork
  s.-f. deformity
  s.-f. fracture
Silver-Simon lengthening
Silverskiöld syndrome
Silver-Thera
  S.-T. stocking electrode
  S.-T. stockings
Simmonds-Menelaus
  S.-M. metatarsal osteotomy

NOTES

S

641

Simmonds-Menelaus (*continued*)
  S.-M. proximal phalangeal
    osteotomy
Simmonds test
Simmons
  S. cervical spine fusion
  S. chisel
  S. crimper
  S. double-hole spinal screw
  S. Multi-Matic orthopedic bed
  S. osteotome
  S. osteotomy
  S. plate
  S. plating system
  S. and Segil classification system
  S. spinal arthrodesis
  S. Vari-Hite orthopedic bed
Simmons-Martin screw
Simonart band
simple
  s. bone cyst
  s. button patellar implant
  S. Calculated Osteoporosis Risk
    Estimation (SCORE)
  s. dislocation
  s. fracture
  s. joint
  s. knee test (SKT)
  s. metatarsus adductus
  S. Shoulder Test patient
    questionnaire
  s. shoulder test thermal alteration
    Thomas traction
  s. suture
  s. syndactyly
  s. synovitis
simplex
  S. cement adhesive
  herpes s.
  hidroacanthoma s.
  S. P bone cement
SimplyStable trace
Simpson
  S. arthrectomy catheter
  S. sugar-tong splint
Simpulse
  S. pulsing lavage
  S. S/I lavage
Sims
  S. position
  S. retractor
simulator
  Baltimore Therapeutic Equipment
    Work S.
  BTE Work S.
  ERGOS work s.
  Lido WorkSET work s.

  Spinal Physiotherapy S.
  Work Seat driving s.
Simultaneous Interview Technique (SIT)
S incision
Sinding-Larsen-Johansson
  S.-L.-J. disease
  S.-L.-J. lesion
  S.-L.-J. syndrome
Singh
  S. index of osteoporosis
  S. osteoporosis classification
  S. osteoporosis index
  trabecular index of S.
single
  s. axis
  s. clamp
  s. cross-slot screwdriver
  s. fiber EMG
  s. fiber needle electrode
  s. heel rise
  s. pearl-face hip joint
  s. photon emission computed
    tomography (SPECT)
  s. plantar verruca
  s. proximal portal technique
  s. reference point (SRP)
  s. reference point instrument
  s. smooth-face hip joint
single-action rongeur
single-axis
  s.-a. ankle joint
  s.-a. ankle prosthesis
  s.-a. friction knee (SAFK)
  s.-a. knee unit
  s.-a. locking knee (SALK)
  s.-a. Syme DYCOR foot
single-blade saw
single-cannula system
single-channel
  MyoTrac s.-c.
  s.-c. surface EMG
single-column fracture
single-condylar graft
single-contrast arthrogram
single-fiber electromyography (SFEMG)
single-heel rise test
single-incision fasciotomy
single-leg
  s.-l. spica cast
  s.-l. toe raise
single-level spinal fusion
single-limb stance
single-lobed skin flap
single-onlay cortical bone graft
single-organ athlete
single-panel knee immobilizer
single-photon electrospinal orthosis
single-point cane

single-prong broad acetabular retractor
single-rod construct
single-row exercise
single-sided bone saw
single-slot screwdriver
single-stage
    s.-s. tendon graft
    s.-s. tissue transfer
single-stemmed
    s.-s. silicone hemiprosthesis
    s.-s. toe implant
single-unit pattern
sink
    counter s.
sinogram
sinography
sintered
    s. implant prosthesis
    s. titanium mesh
sintering
    s. of cobalt-chrome powder coating
    cobalt-chrome power s.
Sinterlock
    S. implant
    S. implant metal
    S. implant metal prosthesis
sinus
    air s.
    cervical ligament of tarsal s.
    coccygeal s.
    dermal s.
    s. histiocytosis
    lunate s.
    osteomyelitic s.
    peroneal s.
    talar s.
    tarsal s.
    s. tarsi
    s. tarsi syndrome
    tentorial s.
    s. tract
    traumatic s.
sinusoidal
sinuvertebral nerve
SIO
    sacroiliac orthosis
Sir Henry Platt transverse approach
sismotherapy
sisomicin
Sisson fracture reducing elevator
Sistron scissors
Sistrunk scissors

SIT
    Simultaneous Interview Technique
sit-and-reach
    s.-a.-r. box
    s.-a.-r. test
site
    donor s.
    Evan calcaneal lengthening
      osteotomy s.
    fracture s.
    harvest s.
    hook s.
    nerve entrapment s.
    nonunion of fracture s.
    operative s.
    pin s.
    recipient s.
sit/stand chair
Sit-Straight wheelchair cushion
sitter
    floor s.
sitting
    s. flexion
    s. flexion test
    s. knee extension
    s. position
    s. root test
    s. side bend
sit-to-stand test
sit-up test
Sivash hip prosthesis
six-degrees-of-freedom electrogoniometer
six-hole plate
six-minute walk test
six-pack hand exercise
six-point knee brace
six-portal synovectomy
size
    crosslink plate s.
sizer
    Brannock Device shoe s.
SJA
    subtalar joint axis
SJF
    subtalar joint function
SJK
    Scheuermann juvenile kyphosis
Sjögren syndrome
skate
    arm s.
skateboard
skater's gait

S

NOTES

skeletal
  s. age (SA)
  s. amyloidosis
  s. bed
  s. defect
  s. deformity
  s. disruption
  s. dysplasia
  s. extension
  s. growth factor
  s. hyperostosis syndrome
  s. hypoplasia
  s. hypoplasia disease
  idiopathic s.
  s. injury score
  s. limb deficiency
  s. maturation
  s. maturity
  s. muscle
  s. muscle fiber
  s. muscle relaxant
  s. pin
  s. repair system (SRS)
  s. stabilization
  s. tissue
  s. traction
  s. tuberculosis
  s. wry neck
skeletal-extraskeletal angiomatosis
skeletally immature
skeleton
  appendicular s.
  articulated s.
  bony s.
  s. hand
  s. shortening
  spidering s.
skeletonize
skew
  s. flap
  s. foot
skewer
skewering
skewfoot
  complex s.
  s. deformity
ski
  impact-release binding on s.
  walker s.'s
skid
  bone s.
  hip s.
  s. humeral head retractor
  Meyerding bone s.
  Murphy s.
  Murphy-Lane bone s.
skier's
  s. fracture

  s. injury
  s. thumb
skijump view
Skil-Care
  S.-C. cushion
  S.-C. cushion grip
  S.-C. reclining wheelchair
skill
  ambulation s.'s
  articulatory s.
  bed mobility s.
  donning-doffing s.
  palpatory s.
  physical daily living s.'s (PDLS)
Skillbuilder half roll
Skillern fracture
Skil Saw
skin
  s. adherence
  s. blood flow determination
  s. breakdown
  s. bridge
  S. Care kit
  s. closure
  s. coverage
  s. creaking
  s. crease
  dorsal s.
  s. flap
  s. glue
  s. hook
  s. incision
  s. marker
  s. necrosis
  nonglabrous s.
  s. pencil
  perianal s.
  s. plasty
  s. preparation
  s. resistance test
  s. restriction
  s. rolling
  s. slough
  s. staple
  s. stroker
  s. tag
  s. tape
  s. temperature monitoring probe
  s. traction
  undermined s.
skin-contact instrumentation
skinfold
  s. caliper
  s. measurement
skin-gliding test
Skinner line
skin-slough
  incisional s.-s.

SkinTemp collagen skin dressing
skin-tight cast
skive
skived incision
skiving knife
Sklar
- S. bone drill
- S. bone saw
- S. ligature needle
- S. pin cutter
- S. wire tightener

Skoog
- S. fasciotomy
- S. procedure for release of Dupuytren contracture
- S. technique

S-K reconstruction of distal radioulnar joint
SKT
- simple knee test

skull
- base of s. (BOS)
- hot-cross-bun s.
- s. plate screwdriver
- s. tongs

skull-occiput-mandibular immobilization orthosis
skyline
- s. radiograph
- s. view
- s. x-ray view of patella

Skytron
- S. bed
- S. operating room table

SL
- scapholunate
- stereolithography
- SL cage

SLAC
- scapholunate advanced collapse
- scapholunate arthritis collapse

slack
- motion s.
- tissue s.
- s. wrist

Slam'r wheelchair
slant
- foam s.
- OPTP S.

SLAP
- superior labrum anterior and posterior
- SLAP lesion

slap
- foot s.
- s. foot gait
- s. hammer

slapping gait
Slatis
- S. fixation
- S. pelvic fracture frame

slatted plinth table
Slattery-McGrouther dynamic flexion splint
SLC
- short leg cast

SLE
- systemic lupus erythematosus
- SLE arthropathy

sled
- Penco Walker S.'s
- walker s.'s

Sleeper Gripper prosthetic device
sleeve
- arthroscopic monopolar thermal stabilization forefoot compression s.
- BioCompression Pneumatic S.
- circumferential ligamentous s.
- cylindrical s.
- drill s.
- Edwards-Levine s.
- Edwards modular system spinal s.
- Edwards polyethylene s.
- elbow s.
- Electro-Mesh s.
- epX suspension s.
- excursion amplifier s.
- s. fracture
- gel suspension s.
- heel s.
- Iceflex Endurance suction suspension s.
- knee s.
- Knit-Rite suspension s.
- malleolar gel s.
- MICA 3x s.
- neoprene elbow s.
- neoprene knee s.
- obturator s.
- Pedifix forefoot compression s.
- periosteal s.
- pin s.
- pneumatic compression s.
- polyethylene s.

NOTES

S

sleeve *(continued)*
    rod s.
    Silipos suspension s.
    Silopad body s.
    Silopad toe s.
    Super Grip s.
    s. type
slide
    flexor pronator s.
    Glassman-Engh-Bobyn
      trochanteric s.
    head-first s.
    muscle s.
    s. plate
    trochanteric s.
slideboard
    Activ s.
slider crank mechanism
sliding
    s. AFO
    s. arthrodesis
    s. barrel hook
    s. bone graft
    s. compression hip screw
    s. compression screw with sideplate
    s. fixation device
    s. flap
    s. hammer
    s. knot
    s. nail
    s. nail device
    s. plane osteotomy of   Samilson
    s. tenotomy
    s. Z-plasty
slightly movable articulation
SlimLine cast boot
Slim Option shoe orthosis
Slimrest
    Core S.
Slimthetics orthotic
sling
    Action thumb s.
    AliMed hemi arm s.
    Ampoxen s.
    arm elevator s.
    Barton s.
    Böhler-Braun leg s.
    collar-and-cuff s.
    cradle arm s.
    CVA S.
    s. dressing
    envelope arm s.
    finger s.
    Fits-All s.
    foot s.
    s. frame
    Glisson s.
    Haacker s.

hanging cast s.
Harris Hemi Arm S.
Harris splint s.
s. immobilization
s. immobilizer
Jacksonville s.
Kenny-Howard shoulder s.
knee s.
Kodel knee s.
leg s.
Legg-Perthes s.
lymphedema s.
Mersilene s.
Murphy s.
muslin s.
Nada-Chair Back-Up portable
  back s.
Pavlik s.
pelvic s.
Posey s.
pouch-type s.
s. procedure
Rauchfuss s.
s. and reef technique
resting foot s.
rubber s.
Salter s.
s. seat sag
s. seat wheelchair
shoulder saddle s.
sling-and-swathe s.
Slingers arm s.
slinger-style envelope s.
soft tissue coaptation s.
stockinette s.
strap s.
s. suspension range of motion
s. suture
swathe and s.
Teare s.
Thomas buckle s.
Thomas Kodel s.
triangular arm s.
universal s.
Uni-Versatil s.
Velpeau shoulder s.
Vogue arm s.
volar ulnar s.
Weil pelvic s.
Westfield-style envelope s.
sling-and-swathe
    s.-a.-s. bandage
    s.-a.-s. sling
sling-dressing
    Velpeau s.-d.
Slingers arm sling
slinger-style envelope sling
Slingshot shoulder immobilizer

slip

    s. angle
    s. angle spondylolisthesis
    central s.
    conjoined gastrocnemius soleus
      fascial s.
    flexor digitorum s.
    s. joint
    lateral s.
    s. of tendon

slip-joint pliers
Slip-N-Snip scissors
slip-on finger splint
slipped

    s. capital femoral epiphysis (SCFE)
    s. disk
    s. elbow
    s. under femoral epiphysis (SUFE)
    s. vertebral apophysis

slipper

    Acu-Pressure s.
    s. cast
    Kite s.

slipping

    s. patella
    s. rib
    s. rib cartilage

slit catheter technique
sliver of bone
Slocum

    S. ALRI test
    S. anterior rotary drawer test
    S. fusion technique
    S. knee procedure
    S. lateral pivot-shift test
    S. maneuver
    S. meniscal clamp
    S. nail
    S. pes anserinus transplant
    S. rotary instability test
    S. splint

Slo-Mo ball
slope

    dorsal radial s.
    tibial s.

slot

    acetabular s.
    S. distraction device
    glenoid s.
    s. table

slot-graft

slotted

    s. acetabular augmentation
    s. bolt
    s. femur plate
    s. mallet
    s. nail
    s. obturator-cannula system
    s. tendon stripper

slough

    skin s.

slow

    s. cautery
    s. distraction
    s. muscle
    s. stretch
    s. stretch reflex
    s. union

slow-acting antirheumatic drug (SAARD)
SL-Plus stem
SLR

    straight leg raising
      SLR with Bragard test
      SLR with external rotation test
      SLR with Kernig test

SLRT

    straight leg raising test

slump test
slurry

    autogenous bone s.
    bone s.
    matrix-bone marrow s.

SLWC

    short leg walking cast

Sly syndrome
SMA

    spinal muscular atrophy
      SMA prosthesis

SMALL

    same-day microsurgical arthroscopic
    lateral-approach laser-assisted
    SMALL fluoroscopic diskectomy

small

    s. cell osteogenic sarcoma
    s. egress cannula
    s. fracture
    s. fragment screw
    s. lamina spreader
    s. nail spicule bur
    s. patella syndrome
    s. plate forceps
    s. step distraction

S

NOTES

small-base quad cane
small-headed screw
small-joint stiffness
smart
    S. Pin
    S. Screw bioabsorbable implant
SMART Balance Master
SmartBrace
    S. brace
    S. wrist splint
SmartKnit seamless sock
SmartPin instrument set
SmartTack fixation
SmartWrap elbow brace
Smedberg
    S. brace
    S. hand drill
    S. twist drill
Smedley dynamometer
SMFA
    Short Musculoskeletal Function
    Assessment
SMI 3000, 5000 bed
SMIC sternal drill
smile
    inverted s.
Smillie
    S. cartilage chisel
    S. cartilage knife
    S. knee retractor
    S. meniscal knife
    S. meniscal scissors
    S. meniscectomy chisel
    S. nail
    S. pin
Smillie-Beaver
    S.-B. blade
    S.-B. knife
Smith
    S. ankle fracture
    S. ankle prosthesis
    S. automatic perforated drill
    S. bone clamp
    S. cartilage knife
    S. dislocation
    S. flexor pollicis longus abductor-
    plasty
    S. maneuver
    S. & Nephew bracing and support
    system
    S. & Nephew medium barbed
    staple
    S. & Nephew reflection acetabular
    cup implant component
    S. & Nephew small barbed staple
    S. physical capacities evaluation
    (PCE)

    S. and Ross test
    S. scissors
    S. STA-peg
    S. subtalar joint arthroereisis peg
    (STA-peg)
    S. technique
Smith-Brown long-stem prosthesis
Smith-Davis Converta-Hite orthopedic
bed
Smith-Lemli-Opitz syndrome
Smith-Petersen
    S.-P. approach
    S.-P. chisel
    S.-P. cup
    S.-P. cup arthroplasty
    S.-P. curved gouge
    S.-P. curved osteotome
    S.-P. femoral neck nail
    S.-P. fracture pin
    S.-P. gooseneck gouge
    S.-P. hemiarthroplasty
    S.-P. hip cup prosthesis
    S.-P. impactor
    S.-P. intertrochanteric plate
    S.-P. nail with Lloyd adapter
    S.-P. osteotomy
    S.-P. reamer
    S.-P. rongeur
    S.-P. sacroiliac joint fusion
    S.-P. straight gouge
    S.-P. straight osteotome
    S.-P. synovectomy
    S.-P. technique
    S.-P. transarticular nail
Smith-Petersen-Cave-Van Gorder
    anterolateral approach
Smith-Richards instrumentation
Smith-Robinson
    S.-R. anterior cervical diskectomy
    S.-R. anterior fusion
    S.-R. cervical disk approach
    S.-R. cervical interbody fusion
    S.-R. interbody arthrodesis
    S.-R. operation
    S.-R. technique
Smithwick clip-applying forceps
SMO
    stainless steel and molybdenum
    supramalleolar orthosis
    SMO Moore pin
    SMO plate
    SMO prosthesis
smooth
    s. broach
    s. cobalt-chromium
    s. endoprosthesis

s. muscle
s. Steinmann pin
s. transfixion wire

smoother

Gore s.

smoothie junior bur

smooth-tipped jeweler's forceps

SMPS

sympathetic maintained pain syndrome

SMT

spinal manipulative therapy

SNAGS

sustained natural apophysial glides

SNAP

sensory nerve action potential

snap

s. finger
s. fit
S. fixation pin
S. Lock wire/pin extractor

snap-fit

s.-f. apparatus
s.-f. device

snap-lock brace

Snap-Pak

Mitek GII S.-P.

snapping

s. hip
s. knee syndrome
s. scapula
s. scapula syndrome
tendon s.
s. tendon
s. thumb flexor

snare

Zimmer s.

Sneppen talar fracture

sniffer's position

snooze pillow

snowboarder's

s. ankle
s. fracture

snowboarding injury

Snow-Littler release

snowstorm knee

SNS

sympathetic nervous system

S'n'S

Mauch S'n'S

snuffbox

anatomic s.

snug

S. seat
s. traction
S.'s wrap

SO

shoulder orthosis
spinal orthosis

soak

Betadine s.
Epsom salts s.

soap

Betadine s.

social integration World Health Organization Handicap Scale

society

American Knee S.
American Orthopaedic Foot and Ankle s. (AOFAS)
Musculoskeletal Tumor S.

sock

active s.
AFO brace s.
s. aid
ankle-foot orthosis brace s.
arthritis s.
Bio-Wick s.
Carolon AFO s.
cast s.
Comfort Ag prosthetic s.
Dero hole-in-one prosthetic s.
diabetic s.
edema s.
electrode s.
gel stump s.
molding s.
Orlon with Lycra stump s.
Regal Acrylic/Stretch prosthetic s.
Rx Comfort s.
Silosheath s.
SmartKnit seamless s.
Soft Walk gel s.
Spandex Lycra three-ply stump s.
Strassburg s.
STS molding s.
stump s.
Venosan support s.

Sock-Assist device

socket

adjustable postoperative protective prosthetic s. (APOPPS)
all-alumina s.
all-polyethylene s.

S

NOTES

socket *(continued)*
    AML s.
    Arthropor II porous s.
    check s.
    Clearpro suction s.
    concave loading s.
    endoskeletal s.
    flexible s.
    Flo-Tech prosthetic s.
    s. gauge
    hard s.
    ICEX s.
    intermediate s.
    ischial containment s.
    ischial-gluteal weightbearing s.
    metal-backed s.
    modular s.
    patellar tendon s. (PTS)
    s. pin
    Poly-Dial s.
    polyethylene s.
    preassembled metal-backed s.
    prosthetic s.
    s. purchase
    quadrilateral ischial weight-
      bearing s.
    standard s.
    supracondylar s.
    suspension-type s.
    temporary s.
    total contact s.
    universal frame outer s. (UFOS)
    University of California cuff
      suspension PTB s.
    variable circumference
      suprapatellar s. (VCSPS)
    s. wrench
Socon spinal system
SOCS
    SOCS AFO system
    SOCS pad system
Sof
    S. Gel HeelCup
    S. Matt pressure relieving mattress
    S. Sole motion control orthotic
    S. Sole Sof Gel heel pad
Sofamor spinal device
Sofflex
    S. mattress
    S. mattress system
Sof-Gel palm shield
Sofield
    S. femoral deficiency operation
    S. femoral deficiency technique
    S. osteotomy
    S. pinning
    S. retractor

Sof-Rol
    S.-R. cast pad
    S.-R. dressing
SofSole Airr insole
soft
    s. bulky dressing
    s. callus stage
    s. collar
    s. collar cervical orthosis
    s. corn
    s. corset
    s. cosmetic cover
    s. fibroma
    S. Silicones Wonderzorb
    s. socket insert
    S. Super Sport orthotic
    S. Support Preforms orthotic
    s. tissue
    s. tissue abnormality
    s. tissue abscess
    s. tissue biomechanics
    s. tissue blade retractor
    s. tissue calcification
    s. tissue coaptation sling
    s. tissue contracture
    s. tissue envelope
    s. tissue flap
    s. tissue healing
    s. tissue hinge
    s. tissue injury
    s. tissue integrity
    s. tissue interface
    s. tissue interposition
    s. tissue irritability
    s. tissue lesion
    s. tissue maladaptation
    s. tissue manipulation
    s. tissue mass
    s. tissue massage
    s. tissue mobilization
    s. tissue myxoma
    s. tissue plication
    s. tissue release
    s. tissue restriction
    s. tissue sarcoma
    s. tissue stretching
    s. tissue tumor
    s. touch hand exerciser
    S. Touch stockings
    S. Walk gel sock
softball sliding injury
SofTec rigid brace
Softeze water pillow
SoftFlex
    S. computer glove
    S. Wrist Wear
Softie shoe
Softip monofilament

Softouch Cold/Hot Pack
Softsplint foot splint
soft-vamp shoe
software
    Image-I analysis s.
    osteotomy analysis simulation s.
    (OASIS)
    Stat Graphics s.
    Yochum chiropractic s.
Sof-Wick dressing
Sofwire cable system
Solcotrans
    S. autotransfusion system
    S. orthopedic drainage-refusion
    system
sole
    Ambulator Bio-Rocker s.
    s. of foot
    s. insert
    plaster s.
    Poro-in-between s.
    s. reflex
    rocker bottom s.
    shock-absorbent s.
    shoe s.
    Texon s.
    Vibram s.
sole-tap reflex
soleus
    accessory s.
    s. complex
    gastrocnemius s.
    s. muscle
    s. syndrome
SOLEutions
    S. custom orthosis
    S. custom orthotic device
    S. Prefab orthotic device
    S. soft plus orthotic
    S. sport shell orthotic
solid
    s. ankle, cushioned heel (SACH)
    s. ankle, cushioned heel foot
    s. ankle, cushioned heel orthotic
    s. ankle, cushioned heel prosthesis
    s. ankle flexible endoskeletal
    (SAFE)
    s. ankle joint
    s. buckling implant material
    s. hex bolt
    s. silicone exoplant implant
    material

solitary
    s. bone cyst
    s. enchondroma
    s. fibromatosis
    s. myeloma
    s. osteoma
Solitens transcutaneous electrical nerve
    stimulation unit
Soluspan
solution
    antibiotic and saline s.
    antiseptic s.
    bacitracin s.
    Betadine scrub s.
    Bunnell s.
    colloid s.
    crystalloid s.
    dextrose s.
    extravasation irrigation s.
    ferumoxide injectable s.
    heparinized Ringer lactate s.
    Hibiclens s.
    iodophor s.
    irrigating s.
    irrigation s.
    S. prosthesis
    saline s.
    sterile saline s.
somatectomy
    subtotal s.
somatic
    s. dysfunction
    s. innervation
    s. muscle
    s. nerve
    s. sign
    s. therapy
somatization
somatoautonomic
somatomedin-C
somatoprosthetics
somatosensory
    s. deficit
    s. evoked potential (SEP, SSEP)
    s. evoked potential monitoring
    s. test
somatosomatic reflex
somatovisceral correction
Somerville
    S. anterior approach
    S. procedure
    S. technique

S

NOTES

SOMI
    sternal-occipital-mandibular
      immobilization
        SOMI brace
        SOMI orthosis
Songer cable
sonic-accelerated fracture-healing system
    (SAFHS)
Sonocut ultrasonic aspirator
sonographic abnormality
sonography
sonometer
    clinical bone s.
    Sahara clinical bone s.
    SoundScan 2000 bone s.
    SoundScan Compact bone s.
    ultrasound bone imaging s. (UBIS)
Sontec pliers
Sony CCD/RGB DXC-151 color video
    camera
Sorbie calcaneal fracture classification
Sorbie-Questor
    S.-Q. elbow
    S.-Q. total elbow prosthesis system
sorbitol level
Sorbothane
    S. antivibration glove
    S. heel cushion
    S. II heel cup
    S. insole
    S. orthotic device
    S. recoil pad
    S. rice sheller roller
    S. wrap
sore
    plaster s.
    pressure s.
Soren
    S. ankle fusion
    S. arthrodesis
soreness
    delayed-onset muscle s.
Sorondo-Ferré hindquarter amputation
Sorrells hip arthroplasty retractor
    system
Sorrel-type snowboard boot
SOS
    silicone-only suspension
      SOS total hip system
      SOS total knee system
SOT
    sacrooccipital technique
SOTO
    step out, turn out
      SOTO technique
Soto-Hall
    S.-H. bone graft
    S.-H. maneuver

    S.-H. sign
    S.-H. test
Soudre autogéné
sound
    flexible s.
    radiolucent s.
    rigid s.
    tearing s.
sounder
    pedicle s.
SoundScan
    S. 2000 bone sonometer
    S. Compact bone sonometer
source
    fiberoptic light s.
    light s.
    Wolf light s.
Souter
    S. hip operation
    S. hip procedure
    S. Strathclyde total elbow system
    S. unconstrained elbow prosthesis
Souter-Strathclyde elbow prosthesis
southern
    s. access
    S. California Orthopedic Institute
      (SCOI)
Southwick
    S. biplane trochanteric osteotomy
    S. clamp
    S. lateral slip angle
    S. pin-holding apparatus
    S. pin-holding device
    S. screw extractor
    S. slide procedure
    S. two-tined retractor
Southwick-Robinson anterior cervical
    approach
Sox
    Champion Power S.
SP
    suprapatellar
SpA
    spondyloarthropathy
Spa Bed
space
    s. available for the cord (SAC)
    Barouk button s.
    cartilage s.
    costoclavicular s.
    dead s.
    disk s.
    epidural s.
    fascial s.
    first web s.
    haversian s.
    hypoplastic disk s.
    increased lateral joint s.

intercondylar s.
intercostal s. (ICS)
interdigital web s.
intermetatarsal s.
interpeduncular s.
interphalangeal joint s.
joint s.
lateral joint s.
medial clear s.
midpalmar s.
narrowed joint s.
palm s.
Parona s.
s. of Poirier
popliteal s.
position in s.
prevertebral s.
properitoneal s.
retroperitoneal s.
retropharyngeal s.
s. shoe
subacromial s.
subcoracoid s.
suprasternal s.
thenar s.
tibiocalcaneal s.
tibiofibular clear s.
tibiotalar clear s.
web s.

spacer
acetabular s.
s. bar
Barouk s.
bayonet s.
s. between toes
bone s.
Button S.
ceramic vertebral s.
s. inserter
joint s.
Kinemax s.
passive s.
Plexiglas s.
prosthetic s.
proximal cement s.
rubber s.
silicone s.
telescopic plate s.
temporary articulating
methylmethacrylate antibiotic s.
(TAMMAS)
tibial s.

toe s.
trial s.
true s.
spacer-tensor jig
spade
s. finger
s. hand
Spahr metaphysial dysostosis
Spälteholz
S. preparation
S. technique
Spandex Lycra three-ply stump sock
spanner gauge
spanning external fixator
sparing
glycogen s.
sacral nerve root s.
Spark handheld dynamometer
Spartan jaw wire cutter
spasm
arterial s.
carpal pedal s.
muscle s.
paraspinal muscle s.
paraspinous muscular s.
paravertebral muscle s.
peroneal muscle s.
spasmodic torticollis
spastic
s. cerebral palsy
s. diparesis
s. diplegia
s. disorder
s. equinovalgus
s. equinus
s. equinus gait
s. flat foot
s. flatfoot
s. gait
s. hand
s. hemiplegia
s. hindfoot valgus deformity
s. intrinsic contracture
s. paralysis
s. paraplegia
s. quadriplegia
s. thumb-in-palm deformity
s. varus hindfoot
spasticity
Ashworth score of muscle s.
s. measurement

S

NOTES

spasticity *(continued)*
    s. treatment
    wrist s.
spatula
    cement s.
    s. foot
    s. forceps
spatulate thumb
SPC
    suprapatellar cuff
spear
    s. tackle
    s. tackler's spine
spearing
    injurious energy input s.
special
    s. Colles splint
    Heel Spur S.
    S. Seat
specialized nail
specific
    s. adaptation to imposed demand (SAID)
    s. adjustment
    s. curve
    s. thrust manipulation
SPECT
    single photon emission computed tomography
Spectron
    S. EF total hip system
    S. hip prosthesis
spectroscopy
    Fourier transform infrared s.
    magnetic resonance s.
Spectrum tissue repair system
speech aid
speed
    S. arthroplasty
    S. brace
    S. hand splint
    S. open reduction
    S. osteotomy
    s. play training
    S. radial head fracture classification
    S. radius cap prosthesis
    S. sign
    S. sternoclavicular repair
    S. test
    S. V-Y muscle-plasty
Speed-Boyd
    S.-B. open reduction
    S.-B. radial-ulnar technique
speed-lock clamp
Spelcast car seat
Spence rongeur forceps
Spencer tendon lengthening

Spenco
    S. arch support
    S. boot
    S. insole
    S. liner
    S. orthotic device
    S. Second Skin dressing
    S. shoe insert
Spetzler anterior transoral approach
SpF spinal fusion stimulator
sphenoid
    wing of s.
sphenoidal fossa
sphenoiditis
sphenoidostomy
sphenoidotomy
sphenopalatine ganglion block
sphere
    silicone rubber s.
spherical
    s. bur
    s. gliding principle
    s. reamer
spherical-headed screw
spherocentric
    s. fully constrained tricompartmental knee prosthesis
    s. knee system
spheroidal joint
sphincter
    s. muscle
    s. tone
sphygmomanometer
spica
    s. bandage
    s. cast
    Freedom thumb s.
    hip s.
    Schmeisser s.
    s. splint
    thumb s.
spicule
    bone s.
spider finger
spidering skeleton
Spiegleman acromioclavicular splint
Spier elbow arthrodesis
Spiessel internal screw fixation
spike
    ball-tip s.
    s. of bone
    endplate s.
    Gaenslen s.
    Gissane s.
    heel s.
    metaphysial s.
    s. osteotomy

supracollicular s.

s. washer implant

spiked

s. Darrach-type elevator

s. ligament washer

spilled

s. cup sign

s. teacup sign

spina

s. bifida

s. bifida aperta

s. bifida occulta (SBO)

spinae

erector s.

thoracolumbar erector s.

spinal

s. abscess

s. accessory nerve

s. accessory nerve injury

s. analysis

s. analysis machine (SAM)

s. anesthesia

s. angulation

s. arteriography

s. artery

s. arthritis

s. arthrodesis

s. axial load

s. axis

s. brucellosis

s. canal stenosis (SCS)

s. column

s. contour

s. cord

s. cord angiography

s. cord atrophy

s. cord block

s. cord canal

s. cord compression

s. cord function intraoperative
monitoring

s. cord injury (SCI)

s. cord injury without radiographic
abnormality (SCIWORA)

s. cord-meningeal complex

S. Cord Motor Index and Sensory
Indices

s. cord syndrome

s. cord tract

s. coronal plane deformity

s. curvature

s. decompression

s. deformity instability

s. degeneration

s. distraction

s. dysarthria

s. dysraphism

s. evoked potential

s. fascial release

s. fixation

s. fixation rigidity

s. fixation rod

s. fracture

s. fusion

s. fusion pathomechanics

s. fusion position

s. fusion stimulator

s. fusion technique

s. hitch

s. implant load to failure

s. infection

s. infection biopsy

s. injection therapy

s. injury operative stabilization

s. instability

s. instrumentation

s. joint mobilization

s. learning

s. level

s. load bearing

s. locking procedure

s. malignancy

s. manipulation

s. manipulative therapy (SMT)

s. manual therapy

s. metastasis

s. mobilization technique

s. muscular atrophy (SMA)

s. muscular atrophy (type I–III)

s. myoclonus

s. needle

s. orthosis (SO)

s. osteoblastoma

s. osteomyelitis

s. osteosarcoma

s. osteotomy

s. osteotomy stabilization

S. Physiotherapy Simulator

s. posterior ligament

s. process apophysis

s. puncture

s. rod cross-bracing

s. segment

s. shock

S

NOTES

655

spinal (*continued*)
    s. stenotic myelopathy
    S. Technology bivalve TLSO brace
    s. transverse ligament
    s. tuberculosis
    s. tumor
    s. turning frame
spinale
    filum s.
SpinalPak fusion stimulator
spindle
    anulospiral ending of muscle s.
    s. cell lipoma
    s. effect
    muscle s.
    s. neuroma
spine
    adjustment of s.
    alar s.
    angular s.
    anterior column of s.
    anterior inferior iliac s. (AIIS)
    anterior maxillary s.
    anterior occipitocervical s.
    anterior superior iliac s. (ASIS)
    anterior tibial s.
    anterior upper s.
    s. apparatus
    axial loading of s.
    bamboo s.
    s. board
    cervical s. (C-spine)
    Chance fracture thoracolumbar s.
    Charcot s.
    chiropractic manual manipulation
      of s.
    Civinini s.
    cleft s.
    coccygeal s.
    convexity of the s.
    s. deformity
    fixation dysfunction of the
      lumbar s.
    s. flexion
    s. frame
    full cervical s. (FCS)
    Gait, Arms, Legs, and S. (GALS)
    gibbus deformity of the s.
    iliac s.
    ischial s.
    kinetic cervical s.
    kissing s.'s
    laminectomized s.
    lower cervical s.
    lower lumbar s.
    lower thoracic s.
    lumbar s.
    lumbosacral s.
    mandibular s.
    maxillary s.
    nasal s.
    osteoporotic s.
    palpation of anterior superior
      iliac s.
    palpation of posterior superior
      iliac s.
    poker s.
    posterior-inferior s.
    posterior sacroiliac s. (PSIS)
    posterior superior iliac s. (PSIS)
    posterior tibial s.
    S. Power pelvic stabilizer belt
    s. rotation
    rugger jersey s.
    sacral s.
    s. sign
    spear tackler's s.
    thoracic s. (T-spine)
    thoracolumbar s.
    thoracolumbosacral s.
    three-column s.
    trochanteric s.
    upper thoracic s.
    variable screw placement system-
      instrumented lumbar s.
SpineCor nonrigid brace
SpineScope
    Clarus S.
spinning probe
spinocerebellar
    s. ataxia
    s. degeneration
    s. tract
spinoglenoid notch
spinographic angle
spinography
spinolaminar line
spinomuscular paralysis
spinopelvic
    s. transiliac fixation (STIF)
    s. transiliac fixation system
Spinoscope noninvasive imaging system
spinothalamic tract
spinous
    s. plane
    s. process
    s. process fracture
    s. process plate
    s. process wire
    s. process wiring
    s. pull
    s. push
spiral
    s. bandage
    s. cortical reamer
    s. drill

s. groove syndrome
s. humeral groove
s. joint
s. line of femur
s. oblique fracture
s. oblique retinacular ligament
s. oblique retinacular ligament
  reconstruction splint
s. sulcus
s. technique
s. trochanteric reamer
Spira procedure
Spirec drill
spiritual healing
spirometer
  Buhl s.
Spittler procedure
Spitz-Holter valve implant material
SPL
  short plantar ligament
SPLATT
  split anterior tibialis tendon transfer
  SPLATT procedure
splayfoot deformity
splaying
  forefoot s.
  s. of toe
splint
  Abbott s.
  abduction finger s.
  abduction humeral s.
  abduction pillow cover s.
  abduction thumb s.
  abouna s.
  abutment s.
  acrylic cap s.
  acrylic template s.
  active s.
  Adam and Eve rib belt s.
  Adams s.
  adjustable s.
  Adjusta-Wrist s.
  aeroplane s.
  A-Force dorsal night s.
  Agnew s.
  Ainslie acrylic s.
  air s.
  AirFlex carpal tunnel s.
  Airfoam s.
  airplane s.
  air pressure s.
  Air-Soft S.

AliMed diabetic night s.
AliMed turnbuckle elbow s.
Alumafoam s.
aluminum bridge s.
aluminum fence s.
aluminum finger cot s.
aluminum foam s.
aluminum hand s.
aluminum wire s.
anchor s.
Anderson s.
angle s.
ankle-foot orthotic s.
anterior acute flexion elbow s.
anterior shin s.
any-angle s.
Aquaplast s.
armchair s.
Asch s.
Ashhurst leg s.
s. attachment
backboard s.
balanced s.
Baldan fracture s.
Balkan femoral s.
ball-peen s.
banana finger extension s.
banjo s.
Barlow cruciform infant s.
baseball finger s.
basic hand s.
Basswood s.
Bavarian s.
Baylor adjustable cross s.
Baylor metatarsal s.
Bend-A-Boot foot s.
Bennett basic hand s.
birdcage s.
Bloom s.
Blount s.
board s.
Böhler-Braun s.
Böhler wire s.
Bond arm s.
s. bone
Boston thoracic s.
Bosworth s.
boutonnière s.
Bowlby arm s.
bracketed s.
Brady balanced-suspension s.
Brady leg s.

NOTES

splint *(continued)*
Brant aluminum s.
Brooke Army Hospital s.
Browne s.
Buck extension s.
Buck traction s.
buddy s.
Budin hammertoe s.
Budin toe s.
Bunnell active hand and finger s.
Bunnell finger extension s.
Bunnell gutter s.
Bunnell knuckle-bender s.
Bunnell outrigger s.
Bunnell reverse knuckle bender s.
Bunnell safety-pin s.
Bunny boot foot s.
Burnham finger s.
Burnham thumb s.
Cabot leg s.
Cabot posterior s.
calibrated clubfoot s.
Campbell traction s.
cap s.
Capener coil s.
Capener finger s.
Carl P. Jones traction s.
Carpal Lock cock-up s.
Carpal Lock wrist s.
Carter s.
cartilage elastic pullover kneecap s.
Chandler felt collar s.
Chatfield-Girdlestone s.
clavicular cross s.
Clayton greenstick s.
clubfoot s.
CMC s.
coaptation s.
cock-up arm s.
cock-up hand s.
cock-up wrist s.
Colles s.
Comforfoam s.
Comfy elbow s.
composite spring elastic s.
compression sleeve shin s.
Comprifix ankle s.
Cone s.
constant tension s.
Converse s.
cool IROM s.
cool TROM s.
Cordon-Colles fracture s.
Cosmolon closure for s.
counterrotational s.
countertraction s.
Craig abduction s.
Cramer wire s.

CTS Gripfit s.
cubital tunnel s.
Culley ulnar s.
Curry walking s.
Darco foot s.
Darco medical surgical shoe and toe alignment s.
Davis metacarpal s.
Delbet s.
Denis Browne s. (DBS)
Denis Browne clubfoot s.
Denis Browne hip s.
Denis Browne talipes hobble s.
DePuy aeroplane s.
DePuy any-angle s.
DePuy coaptation s.
DePuy open-spindle s.
DePuy open-thimble s.
DePuy-Pott s.
DePuy rocking leg s.
DePuy rolled Colles s.
dermal interposition s.
derotator s.
DeRoyal LMB finger s.
digit s.
Digit-Aide fifth toe s.
DonJoy knee s.
DonJoy wrist s.
dorsal extension block s.
dorsal wrist s.
dorsiflexion foot s.
Dorsiwedge night s.
double-occlusal s.
drop-foot s.
drop wrist s.
Dupuytren s.
Duran-Houser wrist s.
Dyna knee s.
dynamic s.
Early Fit night s.
Easton cock-up s.
Easy Access foot s.
Eaton s.
Eggers contact s.
Elastomull s.
elbow extension s.
elbow flexion s.
elephant-ear clavicular s.
Engelmann thigh s.
Engen palmar wrist s.
Erich s.
Extend-It finger s.
extension block s.
Ezeform s.
felt collar s.
fence s.
Ferciot tiptoe s.
fiberglass s.

Fillauer night s.
finger cot s.
finger extension clockspring s.
finger flexion s.
Finger-Hugger s.
Firm D-Ring wrist support s.
flat s.
flexor hinge s.
fold-over finger s.
footdrop night s.
forearm s.
Formatray mandibular s.
Forrester s.
Foster s.
four-point IROM s.
four-prong finger s.
Fox clavicular s.
Fractomed s.
fracture s.
Framer s.
Freedom neutral position s.
Freedom omni progressive s.
Freedom Progressive Resting s.
Freedom sportsfit s.
Freedom ultimate grip s.
Frejka pillow s.
Friedman s.
frog-leg s.
Froimson s.
Fruehevald s.
full-hand s.
full-occlusal s.
functional s.
Funsten supination s.
Futuro s.
gait lock s. (GLS)
Gallows s.
Galveston s.
Ganley s.
Gibson s.
Gilchrist s.
Gilmer s.
Gordon s.
Granberry s.
Gunning s.
gutter s.
hairpin s.
half ring leg s.
half-shell s.
hallux valgus night s.
Hammond s.
hand cock-up s.

Hanna night s.
Hare compact traction s.
Harrington outrigger s.
Harris s.
Hart extension finger s.
Haynes-Griffin mandibular s.
Heal Well night s.
Heel Free s.
Hexcelite sheet s.
hinged cylinder s.
hinged Thomas s.
HIPciser abduction s.
Hirschtick utility shoulder s.
Hodgen hip s.
Hodgen leg s.
humeral fracture abduction s.
HV NightSplint s.
HV SoftSplint s.
Ilfeld s.
Ilfeld-Gustafson s.
infant abduction s.
inflatable elbow s.
IROM bilateral s.
IROM Regal s.
Isoprene plastic s.
Jacoby bunion s.
Jacoby heel s.
James s.
Jelanko s.
Jet-Air s.
Joint-Jack finger s.
Jonell countertraction finger s.
Jonell thumb s.
Jones arm s.
Jones metacarpal s.
Jones traction s.
Joseph s.
Kanavel cock-up s.
Karfoil s.
Kazanjian s.
Keller-Blake half-ring s.
Keller-Blake leg s.
Kenny-Howard s.
Kerr abduction s.
Keystone s.
kinetic s.
Kleinert s.
Klenzak double-upright s.
knee brace s.
knee immobilizer s.
knuckle-bender s.
ladder s.

NOTES

splint *(continued)*

Lambrinudi s.
leaf s.
Levis arm s.
Lewin finger s.
Lewin-Stern finger s.
Lewin-Stern thumb s.
Liberty One s.
s. liner
Link toe s.
Liston s.
live s.
LMB finger s.
LMB wire-foam economical resting s.
Lockhart toe s.
long arm s.
long leg s. (LLS)
loop-lock cock-up s.
Love s.
Lynx wrist, hand, finger orthosis arm positioner s.
Lytle metacarpal s.
magnet s.
Magnuson abduction humeral s.
malleable metal finger s.
Mason s.
Mason-Allen Universal hand s.
Mayer s.
McGee s.
McIntire s.
McLeod padded clavicular s.
memory s.
metal s.
Middeldorpf s.
MindSet toe s.
Moberg s.
modified Oppenheimer s.
Mohr finger s.
molded posterior plaster s.
Murphy s.
Murray-Jones arm s.
Murray-Thomas arm s.
Neubeiser adjustable forearm s.
neutral position s.
New Mind Set toe s.
N'ice Stretch night s.
night s. *night fighter*
occlusal s.
OCL volar s.
O'Donoghue knee s.
O'Donoghue stirrup s.
OEC s.
O'Malley jaw fracture s.
open-air s.
Oppenheimer spring-wire s.
Oppenheimer with reverse knuckle-bender s.

opponens s.
Orfit s.
Ortho-Glass s.
Ortho-last s.
Orthomedics Stretch and Heel s.
Ortho-Mold s.
orthopaedic strap clavicular s.
Orthoplast isoprene s.
outrigger s.
padded aluminum s.
padded board s.
padded plywood s.
padded tongue blade s.
s. padding
palmar cock-up s.
palmar wrist s.
pan s.
s. pan netting
passive night stretch s.
Pavlik harness s.
Peabody s.
Pearson attachment to Thomas s.
pelvic s.
PF Night Splint II s.
PFO night s.
Phelps s.
Phillips s.
Phoenix Outrigger s.
pillow s.
Pil-O-Splint wrist s.
plantar fasciitis night s.
Plastalume bulb-ended s.
Plastalume straight s.
plaster of Paris s.
plaster slab s.
pneumatic s.
Polyform s.
polyvinyl alcohol s.
Pond adjustable s.
Ponseti s.
poroplastic s.
Porzett s.
Postalume finger s.
posterior mold s.
Potts s.
Pro-glide s.
Progress s.
Protecto s.
Pucci s.
Puth abduction s.
Putti s.
QualCraft s.
QuickCast s.
Quik s.
radial slab s.
radiolucent s.

ratchet flexor tenodesis s.
Redi-Around finger s.
resting pan s.
reverse knuckle-bender s.
Robert Jones s.
Roger Anderson s.
Rolyan AquaForm wrist and thumb
  spica s.
Rolyan Gel Shell spica s.
Rosen s.
Rowland-Hughes s.
Rumel aluminum bridge s.
Russell s.
safety pin s.
Sager traction s.
SAM s.
Sam s.
Saturn carpal tunnel s.
Sayre s.
Scott ankle s.
Scott humeral s.
Scottish Rite s.
Scott Uniform tennis elbow s.
Seattle s.
shin s.
short arm s. (SAS)
short arm sugar-tong s.
short leg s.
shoulder spica s.
Simpson sugar-tong s.
Slattery-McGrouther dynamic
  flexion s.
slip-on finger s.
Slocum s.
SmartBrace wrist s.
Softsplint foot s.
special Colles s.
Speed hand s.
spica s.
Spiegleman acromioclavicular s.
spiral oblique retinacular ligament
  reconstruction s.
spreading hand s.
spring cock-up s.
spring-wire safety pin s.
Stack s.
Stader s.
static s.
Stax fingertip s.
stirrup plaster s.
Stock finger s.
Strampelli s.

strap clavicular s.
Stretch and Heel night s.
Stromeyer s.
Stuart Gordon hand s.
Stubbs acromioclavicular s.
Stulberg HIPciser abduction s.
sugar-tong plaster s.
surgical s.
suspension s.
swan-neck s.
Swanson dynamic toe s.
Swanson hand s.
synergistic wrist motion s.
Synergy s.
Tauranga s.
Taylor s.
Teare arm s.
tennis elbow s.
tension night s. (TNS)
T-finger s.
therapeutic s.
thermoplastic s.
Thomas full-ring s.
Thomas hinged s.
Thomas knee s.
Thomas leg s.
Thomas posterior s.
Thomas suspension s.
Thompson modification of Denis
  Browne s.
thumb web s.
ThumZ'Up thumb s.
Ticonium s.
Titus forearm s.
Titus wrist s.
Toad finger s.
Tobruk s.
Tomberlin-Alemdaroglu s.
Toronto s.
torsion bar s.
traction s.
triangular pillow s.
turnbuckle elbow s.
type 501, 502, 504, 602 finger s.
ulnar gutter s.
Universal acromioclavicular s.
Universal gutter s.
Universal support s.
Urias air s.
Urias pressure s.
U-splint s.
U-stirrup s.

NOTES

splint *(continued)*
    Valentine s.
    Van Arsdale triangular s.
    Van Rosen s.
    Velcro extenders s.
    VersaWrist wrist s.
    Vesely-Street s.
    volar plaster s.
    Volkmann s.
    von Rosen abduction s.
    von Rosen cruciform s.
    Wanchik neutral position s.
    Weil s.
    well-leg s.
    Wertheim s.
    Wheaton bunion s.
    Wilson s.
    Winter s.
    wire grip finger s.
    wire grip toe s.
    wraparound s.
    WristJack wrist s.
    wrist rest s.
    yucca wood s.
    Zimfoam s.
    Zimmer airplane s.
    Zimmer clavicular cross s.
    Zim-Trac traction s.
    Zim-Zip rib belt s.
    Zollinger s.
    Zucker s.
splintage
splinted in position of function
splintered fracture
splinting
    dynamic s.
    s. material
    night s.
    pelvic s.
    silicone thermoplastic s. (STS)
    Strong dorsal extension block s.
    s. therapy
splint-like pain
split
    s. anterior tibialis tendon transfer
      (SPLATT)
    s. anterior tibial tendon
    s. anterior tibial tendon procedure
    s. calvarial bone graft
    s. foot
    s. fracture
    s. hand
    s. incision
    Link Stack S. Splint
    longitudinal tendon s.
    s. patellar approach
    s. pelvis
    peroneus brevis s. (PBS)

    s. Russell skeletal traction
    s. screen
    s. stirrup
split-finger hook
split-hand deformity
split-heel
    s.-h. approach
    s.-h. fracture
    s.-h. incision
split-nail deformity
split-thickness
    s.-t. skin excision (STSE)
    s.-t. skin graft (STSG)
Sponastrine dysplasia
spondylalagia
spondylalgia
spondylarthritis
spondylectomy
spondylexarthrosis
spondylitis
    ankylosing s.
    Bekhterev rheumatoid s.
    Bekhterev-Strümpell s.
    s. deformans
    hypertrophic s.
    juvenile-onset ankylosing s.
    Kümmell s.
    Marie-Strümpell s.
    rheumatoid s.
    tuberculous s.
spondylizema
spondyloarthropathy (SpA)
    inflammatory s.
    sacroiliac joint inflammatory s.
spondyloarthrosis
spondylodesis
    ventral derotation s. (VDS)
spondylodiscitis
spondylodynia
spondyloepiphysial
    s. dysplasia
    s. dysplasia of Maroteaux
spondylogenic
spondylolisthesis
    anteroinferior s.
    congenital s.
    degenerative s.
    doweling s.
    dysplastic s.
    five classifications of s.
    Gill-Manning-White s.
    high-grade s.
    isthmic s.
    lumbosacral s.
    pathologic s.
    postlaminectomy two-level s.
    s. reduction
    s. reduction fixation

sagittal roll s.
slip angle s.
symptomatic s.
traumatic s.
Winter s.
spondylolisthetic pelvis
spondyloloptosis
spondylolysis
cervical s.
contralateral s.
spondylomalacia
spondylometer
spondylopathy
spondylophyte
spondyloptosis
spondylopyosis
spondyloschisis
spondylosis
central spine s.
cervical s.
degenerative s.
hyperostotic s.
lumbar s.
Nurick classification of s.
rhizomelic s.
Scheuermann dystrophic s.
thoracolumbar s.
spondylosyndesis
spondylotherapy
spondylotic
s. bar
s. spur
spondylotomy
sponge
Adaptic s.
bone wax gelatin s.
buffing s.
s. clamp
EZ Bend s.
gauze s.
Instat collagen s.
laparotomy s.
Mediskin hemostatic s.
Mikulicz s.
Pedic s.
Ray-Tec s.
s. stick
Telfa s.
s. test
Vistec x-ray detectable s.
sponge-holding forceps
spongialization

spongiosa
primary s.
s. screw
spongiosum
osteoma s.
spongoide
spongy
s. appearance
s. bone
Sponsel oblique osteotomy
spontaneous
s. activity
s. amputation
s. fracture
s. hyperemic dislocation
s. median neuropathy
s. postfracture epiphysiodesis
s. rupture
s. wrist clunk
spoon
maroon s.
meniscal s.
s. plate
sporotrichosis
S'port
S. Max back support
S. Max sacroiliac belt
S. Max stabilization pad
Posture S.
Scully Hip S.
sport
S.'s Activity Scale
s.'s anemia
s.'s anemia exercise
s.'s chiropractic
S. Cord
s.'s injury
lateral motion racket s.
s.'s medicine
s.'s medicine law
s.'s participation
pivoting s.'s
S.'s Plus II back belt
S. Preforms orthotic
stop-and-go s.'s
s.'s terminal device
SportCord exercise and rehabilitation system
Sportelli system collimator mounted contact shield
Sporthotics orthotic

NOTES

S

Sportono
    cementless S. (CLS)
Sport-Rite
    S.-R. Olympian device
    S.-R. Runner device
Sports-Caster I, II knee brace
Sports-Grip Bar
sportsman's
    s. hernia
    s. toe
sportstape
    Leukotape P s.
Sport-Stirrup orthosis
SporTX
    S. pulsed direct current stimulator
    S. stimulation device
spot
    café au lait s.
    Carleton s.
    de Morgan s.
    s. film
    s. radiograph
    s. view
    s. weld
spot-face reamer
Spotorno
    S. cementless hip arthroplasty stem
    S. hip prosthesis
    S. index
SPR
    selective posterior rhizotomy
    superior peroneal retinaculum
Sprague arthroscopic technique
sprain
    acromioclavicular s.
    ankle s.
    anterior cruciate s.
    anterior talofibular s.
    calcaneofibular s.
    chronic ankle s.
    chronic foot s.
    deltoid s.
    fibular collateral s.
    s. fracture
    inversion ankle s.
    joint s.
    lateral ankle s.
    lateral collateral s.
    ligament rupture s.
    medial collateral s.
    postacute s.
    posterior cruciate s.
    posterior oblique s.
    relapsing ankle s.
    rider's s.
    syndesmotic s.
    talocrural s.

    talonavicular s.
    tibiofibular s.
sprained ankle syndrome
Spratt
    S. bone curette
    S. mastoid curette
spray
    air plasma s. (APS)
    AliCool splint s.
    Aqua S.
    HandClens ultra antiseptic s.
    L'Aprina topical s.
    low-pressure plasma s. (LLPS)
    Proderm topical s.
    s. and stretch
    s. and stretch technique
    vasocoolant s.
spread
    s. foot
    Fowler s.
    s. hand
spreader
    Assistant Free calibrated femoral
        tibial s.
    Bailey rib s.
    s. bar
    Beeson cast s.
    Beeson plaster s.
    Blount bone s.
    Blount laminar s.
    Bobechko s.
    bone s.
    Burford-Finochietto rib s.
    Burford rib s.
    calcaneal s.
    Cloward s.
    Feochetti rib s.
    Haglund-Stille plaster s.
    Haight-Finochietto rib s.
    Harrington s.
    Henning cast s.
    Henning plaster s.
    Hoffer-Daimler cast s.
    Inge s.
    laminar s.
    Lemmon sternal s.
    Lilienthal rib s.
    M-Pact cast s.
    Nelson rib s.
    small lamina s.
    TSRH eyebolt s.
spreading
    s. forceps
    s. hand splint
Sprengel deformity
spring
    S. angled adjustable barbell
    s. cock-up splint

compression s.
s. finger
s. fixation
Gruca-Weiss s.
internal fixation s.
s. ligament
s. ligament complex
s. pin
s. plate
s. swivel thumb
s. test
Weiss s.

Springer fracture
Springlite
S. Advantage DP
S. II foot component
S. G foot component
S. lower limb prosthesis
S. low profile Symes II
S. polyolefin BK cover
S. polyurethane AK, BK conical cover
S. super low profile Symes II
S. toe filler

spring-loaded
s.-l. knee lock
s.-l. lock orthosis
s.-l. nail

spring-mounted electromagnet
spring-wire
s.-w. ankle-foot orthosis
s.-w. safety pin splint

sprint
S. Climber
S. cross trainer
S. Runner

sprinter's fracture
Spri Xercise board
S.P. 100 transcutaneous electrical neural stimulator
spur
acromial s.
anterior impingement s.
bone s.
calcaneal s.
calcific s.
cartilaginous s.
chondroosseous s.
degenerative s.
fibrous s.
s. formation
heel s.

impingement s.
inferior s.
osteophytic s.
s. pad
painful s.
plantar calcaneal s.
posterior s.
prominent s.
retrocalcaneal s.
s. sign
spondylotic s.
subacromial s.
traction s.
uncovertebral s.

spur-crushing clamp
spuria
pelvis s.
spurious
s. ankylosis
s. articular process
s. rib
s. torticollis
Spurling
S. maneuver
S. rongeur
S. test
Spurling-Kerrison
S.-K. rongeur forceps
S.-K. upbiting and downbiting rongeur
spurring
anterior s.
bony s.
degenerative s.
inferior s.
spurt muscle
squamooccipital bone
squamous cell
squamous-type bone
square
S. Module Seating System
rocker balance s.
square-ended
s.-e. distraction rod
s.-e. hook
square-end pliers
square-hole broach
square-hollow chisel
square-shaped
s.-s. awl
s.-s. wrist test

NOTES

S

squat
    s. jump
    s. lift
    s. test
squatting
    s. ability
    s. test
squeeze
    s. ball
    s. dynamometer
    s. exerciser
    Schaffer s.
    s. test
squinting patella
SR
    stabilizing reversal
SRF
    semirigid fiberglass cast
SRL
    short radiolunate
    SRL ligament
SRN
    superficial radial nerve
S-ROM
    S-ROM acetabular cup
    S-ROM Arthropor I–III prosthesis
    S-ROM Arthropor oblong prosthesis
    S-ROM contained shell
    S-ROM femoral stem prosthesis
    S-ROM hip prosthesis
    S-ROM hip replacement system
    S-ROM modular femoral
      component
    S-ROM modular stem
    S-ROM modular total knee system
    S-ROM Poly-Dial insert
    S-ROM proximally modular total
      hip system
    S-ROM Super Cup
    S-ROM super cup prosthesis
    S-ROM ZZT I, II prosthesis
SRP
    single reference point
    SRP instrument
SR-PLLA
    self-reinforcing polylevolactic acid
SRS
    skeletal repair system
    SRS injectable cement
SS
    suture system
SSCS
    segmental spinal correction system
SSEP
    somatosensory evoked potential
S-shaped
    S-s. deformity

    S-s. foot
    S-s. incision
SSHR
    steady state heart rate
SSI
    segmental spinal instrumentation
    shoulder subluxation inhibitor
    anterior-posterior fusion with SSI
    SSI brace
S-Soles insole
St.
    St. Georg-Buchholz ankle prosthesis
    St. Georg fully constrained
      prosthesis
    St. Georg sledge unicompartment
      prosthesis
    St. John's Wort
    St. Jude prosthesis
stab
    s. incision
    s. wound
    s. wound arthroscopy entry portal
stabilimetry
stability
    ankle s.
    elbow s.
    glenohumeral joint s.
    immediate postoperative s. (IPS)
    knee s.
    lateral s.
    ligamentous s.
    lumbar spine rotational s.
    posterior s.
    rotary s.
    tibiotalar s.
    S. total hip system
stabilization
    anterior short-segment s.
    s. approach
    atlantoaxial s.
    cervical spine s.
    cervicothoracic junction s.
    s. of the chevron procedure
    definitive s.
    distal radioulnar joint s.
    Dunn-Brittain foot s.
    dynamic lumbar s.
    flexion compression spine injury s.
    fracture s.
    Gruca s.
    iliac crest bone graft s.
    lower cervical spine posterior s.
    myoplastic muscle s.
    occipitocervical s.
    odontoid fracture s.
    patellar tendon s. (PTS)
    s. plate
    posterior lower cervical spine s.

prophylactic operative s.
provisional s.
rhythmic s.
sacral spine s.
screw s.
skeletal s.
spinal injury operative s.
spinal osteotomy s.
subluxation s.
thoracolumbar spine s.
s. training
TSRH crosslink s.
wire s.

stabilizer
ankle s.
Dynamic foot s.
foot s.
forearm s.
Freedom thumb s.
Heel Hugger therapeutic heel s.
kneecap s.
KT-1000 foot s.
Palumbo ankle s.
patellar s.
secondary s.
Verteflex arthrotonic s.

stabilizing
s. bar
s. hinge
s. reversal (SR)

stable
s. burst fracture
s. cervical spine injury
s. gait
s. hinge joint
s. to motion
s. reduction
s. vertebra

Stablecut sawblade
Stableloc
S. Colles fracture external fixator
S. II external fixation
S. II external fixation system
S. external wrist fixation system

stack
S. shoulder procedure
S. splint

stacking cone
Stader
S. pin
S. pin guide
S. splint

stage
distraction-flexion s. (DFS)
Eichenholz s.
Enneking disease s.
Ficat and Arlet disease s.
Greulich and Pyle skeletal
  maturation s.
hard callus s.
implant s.
S. model of industrial rehabilitation
Risser s.
silent hip s.
soft callus s.

staggering gait
staghorn calculus
staging
Functional Assessment S. (FAST)
Lichtman s.
Outerbridge degenerative arthritis s.
Waldenström s.

Stagnara
S. gouge
S. wake-up test

stagnation
foot s.
qi s.

Staheli
S. rotational profile
S. shelf procedure
S. technique
S. test

Stahl
S. index
S. Kienbock disease classification
S. staging system

stain
Gram s.
port-wine s.
reticulin s.
Stevenel blue s.
van Gieson picrofuchsin s.

stainless
s. steel
s. steel alloy
s. steel clamp
s. steel equipment
s. steel implant metal prosthesis
s. steel mesh
s. steel and molybdenum (SMO)
s. steel plate
s. steel screw

NOTES

667

stainless (*continued*)
    s. steel staple
    s. steel wire
stair
    s. running test
    s. sign
staircase phenomenon
StairClimber assist device
stairclimber's foot
stair-climbing exercise
StairMaster exercise system
stairstep
    cervical s.
    s. fracture
stall bar
Stamm
    S. metatarsal osteotomy
    S. method
    S. procedure for intraarticular hip fusion
    S. and Wilson overlapping toe management procedure
stamp
    Gelfoam s.
stamping gait
stance
    calcaneal s.
    frontside snowboard s.
    initial s.
    late s.
    s. phase
    s. phase of gait
    s. phase walking
    single-limb s.
    terminal s.
    through s.
stand
    Atlas adjustable s.
    Cherf cast s.
    Grand Stand support s.
    heel s.
    IMP turnstile casting s.
    stork s.
    turnstile casting s.
    Versa-Helper floor s.
standard
    s. deviation
    S. E-Z-On Vest
    s. goniometric measure
    s. 2-inch blade retractor
    s. 4-inch blade retractor
    s. medullary nail
    s. shell ankle-foot orthosis
    s. socket
    s. thoracotomy
    s. U patellar support
standardized growth curve

standing
    s. apprehension test
    s. dorsoplantar view
    s. flexion
    s. flexion test
    s. frame orthosis
    s. Gillet test
    s. knee bend PSIS-sacrum contact
    s. lateral view
    s. side bend
    s. stability walking component
    s. weightbearing view
Stanford Hypnotic Clinical Scale
Stanisavljevic technique
Stanmore
    S. knee replacement
    S. shoulder arthroplasty
    S. shoulder prosthesis
    S. total hip replacement
    S. totally constrained elbow prosthesis
Staodyne EMS+2 neurostimulator
stapedial tenotomy
STA-peg
    Smith subtalar joint arthroereisis peg
    STA-peg implant
    STA-peg procedure
    Smith STA-peg
STA-Pen writer pen
Staph-Chek
    S.-C. pad
    S.-C. Synergy fabric
staphylococcal
    s. arthritis
    s. pyomyositis
staphylorrhaphy elevator
staple
    s. arthroereisis
    automatic s.
    barbed s.
    Biomet s.
    Blount fracture s.
    Bostick s.
    s. capsulorrhaphy
    capsulorrhaphy s.
    Coventry s.
    Day fixation s.
    DePalma s.
    Downing s.
    s. driver
    duToit shoulder s.
    Ellison fixation s.
    epiphysial s.
    s. extractor
    Fastlok implantable s.
    s. fixation
    GIA s.
    s. gun

Hernandez-Ros bone s.
s. holder
Howmedica Vitallium s.
s. inserter
s. introducer
Johannesberg s.
Krackow HTO blade s.
3M s.
meniscal s.
s. migration
Nakayama s.
O'Brien s.
osteoclast tension s.
Richards fixation s.
SD sorb s.
skin s.
Smith & Nephew medium
  barbed s.
Smith & Nephew small barbed s.
stainless steel s.
Stone four-point s.
Stryker soft tissue s.
s. suture
tabletop Stone s.
TA metallic s.
TA Premium 30, 55, 90 s.
Uni-Clip s.
Vitallium s.
Wiberg fracture s.
Zimaloy s.

stapler
Auto Suture s.
Biologically quiet s.
Closer s.
Dwyer spinal mechanical s.
GIA s.
Hall double-hole spinal s.
metaphysial s.
Oswestry-O'Brien spinal s.
powered metaphysial s.
Wiberg fracture s.

Staples
S. elbow arthrodesis
S. repair
S. technique

Staples-Black-Broström ligament repair
stapling
Blount s.
epiphysial s.
percutaneous s.
physial s.

STAR
Scandinavian total ankle replacement
  STAR technique
starch
s. bandage
s. test
Stardox wrist brace
star gait
stark
S. arthrodesis
S. graft
Stark-Moore-Ashworth-Boyes technique
Starrett pin vise
starter
nail s.
stasimorphia
stasis ulcer
Statak
S. anchor system
S. curette
S. soft tissue attachment device
state
pathomechanical s.
proinflammatory s.
prothrombotic s.
Stat Graphics software
static
s. alignment
s. arthropathy
s. back
s. compression
s. compression plate
s. evaluation
s. fixation
s. foot deformity
s. foot pain
s. footprint
s. listing
s. listing nomenclature
s. locking nail
s. lock nailing
s. orthosis
s. palpation
s. scoliosis
s. splint
s. stretch
s. stretching
s. tendon transfer
s. traction
statically
station
Aquatrend water workout s.

S

NOTES

station *(continued)*
> s. and gait
> gait and s.
> s. test
> unsteadiness of gait and s.

stationary
> s. angle guide
> s. arthropathy
> s. attachment flexible endoskeletal (SAFE)
> s. attachment flexible endoskeletal orthotic

stature
> short s.

status
> ambulatory s.
> hydration s.
> intact neurovascular s.
> s. loading
> neurovascular s.
> s. post

Stauffer modification
Stax fingertip splint
stay
> length of s. (LOS)

stay-retractor
> Freebody s.-r.

STC 900-series travel chair
steady state heart rate (SSHR)
steal
> s. effect
> s. syndrome

Stealth
> S. anchor
> S. frame
> S. image-guided system
> S. knee brace

Stedman awl
steel
> austenitic stainless s.
> S. correction
> S. maneuver
> martensitic stainless s.
> S. rule of thirds
> s. shank
> s. sole plate orthosis
> stainless s.
> S. triple innominate osteotomy
> S. triradiate osteotomy

steering wheel injury
Steffee
> S. instrument
> S. instrumentation technique
> S. pedicle plate
> S. pedicle screw-plate system
> S. plate and screw
> S. screw plate
> S. spinal instrumentation

> S. thumb arthroplasty
> S. variable spine plating system

Steffensmeier board
Steichen neurovascular free flap
Steida
> S. bony process
> S. fracture

Steinbach mallet
Steinberg
> S. infiltration block
> S. rating scale

Steinbrocker rheumatoid arthritis classification
Steindler
> S. effect
> S. elbow arthrodesis
> S. flexorplasty
> S. matrixectomy
> S. procedure
> S. stripping

Steinert
> S. disease
> S. epiphysial fracture classification

Steinhauser bone clamp
Steinmann
> S. extension nail
> S. fixation pin
> S. pin fixation
> S. pin with ball bearing
> S. pin with Crowe pilot point
> S. pin with pin chuck
> S. tendon forceps
> S. test
> S. traction

stellate
> s. fracture
> s. nail bed laceration
> s. sympathetic ganglion block

Stellbrink fixation device
Stelling and Tucker polydactyly classification
stem
> Aequalis s.
> APR hip s.
> APR I femoral s.
> Aufranc-Turner s.
> s. base plate
> Biomet revision hip s.
> calcar replacement s.
> collarless s.
> Continuum hip s.
> contoured femoral s. (CFS, CSF)
> Corail HA-coated s.
> CRM s.
> s. deformation
> Engh-Glassman femoral s.
> Exeter s.
> Extend s.

s. extractor
s. failure
fenestrated s.
F2L Multineck femoral s.
Harris-Galante s.
HG multilock hip s.
hydroxyapatite-coated s.
implant s.
intramedullary s.
Iowa s.
Kirschner s.
KMP femoral s.
Linear hip s.
Link MP microporous hip s.
long s. (LS)
Mallory-Head femoral s.
modular Moniflex hip s.
Moniflex hip s.
Moore s.
Natural-Hip titanium hip s.
nonfenestrated s.
Opti-Fix hip s.
Osteonics Omnifit-HA hip s.
PCA hip s.
Perfecta femoral s.
PFC hip s.
Precision hip s.
press-fit s.
primary s. (PS)
Profile hip s.
Profix metaphysial tibial s.
Ranawat-Burstein porous s.
regular s.
s. removal
Revision hip s.
Richards modular s.
roundback s.
SL-Plus s.
Spectric EF s.
Spotorno cementless hip
  arthroplasty s.
S-ROM modular s.
straight femoral s.
Taperloc femoral s.
trial s.
Ultima calcar s.'s
Ultima Fx s.'s
Zimmer bone s.
stemmed tibial prosthesis
Stener-Gunterberg
S.-G. hip operation
S.-G. resection

Stener lesion
stenosans
tenosynovitis serosa s.
stenosed
stenosing tenosynovitis
stenosis, pl. **stenoses**
achondroplastic s.
ankylosing spinal s.
central canal s.
cervical s.
combined s.
congenital s.
constitutional s.
degenerative s.
foraminal s.
lateral recess s. (LRS)
multisegmental spinal s.
neural foraminal s. (NFS)
spinal canal s. (SCS)
stent
Carcon s.
Dacron s.
s. dressing
Omnifit HA hip s.
synthetic s.
stenting
Stenver view
Stenzel
S. rod
S. rod prosthesis
step
CUBEx multifunctional s.
s. defect
s. drill
equinus s.
s. exercise
s. length
s. osteotomy
s. out, turn out (SOTO)
s. screw
s. time
s. width
step-cut
s.-c. lengthening
s.-c. osteotomy
s.-c. reamer
s.-c. transection
step-down
s.-d. drill
s.-d. osteotomy

NOTES

Stephen
    S. scissors
    S. spreader bar
stepladder sign
step-off
    s.-o. between bone fracture
      fragments
    s.-o. of fracture
steppage gait
stepper
    Diamondback 1100 recumbent s.
    Diamondback 1100 self-generated s.
    Diamondback 100 upright s.
    NuStep total body recumbent s.
step-up
    lateral s.-u.
stereoarthrolysis
stereognosis
stereolithography (SL)
    s. cage
stereophotogrammetry
    optical s.
    roentgen s.
stereotaxic anterior capsulotomy
Steri-Clamp
    S.-C. clamp
    IMP S.-C.
    Innovative Medical Products S.-C.
Steri-Cuff
    S.-C. disposable tourniquet cuff
    S.-C. Plus
sterile
    s. condition
    s. dry dressing (SDD)
    s. loosening
    s. matrix
    s. pencil
    s. saline solution
    s. sheet
    s. sheeting
    s. towel
sterilization
    ethylene oxide s.
Steri-Strips
Sterivap cement gun
sterna (*pl. of* sternum)
sternal
    s. approximator
    s. attachment component
    s. rib
sternal-occipital-mandibular
    s.-o.-m. immobilization (SOMI)
    s.-o.-m. immobilizer
    s.-o.-m. immobilizer orthosis
sternal-occipital-manubrial immobilizer
sternochondral articulation
sternoclavicular (SC)
    s. angle

    s. articulation
    s. disk
    s. joint (SCJ)
    s. joint dislocation
    s. joint injury
    s. joint reconstruction
    s. joint reduction
    s. joint separation
    s. ligament
sternocleidomastoid
    s. muscle
    s. muscle fibromatosis
sternocostal
    s. joint
    s. ligament
sternohyoid muscle
sternomastoid muscle
sternooccipital mandibular immobilizer orthosis
sternothyroid muscle
sternotomy
sternoxiphoid plane
sternum, pl. **sterna**
    duplicate s.
    s. fracture
sternum-splitting approach
steroid
    epidural s.
    s. Injection
    s. myopathy
    performance-enhancing s.
    tapering dose s.
    s. therapy
steroid-induced
    s.-i. avascular necrosis
    s.-i. bone disease
    s.-i. osteonecrosis
Stevenel blue stain
Stevenson
    S. alligator forceps
    S. grasping forceps
Stevens-Street
    S.-S. elbow prosthesis
    S.-S. elbow prosthesis template
Steward-Milford fracture classification
Stewart
    S. arm operation
    S. distal clavicular excision
    S. styloidectomy
Stewart-Harley transmalleolar ankle arthrodesis
Stewart-Morel syndrome
Steytler-Van Der Walt procedure
STH-2 hip prosthesis
sthenometry
stick
    Back Revolution S.
    dressing s.

FMS Intracell s.
Intracell Sprinter s.
sponge s.
switching s.
s. tie ligature
weighted walking s.
Stickler syndrome
Stieda
S. fracture
S. process
S. tubercle
STIF
spinopelvic transiliac fixation
STIF system
stiff
s. gait
s. man syndrome
s. ray
s. ribbon retractor
s. toe
stiff-knee gait
stiff-legged gait
stiffness
axial s.
fusion s.
joint s.
resting shear s.
shear s.
small-joint s.
torsional s.
stiff-soled shoe
stifle joint
stigmatic electrode
Stiles-Bunnell transfer technique
Still disease
Stille
S. bone biter
S. bone chisel
S. bone drill
S. bone drill set
S. bone gouge
S. brace
S. bur
S. hand drill
S. osteotome
S. plaster shears
S. rongeur
Stille-Horsley
S.-H. bone forceps
S.-H. bone rongeur
S.-H. rib forceps

Stille-Liston
S.-L. bone-cutting forceps
S.-L. bone rongeur
Stille-Luer
S.-L. bone rongeur
S.-L. duckbill rongeur
S.-L. rongeur forceps
Stille-Luer-Echlin rongeur
Stille-pattern trephine and bone drill set
Stiller rib
Stille-Ruskin bone rongeur
Stille-Sherman bone drill
Stimoceiver implant material
Stimprene
S. electrotherapy brace
S. wrap
Stimson
S. anterior shoulder reduction technique
S. dressing
gravity method of S.
S. gravity method
S. maneuver
S. reduction
stimulated graciloplasty
stimulating
s. electrode
s. massage
stimulation
antidromic s.
cranial electrical s. (CES)
direct electrical nerve s. (DENS)
double simultaneous sensory s.
electrical bone-growth s. (EBGS)
electrical nerve s.
electrical surface s.
electronic bone s. (EBI)
electrotherapeutic point s. (ETPS)
external-coil electrical s.
functional electrical s. (FES)
functional neuromuscular s.
galvanic s.
high-voltage pulsed s. (HVPS)
high-voltage pulsed galvanic s. (HVPGS)
interferential s. (IFC)
interferential electrical s.
lateral electrical surface s. (LESS)
magnetic s.
marrow s.

NOTES

stimulation *(continued)*
    microamperage electrical nerve s. (MENS)
    microamperage neural s. (MNS)
    neuromuscular electrical s. (NMES)
    OrthoLogic 1000 bone growth s.
    OsteoGen bone growth s.
    Osteo-Stim implantable bone growth s.
    PEMF bone growth s.
    pulsed electric magnetic field bone growth s.
    repetitive nerve s.
    transcutaneous electrical nerve s. (TENS)

stimulation-ultrasound
    Amrex SynchroSonic muscle s.-u.

stimulator
    Acupoint s.
    AME bone growth s.
    Amrex muscle s.
    Back Hammer muscle s.
    battery-pack Osteo-Stim bone s.
    Biolectron bone growth s.
    bone growth s.
    constant direct current s.
    dorsal column s. (DCS)
    EBI Medical OsteoGen bone growth s.
    EBI SpF-2 implantable bone s.
    EBI SpF-T implantable bone s.
    electrical bone-growth s. (EBGS)
    Electro-Acuscope 85 s.
    EMS 2000 neuromuscular s.
    Endo Multi-Mode s.
    Freedom Micro Pro s.
    galvanic electrode s.
    G5 Porta-Plus muscle s.
    implanted bone growth s.
    Intelect electric s.
    Intelect Legend s.
    Intelect 600MP microcurrent s.
    interferential s.
    Magnum 100 s.
    Magnum 101 Plus s.
    Master-Stim interferential s.
    Maxima II transcutaneous electrical nerve s.
    Medi-Stim s.
    Mettler Trio neuromuscular electrical s.
    Micro-Z neuromuscular s.
    MS322 muscle s.
    neuromuscular III s.
    Nuwave transcutaneous electrical nerve s.
    Ortho DX electromedical s.
    Orthofix Cervical-Stim bone growth s.
    Orthofuse implantable growth s.
    OrthoGen bone growth s.
    OrthoLogic 1000 bone growth s.
    OrthoPak II bone growth s.
    OsteoGen implantable bone growth s.
    Osteo-Stim implantable bone growth s.
    PGS-3000 pulsed galvanic s.
    Physio-Stim bone growth s.
    Physio-Stim Lite bone growth s.
    Piezo electro-needleless s.
    prizm Electro-Mesh Z-Stim-II s.
    pulsed galvanic s.
    Respond II muscle s.
    SpF spinal fusion s.
    spinal fusion s.
    SpinalPak fusion s.
    SporTX pulsed direct current s.
    S.P. 100 transcutaneous electrical neural s.
    Stimuplex-S nerve s.
    Super Stimm MF s.
    SynchroSonic s.
    SysStim 226 muscle s.
    Theramini 1, 2 electrotherapy s.
    Theratouch 4.7 s.
    ThermaStim muscle s.
    Trio-Stim neuromuscular s.
    Zimmer Osteo Stim bone growth s.
    Z-Stim IF 250 microprocessor controlled s.
    Z-Stim 100 microprocessor controlled s.

stimulator/ultrasound
    Intelect Combo s./u.

Stimulite honeycomb mattress overlay

stimulus, pl. **stimuli**
    s. artifact
    conditioned s. (CS)
    maximal s.
    paired s.
    submaximal s.
    subthreshold s.
    supramaximal s.
    test s.
    threshold s.
    unconditional s. (US)

Stimuplex block needle

Stimuplex-S nerve stimulator

Stinchfield test

sting mat

stippled epiphysis

stippling

stirrup
Aircast pneumatic air s.
Allen s.
Böhler s.
s. brace
Comfort Cast s.
s. plaster splint
split s.
Swivel-Strap ankle s.
traction s.
walking s.

stitch
Allgöwer s.
apical s.
baseball s.
Bunnell s.
Frost s.
intracuticular s.
Kessler s.
Mersilene Kessler s.
Pulvertaft fish-mouth s.
roll s.

stitcher
Acufex meniscal s.

Stiwer
S. bone-holding forceps
S. hand drill

STJ
subtalar joint

STNP
subtalar joint neutral position

stock
bone s.
S. finger splint
osteopenic bone s.
poor bone s.

Stockholm hand arm vibration syndrome staging system

stockinette
s. bandage
basket s.
bias-cut s.
Buck traction s.
orthopaedic s.
s. sling
s. tube
tubular s.
Velpeau s.

stocking-glove distribution

stockings
antiembolic s.

compression s.
drop-foot redression s.
elastic s.
Jobst s.
long leg s.
MEDI Plus compression s.
Orthawear antiembolism s.
Planostretch s.
pneumatic compression s.
SCD s.
Sigvaris s.
Silver-Thera s.
Soft Touch s.
TED s.
thromboembolic s.
Zimmer antiembolism s.

Stokes amputation

stone
s. arthrodesis
s. basket screw mounted handle
S. bunionectomy
S. clamp-locking device
S. four-point staple
S. procedure
pumice s.

Stookey reflex

stool
foot s.
nested step s.
Swedish support s.

stop
s. action brace
Elite posterior adjustable s.

stop-and-go sports

stopwatch

storiform pattern

stork
s. leg
s. stand

Storz
S. meniscotome
S. Microsystems drill bit
S. Microsystems plate cutter
S. Microsystems plate-holding forceps
S. Microsystems pliers
S. oblique arthroscope
S. screw

stout-neck curette

stove-in pelvis

stovepipe leg

S

NOTES

straddle
- s. fracture
- s. injury

StraddleSitter seating aid

straight
- s. basket forceps
- s. bone rongeur
- s. chisel
- s. curette
- s. femoral stem
- s. gouge
- s. hex screwdriver
- s. incision
- s. last shoe
- s. lateral instability
- s. leg raising (SLR)
- s. leg raising exercise
- s. leg raising test (SLRT)
- s. osteotome
- s. periosteal elevator
- s. pituitary rongeur
- s. posterior portal
- s. power reamer
- s. scissors
- s. spine syndrome
- s. stem femoral component
- s. threaded rod
- s. walker brace

strain
- acute foot s.
- articular s.
- back s.
- Brunhilde s.
- compression s.
- elastic s.
- s. energy
- foot s.
- s. fracture
- s. gauge
- muscle s.
- plastic s.
- postural s.
- shear s.
- tensile s.
- thoracolumbosacral s. (TLS)
- TLS s.

strain/counterstrain technique
strain-gauge extensometer
strain-sprain injury
strain-stress curve
Strampelli splint
strap
- Band-It tennis elbow s.
- Beta Pile II, III splint s.
- buddy s.
- Butterfly cushion with s.
- capsular s.
- Cho-Pat Achilles tendon s.
- Cho-Pat Dual Action Knee S.
- Cho-Pat elbow s.
- Cho-Pat ITB S.
- s. clavicular splint
- counterforce s.
- crotch s.
- D-ring s.
- Eclipse Gel elbow s.
- external elastic s.
- extremity mobilization s.
- fork s.
- Gel-Bank patellar s.
- infrapatellar s.
- Lema s.
- Levine patellar tendon s.
- S. Lok ankle brace
- Meek clavicular s.
- s. muscle
- neoprene wrist s.
- Nylatex s.
- Partridge s.
- Pebax fastening s.
- PIP/DIP s.
- Pro-Tec patellar tendon s.
- QualCraft s.
- Scott elastic ankle s.
- s. sling
- stretch-out s.
- suprapatellar s.
- suspension s.
- Synergistic suspension s.
- valgus corrective ankle s.
- varus corrective ankle s.
- Velcro s.

Strap-Pad
- DAW S.-P.

strapping
- adhesive s.
- garter s.
- loop & hook s.
- LowDye s.

Strassburg sock
Strata hip system
strategy
- cuing s.
- diagnostic s.

Stratos orthotic
stratum corneum
Stratus impact-reducing pylon
Straub technique
Strayer
- S. Achilles lengthening procedure
- S. gastrocnemius recession
- S. gastrocnemius-soleus recession
- S. lengthening
- S. tendon technique

streaming potential
streblodactyly

street
> S. forearm nail
> S. medullary pin

Streeter dysplasia

Street-Stevens humeral prosthesis

strength
> 5/5 s.
> s. against resistance
> axial gripping s.
> bending s.
> bone s.
> bone-screw interface s.
> BUE s.
> C-D instrumentation fixation s.
> cervical extension s.
> Cotrel pedicle screw fixation s.
> s. curve
> extensor hallucis longus s.
> extrinsic muscle s.
> fatigue s.
> graft s.
> grip s.
> hand grasp s.
> hand grip s.
> intrinsic muscle s.
> isometric cervical extension s.
> Lovett clinical scale of s.
> motor s.
> pedicle screw pull-out s.
> pinch s.
> pull-out s.
> tensile s.
> s. test eccentric bilateral
> s. testing
> torsional gripping s.
> s. training
> ultimate s.
> yield s.

strength-duration curve

strengthened
> gas atomized dispersion s. (GADS)

strengthening
> s. exerciser
> rehabilitation muscle s.
> wrist extensor s.
> wrist flexor s.

Stren intraepiphyseal osteotomy

streptococcal myositis

stress
> bending s.
> biomechanical s.
> s. distribution
> s. dorsiflexion projection
> s. examination
> fatigue s.
> s. film
> s. fracture
> heat s.
> hyperextension s.
> s. injury
> laxity to varus s.
> low-contact s. (LCS)
> measured s.
> mediolateral s.
> principal s.
> s. radiograph
> s. radiography
> s. riser
> s. roentgenography
> s. rupture
> shear s.
> s. shielding
> tensile s.
> s. test
> s. testing
> torsional s.
> s. transfer
> valgus s.
> s. view
> Von Mises s.

stress-corrosion cracking

stressor

Stress-Ray varus-valgus device

stress-relaxation
> intraoperative s.-r.

stress-strain curve

stress-testing arthrometer

stretch
> carpal tunnel s.
> diagonal s.
> elastic s.
> general capsular s.
> heel cord s.
> S. and Heel night splint
> s. injury
> low-load prolonged s. (LLPS)
> passive s.
> s. pattern
> quick s.
> s. receptor
> s. reflex
> repeated quick s. (RQS)
> slow s.
> spray and s.

NOTES

S

stretch (continued)
    static s.
    s. test
    Vapo coolant spray and s.
    wrist extensor s.
    wrist and finger flexor s.
stretcher
    hamstring s.
    shoe s.
stretching
    bullet s.
    s. contraindication
    gastrocnemius-soleus s.
    nerve s.
    s. program
    range of motion therapeutic s.
    soft tissue s.
    static s.
stretch-out strap
Stretch-Rite exerciser system
striata
    osteopathia s.
striatal
    s. lesion
    s. toe
striated
    s. muscle
    s. nail
Strickland
    S. modification
    S. technique
    S. tendon repair
stride
    S. Analyzer
    s. length
    s. length of gait
    s. time
strike
    heel s.
    knee s.
    s. phase of gait
striker
    forefoot s.
    forefoot-to-rearfoot s.
string drawing board
stringiness
stringing peg
strip
    corticocancellous bone s.
    Fas-Trac s.
    gastrocnemius-soleus fascial s.
    s. posting
    Thera-Band s.
stripe
    vertebral s.
striped muscle
stripout
    screw s.

stripper
    Acufex microsurgical tendon s.
    Brand tendon s.
    Bunnell tendon s.
    cartilage s.
    Fischer tendon s.
    Furlong tendon s.
    Grierson tendon s.
    orthopaedic surgical s.
    pigtail tendon s.
    slotted tendon s.
    tendon s.
stripping
    Steindler s.
stroke
    heat s.
    s. test
    s. volume
stroker
    skin s.
stroke-related deconditioning
stroller
    adapted s.
stroma, pl. stromata
    fibrovascular connective tissue s.
Stromeyer
    S. Achilles tenotomy procedure
    S. splint
Stromgren
    S. ankle brace
    S. support
Stromqvist hook pin system
Strong dorsal extension block splinting
Stronghands hand exerciser
strontium-85 resorption rate
Stroop test
structural
    s. aluminum malleable (SAM)
    s. bone graft
    s. component
    s. congenital myopathy
    s. curve
    s. derangement
    s. intersegmental distortion
    s. scoliosis
structure
    articular s.
    contiguous vertebral s.
    cordlike s.
    extraarticular s.
    graft s.
    Hedrocel tantalum metal s.
    intraarticular s.
    keystone s.
    ligamentous s.
    neurovascular s.
    osseous s.
    posterolateral s.

ring s.
uniaxial s.
waist of anatomical s.
Wolff law of bone s.
strumming
perpendicular s.
Strümpell
S. disease
S. sign
Strümpell-Marie disease
Strunsky sign
strut
s. bone graft
fibrotic s.
s. fusion technique
Littig s.
s. plate fixation
Struthers
arcade of S.
ligament of S.
strut-type pin
Stryker
S. bed
S. camera
S. cartilage knife
S. CPM exerciser
S. dermatome
S. drill
S. fracture frame
S. Howmedica Osteonics
S. Intracompartmental Pressure
Monitor System
S. knee joint laxity device
S. knee laxity arthrometer
S. lag screw
S. leg exerciser
S. power instrumentation
S. saw
S. screwdriver
S. SE3 drive system
S. soft tissue staple
S. surgical hand table
S. turning frame
S. viewing arthroscope
Stryker-Notch view
STS
silicone thermoplastic splinting
STS molding sock
STSE
split-thickness skin excision
STSG
split-thickness skin graft

STT
scaphotrapezoid-trapezial
superficial tibiotalar
STT joint
STT ligament
Stuart Gordon hand splint
stubbed shoulder
Stubbs
S. acromioclavicular splint
S. elastic wrist support
S. 4-way clavicle brace
stucco keratosis
stuck finger
student's elbow
studio cycling
study
air-contrast s.
anatomopathological s.
bone density s.
cinematographic gait s.
cohort s.
Copenhagen Stroke s.
Cornwall hip fracture s.
Doppler s.
double-contrast s.
electrophysiologic s.
evoked potential s.
fluorescein s.
injection s.
Johns Hopkins National Low Back
Pain S.
kinematic s.
Michigan Bone Health S.
nerve conduction s. (NCS)
radiodiagnostic s.
roentgen-stereophotogrammatic s.
sudomotor s.
in vivo s.
Stulberg
S. HIPciser abduction splint
S. hip classification
S. hip positioner
S. Mark II leg positioner
S. method
stump
amputation s.
s. of bone
s. edema
s. hallucination
s. neuralgia
painful s.
s. revision

NOTES

S

stump (*continued*)
   s. shrinker
   s. sock
   s. wrapping
stuttering of gait
STx
   STx lumbar traction device
   STx Saunders lumbar disc device
stylet
   blunt s.
stylohyoid
styloid
   s. fracture
   s. process
styloidectomy
   Stewart s.
styloidium
stylus
   tibial s.
Styrofoam filler block
subacromial
   s. bursa
   s. bursal adhesion
   s. bursitis
   s. bursography
   s. decompression
   s. impingement syndrome
   s. portal
   s. space
   s. spur
subacromiodeltoid bursa
subacute
   s. hematogenous osteomyelitis
   s. subperiosteal hemorrhage
subaponeurotic abscess
subarachnoid block
subarticular
   s. cyst
   s. screw
subastragalar
   s. amputation
   s. dislocation
   s. fusion
subaxial
   s. posterior cervical spinal fusion
   s. subluxation
subcalcaneal bursitis
subcapital
   s. fracture
   s. osteotomy
subchondral
   s. bone
   s. bone cyst
   s. lesion
   s. lucency
   s. plate
   s. sclerosis

subclavian
   s. artery
   s. artery injury
   s. steal syndrome
   s. vein
   s. vein injury
subclavicular approach
subclavius
   s. muscle
   s. tendon graft
subcondylar
   s. deformity
   s. osteotomy
subcoracoid
   s. bone
   s. shoulder dislocation
   s. space
subcortical defect
subcostal
   s. muscle
   s. plane
subcutaneous
   s. abscess
   s. anterior transposition
   s. drain
   s. fracture
   s. granuloma annulare
   s. intracompartmental soft tissue
     sarcoma
   s. operation
   s. palmar fasciotomy
   s. pseudosarcomatous fibromatosis
   s. soft tissue sarcoma
   s. tenotomy
   s. tissue
subcuticular suture
subdeltoid
   s. bursa
   s. bursal adhesion
   s. bursitis
subdermal plexus
subdural button
subfascial
   s. abscess
   s. incision
   s. transposition
subgaleal abscess
subglenoid shoulder dislocation
subgluteal
   s. bursitis
   s. hematoma
subjacent
Subjective Shoulder Rating Scale
   patient questionnaire
sublaminar
   s. fixation
   s. wire
   s. wiring

S

sublesional ulceration
subligamentous dissection
sublimis
    s. bridge syndrome
    flexor digitorum s. (FDS)
    s. tendon
    s. tenodesis
subluxated metatarsophalangeal joint
subluxation
    AS s.
    ASEx s.
    ASIn s.
    atlantoaxial s. (AAS)
    atlantoaxial rotatory s.
    atlantooccipital s.
    calcaneocuboid s.
    compensatory structural s.
    congenital hip s.
    Crowe s.
    facet s.
    facilitated s.
    fixation s.
    foraminal encroachment s.
    functional s.
    glenohumeral joint s.
    hip s.
    joint s.
    Madelung s.
    metatarsophalangeal s.
    neuroarticular s.
    neurofunctional s.
    patellar s.
    peroneal tendon s.
    PIEx s.
    PIIn s.
    proximal tibiofibular s.
    radial head s.
    radiocapitellar s.
    radioulnar s.
    rotatory atlantoaxial s.
    sacroiliac s.
    shoulder s.
    s. stabilization
    subaxial s.
    talar s.
    tibiofibular s.
    unilateral facet s.
    unilateral interfacetal dislocation
      or s. (UID/S)
    vertebral s.
    Volkmann s.

    wrist s.
    Yergason test of shoulder s.
subluxed vertebra
subluxing patella
submandibular
submaximal stimulus
subneural apparatus
suboccipital muscle
subperiosteal
    s. abscess
    s. amputation
    s. cortical defect
    s. dissection
    s. exposure
    s. fracture
    s. giant-cell reparative granuloma
    s. new bone
    s. new bone formation
subperiosteal-paraarticular–type osteoid
  osteoma
subphrenic abscess
subplatysmal abscess
subsartorial tunnel
subscapular
    s. angle
    s. artery injury
    s. nerve injury
    s. tendinitis
subscapularis
    s. bursitis
    s. muscle
    s. rupture
    s. tendon
    s. tendon transfer
subscapularis-capsular lengthening
subsidence
    benign s.
    component s.
    prosthesis component s.
    vertical s.
subspinous dislocation
substance
    bone s.
    metachromatic mucoid s.
    s. P
substitute
    bone s.
    Boplant Surgibone bovine bone s.
    Healos bone graft s.
    OsteoSet bone graft s.
    OsteoSet-T medicated bone graft s.

NOTES

substitute *(continued)*
    Pro Osteon 500 bone graft s.
    protein-based bone graft s.
substituting knee prosthesis
substitution
    arthroscopy-assisted patellar
      tendon s.
    Carrell fibular s.
    creeping s.
    extensor s.
    Marshall patelloquadriceps tendon s.
    patellar tendon s.
    patelloquadriceps tendon s.
    tendon s.
subsulfate
subsurface white band
subtalar
    s. arthralgia
    s. arthrodesis
    s. arthroereisis
    s. arthrosis
    s. arthrotomy
    s. articulation
    s. capsulotomy
    s. coalition
    s. distraction bone block fusion
    s. interosseous ligament
    s. inversion test
    s. joint (STJ)
    s. joint arthritis
    s. joint axis (SJA)
    s. joint dislocation
    s. joint function (SJF)
    s. joint incongruency
    s. joint instability
    s. joint neutral position (STNP)
    s. laxity
    s. MBA implant
    s. motion
    s. pronation
    s. supination
    s. tilt
    s. varus
subtendinous
    s. iliac bursa
    s. prepatellar bursa
subthreshold
    s. force
    s. stimulus
subtotal
    s. lateral meniscectomy
    s. maxillectomy
    s. plantar fasciectomy
    s. somatectomy
subtraction osteotomy
subtrochanteric
    s. femoral fracture
    s. osteotomy

subungual
    s. abscess
    s. exostosis
    s. fibroma
    s. granuloma
    s. hematoma
    s. onychomycosis
subvertebral muscle
succinate
    methylprednisolone sodium s.
sucker
    KAM Super S.
    s. shaver
suction
    autotransfusion s.
    s. biter
    s. cannula
    s. drainage
    irrigation s.
    s. nozzle
    s. punch
    s. pyramid
    s. sign
    s. socket suspension
    s. suspension prosthesis
    s. tip
    s. tube
suction-irrigation
    s.-i. system
    s.-i. technique
Sudeck
    S. atrophy
    S. disease
    S. syndrome
sudomotor
    s. activity
    s. activity test
    s. function
    s. startle reflex
    s. study
SUFE
    slipped under femoral epiphysis
sugar-tong
    s.-t. cast
    s.-t. plaster splint
    s.-t. traction
Sugioka transtrochanteric rotational osteotomy
suit
    body-exhaust s.
    G s.
Sukhtian-Hughes
    S.-H. fixation
    S.-H. fixation device
sulcus, pl. **sulci**
    s. angle
    bicipital s.
    calcaneal s.

s. calcanei
carpal s.
cuboid s.
gluteal s.
inferior costal s.
interarticular s.
intertubercular s.
lateral bicipital s.
malleolar s.
medial bicipital s.
obturator s.
paraglenoid s.
radial s.
semicanal of humerus s.
semilunar s.
s. sign
spiral s.
supraacetabular s.
talar s.
s. of talus
s. test
s. of wrist

sulfadiazine
silver s.

sulfate
magnesium s.

sulfated mucopolysaccharide
sulfide
sulfoxide
Sully shoulder stabilizer brace
Sulzer
S. Orthopaedics instrument
S. Orthopedic
S. prosthesis

Sunday staphylorrhaphy elevator
Sunderland
S. classification of nerve injury
S. first-degree nerve injury

Sundt shunt
sunrise view
sunset view
super
S. Cut laminectomy rongeur
S. Grip sleeve
S. Jock n' Jill store Superfeet
orthotic
S. Stimm MF stimulator
s. wedge
s. wrap

superabduction
Superblade blade
SuperCup acetabular cup prosthesis

superextension
**Superfeet Custom Pre-Fabricated
Orthotic**
superficial
s. circumflex iliac artery
s. femoral artery (SFA)
s. heat modality
s. infection
s. necrosis
s. palmar arch
s. peroneal nerve
s. posterior compartment
s. radial nerve (SRN)
s. temporal artery
s. temporal vein
s. tibiotalar (STT)
s. varicosity
s. white onychomycosis (SWO)

superficialis
s. arcade
flexor digitorum s. (FDS)
s. tendon

superflexion
Superform Contours orthotic
Superglue adhesive
superincumbent
superior
s. border
s. costotransverse ligament
s. dislocation
s. endplate
s. extensor retinaculum of foot
s. glide
s. gluteal neurovascular bundle
s. labrum anterior and posterior
(SLAP)
s. labrum anterior and posterior
lesion
s. laryngeal artery
s. laryngeal nerve
s. laryngeal nerve external branch
s. leaf
s. peroneal retinaculum (SPR)
s. pole of patella
s. portal
s. process
s. radioulnar joint
S. Sleeprite Hi-Lo orthopedic bed
s. sulcus tumor
s. thoracic pedicle screw
s. thyroid artery
s. thyroid vein

NOTES

superior *(continued)*
    s. tibial articulation
    s. tibiofibular joint
superman back exercise technique
supermarket elbow
supernumerary
    s. bone
    s. digit
    s. lumbar segmentation
    s. thumb
    s. toe
superoinferior tilt
superolateral portal
superomedial
    s. calcaneonavicular ligament
    s. fragment
    s. portal
    s. region
SuperQuad assistive device
supersensitivity
    Cannon Law of Denervation S.
    denervation s.
Super-Seven exercise
SuperSkin thin film dressing
Superstabilizer
    S. cemented stem extender
    S. press-fit stem extender
supertubercular wedge
  osteotomy/bunionectomy
supinate
supination
    s. contracture
    s. deformity
    s. of foot
    hindfoot s.
    s. injury
    pronation and s.
    subtalar s.
    s. torque
supination-adduction
    s.-a. fracture
    s.-a. injury
supination-eversion
    s.-e. fracture
    s.-e. injury
supination-external
    s.-e. rotation (SER)
    s.-e. rotation IV (SER-IV)
    s.-e. rotation IV fracture
    s.-e. rotation injury
supination-inversion rotation injury
supination-outward rotation injury
supination-plantarflexion injury
supinator
    s. fat pad sign
    s. fossa
    s. fossa supraclavicular fossa
  Frenkel exercises

    s. jerk
    s. jerk reflex
    s. longus reflex
    s. muscle
    s. syndrome
supine
    s. chest press
    s. C-Trax traction
    s. C-Trax traction system
    s. iliac gapping test
    s. long sitting test
    s. position
    s. position driver
    s. straight leg raising test
Suppan foot operation
supplement
    oral nutritional s.
supplementation
    zinc s.
supple neck
supplier
    National Association of Medical
      Equipment S.'s
supply
    blood s.
    longitudinal blood s.
    reanastomosis of blood s.
support
    Accommodator arch s.
    Accu-Back back s.
    Achillotrain active Achilles
     tendon s.
    Active Ankle s.
    Act joint s.
    Act knee s.
    AliMed-Freedom arthritis s.
    AliMed wrist/thumb s.
    ankle stabilizing orthosis s.
    ANNA-DOTE Positioning S.
    arch s.
    Arizona universal leg s.
    ASO s.
    Assistant Free foot/ankle s.
    back s.
    Back-Huggar lumbar s.
    BackThing lumbar s.
    Band-It magnetic elbow s.
    base of s.
    Bauerfeind s.
    BIOflex Magnet Back S.
    BioSkin DP wrist s.
    BioWrap lumbosacral/sacral s.
    Birkenstock Blue Footbed arch s.
    Birkenstock high-flange arch s.
    Body Gard neoprene s.
    boomerang wrist s.
    Carabelt lower back s.
    Carpal-Lock wrist s.

Castech extremity s.
Cavus foot s.
cervical s.
ChinUpps cervicofacial s.
ChiroFlow adjustable back s.
Cho-Pat knitted compression s.
cock-up wrist s.
Comfort Cool neoprene s.
Comprifix active ankle s.
Compro Plus Knee s.
Core Reflex wrist s.
Core Universal elastic knee s.
Core Universal elbow s.
Core Universal rib s.
Corfit System 7000 Series
    Lumbosacral S.
Cryo/Cuff compression s.
cutout knee s.
Deltoid-Aid arm s.
DePuy s.
Desk-rest arm s.
Dr. Kho's CMC S.
Epi-Lock elbow s.
Epipoint elbow s.
Epitrain active elbow s.
Epitrain knitted elbow s.
Epitrain Viscoped s.
Ergo Cush back s.
Ergoflex Premiere back s.
external s.
Ezy Wrap lumbosacral s.
Fits-All s.
FlexLite hinged knee s.
Foot Hugger foot s.
fork strap prosthetic s.
Freedom accommodator arch s.
Freedom arthritis s.
Freedom back s.
Freedom elastic long wrist s.
Friedman s.
Futuro wrist s.
Genutrain P3 knee s.
geriatric chair trunk s.
Houston halo cervical s.
Innovation Sports bracing s.
Juzo s.
Kallassy ankle s.
Kerr-Lagen abdominal s.
Knee Sleeve knee s.
Lo Bak spinal s.
Loving Comfort maternity s.
Loving Comfort postpartum s.

Lumbotrain lumbosacral s.
Malleoloc ankle s.
Malleotrain ankle s.
Manutrain active wrist s.
Markwort ankle s.
MKG knee s.
Mold-In-Place back s.
Momma-Too Maternity S.
Monitor Master monitor s.
Morton toe s.
Mother-To-Be abdominal s.
Mother-To-Be Support Maternity S.
neoprene ankle s.
neoprene back s.
Nightimer carpal tunnel s.
Night Splint s.
obese s.
OBUS back s.
OEC wrist/forearm s.
Omotrain active shoulder s.
Ortho-Pal body s.
OSI Well Leg S.
Palumbo knee s.
Parham s.
PattStrap knee s.
Pediatric Advanced Life S. (PALS)
Performance Wrap knee s.
peripatellar retinacular s.
Philadelphia collar cervical s.
Plastizote arch s.
Playmaker s.
Powerstep foot s.
ProFlex wrist s.
prosthetic s.
QualCraft ankle s.
QualCraft short elastic wrist s.
Relax-A-Bac posture s.
Rolyan foot s.
sacral s.
Sacro-Eze lumbar s.
Scott double-strap ankle s.
Scott hinged knee s.
Sheffield s.
ShiatsuBACK back s.
Shoulder Ease abduction s.
Sidekick foot s.
Silesian bandage prosthetic s.
Spenco arch s.
S'port Max back s.
standard U patellar s.
Stromgren s.
Stubbs elastic wrist s.

NOTES

S

685

support *(continued)*
    SureStep ankle s.
    TakeOff elbow s.
    Taylor clavicle s.
    Thera-Back back s.
    therapeutic spinal s.
    tibial fracture brace proximal s.
     (TFB-PS)
    Valeo back s.
    Viscoped S s.
    ViscoSpot s.
    walking with s.
    walking without s.
    well-leg s.
    Whitman arch s.
    WorkMod back s.
    wrist hand extension
     compression s. (WHECS)
    WrisTimer CTS s.
    Wrist Pro wrist s.
supported extension exercise
suppurative
    s. arthritis
    s. flexor tenosynovitis
    s. joint infection
    s. myositis
    s. osteitis
    s. osteomyelitis
    s. periostitis
    s. synovitis
supraacetabular sulcus
supraclavicular
    s. approach
    s. brachial block anesthesia
    s. fossa
    s. fossa artery
supracollicular spike
supracondylar (SC)
    s. amputation
    s. cuff
    s. femoral derotational osteotomy
    s. humeral fracture
    intramedullary s. (IMSC)
    s. medullary nail
    s. nonunion
    patellar tendon-bearing–s.
    s. plate
    s. process
    s. process syndrome
    s. socket
    s. varus osteotomy
    s. Y-shaped fracture
supracondylar-suprapatellar (SCSP, SC-SP)
supraganglionic injury
supraglenoid tuberosity
suprahyoid

Supralen
    S. cradle orthotic
    S. Schaefer orthotic
supralevator abscess
supramalleolar
    s. derotational osteotomy
    s. flap
    s. open amputation
    s. orthosis (SMO)
    s. varus derotation osteotomy
    s. venous ulcer
supramaximal stimulus
supranaviculare
supraoccipital bone
suprapatellar (SP)
    s. cannula
    s. cuff (SPC)
    patellar tendon-
     bearing–supracondylar-s. (PTB-SC-SP)
    s. plica
    s. portal
    s. pouch
    s. reflex
    s. strap
suprapubic
suprascapular
    s. nerve
    s. nerve entrapment test
    s. nerve injury
    s. neuritis
suprasellar capsule
supraspinatus
    s. calcification
    s. implant
    s. muscle
    s. outlet
    s. syndrome
    s. tendinitis
    s. tendon
    s. test
supraspinous
    s. ligament
    s. muscle
suprasternal
    s. bone
    s. notch
    s. plane
    s. space
suprasyndesmotic
    s. fracture
    s. membrane
    s. screw fixation
supratectal transverse fracture
supratubercular
    s. wedge osteotomy
    s. wedge osteotomy bunionectomy

sural
    s. island flap
    s. island flap for foot and ankle
      reconstruction
    s. nerve
    s. neuritis
    s. neuroma
    s. neuropathy
Surbaugh
    S. leg holder
    S. legholder
sure
    S. Sport pad
    S. Step ankle brace
SureClosure
    S. closure
    S. skin stretching system
Sure-Flex
    S.-F. prosthesis
    S.-F. III prosthetic foot
SureStep
    S. ankle support
    S. ankle support system
Suretac
    S. bioabsorbable shoulder fixation
      device
    S. shoulder fixation
surface
    apposing articular s.
    articular s.
    Bazooka support s.
    cancellous s.
    s. cement
    ceramic-on-ceramic bearing s.
    concave articular s.
    contiguous articular s.
    distal concave articular s.
    eburnated bone s.
    s. electrode
    s. electromyography (sEMG)
    endosteal s.
    erosion of articular s.
    facet s.
    freshen the s.
    irregular articular s.
    Micro-Aire débridement of bone s.
    radioulnar s.
    s. replacement
    s. replacement hip arthroplasty
    roughen the s.
    s. shoe interaction
    volar s.

    wear-resistant s.
    weightbearing s.
surfer's knot
Surfit adhesive
Surgairtome air drill
SurgAssist
    S. leg positioner
    S. surgical legholder
surgeon
    American Academy of
      Orthopaedic S.'s (AAOS)
surgeon's thumb
surgery
    ablative s.
    adult scoliosis s.
    anterior cervicothoracic junction s.
    anterior lower cervical spine s.
    arthroscopic laser s.
    bypass s.
    cervical disk s.
    cervicothoracic junction s.
    closed s.
    computer-assisted orthopedic s.
      (CAOS)
    failed s.
    first ray s.
    H-block nail s.
    hypotensive s.
    intradural tumor s.
    joint replacement s.
    lateral column-lengthening s.
    limb-salvage s.
    lower extremity s.
    lower posterior lumbar spine and
     sacrum s.
    McCash hand s.
    minimum incision s. (MIS)
    MRI-directed s.
    open disk s.
    orthopaedic s.
    peripheral vascular s. (PVS)
    posterior lower cervical spine s.
    posterior lumbar interbody fusion s.
    posterior lumbar spine and
     sacrum s.
    posterior upper cervical spine s.
    ProTrac system for knee s.
    scoliosis s.
    traumatic unidirectional Bankart
     lesion s. (TUBS)
    Unilink system for hand s.
    vascular s.

S

NOTES

Surgibone
    Boplant S.
    S. implant
    Unilab S.
surgical
    s. ablation
    s. approach
    s. autoimmunization
    s. corset
    s. dressing room (SDR)
    s. exposure
    s. glove
    s. hand tray
    s. knife handle
    s. leg pedestal
    s. loupe
    s. neck
    s. neck fracture
    S. No Bounce mallet
    s. orthopedic drill
    s. pin driver
    s. prosthesis
    s. reduction
    s. rod
    S. Simplex P adhesive
    S. Simplex P radiopaque bone
      cement
    s. splint
    s. staple applier
    s. technique
    s. treatment
Surgicel
    S. fibrillar hemostat
    S. implant
    S. Nu-Knit absorbable hemostat
Surgilase CO$_2$ laser
Surgilast tubular elastic dressing
Surgitek prosthesis
Surgitube tubular gauze
Surgivac drain
survey
    bone s.
    metastatic bone s.
susceptibility testing
suspension
    balanced s.
    below-knee s.
    corset s.
    cuff s.
    s. feeder
    fingertrap s.
    flexible hinge s.
    Heyman panmetatarsal forefoot
      equinus s.
    hip disarticulation s.
    hip hemipelvectomy s.
    knee disarticulation s.
    panmetatarsal tendon s.

    patellar tendon-bearing s. (PTBS)
    SC s.
    silicone-only s. (SOS)
    s. splint
    s. strap
    suction socket s.
    s. traction
    transfemoral s.
suspension-type socket
suspensory
sustained
    s. ankle clonus
    s. loading
    s. natural apophysial glides
      (SNAGS)
    s. pressure technique
sustentacular fragment
sustentaculum tali fracture
Sutherland
    S. hip operation
    S. hip procedure
    S. lateral transfer
Sutherland-Greenfield osteotomy
Sutherland-Rowe incision
Sutter
    S. device
    S. double-stem silicone implant
      prosthesis
    S. implant
    S. MCP finger joint prosthesis
    S. silicone metacarpophalangeal
      joint
    S. silicone metacarpophalangeal
      joint arthroplasty
Sutter-CPM
    S.-CPM knee apparatus
    S.-CPM knee device
sutural bone
suture
    s. abscess
    Acufex bioabsorbable Suretac s.
    s. anchor
    s. anchor shoulder repair
    s. anchor technique
    baseball s.
    Bell s.
    Bio-FASTak s.
    BioSorb s.
    Biosyn synthetic monofilament s.
    Bondek s.
    braided s.
    bregmatomastoid s.
    bulb s.
    bundle s.
    Bunnell crisscross s.
    Bunnell figure-eight s.
    Bunnell wire pull-out s.
    button s.

Caprolactam s.
Carrel s.
Chinese fingertrap s.
core s.
cotton s.
cottony Dacron s.
Dacron s.
Dafilon s.
Dagrofil s.
Dexon s.
Donati s.
double right-angle s.
Dupuytren s.
end-to-end s.
epitenon s.
Ethibond s.
Ethicon s.
Ethiflex s.
Ethilon s.
fascial s.
figure-of-eight s.
fingertrap s.
fishmouth end-to-end s.
s. fixation
Gillis s.
Gore-Tex nonabsorbable s.
grasping s.
guy s.
s. hole drill
horizontal mattress s.
interrupted s.
intradermal s.
jugal s.
Kessler grasping s.
Kessler-Tajima s.
Krackow s.
s. of Krause
lamboid s.
lashing s.
lateral trap s.
Le Dentu s.
linen s.
locking horizontal mattress s.
lockout s.
Mason-Allen s.
mattress s.
Maxon s.
McLaughlin modification of
  Bunnell pull-out s.
Mersilene s.
MicroMite anchor s.
modified Kessler s.

modified Kessler-Tajima s.
monofilament s.
muscle-to-bone s.
nail s.
Nicoladoni s.
nonabsorbable s.
Nurolon s.
nylon s.
Panacryl s.
s. passer
passing s.
PDS s.
Perma-Hand silk s.
pin s.
polybutester s.
Polydek s.
polydioxanone s. (PDS)
polyester s.
polyethylene s.
polygalactic acid s.
polyglactin s.
polyglycolic acid s.
polyglyconate s.
polypropylene s.
Polysorb s.
popoff s.
Prolene s.
pull-out s.
Pulvertaft end-to-end s.
Pulvertaft interweave s.
pursestring s.
s. pusher talofibular joint
RB1 s.
retention s.
running s.
safety-bolt s.
s. scissors
silk s.
simple s.
sling s.
staple s.
subcuticular s.
s. system (SS)
Tajima modified Kessler s.
Teflon-coated s.
tendon s.
Tevdek s.
transosseous s.
Tycron s.
UltraFix MicroMite anchor s.
undyed s.
USP#2 s.

S

NOTES

suture *(continued)*
    vertical mattress s.
    Vicryl s.
    wire s.
suture-loop technique
Suture-Self dressing
suturing
    Johnson medial meniscal s.
    Morgan-Casscells meniscus s.
SVCPMS
    segmental vertebral
    cellulotenoperiosteomyalgic syndrome
Sven-Johansson
    S.-J. driver
    S.-J. extender
    S.-J. extractor
    S.-J. femoral neck nail
Swafford-Lichtman division
swaged needle
swallow-tail sign
swan-neck
    s.-n. chisel
    s.-n. deformity reduction
    s.-n. facies
    s.-n. finger deformity
    s.-n. gouge
    s.-n. splint
Swann-Morton surgical blade
Swanson
    S. carpal lunate implant
    S. carpal scaphoid implant
    S. classification
    S. convex condylar arthroplasty
    S. dynamic toe splint
    S. elevator
    S. finger joint
    S. finger joint implant
    S. finger joint prosthesis
    S. flexible hallux valgus prosthesis
    S. great toe implant
    S. great toe prosthesis
    S. Grip-X hand exerciser
    S. hand splint
    S. interpositional wrist arthroplasty
    S. lunate awl
    S. mallet
    S. metacarpal prosthesis
    S. metacarpophalangeal implant
    S. metatarsal broach
    S. metatarsal prosthesis
    S. metatarsophalangeal joint
    arthroplasty
    S. osteotome
    S. osteotomy
    S. PIP joint arthroplasty
    S. radial head implant
    S. radial head implant arthroplasty
    S. radiocarpal implant

    S. reamer
    S. reconstruction
    S. scaphoid awl
    S. Silastic elbow prosthesis
    S. silicone wrist arthroplasty
    S. small joint implant
    S. technique
    S. trapezium implant
    S. T-shaped great toe Silastic
    prosthesis
    S. ulnar head implant
    S. wrist joint implant
    S. wrist prosthesis
swathe, swath
    arm s.
    s. and sling
sway
    anteroposterior lateral s.
    s. back
    body s.
    lateral s.
    postural s.
swaying gait
SWD
    shortwave diathermy
sweating
    excessive s.
    plantar s.
sweat test
Swede-O
    S.-O Ankle Loc brace
    S.-O Arch-Lok
Swede-O-Universal
    S.-O.-U. brace
    S.-O.-U. orthosis
Swediauer disease
Swedish
    S. approach
    S. gymnastics
    S. Helparm
    S. knee cage
    S. knee cage orthosis
    S. massage
    S. movement
    S. portal
    S. support stool
swelling
    boggy s.
    joint s.
    postfracture s.
SwimEx
    S. aquatic therapy
    S. aquatic therapy bodyCushion
    S. hydrotherapy system
    S. pool
swimmer's
    s. shoulder
    s. view

swimming pool granuloma
swing
    s. phase
    s. phase of gait
    s. time
Swinger car bed
swing-phase
    s.-p. acceleration
    s.-p. control
swing-through gait
swing-to gait
Swiss
    S. Balance orthotic
    S. ball
    S. ball therapy
    S. cancellous screw
    S. MP joint implant
    S. pattern osteotome
switching stick
swivel
    s. clamp
    s. dislocation
    s. utensil
    s. walker
Swivel-Strap
    Aircast S.-S.
    S.-S. ankle brace
    S.-S. ankle stirrup
SWO
    superficial white onychomycosis
swollen disk
SWT
    shock-wave therapy
Sydney line
Syed-Neblett implant
Syed template implant
symbrachydactyly
Syme
    S. amputation prosthesis
    S. ankle disarticulation amputation
    S. Dycor prosthetic foot
    S. foot prosthesis
    S. operation
    S. procedure
symmetric
    s. sacral plate
    s. thumb duplication
    s. tonicity
    s. vertebral fusion
symmetrical thoracic vertebral plate
symmetry
    weightbearing s.

sympathectomy
    cervical s.
    chemical s.
    lumbar s.
    peripheral chemical s.
    preganglionic s.
sympathetic
    s. block
    s. blockade
    s. chain
    s. component
    s. dysfunction
    s. innervation
    s. maintained pain syndrome
    (SMPS)
    s. nerve
    s. nervous system (SNS)
    s. reflex dystrophy
    s. trunk
sympathetically mediated pain
symphalangism
symphysial mobility
symphysis, pl. **symphyses**
    pubic s.
    s. pubis
    s. pubis diastasis
symptom
    S.'s Checklist 90 Revised (SCL-90R)
    functionally debilitating s.
    irritable s.
    s. magnification syndrome
    Oehler s.
    Pratt s.
    S.'s and Sports Participation Rating Scale
symptomatic
    s. spondylolisthesis
    s. synovial plica
    s. torticollis
symptomatology
Syms traction
Synaptic 2000 pain management system
synarthrodial joint
synarthrophysis
synarthrosis
Synatomic total knee prosthesis
synchondritic fracture
synchondrosis, pl. **synchondroses**
    neurocentral s.
    tibiofibular s.
synchondrotomy

NOTES

synchronized fibrillation
synchronous scapuloclavicular rotation
synchrony
    arm heel-strike s.
SynchroSonic
    S. stimulator
    S. U/HVG50 ultrasound/stimulator
syncope
    heat s.
syndactylization
syndactylized finger
syndactyly
    burn s.
    complete s.
    complex s.
    complicated complex s.
    Diamond-Gould reduction s.
    Hass type s.
    incomplete s.
    Kelikian-Clayton-Loseff surgical s.
    pure s.
    reduction s.
    ring finger–small finger s.
    simple s.
syndesmectomy
syndesmectopia
syndesmitis
syndesmopexy
syndesmophyte
syndesmoplasty
syndesmorrhaphy
syndesmosis, pl. **syndesmoses**
    s. rupture
    s. screw lucency
    tibiofibular s.
syndesmotic
    s. avulsion
    s. diastasis
    s. ligament
    s. screw
    s. sprain
syndesmotomy
syndrome
    Aarskog-Scott s.
    acetabular rim s.
    acute exertional compartment s.
    (AECS)
    acute low back s.
    Adair-Dighton s.
    Adamantiades-Behçet s.
    Albright s.
    Albright-McCune-Sternberg s.
    alcohol fat embolism s.
    algodystrophy s.
    Alpers s.
    altitude s.
    anterior cervical cord s.
    anterior compartment s. (ACS)

anterior tibial compartment s.
anterolateral impingement s.
anteversion s.
anular constricting band s.
Apert s.
Arnold-Chiari s.
arthroonychodysplasia s.
athletic heart s.
Baastrup s.
Babinski-Fröhlich s.
Babinski-Nageotte s.
Bamberger-Marie s.
Barre-Lieou s.
Barsony-Polgar s.
Barsony-Teschendorf s.
Bart-Phumphery s.
Basser s.
Beals s.
Behçet s.
Behr s.
benign hypermobile joint s.
bent-knee s.
Bertolotti s.
bicipital s.
bilateral acute radicular s.
bilateral chronic radicular s.
Bing-Horton s.
bioenergy imbalance s. (BIS)
BK mole s.
black heel s.
Bloom s.
blue foot s.
blue toe s.
body cast s.
Brissaud s.
broad thumb–big toe s.
Brown-Séquard s.
Bruns gait apraxia Bruns s.
burning-feet s.
Cacchione s.
Caffey s.
Caffey-Silverman s.
calcaneal spur s.
Calvé-Legg-Perthes s.
Caplan s.
carpal tunnel s. (CTS)
Carpenter s.
Carter-Wilkinson criteria for
  hypermobility s.
cast s.
cauda equina s.
central cord s.
central heel pad s.
central herniation s.
cervical acceleration/deceleration s.
cervical dorsal outlet s.
cervical rib s.
cervicoencephalic s.

cervicogenic s.
Cestan-Chenais s.
Charcot s.
Charles Bonnet s.
Chiari-Foix-Nicolesco s.
choke s.
chronic anterior exertional
  compartment s. (CAECS)
chronic compartment s. (CCS)
chronic heel pain s. (CHPS)
chronic intractable benign pain s.
  (CIBPS)
chronic musculoskeletal pain s.
  (CMPS)
Claude s.
clenched fist s.
clumsy hand s.
Cobb s.
Cockayne s.
Coffin-Lowry s.
common peroneal nerve s.
compartment s.
complex regional pain s. (CRPS)
compression s.
congenital band s.
Conradi s.
constriction band s.
conus medullaris s.
copper deficiency s.
coracoid impingement s.
cord-traction s.
Cornelia de Lange s.
Costen s.
costoclavicular s.
Cotton-Berg s.
Cowden s.
CREST s.
crossover s.
Crouzon s.
crush s.
cubital tunnel s.
cuboid s.
Cushing s.
cyclops s.
dancing bear s.
dead arm s.
de Barsy s.
deconditioning s.
Dejerine-Sottas s.
de Lange s.
de Quervain s.
derangement s.

diffuse idiopathic skeletal
  hyperostosis s.
DiGeorge s.
DISH s.
disk s.
DOOR s.
dorsi jam s.
double crush s.
Down s.
droopy shoulder s.
drug-related hydantoin s.
Duplay s.
Dyggve-Melchior-Clausen s.
Dyke-Davidoff-Masson s.
dysfunction s.
dysplastic nevus s.
Eagle-Barrett s.
Eaton-Lambert s.
Eddowes s.
Edwards s.
Ehlers-Danlos s. (EDS)
Ekbom restless leg s.
Ellis-van Creveld s.
empty can s.
entrapment s.
eosinophilia-myalgia s.
Erdheim s.
exercise-induced compartment s.
exertional anterior compartment s.
  (EACS)
exertional deep posterior
  compartment s. (EDPCS)
extraarticular pain s.
fabella s.
facet joint s.
failed back s. (FBS)
failed back surgery s. (FBSS)
failed surgery s.
Fanconi s.
Fanconi-Albertini-Zellweger s.
far-out s.
fat embolism s.
fat pad s.
FAV s.
Fazio-Londe s.
fetal alcohol s.
fibromyalgia s. (FMS)
filum terminale s.
flat back s.
flexor carpi ulnaris s.
flexor origin s.
forearm compartment s.

S

NOTES

syndrome *(continued)*
Freeman-Sheldon s.
frozen shoulder s.
Funk tibialis posterior tendon
  dysfunction classification s.
Funston s.
GALOP s.
Gardner s.
Gardner-Diamond s.
General Adaption S. (GAS)
Goldenhar s.
Gowers s.
gracilis s.
Grisel s.
Guillain-Barré s.
Guyon tunnel s.
Haglund s.
Hajdu-Cheney s.
hammer digit s.
hammertoe s. (HTS)
hamstring s.
hand-foot s.
hand-foot-uterus s.
Hand-Schüller-Christian s.
heart-and-hand s.
heel compression s.
heel pain s.
heel spur s.
heel spur/plantar fasciitis s.
Heerfort s.
hip joint s.
HLA B27-related
  spondyloarthropathy intersection s.
Hoffa s.
Hoffmann s.
Hurler s.
Hurler-Scheie s.
hyperflexed toe compartment s.
hypermobile joint s.
hyperostosis s.
hypersensitivity s.
hypothenar hammertoe s.
idiopathic skeletal hyperostosis s.
iliacus s.
iliocostalis lumborum s.
ilioinguinal s.
iliotibial band friction s. (ITBFS)
impingement s.
infrapatellar contracture s. (IPCS)
inguinal ligament s.
internal snapping hip s.
interosseous nerve s.
intersection s.
Isaacs s.
Jaccoud s.
Jackson s.
Jackson-Gorham s.
Jackson-Weiss s.

Jadassohn-Lewandowsky s.
Jarcho-Levin s.
Johanson-Blizzard s.
Karsch-Neugebauer s.
Kast s.
Kast-Maffucci s.
Kearns-Sayre s.
Kenny-Caffey s.
Kinsbourne s.
Kleine-Levin s.
Klippel-Feil s. (KFS)
Klippel-Trenaunay s.
Klippel-Trenaunay-Weber s.
Kniest s.
Kocher-Debré-Semelaigne s.
Kretschmer s.
Kuskokwim s.
Lambert-Eaton myasthenic s.
  (LEMS)
Larsen s.
lateral column s.
lateral gutter s.
lateral hyperpressure s.
lateral patellar compression s.
Laurence-Biedl s.
Laurence-Moon s.
Laurence-Moon-Biedl s.
Lawrence-Seip s.
leg-foot-toe s.
Legg-Calvé-Perthes s.
Legg-Calvé-Waldenström s.
LEOPARD s.
Leri s.
Leriche s.
Leri-Weill s.
levator scapulae s.
Linberg s.
Little s.
Lobstein s.
local adaptation s. (LAS)
Looser-Milkman s.
lumbago-mechanical instability s.
lumbar flat back s.
lumbar thecoperitoneal shunt s.
lumbosacral mechanical s.
Maffucci s.
Marfan s.
Maroteaux-Lamy s.
McArdle s.
McCune-Albright s.
mechanical low back pain s.
medial tibial s. (MTS)
medial tibial stress s. (MTSS)
Meige s.
meningeal s.
metabolic s. (MS)
metatarsal overload s.
Meyer-Betz s.

microgeodic s.
Milch fracture classification s.
milkman's s.
Milwaukee shoulder s.
miserable misalignment s.
mixed cord s.
Morel s.
Morquio s.
Morquio-Brailsford s.
Morquio-Ullrich s.
Morton s.
Mueller Weiss s.
multifidus s.
multiple pterygium s.
multiple synostoses s.
myofascial pain s. (MPF)
Naffziger s.
nail-patella s.
naviculocapitate fracture s.
neck pain s.
nerve entrapment s.
Neumann s.
neuroarticular s.
neurogenic s.
Nievergelt-Pearlman s.
occupational stress s. (OSS)
Ollier s.
Oppenheim s.
Osebold-Remondini s.
Osgood-Schlatter s.
osteoporosis pseudoglioma s.
Ostrum-Furst s.
overtraining s.
overuse s.
Paget juvenile s.
Paget-Schrötter s.
pain-all-over s.
pain dysfunction s.
painful arc s.
Parsonage-Aldren-Turner s.
Parsonage-Turner s.
Patau s.
patellar clunk s.
patellar malalignment s.
patellar pair s.
patellofemoral pain s. (PPS)
patellofemoral stress s.
peroneal compartment s.
pes anserinus s.
Peterson s.
Pfeiffer s.
phalangeal microgeodic s.

phantom limb s.
piriformis s.
plantar fasciitis s.
plica s.
Poland s.
popliteal entrapment s.
popliteal pterygium s.
postcasting s.
postconcussive s.
posterior cord s.
posterior interosseous nerve
  compression s.
posterior joint s.
posterior knee pull s.
postfracture s.
postphlebitis s.
postpolio s.
postpyelomyelitis s.
posttraumatic algodystrophic s.
posttraumatic chronic cord s.
postural s.
Pouteau s.
predislocation s.
pronator teres s.
Proteus s.
prune-belly s.
pseudoradicular s.
psoas tendon s.
punch drunk s.
quadratus lumborum s.
quadrilateral space s.
radial sensory nerve entrapment s.
radial tunnel s.
Raynaud s.
rectus adductor s.
Refsum s.
Reiter s.
repetitive stress s. (RSS)
Rett s.
Riley-Day s.
ring s.
rotator cuff impingement s.
rotatores s.
Rotter-Erb s.
Roussy-Lévy s.
Rubinstein-Taybi s.
Rust s.
sacroiliac hypermobility s.
sacroiliac joint s.
Sanfilippo s.
SAPHO s.
scalenus anterior s.

S

NOTES

syndrome *(continued)*
    scaphocapitate s.
    scapulocostal s.
    scapuloperoneal s.
    Schanz s.
    Scheie s.
    Scheuermann s.
    Schwartz s.
    Schwartz-Jampel s.
    secondary hip-spine s.
    second impact s.
    segmental vertebral
      cellulotenoperiosteomyalgic s.
      (SVCPMS)
    seronegative enthesopathy and
      arthropathy s.
    serotonin s.
    short leg s.
    shoulder-girdle s.
    shoulder-hand s.
    shoulder-hand-finger s.
    Shwachman s.
    Silverskiöld s.
    Sinding-Larsen-Johansson s.
    sinus tarsi s.
    Sjögren s.
    skeletal hyperostosis s.
    Sly s.
    small patella s.
    Smith-Lemli-Opitz s.
    snapping knee s.
    snapping scapula s.
    soleus s.
    spinal cord s.
    spiral groove s.
    sprained ankle s.
    steal s.
    Stewart-Morel s.
    Stickler s.
    stiff man s.
    straight spine s.
    subacromial impingement s.
    subclavian steal s.
    sublimis bridge s.
    Sudeck s.
    supinator s.
    supracondylar process s.
    supraspinatus s.
    sympathetic maintained pain s.
      (SMPS)
    symptom magnification s.
    synovial plica s.
    TAR s.
    tarsal tunnel s. (TTS)
    temporomandibular joint s.
    tensor fascia lata s.
    tethered cord s.
    tethered patellar tendon s.

    thoracic inlet s.
    thoracic outlet s. (TOS)
    thrombocytopenia-absent radius s.
    Tietze s.
    transient bone marrow edema s.
    transversospinalis s.
    traumatic compartment s.
    trigger finger s.
    trochanteric s.
    Turner s.
    Uhthoff s.
    ulnar cubital tunnel s.
    ulnar impaction s.
    ulnar styloid impaction s.
    ulnocarpal abutment s.
    ulnocarpal impaction s.
    unbalanced wrist s.
    unilateral acute radicular s.
    unilateral chronic radicular s.
    valgus extension overload s.
    VATER s.
    vertebral steal s.
    vertebral subluxation s.
    vibration white finger s.
    vibrator hand s.
    volar compartment s.
    von Hippel-Lindau s.
    Wallenberg s.
    washboard s.
    Weber s.
    whiplash s.
    whiplash-shaken infant s.
    whistling face s.
    Wilkie s.
    windblown hand, whistling face s.
    wrist pain s.
    yellow nail s.
synergia
    detrusor-sphincter s.
synergist
synergistic
    s. finger motion
    s. muscle
    S. suspension strap
    s. wrist motion
    s. wrist motion splint
synergy
    S. flexible splinting material
    S. joint rehabilitation
    limb s.
    S. spine rehab system
    S. splint
    S. Therapeutic System
syngraft
synosteosis
synostosis
    cervical s.
    congenital radioulnar s.

fibula protibial s.
phalangeal s.
proximal tibiofibular s.
radioulnar s. (type I, II)
tibiofibular s.
synostotic
Synovator arthroscopic blade
synovectomy
    Albright s.
    arthroscopic s.
    arthroscopically assisted s.
    s. blade
    carpal s.
    dorsal s.
    Inglis-Ranawat-Straub elbow s.
    palmar s.
    Porter-Richardson-Vainio s.
    six-portal s.
    Smith-Petersen s.
    volar s.
    Wilkinson s.
synovia (*pl. of* synovium)
synovial
    s. biopsy
    s. bursa
    s. cavity
    s. cell sarcoma
    s. chondroma
    s. chondromatosis
    s. cyst
    s. disease
    s. fistula
    s. fluid
    s. fold
    s. fringe
    s. frond
    s. hernia
    s. herniation
    s. histopathology
    s. injury
    s. joint
    s. membrane
    s. nodule
    s. nonunion
    s. osteochondromatosis
    s. plica
    s. plica syndrome
    s. pseudarthrosis
    s. resector
    s. rongeur
    s. shaver
    s. sheath

s. stromal cell
s. tag
s. tap
s. tumor
synoviocyte
synoviogram
synovioma
synoviorthesis
synovitis
    boggy s.
    bursal s.
    chronic hemorrhagic villous s.
    chronic purulent s.
    crystal-induced s.
    dendritic s.
    diffuse pigmented villonodular s. (DPVNS)
    disseminated pigmented villonodular s.
    dry s.
    extraarticular pigmented villonodular s.
    filarial s.
    Finkelstein test for s.
    florid s.
    focal pigmented villonodular s.
    fungous s.
    hemorrhagic villous s.
    s. hyperplastica
    hypertrophic s.
    inflammatory s.
    lead s.
    localized nodular s. (LNS)
    metatarsophalangeal joint s.
    monarticular s.
    nontraumatic s.
    parapatellar s.
    particulate s.
    pigmented villonodular s. (PVS)
    postoperative s.
    proliferative s.
    puerperal s.
    purulent s.
    reactive s.
    recurrent s.
    rheumatoid arthritis s.
    scarlatinal s.
    serous s.
    s. sicca
    silicone s.
    simple s.
    suppurative s.

NOTES

synovitis *(continued)*
    tendinous s.
    transient s.
    traumatic s.
    tuberculous s.
    vaginal s.
    vibration s.
    villonodular s.
    villous s.
synovitis-acne-pustulosis-hyperostosis osteomyelitis (SAPHO)
synovium, pl. **synovia**
    cartilage s.
    exuberant s.
    opaque s.
    pannus of s.
synpolydactyly
Synthaderm dressing
Synthes
    S. CerviFix system
    S. compression hip screw
    S. dorsal distal radius plate
    S. drill
    S. fixation system
    S. guidepin
    S. ligament washer
    S. Microsystems drill bit
    S. Microsystems plate cutter
    S. Microsystems plate-holding forceps
    S. Microsystems pliers
    S. mini L-plate
    S. pie plate
    S. Schuhli implant system
    S. wire guide
synthesis, pl. **syntheses**
    activity s.
    s. of continuity
    muscle protein s.
    proteoglycan s.
synthetic
    s. augmentation
    s. bone
    s. bone implant
    s. material
    s. prosthesis
    s. stent
    s. testosterone
syphilitic
    s. abscess
    s. amyotrophy
    s. osteochondritis
Syracuse anterior I plate
syringe
    cement s.
    s. grip
    Terumo s.
syringes (*pl. of* syrinx)

syringohydromyelia
syringoma
    chondroid s.
syringometaplasia
syringomyelia
    posttraumatic s.
    secondary posttraumatic s.
syrinx, pl. **syringes**
SysStim 226 muscle stimulator
Systec irrigation
system
    ABG cement-free hip s.
    above-knee suction enhancement s.
    Accu-Cut osteotomy guide s.
    Accu-Flo ultrafiltration s.
    Acculength arthroplasty measuring s.
    Accusway balance measurement s.
    Ace intramedullary femoral nail s.
    ACET s.
    acetabular cup s.
    achilleocalcaneal-plantar s.
    AcroMed VSP fixation s.
    Acryl-X orthopaedic cement removal s.
    Action traction s.
    Acufex microsurgical rear-entry to front-entry femoral guide s.
    AcuFix anterior cervical plate s.
    AcuMatch integrated hip s.
    Acumed great toe s.
    Acuson imaging s.
    Acustar surgical navigation s.
    Acutrak screw s.
    Acutrak small bone fixation s.
    Adjustaback wheelchair backrest s.
    Advance PS total knee s.
    Advantim revision knee s.
    Advantim total knee s.
    Aequalis s.
    Aesculap ABC cervical plating s.
    AGC Biomet total knee s.
    AGC knee replacement s.
    Agee carpal tunnel release s.
    Agee WristJack fracture reduction s.
    Agility total ankle s.
    AIM femoral nail s.
    Air-Back spinal s.
    Aircast Knee S.
    air inflation s.
    Airtrac ambulatory cervical/lumbar traction s.
    Alcon Closure S.
    AlgoMed infusion s.
    Allen shoulder/wrist arthroscopy traction s.
    Alliance rehabilitation s.

S. Alloclassic hip S.
Allofit acetabular cup s.
Allo-Pro hip s.
Alphatec mini lag-screw s.
Alphatec small fragment s.
Alta modular trauma s.
AMBI compression hip screw s.
American Joint Commission on Cancer staging s.'s
American shoulder and elbow s. (ASES)
American Society of Anesthesiologists physical status classification s.
AMK fixed bearing knee s.
AMK total knee s.
AML total hip s.
Amplatz anchor s.
Amset ALPS anterior locking plate s.
Amset R-F fixation s.
Anametric total knee s.
anatomically based exercise s.
anatomic medullary locking hip s.
Anchorlok soft tissue suture anchor s.
Anderson s.
Andersson hip status s.
AnkleTough ankle rehabilitation s.
AnkleTough Rehab S.
Anspach 65K Universal instrument s.
anterior cervical plate fixation s. (ACFS)
anterior Kostuik-Harrington distraction s.
anterior locking plate s. (ALPS)
anterior plate s. (APS)
antimigration s. (AMS)
AOFAS Hallux Rating s.
Apex Universal Drive and Irrigation S.
Apollo DXA bone densitometry s.
Apollo hip s.
Apollo knee prosthesis s.
Apollo total knee s.
APR II hip s.
APR total hip s.
Aqua-Cel heating pad s.
Aquaciser hydrodynamic measurement s.

Aquaciser 100R underwater treadmill s.
Aquanex hydrodynamic measurement s.
AquaSens fluid monitoring s.
Aqua Spray wet nail débridement s.
Ariel computerized exercise s.
Arthrex instruments and s.'s
ArthroCare arthroscopic s.
Arthro-Flo arthroscopic irrigation s.
ArthroProbe laser s.
articular-ligamentous s.
Artisan cement s.
Ascent total knee s.
Ashhurst fracture classification s.
ASIF s.
Asnis 2 guided-screw s.
Assistant Free self-retaining hip surgery retractor s.
Association Research Circulation Osseous classification s.
Atavi atraumatic spine fusion s.
Atlantis cervical plate s.
Atlas cable s.
AuRA cemented total hip s.
autonomic nervous s.
A-V Impulse s.
axial spinal s.
Axiom modular knee s.
Axiom total knee s.
Axis fixation s.
AxyaWeld bone anchor s.
AxyaWeld J-tip suture welding s.
BacFix s.
Back Bull lumbar support s.
Back Revolution S.
Back Trainer spinal exercise s.
Bad Wildungen Metz spine s.
BAK interbody fusion s.
BAK/T thoracic interbody fusion s.
Balance Master training and assessment s.
BAPS Ankle S.
Bassett electrical stimulation s.
Bateman UPF II bipolar knee s.
Batson vertebral brain s.
Becker orthopaedic spinal s. (BOSS)
Becker orthopaedic thermoformable ankle s.

NOTES

system *(continued)*

bilateral variable screw placement s.
Biodex Balance S.
Biodex Unweighing Support S.
Biodynamic Molding S.
Biofix absorbable fixation s.
Bio Flote air flotation s.
Biomechanical Ankle Platform S. (BAPS)
Biomet M2A metal-on-metal hip articulation s.
Biomet Maxim knee s.
Biomet revision knee s.
Biomet Ultra-Drive ultrasonic revision s.
Bio-Modular total shoulder s.
Bionicare 1000 stimulator s.
bioresorbable drug delivery s.
Biosensor biomechanical testing s.
Blajwas-Schwartz-Marcinko irrigation drainage s.
BMP cabling and plating s.
body logic rehabilitation s.
Body Masters MD 510 hi-lo pulley s.
Body Response s.
Bolin wedge filter s.
bone density and arthritis testing s.
bone staple s.
Boston Classification S.
Boston elbow s.
Bottoms-Up posture s.
Bowden cable suspension s.
Boyer degenerative joint disease grading s.
Bremer halo s.
Bridge Hip s.
Brighton electrical stimulation s.
Browlift bone bridge s.
Buechel-Pappas total ankle replacement s.
Cable-Ready cable grip s.
cable suspension s.
Calandruccio external fixation s.
California soft spinal s. (CASS)
cannula s.
cannulated guided hip screw s.
Cannulated Plus screw s.
CAPIS bone plate s.
capsuloligamentous s.
Carbon Monotube long bone fracture external fixation s.
Cascade Up and About s.
CC Rider closed-chain rehabilitation s.
central nervous s. (CNS)
Ceraver Osteal knee replacement s.

Cervifix s.
Charnley Howorth Exflow s.
Charnley-Merle D'Aubigné disability grading s.
Charnley total hip s.
Chiba spinal s.
C-2 hip s.
Chirotech x-ray s.
Cincinnati Knee Rating S.
CircPlus bandage/wrap s.
Circul'Air shoe process s.
Circulator boot s.
CKS knee s.
Clanton turf toe grading s.
closed drainage s.
CLS hip s.
Coblation spinal surgery s.
Codman ACP s.
Codman anterior cervical plating s.
Codman Ti-frame posterior fixation s.
Cofield total shoulder s.
Cohort anterior plate s.
Combi Multi-Traction S.
combined magnetic field s.
ComfortWalk foot s.
Command hip instrumentation s.
Command joint replacement instrument s.
Compass stereotactic s.
compliant prestress s. (CPS)
Concept arthroscopy power s.
Concept beach chair shoulder positioning s.
Concept Precise ACL guide s.
Concept rotator cuff repair s.
Concept self-compressing cannulated screw s.
Concept Sterling arthroscopy blade s.
Concise compression hip screw s.
concurrent force s.
Conserve hip s.
Constant and Murley shoulder scoring s.
ConstaVac autoreinfusion s.
contact laser delivery s.
Contact SPH cups s.
Continuum knee s. (CKS)
Coombs bone biopsy s.
Coordinate complete revision knee s.
coordinate s. X,Y,Z
Corail hip s.
Corin hip arthroplasty s.
Corkscrew rotator cuff repair s.
Counter Rotation S. (CRS)
CPT hip s.

CRM s.
Crowe congenital hip dysplasia classification s.
CRS Tibial Torsion S.
cruciate condylar knee s.
Cryo/Cuff Knee Compression Dressing S.
C-Tek anterior cervical plate s.
curved Küntscher nail s.
Cybex I, II+ exercise s.
Cybex 340 isokinetic rehabilitation and testing s.
Cybex training s.
Dallas grading s.
Dall-Miles cable/crimp cerclage s.
Dall-Miles cable grip s.
DataHand s.
D'Aubigne hip status s.
deep bonding s. (DBS)
Deknatel orthopedic autotransfusion s.
Diab-A-Foot protection s.
Digital Biofeedback S.
Dimension hip s.
double-cannula s.
double inflow cannula s.
DTT s.
dual-lock total hip replacement s.
Dual Range Limiter S.
Dupont distal humeral plate s.
Duraloc acetabular cup s.
Durasul head s.
Dwyer-Wickham electrical stimulation s.
DynaFix external fixation s.
DynaFlex multilayer compression s.
Dyna-Lok pedicle screw s.
Dyna-Lok plating s.
dynamic stabilizing innersole s. (DSIS)
Dynasplint shoulder s.
EBI Medical Systems bone healing s.
EBI Medical Systems Orthofix fixation s.
ECT internal fracture fixation s.
EDG s.
Edintrak s.
Edwards modular s.
ElastaTrac home lumbar traction s.
Electri-Cool cold therapy s.
electrotherapy s. (ES)

Elite hip s.
Emerald implantation s.
EMG biofeedback s.
Endius endoscopic access s.
Endolite transtibial s.
Endoprothetik CSL-Plus cemented-hip s.
Endoprothetik CS-Plus cemented-hip s.
endoscopic carpal tunnel release s.
endoskeletal alignment s. (EAS)
Endotrac blade s.
Endotrac carpal tunnel release s.
EPIC functional evaluation s.
E-Series hip s.
ESKA modular hip s.
Estraderm estradiol transdermal s.
Evans fracture classification s.
Ewald elbow arthroplasty rating s.
Exact-Fit ATH hip replacement s.
EXAKT-MicroGrinding S.
EX-FI-RE external fixation s.
Exogen 2000 sonic accelerated fracture healing s.
Extend total hip s.
facet screw s.
Facial Grading S. (FGS)
facilitated spinal s.
FASTak suture anchor s.
FAST 1 intraosseous infusion s.
felt apron Bowden cable suspension s.
Fenlin total shoulder s.
Fernandez point-score wrist assessment s.
Fernandez scale posttraumatic wrist assessment s.
Ferno AquaCiser underwater treadmill s.
Ficat-Marcus grading s.
Fillauer endoskeletal alignment s.
Fillauer modular shuttle lock s.
filtration s.
FIN s.
Finn knee s.
Fitnet joint testing s.
Fixateur Interne fixation s.
FlexiTherm Thermographic S.
Flowtron pneumatic compression system BioCryo s.
Foamart foot impression s.
Foot-Station 3-D foot imaging s.

NOTES

system *(continued)*

Foundation total knee and hip s.
four-in-one positioning block s.
Fowler knee s.
FP5000 pump s.
Freehand prosthesis s.
Freeman-Swanson knee s.
F-Scan foot force and gait
  analysis s.
F-Scan in-shoe s.
F-Scan pressure measurement s.
fusimotor s.
GDLH posterior spinal s.
GD Regainer S.
Gem total knee s.
Genesis II foot s.
Genesis II foot/ankle s.
Genesis II total knee s.
genital s.
Genucom ACL laxity analysis s.
Genucom knee flexion analysis s.
Geomedic s.
Gillette double-flexure ankle
  joint s.
Glider II patient transfer s.
Global Fx shoulder fracture s.
Global total shoulder arthroplasty s.
Golden mean testing s.
Golf Exercise S.
Gonstead pelvic marking s.
Graf stabilization s.
Granberg cervical traction s.
gravity extension locking s.
  (GELS)
Gray revision instrument s.
Green-O'Brien evaluation s.
GTS two-piece implant s.
Guardian limb salvage s.
Guldmann Overhead Trac S.
Haid UBP s.
Hajdu staging s.
Hall mandibular implant s.
Hall modular acetabular reamer s.
halo cervical traction s.
Hannover scoring s.
Harrington rod and hook s.
Harris hip status s.
Hausmann Work-Well work
  hardening s.
haversian s.
HCMI Chiropractic S.
Herbert bone screw s.
Heritage hip s.
Hermes Evolution tricompartmental
  knee s.
Hermes total knee s.
Hexcel total condylar knee s.
hipGRIP pelvic positioning s.

Hipokrat bimodular shoulder s.
Histofreezer cryosurgical s.
HJD total hip s.
Hoek-Bowen cement removal s.
Hoffmann external fixation s.
hook probe s.
Howmedica knee s.
Howmedica total ankle s.
Howmedica VSF fixation s.
HybridFit total hip s.
HybridFit total knee s.
hydraulic test s.
HydroFlex arthroscopy irrigating s.
HydroTrack underwater treadmill s.
Hypobaric transfemoral s.
Hypobaric transtibial s.
ICRS arthroscopic staging s.
Ilizarov limb-lengthening s.
immune s.
Impact modular total hip s.
Impingement-Free Tibial Guide S.
Index Chemicus Registry S. (ICRS)
Indiana tome carpal tunnel
  syndrome release s.
In-Fast bone screw s.
Infinity hip s.
InFix interbody fusion s.
Inglis-Pellicci elbow arthroplasty
  rating s.
Innomed arthroplasty measuring s.
Innovative COR/T implant s.
Insall-Burstein II modular total
  knee s.
Insight knee positioning and
  alignment s.
instrumentation s.
In-Tac bone-anchoring s.
Integral hip s.
integrated shape and imaging s.
  (ISIS)
InteliJet fluid management s.
Inteq small joint suturing s.
Interax total knee s.
Intermedics natural hip s.
internal fixation plate-screw s.
International 10-20 s.
International Listing S.
Iowa hip status rating s.
ipos arch support s.
IPS total hip s.
irrigation s.
Isola fixation s.
Isola spinal instrumentation s.
Itrel II, III spinal cord
  stimulation s.
Jacobson s.
joint activated s. (JAS)
Judet hip status s.

Jurgan pin ball s.
J-Vac closed drainage s.
Kaltenborn joint mobilization s.
Kaneda anterior spinal/scoliosis s.
  (KASS)
Kellgren-Lawrence grading s.
Kendall A-V impulse s.
K-Fix Fixator s.
Kinamed Exact-Fit ATH s.
Kin-Con isokinetic exercise s.
Kinematic II condylar and
  stabilizer total knee s.
Kinematic II rotating hinge knee s.
Kinemax modular condylar and
  stabilizer total knee s.
Kinemax Plus total knee s.
Kinemetric guide s.
Kinetik great toe implant s.
Kirschner II-C shoulder s.
Kirschner integrated shoulder s.
knee signature s.
Kofoed scoring s.
Kostuik-Harrington distraction s.
Kurtzke Functional s.
Kyle fracture classification s.
Langenskiöld grading s.
Larson hip status s.
LCR s.
LCS mobile bearing knee s.
LCS total knee s.
Leibinger Profyle hand s.
Liberty spinal s.
Lido Active Multijoint S.
Lidoback isokinetic dynamometry s.
Lido Passive Multijoint S.
Lifeline Wall Gym 2000 fitness s.
Linear total hip s.
Link custom partial pelvis
  replacement s.
Link Endo-Model rotational knee s.
Link Lubinus SP II hip
  replacement s.
Link Saddle Prosthesis Endo-Model
  hip replacement s.
locomotor s.
Lone Star retractor s.
Lordex lumbar spine s.
Lorenz osteosynthesis s.
Lubinus AP hip s.
Lubinus SP II anatomically adapted
  hip s.
Luhr fixation s.

Lumbo 90 home care traction s.
lumbosacral cartilaginous s.
Luque II fixation s.
Lynco biomechanical orthotic s.
Mackinnon-Dellon staging s.
Madajet XL jet-injection
  anesthesia s.
Magerl hook-plate s.
Magerl plate-screw s.
Magna-FX cannulated screw s.
Malcolm-Lynn radiolucent spinal
  retraction s.
Malcolm-Rand radiolucent headrest
  and retraction s.
Mallory-Head modular calcar s.
Maramed Miami fracture brace s.
Mark III halo s.
Mark II Sorrells hip arthroplasty
  retractor s.
Mason fracture classification s.
matrix seating s.
Mattrix spinal cord stimulation s.
Maxim Modular Knee S.
Mayo Clinic hip scoring s.
McCain TMJ arthroscopic s.
Medical Examination and
  Diagnostic Coding S. (MEDICS)
Medical Research Council s.
Medtronic spinal cord
  stimulation s.
Meniscus Mender II s.
Metasul metal-on-metal hip
  prosthesis s.
MG II total knee s.
Microloc knee s.
Micro-Mill knee instrument s.
MicroPhor iontophoretic drug
  delivery s.
Midas Rex instrumentation s.
Miller-Galante I condylar total
  knee s.
Miller-Galante revision knee s.
Miller-Galante total knee s.
Minaar classification s.
Mini-Acutrak small bone fixation s.
Mini-Flap drain s.
mini lag screw s. (MLS)
Mirage Spinal S.
Mitek anchor s.
Mitek GII suture anchor s.
Mitek VAPR tissue removal s.
modified Wagner classification s.

NOTES

S

system *(continued)*

Modular Acetabular Revision S. (MARS)
modular Lenbach hip s.
modular S-ROM total hip s.
MOD unicompartmental knee s.
Moe s.
Monotube external fixator s.
Monticelli-Spinelli circular external fixation s.
Moore hip endoprosthesis s.
Morrey elbow arthroplasty rating s.
MosaicPlasty s.
Moss fixation s.
motorized shaving s.
Mouradian humeral fixation s.
MRI-compatible plate and screw s.
Multi Balance S. (MBS)
Multidex chronic wound treatment s.
Multi Podus boot s.
Multi Podus foot s.
Multitak SS s.
Multitak suture snap s.
musculotendinous s.
Musgrave Footprint S.
M3-X fixation s.
Myobock s.
Natural-Hip s.
Natural-Knee II s.
Navitrack computer-assisted surgery s.
Neer II shoulder s.
Neer II total knee s.
Neff femorotibial nail s.
Newport hip s.
NexGen complete knee s.
Nexus wheelchair seating s.
NoHands Mouse-Foot-Operated Computer Mouse S.
– NordiCare Back Therapy S.
Norm testing and rehabilitation s.
Nucleotome s.
OEC Mini 6600 imaging s.
Ogden fracture classification s.
Ogden plate s.
Ogden tissue reattachment mini s.
Oklahoma cable s.
Olerud pedicle fixation s.
Olerud PSF fixation s.
Omega compression hip screw s.
Omega Plus compression hip s.
Omnifit Plus hip s.
Omnifit total knee s.
open double-decked hook cervical s.
Optetrak comprehensive knee s.
Optetrak total knee replacement s.

Opti-Fix total hip s.
Option hip s.
optoelectric measuring s.
Optotrak motion measurement s.
Orth-evac autotransfusion s.
Orthodoc presurgical planning s.
Ortho-evac postoperative transfusion s.
Ortholoc Advantim revision knee s.
Ortholoc Advantim total knee s.
Orthomerica TC AFO s.
Orthomet Axiom total knee s.
Orthomet Perfecta total hip s.
OrthoPak bone growth stimulator s.
Orthotec pressurized fluid irrigation s.
Osada portable handpiece s.
OSCAR ultrasonic bone cement removal s.
OSI modular table s.
osteochondral autograft transfer s. (OATS)
Osteo-Clage Cable S.
Osteonics Scorpio posterior cruciate retaining total knee s.
Osteopower modular handpiece s.
OsteoView 2000 imaging s.
Palmer-Gonstead-Firth listing s.
Panoview arthroscopic s.
ParaMax ACL guide s.
parasympathetic nervous s. (PNS)
Partnership s.
PCA primary total knee s.
PCA Universal total knee instrument s.
Peak anterior compression plate s.
Peak Fixation S.
Peak Motus Motion Measurement S.
PEC modular total knee s.
PEC total hip s.
Pedar-in-shoe measurement s.
Pedar pressure insole s.
Pedar pressure measurement s.
pediatric s.
pedicle screw s.
Perfecta Interseal total hip s.
PerFixation s.
Performance modular total knee s.
Performance unicompartmental knee s.
peripheral nervous s. (PNS)
peripheral vascular s. (PVS)
PFC modular total knee s.
PFC Sigma knee s.
PFC TC3 modular knee s.
PFC total hip replacement s.
PGP flexible nail s.

Phoenix foot s.
Phoresor II iontophoretic drug delivery s.
Phoresor PM900 iontophoresis s.
pin ball s.
Pinch Gauge and Jackson Strength Evaluation S.
Pinnacle acetabular cup s.
Pinn-ACL guide s.
Pinn anterior cruciate ligament guide s.
Pinwheel S.
Pipkin fracture classification s.
PlastiCast adjustable joint cast s.
plate-screw s.
PlexiPulse DVT prophylaxis s.
PMT halo s.
Podospray nail drill s.
Polarus Plus humeral fixation s.
Polarus positional humeral fixation s.
Polycentric and Wide-Track knee s.
Postel hip status s.
posterior cruciate condylar knee s.
posterior rod s.
Powerbelt exercise s.
PPT insole s.
PPT soft tissue orthotic s.
Precision Osteolock femoral component s.
Precision Strata hip s.
press-fit total condylar knee s.
pressure transducer-monitor s.
pretarget filtration s.
Profile total hip s.
Profix total knee replacement s.
Profore Four-Layer bandage s.
programmable VariGrip II prosthetic control s.
Protector meniscus suturing s.
ProTrac cruciate reconstruction s.
Providence Scoliosis S.
Provisional Fixation TC-100 plating s.
Proxiderm wound closure s.
Pulsavac III wound débridement s.
Pump It Up pneumatic socket volume management s.
Puno-Winter-Byrd s.
PWB transpedicular spine fixation s.
Pylon intramedullary nail s.

Quick-Sil silicone s.
QuickTack periosteal fixation s.
radiolucent wrist fixation s.
Rancho Cube S.
rearfoot stability s. (RSS)
Reebok Slide S.
Reebok Step S.
Reese osteotomy guide s.
ReFlexion first MPJ implant s.
Replica total hip replacement s.
Restoration acetabular s.
Restoration-HA hip s.
Restore ACL guide s.
reticuloendothelial s.
ReUnite resorbable orthopedic fixation s.
Revelation hip s.
Revo rotator cuff repair s.
rHead implant s.
Richards fixator s.
Richards hip endoprosthesis s.
Richards modular hip s.
Richards Solcotrans orthopedic drainage-reinfusion s.
right-handed orthogonal coordinate s. (RHOCS)
Riseborough-Radin fracture classification s.
Rochester compression s.
Rod TAG suture anchor s.
Roger Anderson s.
Rogozinski screw s.
Rogozinski spinal fixation s.
Rogozinski spinal rod s.
ROHO pediatric seating s.
Rolyan Reach N Range Pulley S.
Romano curved drilling s.
Rotaglide total knee s.
Russell-Taylor femoral interlocking nail s.
Sabolich above-knee socket s.
Savastano Hemi-Knee s.
Scaphoid-Microstaple s.
Schwartz-Blajwas-Marcinko irrigation s.
Scorpio total knee s.
Scotchcast length splinting s.
Secure Yet Gentle surgical dressing s.
segmental spinal correction s. (SSCS)

NOTES

system *(continued)*

segmented orthopedic system total hip and knee s.
Selby I, II fixation s.
Select shoulder s.
Shadow-Line ACF spine retractor s.
SharpShooter tissue repair s.
shaving s.
Sherman remote podiatric vacuum s.
shoulder arm s. (SAS)
Shuttle MiniClinic resistance s.
Silhouette spinal s.
Simmons plating s.
Simmons and Segil classification s.
single-cannula s.
skeletal repair s. (SRS)
slotted obturator-cannula s.
Smith & Nephew bracing and support s.
Socon spinal s.
SOCS AFO s.
SOCS pad s.
Sofflex mattress s.
Sofwire cable s.
Solcotrans autotransfusion s.
Solcotrans orthopedic drainage-refusion s.
Soma Gonio s.
Soma pulley s.
sonic-accelerated fracture-healing s. (SAFHS)
Sorbie-Questor total elbow prosthesis s.
Sorrells hip arthroplasty retractor s.
SOS total hip s.
SOS total knee s.
Souter Strathclyde total elbow s.
Spectron EF total hip s.
Spectrum tissue repair s.
spherocentric knee s.
spinopelvic transiliac fixation s.
Spinoscope noninvasive imaging s.
SportCord exercise and rehabilitation s.
Square Module Seating S.
S-ROM hip replacement s.
S-ROM modular total knee s.
S-ROM proximally modular total hip s.
Stability total hip s.
Stableloc external wrist fixation s.
Stableloc II external fixation s.
Stahl staging s.
StairMaster exercise s.
Statak anchor s.
Stealth image-guided s.

Steffee pedicle screw-plate s.
Steffee variable spine plating s.
STIF s.
Stockholm hand arm vibration syndrome staging s.
Strata hip s.
Stretch-Rite exerciser s.
Stromqvist hook pin s.
Stryker Intracompartmental Pressure Monitor S.
Stryker SE3 drive s.
suction-irrigation s.
supine C-Trax traction s.
SureClosure skin stretching s.
SureStep ankle support s.
suture s. (SS)
SwimEx hydrotherapy s.
sympathetic nervous s. (SNS)
Synaptic 2000 pain management s.
Synergy spine rehab s.
Synergy Therapeutic S.
Synthes CerviFix s.
Synthes fixation s.
Synthes Schuhli implant s.
System Alloclassic hip s.
TAG anchor s.
Tamarack flexure joint s.
TEC interface s.
S.'s 2000 TENS unit
The Healthy Back S.
Thera-Band resistive therapy s.
Therabath paraffin heat therapy s.
Thera-Ciser light exercise s.
Thera-Ciser therapeutic exercise s.
Thera-Wedge s.
Thompson hip endoprosthesis s.
Thompson leg check s.
THORP s.
three-point pressure s.
tibia coordinate s.
tibial torsion s.
Ti-Fit total hip s.
titanium hollow screw plate s.
top-loading screw and rod s.
Torus external fixation s.
Total Condylar Knee s.
Total Gym rehabilitation s.
Townley anatomic knee s.
TransFix ACL s.
triangle blade s.
Triax monotube external fixation s.
Trilogy acetabular cup s.
Tri-Motion Knee S.
triple envelope s.
Tri-Wedge total hip s.
True/Fit femoral intramedullary rod s.
True/Flex intramedullary rod s.

True-Lok external fixator s.
Trunkey fracture classification s.
TSRH crosslink s.
TSRH fixation s.
TSRH spinal implant s.
TSRH Universal spinal
  instrumentation s.
TurnAide therapeutic s.
Turning Board Exercise S.
Tylok high-tension cable s.
UBP s.
UCO Quick-Sil silicone s.
UE Tech Weight Well Exercise S.
Ulson fixator s.
Ultima hip replacement s.
Ultima total hip s.
Ultimax distal femoral
  intramedullary rod s.
Ultra-Drive bone cement
  removal s.
Ultra-Drive ultrasonic revision s.
UltraFix RC suture anchor s.
Ultra-Guard FS hip bracing s.
Ultra-Guard hip orthosis s.
UltraPower drill s.
Ultra-X external fixation s.
unicompartmental knee s.
Unicondylar Geomedic hemi-knee s.
Uniflex nailing s.
unilateral variable screw
  placement s.
Uniportal fascial release s.
Universal bone plate s.
Universal Spine S. (USS)
Up and About s.
variable axis knee s.
variable screw placement s.
Vector low back analysis s.
Vermont pedicle fixation s.
Versaback back s.
Versa-Fx femoral hip fixation s.
Versalok low back fixation s.
Versa-Trac lumbar spine
  retractor s.
VerSys hip s.
VertAlign spinal support s.
Vertetrac ambulatory traction s.
Vicon three-dimensional gait
  analysis s.

Vilex cannulated screw s.
VSF fixation s.
VSP s.
Wagner revision hip s.
WalkAide s.
WarmTouch patient warming s.
Warm-Up active wound therapy s.
Wedge TAG suture anchor s.
West Point Ankle Grading S.
Wiltse pedicle screw fixation s.
Wisconsin spinal fracture s.
Wit portable TENS s.
Wrightlock posterior fixation s.
Wrightlock spinal fixation s.
WrisTimer carpal tunnel support s.
Xact ACL graft-fixation s.
Xia hook s.
Xia spinal s.
X-Y sensor s.
Y-knot tying s.
ZAAG Bone Anchoring S.
Zenith Electrotherapy ultrasound s.
Zephir anterior cervical plate s.
Zest Anchor Advanced Generation
  bone anchoring s.
Zest Anchor Advanced Generation
  Bone Anchoring S.
Zickel fracture classification s.
Zimmer anatomic hip s.
Zimmer collarless polished taper
  hip s.
Zimmer crossover instrumentation s.
Zimmer-Hall drive s.
Zimmer hip implant s.
Zimmer Pulsavac wound
  débridement s.
Zimmer THARIES surface
  arthroplasty s.
ZMR hip s.
ZMS intramedullary fixation s.
Zone Specific II meniscal repair s.
Zuni exercise s.
Zweymuller hip s.

systemic
  s. lupus erythematosus (SLE)
  s. sclerosis
systolic blood pressure
systremma

NOTES

T

T buttress plate
T condylar fracture
T fracture
T handle elevator

T28

Trapezoidal-28
T28 hip prosthesis

TA

TA metallic staple
TA Premium 30, 55, 90 staple

TAA

total ankle arthroplasty

tabes dorsalis

tabetic

t. arthropathy
t. foot
t. gait
t. osteoarthropathy

Tab Grabber

table

Adapta physical therapy t.
adjusting t.
Advocate electric flexion
  distraction t.
Air-Drop chiropractic t.
Air-Flex chiropractic t.
Albee-Compere fracture t.
Albee orthopaedic t.
Allen hand/arm surgery t.
AlphaStar t.
American Chiropractic College of
  Radiology adjusting t.
AM-MI orthopaedic t.
Anatomotor traction/massage t.
Andrews SST-3000 spinal
  surgery t.
Apollo TM electric flexion t.
APS Hi-Lo electric lift t.
ATT-300 LAT traction t.
Back Specialist chiropractic t.
Back Specialist electric t.
Back Specialist manual t.
Bell t.
Berstein cast t.
cast t.
Chick CLT operating t.
Chick fracture t.
Chick-Langren orthopedic t.
Chiro-Manis chiropractic t.
circumductor t.
Cobb attachment for Albee-
  Compere fracture t.
craniosacral t.
crank t.

Crystal adjusting t.
cutout t.
DC-101 chiropractic t.
DDP t.
DePuy graft preparation t.
Diamond biomechanical t.
Ergo style flexion t.
Eurotech Diamond t.
Eurotech Emerald t.
Eurotech Platinum t.
Eurotech Sapphire t.
EZ-Up inversion t.
flexion-distraction chiropractic t.
fluoroscopic t.
fracture t.
friction-reduced examination t.
friction-reduced segmented t.
Galaxy 900HS adjusting t.
Galaxy McManis hylo t.
Gemini chiropractic t.
Green-Anderson growth t.
Hercules TM drop-adjusting t.
HESSCO 300, 500 series
  hydrotherapy t.
Hill Air-Drop HA90C t.
hi-lo t.
HLT-405 instrument adjusting t.
horseshoe therapy t.
hydromassage t.
inner t.
intersegmental traction
  chiropractic t.
Jackson spinal surgery and
  imaging t.
knavel t.
knee-chest t.
Leander chiropractic t.
Leander motorized flexion t.
Legend Hy-Lo adjusting t.
Legend stationary adjusting t.
Lloyd chiropractic t.
long axis traction chiropractic t.
Magnum 101 Plus t.
Marquet fracture t.
Massage Time Pro hydromassage t.
mat t.
McKenzie Repex t.
Med-Fit cranial-sacral t.
Meridian Intersegmental t.
Midland tilt t.
Multi-Lock hand operating t.
orthopaedic t.
over-bed t.
Paris manual therapy t.
passive traction t.

T

table *(continued)*
    PET/Eurotech Generation 2000 t.
    physical therapy t.
    Platinum stationary t.
    Powermatic t.
    Protege manual flexion
      distraction t.
    PT tilt t.
    Rath treatment t.
    Re-Lax-O chiropractic t.
    resistive exercise t.
    Roger Anderson t.
    Sapphire t.
    t. short leg
    Side Kick I, II t.
    Sieman t.
    Skytron operating room t.
    slatted plinth t.
    slot t.
    Stryker surgical hand t.
    Telos fracture t.
    t. tie
    tilt t.
    Titan Apollo electric flexion t.
    Titan Meridian Intersegmental
      Traction t.
    Titan Nova manual flexion-
      extension multi flex t.
    Topaz manual flexion t.
    Tri W-G t.
    TX-1, TX-7 traction t.
    VAX-D therapy t.
    Verteflex Intersegmental Traction T.
    Williams Advantage t.
    Williams Model 170 t.
    Winco Folding Treatment T.
    Zenith ACS t.
    Zenith chiropractic t.
    Zenith-Cox flexion/distraction t.
    Zenith Hylos t.
    Zenith stationary t.
    Zenith Thompson t.
    Zenith Verti-Lift t.
    Zodiac TM Manual Flexion-
      Distraction t.
tablet
    bonemeal t.
tabletop Stone staple
taboparesis
TABS Elite mobility monitor
Tab-Strap knee immobilizer
Tachdjian
    T. classification
    T. fractional lengthening
    T. hamstring lengthening
    T. orthosis
    T. pin
    T. procedure

Tacit threaded anchor
TACK
    Translating and Congruent Mobile-
      Bearing Knee
      TACK implant
tack
    Bankart t.
    biodegradable surgical t.
    t. breakage
    membrane t.
tack-and-pin forceps
tackle
    spear t.
tackler's
    t. arm
    t. exostosis
Tacoma sacral plate
Tacticon
    T. peripheral neuropathy kit
    T. peripheral neuropathy screening
      device
    T. quantitative sensory testing
tactile anesthesia
Tae Bo
taenia
    lip of t.
TAG
    tissue anchor guide
      TAG anchor system
tag
    skin t.
    synovial t.
tai
    t. chi
    T. Chi Chuan exercise
tailbone
tailor's
    t. ankle
    t. bunion
    t. bunionectomy
    t. bunionette
Tait
    T. flap
    T. graft
Tajima
    T. metacarpal lengthening
    T. method
    T. modified Kessler suture
    T. suture technique
Takahashi forceps
Takakura index
Take-apart forceps
TakeOff elbow support
Take-Out Extractor
TAL
    tendo Achillis lengthening
talalgia

talar
- t. avulsion fracture
- t. axis–first metatarsal base angle (TAMBA)
- t. beak
- t. beaking
- t. body
- t. body fusion
- t. body nonunion
- t. canal
- t. declination angle
- t. dislocation
- t. dome
- t. head
- t. malunion
- t. neck
- t. neck class I–III injury
- t. neck exostosis
- t. neck fracture
- t. neck osteotomy
- t. neck tunnel
- t. osteochondral fracture
- t. process
- t. ridge
- t. shift
- t. sinus
- t. subluxation
- t. sulcus
- t. tilt (TT)
- t. triple arthrodesis

talar-tilt angle

talectomy
- Trumble t.

Talesnick scapholunate repair

talipes
- t. calcaneocavus
- t. calcaneovalgus
- t. calcaneovarus
- t. calcaneus
- t. cavovalgus
- t. cavovarus
- t. cavus
- t. cavus deformity
- t. convex pes valgus
- t. equinovalgus
- t. equinovarus (TEV)
- t. equinus
- flexible t.
- t. planovalgus
- t. planus
- t. tendinoplasty

- t. transversoplanus
- t. varus

Tall-ette toilet seat

Talma disease

talocalcaneal
- t. angle
- t. coalition
- t. fusion
- t. index
- t. index classification
- t. joint
- t. ligament
- t. ligament disruption
- t. osteotomy

talocalcaneonavicular
- t. complex
- t. joint
- t. ligament articulation

talocrural
- t. alignment
- t. angle
- t. fusion
- t. joint
- t. sprain

talocruralis

talofibular
- t. articulation
- t. joint
- t. ligament

talometatarsal angle

talonavicular (TN)
- t. angle
- t. arthrodesis
- t. articulation
- t. bone
- t. capsule
- t. capsulotomy
- t. dislocation
- t. fusion
- t. joint
- t. ligament
- t. ossicle of Pirie
- t. sprain

talotibial exostosis

talus
- beaking of head of t.
- t. body fracture
- congenital vertical t. (CVT)
- flattop t.
- t. foot deformity
- t. lateral posterior process
- t. lateral tubercle

NOTES

T

talus (*continued*)
  osteochondral fracture of the dome of the t.
  sulcus of t.
  Tricodur T. compression dressing
  truncated wedge tarsometatarsal arthrodesis vertical t.
  valgus tilt of the t.
  vertical t.
TAM
  total active motion
Tamae harvesting
Tamarack
  T. flexure joint
  T. flexure joint system
TAMBA
  talar axis–first metatarsal base angle
TAMMAS
  temporary articulating methylmethacrylate antibiotic spacer
tamp
  bone t.
  Kiene bone t.
  tension band wire t.
tandem
  t. connector
  t. gait
  t. gait test
tangential
  t. hand
  t. incision
  t. layer
  t. standing radiograph
  t. x-ray view
Tang retractor
Tanita Professional Body Composition Analyzer
tank
  Hubbard t. (HT)
  Hubbard physical therapy t.
  therapy t.
Tanner developmental model
Tanner-Whitehouse bone-age reference value
tantalum-ball marker
tantalum mesh
tap
  AO t.
  t. drill
  dynamic condylar screw t.
  screw t.
  Screw-Lok t.
  synovial t.
tape
  anthropometric measuring t.
  benzoin adherent t.
  bias-cut t.
  cast t.

Delta-Lite casting t.
DynaSport athletic t.
Elastikon elastic t.
Expandover athletic t.
foam t.
graded Gore-Tex t.
Gulick II t.
Lightplast athletic t.
MaxCast casting t.
Medipore H surgical t.
Mersilene t.
moleskin traction t.
Powerflex t.
Scotchcast 2 cast t.
skin t.
t. traction
TufStuf II cast t.
Ultra-Light athletic t.
umbilical t.
Zonas porous t.
taper
  collarless polished t.
  t. cut needle
  Eurotaper 12/14 t.
  Morse t.
tapered
  collarless, polished, t. (CPT)
  t. hand reamer
  t. pin
  t. reamer
tapering dose steroid
taper-jaw forceps
Taperloc
  T. femoral component
  T. femoral prosthesis
  T. femoral stem
taping
  basket-weave ankle t.
  buddy t.
  figure-of-eight t.
  Gibney t.
  LowDye t.
  patellar t.
  plantar fasciitis t.
  prophylactic t.
  t. technique
tapir
  bouche de t.
tapotement
tapping test of arm disability
TAR
  thrombocytopenia-absent radius
  total ankle replacement
  TAR syndrome
TARA
  total articular replacement arthroplasty
  total articular resurfacing arthroplasty
  TARA total hip prosthesis

Taratynov disease
tarda
    osteogenesis imperfecta t. (OIT)
Tardieu spasticity measurement scale
tardy ulnar palsy
targeter
    bone screw t.
    IMP bone screw t.
targeting
    t. bead
    distal t.
    t. drill guide
Target prosthesis
tarsal
    t. amputation
    t. arthrodesis
    t. bar
    t. bone
    t. bone fracture
    t. bridge
    t. canal
    t. canal artery
    t. coalition
    t. dislocation
    t. joint
    t. joint infection
    t. medullostomy
    t. navicular
    t. navicular bursitis
    t. plate
    t. pronator shoe
    t. sinus
    t. sinus artery
    t. tunnel
    t. tunnel release (TTR)
    t. tunnel syndrome (TTS)
    t. wedge osteotomy
tarsalgia
tarsectomy
tarsectopia
tarsi (*pl. of* tarsus)
tarsitis
tarsoclasia
tarsoepiphysial aclasis
tarsometatarsal (TMT)
    t. amputation
    t. angle
    t. articulation
    t. dislocation
    t. fracture-dislocation
    t. joint
    t. joint injury

    t. junction
    t. ligament
    t. osteoarthritis
    t. truncated-wedge arthrodesis
tarsophalangeal reflex
tarsotibial amputation
tarsotomy
tarsus, pl. **tarsi**
    ligament of t.
    ossa tarsi
    sinus tarsi
tartrate
    t. resistant acid phosphatase (TRAP)
task
    T. Force on Standards of Physical Therapy
    metabolic equivalent of t. (MET)
    walking t.
Tauranga splint
taut
    t. band
    t. foot
Tavernetti-Tennant knee prosthesis
Taylor
    T. apparatus
    T. back brace
    T. clavicle support
    T. percussion hammer
    T. procedure
    T. retractor
    T. spinal frame
    T. spinal retractor blade
    T. spine brace
    T. splint
    T. technique
    T. thoracolumbosacral orthosis
Taylor-Daniel-Weiland technique
Taylor-Knight brace
Taylor-Townsend-Corlett iliac crest bone graft
T-Bar
    T-B. guide
    T-B. trigger-point massager
TBI
    traumatic brain injury
TCA
    transcondylar axis
TCAT
    Toglia Category Assessment Test
TCC
    total contact casting

NOTES

TCCK unconstrained knee prosthesis
TCFO
Therapy Carrot Finger Orthosis
TCFO placement wand
TC-III
total condylar III
TCL
tibial collateral ligament
T-clamp
Pratt T-c.
Presbyterian Hospital T-c.
Tc-99m
technetium-99m
TCO
total contact orthosis
TCP-III
total condylar prosthesis III
TCP III
total condylar III
TD
temperature differential
terminal device
tea-and-toast diet
teacup fracture
Teale amputation
team
donor t.
recipient t.
tear
anterior horn meniscal t.
anterior oblique meniscal t.
bowstring t.
bucket-handle t.
cleavage t.
complex meniscal t.
degenerative t.
deltoid ligament t.
flap meniscal t.
full-thickness cuff t.
horizontal meniscal t.
horse-tail Achilles tendon t.
iatrogenic dural t.
incomplete t.
interstitial meniscal t.
intraoperative dural t.
Johnson-Jahss classification of
posterior tibial tendon t.
labral t.
lateral t.
longitudinal displaced complete t.
longitudinal incomplete
intrameniscal t.
longitudinal meniscal t.
longitudinal split t.
L-shaped rotator cuff t.
meniscal lateral t.
meniscal radial t.
meniscal transverse t.

meniscocapsular t.
midsubstance t.
mop-end Achilles tendon t.
mop-end mid-substance t.
Neer acromioplasty for rotator
cuff t.
oblique meniscal t.
parrot-beak t.
posterior cruciate ligament t.
posterior horn meniscal t.
posterior oblique meniscal t.
radial meniscal t.
rotator cuff t.
TFC t.
through-and-through t.
transverse t.
triangular fibrocartilage complex t.
vertical longitudinal t.
V-shaped rotator cuff t.
teardrop
t. fracture
t. line
**teardrop-shaped flexion-compression
fracture**
Teare
T. arm splint
T. sling
tearing sound
teaspoon
nylon t.
TEC
Total Environment Control
TEC interface system
TEC liner
Techmedica implant
technetium
technetium-99m (Tc-99m)
t. diphosphonate scan
t. phosphate
t. pyrophosphate scan
t. sulfur colloid scan
technique
abduction traction t.
abductor slide t.
Abumi t.
accessory movement t.
Ace-Colles frame t.
Achilles tendon taping t.
active-release t. (ART)
adduction traction t.
Alexander t.
Allgöwer suture t.
Amspacher-Messenbaugh t.
Amstutz resurfacing t.
Anderson-Hutchins t.
Anderson screw placement t.
Andrews t.
anterior iliofemoral t.

anterior quadriceps musculocutaneous flap t.
AO-ASIF compression t.
AO surgical t.
Armistead t.
Aronson-Prager t.
arthrographic capsular distension and rupture t.
Asher physical build assessment t.
ASIF screw fixation t.
Asnis t.
Atasoy V-Y t.
Avila t.
avulsion t.
axial pin t.
Badgley t.
bag-of-bones t.
Bailey-Badgley t.
Bailey-Dubow t.
Baker t.
Balacescu-Golden t.
Banks-Laufman t.
Barbour t.
barrier t.
Barsky t.
basic t.
Basmajian t.
Batch-Spittler-McFaddin t.
Bauer-Tondra-Trusler t.
Baumgaertel and Gotzen calcaneal fracture reduction t.
Baumgard-Schwartz tennis elbow t.
Beall-Webel-Bailey t.
Beckenbaugh t.
Becker t.
Becton t.
Bell-Tawse open reduction t.
biframed distraction t.
bilateral arm raise back exercise t.
Bircher-Weber t.
Black t.
Black-Broström staple t.
Blackburn t.
Blair t.
Bleck recession t.
Bloom-Raney modification of Smith-Robinson t.
Blount tracing t.
Blundell-Jones t.
Bobath t.
Böhler calcaneal fracture reduction t.

Bohlman cervical fusion t.
Bohlman triple-wire t.
bone marrow stimulating t.
Bonfiglio-Bardenstein t.
Bonfiglio modification of Phemister t.
Bonola t.
Bora t.
Borggreve-Hall t.
Bosworth t.
Bowers t.
Boyd-Anderson t.
Boyd-McLeod tennis elbow t.
Boyes brachioradialis transfer t.
Brackett-Osgood-Putti-Abbott t.
Brady-Jewett t.
Brand tendon transfer t.
Brannon-Wickström t.
bridge back exercise t.
Brooks t.
Brooks-Jenkins atlantoaxial fusion t.
Brooks-Seddon transfer t.
Broström injection t.
Brown t.
Bruser t.
Bryan-Morrey t.
Buck-Gramcko t.
Bugg-Boyd t.
Buncke t.
Bunnell atraumatic t.
Bunnell tendon suturing t.
Bunnell tendon transfer t.
bur-down t.
Burgess t.
Burkhalter modification of Stiles-Bunnell t.
Burkhalter transfer t.
Burow skin flap t.
Burrows t.
Calandruccio t.
Caldwell-Coleman flatfoot t.
Callahan fusion t.
Camino catheter t.
Camitz t.
Campbell t.
Canale t.
cannulated reaming t.
Capello t.
Carnesale t.
Carrell fibular substitution t.

T

NOTES

technique *(continued)*
    Caspar anterior cervical plating t.
    Cave-Rowe shoulder dislocation t.
    CBP t.
    cementless t.
    central slip sparing t.
    central splitting t.
    cervical screw insertion t.
    cervical spondylotic myelopathy fusion t.
    Chaves-Rapp muscle transfer t.
    chevron t.
    Chiari t.
    Childress ankle fixation t.
    chiropractic manipulative reflex t. (CMRT)
    Cho tendon t.
    Chow transbursal carpal tunnel release t.
    Chrisman-Snook ankle t.
    Cierny-Mader t.
    Cincinnati t.
    Clancy ligament t.
    Clark transfer t.
    Clayton-Fowler t.
    Cleveland-Bosworth-Thompson t.
    Cloward t.
    t. of Cobb
    Cobb scoliosis measuring t.
    Codivilla tendon lengthening t.
    Cofield t.
    Cole t.
    Coleman flatfoot t.
    Collis broken femoral stem t.
    Coltart fracture t.
    combination of isotonics t.
    compression t.
    Cone-Grant t.
    Connolly t.
    contoured anterior spinal plate t.
    contract-relax t.
    conventional t.
    Conyers t.
    Coonse-Adams t.
    coracoclavicular t.
    costotransversectomy t.
    cotyloplasty t.
    Cox flexion-distraction t.
    Cozen-Brockway t.
    Craig Handicap Assessment and Reporting T. (CHART)
    craniosacral therapy t.
    Crawford-Marxen-Osterfeld t.
    Crego tendon transfer t.
    Cubbins shoulder dislocation t.
    Cuniard and Campell t.
    Curtis t.
    Curtis-Fisher knee t.
    Cyriax t.
    Darrach-McLaughlin shoulder t.
    Davey-Rorabeck-Fowler decompression t.
    Davis drainage t.
    DeBastiani t.
    decompression t.
    decortication t.
    DePalma modified patellar t.
    Dewar-Barrington clavicular dislocation t.
    Dewar-Harris shoulder t.
    Dewar posterior cervical fusion t.
    Deyerle femoral fracture t.
    Dias-Giegerich fracture t.
    Dickinson calcaneal bursitis t.
    Dickson transplant t.
    Dimon-Hughston t.
    distraction t.
    Doll trochanteric reattachment t.
    Doppler t.
    double-looped semitendinous and gracilis hamstring graft knee reconstruction t.
    double portal t.
    double-rod t.
    dowel graft t.
    doweling spondylolisthesis t.
    DREZ modification of Eriksson t.
    drilling t.
    Drummond spinous wiring t.
    Dunn t.
    Dunn-Brittain foot stabilization t.
    DuVries deltoid ligament reconstruction t.
    Eastwood t.
    Eaton-Littler t.
    Eaton-Malerich fracture-dislocation t.
    Eberle contracture release t.
    Ecker-Lotke-Glazer tendon reconstruction t.
    Eftekhar broken femoral stem t.
    Eggers tendon transfer t.
    Ellis-Jones peroneal tendon t.
    Ellison t.
    Ellis skin traction t.
    Ender femoral fracture t.
    Erickson-Leider-Brown t.
    Eriksson brachial block t.
    Eriksson ligament t.
    Essex-Lopresti axial fixation t.
    Essex-Lopresti calcaneal fracture t.
    European compression t. (ECT)
    Evans ankle reconstruction t.
    excision-curettage t.
    extraarticular t.
    extremity mobilization t.
    facet excision t.

facilitatory t.
Fahey t.
Fahey-O'Brien t.
Fairbanks t.
Farmer t.
Ferkel torticollis t.
Fielding modification of Gallie t.
Fish cuneiform osteotomy t.
fixation t.
flat-cut t.
Flatt t.
Flick-Gould t.
Flynn t.
Forbes modification of Phemister
  graft t.
Ford triangulation t.
Forest-Hastings t.
Fowler t.
Fowles dislocation t.
Freebody-Bendall-Taylor fusion t.
freehand suturing t.
French fracture t.
Fried-Hendel tendon t.
Froimson t.
Frost posterior tibialis t.
functional squats back exercise t.
funnel t.
Furnas-Haq-Somers t.
fusion t.
Gaenslen split-heel t.
Gallie atlantoaxial fusion t.
Gallie wire fixation t.
Gallie wiring t.
Galveston t.
Ganley t.
Garceau tendon t.
Ger t.
Giannestras modification of
  Lapidus t.
Gilbert-Tamai-Weiland t.
Gillies-Millard cocked-hat t.
Gill-Manning-White
  spondylolisthesis t.
Gill sliding graft t.
gliding-hole-first t.
gluteal/hamstring raise back
  exercise t.
Glynn-Neibauer t.
Goldberg t.
Goldner-Clippinger t.
Goldstein spinal fusion t.
Gonstead t.

Gordon-Broström t.
Gordon joint injection t.
Gordon-Taylor t.
great toe arthroplasty implant t.
  (GAIT)
Green-Banks t.
Greulich-Pyle t.
Grice-Green t.
Grosse-Kempf tibial t.
Groves-Goldner t.
Guhl t.
Guttmann t.
Hackethal stacked nailing t.
Hall t.
Hamas t.
hamstring fixation t.
Hardinge t.
Harmon transfer t.
Harriluque t.
Hassmann-Brunn-Neer elbow t.
Hauser patellar realignment t.
Hendler unitunnel t.
Henning inside-to-outside t.
Henry acromioclavicular t.
Hermodsson internal rotation t.
Hey-Groves fascia lata t.
Hey-Groves-Kirk t.
Hey-Groves ligament
  reconstruction t.
Heyman t.
Heyman-Herndon-Strong t.
Hill-Nahai-Vasconez-Mathes t.
HIO t.
hip hinge back exercise t.
Hirschhorn compression t.
Hitchcock tendon t.
Hodgson t.
Hohl-Moore t.
Hoke-Kite t.
hold-relax t.
hole-in-one t.
Hoppenfeld-DeBoer t.
Hori t.
hot dog t.
Houghton-Akroyd fracture t.
Hovanian transfer t.
Howard t.
Hughston-Jacobson t.
Hungerford t.
Huntington tibial t.
Ilizarov ankle fusion t.
Ilizarov limb-lengthening t.

T

NOTES

technique *(continued)*

inferior capsular split t.
Inglis-Cooper t.
Inglis-Ranawat-Straub t.
injection t.
Insall-Hood reconstruction t.
Insall ligament reconstruction t.
inside-to-outside t.
interference screw t.
interspinous segmental spinal
   instrumentation t. (ISSI)
intrafocal reduction t.
inverting knot t.
ischemic tourniquet t.
Isobaric epidural/spinal anesthesia t.
isometric t.
Jacobs locking hook spinal rod t.
Jansey t.
Jeffery t.
Johnson pelvic fracture t.
Johnson staple t.
Jones-Brackett t.
Kapandji pinning t.
Kapel elbow dislocation t.
Kaplan t.
Kashiwagi t.
Kates-Kessel-Kay t.
Kaufer tendon t.
Kaufmann t.
Kelikian-Clayton-Loseff t.
Kelikian-Riashi-Gleason t.
Kellogg-Speed fusion t.
Kendrick-Sharma-Hassler-Herndon t.
Kennedy ligament t.
Kessler suture t.
keyhole tenodesis t.
King t.
King-Richards dislocation t.
King-Steelquist t.
Kite and Lovell t.
Kjolbe t.
Klagsbrun harvesting t.
Klein t.
Klisic-Jankovic t.
Kloehn craniofacial remodeling t.
kneeling reciprocal back exercise t.
Krackow-Cohn t.
Krackow locking loop t.
Krackow locking suture t.
Krackow-Thomas-Jones t.
Krempen-Craig-Sotelo tibial
   nonunion t.
Kumar-Cowell-Ramsey t.
Kumar spica cast t.
Küntscher t.
Lamb-Marks-Bayne t.
Lambrinudi t.
Lapidus hammertoe t.

Larson t.
Leadbetter t.
Lee t.
Lehman t.
Leibolt t.
Lenart-Kullman t.
Lewit stretch t.
Lichtman t.
Liebolt radioulnar t.
Lindholm t.
line-to-line reaming t.
Lipscomb t.
Lister t.
Little t.
Littler t.
Littler-Cooley t.
Lloyd-Roberts fracture t.
local standby anesthesia t.
locking-suture t.
Losee modification of MacIntosh t.
Losee sling and reef t.
Louisiana ankle wrap t.
LowDye taping t.
Ludloff t.
lumbar accessory movement t.
Luque instrumentation concave t.
Luque instrumentation convex t.
Luque sublaminar wiring t.
Lyden t.
Lyden-Lehman t.
Lynn Achilles tendon repair t.
MacIntosh t.
Magerl screw placement t.
Magerl translaminar facet screw
   fixation t.
Magilligan measuring t.
Magnuson t.
Ma-Griffith t.
Maitland t.
Majestro-Ruda-Frost tendon t.
Malawer excision t.
Mallory t.
manipulative t.
Mankin t.
Mann t.
Manske t.
manual push-pull t.
Maquet t.
Marcus-Balourdas-Heiple ankle
   fusion t.
Marshall ligament repair t.
Marshall-McIntosh t.
Martin patellar wiring t.
Matti-Russe t.
Mazet t.
McConnell t.
McElfresh-Dobyns-O'Brien t.
McElvenny t.

McFarland-Osborne t.
McFarlane t.
McKeever-Buck elbow t.
McLaughlin-Hay t.
McReynolds open fracture
    reduction t.
medial cortical overlap t.
medial heel skive t.
Mehn-Quigley t.
Mendelsohn modification of
    matrixectomy suture t.
Mensor-Scheck t.
Meyerding-Van Demark t.
microneurosurgical t.
Milch cuff resection of ulna t.
Milch elbow t.
Milford mallet finger t.
mille pattes t.
Millesi modified t.
Mital elbow release t.
miter t.
Mizuno t.
Mizuno-Hirohata-Kashiwagi t.
modified Crawford Campbell inlaid
    bone-grafting t.
Moe scoliosis t.
Mohs t.
Monticelli-Spinelli distraction t.
Moore t.
Morgan-Casscells meniscus
    suturing t.
Morrison t.
mosaicplasty t.
Mubarak-Hargens decompression t.
Mueller t.
muscle energy t.
Nalebuff-Millender lateral band
    mobilization t.
neural arch resection t.
Neviaser acromioclavicular t.
Neviaser-Wilson-Gardner t.
Nicholas five-in-one
    reconstruction t.
Nicholas ligament t.
Niebauer-King t.
Nimmo receptor-tonus t.
Nirschl t.
noninvasive t.
no-touch t.
OATS t.
Ober-Barr transfer t.
Ober tendon t.

Obwegeser sagittal mandibular
    osteotomy t.
Ogata t.
Ollier t.
Omer-Capen t.
open-bowl cement t.
open palm t.
O'Phelan t.
Osborne-Cotterill elbow t.
Osgood modified t.
Osmond-Clarke t.
Ostrup harvesting t.
outside-in t.
outside-to-outside arthroscopy t.
Pack t.
Palmer t.
Palmer-Widen shoulder t.
pants-over-vest t.
Papineau t.
Parachute t.
Parrish-Mann hammertoe t.
partial sit-ups back exercise t.
Parvin gravity t.
passive gliding t.
Paterson t.
Paulos ligament t.
Pauwels t.
Peacock transposing t.
peg-and-socket t.
Perry t.
Perry-Nickel t.
Perry-O'Brien-Hodgson t.
Perry-Robinson cervical t.
Pheasant elbow t.
Phemister-Bonfiglio t.
Phemister onlay bone graft t.
Pierrot-Murphy tendon t.
PNF t.
Ponseti t.
Porter-Richardson-Vainio t.
posterior flap t.
posterior iliofemoral t.
posterolateral costotransversectomy t.
postganglionic t.
postisometric relaxation traction t.
postisometric stretch t.
Pratt t.
preemptive blockade t.
preganglionic t.
press-fit acetabular implant
    insertion t.
prone blocking t.

T

NOTES

technique *(continued)*

proximal-to-distal dissection t.
Puddu tendon t.
Pulvertaft weave tendon repair t.
quadruped back exercise t.
Quénu nail plate removal t.
Ralston-Thompson pseudarthrosis t.
Ranawat-DeFiore-Straub t.
Ray-Clancy-Lemon t.
Rayhack t.
reciprocal arm raise back
  exercise t.
reduction t.
Reichenheim t.
reverse lunge back exercise t.
reverse wedge t.
rhythmic initiation t.
Rideau t.
Riordan tendon transfer t.
Risser t.
Roberts t.
Robinson-Southwick fusion t.
Rockwood-Green t.
Rogers cervical fusion t.
Rood t.
Royle-Thompson transfer t.
Russe t.
Ryerson t.
sacral bar t.
sacrooccipital t. (SOT)
Sage-Clark t.
Saha transfer t.
Sakellarides-Deweese t.
Salter t.
Sammarco-DiRaimondo modification
  of Elmslie t.
Sarmiento trochanteric fracture t.
Scaglietti closed reduction t.
Schaberg-Harper-Allen t.
Schauwecker patellar wiring t.
Schepsis-Leach t.
Schnute wedge resection t.
Schober t.
Scott glenoplasty t.
screw insertion t.
Scuderi t.
second-generation cementing t.
Seddon t.
Sell-Frank-Johnson extensor shift t.
semi suture-loop t.
semitendinosus t.
Serafin t.
Sever modification of Fairbank t.
SharpShooter tissue repair t.
Sharrard transfer t.
Sherk-Probst t.
shish kebab t.
short lever accessory movement t.

side lunge back exercise t.
side-lying back exercise t.
Silfverskiöld t.
silver dollar t.
Simultaneous Interview T. (SIT)
single proximal portal t.
Skoog t.
sling and reef t.
slit catheter t.
Slocum fusion t.
Smith t.
Smith-Petersen t.
Smith-Robinson t.
Sofield femoral deficiency t.
Somerville t.
SOTO t.
Spälteholz t.
Speed-Boyd radial-ulnar t.
spinal fusion t.
spinal mobilization t.
spiral t.
Sprague arthroscopic t.
spray and stretch t.
Staheli t.
Stanisavljevic t.
Staples t.
STAR t.
Stark-Moore-Ashworth-Boyes t.
Steffee instrumentation t.
Stiles-Bunnell transfer t.
Stimson anterior shoulder
  reduction t.
strain/counterstrain t.
Straub t.
Strayer tendon t.
Strickland t.
strut fusion t.
suction-irrigation t.
superman back exercise t.
surgical t.
sustained pressure t.
suture anchor t.
suture-loop t.
Swanson t.
Tajima suture t.
taping t.
Taylor t.
Taylor-Daniel-Weiland t.
tension band wiring t.
Teuffer t.
third-generation cementing t.
Thomas-Thompson-Straub transfer t.
Thompson-Henry t.
Thompson-Loomer t.
thoracolumbar spondylosis
  surgical t.
threaded-hole-first t.
three-point pressure t.

three-portal t.
Tohen tendon t.
Torg t.
Torgerson-Leach modified t.
transiliac bar t.
Trethowan-Stamm-Simmonds-
  Menelaus-Haddad t.
triangulation t.
triple bundle t.
triple-wire t.
Tullos t.
Turco clubfoot release t.
two-portal t.
two-sleeve t.
two-stage tendon grafting t.
two-strut tibial graft t.
unassisted locking-suture t.
unitunnel t.
unlocking spiral t.
vacuum cement mix t.
vasomotor t.
Vastamäki t.
Veleanu-Rosianu-Ionescu t.
Verdan t.
Vidal-Adrey fracture t.
Viladot surgical t.
Volz-Turner reattachment t.
Vulpius-Compere tendon t.
Wadsworth t.
Wagner open reduction t.
Wagoner cervical t.
Warner-Farber ankle fixation t.
Watkins fusion t.
Watson t.
Watson-Cheyne t.
Weaver-Dunn acromioclavicular t.
Weber-Brunner-Freuler-Boitzy t.
Weber-Vasey traction-absorption
  wiring t.
Weckesser t.
Weinstein-Ponseti t.
Wertheim-Bohlman t.
West and Soto-Hall patella t.
West-Soto-Hall patellar t.
Whitesides t.
Whitesides-Kelly cervical t.
wick t.
Wick catheter t.
Williams flexion back exercise t.
Williams-Haddad t.
Wilson t.

Wilson-Jacobs tibial fracture
  fixation t.
Wilson-McKeever shoulder t.
Windson-Insall-Vince grafting t.
Winograd ingrown nail t.
Winter spondylolisthesis t.
wire removal t.
Wirth-Jager tendon t.
Woodward t.
Wynne-Davis joint laxity t.
Zancolli rerouting t.
Zariczny ligament t.
Zarins-Rowe ligament t.
Zazepen-Gamidov t.
Zeier transfer t.
Zielke t.

TechnoGel insole
technology
  Cascading Tower T.
  GADS t.
  segmentally demineralized bone t.
  VSL t.
  work evaluation systems t. (WEST)
tectal plate
Tectonic magnet
tectoral ligament
TED
  thromboembolic disease
    TED hose
    TED stockings
teeth (*pl. of* tooth)
Teflon
  T. cannula
  T. implant
  T. tri-leaflet prosthesis
Teflon-coated
  T.-c. driver
  T.-c. suture
Tegaderm dressing
Tegner
  T. activity rating scale
  T. knee reconstruction activity
    score
Tegtmeier
  T. elevator
  T. hand board
Tei-Shin
Tekscan in-shoe monitoring device
telangiectasia
  calcinosis, Raynaud, esophageal
    motility disorders, sclerodactyly, t.
    (CREST)

T.

NOTES

telangiectasia-ataxia
telangiectatic osteosarcoma
Telectronics
    T. electrical stimulation apparatus
    T. electrical stimulation device
Teledyne Water Pik misting massage
teleroentgenography
telescopic
    t. plate spacer
    t. view guide
telescoping
    t. brace
    t. medullary rod
    t. nail
telethermometer
Telfa
    T. bolster
    T. gauze
    T. gauze dressing
    T. sponge
Telos fracture table
TEM
    terminal extensor mechanism
temper
    T. Foam
    T. Foam cube
    T. Foam cushion
    t. tantrum elbow
temperature
    capillary refill, sensation, motor
      function, t. (CSMT)
    t. differential (TD)
    wet globe t.
Temperlite saw blade
template
    acetabular cup t.
    Charnley t.
    femoral condylar t.
    malleable t.
    Moore t.
    Mueller t.
    Pedrialle t.
    prosthesis t.
    rod t.
    Stevens-Street elbow prosthesis t.
    thermoplastic t.
    tibial track t.
    transparent t.
templating roentgenogram
temple
    T. University nail
    T. University plate
temporal
    t. bone
    t. bone fracture
    t. dispersion
    t. fascia graft
temporalis fascia flap

temporary
    t. articulating methylmethacrylate
      antibiotic spacer (TAMMAS)
    t. callus
    t. cavity phenomenon
    t. cerclage wire
    t. external fixator
    t. prosthetic fitting
    t. socket
temporomandibular
    t. joint (TMJ)
    t. joint arthralgia
    t. joint dislocation
    t. joint syndrome
Tempur-Pedic
    T.-P. pressure relieving Swedish
      mattress
    T.-P. pressure relieving Swedish
      pillow
tenaculum
tenaculum-reducing forceps
tenalgia crepitans
Tenderlett device
tenderness
    bony t.
    costovertebral angle t. (CVAT)
    joint line t.
    myofascial t.
    percussion t.
    pillar t.
    point t.
    rebound t.
tender point (TeP)
tendinitis, tendonitis
    Achilles t.
    acute calcific t.
    anterior tarsal t.
    biceps t.
    bicipital t.
    birefringent lipid crystals in t.
    calcific t.
    chronic Achilles t.
    de Quervain t.
    digital flexor t.
    infrapatellar t.
    infraspinatus t.
    patellar t.
    peripatellar t.
    peroneal t.
    popliteus t.
    posterior tibial t. (PTT)
    radial wrist extensor t.
    rotator cuff calcific t.
    semimembranosus t.
    subscapular t.
    supraspinatus t.
    ulnar wrist extensor t.

wrist extensor t.
wrist flexor t.

tendinopathy
Achilles t.
Blazina t.
insertion t.
peroneus longus t. (PLT)
primary peroneus longus t.
rotator cuff t.

tendinoplasty
talipes t.

tendinosis
angiofibroblastic hyperplasia t.
calcific t.
insertional Achilles t.
medial tennis elbow t.

tendinosuture
tendinotrochanteric ligament
tendinous
t. attachment
t. fiber
t. sheath
t. synovitis

tendinum
tendo
t. Achillis
t. Achillis lengthening (TAL)
t. Achillis mechanism
t. calcaneus

tendolysis
tendon
abductor digiti quinti t.
abductor hallucis t.
abductor pollicis brevis t.
abductor pollicis longus t.
accessory communicating t.
Achilles t. (AT)
adductor hallucis t.
adductor pollicis brevis t.
adherent profundus t.
t. advancement
anchoring t.
anterior tibial t.
aponeurosis of t.
attenuation of t.
attrition of t.
attrition rupture of t.
biceps brachialis t.
biceps brachii t.
biceps femoris t.
bicipital t.
t. bowing in arthritis

brachialis t.
brachial plexus t.
brachioradialis t.
calcaneal t.
carpi radialis brevis t.
carpi radialis longus t.
t. cartilage
t. centralization
t. checkrein procedure
common extensor t.
conjoined t.
digital extensor t.
digital flexor t.
digiti quinti proprius t.
digitorum communis t.
t. disorder
t. displacement
ECRB t.
ECRL t.
ECU t.
EDB t.
EHL t.
EIP t.
elbow extensor t.
evertor t.
t. excursion
extensor carpi radialis brevis t.
extensor carpi radialis longus t.
extensor carpi ulnaris t.
extensor digiti minimi t.
extensor digiti quinti t.
extensor digitorum brevis t.
extensor digitorum communis t.
extensor digitorum longus t.
extensor hallucis longus t.
extensor indicis proprius t.
extensor pollicis brevis t.
extensor pollicis longus t.
extensor quinti t.
flexor carpi radialis t.
flexor carpi ulnaris t.
flexor digitorum communis t.
flexor digitorum longus t.
flexor digitorum profundus t.
flexor digitorum sublimis t.
flexor digitorum superficialis t.
flexor hallucis brevis t.
flexor hallucis longus t.
flexor pollicis brevis t.
flexor pollicis longus t.
flexor profundus t.
flexor sublimis t.

T

NOTES

tendon *(continued)*
  t. forceps
  gastrocnemius t.
  gastrocnemius-soleus t.
  G-lengthening of semitendinosus t.
  Golgi t.
  t. gouge
  t. grabber
  gracilis t.
  t. graft (TG)
  hamstring t.
  Hector t.
  hilus of t.
  iliopsoas t.
  t. inflammation
  infrapatellar t.
  infraspinatus t.
  interosseous t.
  t. interposition arthroplasty
  t. irregularity
  t. jerk
  t. leader
  t. lengthening
  long head biceps t.
  lumbrical t.
  midpatellar t.
  t. needle
  t. nodularity
  t. nodule
  obturator internus t.
  palmaris longus t.
  t. passer
  patellar t.
  patelloquadriceps t.
  peroneal t.
  peroneus brevis t.
  peroneus longus t.
  peroneus tertius t.
  plantaris t.
  t. plate
  t. plica
  popliteal t.
  popliteus t.
  posterior tibial t. (PTT)
  postoperative flexor t. (PFT)
  ProCol bovine bioprosthesis t.
  profundus t.
  pronator teres t.
  proprius t.
  t. prosthesis
  quadriceps t.
  rectus femoris t.
  t. reflex
  t. release
  t. repair
  rerouted t.
  rider's t.
  t. rod

rotator cuff t.
  t. rupture
  sartorius t.
  semimembranosus t.
  semitendinosus t.
  t. sheath
  slip of t.
  snapping t.
  t. snapping
  split anterior tibial t.
  t. stripper
  sublimis t.
  subscapularis t.
  t. substitution
  superficialis t.
  supraspinatus t.
  t. suture
  t. thickening
  thumb extensor t.
  thumb flexor t.
  tibial t.
  tibialis anterior t.
  tibialis posterior t.
  toe extensor t.
  t. transfer
  t. transplantation
  t. transposition
  t. trapping
  triceps brachii t.
  t. tucker
  t. tunneler
  wrist extensor t.
  Z-lengthening of biceps t.
tendon-bearing
  patellar t.-b. (PTB)
tendon-bone
  t.-b. allograft
  t.-b. attachment
  bone-patellar t.-b. (BPB, BPTB)
  t.-b. bridge
tendon-braiding forceps
tendon-holding forceps
tendonitis *(var. of* tendinitis)
tendon-passing forceps
tendon-pulling forceps
tendon-retrieving forceps
tendon-seizing forceps
tendon-to-bone attachment
tendon-tunneling forceps
tendopathy
  plantar t.
tendosuspension
  Hibbs t.
  Jones t.
tendosynovitis
tendotomy
tendovaginitis
tenectomy

ten-hole blade plate
tennis
    t. elbow
    t. elbow arm band
    t. elbow splint
    t. elbow test
    t. fracture
    t. heel
    t. leg
    t. shoulder
    t. thumb
    t. toe
tenocyte
tenodesis
    Andrews iliotibial band t.
    Andrews lateral t.
    anterolateral femorotibial ligament t.
    band t.
    calcaneal t.
    Chrisman-Snook t.
    t. effect
    Eggers t.
    Ellison iliotibial band t.
    Evans t.
    extensor hallucis longus t.
    femorotibial ligament t.
    Fowler t.
    hallucis brevis t.
    t. of the heel cord
    iliotibial band t.
    interphalangeal t.
    key-grip t.
    keyhole t.
    MacIntosh extraarticular t.
    MacIntosh iliotibial band t.
    Moberg key-grip t.
    modified Watson-Jones ankle t.
    Mueller anterolateral femorotibial
      ligament t.
    Norwood iliotibial band t.
    t. orthosis
    Perry-O'Brien-Hodgson triple t.
    SCOI arthroscopic t.
    semitendinosus t.
    sublimis t.
    t. test
    triple t.
    Watson-Jones ankle t.
    Westin t.
tenodynia
tenography

tenolysis
    flexor t.
    peroneal t.
tenomyoplasty
tenomyotomy
tenonectomy
tenonitis
tenontodynia
tenontomyoplasty
tenontomyotomy
tenontophyma
tenontoplastic
tenontoplasty
tenontothecitis
tenoperiostitis
tenophyte
tenoplastic reconstruction
tenoplasty
tenorrhaphy
tenositis
tenostosis
tenosuspension
tenosuture
tenosynography
tenosynovectomy
    dorsal t.
    flexor t.
tenosynovial
    t. giant cell tumor
    t. injection
    t. sheath
tenosynovitis
    adhesive t.
    bicipital t.
    t. crepitans
    de Quervain stenosing t.
    flexor hallucis longus t.
    gonococcic t.
    gonorrheal t.
    granulomatous t.
    t. hypertrophica
    infectious t.
    localized nodular t.
    nodular t.
    peroneal t.
    t. serosa stenosans
    stenosing t.
    suppurative flexor t.
    tuberculous peroneal t.
    villonodular t.
    villous t.
tenotomized

T

NOTES

tenotomy
Achilles t.
adductor t.
Braun shoulder t.
curb t.
extensor t.
fenestrated t.
flexor t.
Fowler central slip t.
graduated t.
inverted-Y Achilles t.
t. knife
Lichtblau t.
open t.
percutaneous t.
semiopen sliding t.
sliding t.
stapedial t.
subcutaneous t.
transverse t.
Veleanu-Rosianu-Ionescu adductor t.
Z-plasty t.
tenovaginitis
inflammatory t.
TENS
transcutaneous electrical nerve
stimulation
TENS therapy
TENS unit
tensile
t. force
t. strain
t. strength
t. stress
Tensilon
T. test
T. test for myasthenia gravis
tensing test
tensiometer
Acufex t.
tensiometry
tension
t. band
t. band fixation
t. band of knee
t. band plate
t. band wire
t. band wire tamp
t. band wiring technique
capsular-ligamentous t.
t. curve
t. force
t. fracture
graft t.
heel t.
t. isometer
t. loading
t. myositis

neural t.
t. neuralgia
t. night splint (TNS)
oxygen t.
residual t.
tension-band wiring
tensioner
cable t.
Dwyer t.
Kirschner wire t.
tension-free Millesi nerve graft
tensor
t. fascia femoris flap
t. fascia lata (TFL)
t. fascia lata muscle flap
t. fascia lata syndrome
tent frame
tentorial sinus
tenuous vascularity
Tenzel elevator
TeP
tender point
Tepperwedge wedge
Teq-Trode electrode
teratologic dislocation
teres
anterior pronator t.
t. major muscle
t. minor muscle
pronator t. (PT)
terminal
t. device (TD)
t. extensor mechanism (TEM)
t. head
t. J sign
t. knee extension
t. latency
t. overgrowth
t. stance
t. Syme procedure
terrible triad of the shoulder
Terrmocork diabetic shoe
Terry
T. nail
T. Thomas sign
TERT
total end-range time
tertiary amputation
Terumo syringe
TES belt
test
abduction external rotation t.
abduction load and shift t.
abduction stress t.
accordion t.
Achilles squeeze t.
Achilles tendon t.

activated partial thromboplastin
time t. (APTT)
active bending t.
active knee extension t.
actual leg length t.
Adams forward-bending t.
Adams position t.
Adams scoliosis t.
adduction load and shift t.
adduction stress t.
Adson t.
AKE t.
Allen t.
Allis t.
ALRI t.
Anderson medial-lateral grind t.
Andrews anterior instability t.
ankle clonus t.
ankle dorsiflexion t.
anterior drawer t. (ADT)
anteroposterior stress t.
antinuclear antibody t.
anvil t.
AO pseudoisochromatic color
plate t.
Apley compression t.
Apley distraction t.
Apley grinding t.
Apley knee t.
Apley scratch t.
apprehension t.
ARA T.
arch-up t.
arm fossa t.
arthrometer t.
axial compression t.
axial load t.
axial manual traction t.
axon reflex t.
Babinski t.
ballottement t.
Barlow hip instability t.
Barlow provocative t.
Beals t.
Bechterew t.
Beery Visual Motor Integration T.
Bekhterev sitting t.
belly-press t.
bench t.
Berg balance t.
biceps jerk reflex t.
Bielschowsky head tilt t.

big toe t.
Biodex t.
block t.
blot t.
Booth t.
bounce home t.
bowstring t.
Boyes t.
bracelet t.
brachial plexus tension t.
Bragard t.
break t.
British t.
brush t.
Bunnell t.
Bunnell-Littler t.
Burke t.
Burn bench t.
calcidiol t.
calf squeeze t.
Callaway t.
carpal compression t.
Carroll t.
catch and clunk t.
Centinela supraspinatus t.
cerebellar function t.
cervical compaction t.
cervical sidegliding t.
Chaddock t.
chest expansion t.
Chiene t.
Childress duck waddle t.
chin-to-chest t.
circle draw t.
Clarke patellar compression t.
clock balance t.
clunk t.
cold pressor t.
Coleman lateral block t.
Combat Task t.
compression t.
concealed straight leg raising t.
conduction velocity t.
confrontational t.
contralateral straight leg raising t.
costoclavicular syndrome t.
Cotton ankle instability t.
Cotton fibular bone hook t.
cough t.
Cozen t.
Cram t.
crank t.

T

NOTES

test *(continued)*

Crawford small parts dexterity t.
crossover t.
Cybex isokinetic t.
D'Ambrosia t.
Deerfield t.
de Kleyn t.
Deyerle sciatic tension t.
dial t.
digital response t.
dipyridamole handgrip t.
disk diffusion t.
disk space saline acceptance t.
distal compression t.
distraction t.
dorsal drawer t.
dorsiflexion-eversion t.
double leg raise t.
Downey texture discrimination t.
drawer t.
drop-arm t.
dual photon densitometry t.
duck-waddle t.
Dugas t.
Duncan prone rectus t.
Dunn multiple comparison t.
Durkan carpal compression t.
Dvorak t.
Dynatron 2000 muscle t.
Eden t.
eighty-nine-newton t.
elbow flexion t.
elbow jerk reflex t.
Elithorn Maze T.
Elson middle slip t.
Ely heel-to-buttock t.
empty can t.
endpoint of orthopedic t.
eversion stress t.
excessive laxity t.
external rotation-abduction stress t.
  (EAST)
external rotation stress t.
extrinsic entrapment t.
extrinsic tightness t.
FABER t.
fabere t.
FADIR t.
Fastex proprioceptive and agility t.
Feagin shoulder dislocation t.
femoral nerve stretch t.
femoral nerve traction t.
fibular bone hook t.
fibular compression t.
figure-of-eight t.
figure-of-four t.
fingertips-to-floor t.
finger-to-finger t.

finger-to-nose t.
Finkelstein t.
first metatarsus rise t.
Fisher Protected Least Significant
  Difference t.
Fist-Palm-Side T.
Fist-Ring T.
flat-hand t.
flexion-rotation-drawer knee
  instability t.
flexion spinal radiography t.
flip t.
fluctuation t.
foot placement t.
foraminal compression t.
forced adduction t.
forearm supination t.
forefoot adduction correction t.
forefoot block t.
Fortin finger t.
Fournier t.
Fowler t.
FRD t.
Froment ulnar nerve function t.
fulcrum t.
Gaenslen t.
Galant t.
Galeazzi t.
Galveston orientation and
  amnesia t. (GOAT)
Garrick t.
George t.
Gilchrist t.
Gillet marching t.
gluteus maximus tensing t.
golfer's elbow t.
Gordon squeeze t.
gracilis t.
gravity drawer t.
gravity stress t.
grimace t.
grinding t.
grip strength t.
Grooved Pegboard T.
Hamilton ruler t.
Harris Infant Neuromotor T.
  (HINT)
Hautant t.
Hawiva t.
Hawkins t.
heel-palm t.
heel-rise t.
heel-tip t.
heel-to-knee t.
heel-to-shin t.
Helfet t.
hip abduction stress t.
Hoffa t.

Homans t.
Hoover t.
hop t.
Houle t.
Hughston external rotation recurvatum t.
Hughston knee jerk t.
Hughston-Losee jerk t.
Hughston plica t.
Hughston posterolateral drawer t.
Hughston posteromedial drawer t.
hyperabduction syndrome t.
hyperextension t.
iliac compression t.
iliopsoas t.
impingement t.
T. of Infant Motor Performance (TIMP)
Ingram-Withers-Speltz motor t.
inhibition t.
intrinsic tightness t.
inversion stress t.
ischemic forearm exercise t.
Jack t.
jackknife t.
Jackson compression t.
Jacob shift t.
Jakob t.
Jamar t.
Jansen t.
Jebsen hand t.
Jebsen-Taylor hand function t.
jerk t.
Jobe t.
jogging in place t.
Johnson-Zuck-Wingate motor t.
Jolly t.
Kelikian push-up t.
Kemp t.
Kernig t.
Kleiger t.
Kleinman shear t.
knee-drop t.
knee flexion stress t.
knee instability t.
knee jerk reflex t.
knee laxity t.
kneeling bench t.
Kolmogorov-Smirnov t.
Kruskal-Wallis t.
Lachman t.
Lam inversion t.

Lasègue rebound t.
lateral block t.
lateral pivot shift t.
lateral squeeze t.
leaning hop t.
Lewin-Gaenslen t.
Lewin punch t.
Lewin reverse Lasègue t.
Lewin snuff t.
Lewin standing t.
Lewin supine t.
Lewis-Prusik t.
Lichtman t.
lift-off t.
ligamentous instability t.
light touch t.
Lippman t.
load and shift t.
locking-position t.
Losee knee instability t.
Lovett t.
Ludington t.
Luekens wrinkle t.
lumbar extension t.
lumbar lateral flexion t.
lumbar protective mechanism t.
lumbar rotation t.
lunotriquetral shear t.
Lysholm knee t.
MacIntosh lateral pivot shift t.
Maddox rod t.
Maigne t.
manual muscle t.
matchstick t.
McMurray t.
Mennell t.
MicroFET2 muscle t.
middle-finger t.
military posture t.
milk t.
Mills t.
Minnesota Manual Dexterity T.
Minnesota Rate of Manipulation t.
Minnesota Spatial Relations T.
Moberg Picking Up T.
monofilament pressure t.
Morton t.
Murphy punch t.
MyoForce t.
Naffziger t.
navicular drop t.
Neer impingement t.

NOTES

T

test *(continued)*

nerve compression t. (NCT)
nerve conduction velocity t.
Neviaser t.
Nobel t.
Noyes flexion rotation drawer t.
Ober t.
oblique retinacular ligament
   tightness t.
O'Connor finger dexterity t.
O'Connor tweezer dexterity t.
O'Donoghue t.
one-leg hop for distance t.
one-leg stance t.
Oppenheim stroke t.
opposition t.
OsteoGram bone density t.
Osteomark bone-loss urine t.
Osteopatch bone density t.
overhead exercise t.
Paget t.
pain provocation t.
palm-up t.
parachute t.
passive accessory motion t.
passive patellar glide t.
passive patellar tilt t.
passive physiological t.
patellar apprehension t.
patellar glide t.
patellar inhibition test probe-to-
   bone t.
patellar retraction t.
patellar tap t.
Patrick t.
Patrick/fabere t.
peak torque t.
pelvic rock t.
Perkins t.
peroneal tunnel compression t.
Perthes tourniquet t.
Phalen wrist flexion t.
Physical Ability T. (PAT)
pick-up t.
pinprick hyperalgesia t.
pivot-shift t.
plantarflexion-inversion t.
plica t.
posterior apprehension t.
posterior drawer t.
posterior stress t.
posterolateral drawer t.
posteromedial pivot-shift t.
prone extension t.
prone external rotation t.
prone knee-bend t.
prone knee flexion t.
prone rectus t.

proximal compression t.
pseudostability t.
pulse status-pull t.
push-pull t.
push-up t.
quadrant t.
quadriceps active t.
quadriceps contraction t.
quantitative sudomotor axon
   reflex t. (QSART)
Queckenstedt t.
Queckenstedt-Stookey t.
RA t.
recurvatum t.
rekindling t.
relocation t.
reverse Lasègue t.
reverse pivot shift t.
Romberg t.
Roos overhead exercise t.
rotary drawer t.
rotary instability t.
rotation drawer t.
rotation recurvatum t.
sagittal stress t.
saline acceptance t.
scaphoid lift t.
scaphoid shift t.
scapular approximation t.
Scheffé t.
Schober t.
seated root t.
Seddon coin t.
Semmes-Weinstein monofilament
   pressure t.
Sharp-Purser T.
shear t.
Sherman block t.
shift t.
shoulder abduction t.
shoulder depression t.
shuck t.
side-glide t.
side-jump t.
side-lying iliac compression t.
Silfverskiöld t.
Simmonds t.
simple knee t. (SKT)
single-heel rise t.
sit-and-reach t.
sitting flexion t.
sitting root t.
sit-to-stand t.
sit-up t.
six-minute walk t.
skin-gliding t.
skin resistance t.
Slocum ALRI t.

Slocum anterior rotary drawer t.
Slocum lateral pivot-shift t.
Slocum rotary instability t.
SLR with Bragard t.
SLR with external rotation t.
SLR with Kernig t.
slump t.
Smith and Ross t.
somatosensory t.
Soto-Hall t.
Speed t.
sponge t.
spring t.
Spurling t.
square-shaped wrist t.
squat t.
squatting t.
squeeze t.
Stagnara wake-up t.
Staheli t.
stair running t.
standing apprehension t.
standing flexion t.
standing Gillet t.
starch t.
station t.
Steinmann t.
t. stimulus
Stinchfield t.
straight leg raising t. (SLRT)
stress t.
stretch t.
stroke t.
Stroop t.
subtalar inversion t.
sudomotor activity t.
sulcus t.
supine iliac gapping t.
supine long sitting t.
supine straight leg raising t.
suprascapular nerve entrapment t.
supraspinatus t.
sweat t.
tandem gait t.
tennis elbow t.
tenodesis t.
Tensilon t.
tensing t.
thenar weakness t.
Thomas t.
Thomasen t.
Thompson t.

thumbnail t.
thumb-to-forearm t.
tight retinacular ligament t.
tilt-up t.
timed Allen t.
tissue compression t.
Toglia Category Assessment T. (TCAT)
tourniquet t.
transverse humeral ligament t.
treadmill t.
Trendelenburg t.
triceps jerk reflex t.
triceps skinfold t.
triple-jump t.
Trömner t.
trunk incurvation t.
Tukey t.
two-part Apley t.
two-point discrimination t.
ulnar grind t.
Underburger t.
unilateral standing t.
upper limb tension t. (ULTT)
valgus stress t.
Valpar Whole Body Range of Motion T.
Valsalva t.
varus stress t.
vertebral artery t.
vertical compression t.
vibration threshold t.
vibrometer t.
volitional muscle action t.
Voshell t.
wake-up t.
Waldron t.
walk t.
Wallenberg t.
water acceptance t.
Watson t.
Weber t.
Weinstein enhanced sensory t. (WEST)
well leg straight leg raising t.
Wilson t.
wipe t.
Wolf motor function t.
Wright t.
Wright-Adson t.
wrinkle t.
wrist flexion t.

T

NOTES

test *(continued)*
    Wu sole opposition t.
    Yeager t.
    Yergason shoulder subluxation t.

tester
    Cybex t.
    grip t.
    GripTrack Commander strength t.
    Jamar grip t.
    Nicholas manual muscle t.
    OSI laxity t.
    West nerve t.

testing
    active motion t. (AMT)
    active movement t.
    angle isometric t.
    aquatic cardiac evaluation and t. (ACET)
    arthrometer t.
    biomechanical t.
    biothesiometer t.
    blunt pressure t.
    brush-evoked pain t.
    compression t.
    confirmatory t.
    Cybex t.
    Disk-Criminator sensory t.
    dynametric t.
    enzyme-based lactic acid blood t.
    exercise t.
    face validity of rehabilitation t.
    isokinetic t.
    isometric motor t.
    isometric strength t.
    isotonic motor t.
    manual muscle t. (MMT)
    mobility t.
    Model 810 axial closed-loop hydraulic mechanical t.
    motion t.
    motor neglect t.
    MRI t.
    muscle t. (MT)
    nerve involvement t.
    neurological t.
    NUTRI-SPEC t.
    Omnitron exercise t.
    palpation t.
    passive mobility t.
    pincer t.
    PIVM t.
    premanipulative t.
    quantitative mechanical pain t.
    quantitative sensory t. (QST)
    range-of-motion t.
    ratio scale in rehabilitation t.
    reciprocal isokinetic t.
    rotation t.

    segmental mobility t.
    shear t.
    strength t.
    stress t.
    susceptibility t.
    Tacticon quantitative sensory t.

tetanic contraction
tetanolysin
tetanospasmin
tetanus
tetany
tethered
    t. cord syndrome
    t. patellar tendon syndrome
    t. spinal cord
tethering effect
tetracalcium phosphate
tetraphasic action potential
tetraplegia
    International Classification for Surgery of the Hand in T.
    traumatic t.
Tetrapolar
    Electro-Diagnostic Instruments Model 720 Bilateral T.
Teufel cervical brace
Teuffer
    T. technique
    T. tendo calcaneus repair
Teurlings wrist brace
TEV
    talipes equinovarus
Tevdek suture
Texas
    T. Scottish Rite Hospital (TSRH)
    T. T incision
Texon sole
TFA
    thigh-foot angle
    tibiofemoral angle
TFB-PS
    tibial fracture brace proximal support
TFC
    threaded fusion cage
    triangular fibrocartilage complex
        TFC tear
TFCC
    triangular fibrocartilage complex
T-finger splint
T-Fix absorbable meniscal repair device
TFL
    tensor fascia lata
T-Foam
    T-F. bed pad
    T-F. cushion
    T-F. mattress
    T-F. pillow

TG
    tendon graft
T-Gel cushion
TGF
    transforming growth factor
THA
    total hip arthroplasty
Thackray
    T. hip prosthesis
    T. low friction arthroplasty
thalamic
    t. fracture
    t. fragment
thalamotomy
thalassemia
thallium
    radioisotope t.
    t. scan
Than anaerobic threshold
T-handle
    T-h. curette
    ratcheting T-h.
    T-h. Zimmer chuck
T-handled
    T-h. awl
    T-h. hook
    T-h. nut wrench
    T-h. reamer
    T-h. screw wrench
    T-h. trocar
THARIES
    total hip articular replacement by internal eccentric shells
Tharies
    T. femoral resurfacing component
    T. hip component
    T. hip replacement
    T. hip replacement operation
    T. hip replacement prosthesis
Thatcher
    T. nail
    T. screw
theater
    t. ache
    t. sign
theca
    digital t.
thecal
    t. abscess
    t. injection
    t. sac
    t. whitlow

themoplastic ankle-foot orthosis
thenar
    t. area
    t. atrophy
    t. branch
    t. creaking
    t. eminence
    t. fascia
    t. flap
    t. muscle
    t. palmar crease (TPC)
    t. palsy
    t. space
    t. weakness test
theory
    Denis Browne three-column spine t.
    kinetic energy t.
    Maisel suppression t.
    Neviaser t.
    three-column spine t.
Thera
    T. cane
    T. Cane massager
    T. Cane shoulder exerciser
    T. Pulse bed
Thera-Back back support
Thera-Band
    T.-B. Aqua Belt
    T.-B. ASSIST
    T.-B. ASSIST exerciser
    T.-B. exercise ball
    T.-B. Exercise System for Golfers
    T.-B. hand exerciser
    T.-B. handle
    T.-B. Max
    T.-B. Max resistive exercise
    T.-B. progressive weight
    T.-B. resistive exerciser
    T.-B. resistive therapy system
    T.-B. strip
    T.-B. System of Progressive Resistance
    T.-B. tubing
Therabath paraffin heat therapy system
TheraBeads microwaveable moist heat pack
Thera-Boot bandage
Thera-Ciser
    T.-C. light exercise system
    T.-C. therapeutic exercise system
Theracloud pillow

NOTES

TheraCool cold therapy
Thera-Fit
Theraflex wrist exerciser
Therafoam padding
Theraform Selectives
Thera-Gesic cream
Theragloves
Theragym ball
Ther-A-Hoop exerciser
TheraKnit electrode glove
Thera-Loop exerciser
Thera-Med cold pack
Thera-Medic shoe
Theramini 1, 2 electrotherapy
  stimulator
therapeutic
  t. exercise
  t. lifestyle change (TLC)
  t. light
  t. orthosis
  t. shoe
  t. spinal support
  t. splint
  t. ultrasound
  t. ultrasound for tendon healing
Therapeutica Sleeping Pillow
Thera-P exercise bar
Thera-Plast putty
Therap-Loop
  T.-L. door anchor
  T.-L. door handle
Thera-Pos elbow orthosis
Therapress pressure point release tool
Thera-Putty CTS exerciser
therapy
  ablative laser t.
  active-assistive motion t.
  Acu-Magnet t.
  amplitude-summation interferential
    current t. (ASICT)
  animal-assisted t. (AAT)
  anticoagulant t.
  anticonvulsant t.
  antithrombotic t.
  bee venom t.
  Biodex Unweighing System partial
    weight t.
  Bragg-peak photon-beam t.
  brisement t.
  carpal tunnel syndrome injection t.
  T. Carrot Finger Orthosis (TCFO)
  cell t.
  chelation t.
  cold t.
  compression t.
  conservative t.
  Cool-Aid continuous controlled
    cold t.

corrective t.
corticosteroid t. (CS)
craniosacral t. (CST)
diet t.
Diversified chiropractic
  manipulative t.
dry heat t.
edema heat t.
electrical stimulation t.
electric differential t. (EDit)
Electri-Cool continuous controlled
  cold t.
electron beam t.
ETPS t.
Exogen 2000+ noninvasive
  ultrasound t.
extracorporeal shock wave t.
  (ESWT)
fad t.
flexion-distraction t.
fomentation t.
frequency-difference interferential
  current t. (FDICT)
HBO t.
heat t.
herbal t.
high-voltage t. (HVT)
hot fomentation t.
hyperbaric oxygen t.
hypnotic t.
immunosuppressive t.
inferential t.
InFerno moist heat t.
infrared t.
injection t.
interferential t.
intradiskal electrothermal t. (IDET)
intraosseous t.
intravenous t.
Kelsey unloading exercise t.
LaserPen laser t.
Livingstone t.
magnetic t.
manipulative t.
manual t.
massage t.
meridian t.
microcurrent t.
mind-body t.
moist heat t.
motion t.
moxa heat t.
moxibustion heat t.
neuromuscular electrical
  stimulation t.
NMES t.
occupational t. (OT)

orthomolecular
  medicine/megavitamin t.
osteomanipulative t. (OMT)
osteopathic manipulative t. (OMT)
outpatient physical t.
oxygen t.
pancreatic enzyme t.
parachute t.
paraffin heat t.
perioperative antibiotic t.
physical t. (PT)
piperacillin/tazobactam t.
pneumatic compression t.
Polar Wrap cold t.
pool t.
positional release t.
postoperative t.
pressure t.
ProFlo vascular compression t.
proliferation t.
prophylactic antibiotic t.
pulsed short-wave t.
T. Putty
qi gong t.
radiation t.
range of motion t., ROM t.
recreational t. (RT)
reflex t.
rolfing t.
sedation t.
shock-wave t. (SWT)
Silastic ball t.
somatic t.
spinal injection t.
spinal manipulative t. (SMT)
spinal manual t.
splinting t.
steroid t.
SwimEx aquatic t.
Swiss ball t.
t. tank
Task Force on Standards of
  Physical T.
TENS t.
TheraCool cold t.
therapy electroconvulsive t.
tonification t.
transfusion t.
transverse friction t.
trial of conservative t.
trigger point t. (TPT)
tumor t.

ultrasound t.
vasoconstrictive t.
whirlpool t.
TheraSeed implant
Ther-A-Shapes positioner
Therasleep Cervical Pillow
Therasound transducer
Theratotic
  T. firm foot orthosis
  T. soft foot orthosis
Theratouch 4.7 stimulator
Thera-Wedge system
thermal
  t. agent
  t. anesthesia
  t. capsulorrhaphy
  t. modality
  T. Pack
thermalator
  Whitehall t.
Thermalator heating unit
ThermalSoft hot & cold packs
Thermapad pad
Thermasonic gel warmer
Thermassage
  Aqua T.
ThermaStim
  T. muscle stimulator
  T. muscle warming device
Thermo
  T. hand comforter
  T. HK/Rohadur orthotic
  T. HK/Tepefom orthotic
  T. knee comforter
ThermoCork orthotic
thermocouple
  t. instrument
  low impedance t.
  t. skin temperature device
ThermoFlex
  Maramed T.
thermogram
thermographic
  t. examination
  t. finding
  t. scanner
thermography
  chiropractic t.
  infrared t.
  liquid crystal t. (LCT)
thermolabile plastic
Thermold heat moldable shoe lining

NOTES

thermomassage
thermomechanical implant metal
   prosthesis
thermomoldable
   t. insert
   t. material
Thermophore
   T. hot pack
   T. moist heat pad
thermoplastic
   DynaPrene splinting t.
   t. elastomer (TPE)
   t. heating unit
   t. splint
   t. template
thermoregulate
thermoregulation
thermoregulatory sign
Thermoskin
   T. arthritic knee wrap
   T. brace
   T. heat retainer
ThermoSKY orthotic material
Thermosport hot/cold wrap
thermotherapy
Thero-Skin gel padding
thickened synovial membrane
thickening
   cortical t.
   heel pad t.
   lamellar t.
   ligamentous t.
   tendon t.
thickness
   cortical t.
   t. of heel pad
thick patella sign
Thiemann disease
Thiersch
   T. medium split free graft
   T. thin split free graft
   T. wire
thigh
   t. atrophy
   t. corset
   t. cuff
   t. holder
   t. shell
   t. tourniquet
thigh-foot angle (TFA)
thigh-shank plane
thin
   t. disk
   t. glenoid retractor
   t. osteotome
   t. pin fixation
Thinline uncovered orthotic
THINSite dressing

thin-wire Ilizarov fixator
thiomalate
thiopental sodium
thiosulfate
third
   distal t. (D/3, distal/3)
   t. fibular muscle
   middle t. (M/3)
   proximal t. (P/3)
   Steel rule of t.'s
third-generation cementing technique
THKAFO
   trunk-hip-knee-ankle-foot orthosis
Thomas
   T. buckle sling
   T. cervical collar brace
   T. classification
   T. collar cervical orthosis
   T. extrapolated bar graft
   T. fixator
   T. frame
   T. full-ring splint
   T. heel
   T. heel orthosis
   T. hinged splint
   T. knee splint
   T. Kodel sling
   T. leg splint
   T. needle
   T. posterior splint
   T. procedure
   T. rigid collar
   T. sign
   T. splint with Pearson attachment
   T. suspension splint
   T. test
   T. traction
   T. walking brace
   T. walking caliper
   T. wrench
Thomasen test
Thomas-Thompson procedure
Thomas-Thompson-Straub
   T.-T.-S. transfer
   T.-T.-S. transfer technique
Thompson
   T. anterolateral approach
   T. anteromedial approach
   T. arthroplasty
   T. excision
   T. femoral neck prosthesis
   T. frame
   T. hemiarthroplasty hip prosthesis
   T. hip endoprosthesis system
   T. hip prosthesis forceps
   T. leg check system
   T. modification of Denis Browne
   splint

T. nail
T. posterior radial approach
T. quadricepsplasty
T. rasp
T. resection
T. sign
T. telescoping V osteotomy
T. test
Thompson-Epstein classification
Thompson-Henry
T.-H. approach
T.-H. technique
Thompson-Loomer technique
Thompson-Parkridge-Richards (TPR)
T.-P.-R. ankle prosthesis
Thomsen disease
thoraces (*pl. of* thorax)
thoracic
t. approach
t. bone
t. curve
t. curve scoliosis
t. duct
t. duct injury
t. epidural injection
t. extension component
t. facet fusion
t. hypokyphosis
t. inlet syndrome
t. kyphosis
t. manual traction
t. microtrauma
t. nerve
t. nerve injury
t. nerve palsy
t. orthosis (TO)
t. outlet syndrome (TOS)
t. pedicle
t. pedicle marker
t. plane
t. spinal fusion
t. spine (T-spine)
t. spine biopsy
t. spine decompression
t. spine fracture
t. spine kyphotic deformity
t. spine lordosis
t. spine orthosis
t. spine pedicle diameter
t. spine scoliotic deformity
t. spine vertebral osteosynthesis
t. vertebra

thoracoabdominal
t. approach
t. artery injury
t. incision
thoracoacromial artery
thoracodorsal
t. artery transfer
t. nerve
t. nerve injury
thoracoepigastric flap
thoracolumbar
t. burst fracture
t. corset
t. curve
t. erector spinae
t. idiopathic scoliosis
t. junction
t. junction surgical exposure
t. kyphoscoliosis
t. kyphosis
t. orthosis
t. pedicle screw
t. retroperitoneal approach
t. spinal injury
t. spine
t. spine anterior exposure
t. spine decompression
t. spine flexion-distraction injury
t. spine fracture-dislocation
t. spine scoliosis
t. spine stabilization
t. spine vertebral osteosynthesis
t. spondylosis
t. spondylosis surgical technique
t. standing orthosis brace
t. trauma
thoracolumbosacral
t. orthosis (TLSO)
t. orthosis—flexion, extension, lateral bending, and transverse rotation (TLSO-FELR)
t. plate
t. spine
t. strain (TLS)
thoracoscapular arthrodesis
thoracotomy
t. approach
left-sided t.
right-sided t.
standard t.
thorax, pl. **thoraces**
thorn sign

NOTES

T

Thornton
- T. bar
- T. nail
- T. nail plate
- T. screw

Thornwald antral drill

THORP
- titanium hollow screw osseointegrating reconstruction plate
- THORP system

THR
- total hip replacement

threaded
- t. cancellous screw
- t. cortical dowel
- t. fusion cage (TFC)
- t. guidepin
- t. rod
- t. Steinmann pin
- t. titanium acetabular prosthesis (TTAP)
- t. wire

threaded-hole-first technique

three-beat clonus

three-body wear

three-bone forearm

Three Color Concept of Wound classification

three-column
- t.-c. cervical spine injury
- t.-c. concept
- t.-c. spine
- t.-c. spine theory

three-cornered bone

three-dimensional (3D)
- t.-d. analysis

three-edge cutting forceps

three-finger spica cast

three-hole
- t.-h. plate
- t.-h. suture tendon fixation

three-in-one diamond bur

three-jaw chuck

three-joint complex

three-part fracture

three-phase bone scan

three-plane deformity

three-point
- t.-p. bending moment
- t.-p. gait
- t.-p. pressure cast
- t.-p. pressure system
- t.-p. pressure technique
- t.-p. skeletal traction

three-portal technique

three-prong
- t.-p. headrest
- t.-p. rake blade retractor

three-quarters prone position

three-two Weitlaner self-retaining retractor

three-wheel walker

threshold
- anaerobic t. (AT)
- bone conduction t.
- cutaneous pressure t.
- experimental t.
- lactate t. (LT)
- lactic acidosis t.
- mechanical pain t. (MPTh)
- pressure t.
- reflex t.
- t. stimulus
- Than anaerobic t.
- vibration perception t. (VPT)

thrombectomy

thrombin powder

thrombin-soaked Gelfoam

thrombocytopenia

thrombocytopenia-absent
- t.-a. radius (TAR)
- t.-a. radius syndrome

thromboembolic
- t. disease (TED)
- t. stockings

thromboembolism

thromboembolus

thrombogenesis

thrombophilia

thrombophlebitis
- femoroiliac t.

thrombosed

thrombosis, pl. **thromboses**
- deep venous t. (DVT)
- effort t.
- effort-induced t.
- iliofemoral t.
- t. radial artery
- silent t.
- venous t.

Thrombostat

through-and-through
- t.-a.-t. fracture
- t.-a.-t. tear
- t.-a.-t. V-shaped horizontal osteotomy

through stance

through-the-knee amputation

thrower's
- t. elbow
- t. fracture

throwing
- t. function
- t. injury

thrust
- adjustive t.

double-thumb t.
lateral-to-medial t.
t. manipulation
pattern of t.
t. plate prosthesis (TPP)

thumb
abducted t.
adducted t.
adductor sweep of t.
Bennett fracture of t.
bifid t.
bowler's t.
breakdancer's t.
clasped t.
congenital clasped t.
cortical t.
t. deformity
duplicate t.
t. duplication
t. extensor tendon
t. flexor tendon
floating t.
Flotan t.
t. forceps
gamekeeper's t.
hypoplastic t.
t. instability
t. interphalangeal extension assist
jeweler's t.
laparoscopic surgeon's t.
t. loop
low-set t.
mallet t.
t. metacarpal
t. metacarpophalangeal joint
  approach
t. opposition
t. pinch power
t. polydactyly
t. post
proximal annular pulley of the t.
t. reconstruction
t. screw
short t.
skier's t.
spatulate t.
t. spica
t. spica cast
spring swivel t.
supernumerary t.
surgeon's t.
tennis t.

trigger t.
triphalangeal t.
t. web
t. web splint
thumb-in-palm deformity
Thumbkeeper
Freedom T.
thumbnail test
thumb-pinch grasp
thumb-to-forearm test
Thumper device
ThumZ'Up thumb splint
Thurston-Holland
T.-H. flag sign
T.-H. fracture
T.-H. fragment
thyroid
t. cartilage
t. gland
thyrotropin-releasing hormone
Ti-Bac
T.-B. acetabular component
T.-B. II hip prosthesis
tibia, pl. **tibiae**
absent t.
t. bone
t. coordinate system
corticotomy of proximal t.
distal t.
dysplastic t.
groove distal t.
lip of t.
malleolus tibiae
malleolus medialis tibiae
medial malleolus of t.
osteochondrosis deformans tibiae
Phemister medial approach to t.
proximal t.
saber t.
transmetaphyseal amputation of t.
t. valga
t. vara
tibial
t. acceleration
t. adamantinoma
t. aimer
t. aligner
t. artery
t. axial load injury
t. base plate
t. bolt
t. bone defect regeneration

T

NOTES

tibial *(continued)*
t. bone graft
t. bowing
t. channel
t. collateral ligament (TCL)
t. collateral ligament bursitis
t. Collet
t. component
t. condyle
t. cutting block
t. cutting guide
t. defect
t. diaphysial shortening
t. drill guide
t. driver
t. eminence
t. endoprosthesis
t. epiphysis
t. footprint
t. fracture brace proximal support (TFB-PS)
t. guidepin
t. hallux sesamoid
t. head screw
t. hemimelia
t. hindfoot osteomusculocutaneous rotationplasty
t. insert
t. jig
t. lengthening
t. lift-off
t. longitudinal deficiency
t. malleolus
t. medullary canal
t. metaphysis
t. mortise
t. muscle
t. nerve
t. nerve injury
t. phenomenon
t. pin
t. plafond
t. plateau
t. plateau fracture-dislocation
t. plateau prosthesis
t. pseudarthrosis
t. punch
t. resector
t. retractor
t. retroflexion
t. retrotorsion
t. retroversion
t. rim
t. sesamoid
t. sesamoid ligament
t. sesamoid position (TSP)
t. slope
t. spacer

t. stylus
t. talar tilt/tibiotalar tilt (TTT)
t. tendon
t. torsion
t. torsion system
t. track holder
t. track template
t. tray
t. tubercle
t. tubercle avulsion
t. tubercle prominence
t. tuberosity
t. tuberosity fractures in children classification
t. tuberosity osteotomy
t. tunnel
t. tunnel enlargement
t. tunnel widening
t. varus
t. vein
t. wedge

tibialis
t. anterior
t. anterior muscle
t. anterior tendon
apophysitis t.
t. posterior dislocation
t. posterior function
t. posterior muscle
t. posterior tendon
t. sign

tibioadductor reflex
tibioastragalocalcaneal Richet canal
tibiocalcaneal
t. arthrodesis
t. fusion
t. joint complex
t. ligament
t. medullary nailing
t. space

tibiofemoral
t. alignment
t. angle (TFA)
t. articulation
t. interaction
t. joint

tibiofibular
t. articulation
t. clear space
t. cyst
t. diastasis
t. fracture
t. fusion
t. joint
t. joint dislocation
t. joint instability
t. joint reduction
t. ligament

t. line
t. overlap
t. overlap measurement
t. rotation
t. sprain
t. subluxation
t. synchondrosis
t. syndesmosis
t. synostosis
tibionavicular ligament
tibiotalar
t. angle
t. arthritis
t. clear space
deep anterior t. (DATT)
deep posterior t. (DPTT)
t. diastasis
t. fusion
t. impingement
t. instability
t. joint
t. joint primary arthrodesis
t. stability
superficial t. (STT)
tibiotalocalcaneal
t. arthrodesis
t. fusion
Tibone posterior capsulorrhaphy
Tib-Transformer orthosis
tic
articulatory t.
ticlike pain
Ti/CoCr hip prosthesis
Ticonium splint
Ti-Con prosthesis
tie
free t.
table t.
Tiemann nail
tie-over bolster
tier
Harris wire t.
Tietze syndrome
Ti-Fit total hip system
Tiger blade
tight
t. retinacular ligament test
t. spinal canal trefoil canal
tightener
Charnley wire t.
Kirschner t.

Sklar wire t.
wire t.
tightness
adductor hamstring t.
hamstring t.
Tikhoff-Linberg
T.-L. radical arm procedure
T.-L. shoulder girdle resection
Tilastin hip prosthesis
tile
T. classification
t. plate facet replacement
T. polytrauma algorithm
T. view
Tillaux-Chaput
T.-C. fracture
T.-C. tubercle
Tillaux fracture
Tillaux-Kleiger fracture
Tillman prosthesis
tilt
angular t.
anterior pelvic t.
anteroposterior t.
cock-robin head t.
manual talar t.
mediolateral t.
palmar t.
pelvic lateral t.
posterior pelvic t.
sacral t.
subtalar t.
superoinferior t.
t. table
talar t. (TT)
tibial talar tilt/tibiotalar t. (TTT)
T. and Turn Paragon bed
varus t.
t. wrist
4XP T. System wheelchair
tilting
coronal t.
t. frame wheelchair
t. reflex
Tilt-In-Space wheelchair conversion
tilt-up test
TIME
toddler and infant motor evaluation
time
capillary refill t.
conduction t.
cycle t.

NOTES

time *(continued)*
    double support t.
    echo t.
    floating t.
    intercritical t.
    loading t.
    operating t.
    partial thromboplastin t. (PTT)
    procedure t.
    prothrombin t. (PT)
    reaction t.
    repetition t. (TR)
    rise t.
    step t.
    stride t.
    swing t.
    tincture of t. (TOT)
    total end-range t. (TERT)
    total tourniquet t.
    tourniquet t.
    warm ischemic t.
timed Allen test
TiMesh implantable hardware fixation
timing
    right/left t.
TIMP
    Test of Infant Motor Performance
    tissue inhibitor of metalloproteinase
tincture
    t. of belladonna
    t. of benzoin
    t. of time (TOT)
tinea
    t. cruris
    t. gladiatorum
    t. pedis
    t. versicolor
Tinel-Hoffmann sign
Tinel sign
Tinetti gait assessment
Ti-Nidium alloy
Tiobi transfer
tip
    acromionizer t.
    Cloward cervical drill t.
    Fragmatome t.
    Frazier suction t.
    t. of medial malleolus
    sacral bone t.
    screw t.
    suction t.
    Woodruff t.
tip-pinch dynamometry
tiptoe gait
TIRR
    The Institute for Rehabilitation Research
    TIRR foot-ankle orthosis

Ti-spacer
    Cohort T.-s.
Tisseel fibrin glue
Tissucol
tissue
    adipose t.
    t. anchor guide (TAG)
    bursal t.
    capsular support t.
    capsuloligamentous t.
    cartilaginous t.
    t. compression test
    connective t.
    Conrad-Bugg trapping of soft t.
    t. debris
    devitalized t.
    t. elongation
    t. expander
    exuberant granulation t.
    fatty t.
    fibroadipose t.
    fibrocartilaginous t.
    fibroconnective t.
    fibrofatty t.
    fibrous scar t.
    t. forceps
    granulation t.
    hypertrophic granulation t.
    t. inhibitor of metalloproteinase (TIMP)
    intervening connective t.
    ligamentous support t.
    t. mandrel implant material
    muscular t.
    necrotic t.
    neural t.
    t. nutrition
    osseous t.
    periarticular t.
    perineural t.
    periosteal t.
    pharyngeal t.
    t. pressure
    t. pressure measurement
    pressure-sensitive t.
    pressure-tolerant t.
    t. protector
    t. repair
    revascularized t.
    scar t.
    t. scissors
    skeletal t.
    t. slack
    soft t.
    subcutaneous t.
    t. texture abnormality (TTA)
    t. transfer
    t. transplant

t. transplantation
vascular t.
viable t.
viscoelastic t.
TissueTak corkscrew implant
tissue-type plasminogen activator
Titan
T. Apollo electric flexion table
T. cemented hip prosthesis
T. Meridian Intersegmental Traction table
T. Nova manual flexion-extension multi flex table
titanium
t. alloy
t. cable
t. circumferential grommet
t. half pin
t. hip prosthesis
t. hollow screw osseointegrating reconstruction plate (THORP)
t. hollow screw plate system
t. implant
t. implant material
t. implant prosthesis
t. mandibular plate
t. microsurgical bipolar forceps
t. nail
plasma-sprayed t.
t. screw
titanium-alloy implant
titer
antistreptolysin-O t. (ASOT)
Ti-Thread prosthesis
Titian hip prosthesis
Titus
T. forearm splint
T. wrist splint
Tivanium
T. cancellous bone screw
T. hip prosthesis
T. implant metal
T. implant metal prosthesis
TJ
triceps jerk
TJA
total joint arthroplasty
TJR
total joint replacement
TKA
total knee arthroplasty
trochanter-knee-ankle

TKR
total knee replacement
TLC
therapeutic lifestyle change
TLS
thoracolumbosacral strain
TLS strain
TLSO
thoracolumbosacral orthosis
TLSO brace
TLSO-FELR
thoracolumbosacral orthosis—flexion, extension, lateral bending, and transverse rotation
TMA
transmalleolar axis
transmetatarsal amputation
true metatarsus adductus
TMA prosthesis
TMJ
temporomandibular joint
TMJ halter
TMT
tarsometatarsal
TN
talonavicular
TN joint
T-nail
TNS
tension night splint
TO
thoracic orthosis
Toad finger splint
tobramycin-impregnated PMMA implant
Tobruk splint
Todd gait
toddler and infant motor evaluation (TIME)
toddler's fracture
Todd-Wells guide
toe
t. alignment
t. amputation
Astroturf t.
t. block anesthesia
t. box
Butler procedure to correct overlapping t.'s
t. cap
Clanton turf t.
claw t.
t. clawing

NOTES

toe *(continued)*
    clubbed t.
    cock-up deformity of t.
    t. comb
    t. crest
    crossover second t.
    curly t.
    distal tuberosity of t.
    downgoing t.'s
    DuVries technique for
      overlapping t.
    t. extensor
    t. extensor muscle
    t. extensor tendon
    extra t.
    flail t.
    t. flexion
    t. flexor
    t. flexor muscle
    floating t.
    floppy t.
    t. gait
    great t.
    t. gripping exercise
    hammer t.
    t. implant
    t. index
    jogger's t.
    lesser t.
    t. loop
    mallet t.
    marathoner's t.
    medial crossover t.
    medial deviation of the second t.
    Morton t.
    overlapping fifth t.
    overriding fifth t.
    over-straight t.
    painful t.
    t. phenomenon
    t. plate
    t. plate extension
    t. pressure
    Primus flexible great t.
    t. prosthesis
    push-off by great t.
    t. raise exercise
    t. range of motion
    t. reflex
    runner's t.
    sausage t.
    searching big t.
    t. separator
    set angle of t.
    t. spacer
    spacer between t.'s
    t. spica cast
    splaying of t.

    sportsman's t.
    t. spread sign
    stiff t.
    striatal t.
    supernumerary t.
    tennis t.
    turf t.
    underlapping t.
    unilaterally upgoing t.
    upgoing t.'s
    V-Y plasty correction of varus t.
    t. walk
    t. walking
    webbed t.
    t. wedge
Toe-Aid dressing
toe-drop brace
toe-ground purchase
toe-heel gait
toeing-in gait
toeing out
toeing-out gait
toenail
    dystrophic t.
    ingrowing t.
    ingrown t.
    onychomycotic t.
Toennis tumor forceps
ToeOFF orthosis
toe-off phase of gait
toe-out angle
toe-phalanx transplantation
toe-straight device
toe-toe gait
toe-to-groin
    t.-t.-g. cast
    t.-t.-g. modified Jones dressing
toe-to-hand transfer
toe-to-midthigh cast
toe-touch weightbearing
toe-walker
    idiopathic t.-w. (ITW)
toe-walking gait
toggle
    screw t.
    t. sign
toggle-recoil adjustment
Toglia Category Assessment Test (TCAT)
Tohen-Carmona-Barrera transfer
Tohen tendon technique
tolerance
    fatigue t.
    pressure t.
tolerated
    weightbearing as t. (WBAT)
Tomasini brace
Tomberlin-Alemdaroglu splint

Tommy trapeze bar
tomogram
tomography
    computed t. (CT)
    computerized axial t. (CAT)
    conventional t.
    emission t.
    helical computed t.
    hypocycloidal ankle t.
    positron emission t. (PET)
    preoperative t.
    quantitative computed t. (QCT)
    single photon emission computed t.
     (SPECT)
    transpiral t.
    trispiral t.
Tom Smith arthritis
tone
    muscle t.
    sphincter t.
tone-inhibiting leg cast
tone-reducing ankle-foot orthosis
  (TRAFO)
tongs
    Barton t.
    Barton-Cone t.
    Böhler t.
    cervical fracture t.
    Cherry traction t.
    cranial t.
    Crutchfield-Raney t.
    Gardner-Wells t.
    Raney-Crutchfield t.
    skull t.
    traction t.
    Trippi-Wells traction t.
    Vinke skull traction t.
tongue fracture
tongue-in-groove
    t.-i.-g. advancement
    t.-i.-g. recession
tonic
    t. muscle
    t. neck reflex
tonicity
    symmetric t.
tonification therapy
tonus
    myogenic t.
tool
    Acuforce 7.0 therapy t.
    AcuPressor myotherapy t.

    Adolescent and Pediatric Pain T.
     (APPT)
    ArthroWand t.
    Backnobber II massage t.
    Gore smoother crucial t.
    Index Knobber II massage t.
    Magnassager massage t.
    one-handed kitchen t.
    Original Backnobber massage t.
    Original Index Knobber II
     massage t.
    OsteoStat disposable power t.
    Therapress pressure point release t.
too-many-toes sign
tooth, pl. teeth
    Hutchinson teeth
toothed
    t. cutter
    t. tissue forceps
    t. washer
top
    circular laminar hook with offset t.
Topaz manual flexion table
top-entry (open body) hook
tophaceous
    t. deposit
    t. gout
tophectomy
tophus, pl. tophi
    gouty t.
topical
top-loading screw and rod system
topography
    internal t.
Toradol
Torg
    T. classification
    T. fracture
    T. knee reconstruction
    T. technique
Torgerson-Leach modified technique
torn
    t. ligament
    t. meniscus
tornado injury
Tornwaldt bursitis
Torode-Zieg classification
Toronto
    T. brace
    T. Medical CPM exerciser
    T. parapodium orthosis

T

NOTES

Toronto *(continued)*
    T. pelvic fracture classification
    T. splint
TORP
    total ossicular replacement prosthesis
    Plastiport TORP
    TORP prosthesis
torque
    t. curve
    t. force
    frictional t.
    t. heel shoe
    t. load
    peak t.
    t. production
    rotatory t.
    screw t.
    t. screwdriver
    supination t.
    t. wrench
torque-meter
    Compudriver digital t.-m.
torsion
    angle of t.
    t. bar
    t. bar splint
    t. dystonia
    external tibial t.
    femoral t.
    femorotibial t.
    internal tibial t. (ITT)
    internal tibiofibular t.
    medial t.
    t. neurosis
    tibial t.
    t. unit
    t. wedge fracture nonunion
torsional
    t. abnormality
    t. alignment
    t. deformity
    t. fracture
    t. gripping strength
    t. load
    t. overload
    t. stiffness
    t. stress
torsionometer
torticollis
    acquired t.
    congenital t.
    dermatogenic t.
    fixed t.
    intermittent t.
    mental t.
    muscular t.
    myogenic t.
    neurogenic t.

    nonspasmodic t.
    spasmodic t.
    spurious t.
    symptomatic t.
tortipelvis
torus
    T. external fixation system
    t. fracture
    regeneration t.
TOS
    thoracic outlet syndrome
TOT
    tincture of time
total
    t. active motion (TAM)
    t. anatomical hinge knee brace
    t. ankle arthroplasty (TAA)
    t. ankle replacement (TAR)
    t. arthrodesis of the wrist
    t. articular replacement arthroplasty
      (TARA)
    t. articular replacement arthroplasty
      prosthesis
    t. articular resurfacing arthroplasty
      (TARA)
    t. body movement
    t. body water
    T. Concept ankle/foot prosthesis
    t. condylar III (TC-III, TCP III)
    t. condylar III fully constrained
      prosthesis
    t. condylar knee
    t. condylar knee prosthesis
    T. Condylar Knee system
    t. condylar prosthesis III (TCP-III)
    t. condylar semiconstrained
      tricompartmental prosthesis
    t. contact bivalve ankle-foot
      orthosis
    t. contact cast
    t. contact casting (TCC)
    t. contact orthosis (TCO)
    t. contact shell ankle-foot orthotic
    t. contact socket
    t. elbow arthroplasty
    t. end-range time (TERT)
    T. Environment Control (TEC)
    t. eversion range of motion
    T. Gym
    T. Gym rehabilitation system
    t. hip arthroplasty (THA)
    t. hip articular replacement by
      internal eccentric shells
      (THARIES)
    t. hip replacement (THR)
    t. hip replacement prosthesis
    t. hip stabilization orthosis
    t. joint arthroplasty (TJA)

t. joint replacement (TJR)
t. joint replacement prosthesis
t. knee arthroplasty (TKA)
T. Knee for Children
t. knee implant
t. knee instrumentation
T. Knee prosthesis
T. Knee 2100 prosthetic knee
t. knee replacement (TKR)
t. knee replacement prosthesis
t. matrixectomy
t. maxillary osteotomy
t. meniscectomy
t. mesenteric apron method
t. necrosis
t. ossicular replacement prosthesis
  (TORP)
t. parenteral nutrition (TPN)
t. passive motion (TPM)
t. patellectomy
t. patellofemoral joint arthroplasty
t. range of motion (TROM)
t. replacement joint
t. rotating knee (TRK)
T. Shock prosthesis
t. shoulder arthroplasty
t. talus fracture
t. tourniquet time
t. transfer (TT)
t. wrist arthroplasty
TotalGym Exercise Program
Totallift-II
Toti trephine drill
toto
  in t.
tottering gait
touchdown weightbearing
touch sensation
Touch-Test sensory evaluator
tourniquet
  Accuflate t.
  arthroscopic t.
  Bodenstab t.
  t. control
  Digikit finger t.
  digital t.
  double t.
  Esmarch t.
  finger t.
  forearm t.
  t. gauge
  t. ischemia

t. palsy
t. paralysis
pneumatic ankle t.
t. pressure
Profex arthroscopic t.
t. test
thigh t.
t. time
upper arm t.
towel
  Charnley t.
  t. clamp
  t. clip
  t. exercise
  t. roll
  sterile t.
Townley
  T. anatomic knee system
  T. bone graft screw
  T. femur caliper
  T. TARA prosthesis
  T. tibial plateau plate
  T. total knee prosthesis
Townley-horizontal platform prosthesis
Townsend
  T. Rebel convertible brace
Townsend-Gilfillan
  T.-G. plate
  T.-G. screw
toxemia
toxicity
  aluminum t.
  methotrexate t.
Toygar angle
TPC
  thenar palmar crease
TPE
  thermoplastic elastomer
  TPE ankle-foot orthosis
  TPE biomechanical foot orthosis
T-pin
  Delitala T-p.
  T-p. handle
T-plasty modification of Bankart
  shoulder operation
TPM
  total passive motion
TPN
  total parenteral nutrition
TPP
  thrust plate prosthesis
  TPP hip endoprosthesis

T

NOTES

747

TPR
    Thompson-Parkridge-Richards
    TPR ankle prosthesis
TPT
    trigger point therapy
TR
    repetition time
TR-28
    TR-28 hip prosthesis
    TR-28 total hip replacement
trabecula, pl. trabeculae
    partially necrotic osseous t.
trabecular
    t. bone
    t. index of Singh
    t. traction
Trac
    T. II knee implant
    T. II knee prosthesis
trace
    SimplyStable t.
tracer catheter
tracheal injury
trachelomastoid muscle
tracheostomy
tracheotomy tube
tracing
    nerve t.
track
    Frenkel t.
    pin t.
track-bound joint
tracker
    T. knee brace
    Palumbo patella t.
    patella t.
tracking
    patellar t.
tract
    anterior spinocerebellar t.
    anterior spinothalamic t.
    gastrointestinal t.
    iliotibial t.
    lateral corticospinal t.
    pyramidal t.
    sinus t.
    spinal cord t.
    spinocerebellar t.
    spinothalamic t.
    urinary t.
    vestibulospinal t.
traction
    90-90 t.
    ambulatory t.
    t. anchor
    Anderson t.
    AOA halo cervical t.
    Apley t.

    t. application
    t. atrophy
    autologous t.
    axial t.
    axis t.
    Baker trabecular t.
    balanced skeletal t.
    balanced suspension t.
    banjo t.
    t. bar
    Barton-Cone tong t.
    Bendixen-Kirschner t.
    bidirectional t.
    bipolar vertebral t.
    Blackburn t.
    Böhler tong t.
    Borchgrevin t.
    t. bow
    t. bow nut
    Bremer halo cervical t.
    Bryant t.
    Buck t.
    calcaneal pin t.
    Carpal Trac t.
    t. cast
    cervical AOA halo t.
    cervical halter t.
    cervical manual t.
    C-Flex supine cervical t.
    Chattanooga t.
    Cherry tong t.
    Cotrel t.
    Crego-McCarroll t.
    Crile head t.
    Crutchfield skeletal tong t.
    device for transverse t. (DTT)
    Dunlop t.
    Econo-Cerv supine cervical t.
    Econo 90 lumbar home t.
    ElastaTrac lumbar t.
    elastic t.
    t. epiphysis
    t. epiphysitis
    Exo-Static t.
    t. exostosis
    external t.
    fingertrap t.
    floating t.
    t. footpiece
    t. fracture
    Freiberg t.
    Frejka t.
    Gallo t.
    Gardner-Wells tong t.
    gentle t.
    Georgiade visor cervical t.
    Graham t.
    Granberry t.

halo t.
halo-dependent t.
halo-extension t.
halo-femoral t.
halo-hyperextension t.
halo-pelvic t.
halo-wheelchair t.
halter t.
Hamilton t.
t. handle
Handy-Buck t.
Hare t.
head-halter t.
Hoke-Martin t.
Holter t.
HomeStretch lumbar t.
t. hook
Houston halo cervical t.
Hoyer t.
Ingebrightsen t.
inhibitive t.
intermittent cervical t. (ICT)
isometric t.
isotonic t.
Jones suspension t.
Kessler t.
Keys-Kirschner t.
King cervical t.
Kirschner skeletal t.
Kuhlman t.
leg t.
Logan t.
longitudinal t.
low-profile halo t.
lumbar t.
lumbosacral t.
Lyman-Smith t.
lympha press t.
manual t.
McBride tripod pin t.
metatarsal t.
Miami Acute collar cervical t.
Miami J collar cervical t.
Necktrac t.
Neufeld roller t.
t. neurapraxia
ninety-ninety t.
Orr-Buck t.
Ortho-Vent t.
overhead olecranon t.
Pease-Thomson t.
pelvic hyperextension t.

Perkins t.
Peterson t.
Philadelphia collar cervical t.
t. pin
pounds of t.
Pronex home t.
Pronex pneumatic cervical t.
Pugh t.
pulp t.
Quantum 400 t.
Quigley t.
Raney-Crutchfield tong t.
Roger Anderson t.
rubber band t.
Russell skeletal t.
Saunders t.
Sayre suspension t.
sequential pneumatic pump t.
simple shoulder test thermal
  alteration Thomas t.
skeletal t.
skin t.
snug t.
t. splint
split Russell skeletal t.
t. spur
static t.
Steinmann t.
t. stirrup
sugar-tong t.
supine C-Trax t.
suspension t.
Syms t.
tape t.
Thomas t.
thoracic manual t.
three-point skeletal t.
t. tongs
t. tongs screw
trabecular t.
transverse t.
vertical t.
Vinke tong t.
Watson-Jones t.
weight t.
well-leg t.
Wells t.
Whitman t.
Zimfoam splint t.
traction-absorption
  Weber-Vasey t.-a.

T

NOTES

tractograph
    MOM t.
Tracto-Halter
    T.-H. gait
    T.-H. training
tractor
    Hamilton pelvic traction screw t.
    Zim-Trac traction splint t.
tractotomy
TRAFO
    tone-reducing ankle-foot orthosis
    TRAFO orthosis
Trager method
Tragerwork
trailer
    leaders and t.'s
train
    near-constant frequency t.'s
trainer
    athletic t.
    Biodex Gait T.
    Biodex target balance t.
    dynamic stabilization t.
    impulse inertial exercise t.
    Kinesthetic Ability T. (KAT)
    Monark Rehab T.
    Posture Pump Spine T.
    Shuttle Balance t.
    Sprint cross t.
training
    activity t. (AT)
    ankle disk t.
    balance board t.
    bowel t.
    DAPRE strength t.
    t. diet
    eccentric muscle t.
    endurance t.
    Fartlek t.
    flexibility t.
    functional t.
    gait t.
    hypertrophic strength t.
    interval t.
    isometric t.
    isotonic t.
    light intensity t.
    neural strength t.
    neurodevelopmental t.
    periodization of t.
    physical t. (PT)
    progression of t.
    proprioceptive t.
    propriosensory t.
    prosthetic t.
    prosthetic gait t.
    relaxation t.
    resistance t.

    t. room
    sensory-motor t.
    speed play t.
    stabilization t.
    strength t.
    Tracto-Halter t.
    variable resistance t.
    weight t.
trampoline injury
transacromial
    t. approach
    t. coracoacromial ligament repair
transaminase
    glutamic-oxaloacetic t.
    glutamic-pyruvic t.
transarticular
    t. pin
    t. screw
    t. screw fixation
    t. wire fixation
transaxillary approach
trans-bone plasty
transbrachioradialis approach
transcalcaneal approach
transcapitate
    t. fracture
    t. fracture-dislocation
transcapitellar
    t. pin
    t. wire fixation
transcarpal amputation
transcervical femoral fracture
transchondral fracture
transclavicular approach
transcondylar
    t. amputation
    t. axis (TCA)
    t. fracture
transcutaneous
    t. crush injury
    t. electrical nerve stimulation
        (TENS)
    t. oxygen
    t. oxygen tension determination
transducer
    ergonomically designed t.
    force t.
    FT03C t.
    Hall-effect strain t.
    in-shoe t.
    linear-variable-differential t.
    magnetic motion t.
    pressure t.
    rotatory-variable-differential t.
    Therasound t.
transection
    step-cut t.
transepicondylar axis

transepiphysial
    t. fracture
    t. separation
transfemoral
    t. alignment
    t. amputation
    t. amputee
    t. suspension
transfer
    anterior t.
    anteromedial tubercle t.
    autogenous osteocartilage t.
    Baker lateral semitendinosus t.
    Barr anterior t.
    bed-to-chair t.
    biceps brachialis muscle t.
    t. board
    bone t.
    Boyes t.
    Boyle-Thompson tendon t.
    brachioradialis t.
    Brooks-Jones tendon t.
    Brooks-Seddon pectoralis major
      tendon t.
    Brooks-Seddon tendon t.
    Brown fibular t.
    Buncke t.
    Bunnell posterior tibial tendon t.
    Caldwell-Durham tendon t.
    Camitz tendon t.
    Campbell t.
    Chandler tendon t.
    Chaves muscle t.
    Chaves-Rapp muscle t.
    Clark pectoralis major t.
    Columbus McKinnon assist for
      lifting or t.
    composite free tissue t.
    coracoacromial ligament t.
    Couch-Derosa-Throop t.
    crossed intrinsic t.
    Dickson muscle t.
    distal t.
    double tendon t.
    Drennan posterior t.
    dynamic muscle t.
    Eggers t.
    extensor digitorum t.
    extensor hallucis longus t.
    extensor tendon t.
    fibular t.
    Flatt tendon t.

flexor digitorum longus tendon t.
flexor to extensor tendon t.
flexor-to-extensor tendon t.
Fowler tendon t.
free flap t.
free gracilis muscle t.
free tissue t.
free toe t.
Gage distal t.
Ganley tendon t.
gastrocnemius tendon t.
Girdlestone tendon t.
Green t.
Green-Banks t.
T. Handle support handle
Harmon t.
Henry muscle t.
Hiroshim t.
His-Haas muscle t.
Hoffer split t.
Hovanian latissimus dorsi muscle t.
Huber abductor digiti quinti t.
Ikuta pectoralis major t.
iliopsoas t.
iliotibial band t.
independent t.
ion t.
Johnson-Spiegl tendon t.
Jones t.
Kessler posterior tibial tendon t.
Lamb muscle t.
lateral t.
t. lesion
Littler-Cooley abductor digiti
  quinti t.
Littler-Cooley muscle t.
magnetization t.
Manktelow pectoralis major t.
McLaughlin subscapularis t.
Menelaus triceps t.
t. metatarsalgia
microvascular osseous t.
Moberg deltoid muscle t.
Moberg deltoid-to-triceps t.
muscle t.
Mustard iliopsoas t.
neuromuscular t.
Neviaser-Wilson-Gardner t.
Ober anterior t.
Ober-Barr procedure for
  brachioradialis t.
opponens t.

T

NOTES

transfer *(continued)*
    patellar tendon t. (PTT)
    pedicled fibular t.
    peroneus brevis t.
    posterior deltoid-to-triceps t.
    posterior tibial tendon t.
    semitendinosus tendon t.
    Sharrard posterior t.
    single-stage tissue t.
    split anterior tibialis tendon t.
        (SPLATT)
    static tendon t.
    stress t.
    subscapularis tendon t.
    Sutherland lateral t.
    tendon t.
    Thomas-Thompson-Straub t.
    thoracodorsal artery t.
    Tiobi t.
    tissue t.
    toe-to-hand t.
    Tohen-Carmona-Barrera t.
    total t. (TT)
    vascularized osseous t.
    Vastamäki muscle t.
    Whitman muscle t.
    wraparound neurovascular composite
        free tissue t.
    wrap-around toe t.
transfer/augmentation
    FHL tendon t.
transfibular
    t. approach
    t. arthrodesis
    t. fusion
TransFix
    T. ACL system
    T. ACL system fixation
transfixation amputation
transfixing pin
transfixion
    t. bolt
    t. screw
transformation
transforming growth factor (TGF)
transfusion
    autologous blood t.
    blood t.
    t. therapy
transglenoid suture repair
transhamate
    t. fracture
    t. fracture-dislocation
transhumeral amputation
transient
    t. bone marrow edema
    t. bone marrow edema syndrome
    t. clonus

    t. epiphysitis
    t. lesion
    t. neurapraxia
    t. osteopenia
    t. osteoporosis
    t. quadriplegia
    t. synovitis
transiliac
    t. amputation
    t. bar technique
    t. fracture
    t. lengthening
    t. rod fixation
transition
    cervicothoracic t.
transitional vertebra
**Translating and Congruent Mobile-
    Bearing Knee (TACK)**
translation
    anterior t.
    anterior talar t. (ATT)
    anteroposterior t.
    caudal t.
    cephalad t.
    coronal plane deformity sagittal t.
    dorsal t.
    t. injury
    t. mobility
    t. motion
    obligate t.
    posterior t.
    ulnar t.
    vertical t.
translational
    t. displacement
    t. osteotomy
    t. position
translatory
    t. force
    t. motion
translocation
    ulnar t.
translumbar amputation
transmalleolar
    t. ankle
    t. ankle arthrodesis
    t. axis (TMA)
    t. portal
transmetacarpal amputation
transmetaphyseal amputation of tibia
transmetatarsal
    t. amputation (TMA)
    t. capsulotomy
transmission
    t. electron microscopy
    impulse-based nerve t.
    nerve t.

nociceptive t.
nonimpulsed base nerve t.
transmitter
chest-band t.
transmitter-receiver
Itrel programmed t.-r.
transolecranon approach
transoral odontoid resection
transosseous suture
transparent
t. adhesive dressing
t. template
transpatellar tendon portal
transpedal
t. multiplanar wedge fusion
t. multiplanar wedge osteotomy
transpedicular
t. approach
t. fixation
t. fixation effective pedicle
diameter
t. screw
transpedicularly implanted anterior
spinal support device
transpelvic amputation
transperitoneal
t. approach
t. exposure
transphalangeal amputation
transpiral tomography
Transpire wrist orthosis
transplant
Bosworth femoroischial t.
D'Aubigne patellar t.
Elmslie-Trillat t.
fibular t.
free vascularized bone t.
one-half patellar tendon t.
patellar t.
pedicled t.
pes anserinus t.
Slocum pes anserinus t.
tissue t.
vascularized bone t.
whole bone t.
whole fibular t.
transplantation
allograft t.
t. antigen
autogenous cartilage t.
Bosworth femoroischial t.
Cowen-Loftus toe-phalanx t.

femoroischial t.
meniscal autograft t.
muscle-tendon t.
osteoarticular allograft t.
tendon t.
tissue t.
toe-phalanx t.
transposing index ray
transposition
dorsal subcutaneous nerve t.
t. flap
intermuscular neuroma t.
intramuscular nerve t.
intraosseous nerve t.
plantar t.
subcutaneous anterior t.
subfascial t.
tendon t.
transpositional
transsacral
t. block
t. fracture
transscaphoid
t. dislocation fracture
t. perilunate dislocation
transsphenoidal dissector
transsternal approach
transsyndesmotic screw fixation
transtendocalcaneus portal
transtentorial brainstem
transthoracic
t. approach
t. lateral view
transtibial
t. amputation
t. immediate postoperative
prosthesis
transtriquetral
t. fracture
t. fracture-dislocation
transtrochanteric
t. approach
t. rotational osteotomy
t. valgus osteotomy (TVO)
transversalis fascia
transversarium
foramen t.
transverse (TV)
t. amputation
t. approach
t. axis
t. axis knee flexion

T

NOTES

transverse *(continued)*
  t. capsulotomy
  t. connector
  t. deficiency
  t. disk
  t. fixation
  t. fixator application
  t. friction massage
  t. friction therapy
  t. humeral ligament test
  t. incision
  t. ligament of knee
  t. ligament rupture
  t. line of Park
  t. loading device
  t. myelopathy
  t. pedicle angle
  t. pedicle diameter
  t. plane
  t. plane motion insufficiency
  t. process
  t. process fracture
  t. process of sacrum
  t. process of vertebra
  t. screw
  t. tarsal articulation
  t. tarsal joint
  t. tear
  t. tenotomy
  t. traction
transversectomy
transversely
transversoplanus
  talipes t.
transversospinalis syndrome
transversum
transversus abdominis muscle
TRAP
  tartrate resistant acid phosphatase
trapdoor
trapeze bar
trapezia (*pl. of* trapezium)
trapezial
  t. area
  t. arthrosis
  t. prosthesis
  t. ridge
trapeziectomy
trapeziodeltoid interval
trapeziometacarpal
  t. capsule
  t. fusion
  t. joint
  t. joint replacement prosthesis
trapeziotrapezoidal joint
trapezium, pl. **trapezia**
  t. bone
  Burton-Pelligrini excising t.

  t. fracture
  t. implant prosthesis
  t. ossification
trapezius
  t. fiber analysis
  t. muscle
trapezoid
  t. bone
  t. bone of Henle
  t. bone of Lyser
  t. ligament
  t. line
  t. ossification
Trapezoidal-28 (T28)
  T.-28 hip prosthesis
  T.-28 internal prosthesis
trapezoidal resection osteotomy
trapezoideum
trapped meniscus
trapping
  Conrad-Bugg t.
  optical t.
  tendon t.
trauma
  arterial t.
  awakening t.
  birth t.
  cervical spine t.
  craniospinal t.
  high-energy t.
  hyperextension t.
  hyperflexion t.
  lumbar spine t.
  multiple t.
  musculoskeletal t.
  nonosseous tissue t.
  nonunion fracture t.
  repetitive t.
  t. score
  thoracolumbar t.
  t. view
trauma-induced membrane
traumatic
  t. abscess
  t. amputation
  t. anterior instability
  t. arthritis
  t. bone cyst
  t. brain injury (TBI)
  t. brain injury-related ataxia
  t. brain injury-related neglect
  t. burn injury
  t. cervical discopathy
  t. cervical disk herniation
  t. compartment syndrome
  t. dislocation
  t. displacement
  t. hemiplegia

t. neuroma
t. osteoarthritis
t. paraplegia
t. prepatellar neuralgia
t. sinus
t. spondylolisthesis
t. synovitis
t. tetraplegia
t. unidirectional Bankart lesion
   surgery (TUBS)
traumatic, unidirectional instability and Bankart lesion
traumatized ligament
Trautman Locktite prosthetic hook
Trautmann chisel
traverse amputation
tray
Alcon Instrument Delivery
   System t.
Bucky x-ray t.
CAPIS screw assortment t.
Denis Browne t.
glenoid metal t.
one-time sharp débridement t.
PFC offset tibial t.
surgical hand t.
tibial t.
x-ray t.
Treace stapes drill
treatment
acid t.
active t.
adjustive t.
bone cyst t.
Boyd-Ingram-Bourkhard t.
Carrel t.
closed t.
cold laser t.
compression rod t.
distraction-compression scoliosis t.
dual compression scoliosis t.
IonGuard orthopedic surface t.
Keesay t.
Kenny t.
low-friction ion t. (LFIT)
manual t.
neurodevelopmental t.
neuromuscular reflex t.
neuromuscular scoliosis orthotic t.
nonoperative t.
osteopathic manipulative t.
Parabath paraffin heat t.

paraffin t.
poliomyelitis t.
rehabilitation t.
ReJuveness scar t.
SB+ testing and t.
SB− testing and t.
shock t.
spasticity t.
surgical t.
ulcer t.
Tredex
Universal T.
tree
BTE Assembly T.
Finger Blocking T.
pinch t.
pipe t.
trellis formation
tremor
action t.
contraction t.
essential t.
intention t.
pill rolling t.
postural t.
resting t.
tremulor
tremulousness
trench foot
Trendelenburg
T. gait
T. limp
T. lurch
T. position
T. sign
T. test
trephine
bone t.
Castroviejo t.
t. drill
hollow bone t.
Michele vertebral t.
t. needle biopsy
Phemister biopsy t.
Trethowan metatarsal osteotomy
Trethowan-Stamm-Simmonds-Menelaus-Haddad technique
Trevor disease
triad
Charcot t.
female athletic t.
t. knee repair

NOTES

triad (*continued*)
    t. of O'Donoghue
    T. prosthesis
    Virchow t.
    Waddell t.
triage
    sidelines t.
trial
    t. acetabular cup
    t. base plate
    clinical t.
    component t.
    t. of conservative therapy
    t. driver
    t. femoral component
    t. fit
    Fracture Intervention T. (FIT)
    t. implant
    lower hook t.
    t. prosthesis
    radial t.
    t. range of motion
    t. reduction
    t. seating
    t. spacer
    t. stem
    ulnar t.
    upper hook t.
    VIGOR t.
    Vioxx Gastrointestinal Outcomes
        Research t.
trialkylphosphine gold complex
triangle
    Alsberg t.
    anal t.
    anterior t.
    aponeurotic t.
    t. blade system
    Bryant t.
    Burow t.
    Burrow t.
    cervical t.
    clavipectoral t.
    Codman t.
    Hardy-Joyce t.
    iliofemoral t.
    IMP knee positioning t.
    infraclavicular t.
    Kager t.
    Kanavel t.
    knee positioning t.
    Langenbeck t.
    metal measuring t.
    Middeldorpf t.
    neutral t.
    Petit t.
    posterior t.
    Rauchfuss t.

    sacral t.
    Volkman t.
    von Weber t.
    Ward t.
    Weber t.
Tri-angle shoulder abduction brace
triangular
    t. advancement flap
    t. ankle fusion frame
    t. arm sling
    t. bandage
    t. base transverse bar configuration
    t. bone reamer
    t. compression device
    t. defect
    t. disk of wrist
    t. external ankle fixation
    t. fibrocartilage
    t. fibrocartilage complex (TFC,
        TFCC)
    t. fibrocartilage complex tear
    t. ligament
    t. medullary nail
    t. muscle
    t. pillow splint
    t. rasp
    t. working zone
    t. wrist bone
triangulated pedicle screw
triangulate triple frame
triangulating
triangulation
    indirect t.
    t. technique
    t. technique for arthroscope
triaxial
    t. motion
    t. semiconstrained elbow prosthesis
    t. total elbow arthroplasty
Tri-Axial prosthesis
**Triax monotube external fixation
    system**
tricalcium phosphate
triceps
    t. brachii tendon
    t. jerk (TJ)
    t. jerk reflex test
    t. skinfold test
    t. surae jerk
    t. surae muscle
    t. surae reflex
    t. surae release
tricepsplasty
trichterbrust
tricipital muscle
trick
    t. knee
    t. movement

Tricodur
- T. compression support bandage
- T. Epi compression bandage
- T. Epi compression dressing
- T. Omos compression bandage
- T. Omos compression dressing
- T. Talus compression bandage
- T. Talus compression dressing

tricompartmental
- t. implant
- t. knee prosthesis

Tri-Con component

Tricon-M
- T.-M component
- T.-M cruciate-sparing prosthesis
- T.-M patellar prosthesis

Tri-Core cervical support pillow

tricorrectional bunionectomy

tricortical
- t. iliac crest bone graft
- t. ilial strip graft

trident hand

triethiodide

triflanged
- t. Lottes nail
- t. medullary nail

Tri-Flex auxiliary suspension belt

Tri-Float pressure reduction mattress

trifurcation

trigeminal neuralgia

trigger
- t. digit
- t. finger
- t. finger release
- t. finger syndrome
- t. point
- t. point injection
- t. point therapy (TPT)
- t. thumb
- t. thumb release

TriggerWheel
- T. device
- T. Wand

trigonum

trilaminate cushion

trilateral knee-ankle-foot orthosis

trileaflet prosthesis

Trillat
- T. arthroplasty
- T. osteotomy
- T. procedure

Tri-Lock
- T.-L. press-fit prosthesis
- T.-L. total hip prosthesis with Porocoat

trilogy
- T. acetabular cup system
- T. prosthesis

trimalleolar ankle fracture

Trimedyne Omnipulse holmium laser

Trimline knee immobilizer

trimmer
- motorized t.

Tri-Motion Knee System

trinkle
- T. bone drill
- T. brace
- T. brace and adapter
- T. chuck adapter
- T. power drill
- T. screwdriver
- T. Super-Cut twist drill

Trio arthroscope

triode

Trio-Stim neuromuscular stimulator

tri-panel knee immobilizer

tripartite
- t. bone
- t. muscle origin

triphalangeal
- t. thumb
- t. thumb deformity

triphase technetium scintigraphy

triphasic action potential

Tripier amputation

triplanar
- t. protractor
- t. protractor apparatus

triplane
- t. construct
- t. motion
- t. osteotomy
- t. tibial fracture

triple
- t. arthrodesis
- t. bundle technique
- t. discharge
- t. envelope system
- t. frame
- t. hemisection
- t. innominate osteotomy
- t. ligamentous repair
- t. reamer

NOTES

T

triple *(continued)*
    t. tarsal fusion
    t. tenodesis
triplegia
triple-injection cinearthrography
triple-jump test
triple-phase
    t.-p. bone scan
    t.-p. isotope bone scan
triple-wire
    t.-w. fusion
    t.-w. procedure
    t.-w. technique
triploscope
tripod
    t. cane
    t. foot
    McBride t.
    t. sign
tripoding gait
Trippi-Wells traction tongs
tripsis
triquetral fracture
triquetrolunate
    t. dislocation
    t. instability
triquetrum
    t. bone
    t. ossification
triquetrum-lunate arthrodesis
triradial
    t. cartilage
    t. resector blade
triradiate
    t. acetabular extensile approach
    t. cartilage
    t. incision
    t. transtrochanteric approach
trisalicylate
triscaphe
    t. arthrodesis
    t. fusion
    t. joint
trismus
trispiked
trispiral tomography
TriStander
triton tumor
trivector retaining approach
Tri-Wedge total hip system
Tri W-G table
TRK
    total rotating knee
trocar
    blunt t.
    sharp t.
    T-handled t.

trochanter
    greater t.
    t. holder
    lesser t.
trochanter-holding clamp
trochanteric
    t. advancement
    t. band
    t. bolt
    t. bursa
    t. bursitis
    t. migration
    t. osteotomy
    t. pin
    t. reamer
    t. shift
    t. slide
    t. spine
    t. syndrome
    t. wire
trochanter-knee-ankle (TKA)
trochanterplasty
trochlea peronealis
trochlear
    t. defect
    t. groove
    t. notch
trochoid
    t. articulation
    t. joint
Troemner percussion hammer
troika
    aponeurotic t.
trolley
    Bolero lift bath t.
    Tupper t.
TROM
    total range of motion
    TROM knee brace
Trömner
    T. percussion
    T. test
Tronzo
    T. elevator
    T. intertrochanteric fracture
      classification
    T. prosthesis
trophic
    t. change
    t. fracture
    t. joint disorder
    t. ulcer
    t. ulceration
trophoneurosis
    muscular t.
tropism
    facet t.
tropometer

trough
- bone t.
- t. line
- t. sign

trousers
- military antishock t. (MAST)

Trousseau point

Trow Bridge
- T. Terra-Round all-terrain prosthesis
- T. TerraRound foot
- T. TerraRound sports limb
- T. triple-speed drill

Trowbridge-Campau bone drill

true
- t. acetabular region
- t. acetabulum
- t. ankylosis
- T. Blue exercise band
- t. lateral view
- t. metatarsus adductus (TMA)
- t. rib
- t. spacer
- t. vertebra

True/Fit femoral intramedullary rod system

True/Flex
- T. intramedullary nail
- T. intramedullary rod system

True-Lok
- T.-L. external fixation
- T.-L. external fixator system

Tru-Fit
- T.-F. brace
- T.-F. custom molded shoe

Trumble
- T. arthrodesis
- T. talectomy

Trümmerfeld
- T. line
- T. zone

Tru-Mold shoe

truncal dysmetria

truncated
- t. tarsometatarsal wedge arthrodesis
- t. wedge tarsometatarsal arthrodesis vertical talus

trunk
- anatomic nerve t.
- t. control
- t. curl
- t. incurvation test
- t. righting

- t. shift
- t. stabilization rehabilitation program
- sympathetic t.

Trunkey
- T. fracture classification
- T. fracture classification system

trunk-hip-knee-ankle-foot orthosis (THKAFO)

trunnion-bearing hip prosthesis

TruStep foot prosthesis

Tru-Support
- T.-S. EW bandage
- T.-S. SA bandage

Tsai-Stillwell procedure

Tscherne classification

Tscherne-Gotzen tibial fracture classification

T-shaped
- T-s. AO plate
- T-s. capsulotomy
- T-s. fracture
- T-s. incision
- T-s. inserter

TSP
- tibial sesamoid position

T-spine
- thoracic spine

TSRH
- Texas Scottish Rite Hospital
  - TSRH buttressed laminar hook
  - TSRH circular laminar hook
  - TSRH corkscrew device
  - TSRH crosslink
  - TSRH crosslink stabilization
  - TSRH crosslink system
  - TSRH double-rod construct
  - TSRH eyebolt spreader
  - TSRH fixation system
  - TSRH hook holder
  - TSRH hook inserter
  - TSRH hook-rod
  - TSRH implant
  - TSRH instrumentation
  - TSRH L-bolt
  - TSRH mini-corkscrew device
  - TSRH pedicle hook
  - TSRH pedicle screw
  - TSRH plate
  - TSRH rod fixation
  - TSRH spinal implant system
  - TSRH trial hook

NOTES

TSRH (continued)
    TSRH Universal spinal
      instrumentation system
    TSRH wrench
T-Stick adhesive
T-strap
    medial T-s.
Tsuge
    T. debulking
    T. tendon repair
Tsuji laminaplasty
TT
    talar tilt
    total transfer
    TT Pylon prosthesis
TTA
    tissue texture abnormality
TTAP
    threaded titanium acetabular prosthesis
    TTAP prosthesis
TTAP-ST acetabular prosthesis
TTR
    tarsal tunnel release
TTS
    tarsal tunnel syndrome
TTT
    tibial talar tilt/tibiotalar tilt
tube
    Adson suction t.
    Baron suction t.
    chest t.
    Dawson-Yuhl suction t.
    digit t.
    Dynamic digit extensor t.
    endoneural t.
    Esmarch t.
    Exerband Pak bilateral t.
    Exerband Pak unilateral t.
    Ferguson-Frazier suction t.
    t. flap graft
    t. foam
    Gillquist suction t.
    t. guide
    Hemovac suction t.
    irrigation t.
    Jergesen t.
    stockinette t.
    suction t.
    tracheotomy t.
    vent t.
TubeGauz bandage
tuber angle
tubercle
    adductor t.
    anterior tibial t.
    articular bone t.
    t. avulsion
    Chaput t.

    Chassaignac t.
    conoid t.
    Gerdy t.
    Ghon t.
    lateral tibial t.
    Lisfranc t.
    Lister t.
    medial t.
    t. osteotomy
    Stieda t.
    talus lateral t.
    tibial t.
    Tillaux-Chaput t.
    Wagstaff t.
tubercular granuloma
tuberculoma
    bone t.
tuberculosis
    diaphysial t.
    extraarticular t.
    t. of hip
    metaphysial t.
    osteoarticular t.
    skeletal t.
    spinal t.
tuberculous
    t. arthritis
    t. dactylitis
    t. lesion
    t. peroneal tenosynovitis
    t. rheumatism
    t. sequestrum
    t. spinal osteomyelitis
    t. spondylitis
    t. synovitis
    t. trochanteric bursitis
    t. vertebral osteomyelitis
tuber-joint angle
tuberosity
    adductor t.
    t. avulsion fracture
    bicipital t.
    calcaneal t.
    t. of calcaneus
    t. of clavicle
    coracoid t.
    cuboidal t.
    femoral t.
    t. fracture
    t. fragment
    greater t.
    iliac t.
    infraglenoid t.
    ischial t.
    t. joint angle
    lateral t.
    lesser t.
    navicular t.

parietal t.
patellar t.
posterior t.
radial t.
sacral t.
supraglenoid t.
tibial t.
ulnar t.
ungual t.
ununited tibial t.
tuberous xanthoma
Tubersitz amputee gait
Tubex gauze dressing
Tubigrip
T. bandage
T. dressing
T. glove
tubing
Dakin t.
elastic t.
Fit-Lastic therapy t.
foam t.
gel t.
medullary vent t.
PVC t.
Silipos mesh t.
Thera-Band t.
TUBS
traumatic unidirectional Bankart lesion surgery
TUBS procedure
Tubsider Kneeling Seat
tubular
t. bone plate
t. elastic bandage
t. punch
t. stockinette
tubularization of the graft
tubulization
tucker
Bishop-Black tendon t.
Bishop-DeWitt tendon t.
Bishop-Peter tendon t.
Burch-Greenwood tendon t.
tendon t.
tuck sign
Tudor-Edwards bone-cutting forceps
Tuf Nex neck exerciser
Tuf-Skin tape adherent
TufStuf II cast tape
tuft
distal t.

finger t.
t. fracture
tuftal resorption
tufted phalanx
Tuke saw
Tukey test
Tuli
T. Pro Heel Cup
T. rubber heel cup
TuliGel heel cup
tulip pedicle screw
Tullos technique
tumble
T. Forms feeder
T. Forms roll
tumbler graft
tumefaction
tumor
Abrikossoff t.
aggressive t.
ball-valve t.
Bednar t.
benign t.
blood vessel t.
bone-forming t.
bone marrow t.
brown fat t.
cartilaginous t.
cerebellopontine angle t.
Codman t.
cortical desmoid t.
cystic t.
desmoid t.
dumbbell t.
Enneking staging of malignant soft tissue t.
epidermal cell t.
epiphysial chondromatous giant cell t.
Ewing t.
extraabdominal desmoid t.
fatty tissue t.
fibroblastic t.
fibroid t.
fibrous t.
giant cell t. (GCT)
glomus t.
Gubler t.
histiocytic t.
hyperparathyroidism t.
intraosseous t.
lipid t.

NOTES

T

tumor *(continued)*
    lumbar t.
    mesenchymal t.
    metastatic spinal t.
    nerve sheath t.
    neural t.
    neuroectodermal t.
    occult primary malignant t.
    plexiform fibrohistiocytic t.
    pluripotential mesenchymal t.
    Pott puffy t.
    primary t.
    t. resection
    Schwann t.
    soft tissue t.
    spinal t.
    superior sulcus t.
    synovial t.
    tenosynovial giant cell t.
    t. therapy
    triton t.
    vascular t.
    vertebral body t.
    t. vessel
    xanthomatous giant cell t.
tumoral calcinosis
tumor-bearing bone
tumor-grasping forceps
tumorous
    t. condition
    t. involvement
tumor-replacement endoprosthesis
tunnel
    bone t.
    carpal t. (CT)
    cubital t.
    t. drill guide
    femoral t.
    fibroosseous t.
    Gaynor-Hart x-ray position of
      carpal t.
    t. locator guide
    osseous t.
    peroneal t.
    radial t.
    subsartorial t.
    talar neck t.
    tarsal t.
    tibial t.
    ulnar t.
    t. view
tunnel-and-sling fixation
tunneler
    tendon t.
Tunneloc bone mulch screw
Tunturi hand exerciser
Tuohy lumbar puncture needle
Tupman plate

Tupper
    T. arthroplasty
    T. hand-holder and retractor
    T. trolley
Turco
    T. clubfoot release
    T. clubfoot release technique
    T. oblique posteromedial incision
    T. posteromedial release
    T. repair of talipes equinovarus
Turco-Spinella tendo calcaneus repair
turf
    t. toe
    t. toe grading
    t. toe injury
turgor
Turkel bone biopsy
TurnAide therapeutic system
turnbuckle
    t. ankle brace
    t. cast
    t. distractor
    t. elbow splint
    t. jack
    t. knee brace
    t. wrist orthosis
turn-down tendon flap
Turn-Easy transfer aid
turned-up pulp deformity
turner
    T. pin
    T. prosthesis
    rotating t.
    T. syndrome
Turning Board Exercise System
turnstile casting stand
turret exostosis
turtle neck nail
Turvy internal screw fixation
Turyn sign
Tutofix cortical pin
Tuxedo collar
TV
    transverse
TVO
    transtrochanteric valgus osteotomy
tweezers
    Kaprelian easy-access t. (KEAT)
twin-blade oscillating saw
Twin Cities Lo-Profile halo
twist
    t. drill
    t. drill point
    t. hook
twisted plate
twister
    Axel wire t.
    Batzdorf cervical wire t.

t. cable
cerclage wire t.
Cooley-Baumgarten wire t.
Miltex wire t.
orthotic coiled spring t.
Shifrin wire t.
twitch muscle
two-arm goniometer
two-column cervical spine injury
two-hole plate
two-inclinometer method
two-part
t.-p. Apley test
t.-p. fracture
two-plane
t.-p. bilateral external fixator
t.-p. bilateral frame
t.-p. deformity
t.-p. fluoroscopy
t.-p. roentgenogram
t.-p. unilateral external fixator
t.-p. unilateral frame
two-point
t.-p. discrimination
t.-p. discrimination test
t.-p. gait
t.-p. nerve block
t.-p. step-to gait pattern
two-portal technique
two-poster
t.-p. brace
t.-p. cervical orthosis

two-prong
t.-p. rake retractor
t.-p. stem finger prosthesis
Tworek screw guide
two-sleeve technique
two-stage
t.-s. hip fusion
t.-s. tendon grafting technique
t.-s. tendon graft reconstruction
two-strut tibial graft technique
TX-1, TX-7 traction table
Tycron suture
tying forceps
Tylok high-tension cable system
tyloma
tympanic bone
type
T. C-50, C-90 AFO
contraction t.
t. II curve pattern
t. 501, 502, 504, 602 finger splint
foot t.
frequency, intensity, time, t. (FITT)
t. I, II, III, IIIA, IIIB, IIIC open
   fracture
rectus foot t.
Sanders t.
sleeve t.
typhoid osteomyelitis
Tyrell hook

T

NOTES

U

U Luque vertebral rod
U osteotomy
U wrench

UBC

University of British Columbia
UBC brace

UBE

uniaxial balance evaluation
upper body ergometer

UBIS

ultrasound bone imaging sonometer

UBP

universal bone plate
UBP system

UCB

unilateral calcaneal brace
University of California, Berkeley
UCB foot orthosis
UCB shoe insert

UCBL

University of California, Berkeley
Laboratory
UCBL foot plate
UCBL orthosis

UCI

University of California, Irvine
UCI ankle prosthesis
UCI unconstrained prosthesis

UCL

ulnar collateral ligament

UCLA

University of California, Los Angeles
UCLA anatomic shoulder
arthroplasty
UCLA CAPP TD hook
UCLA functional long leg brace
UCLA Shoulder Rating scale

UCOheal orthotic
UCOlite orthosis
UCO Quick-Sil silicone system
UE

upper extremity
UE Tech Weight Well Exercise
System

Ueba release
Uematsu shoulder arthrodesis
UFO

Universal plantar fasciitis orthotic
Orthomerica UFO

UFOS

universal frame outer socket

UHMWPE

ultrahigh molecular weight polyethylene
UHMWPE prosthesis

UHR locking ring mechanism
Uhthoff

U. sign
U. syndrome

UID/S

unilateral interfacetal dislocation or
subluxation

UKA

unicompartmental knee arthroplasty

ulcer

decubitus u.
diabetic neurotrophic u.
ischemic u.
mal perforans u.
neuropathic u.
neurotrophic food u.
peptic u.
pressure u.
recalcitrant neuropathic u.
stasis u.
supramalleolar venous u.
u. treatment
trophic u.
Wagoner u.

ulceration

neuropathic forefoot u.
neurotrophic u.
sublesional u.
trophic u.

ulcerative mutilating acropathy
Ullmann line
Ullrich

U. drill
U. drill guard

ulna

absent u.
u. bone
distal u.
Monteggia fracture-dislocation of u.
proximal u.

ulnar

u. anlage
u. antebrachial region
u. artery
u. artery injury
u. bearing
u. bursa
u. carpal collateral ligament
u. clubhand
u. collateral ligament (UCL)
u. collateral ligament injury
u. collateral ligament rupture
u. collateral nerve of Krause
u. column
u. convexity

U

ulnar *(continued)*
- u. creaking
- u. cubital tunnel syndrome
- u. deviation
- u. deviation deformity
- u. dimelia
- u. drift
- u. drift deformity
- u. extensor
- u. grind test
- u. gutter splint
- u. head
- u. head excision
- u. head implant prosthesis
- u. hemiresection interposition arthroplasty
- u. impaction syndrome
- u. lengthening
- u. malleolus
- midcarpal u. (MCU)
- u. minus variance
- u. motor neurectomy
- u. nerve (UN)
- u. nerve block
- u. nerve entrapment
- u. nerve injury
- u. nerve motor/sensory electromyogram
- u. nerve palsy
- u. nerve paralysis
- u. nerve release
- u. neuropathy
- u. notch
- u. rasp
- u. recession
- u. reflex
- u. ruler
- u. sesamoid bone
- u. side grip
- u. styloid bone
- u. styloid fracture
- u. styloid impaction syndrome
- u. synovial recess
- u. translation
- u. translocation
- u. trial
- u. tuberosity
- u. tunnel
- u. wrist extensor tendinitis

ulnaris
- extensor carpi u. (ECU)
- flexor carpi u. (FCU)
- malleolus u.

ulnarward

ulnocarpal
- u. abutment

- u. abutment syndrome
- u. arthrodesis
- u. impaction syndrome
- u. impingement
- u. joint
- u. ligament

ulnohumeral
- u. angle
- u. joint

ulnolunate
- u. articulation
- u. ligament

ulnotriquetral ligament

ulnotriquetrum articulation

ULO
- upper limb orthosis

ULP
- upper limb prosthesis

Ulrich
- U. bone-holding clamp
- U. bone-holding forceps

Ulrich-St. Gallen forceps

Ulson fixator system

Ultec thin dressing

Ultima
- U. calcar stems
- U. C femoral component
- U. Fx stems
- U. hip replacement system
- U. total hip system

ultimate
- U. Cold N' Hot Pack
- U. Hand Helper strengthening program
- U. knee prosthesis
- u. strength

Ultimax distal femoral intramedullary rod system

Ultrabrace
- U. brace
- U. knee orthosis

Ultra-Cut instrument

Ultra-Drive
- U.-D. bone cement removal system
- U.-D. plug puller
- U.-D. ultrasonic revision system

ultraendurance

UltraFix
- U. MicroMite anchor suture
- U. MicroMite suture anchor
- U. RC suture anchor
- U. RC suture anchor system
- U. rotator cuff repair implant

Ultraflex
- U. Dynamic Joint
- U. orthopedic bed

Ultra-Guard
    U.-G. FS hip bracing system
    U.-G. hip orthosis system
ultrahigh molecular weight polyethylene (UHMWPE)
Ultra-Light athletic tape
UltraPower drill system
UltraSling
ultrasonic
    u. mobility aid
    u. probe
ultrasonography
    compression u.
    duplex Doppler u.
UltraSorb suture anchor
ultrasound (US)
    Amrex therapeutic u.
    u. bone imaging sonometer (UBIS)
    compression u.
    Doppler u.
    duplex u.
    u. electrotherapy
    u. phonophoresis
    pulsed u.
    quantitative u. (QUS)
    therapeutic u.
    u. therapy
ultrasound-guided
    u.-g. echo biopsy
    u.-g. stereotactic biopsy
ultrasound/stimulator
    SynchroSonic U/HVG50 u.
UltraStep orthotic
Ultra Stim silver electrode
ultraviolet (UV)
    u. light
    u. light pressure
Ultra-X external fixation system
ULTT
    upper limb tension test
umbau zone
umbilical tape
UMS
    upper fossa active, medial knee pain, and short leg on the side ipsilateral to the weak fossa
UN
    ulnar nerve
unassisted locking-suture technique
unbalanced
    u. depolymerization

    u. hemivertebra
    u. wrist syndrome
uncemented femoral component
unciform
    u. bone
    u. fracture
    u. process
uncinate
    u. bone
    u. hypertrophy
    u. process fracture
uncommitted metaphysial lesion
uncompensated rotary scoliosis
unconditional stimulus (US)
unconstrained
    u. shoulder arthroplasty
    u. tricompartmental knee prosthesis
uncoordinated gait
uncovertebral
    u. arthrosis
    u. joint
    u. spur
undecylenic
underarm
    u. body jacket
    u. brace
    u. cast
    u. orthosis
Underburger test
under direct vision
undergrowth
underlapping toe
undermined skin
underscoring
undersurface of patella
underwater Bovie
underwear
    HipSaver protective u.
undetermined
    etiology u.
undifferentiated oligoarthritis
undisplaced fracture
undyed suture
ungual
    u. process
    u. tuberosity
unguarded osteotome
unhappy triad of O'Donoghue
uniarticular
uniaxial
    u. balance evaluation (UBE)
    u. joint

U

NOTES

uniaxial *(continued)*
   u. strain gauge
   u. structure
unicameral bone cyst
Uni-Clip staple
unicompartmental
   u. knee arthroplasty (UKA)
   u. knee implant
   u. knee prosthesis
   u. knee system
unicondylar
   u. fracture
   U. Geomedic hemi-knee system
   u. prosthesis
unicortical screw
Uniflex
   U. calibrated step drill
   U. dressing
   U. drill bushing
   U. humeral nail
   U. intramedullary nail
   U. nailing system
Unilab
   U. Surgibone
   U. Surgibone bone replacement
    material
   U. Surgibone surgical implant
unilateral
   u. acute radicular syndrome
   u. calcaneal brace (UCB)
   u. chronic radicular syndrome
   u. facet subluxation
   u. interfacetal dislocation
   u. interfacetal dislocation or
    subluxation (UID/S)
   u. pedicle cannulation
   u. posterior-anterior movement
   u. sacroiliac approach
   u. spastic leg
   u. standing test
   u. variable screw placement system
unilaterally upgoing toe
Unilink system for hand surgery
unilocular joint
uninhibited
   u. ankle motion
   u. flexion
union
   bony u.
   u. broach retention drill
   u. broach retention pin
   callous bone u.
   delayed fracture u.
   European Chiropractic U.
   faulty u.
   fibrous u.
   osteonal bone u.
   Osteotron stimulator for bone u.

   primary bone u.
   secondary bone u.
   slow u.
   vicious u.
Unipen
unipennate muscle
Uniplane rocker
unipolar
   u. bearing
   u. cauterization
   u. cautery
   u. needle electrode
   u. release
uniportal
   u. arthroscopic microdiskectomy
   U. fascial release system
unisegmental mobility
unit
   AME microcurrent TENS u.
   Autoflex II, III CPM u.
   Back Bubble gravity traction u.
   Back Revolution traction/exercise u.
   basic multicellular remodeling u.
   BioMed TENS u.
   bone metabolic u.
   bone remodeling u.
   Bovie coagulating u.
   C-arm fluoroscopy u.
   Cybex Torso Rotation Testing and
    Rehabilitation U.
   Cybex Trunk Extension Flexion u.
   Dynasplint knee extension u.
   Eclipse TENS u.
   Econo 90 traction u.
   E-2 hydrocollator heating u.
   ElastaTrac home lumbar traction u.
   EMG retrainer biofeedback u.
   Exo-Bed traction u.
   Exo-Overhead traction u.
   functional spinal u. (FSU)
   G5 Fleximatic
    massage/percussion u.
   G5 Vibramatic
    massage/percussion u.
   home cervical traction u. (HCTU)
   Hydra-Cadence gait-control u.
   hydraulic knee u.
   Hydrocollator heating u.
   intervertebral motor u.
   JACE hand continuous passive
    motion u.
   JACE-STIM electrotherapy
    stimulation u.
   Magnatherm SSP electromagnetic
    therapy u.
   MENS u.
   motor u.
   musculotendinous u.

myofascial u.
myotatic u.
Orthodyne Enhancer u.
Orthotic Research and Locomotor
    Assessment U. (ORLAU)
over-the-door traction u.
Pebax counter u.
postanesthesia care u. (PACU)
rotator u.
single-axis knee u.
Solitens transcutaneous electrical
    nerve stimulation u.
u. spinal rod
Systems 2000 TENS u.
TENS u.
Thermalator heating u.
thermoplastic heating u.
torsion u.
vertebral motion u. (VMU)
wrist flexion u.

unitary plastic
United States (U.S.)
    U.S. Manufacturing Company
        (USMC)
Unitek steel crown
unitunnel technique
univalve cast
univalved
universal
    U. acromioclavicular splint
    U. AerobiCycle
    u. bone plate (UBP)
    U. bone plate system
    u. canvas body restraint
    u. coronal movement
    U. distal radius fracture
        classification
    U. drill point
    U. femoral head prosthesis
    U. Fitstep
    U. fixation screw
    u. frame outer socket (UFOS)
    u. full-circle manual goniometer
    U. gutter splint
    U. hex screwdriver
    U. hip prosthesis
    u. incision
    U. knee positioner
    U. lateral positioner
    U. modular femoral hip component
        extractor
    U. nail

U. plantar fasciitis orthotic (UFO)
u. precautions
U. I, II prosthesis
U. radial component
U. sacral spine instrumentation
u. sling
U. sling and swathe shoulder
    immobilizer
U. Spine Classification
U. Spine System (USS)
U. support splint
U. Tredex
u. tri-panel knee immobilizer
U. two-speed hand drill
U. wire clamp

Uni-Versatil sling
University
    U. of British Columbia (UBC)
    U. of British Columbia brace
    U. of California, Berkeley (UCB)
    U. of California, Berkeley
        Laboratory (UCBL)
    U. of California Berkeley
        Laboratory orthosis
    U. of California Biomechanics
        Laboratory heel cup
    U. of California cuff suspension
        PTB socket
    U. of California, Irvine (UCI)
    U. of California, Los Angeles
        (UCLA)
    U. of Florida LINAC
    Louisiana State U. (LSU)
unknown
    etiology u.
unleveling
    pelvic u.
Unloader
    U. ADJ Unloader brace
    U. Bi-ComPF knee brace
    U. Express Unloader brace
    U. Select Unloader brace
    U. Spirit knee brace
    The U
unlocking spiral technique
unmineralized osteoid
unmyelinated
Unna
    U. boot cast
    U. boot wrap
    U. paste

NOTES

U

Unna *(continued)*
    U. paste boot
    U. paste shell
Unna-Flex Plus venous ulcer kit
unopposed
unplanned valgus osteotomy
unreduced dislocation
unremodeled defect
unrestricted closed and open chain
  knee extension exercise
unscher wire
unsegmented vertebral bar
unsound ankylosis
unstable
    u. cervical spine injury
    u. fracture
    u. fracture-dislocation
    u. joint
unsteadiness of gait and station
unsteady gait
unstriated muscle
unsustained clonus
unthreaded wire
ununited
    u. fracture
    u. tibial tuberosity
unwinding
up
    U. and About system
    press u.
up-angle hook
upbiting
    u. basket forceps
    u. rongeur
upcurved punch forceps
upcut rongeur
upgoing toes
6U portal
upper
    u. arm tourniquet
    u. body cycle
    u. body ergometer (UBE)
    u. cervical spine anterior construct
    u. cervical spine anterior exposure
    u. cervical spine fusion
    u. cervical spine posterior construct
    u. cervical spine procedure
    u. extremity (UE)
    u. extremity myoelectric prosthesis
    u. fossa active, medial knee pain,
    and short leg on the side
    ipsilateral to the weak fossa
    (UMS)
    u. hand retractor
    U. 7 head halter
    u. hook trial
    u. limb orthosis (ULO)
    u. limb prosthesis (ULP)

    u. limb tension test (ULTT)
    u. limits of normal
    u. motor neuron disease
    u. motor neuron lesion
    u. thoracic spine
Uppsala screw
upright
    orthosis overlapped u.
    u. skeletal radiography
    u. view
upright-Y incision
uptake
    maximal oxygen u.
    maximum oxygen u.
upward-cutting triangular knife
urarthritis
Urbaniak
    U. neurovascular free flap
    U. scapular flap
Urban Walkers shoe
Ureacin-20
urethane
    Poron cellular u.
Urias
    U. air splint
    U. pressure splint
uric acid crystal
uricosuric agent
urinary
    u. incontinence
    u. nitrogen
    u. output
    u. tract
urine culture
urist view
urogenital diaphragm
urologic complication
US
    ultrasound
    unconditional stimulus
    US Manufacturing Air Castaway
U.S.
    United States
    U.S. Army bone chisel
    U.S. Army gouge
    U.S. Army osteotome
U-shaped
    U-s. incision
    U-s. retractor
Uslenghi
    U. drill guide
    U. plate
USMC
    United States Manufacturing Company
    USMC luxury liner
    USMC multiaxis ankle
    USMC stance locking safety knee
USP#2 suture

U-splint splint
USS
    Universal Spine System
ustilaginea
    necrosis u.
U-stirrup splint
Utah
    U. artificial arm
    U. artificial limb

utensil
    Good Grips u.
    swivel u.
Utrata forceps
UV
    ultraviolet

NOTES

U

V

  V blade plate
  V capsulotomy
  V nail plate
  V osteotomy
  V sign

V40

  V40 femoral head implant
    component
  V40 forged femoral head

V-A alignment rod

Vac

  Sani V.

vacant glenoid sign

Vac-Lok immobilization cushion

Vac-Pac

  V.-P. pad
  V.-P. positioner

Vacumix vacuum pump

vacuolar myelopathy

vacuum

  v. cement mix technique
  v. disk
  facet joint v.
  M-Pact cast v.

vagal reaction

vaginal

  v. hand ligament
  v. ligament of hand
  v. pack
  v. synovitis

vagoglossopharyngeal neuralgia

vagus nerve

Vainio arthroplasty

Valenti

  V. arthroereisis device
  V. arthroplasty
  V. procedure

Valentine splint

Valeo back support

valga

  coxa v.
  manus v.
  tibia v.

valgoid

valgum

  genu v.
  idiopathic genu v. (IGV)

valgus

  v. angle
  v. angulation
  v. bar
  calcaneal v.
  congenital convex pes plano v.
  v. contracture

convex pes v.
v. corrective ankle strap
cubitus v.
digitus v.
v. extension overload syndrome
flexible pes v.
v. foot
forefoot v.
genu v.
hallux v.
heel v.
v. heel deformity
hindfoot v.
idiopathic hallux v.
v. instability
juvenile hallux v.
v. knee
v. knee control pad
v. knee motion
McBride bunion hallux v.
metatarsus v.
pes plano v.
physiologic v.
rearfoot v.
senile hallux v.
v. stress
v. stress test
talipes convex pes v.
v. tilt of the talus

Valleix

  V. phenomenon
  V. sign

Valls hip prosthesis

Valls-Ottolenghim-Schajowicz needle
  biopsy

Valpar

  V. component work sample series
  V. Whole Body Range of Motion
    Test

Valrelease

Valsalva

  V. maneuver
  V. test

value

  mean v.
  Tanner-Whitehouse bone-age
    reference v.
  V. Walker brace

valve

  bulb and thumb screw v.
  Heyer-Schulte bur hole v.
  Quadtro cushion with Isoflap v.

vamp of shoe

Van

  V. Arsdale triangular splint

V

Van *(continued)*
    V. Beek nerve approximator
    V. Buren sequestrum forceps
    V. der Hoeve disease
    V. Neck disease
    V. Ness procedure
    V. Ness rotational arthroplasty
    V. Ness rotationplasty
    V. Rosen splint

van
    v. Gieson picrofuchsin stain

vanadium
Vanderbilt Pain Management Inventory
Vanghetti limb prosthesis
Vanore osteotomy
Vantage Performance monitor (VPM)
Vanzetti sign
VAPC
    Veterans Administration Prosthetic
    Center

VAPC dorsiflexion assist orthosis
Vapo coolant spray and stretch
vapor
    Mitek v.

vara
    adolescent tibia v.
    coxa v.
    developmental coxa v.
    false coxa v.
    infantile tibia v. (ITV)
    manus v.
    tibia v.

variable
    v. axis knee system
    v. circumference suprapatellar
      socket (VCSPS)
    v. flexion overhinge (VFO)
    metabolic v.
    v. resistance training
    v. screw placement (VSP)
    v. screw placement system
    v. screw placement system
      instrumentation
    v. screw placement system-
      instrumented lumbar spine
    v. screw plate (VSP)
    v. spinal plating (VSP)

variance
    negative ulnar v. (NUV)
    positive ulnar v. (PUV)
    ulnar minus v.

Vari-Angle
    V.-A. clip applier
    V.-A. screw

variant
    four-part v.

variation
    hindfoot anatomic v.
    postural v.

vari-balance board set
varices (*pl. of* varix)
varicosity
    superficial v.

Vari-Duct hip and knee orthosis
Vari-Firm Medicine Ball
VariFix spinal implant device
Vari-Flex prosthetic foot
VariGrip spinal implant device
Varikopf hip prosthesis
VariLock socket lock
varix, pl. **varices**
Varney
    V. acromioclavicular brace
    V. pin

Varni-Thompson Pediatric Pain
  Questionnaire
varum
    genu v.

varus
    calcaneal v.
    v. contracture
    v. corrective ankle strap
    cubitus v.
    digitus v.
    dynamic hallux v.
    forefoot v.
    genu v.
    hallux v.
    heel v.
    v. hindfoot
    v. hindfoot deformity
    v. knee
    v. knee control pad
    v. malalignment
    v. malunion
    metatarsus v. (MTV)
    metatarsus primus v. (MPV)
    metatarsus primus adductus (MPA)
    v. MTP angle
    pes v.
    v. plafond
    rearfoot v.
    v. rotational osteotomy (VRO)
    v. rotation shortening osteotomy
    v. stress test
    subtalar v.
    talipes v.
    tibial v.
    v. tilt

varus-valgus
    v.-v. adjustment screw
    v.-v. angulation
    v.-v. instability
    knee v.-v.

v.-v. lift-off
v.-v. plane
v.-v. stress of the elbow
vascular
v. accident
v. assessment
v. bundle implantation into bone
v. endothelium
v. forceps
v. gangrene
v. inflow
v. injury
v. invasion
v. metaphysial bone
v. nonunion
v. surgery
v. tissue
v. tumor
vascularity
femoral head v.
tenuous v.
vascularized
v. bone graft
v. bone transplant
v. fibular graft
v. free flap
v. osseous transfer
v. osteoseptocutaneous fibular
autogenous graft
v. rib strut graft
vasculature
vasculitis
mesenteric v.
rheumatoid v.
vasculopathy
vasoconstriction
vasoconstrictive therapy
vasocoolant spray
vasodilation
flow-mediated v. (FMD)
vasodilator
vasogenic shock
vasomotor
v. disorder
v. technique
vasopneumatic intermittent compression
vasopressor
vasospasm
vasospastic ischemia
Vastamäki
V. muscle transfer

V. paralysis
V. technique
vastus
v. intermedius
v. intermedius muscle
v. lateralis (VL)
v. lateralis muscle
v. lateralis ridge
v. medialis
v. medialis advancement (VMA)
v. medialis muscle
v. medialis obliquus (VMO)
v. medialis obliquus:vastus lateralis
(VMO:VL)
VATER
vertebral abnormality, anal imperforation,
tracheoesophageal fistula, and radial,
ray, or renal anomalies
vertebral (defects), (imperforate) anus,
tracheoesophageal (fistula), radial and
renal (dysplasia) anomalies
VATER syndrome
vault
plantar v.
VAX-D
vertebra axial decompression
VAX-D therapy table
VBI
vertebrobasilar insufficiency
VC
voluntary closing
voluntary control
VCSPS
variable circumference suprapatellar
socket
VD
video densitometry
VDA
video-dimensional analysis
VDDR
vitamin D-dependent rickets
VDRR
vitamin D-resistant rickets
VDS
ventral derotation spondylodesis
VDS compression rod
VDS hex nut
VDS screw
VDS screwdriver
VDS wrench
VE
vocational evaluation

V

NOTES

vector
    V. low back analysis system
    major injury v. (MIV)
    v. point
    v. quantity
vectored adjustment
vehicle
vein
    anterior jugular v.
    axillary v.
    v. of Batson
    Boyd communicating perforation v.
    brachiocephalic v.
    carotid v.
    cephalic v.
    Cockett communicating
      perforating v.'s
    common iliac v.
    grafting v.
    iliac v.
    iliolumbar v.
    innominate v.
    intercostal v.
    intermetatarsal v.
    internal iliac v.
    internal jugular v.
    lingual v.
    lumbar v.
    middle sacral v.
    middle thyroid v.
    peroneal v.
    popliteal v.
    saphenous v.
    subclavian v.
    superficial temporal v.
    superior thyroid v.
    tibial v.
    vertebral v.
vela (*pl. of* velum)
velar
    fronting of v.
Velcro
    V. extenders splint
    V. fitting
    V. Hand Exerboard
    V. immobilization
    V. immobilizer
    V. strap
Veleanu-Rosianu-Ionescu
    V.-R.-I. adductor tenotomy
    V.-R.-I. technique
velocity
    angular v.
    conduction v.
    free-walking v.
    maximum conduction v.
    maximum eversion v.
    maximum inversion v.

    mean flow v.
    motion v.
    motor conduction v.
    motor nerve conduction v.
      (MNCV)
    muscle fiber conduction v.
    nerve conduction v. (NCV)
    orthodromic v.
    peak height v. (PHV)
    propagation v.
    push-off v.
    sensory nerve conduction v.
Velpeau
    V. axillary lateral view
    V. axillary radiograph
    V. bandage
    V. cast
    V. deformity
    V. dressing
    V. plaster
    V. shoulder immobilizer
    V. shoulder sling
    V. sling-dressing
    V. stockinette
    V. wrap
velum, pl. **vela**
Venable
    V. plate
    V. screw
Venable-Stuck
    V.-S. fracture pin
    V.-S. nail
    V.-S. screw
Venn-Watson classification
Venodyne boot
venography
    epidural v.
    intraosseous v.
    magnetic resonance v.
Venosan
    V. support hose
    V. support sock
venous
    v. cleft
    v. compression
    v. foot pump
    v. thromboembolic disease (VTED)
    v. thrombosis
ventral
    v. derotating spinal wrench
    v. derotation spondylodesis (VDS)
ventriculography
ventriculoperitoneal shunt
vent tube
Verbrugge
    V. bone clamp
    V. bone-holding forceps
    V. needle

Verbrugge-Hohmann bone retractor
Verdan
    V. osteoplastic thumb reconstruction
    V. technique
Verebelyi-Ogston decancellation
  procedure
Veress needle
Verlow brace
Vermont
    V. pedicle fixation system
    V. spinal fixator (VSF)
    V. spinal fixator articulation
    V. spinal fixator clamp
Vernier
    V. caliber gauge
    V. caliper
Verocay body
verruca, pl. **verrucae**
    v. cryotherapy
    mosaic plantar v.
    single plantar v.
    v. vulgaris
verruciformis
    epidermodysplasia v.
verrucous lesion
Versaback back system
VersaBond medium viscosity bone
  cement
VersaClimber RX exercise machine
VersaFlex tubing kit
Versa-Fx
    V.-F. femoral fixation
    V.-F. femoral hip fixation system
Versa-Helper floor stand
Versalok low back fixation system
VersaPulse holmium laser
Versa-Stim self-adhering electrode
versatility
    attachment v.
Versa-Trac lumbar spine retractor
  system
Versa-Trainer exerciser
VersaWrist wrist splint
versicolor
    tinea v.
version
    external v.
    femoral neck v.
    Gait Abnormality Rating Scale
      Modified v. (GARS-M)
    internal v.

Versi-Splint carry bag
VerSys
    V. hip system
    V. prosthesis
VertAlign spinal support system
vertebra, pl. **vertebrae**
    apex v.
    apical v.
    v. axial decompression (VAX-D)
    basilar v.
    biconcave v.
    block v.
    body of v.
    butterfly v.
    caudal v.
    cervical v.
    cleft v.
    coccygeal v.
    codfish v.
    displaced v.
    dorsal v.
    end v.
    false v.
    first cervical v.
    fish v.
    fractured v.
    fused v.
    hourglass v.
    last normal v. (LNV)
    lumbar v.
    lumbosacral v.
    malposed v.
    midbody of v.
    neural tube defect-related anomaly
      of v.
    olisthetic v.
    pear-shaped v.
    v. plana
    v. prominens reflex
    sacral v.
    scalloping of v.
    second cervical v.
    stable v.
    subluxed v.
    thoracic v.
    transitional v.
    transverse process of v.
    true v.
    wasp-waist v.
    wedge-shaped v.
    wedging of olisthetic v.

V

NOTES

vertebral
- v. abnormality, anal imperforation, tracheoesophageal fistula, and radial, ray, or renal anomalies (VATER)
- v. adjustment
- v. angiography
- v. ankylosis
- v. arch
- v. arteriography
- v. artery
- v. artery test
- v. arthritis
- v. block
- v. body
- v. body anterior cortex
- v. body collapse
- v. body corpectomy
- v. body decompression
- v. body endplate
- v. body fracture
- v. body impactor
- v. body stapling wedge resection
- v. body tumor
- v. border
- v. canal
- v. column
- v. column cleft
- v. compression
- v. (defects), (imperforate) anus, tracheoesophageal (fistula), radial and renal (dysplasia) anomalies (VATER)
- v. derangement
- v. end plate
- v. exposure
- v. fascia
- v. formula
- v. fusion
- v. instability
- v. lesion
- v. level
- v. medicine
- v. motion segment
- v. motion unit (VMU)
- v. nerve
- v. neural reflection
- v. notch
- v. osteomyelitis
- v. osteosynthesis
- v. osteosynthesis fusion rate
- v. plana fracture
- v. polyarthritis
- v. rib
- v. ring apophysis
- v. rotation
- v. scalloping
- v. segmentation anomaly

- v. stable burst fracture
- v. steal phenomenon
- v. steal syndrome
- v. stripe
- v. subluxation
- v. subluxation complex (VSC)
- v. subluxation syndrome
- v. vein
- v. wedge compression fracture
- v. wedging

vertebrectomy
- Bohlman anterior cervical v.
- cervical spondylotic myelopathy v.
- microsurgical thoracoscopic v.

vertebrobasilar
- v. injury
- v. insufficiency (VBI)

vertebrocostal rib

vertebrogenic interference

vertebropelvic ligament

vertebroplasty

vertebrosternal rib

Verteflex
- V. arthrotonic stabilizer
- V. Intersegmental Traction Table

Vertetrac ambulatory traction system

vertical
- anatomical v.
- v. axis
- v. capsulotomy
- v. compression
- v. compression test
- v. foot board
- v. fracture
- v. loading
- v. longitudinal tear
- v. loop suture technique for meniscus repair
- v. mattress suture
- v. pedicle diameter
- v. plane
- v. sacral compaction
- v. sagittal split osteotomy (VSO)
- v. shear (VS)
- v. shear fracture
- v. shock pylon
- v. subsidence
- v. suspension reflex
- v. symphysial mobility
- v. talus
- v. talus foot deformity
- v. traction
- v. translation

verticality control

Vertstreken closed medullary nailing

very low calorie diet (VLCD)

vesalian bone

vesalianum

Vesalius bone
Vesely-Street
    V.-S. splint
    V.-S. split nail
vesicocutaneous fistula
vesicostomy
Vess chair
vessel
    v. clamp
    v. dilator
    endosteal v.
    great v.
    haversian v.
    v. hook
    humeral circumflex v.
    lymph v.
    milking of v.
    periosteal v.
    popliteal v.
    v. shifting
    tumor v.
vest
    Bremer AirFlo halo v.
    halo v.
    Little cargo v.
    Minerva v.
    Ortho-Trac pneumatic v.
    Standard E-Z-On V.
    Vitrathene v.
    weighted v.
vestibular ball
Vestibulator positioning tumble form
vestibulocerebellar ataxia
vestibulospinal
    v. reflex
    v. tract
vestigial muscle
Veterans Administration Prosthetic Center (VAPC)
VFO
    variable flexion overhinge
V1 halo ring
viability
viable tissue
Vibram
    V. rockerbottom shoe
    V. sole
Vibramat
vibration
    v. glove
    v. perception threshold (VPT)
    v. sensation

    v. sense
    v. sensitivity
    v. synovitis
    v. threshold test
    v. white finger syndrome
    whole-body v.
vibrative
vibrator
    v. hand syndrome
    Magic Wand v.
vibratory massage
vibrogram
    digital v.
vibromasseur
vibrometer test
vibrotherapeutics
vice
    mechanic pin v.
vicious union
Vicon three-dimensional gait analysis system
Vicryl suture
Victorian brace
Vidal-Adrey
    V.-A. fracture technique
    V.-A. modified Hoffman external fixation device apparatus
    V.-A. modified Hoffmann external fixation device
    V.-A. modified Hoffmann fixation
video densitometry (VD)
video-dimensional analysis (VDA)
videofluoroscopy
video-gate analysis
videoradiography
vidian neuralgia
Vidicon vacuum chamber pickup tube for video camera
Vi-Drape
    V.-D. dressing
    Ioban V.-D.
view
    abdominal v.
    Adams v.
    Alexander v.
    anterior v.
    anteroposterior v.
    apical lordotic v.
    AP supine v.
    Arcelin v.
    axial calcaneus v.
    axial sesamoid v.

V

NOTES

779

view *(continued)*
    axillary lateral v.
    baseline v.
    Beath v.
    bicipital tuberosity v.
    Böhler calcaneal v.
    Böhler lumbosacral v.
    Breuerton v.
    Broden v.
    Bucky v.
    Burnham v.
    calcaneal axial v.
    Canale v.
    Canale-Kelly v.
    carpal tunnel v.
    Carter-Rowe v.
    charger v.
    cine v.
    clenched fist v.
    coalition v.
    coned-down v.
    cross-table lateral v. (CTLV)
    dens x-ray v.
    Didiee v.
    dorsiflexion v.
    dorsoplantar radiographic v.
    Dunlop-Shands v.
    dynamic stress x-ray v.
    erect v.
    false profile v.
    FCS v.
    Ferguson v.
    Ficat v.
    frog-leg lateral v.
    Garth v.
    Grashey v.
    Harris v.
    Harris-Beath axial calcaneus v.
    Hermodsson tangential v.
    Hill-Sachs v.
    hip-to-ankle v.
    Hobb v.
    Hughston v.
    iliac oblique v.
    infrapatellar v.
    inlet v.
    intraoperative v.
    inversion ankle stress v.
    Jones v.
    Judet pelvic x-ray v.
    Knuttsen bending v.
    lateral bending v.
    lateral monopodal stance v.
    lateral oblique v.
    lateral tilt stress ankle v.
    Lauren v.
    Lowell v.
    Löwenstein v.
    magnification v.
    Merchant v.
    mortise v.
    Neer lateral v.
    Neer transscapular v.
    nonstanding lateral oblique v.
    nonweightbearing v.
    notch v.
    oblique v.
    obturator oblique v.
    odontoid x-ray v.
    outlet v.
    patellar skyline v.
    plantar axial v.
    plantarflexion stress v.
    prayer v.
    push-pull ankle stress v.
    push-pull hip v.
    Robert v.
    Rosenberg v.
    scapulolateral v.
    serendipity v.
    skijump v.
    skyline v.
    spot v.
    standing dorsoplantar v.
    standing lateral v.
    standing weightbearing v.
    Stenver v.
    stress v.
    Stryker-Notch v.
    sunrise v.
    sunset v.
    swimmer's v.
    tangential x-ray v.
    Tile v.
    transthoracic lateral v.
    trauma v.
    true lateral v.
    tunnel v.
    upright v.
    urist v.
    Velpeau axillary lateral v.
    von Rosen v.
    weightbearing dorsoplantar v.
    West Point axillary lateral v.
    White leg length v.
    x-ray v.
    Y scapular v.
    Zanca v.

Vigilon dressing
VIGOR
    Vioxx Gastrointestinal Outcomes
    Research
vigorimeter
VIGOR trial
Viking postoperative shoe

Viladot
- V. arthroereisis device
- V. implant
- V. prosthesis
- V. surgical technique

Vilex
- V. cannulated screw system
- V. Ouchless Hook

villonodular
- v. synovitis
- v. tenosynovitis

villous
- v. lipomatous proliferation
- v. synovitis
- v. tenosynovitis

villusectomy
vinblastine
vinculum, pl. **vincula**
- v. breve
- intertendinous v.
- vincula longa connection

Vinertia
- V. implant metal
- V. implant metal prosthesis

Vinke
- V. skull traction tongs
- V. tong traction

viral
- v. monarthritis
- v. myositis

viral-associated arthritis
Virchow triad
Virgin hip screw
Virtual hip joint
Virtullene brace material
visceral tendon sheath
visceroptosis
viscerosomatic reflex
viscoelastic
- v. creep
- v. heel insert
- v. insole
- v. material
- v. polymer
- v. tissue

viscoelasticity
Viscoheel
- V. K heel cushion
- V. K, N orthosis
- V. N cushion
- V. SofSpot orthosis

- V. SofSpot viscoelastic heel cushion

Viscolas
- V. heel cushion
- V. heel pain and disability benefit
- V. orthosis

Viscoped
- V. S insole
- V. S support

viscosity
- blood v.

ViscoSpot
- V. heel cushion
- V. support

viscosupplementation
viscous
vise
- allograft bone v.
- AlloGrip bone v.
- pin v.
- Starrett pin v.

vise-like pain
VISI
- volar flexed intercalated segment instability

vision
- V. Epic wheelchair
- under direct v.

visor
- v. halo fixation device
- v. osteotomy

visor/sandwich osteotomy
Vistec x-ray detectable sponge
visual
- v. analog scale
- V. Analog Scale of Handicap
- v. closure
- v. evoked potential
- v. evoked response
- v. neglect
- V. Neglect Board
- v. orientation
- v. perception

visual-spatial ability impairment
Vitallium
- V. alloy
- V. cup arthroplasty
- V. drill
- V. equipment
- V. humeral replacement prosthesis
- V. implant
- V. implant material

V

NOTES

Vitallium *(continued)*
 V. implant metal
 V. Küntscher nail
 V. Luhr plate
 V. screw
 V. staple
Vitallium-W implant metal prosthesis
Vitalock
 V. cluster acetabular component
 V. solid-back acetabular component
vitamin
 v. C, D, K deficiency
 v. D-dependent rickets (VDDR)
 v. D receptor gene serum assay
 v. D-resistant rickets (VDRR)
Vitox
 V. alumina ceramic material
 V. femoral head
Vitrathene
 V. jacket
 V. vest
Viva shoe
Vivatek ultimate healing machine
in vivo study
VL
 vastus lateralis
Vladimiroff-Mikulicz amputation
VLC compression screw
VLCD
 very low calorie diet
VMA
 vastus medialis advancement
VMC
 void metal composite
V-medullary nail
VMO
 vastus medialis obliquus
 VMO exercise
 VMO retraining
VMO:VL
 vastus medialis obliquus:vastus lateralis
 VMO:VL EMG ratio
VMU
 vertebral motion unit
VO
 voluntary opening
vocal cord
vocational
 v. assessment
 v. evaluation (VE)
 v. feasibility
 v. rehabilitation (VR)
Vogue arm sling
void
 v. metal composite (VMC)
 signal v.
volar
 v. angulation deformity

 v. antebrachial region
 v. approach
 v. aspect
 v. capsule
 v. compartment syndrome
 v. condyle
 v. digital artery
 v. epineurolysis
 v. flexed intercalated segment instability (VISI)
 v. glide
 v. intercalary wrist instability
 v. midline oblique incision
 v. plaster splint
 v. plate
 v. plate arthroplasty
 v. plate repair
 v. semilunar wrist dislocation
 v. shear fracture
 v. surface
 v. synovectomy
 v. ulnar sling
 v. wrist
 v. zigzag finger incision
volarly
volarward approach
volitional
 v. activation
 v. activity
 v. contraction
 v. exercise
 v. fatigue
 v. muscle action test
 v. resisted flexion
 v. resisted flexion and extension
volitionally
Volkmann
 V. bone curette
 V. bone hook
 V. canal
 V. claw hand
 V. clawhand deformity
 V. contracture
 V. disease
 V. fracture
 V. ischemia
 V. ischemic paralysis
 V. rake retractor
 V. splint
 V. subluxation
Volkman triangle
Volkov-Oganesian
 V.-O. elbow distraction device
 V.-O. external fixation
 V.-O. external fixation apparatus
 V.-O. external fixation device
Volkov-Oganesian-Povarov hinged distraction apparatus

volley of pain
Volpicelli functional ambulation scale
volume
    cartilage v.
    v. conduction
    stroke v.
volumeter
    Ableware V.
    foot v.
    hand v.
    v. set
voluntary
    v. activity
    v. closing (VC)
    v. closing terminal device
    v. control (VC)
    v. control 4-bar knee
    v. muscle
    v. opening (VO)
    v. opening terminal device
Volz
    V. total wrist arthroplasty
    V. wrist
    V. wrist prosthesis
Volz-Turner
    V.-T. reattachment
    V.-T. reattachment technique
vomer bone
von
    v. Bekhterev reflex
    v. Gies joint
    v. Hippel-Lindau syndrome
    v. Lackum transection shift jacket
    v. Lackum transection shift jacket brace
    v. Langenbeck periosteal elevator
    V. Mises stress
    v. Recklinghausen disease
    v. Rosen abduction splint
    v. Rosen cruciform splint
    v. Rosen splint hip orthosis
    v. Rosen view
    v. Saal medullary pin
    v. Schwann law
    v. Weber triangle
Voorhoeve disease
Voshell
    V. bursa
    V. sign
    V. test

Vostal
    V. classification of radial fracture
    V. radial fracture classification
V-osteotomy
    Japas V-o.
    midtarsal V-o.
    offset V-o.
VPM
    Vantage Performance monitor
VPT
    vibration perception threshold
VR
    vocational rehabilitation
VRO
    varus rotational osteotomy
Vrolik disease
VS
    vertical shear
VSC
    vertebral subluxation complex
VSF
    Vermont spinal fixator
    VSF clamp
    VSF fixation system
    VSF rod
    VSF screw
V-shaped
    V-s. fracture
    V-s. incision
    V-s. osteotomy
    V-s. rotator cuff tear
VSL technology
VSO
    vertical sagittal split osteotomy
VSP
    variable screw placement
    variable screw plate
    variable spinal plating
    VSP fixation
    VSP plate
    VSP plate instrumentation
    VSP system
VTED
    venous thromboembolic disease
vulgaris
    verruca v.
Vulpian atrophy
Vulpian-Bernhardt spinal muscular atrophy
Vulpius
    V. Achilles tendon reconstruction
    V. equinus deformity operation

V

NOTES

Vulpius (*continued*)
    V. lengthening
    V. procedure
Vulpius-Compere
    V.-C. gastrocnemius lengthening
    V.-C. tendon technique
Vulpius-Stoffel procedure
VuRyser monitor lift

V-Y
    V-Y advancement flap
    V-Y Kutler flap
    V-Y plasty
    V-Y plasty correction
    V-Y plasty correction of varus toe
    V-Y quadricepsplasty

WACH
    wedge adjustable cushioned heel
    WACH orthopedic shoe
wad
    flexor w.
    mobile w.
Waddell
    W. Chronic Back Pain Disability
      index
    W. sign
    W. triad
wadding
    cotton sheet w.
    shot w.
waddle
    duck w.
waddling gait
Wadsworth
    W. posterolateral approach
    W. technique
    W. unconstrained elbow prosthesis
wafer
    w. distal ulna resection
    w. procedure
Wagdy double-V osteotomy
Wagner
    W. acetabular reamer
    W. approach
    W. classification
    W. closed pinning
    W. device external fixator
    W. disease
    W. distraction device
    W. distractor
    W. external fixation apparatus
    W. external fixation device
    W. external fixator
    W. femoral lengthening
    W. femoral metaphysial shortening
    W. fixation
    W. fixer
    W. frame
    W. grade
    W. leg-lengthening apparatus
    W. limb lengthening method
    W. line
    W. modification of Syme
      amputation
    W. multiple K-wire osteosynthesis
    W. open reduction technique
    W. profundus advancement
    W. prosthesis
    W. retractor
    W. revision hip system
    W. skin incision

    W. tibial lengthening
    W. trochanteric advancement
    W. two-stage Syme amputation
Wagner-Schanz
    W.-S. screw
    W.-S. screw apparatus
    W.-S. screw device
wagon
    dumbbell w.
    w. wheel fracture
Wagoner
    W. cervical technique
    W. posterior approach
    W. ulcer
Wagstaffe fracture
Wagstaffe-Le Fort fracture
Wagstaff tubercle
Wainwright plate
waist
    w. of anatomical structure
    w. fracture
    w. of the phalanx
    w. of scaphoid
    w. suspension belt
waist-to-hip ratio
wake-up test
Waldenström
    W. classification
    W. disease
    W. sign
    W. staging
Waldron test
WALK
    weight-activated locking knee
walk
    heel w.
    heel-and-toe w.
    lift-off of heel in w.
    nonweightbearing crutch w.
    w. test
    toe w.
Walkabout walker
WalkAide system
Walk-A-Matic walker
walker
    air w.
    Aircast pneumatic w.
    ATO w.
    w. basket
    Body Armor short leg w.
    Cam Walker ankle w.
    cast w.
    Castaway ankle w.
    Castaway leg w.

W

walker *(continued)*
Charcot restraint orthotic w. (CROW)
Comfy w.
controlled ankle w.
Delta w.
DH pressure relief w.
EasyStep pressure relief w.
Equalizer air w.
four-point w.
Guardian Red Dot w.
Hi-Top II adjustable w.
Hi-Top foot/ankle w.
W. hollow quill pin
Lumex w.
Merry W.
Moon W.
obese w.
ORLAU swivel w.
Rollator Nova w.
rubber sole cast w.
rubber wedge w.
W. ruptured disk curette
Sabel cast w.
short leg w.
w. skis
w. sleds
swivel w.
three-wheel w.
Walkabout w.
Walk-A-Matic w.
Zimmer w.
Walker-Murdoch wrist sign
walking
w. adjunct
aerobic w.
w. aid
w. biomechanics
bipedal w.
w. boot cast
w. brace
crutch w.
w. cycle
w. footprints classification
w. heel
heel-and-toe w.
idiopathic toe w.
w. mechanics
nonweightbearing crutch w.
w. pole
w. program
stance phase w.
w. stirrup
w. task
toe w.
w. without support
w. with support
Walk-'n-Tone exerciser

Walk-Rite device
wall
medial w.
Walldius Vitallium mechanical knee prosthesis
Wallenberg
W. procedure
W. syndrome
W. test
wallerian degeneration
wallet neuritis
wall-slide exercise
Wal-Pil-O neck pillow
Walsh
protocol of W.
Walter-Liston forceps
Walther fracture
Walton
W. cartilage clamp
W. maneuver
W. meniscal clamp
W. scissors
W. wire-pulling forceps
Walton-Liston bone rongeur
Walton-Ruskin
W.-R. bone rongeur
W.-R. forceps
Wanchik
W. neutral position splint
W. writer
wand
ArthroCare w.
Essential Energy Whole House W.
extensor w.
TCFO placement w.
TriggerWheel W.
Wangensteen
W. needle
W. needle holder
Wanger leg lengthening device
waning discharge
Ward
W. periosteal elevator
W. triangle
Ward-Tomasin-Vander-Griend fixation
warm
w. ischemia
w. ischemic time
W. 'n' Form lumbosacral corset
W. Springs brace
warm-and-form
w.-a.-f. cast
w.-a.-f. insert
warmer
gel w.
Thermasonic gel w.
warmth
joint w.

WarmTouch patient warming system
Warm-Up active wound therapy system
Warner-Farber
    W.-F. ankle fixation
    W.-F. ankle fixation technique
Warren-Mack rotating drill
Warren-Marshall classification
Warren White Achilles tendon
  lengthening
Warsaw hip prosthesis
wart
    mosaic w.
    plantar w. (PW)
Wartenberg
    W. pinwheel
    W. sign
washboard syndrome
washer
    C w.
    contoured w.
    w. crimper
    female w.
    w. holder
    male w.
    oval w.
    plate spacer w.
    spiked ligament w.
    Synthes ligament w.
    toothed w.
wash mitt
wasp-waist vertebra
Wassel
    W. classification of thumb
      polydactyly
    W. thumb duplication classification
    W. type IV thumb duplication
Wasserstein
    W. fixation
    W. fixation device
wasting
    quadriceps w.
Watanabe
    W. discoid meniscus classification
    W. pin
    W. pin holder
    W. retractor
watch crystal nail
Watco
    W. brace
    W. knee immobilizer
water
    w. acceptance test

    Essential Energy W.
    total body w.
water-cooled power bur
Waterman osteotomy
WaterPik irrigation
Waterpillow
    Mediflow W.
water-soluble contrast agent
Watkins
    W. fusion
    W. fusion technique
Watson
    W. maneuver
    W. scaphotrapeziotrapezoidal fusion
    W. technique
    W. test
Watson-Cheyne-Burghard procedure
Watson-Cheyne technique
Watson-Jones
    W.-J. ankle tenodesis
    W.-J. anterior approach
    W.-J. arthrodesis
    W.-J. bone gouge
    W.-J. fracture repair
    W.-J. frame
    W.-J. guidepin
    W.-J. incision
    W.-J. lateral approach
    W.-J. nail
    W.-J. navicular fracture
    W.-J. navicular fracture
      classification
    W.-J. procedure
    W.-J. reconstruction
    W.-J. spinal fracture classification
    W.-J. tibial fracture classification
    W.-J. traction
Watson-Williams intervertebral disk
  rongeur
Waugh
    W. knee prosthesis
    W. total ankle replacement
      prosthesis
wave
    A w.
    double flexion w.
    F w.
    H w.
    w. keyboard
    M w.
    OssaTron shock w.

W

NOTES

wave *(continued)*
    positive sharp w.
    W. Web
waveform
    biphasic w.
    bipolar IF w.
    electrical stimulator w.
    micro w.
    monophasic w.
    quadpolar IF w.
    Russian w.
wax
    bone w.
    Horsley bone w.
way
    W.'s of Coping checklist
    giving w.
Wayfarer
    W. modifiable foot prosthesis
Wayne County reduction
WBAT
    weightbearing as tolerated
WC, W/C, WCh
    wheelchair
WD
    wrist disarticulation
WD, WN
    well developed, well nourished
weak foot
weakness
    breakaway w.
    give-way w.
    motor w.
    overstretch w.
    ratchety w.
wear
    abnormal shoe w.
    accelerated chondral w.
    asymmetric w.
    backside w.
    w. debris
    eccentric w.
    shoe w.
    SoftFlex Wrist W.
    three-body w.
wear-and-tear degeneration
wear-resistant surface
weather-ache
weave
    bob and w.
weaver
    w. bottom
    W. rockerbottom shoe
Weaver-Dunn
    W.-D. acromioclavicular operation
    W.-D. acromioclavicular technique
    W.-D. procedure
    W.-D. resection

web
    w. area of hand
    w. border of hand
    w. contracture
    w. corn
    finger w.
    w. space
    w. space creep
    w. space flap
    w. space infection
    thumb w.
    Wave W.
Webb
    W. bolt nail
    W. fixation
    W. pin
    W. procedure
    W. stove bolt
Webb-Andreesen condylar bolt
webbed
    w. finger
    w. toe
Weber
    W. antiglide plate
    W. B, C fracture
    W. classification of physial injury
    W. fracture classification
    W. frame
    W. hip implant
    W. humeral osteotomy
    W. Permalock
    W. procedure
    W. static two-point discrimination
    W. subcapital osteotomy
    W. syndrome
    W. test
    W. triangle
    W. zone
Weber-Brunner-Freuler-Boitzy technique
Weber-Brunner-Freuler open reduction
Weber-Danis ankle injury classification
Weber-Vasey
    W.-V. traction-absorption
    W.-V. traction-absorption wiring
      technique
Webril
    W. bandage
    W. cotton padding
    W. dressing
    W. immobilization
webspace incision
Webster
    W. meniscectomy scissors
    W. needle
    W. needle holder
Wechsler
    W. Adult Intelligence scale
    W. Memory scale

Weck
- W. clip
- W. knife
- W. microsuture cutting scissors
- W. osteotome

Weckesser technique
Wedeen wire passer
wedge
- abduction w.
- w. adjustable cushioned heel (WACH)
- w. adjustable cushioned heel shoe
- bed w.
- bone w.
- bumper w.
- cast w.
- closing base w.
- compensatory w.
- w. compression fracture
- Duo-Cline Dual Support contoured bed w.
- w. fixation
- w. flexion-compression fracture
- Good 'N Bed w.
- w. graft
- Hapad heel w.
- heel w.
- heel-to-toe medial shoe w.
- inner heel w. (IHW)
- lateral w.
- w. matrix resection (WMR)
- medial heel w. (MHW)
- medial heel-and-sole w.
- medial sole w.
- metaphysial w.
- w. nonunion
- open w. (OW)
- w. osteotomy
- Positex knee w.
- w. posting
- w. resection
- roof w.
- Saunders mobilization w.
- seating w.
- self-adhering varus/valgus w.
- shoe w.
- super w.
- W. TAG suture anchor system
- Tepperwedge w.
- The W. implant
- tibial w.

- toe w.
- Yancy cast w.

wedge-and-groove joint
wedged shoe
wedge-shaped
- w.-s. uncomminuted fragment
- w.-s. uncomminuted tibial plateau fracture
- w.-s. vertebra

wedging
- w. cast
- navicular w.
- w. of olisthetic vertebra
- vertebral w.
- w. of vertebral interspace

WeeFIM instrument
weekend athlete
Wegener granulomatosis
Wegner
- W. disease
- W. line

weight
- w. acceptance
- ankle w.
- body w.
- w. boot
- cutting w.
- distal segment w.
- handheld w. (HHW)
- lean body w. (LBW)
- progressive w.
- w.'s and pulleys
- Thera-Band progressive w.
- w. traction
- w. training

weight-activated locking knee (WALK)
weightbearing
- w. acetabular dome
- w. as tolerated (WBAT)
- w. axis
- w. brace
- w. crutch
- w. dorsoplantar view
- full w. (FWB)
- w. ground reaction force
- w. joint
- pain with w.
- partial w. (PWB)
- progression to full w.
- progressive w.
- protective w.
- w. rotational injury

NOTES

W

weightbearing *(continued)*
    w. surface
    w. symmetry
    w. tangential radiograph
    toe-touch w.
    touchdown w.
    w. x-ray
weight/composition
    body w.
weighted
    w. glove
    w. pen
    w. vest
    w. walking stick
weightlifter's
    w. clavicle
    w. shoulder
weightlifting
weight-relieving
    w.-r. caliper
    w.-r. Forte harness
    w.-r. orthosis
weight-training program
Weil
    W. implant
    W. osteotomy
    W. pelvic sling
    W. splint
Weiland
    W. classification
    W. harvesting
    W. iliac crest bone graft
Weil-Blakesley intervertebral disk rongeur
Weil-modified Swanson implant
Weil-type Swanson-design hammertoe implant
Weinstein enhanced sensory test (WEST)
Weinstein-Ponseti technique
Weinstock desyndactylization
Weise jack screw
Weiss
    W. amputation saw
    W. spring
Weissman classification
Weit-Arner retractor
Weitbrecht
    W. foramen
    W. ligament
    W. retinaculum
Weitlaner retractor
Welander distal myopathy
weld
    callus w.
    cold w.
    hot w.
    spot w.

well
    w. developed, well nourished (WD, WN)
    w. leg straight leg raising test
well-differentiated myxoid liposarcoma
Weller
    W. cartilage forceps
    W. cartilage scissors
    W. total hip joint prosthesis
well-leg
    w.-l. cast
    w.-l. holder
    w.-l. raising
    w.-l. splint
    w.-l. support
    w.-l. traction
Wellmerling maneuver
Wells
    W. pedicle clamp
    W. traction
well-seated prosthesis
Wenger plate
Werdnig-Hoffmann
    W.-H. disease
    W.-H. spinal muscular atrophy
Werenskiold sign
Wernicke aphasia
Wertheim-Bohlman technique
Wertheim splint
WEST
    Weinstein enhanced sensory test
    work evaluation systems technology
West
    W. bone chisel
    W. bone gouge
    W. hand dissector
    W. nerve tester
    W. osteotome
    W. Point Ankle Grading System
    W. Point axillary lateral radiograph
    W. Point axillary lateral view
    W. Shur cartilage clamp
    W. and Soto-Hall patella operation
    W. and Soto-Hall patella technique
Westcott Pyramid Program
Westergren sedimentation rate
Wester meniscal clamp
Western
    W. Ontario Instability Index (WOSI)
    W. Ontario and McMaster University osteoarthritis index
    W. Ontario Rotator Cuff (WORC)
    W. Ontario Rotator Cuff Index
Westfield acromioclavicular immobilizer
Westfield-style envelope sling
Westhaven Yale Multidimensional Pain Inventory (WHYMPI)

Westin-Hall incision
Westin tenodesis
Westin-Turco category
Weston shelf procedure
Westphal phenomenon
West-Soto-Hall

W.-S.-H. patellar technique
W.-S.-H. patellectomy

wet

w. gangrene
w. globe temperature
w. leather sign

wet-to-dry dressing
WFE

Williams flexion exercise

WFL

within functional limits

Wheaton

W. bunion splint
W. Pavlik harness
W. Pavlik Harness brace

WHECS

wrist hand extension compression support

wheel

Carborundum grinding w.
w. chair seating component
pin w.
shoulder w.

wheelchair (WC, W/C, WCh)

Action Jr. w.
Amigo mechanical w.
antitipper w.
Applause Super-Hemi w.
w. chain
w. confinement
w. cushion
electric w.
Epic w.
folding frame w.
Gendron bariatric w.
Invacare manual w.
Jay J2 w.
Kuschkin Ace w.
Landeez all-terrain w.
Lumex lightweight w.
manual w.
Navigator power w.
Nitro w.
power w.
Quickie Carbon w.
Quickie EX w.

Quickie GPS w.
Quickie GP Swing-Away w.
Quickie GPV w.
Quickie Kidz w.
Quickie Recliner w.
Quickie Ti w.
reclining frame w.
rigid frame w.
self-propelling w.
Shark pediatric w.
Skil-Care reclining w.
Slam'r w.
sling seat w.
tilting frame w.
Vision Epic w.
4XP Tilt System w.
Zippie 2 w.
Zippie P500 w.

whettle bone
whiplash

acute w.
chronic w.
w. injury
reflex rebound component of w.
w. syndrome

whiplash-shaken infant syndrome
whirlpool

w. bath (WPB)
w. therapy

whiskering
whistling face syndrome
white

w. band on degenerated implant
w. blood cell count
w. blood cell scan
W. chisel
W. epiphysiodesis
w. fixation
W. leg length view
w. matter
w. muscle
W. and Panjabi cervical spine
  criteria
W. posterior ankle fusion
W. posterior arthrodesis
W. screwdriver
W. slide procedure
w. tendo calcaneus lengthening

Whitecloud-LaRocca

W.-L. cervical arthrodesis
W.-L. fibular strut graft

W

NOTES

Whitehall
    W. Glacier Pack
    W. thermalator
White-Kraynick tendo calcaneus
Whitesides
    W. line
    W. Ortholoc II condylar femoral prosthesis
    W. technique
    W. tissue pressure determination
    W. total knee prosthesis
Whitesides-Kelly cervical technique
whitlow
    herpetic w.
    thecal w.
Whitman
    W. arch support
    W. femoral neck reconstruction
    W. frame
    W. maneuver
    W. muscle transfer
    W. osteotomy
    W. paralysis
    W. plate
    W. talectomy procedure
    W. traction
Whitman-Thompson procedure
Whitney single-use plastic curette
WHO
    wrist-hand orthosis
WHO/LAR
    World Health Organization/International League Against Rheumatism
    WHO/LAR Response Criteria for Rheumatoid Arthritis
    WHO/LAR Response Criteria for Rheumatoid Arthritis growth plate widening
whole
    w. bone transplant
    w. fibular transplant
whole-body vibration
whorled pattern
WHYMPI
    Westhaven Yale Multidimensional Pain Inventory
Wiberg
    angle of W.
    center-edge angle of W.
    W. center edge angle
    W. fracture angle
    W. fracture staple
    W. fracture stapler
    W. patellar classification
    W. periosteal elevator
    W. type II patellar contour
Wichman retractor

wick
    W. catheter technique
    w. technique
wicking catheter
wide
    w. excision
    w. periosteal elevator
    w. toe box
    w. toebox shoe
wide-based gait
wide-mesh petroleum gauze dressing
widening
    ankle mortise w.
    interpedicular distance widening
    joint w.
    tibial tunnel w.
    WHO/LAR Response Criteria for Rheumatoid Arthritis growth plate w.
width
    step w.
Wiet
    W. cup forceps
    W. graft-measuring instrument
Wikco ankle machine
Wilco ankle exerciser
Wilde
    W. ethmoid forceps
    W. intervertebral disk rongeur
    W. rongeur forceps
Wiley-Galey classification
Wilke
    W. boot
    W. boot brace
Wilkie syndrome
Wilkinson synovectomy
Willauer-Gibbon periosteal elevator
William
    W. Harris hip prosthesis
    W. microlumbar disk excision
Williams
    W. Advantage table
    W. brace
    W. diskectomy
    W. diskography
    W. exercise program
    W. flexion back exercise technique
    W. flexion exercise (WFE)
    W. interlocking Y-nail
    W. Model 170 table
    W. nail
    W. orthosis
    W. procedure
    W. rod
    W. screwdriver
    W. self-retaining retractor

Williams-Haddad
    W.-H. release
    W.-H. technique
Williger
    W. bone curette
    W. bone mallet
    W. periosteal elevator
willow fracture
Wilmington
    W. arthroscopic portal
    W. plastic jacket
    W. scoliosis brace
Wilson
    W. ankle fusion
    W. approach
    W. bolt
    W. bone graft
    W. bunionectomy
    W. cone arthrodesis
    W. convex frame
    W. double oblique osteotomy
    W. fracture
    W. gonad retractor
    W. muscle
    W. oblique displacement osteotomy
    W. plate
    W. procedure for extraarticular
      fusion of elbow
    W. sign
    W. splint
    W. technique
    W. test
Wilson-Burstein hip internal prosthesis
Wilson-Cook prosthesis repositioner
Wilson-Jacobs
    W.-J. patellar graft
    W.-J. tibial fixation
    W.-J. tibial fracture fixation
      technique
Wilson-Johansson-Barrington cone
  arthrodesis
Wilson-McKeever
    W.-M. arthroplasty
    W.-M. shoulder technique
Wiltberger anterior cervical approach
Wiltse
    W. ankle osteotomy
    W. approach
    W. bilateral lateral fusion
    W. diskectomy
    W. fixator
    W. osteotomy of ankle

    W. pedicle screw
    W. pedicle screw fixation system
    W. screw-rod
    W. system aluminum master rod
    W. system cross-bracing
    W. system double-rod construct
    W. system H construct
    W. system single-rod construct
    W. system spinal rod
    W. varus supramalleolar osteotomy
Wiltse-Spencer paraspinal approach
Wiltze angle
Wimberger sign
Winberger line
Winco
    W. Adjusting Bench
    W. Folding Treatment Table
windblown
    w. deformity
    w. hand, whistling face syndrome
    w. hip
    w. knee
wind-cold
wind-heat
windlass
    reverse w.
Windlass mechanism
window
    cast w.
    cortical w.
    femoral cortical w.
windowed cast
windowing
    cortical w.
windshield wiper sign
Windson-Insall-Vince
    W.-I.-V. bone graft
    W.-I.-V. grafting technique
windswept
    w. deformity
    w. hip
wind-up
    w.-u. injury
    w.-u. phenomenon
wing
    angel w.
    Badgley resection of iliac w.
    dorsal w.
    w. excision of Littler
    iliac w.
    w. of ilium

NOTES

W

wing (continued)
   w. plate
   w. of sphenoid
Wingfield frame
winging
   w. motion
   w. of scapula
   scapular w.
wink
   anal w.
   W. retractor
   w. sign
Winkelmann rotationplasty
winking
   Gunn jaw w.
   w. owl sign
Winograd
   W. ingrown nail technique
   W. nail plate removal
   W. partial matrixectomy
   W. technique for ingrown nail
Winquist femoral shaft fracture classification
Winquist-Hansen
   W.-H. classification of femoral fracture
   W.-H. femoral fracture classification
   W.-H. fracture comminution classification
Winquist-Hansen-Pearson closed femoral diaphysial shortening
winter
   W. convex fusion
   W. splint
   W. spondylolisthesis
   W. spondylolisthesis technique
winterize body
Winter-King-Moe scoliosis
wipe test
wire
   Babcock stainless steel w.
   band w.
   bayonet-point w.
   beaded transfixion w.
   bead-loaded w.
   w. bending pliers
   bind w.
   bone suturing wire chisel-tip w.
   Brooker w.
   Bunnell pullout w.
   calibrated guide w.
   cerclage w.
   chisel-tip w.
   circular w.
   circumferential w.
   Compere fixation w.
   compression w.
   conical-point w.

   w. contour preparation
   w. crimper
   crossed Kirschner w.
   w. cutter
   Dall-Miles cerclage w.
   definitive cerclage w.
   diamond-point wire double-strand w.
   diamond tip w.
   double-stranded wire double-twisted w.
   w. drill
   w. and drill guide
   w. driver
   Drummond w.
   encircling w.
   figure-of-eight w.
   w. fixation bolt
   w. frame collar
   w. grip finger splint
   w. grip toe splint
   Ilizarov w.
   interfragmentary w.
   intraosseous w.
   Isola w.
   Kirschner w. (K-wire)
   w. knot
   Lengemann w.
   w. loop
   loop circumferential w.
   w. loop fixation
   Luque cerclage w.
   Magnuson w.
   Martin loop circumferential w.
   monofilament w.
   ninety-ninety intraosseous wire Nitinol flexible w.
   nonthreaded w.
   oblique w.
   olive w.
   Oppenheimer spring w.
   Outrigger w.
   over-tying w.
   w. passage
   w. passer
   w. penetration depth
   w. prosthesis-crimping forceps
   w. removal technique
   Schauwecker patellar tension band w.
   sharp-pointed w.
   smooth transfixion w.
   spinous process w.
   w. stabilization
   stainless steel w.
   sublaminar w.
   w. suture
   temporary cerclage w.

tension band w.
Thiersch w.
threaded w.
w. tightener
trochanteric w.
unscher w.
unthreaded w.
Wisconsin button w.
Wisconsin interspinous w.
Wisconsin spinous w.
wire-cutting
  w.-c. forceps
  w.-c. scissors
wire-extracting forceps
wire-fixation buckle
Wire-Foam Orthotic
wire-holding forceps
wire-pulling forceps
wire-tightening
  w.-t. clamp
  w.-t. forceps
wire-twisting forceps
wiring
  cervical oblique facet w.
  circumferential w.
  compression w.
  facet fracture stabilization w.
  facet subluxation stabilization w.
  figure-of-eight w.
  interfacet w.
  interspinous w.
  intraosseous w.
  Luque w.
  oblique facet w.
  posterior interspinous w.
  Schauwecker patellar w.
  spinous process w.
  sublaminar w.
  tension-band w.
  Wisconsin w.
Wirth-Jager tendon technique
Wisconsin
  W. button
  W. button wire
  W. interspinous segmental spinal instrumentation
  W. interspinous wire
  W. spinal fracture system
  W. spinous wire
  W. wire fixation
  W. wiring
Wissinger rod

Wister wire/pin cutter
within functional limits (WFL)
Wit portable TENS system
Wixson hip positioner
WMR
  wedge matrix resection
wobble
  w. board
  Wooden W.
Wohlfart-Kugelberg-Welander disease
Wolf
  W. arthroscope
  W. blade plate ankle arthrodesis
  W. full-thickness free graft
  W. light source
  W. motor function test
Wolfe-Böhler
  W.-B. cast breaker
  W.-B. mallet
Wolfe hand surgery graft
Wolfe-Kawamoto bone graft
Wolferman drill
Wolff
  W. law
  W. law of bone structure
Wolfson frame
Wolin meniscoid lesion
Wolvek sternal approximation fixation
Wonder-Cup heel cup
Wonderflex silicone
Wonder-Spur heel cup
Wonderzorb
  W. heel cup
  Soft Silicones W.
wood
  W. alloy
  w. probe reflexology device
  w. screw
wooden
  w. postoperative clogs
  w. shoe
  W. Wobble
wooden-soled shoe
Woodruff
  W. screw
  W. screwdriver
  W. tip
Woodson
  W. elevator
  W. probe
Woodward
  W. arthroplasty

W

NOTES

Woodward *(continued)*
    W. operation wound
    W. procedure
    W. technique
Woofry-Chandler classification of Osgood-Schlatter lesion
wool
    lamb's w.
WORC
    Western Ontario Rotator Cuff
Woringer-Kolopp disease
work
    concentric w.
    w. conditioning
    eccentric w.
    w. evaluation systems technology (WEST)
    w. hardening
    w. hardening exercise
    w. hardening program
    manual w.
    negative w.
    physical w.
    rhythmic handgrip w.
    W. Seat driving simulator
    sedentary w.
Workgroup
    National Arthritis Data W.
working orthopedic surgery film
WorkMod back support
World Health Organization/International League Against Rheumatism (WHO/LAR)
worm drive
wormian bone
WOSI
    Western Ontario Instability Index
wound
    w. cleanser
    closed w.
    w. closure
    w. culture
    w. dehiscence
    foot puncture w.
    w. gel
    gunshot w.
    Gustilo classification of puncture w.
    incised w.
    w. irrigation
    joint w.
    w. measuring guide
    open w.
    w. packing
    puncture w.
    stab w.
    Woodward operation w.
Wound-Evac drain

woven
    w. bone
    w. gastrocnemius aponeurosis
WPB
    whirlpool bath
W-plasty
wrap
    Ace w.
    Action elbow w.
    Action wrist w.
    BodyIce cold pack w.
    boot w.
    Champ CTS cold therapy w.
    Coban elastic w.
    Co-Flex adherent w.
    Coopercare Lastrap support w.
    digit w.
    Dura-Kold reusable compression ice w.
    Dura-Soft soft-compression reusable ice or heat w.
    Elasto-Gel hot/cold w.
    Elasto-Gel shoulder therapy w.
    Elasto-Link joint w.
    Electro-Link joint w.
    gauze w.
    gel w.
    Gelocast Unna boot compression w.
    Goode w.
    Heat Plus Massage lower body w.
    Ice Wedge hot/cold therapy w.
    joint w.
    Kerlix w.
    kneeRAP w.
    Kold W.
    loop-over w.
    neck w.
    Nylatex w.
    orthoRaps postsurgical wound w.
    Scott wrist w.
    shoulderRAP w.
    Snugs w.
    Sorbothane w.
    Stimprene w.
    super w.
    Thermoskin arthritic knee w.
    Thermosport hot/cold w.
    Unna boot w.
    Velpeau w.
wraparound
    w. flap bone graft
    w. neurovascular composite free tissue transfer
    w. neurovascular free flap
    w. splint
wrap-around toe transfer

wrapping
    compressive centripetal w.
    nerve w.
    stump w.
wrench
    Allen w.
    beaded-pin w.
    box-end w.
    cannulated w.
    conical nut w.
    Fox w.
    Harrington flat w.
    hex w.
    Key-loc w.
    locknut w.
    Mueller w.
    open-end w.
    w. pin
    socket w.
    T-handled nut w.
    T-handled screw w.
    Thomas w.
    torque w.
    TSRH w.
    U w.
    VDS w.
    ventral derotating spinal w.
wrenched knee
wrestler's elbow
Wright
    W. knee prosthesis
    W. maneuver
    W. Medical bone anchor
    W. monoblock titanium implant
    W. plate
    W. test
    W. titanium prosthesis
    W. Universal brace
Wright-Adson test
Wrightlock
    W. posterior fixation system
    W. spinal fixation system
wringer
    w. arm
    w. injury
wrinkle test
Wrisberg
    W. lesion
    ligament of W.
wrist
    w. arthroscopy
    w. capsule

    w. contracture
    w. creaking
    w. curl
    w. deformity
    w. disarticulation (WD)
    dorsal arch of w.
    w. drop
    w. extensor
    w. extensor strengthening
    w. extensor stretch
    w. extensor tendinitis
    w. extensor tendon
    w. and finger flexor stretch
    w. first
    w. flexion reflex
    w. flexion test
    w. flexion unit
    w. flexor strengthening
    w. flexor tendinitis
    w. gauntlet
    golfer's w.
    gymnast's w.
    w. hand extension compression
      support (WHECS)
    w. instability
    w. joint implant prosthesis
    oarsman's w.
    w. pain syndrome
    palmar w.
    W. Pro wrist support
    W. Pro wrist support device
    w. rest splint
    slack w.
    w. spasticity
    w. speed profile
    w. stretch exercise
    w. subluxation
    sulcus of w.
    tilt w.
    total arthrodesis of the w.
    triangular disk of w.
    volar w.
    Volz w.
wrist-driven
    w.-d. flexor hinge orthosis
    w.-d. lateral prehension orthosis
    w.-d. wrist-hand orthosis
wrist-hand orthosis (WHO)
Wristiciser exerciser
WrisTimer
    W. carpal tunnel support system
    W. CTS support

W

NOTES

WristJack wrist splint
wristlet
    elastic w.
    Freedom USA w.
writer
    w. paralysis
    Wanchik w.
writing hand
WRUN-N equipment reflective safety belt

wry neck, wryneck
Wu
    Wu bunionectomy
    Wu sole opposition test
Wullstein drill
Wurzburg
    W. plate
    W. screw
Wylie lumbar bulldog clamp
Wynne-Davis joint laxity technique

X

X axis
X clamp
X plate

Xact ACL graft-fixation system
X-Act podiatric marker
xanthogranuloma

juvenile x.

xanthoma

Achilles tendon x.
fibrous x.
malignant fibrous x.
tuberous x.

xanthomatous giant cell tumor
Xenophor femoral prosthesis
Xercise

X. band
X. Band exercise device
X. tube resistive device

Xeroform gauze dressing
xerography
xeroradiography
xerotic
Xertube
Xia

X. hook system
X. spinal system

XIP

x-ray in plaster

xiphisternal joint
xiphoid

x. bone
x. process

XiScan

X. fluoroscopy
X. mini-C-arm

X-long cement forceps
Xomed drill
XOP

x-ray out of plaster

XO-soft-sole orthotic
XPE foot orthosis
x-ray

artifact on x-r.
Cedell-Magnusson classification of
    arthritis on x-r.
dorsal planar x-r.
dorsiflexion stress ankle x-r.
dynamic motion x-r.
FCS x-r.
Harris-Beath axial hindfoot x-r.
hip-to-ankle x-r.
intraoperative x-r.
lateral tilt stress ankle x-r.
nonweightbearing x-r.
x-r. out of plaster (XOP)
x-r. overlay
penciling of ribs on x-r.
x-r. photogrammetry
plantar stress ankle x-r.
x-r. in plaster (XIP)
postreduction x-r.
sagittal stress x-r.
x-r. tray
x-r. view
weightbearing x-r.

Xsensibles shoe
X-shaped plate
XTB knee extension device
X-TEND-O knee flexor
Xtra Depth shoe
X-Y

X-Y plotter
X-Y sensor system

XY

frontal plane XY

X,Y,Z

cardinal axes X,Y,Z
coordinate system X,Y,Z

X

Y

Y axis
Y bone plate
Y B Sore cushion
Y fracture
Y incision
Y line
Y osteotomy
Y scapular view

Yale brace
Yamanda myelotomy knife
Yancey osteotomy
Yancy cast wedge
Yankauer periosteal elevator
Yasargil

Y. elevator
Y. Leyla retractor arm
Y. ligature carrier
Y. ligature guide
Y. micro rasp
Y. needle holder
Y. spring hook

Y-axis translatory displacement
Yeager test
year

Disability Adjusted Life Y.'s
(DALYs)

Yee posterior shoulder approach
yellow

y. cartilage
y. ligament
y. marrow
y. nail syndrome

Yergason

Y. shoulder subluxation test

Y. sign
Y. test of shoulder subluxation

yield strength
Y-knot tying system
Y-nail

Williams interlocking Y-n.

Yochum chiropractic software
yoga
yoked muscle
Yoke transposition procedure
Y-osteotomy
Young

Y. hinged knee prosthesis
Y. medial approach
Y. modulus
Y. pelvic fracture classification
Y. procedure

Youngswick-Austin procedure
Young-Vitallium hinged prosthesis
Youngwhich modification
Yount

Y. fasciotomy
Y. procedure

Y-shaped

Y-s. incision
Y-s. plate

Y-strap knee immobilizer
Y-T fracture
Yuan screw
yucca

Y. board
y. wood splint

Yu osteotomy
Y-V plasty
Y-V-plasty incision

Y

Z

Z axis
Z band
Z bunionectomy
Z disk
Z fixation nail
Z foot
Z foot deformity
Z line
Z pin
Z retractor

ZAAG

Zest Anchor Advanced Generation
ZAAG Bone Anchoring System

Zachary sensory grade

Zadik

Z. foot operation
Z. foot procedure
Z. total matrixectomy
Z. total nailbed ablation

Zahn

line of Z.

Zaias nail biopsy

Zanca view

Zancolli

Z. biceps tendon rerouting
Z. capsuloplasty
Z. clawhand deformity procedure
Z. flexion capsulodesis
Z. procedure for clawhand
deformity
Z. reconstruction
Z. rerouting technique
Z. static lock procedure

Zancolli-Lasso procedure

Zang

Z. metatarsal cap
Z. metatarsal cap implant

Zaricznyj procedure

Zariczny ligament technique

Zarins-Rowe

Z.-R. ligament technique
Z.-R. procedure

Zazepen-Gamidov technique

zebra body myopathy

Zeichner implant

Zeier transfer technique

Zelicof orthopedic awl

Zenith

Z. ACS table
Z. chiropractic table
Z. Electrotherapy ultrasound system
Z. Hylos table
Z. stationary table

Z. Thompson table
Z. Verti-Lift table

Zenith-Cox flexion/distraction table

Zenker

Z. degeneration
Z. necrosis

Zenotech biomaterial-synthetic ligament

Zephir anterior cervical plate system

Zest

Z. Anchor Advanced Generation
(ZAAG)
Z. Anchor Advanced Generation
bone anchoring system
Z. Anchor Advanced Generation
Bone Anchoring System

Zickel

Z. classification
Z. fracture
Z. fracture classification system
Z. medullary apparatus
Z. nail fixation
Z. nailing
Z. rod
Z. subcondylar nail
Z. subtrochanteric fracture fixation
Z. subtrochanteric fracture operation
Z. subtrochanteric nail
Z. supracondylar device
Z. supracondylar fixation apparatus
Z. supracondylar medullary nail

zidovudine-induced myopathy

Ziehen-Oppenheim disease

Zielke

Z. bifid hook
Z. derotator bar
Z. distraction device
Z. gouge
Z. instrumentation for scoliosis
spinal fusion
Z. pedicular instrumentation
Z. rod
Z. technique

zigzag

z. approach
z. compensatory deformity
z. finger incision

Zimaloy

Z. femoral head prosthesis
Z. implant metal
Z. implant metal prosthesis
Z. staple

Zimfoam

Z. head halter
Z. pad
Z. pin

Z

Zimfoam *(continued)*
    Z. splint
    Z. splint traction
Zimmer
    Z. airplane splint
    Z. anatomic hip system
    Z. antiembolism stockings
    Z. bone cement
    Z. bone stem
    Z. cartilage clamp
    Z. Cebotome bone cement drill
    Z. Centralign Precoat hip prosthesis
    Z. Cibatome cement eater
    Z. clavicular cross splint
    Z. collarless polished taper hip system
    Z. compression hip screw
    Z. continuous anatomical passive exerciser
    Z. crossover instrumentation system
    Z. dermatome
    Z. electrical stimulation apparatus
    Z. electrical stimulation device
    Z. extractor
    Z. femoral canal broach
    Z. femoral condyle blade plate
    Z. fracture frame
    Z. goniometer
    Z. gouge
    Z. hand drill
    Z. head halter
    Z. hip implant system
    Z. hip prosthesis
    Z. impaction screw-plate
    Z. knee immobilizer
    Z. laminectomy frame
    Z. low-viscosity adhesive
    Z. low-viscosity cement
    Z. microsaw
    Z. NexGen LPS knee femoral component
    Z. Orthair ream driver
    Z. orthopedic device
    Z. oscillating saw
    Z. Osteo Stim bone growth stimulator
    Z. pin
    Z. PMMA precoat process
    Z. postoperative shoe
    Z. protractor
    Z. Pulsavac wound débridement system
    Z. reamer brace
    Z. rotary bur
    Z. screwdriver
    Z. shoulder prosthesis
    Z. side plate
    Z. skin graft mesher

    Z. snare
    Z. telescoping nail
    Z. THARIES surface arthroplasty system
    Z. tibial bolt
    Z. tibial nail cap
    Z. tibial prosthesis
    Z. Universal drill
    Z. walker
    Z. Y plate
Zimmer-Gigli saw blade
Zimmer-Hall drive system
Zimmer-Hoen forceps
Zimmer-Hudson shank
Zimmer-Kirschner hand drill
Zimmerlin atrophy
Zimmerman pericyte
Zimmer-Schlesinger forceps
Zimmer-Statak anchor
Zim-Trac
    Z.-T. traction splint
    Z.-T. traction splint tractor
Zim-Zip rib belt splint
Zinco
    Z. Air Cam brace
    Z. Airprene brace
    Z. ankle orthosis
    Z. Cam Walker brace
    Z. Castaway D brace
    Z. Hi-Top brace
    Z. Minerva cervical brace
    Z. Multi-Lig knee brace
    Z. Pin Cam Walker brace
    Z. thumb-wrist immobilizer
zinc supplementation
zipper
    Z. antidisconnect device
    z. cast
Zippie
    Z. P500 wheelchair
    Z. 2 wheelchair
Ziramic femoral head
Zirconia
    Z. femoral head prosthesis
    Z. orthopedic prosthesis
    Z. orthopedic prosthetic head
zirconium
    z. oxide arthroplasty material
    z. oxide ceramic prosthesis
    oxidized z.
Z-lengthening
    Achilles tendon Z-l.
    Z-l. of biceps tendon
Zlotsky-Ballard
    Z.-B. acromioclavicular injury classification
    Z.-B. classification of acromioclavicular injury

ZMC
    zygomatic-malar complex
      ZMC fracture
ZMR hip system
ZMS intramedullary fixation system
Zodiac TM Manual Flexion-Distraction table
Zohar shoe
Zollinger
      Z. legholder
      Z. splint
Zollner rasp
zonal sclerosis
Zonas porous tape
zone
      autonomous z.
      cornuradicular z.
      cut-back z.
      dorsal root entry z. (DREZ)
      elastic z.
      endplate z.
      fracture z.
      growth z.
      Gruen z.
      hyperintense z.
      hypertrophic z.
      isolated z.
      Kambin triangular working z.
      Lissauer z.
      maturation z.
      neutral z. (NZ)
      orbicular z.
      paraphysiologic z.
      peripolar z.
      polar z.
      proliferating z.
      z. of Ranvier
      resting z.
      Z. Specific II meniscal repair
      Z. Specific II meniscal repair system
      triangular working z.
      Trümmerfeld z.
      umbau z.
      Weber z.
zone-specific cannula
zonography
Zorbacel shock-absorbing material
Zoroc plaster
Z-osteotomy
      inverted scarf Z-o.

Z-plasty
      Z-p. approach
      Broadbent-Woolf four-limb Z-p.
      Cozen-Brockway Z-p.
      four-limb Z-p.
      frontal plane Z-p.
      Gudas scarf Z-p.
      Z-p. incision
      Z-p. local flap graft
      Peet Z-p.
      Z-p. release
      scarf Z-p.
      sliding Z-p.
      Z-p. tenotomy
Z-shaped plate
Z-slide
      Z-s. lengthening
      Z-s. lengthening in hallux limitus
Z-stent prosthesis
Z-step cut
Z-Stim
      Z-S. IF 250 microprocessor controlled stimulator
      Z-S. 100 microprocessor controlled stimulator
ZTT
      ZTT acetabular cup
      ZTT I, II acetabular cup prosthesis
      ZTT I, II cup
Zuckerkandl dehiscence
Zucker splint
Zuelzer
      Z. awl
      Z. hook
      Z. hook plate
      Z. screw
Zuni
      Z. exercise system
      Z. gym
      Z. harness
Zweymuller
      Z. cementless hip prosthesis
      Z. hip system
Zwipp
      Z. classification
      Z. method
      Z. subtalar joint instability measurement
zygapophysial, zygapophyseal
      z. articulation
      z. joint
      z. joint injection

NOTES

zygodactyly
zygomatic bone
zygomatic-malar complex (ZMC)

Zymderm collagen implant
Zyranox femoral head

Appendix 1
Anatomical Illustrations

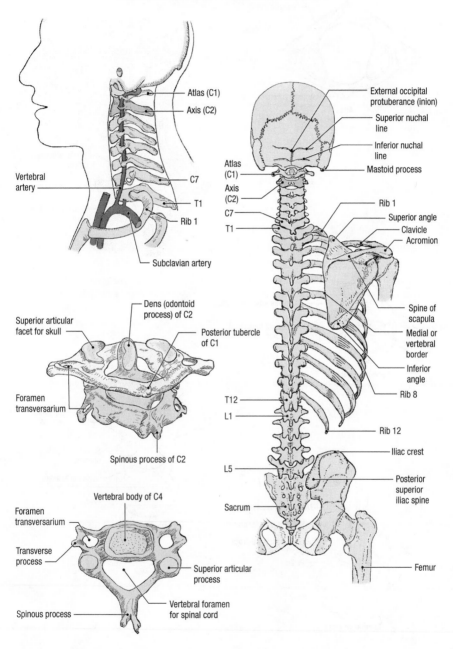

Figure 1. Bony landmarks of the back and vertebral column.

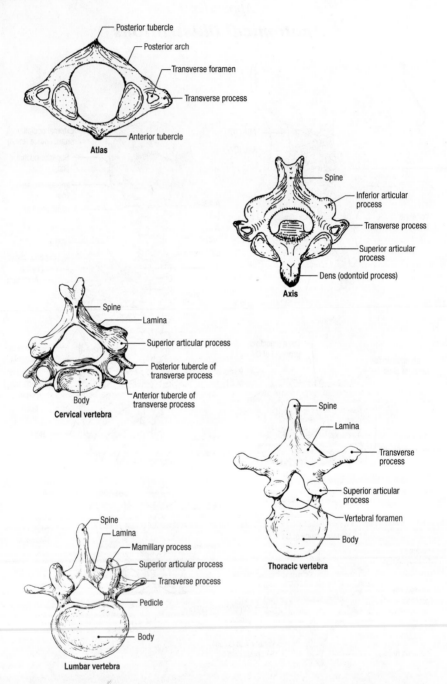

Figure 2. Typical cervical, thoracic, and lumbar vertebrae.

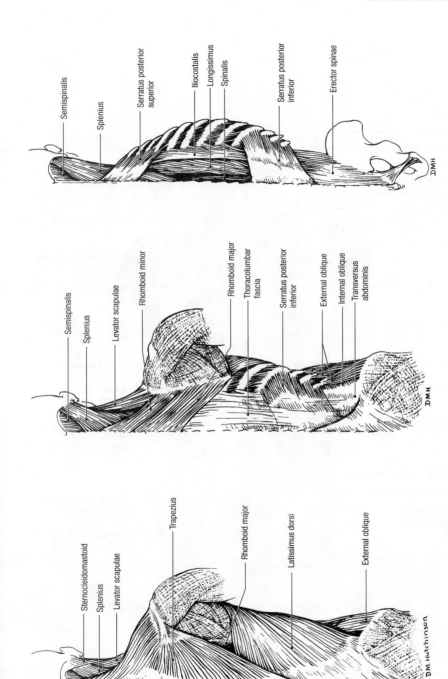

Figure 3. Extrinsic and intrinsic muscles of the back.

A3

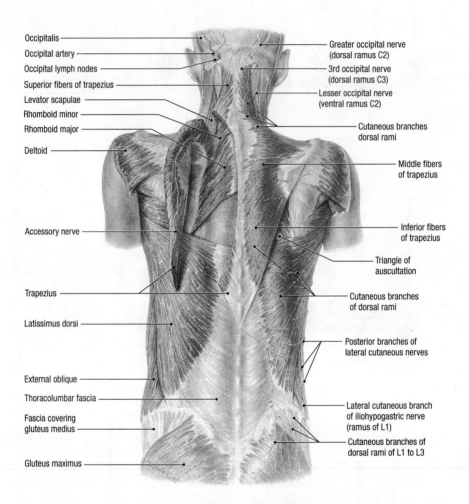

Occipitalis

Occipital artery

Occipital lymph nodes

Superior fibers of trapezius

Levator scapulae

Rhomboid minor

Rhomboid major

Deltoid

Accessory nerve

Trapezius

Latissimus dorsi

External oblique

Thoracolumbar fascia

Fascia covering
gluteus medius

Gluteus maximus

Greater occipital nerve
(dorsal ramus C2)

3rd occipital nerve
(dorsal ramus C3)

Lesser occipital nerve
(ventral ramus C2)

Cutaneous branches
dorsal rami

Middle fibers
of trapezius

Inferior fibers
of trapezius

Triangle of
auscultation

Cutaneous branches
of dorsal rami

Posterior branches of
lateral cutaneous nerves

Lateral cutaneous branch
of iliohypogastric nerve
(ramus of L1)

Cutaneous branches of
dorsal rami of L1 to L3

Figure 4.   Superficial muscles of the back, posterior view.

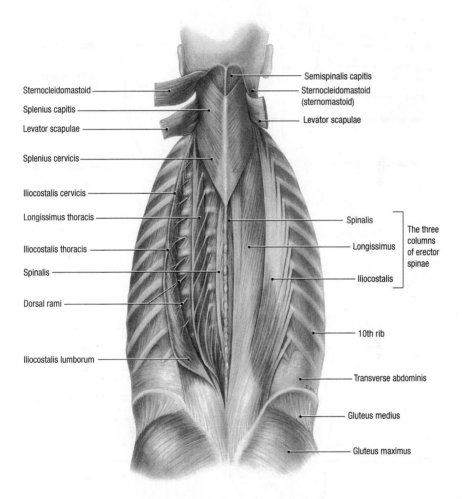

Figure 5. Deep muscles of the back, posterior view.

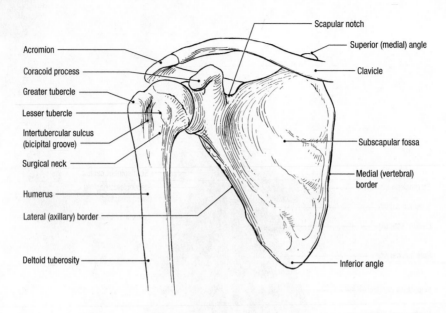

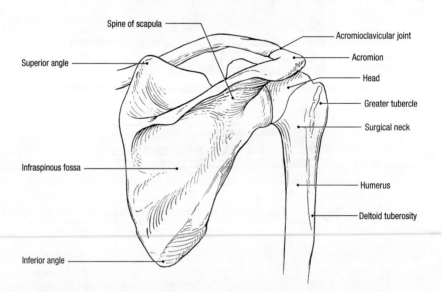

Figure 6. Pectoral girdle and humerus. Anterior view (top), posterior view (bottom).

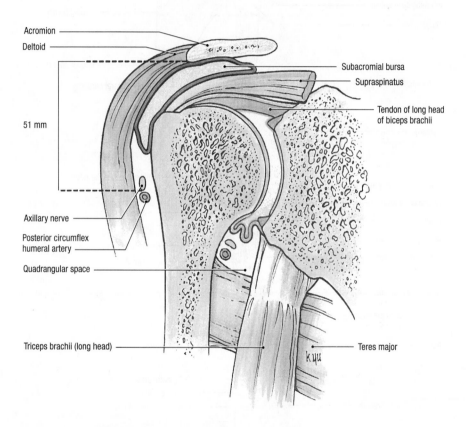

Acromion

Deltoid

Subacromial bursa

Supraspinatus

Tendon of long head
of biceps brachii

51 mm

Axillary nerve

Posterior circumflex
humeral artery

Quadrangular space

Triceps brachii (long head)

Teres major

Figure 7. Coronal section of the shoulder joint, posterior view.

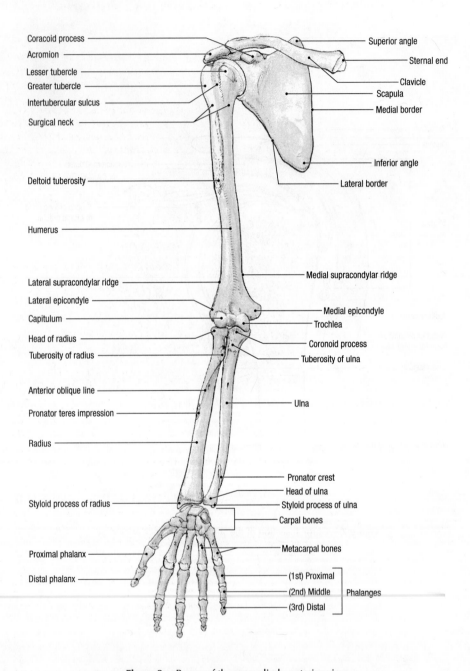

Figure 8. Bones of the upper limb, anterior view.

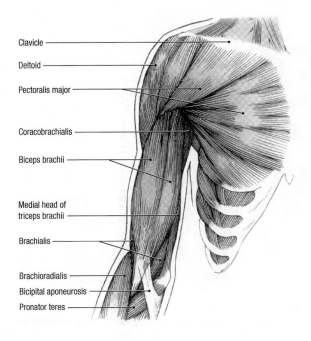

Clavicle

Deltoid

Pectoralis major

Coracobrachialis

Biceps brachii

Medial head of
triceps brachii

Brachialis

Brachioradialis

Bicipital aponeurosis

Pronator teres

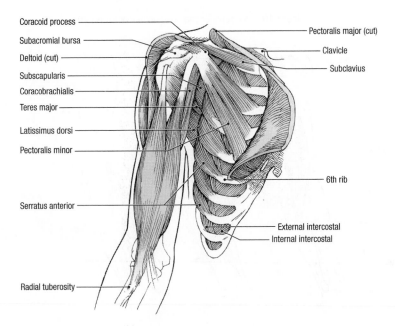

Coracoid process

Subacromial bursa

Deltoid (cut)

Subscapularis

Coracobrachialis

Teres major

Latissimus dorsi

Pectoralis minor

Serratus anterior

Radial tuberosity

Pectoralis major (cut)

Clavicle

Subclavius

6th rib

External intercostal
Internal intercostal

Figure 9. Superficial (top) and deep (bottom) muscles of the shoulder and chest.

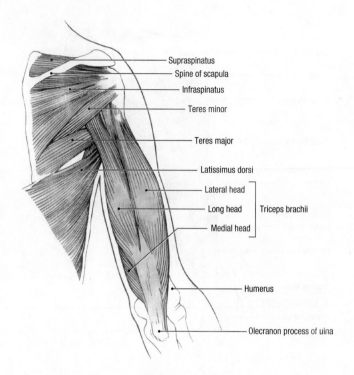

Supraspinatus
Spine of scapula
Infraspinatus
Teres minor
Teres major
Latissimus dorsi
Lateral head
Long head — Triceps brachii
Medial head
Humerus
Olecranon process of ulna

Figure 10. Muscles of the arm, posterior view.

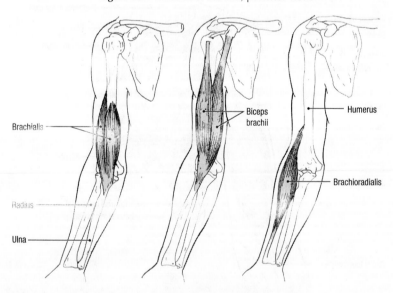

Brachialis

Biceps brachii

Humerus

Brachioradialis

Radius

Ulna

Figure 11. Muscles of the arm, anterior view.

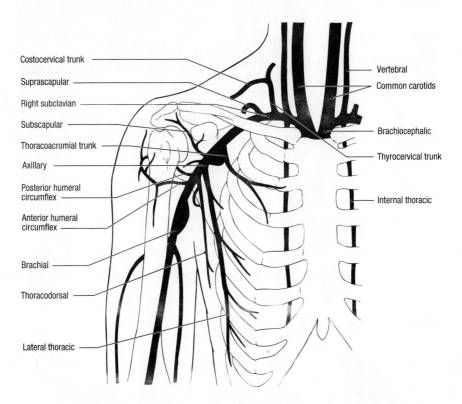

Figure 12. Blood supply to the shoulder.

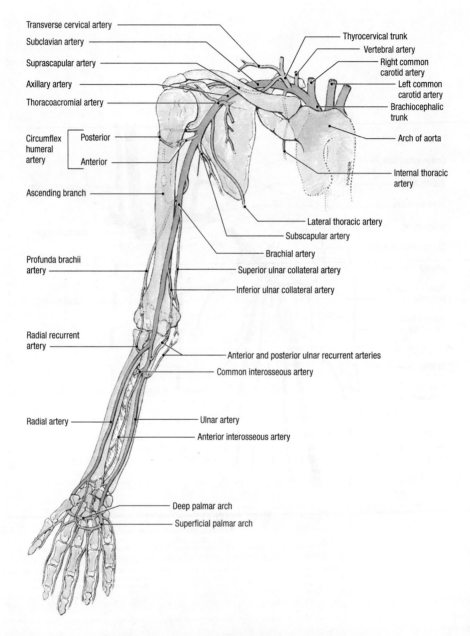

Figure 13. Arteries of the upper limb, anterior view.

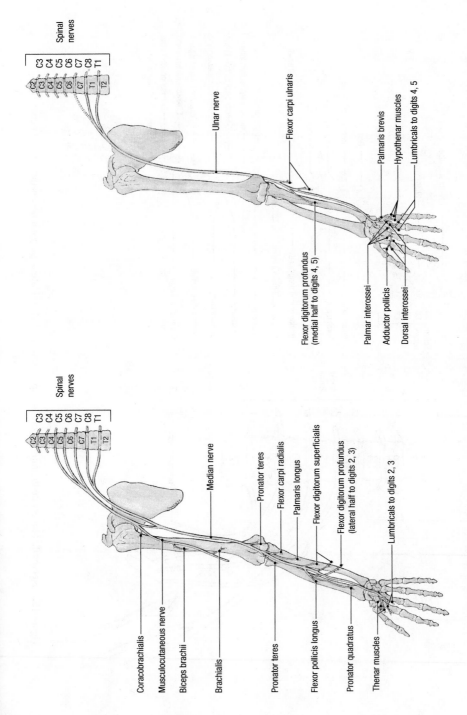

Figure 14. Nerves that innervate the muscles of the upper limb. Median and musculocutaneous nerves (left), ulnar nerve (right).

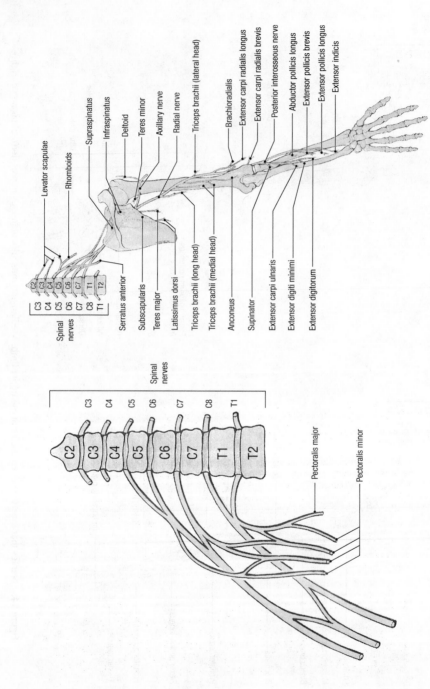

Figure 15. Nerves that innervate the muscles of the upper limb. Medial and lateral pectoral nerves (left), radial nerve (right).

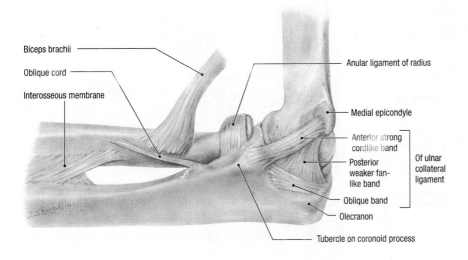

Biceps brachii

Oblique cord

Interosseous membrane

Anular ligament of radius

Medial epicondyle

Anterior strong cordlike band

Posterior weaker fan-like band

Oblique band

Olecranon

Tubercle on coronoid process

Of ulnar collateral ligament

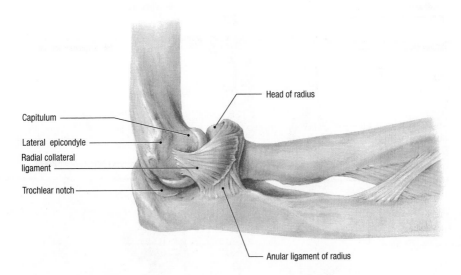

Head of radius

Capitulum

Lateral epicondyle

Radial collateral ligament

Trochlear notch

Anular ligament of radius

Figure 16. Collateral ligaments of the elbow. Medial view (top), lateral view (bottom).

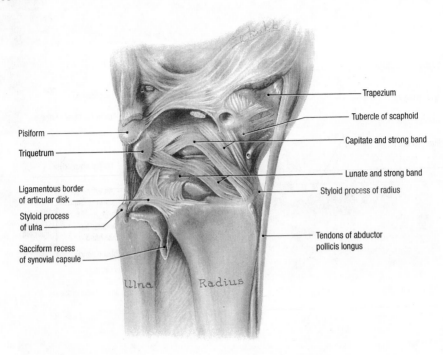

Trapezium

Tubercle of scaphoid

Capitate and strong band

Pisiform

Triquetrum

Lunate and strong band

Styloid process of radius

Ligamentous border of articular disk

Styloid process of ulna

Sacciform recess of synovial capsule

Tendons of abductor pollicis longus

Ulna   Radius

Figure 17. Ligaments of the distal radioulnar, radiocarpal, and intercarpal joints.

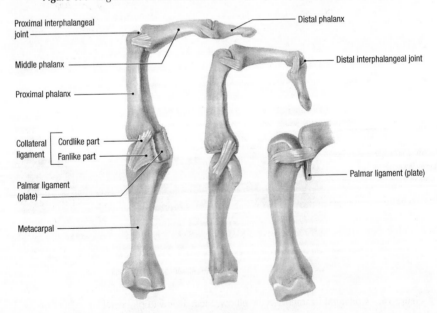

Proximal interphalangeal joint

Distal phalanx

Middle phalanx

Distal interphalangeal joint

Proximal phalanx

Collateral ligament — Cordlike part / Fanlike part

Palmar ligament (plate)

Palmar ligament (plate)

Metacarpal

Figure 18. Ligaments of metacarpophalangeal and interphalangeal joints.

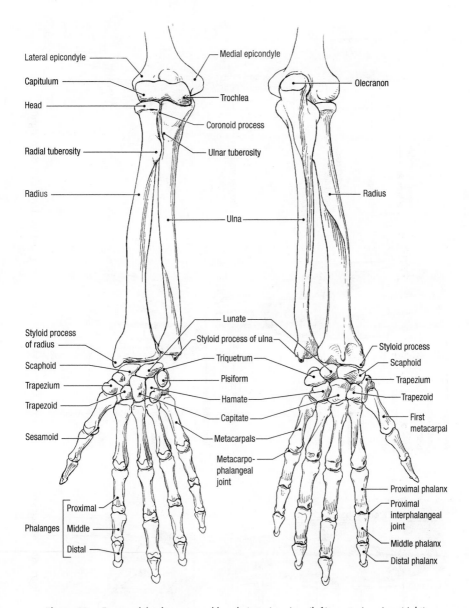

Figure 19. Bones of the forearm and hand. Anterior view (left), posterior view (right).

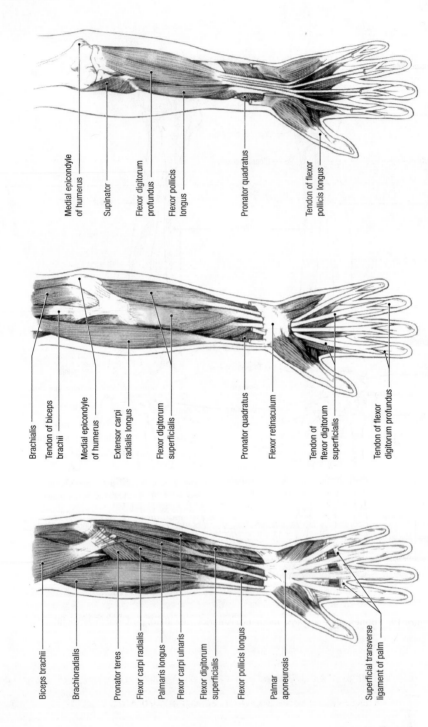

Figure 20. Muscles of the wrist and hand, anterior view. Superficial (left), mid-level (middle), deep (right).

Medial epicondyle of humerus

Supinator

Flexor digitorum profundus

Flexor pollicis longus

Pronator quadratus

Tendon of flexor pollicis longus

Brachialis

Tendon of biceps brachii

Medial epicondyle of humerus

Extensor carpi radialis longus

Flexor digitorum superficialis

Pronator quadratus

Flexor retinaculum

Tendon of flexor digitorum superficialis

Tendon of flexor digitorum profundus

Biceps brachii

Brachioradialis

Pronator teres

Flexor carpi radialis

Palmaris longus

Flexor carpi ulnaris

Flexor digitorum superficialis

Flexor pollicis longus

Palmar aponeurosis

Superficial transverse ligament of palm

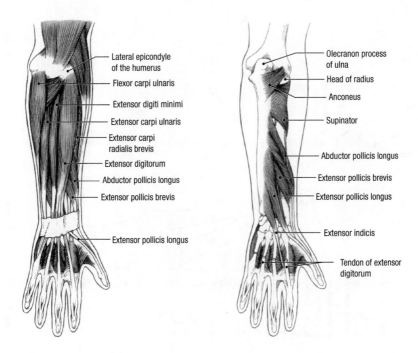

Figure 21. Muscles of the wrist and hand, posterior view. Superficial (left), deep (right).

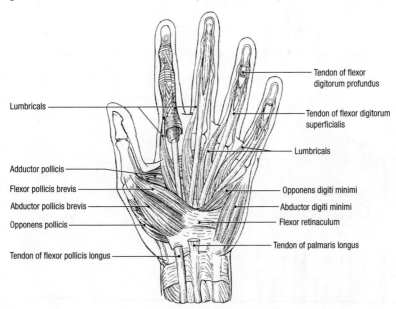

Figure 22. Muscles of the hand, anterior (palmar) view.

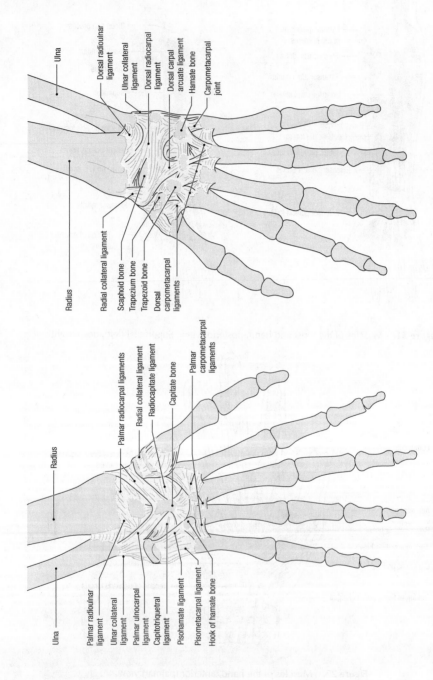

Figure 23. Wrist joint showing relative positions of skeletal structures and ligaments. Anterior (palmar) view of left hand (left), posterior (dorsal) view of left hand (right).

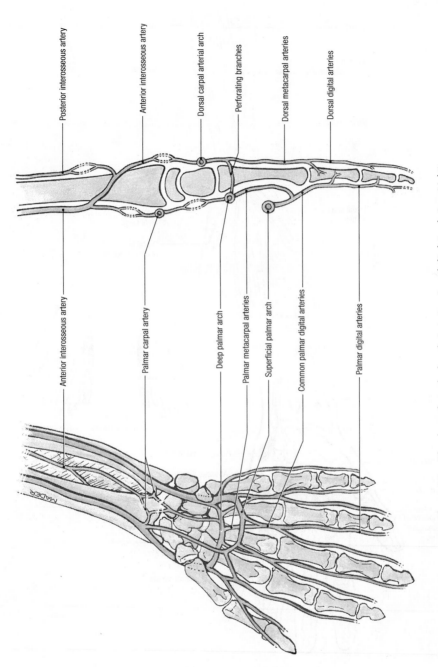

Figure 24. Blood supply to the hand. Anterior view (left), lateral view (right).

Posterior interosseous artery

Anterior interosseous artery

Dorsal carpal arterial arch

Perforating branches

Dorsal metacarpal arteries

Dorsal digital arteries

Anterior interosseous artery

Palmar carpal artery

Deep palmar arch

Palmar metacarpal arteries

Superficial palmar arch

Common palmar digital arteries

Palmar digital arteries

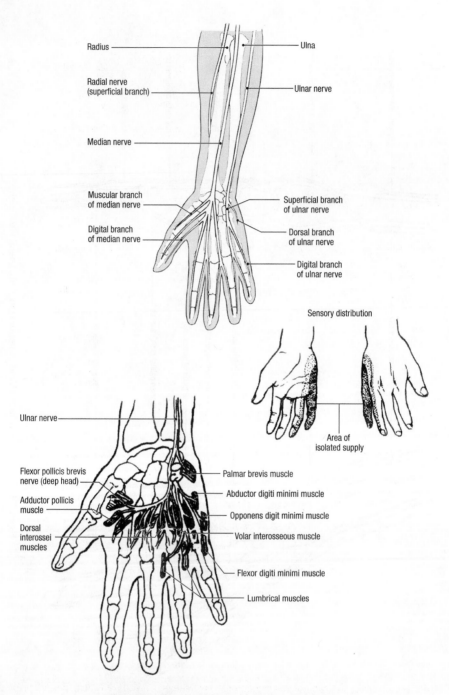

Radius

Ulna

Radial nerve
(superficial branch)

Ulnar nerve

Median nerve

Muscular branch
of median nerve

Superficial branch
of ulnar nerve

Digital branch
of median nerve

Dorsal branch
of ulnar nerve

Digital branch
of ulnar nerve

Sensory distribution

Area of
isolated supply

Ulnar nerve

Flexor pollicis brevis
nerve (deep head)

Palmar brevis muscle

Abductor digiti minimi muscle

Adductor pollicis
muscle

Opponens digit minimi muscle

Dorsal
interossei
muscles

Volar interosseous muscle

Flexor digiti minimi muscle

Lumbrical muscles

Figure 25. Nerves of the hand, sensory distribution.

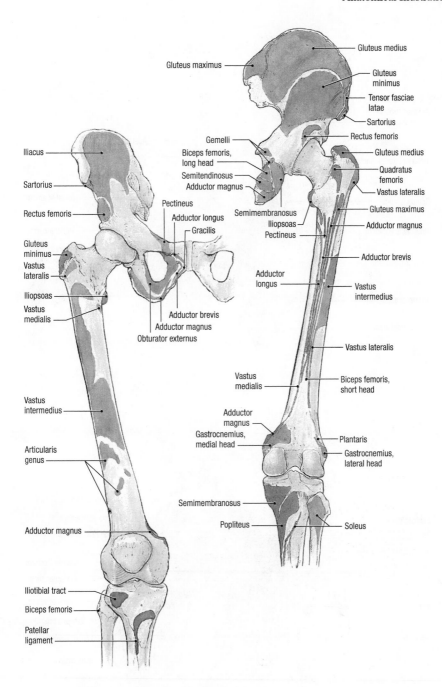

Figure 26. Bones of lower limbs showing muscle attachments. Anterior view (left), posterior view (right).

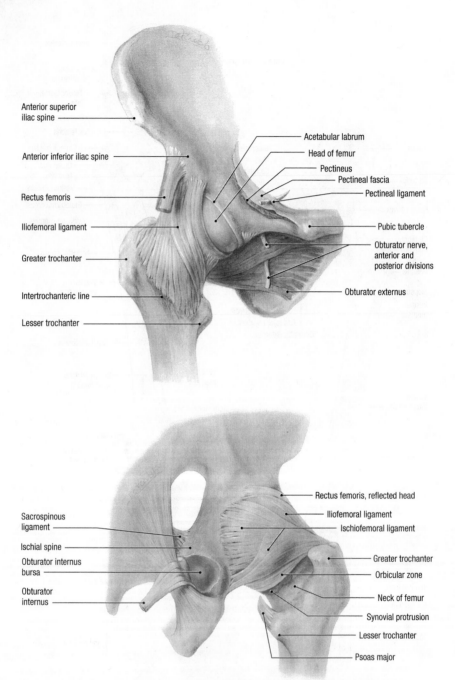

Figure 27. Hip joint. Anterior view (top), posterior view (bottom).

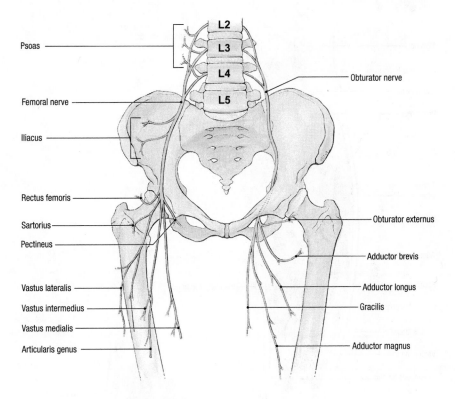

Figure 28.   Femoral and obturator nerves.

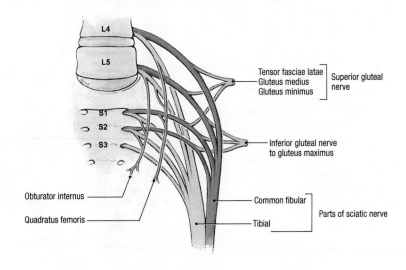

Figure 29.   Formation of the sciatic nerve in the pelvis.

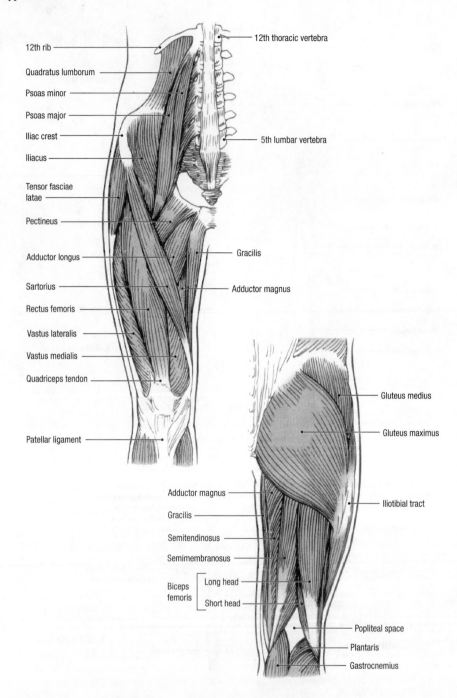

Figure 30. Superficial muscles of the hip and thigh. Anterior view (left), posterior view (right).

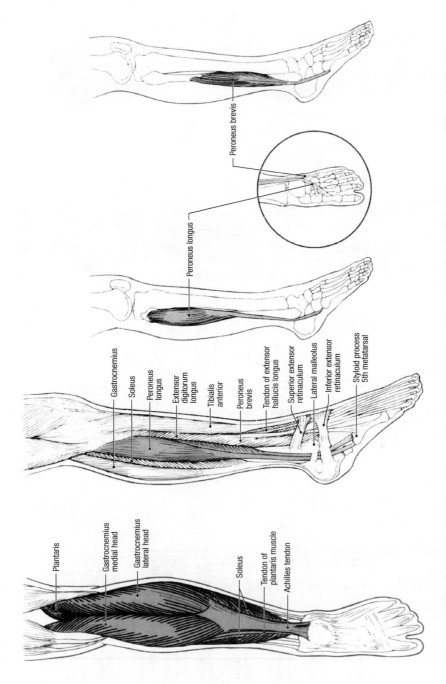

Figure 31. Muscles of the lower leg. Superficial compartment, posterior view (left), lateral compartment (middle and right).

Peroneus brevis

Peroneus longus

Gastrocnemius

Soleus

Peroneus longus

Extensor digitorum longus

Tibialis anterior

Peroneus brevis

Tendon of extensor hallucis longus

Superior extensor retinaculum

Lateral malleolus

Inferior extensor retinaculum

Styloid process 5th metatarsal

Plantaris

Gastrocnemius medial head

Gastrocnemius lateral head

Soleus

Tendon of plantaris muscle

Achilles tendon

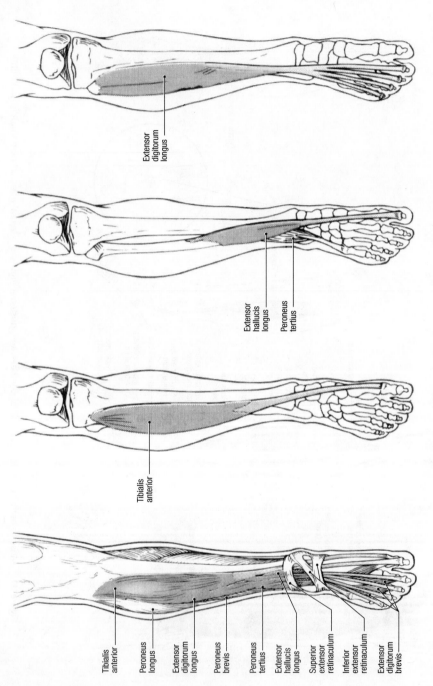

Figure 32. Muscles of the lower leg, anterior compartment.

Extensor
digitorum
longus

Extensor
hallucis
longus

Peroneus
tertius

Tibialis
anterior

Tibialis
anterior

Peroneus
longus

Extensor
digitorum
longus

Peroneus
brevis

Peroneus
tertius

Extensor
hallucis
longus

Superior
extensor
retinaculum

Inferior
extensor
retinaculum

Extensor
digitorum
brevis

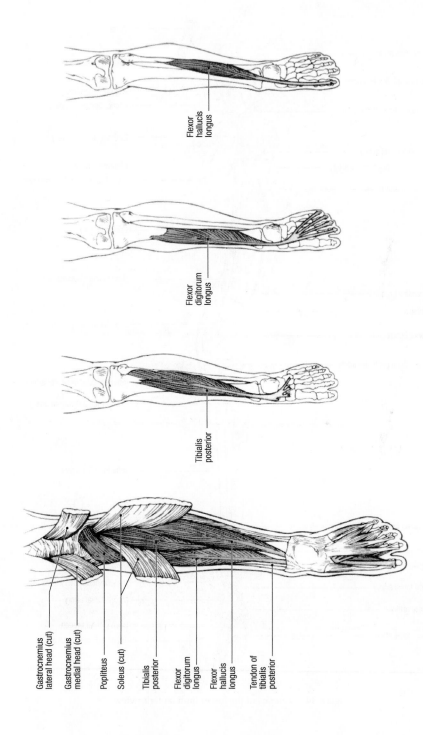

Figure 33. Muscles of the lower leg, deep compartment, posterior view.

Flexor hallucis longus

Flexor digitorum longus

Tibialis posterior

Gastrocnemius lateral head (cut)

Gastrocnemius medial head (cut)

Popliteus

Soleus (cut)

Tibialis posterior

Flexor digitorum longus

Flexor hallucis longus

Tendon of tibialis posterior

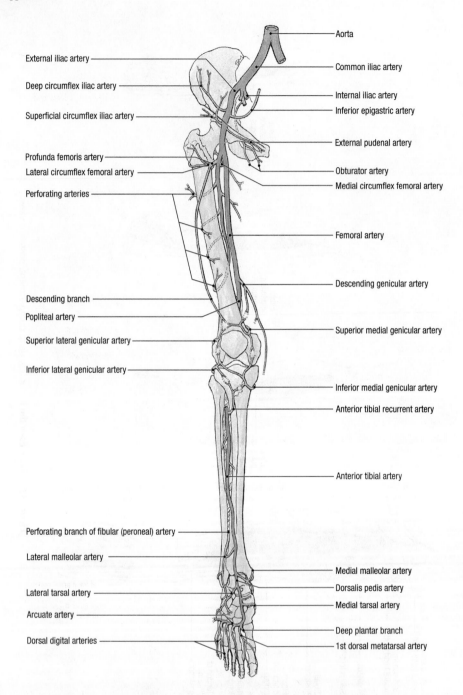

External iliac artery

Deep circumflex iliac artery

Superficial circumflex iliac artery

Profunda femoris artery

Lateral circumflex femoral artery

Perforating arteries

Descending branch

Popliteal artery

Superior lateral genicular artery

Inferior lateral genicular artery

Perforating branch of fibular (peroneal) artery

Lateral malleolar artery

Lateral tarsal artery

Arcuate artery

Dorsal digital arteries

Aorta

Common iliac artery

Internal iliac artery

Inferior epigastric artery

External pudenal artery

Obturator artery

Medial circumflex femoral artery

Femoral artery

Descending genicular artery

Superior medial genicular artery

Inferior medial genicular artery

Anterior tibial recurrent artery

Anterior tibial artery

Medial malleolar artery

Dorsalis pedis artery

Medial tarsal artery

Deep plantar branch

1st dorsal metatarsal artery

Figure 34. Arteries of the lower limb, anterior view.

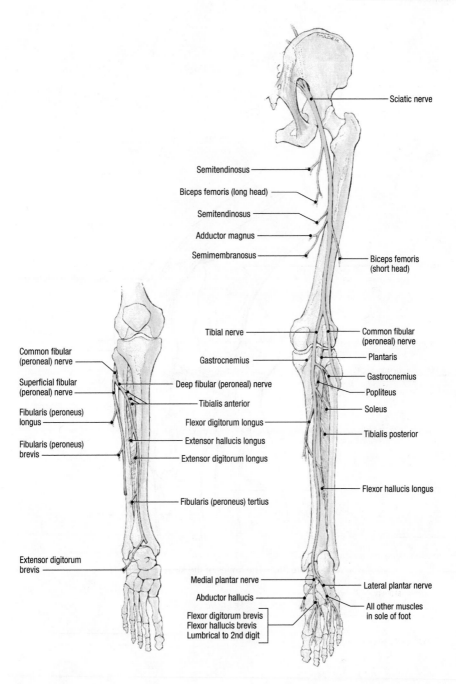

Figure 35. Motor distribution of the nerves of the lower limb. Common fibular (peroneal) nerve (left), sciatic nerve (right).

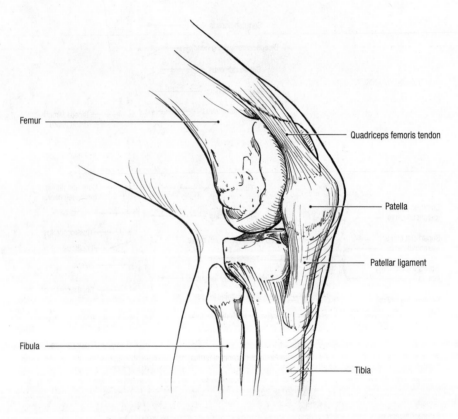

Femur

Quadriceps femoris tendon

Patella

Patellar ligament

Fibula

Tibia

Figure 36.   The bones of the knee joint.

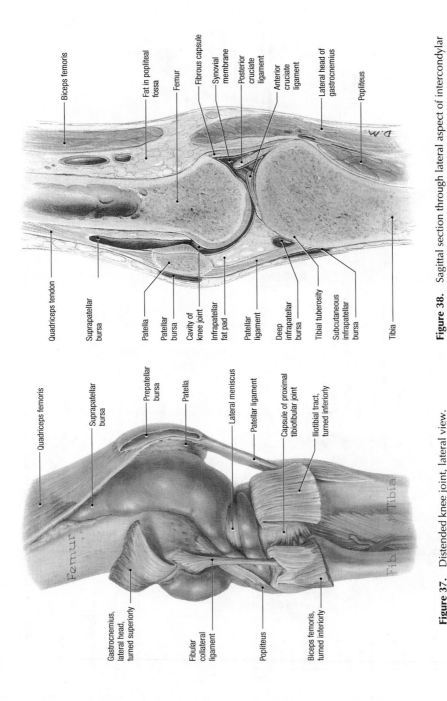

Figure 38. Sagittal section through lateral aspect of intercondylar notch of femur.

Figure 37. Distended knee joint, lateral view.

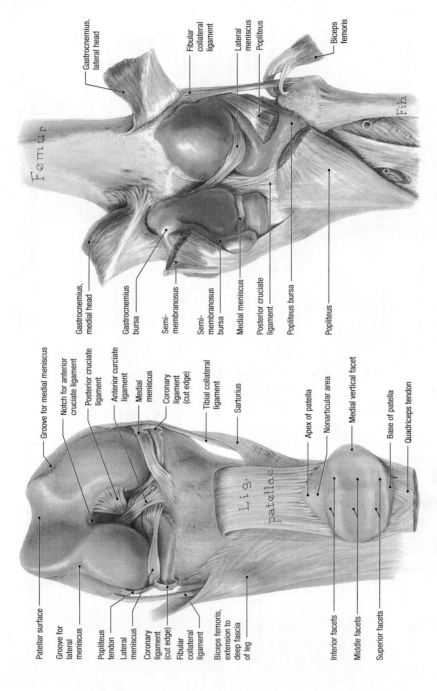

Figure 39. Articular surfaces and ligaments of the knee joint. Anterior view (left), posterior view (right).

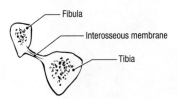

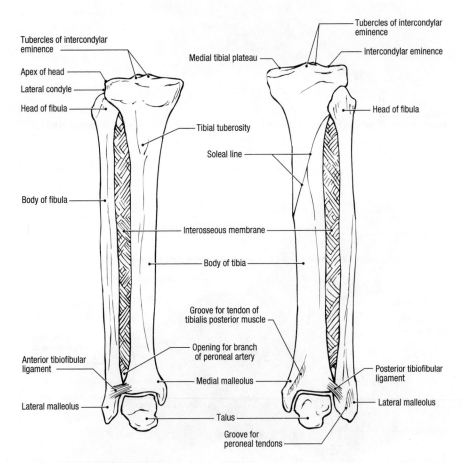

Figure 40. Bones of lower leg. Anterior view (left), posterior view (right), cross-section (top).

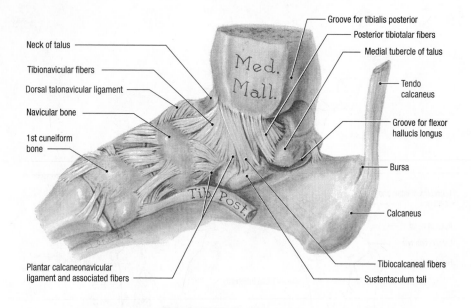

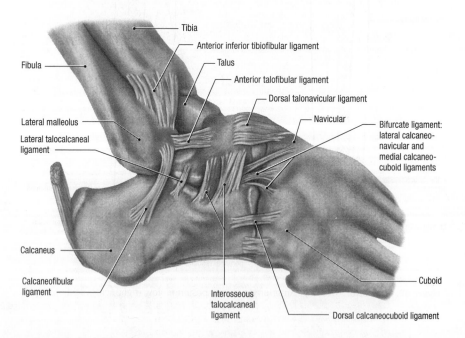

Figure 41. Ligaments of the ankle. Medial view (top), lateral view (bottom).

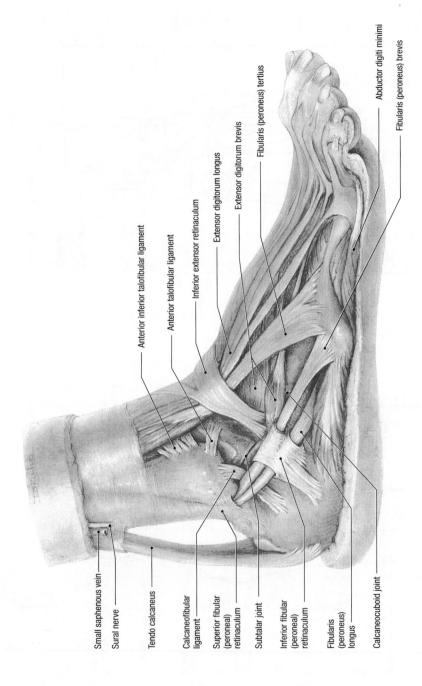

Figure 42. Tendons of the ankle, lateral view.

Small saphenous vein

Sural nerve

Tendo calcaneus

Calcaneofibular ligament

Superior fibular (peroneal) retinaculum

Subtalar joint

Inferior fibular (peroneal) retinaculum

Fibularis (peroneus) longus

Calcaneocuboid joint

Anterior inferior talofibular ligament

Anterior talofibular ligament

Inferior extensor retinaculum

Extensor digitorum longus

Extensor digitorum brevis

Fibularis (peroneus) tertius

Abductor digiti minimi

Fibularis (peroneus) brevis

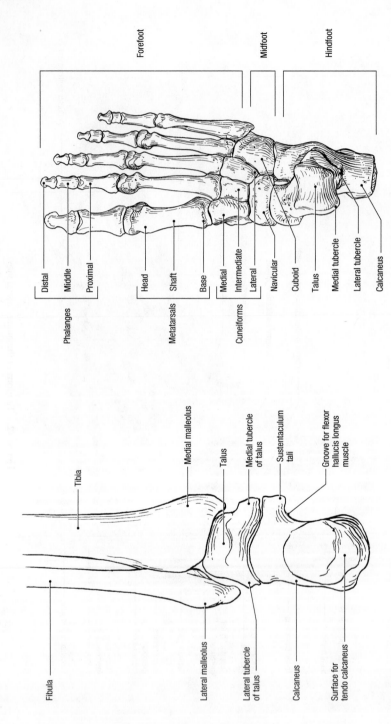

Figure 43. Bones of the ankle and foot. Posterior view (left), dorsal view (right).

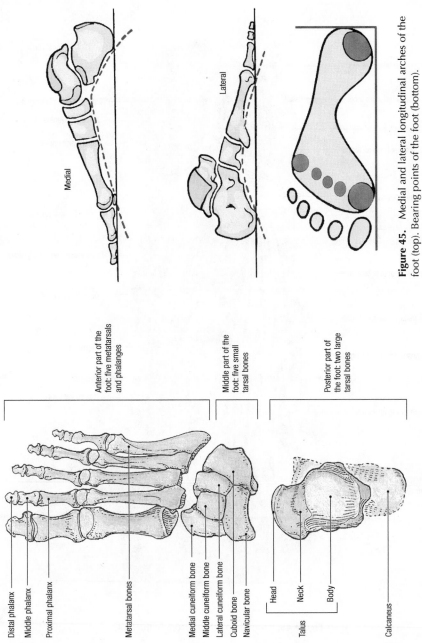

Medial

Lateral

Figure 45. Medial and lateral longitudinal arches of the foot (top). Bearing points of the foot (bottom).

Anterior part of the foot: five metatarsals and phalanges

Middle part of the foot: five small tarsal bones

Posterior part of the foot: two large tarsal bones

Distal phalanx
Middle phalanx
Proximal phalanx

Metatarsal bones

Medial cuneiform bone
Middle cuneiform bone
Lateral cuneiform bone
Cuboid bone
Navicular bone

Head
Neck
Body

Talus

Calcaneus

Figure 44. Bones of the foot, dorsal view.

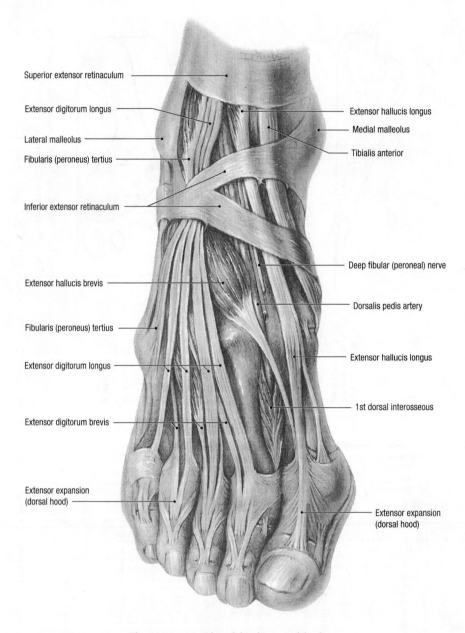

Superior extensor retinaculum

Extensor digitorum longus

Lateral malleolus

Fibularis (peroneus) tertius

Inferior extensor retinaculum

Extensor hallucis brevis

Fibularis (peroneus) tertius

Extensor digitorum longus

Extensor digitorum brevis

Extensor expansion
(dorsal hood)

Extensor hallucis longus

Medial malleolus

Tibialis anterior

Deep fibular (peroneal) nerve

Dorsalis pedis artery

Extensor hallucis longus

1st dorsal interosseous

Extensor expansion
(dorsal hood)

Figure 46. Muscles of the dorsum of the foot.

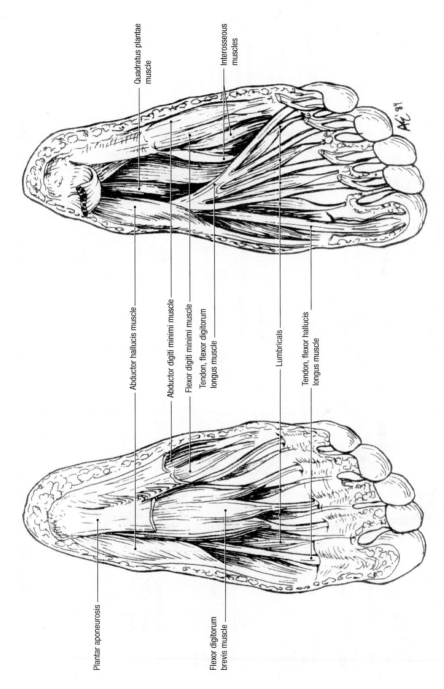

Quadratus plantae muscle

Interosseous muscles

Abductor hallucis muscle

Abductor digiti minimi muscle

Flexor digiti minimi muscle

Tendon, flexor digitorum longus muscle

Lumbricals

Tendon, flexor hallucis longus muscle

Plantar aponeurosis

Flexor digitorum brevis muscle

Figure 47. Superficial muscles of the plantar foot. First layer (left), second layer (right).

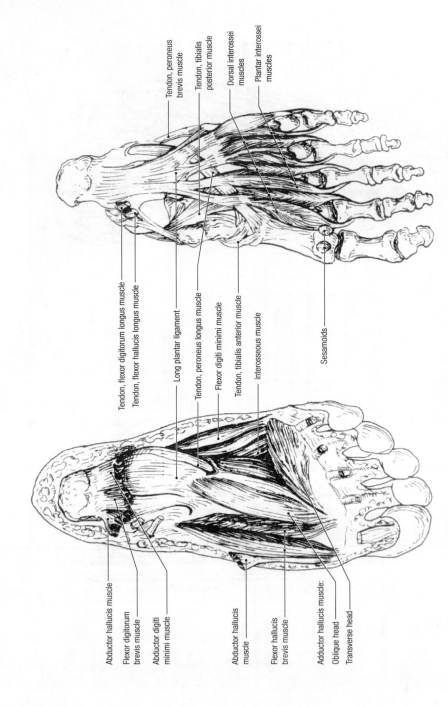

Figure 48. Deep muscles of the plantar foot. Third layer (left), fourth layer (right) with the deep ligaments.

Tendon, peroneus brevis muscle

Tendon, tibialis posterior muscle

Dorsal interossei muscles

Plantar interossei muscles

Tendon, flexor digitorum longus muscle

Tendon, flexor hallucis longus muscle

Long plantar ligament

Tendon, peroneus longus muscle

Flexor digiti minimi muscle

Tendon, tibialis anterior muscle

Interosseous muscle

Sesamoids

Abductor hallucis muscle

Flexor digitorum brevis muscle

Abductor digiti minimi muscle

Abductor hallucis muscle

Flexor hallucis brevis muscle

Adductor hallucis muscle:

Oblique head

Transverse head

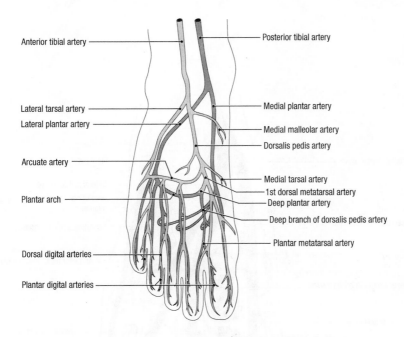

Figure 49. Dorsum of the foot showing the arterial circulation.

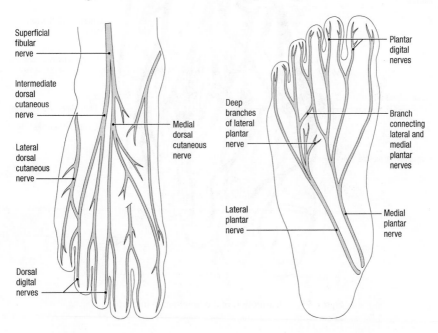

Figure 50. Innervation of the foot. Dorsal view (left), plantar view (right).

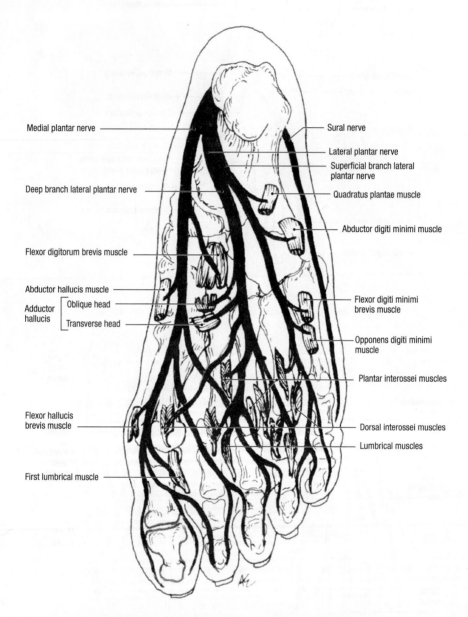

Medial plantar nerve

Sural nerve

Lateral plantar nerve

Superficial branch lateral plantar nerve

Deep branch lateral plantar nerve

Quadratus plantae muscle

Abductor digiti minimi muscle

Flexor digitorum brevis muscle

Abductor hallucis muscle

Adductor hallucis
Oblique head
Transverse head

Flexor digiti minimi brevis muscle

Opponens digiti minimi muscle

Plantar interossei muscles

Flexor hallucis brevis muscle

Dorsal interossei muscles

Lumbrical muscles

First lumbrical muscle

Figure 51. Distribution of the tibial nerve in the foot.

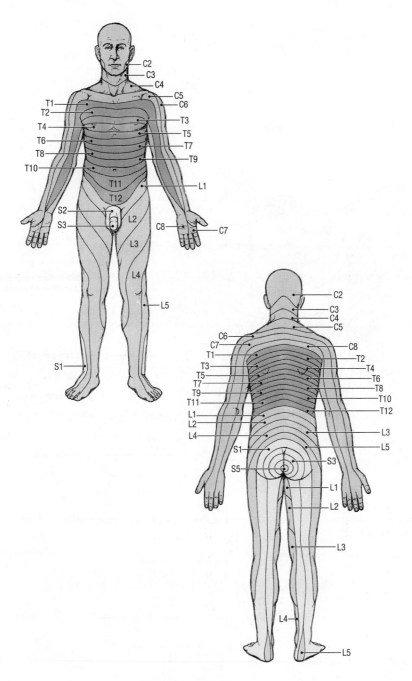

Figure 52. Dermatomes.

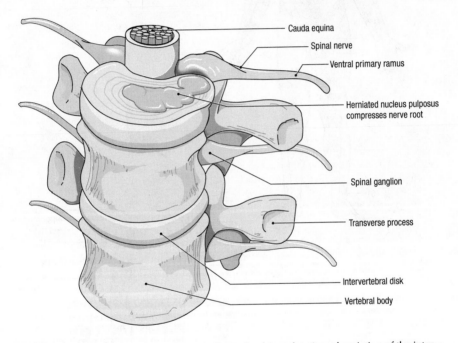

Figure 53. Anterosuperior view of portion of spinal column showing a herniation of the intervertebral disk.

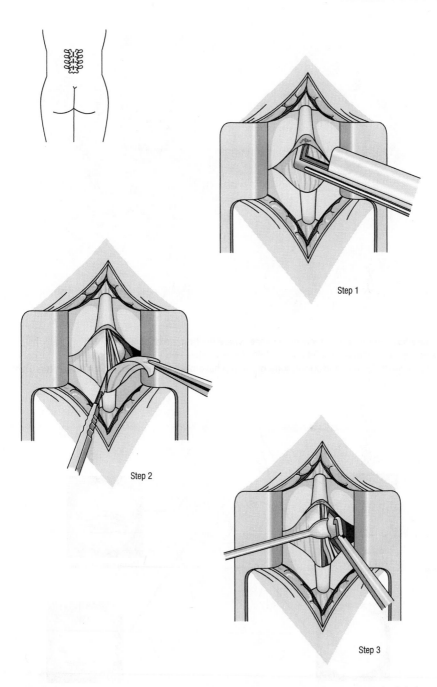

Figure 54. Surgical procedure, shown in three steps, of the excision of an intervertebral disk during diskectomy.

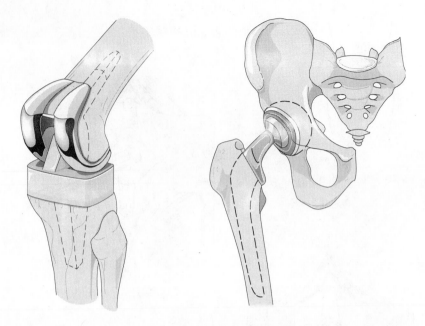

Figure 55. Anterolateral view of the knee where the bones that comprise the hinge joint have been replaced with a prosthetic knee (left). Anterior view of the pelvic skeleton where the bones that comprise the ball and socket joint of the hip have been replaced with a prosthetic hip (right).

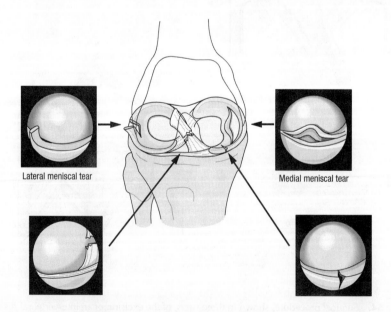

Lateral meniscal tear

Medial meniscal tear

Figure 56. Anterior view of the knee joint surrounded by arthroscopic views of tears.

Appendix 2
Fracture Illustrations

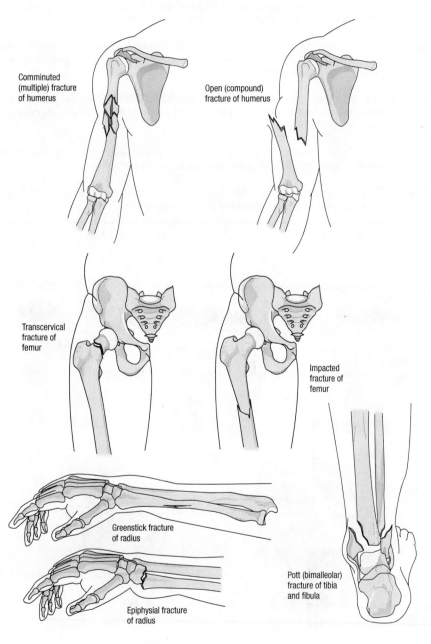

Comminuted (multiple) fracture of humerus

Open (compound) fracture of humerus

Transcervical fracture of femur

Impacted fracture of femur

Greenstick fracture of radius

Epiphysial fracture of radius

Pott (bimalleolar) fracture of tibia and fibula

Figure 1. Types of fractures.

Salter-Harris Classification Table

Type I   A Type I epiphysial separation occurs when the fracture extends through the epiphysial plate, resulting in displacement of the epiphysis.

Type II   In this injury, the direction of the fracture is similar to the Type I injury; however, a triangular segment of metaphysis is fractured and accompanies the separated epiphysial fragment.

Type III In a Type III epiphysial fracture, the fracture line extends from the joint through the epiphysis to the epiphysial plate, and then along the plate, dislodging a segment of epiphysis.

Type IV   In the Type IV injury, the fracture line passes from the joint surface, through the epiphysis, the epiphysial plate, and the adjacent metaphysis.

Type V   This variety of epiphysial injury results from a crushing type of force applied to the epiphysis, and the epiphysial plate is injured.

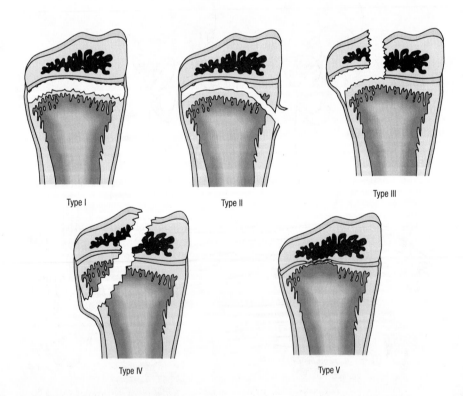

Figure 2. Five groups of the Salter-Harris classification of epiphysial plate injuries.

Direction of Fracture Lines

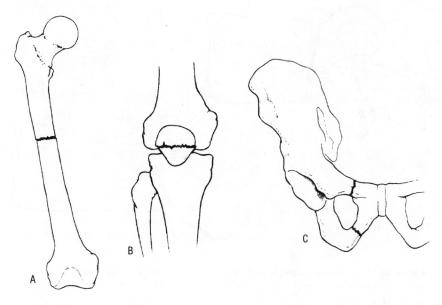

Figure 3. Transverse fractures. (A) Transverse fracture of the middle third of the femur. (B) Transverse fracture of the midpatella. (C) Transverse fracture of the superior and inferior pubic rami.

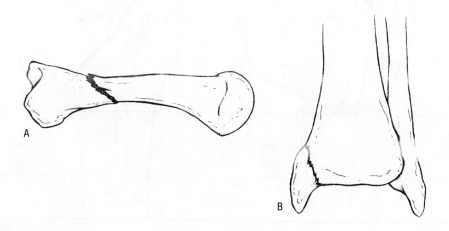

Figure 4. Oblique fractures. (A) Oblique fracture of the proximal third of metacarpal. (B) Oblique fracture of the medial malleolus.

Appendix 2

Spinal Fractures

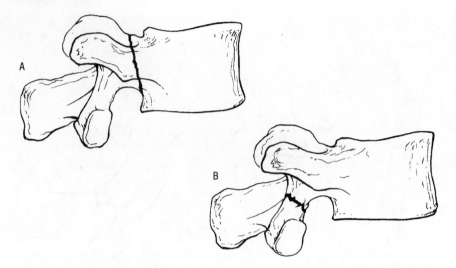

Figure 5. (A) Fracture through the pedicle. (B) Fracture through the pars interarticularis.

Shoulder Fractures

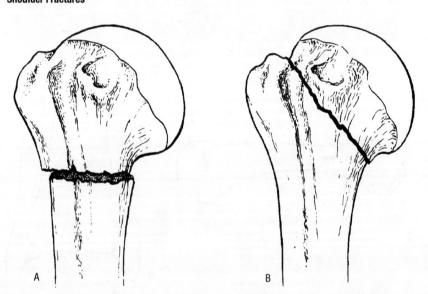

Figure 6. (A) Transverse fracture of the surgical neck of the humerus. (B) Fracture of the anatomic neck of the humerus.

Elbow Fractures

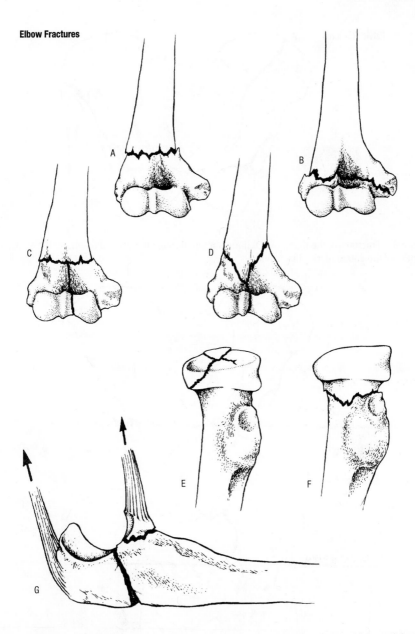

Figure 7. (A) Supracondylar fractures are fractures that occur above the level of the condyles. (B) Transcondylar fracture. Note that the fracture extends through both condyles. Comminuted intraarticular fractures of the distal humerus. (C) T-shaped fracture. (D) Y-shaped fracture. (E) Comminuted fracture of the head of the radius. (F) Transverse nondisplaced fracture of the neck of the radius. (G) Fracture of the olecranon and coronoid process. Muscle contraction can cause distraction of fracture fragments.

Pelvic Fractures

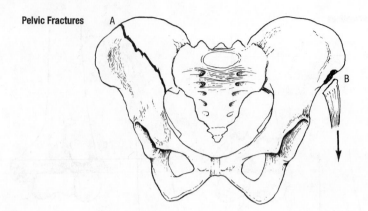

Figure 8. Fractures of the ilium. (A) Oblique fracture through the wing of the ilium. (B) Avulsion fracture of the anteroinferior iliac spine.

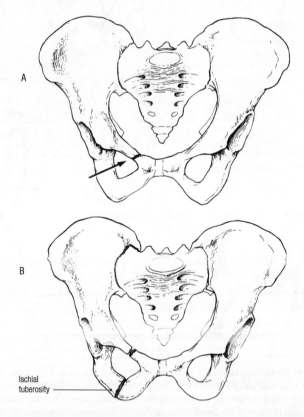

Ischial tuberosity

Figure 9. (A) Oblique fracture of the superior pubic ramus. (B) Transverse fractures of the inferior ischial ramus and superior pubic ramus.

Hip Fractures

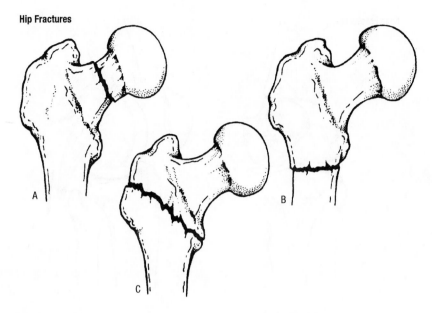

Figure 10. Fractures of the hip are described by the location in which they occur. (A) Transverse intracapsular fracture. (B) Oblique intertrochanteric fracture. (C) Transverse subtrochanteric fracture.

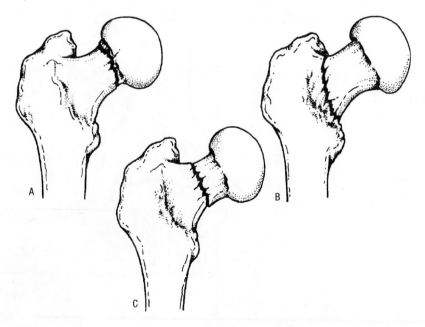

Figure 11. Subclassification of intracapsular fractures. (A) Subcapital fracture. (B) Transcervical fracture. (C) Base of neck fracture.

Knee Fractures

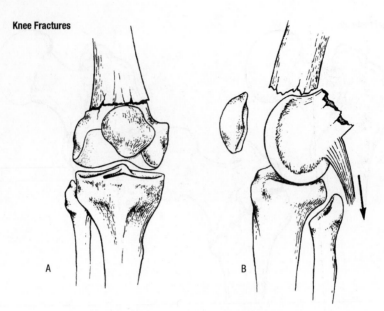

Figure 12. Supracondylar fracture. Transverse supracondylar fracture of the femur. Note the pull of the gastrocnemius muscle, causing the distal fragment to be rotated posteriorly.

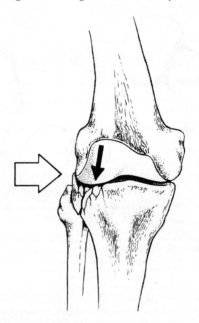

Figure 13. A valgus force applied to the knee causes the hard femoral condyle to be driven into the softer tibial plateau, resulting in depression of the tibial plateau.

Ankle Fractures

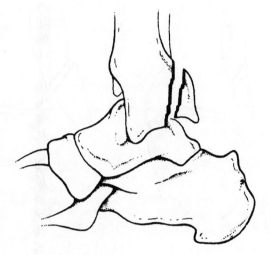

Figure 14. Fracture of the posterior malleolus.

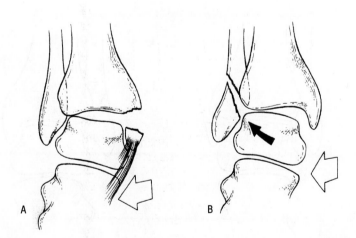

Figure 15. (A) Avulsion fracture of the medial malleolus. (B) Oblique fracture of the lateral malleolus.

Ankle Fractures

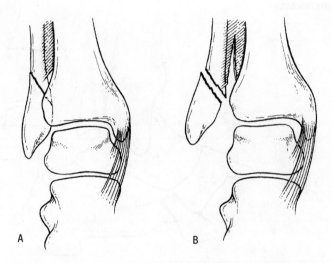

Figure 16. (A) Fracture of the lateral malleolus occurring above its articular surface; thus, the ankle mortise is not involved. (B) Similar fracture as in A, above the articular surface with disturbance of the mortise due to separation of the syndesmosis.

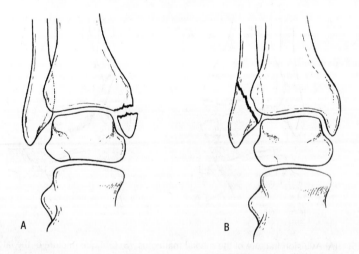

Figure 17. Fractures of the malleoli. (A) Transverse fracture of the medial malleolus. (B) Oblique fracture of the lateral malleolus.

Ankle Fractures

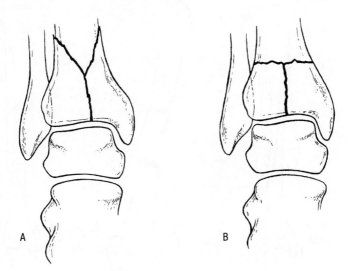

Figure 18. (A) Y-shaped comminuted intraarticular fracture of the distal tibia. (B) T-shaped comminuted intraarticular fracture of the distal tibia.

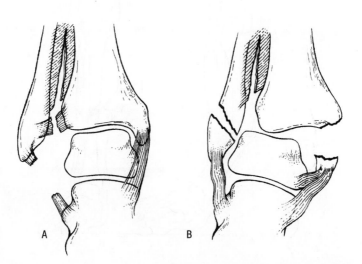

Figure 19. Separation of the distal tibiofibular syndesmosis. (A) Separation of the tibiofibular syndesmosis without an accompanying fracture. (B) Separation of the syndesmosis associated with fracture of the medial and lateral malleoli.

Leg Fractures

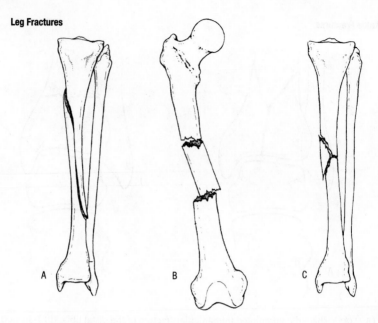

Figure 20. (A) Spiral fractures of the middle third of the tibia. (B) Segmental fracture of the femur. (C) Butterfly fragment.

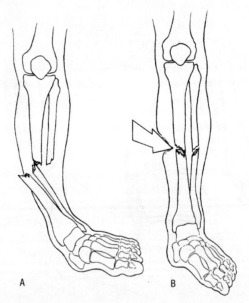

Figure 21. (A) Compound fracture caused by an inside-out injury. The skin defect is caused, following the fracture, by the bone perforating the skin from within. (B) Outside-in compound fracture. In this injury, the skin defect is produced by the fracturing agent entering from without.

Foot Fractures

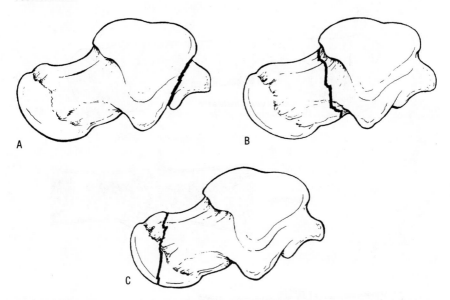

Figure 22. Fractures of the talus can be described by the anatomic area involved. (A) Fracture of the posterior process. (B) Fracture of the body. (C) Fracture of the head.

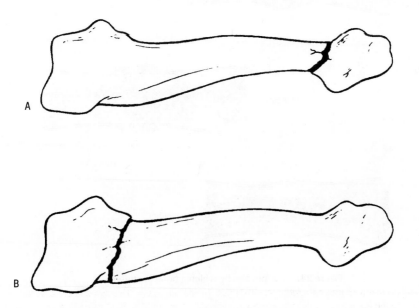

Figure 23. (A) Fracture of the head of a metatarsal. (B) Fracture of the base of a metatarsal.

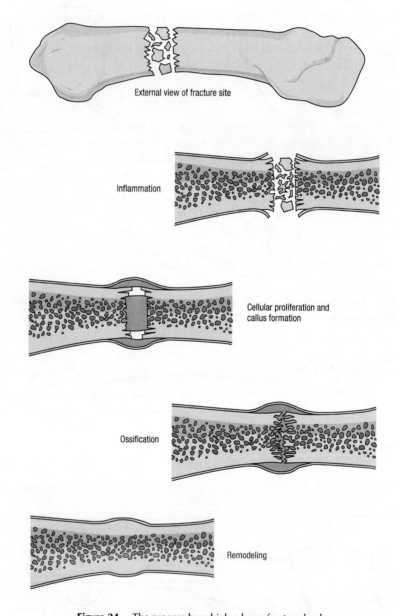

External view of fracture site

Inflammation

Cellular proliferation and
callus formation

Ossification

Remodeling

Figure 24. The process by which a bone fracture heals.

Appendix 3

Table of Muscles

1. Muscles of the Shoulder

Muscle	Origin	Insertion	Nerve	Action
Deltoid	Lateral third of clavicle, acromion, and spine of scapula	Deltoid tuberosity of humerus	Axillary, C5, C6	Abducts, adducts, flexes, extends, and rotates arm medially
Infraspinatus	Infraspinous fossa of scapula	Middle facet of greater tubercle of humerus	Suprascapular, C5, C6	Rotates arm laterally; helps to hold humeral head in glenoid cavity of scapula
Latissimus dorsi	Spines of T7-T12 thoracolumbar fascia, iliac crest, ribs 9–12	Floor of bicipital groove of humerus	Thoracodorsal, C6, C7, C8	Extends, adducts, and medially rotates humerus; raises body towards arms during climbing
Pectoralis major	Clavicular head: anterior surface of medial half of clavicle	Lateral lip of intertubercular groove of humerus	Lateral and medial pectoral nerves; clavicular head C5 and C6, sternocostal head C7, C8, and T1	Abducts, medially rotates humerus; draws scapula anteriorly and inferiorly
Pectoralis minor	3rd to 5th ribs near the costal cartilages	Medial border and superior surface of coracoid process of scapula	Medial pectoral nerve C8 and T1	Stabilizes scapula against thoracic wall
Subscapularis	Subscapular fossa	Lesser tubercle of humerus	Upper and lower subscapular, C5, C6, C7	Medially rotates arm and adducts it; helps to hold humeral head in glenoid cavity

(continued)

Muscle	Origin	Insertion	Nerve	Action
Supraspinatus	Supraspinous fossa of scapula	Superior facet of greater tubercle of humerus	Suprascapular, C4, C5, C6.	Initiates and assists deltoid in abduction of arm and acts with rotator cuff muscles
Teres minor	Superior portion of lateral border of scapula	Inferior facet of greater tubercle of humerus	Axillary, C5, C6	Laterally rotates arm; helps to hold humeral head in glenoid cavity of scapula
Teres major	Dorsal surface of inferior angle of scapula	Medial lip of intertubercular groove of humerus	Lower subscapular, C6, C7	Adducts and rotates arm medially

2. Muscles of the Arm

Muscle	Origin	Insertion	Nerve	Action
Anconeus	Lateral epicondyle of humerus	Lateral surface of olecranon and superior part of posterior surface of ulna	Radial, C7, C8, and T1	Assists triceps in extending forearm; abducts ulna during pronation
Biceps brachii	Long head, supraglenoid tubercle; short head, coracoid process	Radial tuberosity of radius	Musculocutaneous, C5, C6	Flexes arm and forearm, supinates forearm
Brachialis	Distal anterior surface of humerus	Coronoid process of ulna and ulnar tuberosity	Musculocutaneous, C5, C6	Flexes forearm in all positions
Coracobrachialis	Tip of coracoid process of scapula	Middle third of medial surface of humerus	Musculocutaneous, C5, C6, C7	Flexes and adducts arm

(continued)

Muscle	Origin	Insertion	Nerve	Action
Triceps	Long head, infraglenoid tubercle; lateral head, superior to radial groove of humerus; medial head to radial groove	Posterior surface of olecranon process of ulna	Radial, C6, C7, C8	Chief extensor of forearm at elbow

3. Muscles of the Anterior Forearm

Muscle	Origin	Insertion	Nerve	Action
Flexor carpi radialis	Medial epicondyle of humerus	Bases of second and third metacarpals	Median, C6, C7	Flexes forearm; flexes and abducts hand
Flexor carpi ulnaris	Humeral head medial epicondyle of humerus; ulnar head; olecranon and posterior border of ulna	Pisiform bone, hook of hamate, and base of fifth metacarpal	Ulnar, C7, C8	Flexes and adducts hand, flexes forearm
Flexor digitorum profundus	Anteromedial surface of ulna, interosseous membrane	Base of distal phalanges of medial four fingers	Ulnar and median, C8, T1	Flexes distal interphalangeal joints and hand
Flexor digitorum superficialis	Medial epicondyle, coronoid process of ulna, superior anterior border of radius	Middle phalanges of finger	Median, C7, C8, T1	Flexes proximal interphalangeal joints; flexes hand at wrist
Flexor pollicis longus	Anterior surface of radius and adjacent interosseus membrane	Base of distal phalanx of thumb	Median, C8, T1	Flexes thumb
Palmaris longus	Medial epicondyle of humerus	Distal half of flexor retinaculum, palmar aponeurosis	Median, C7, C8	Flexes hand at wrist and forearm

(continued)

Muscle	Origin	Insertion	Nerve	Action
Pronator quadratus	Anterior surface of distal ulna	Anterior surface of distal radius	Anterior interosseous nerve from median, C8, and T1	Pronates forearm; helps hold radius and ulna together
Pronator teres	Medial epicondyle of humerus and coronoid process of ulna	Middle of lateral surface of radius	Median, C6, C7	Pronates and flexes arm at elbow

4. Muscles of the Posterior Forearm

Muscle	Origin	Insertion	Nerve	Action
Abductor pollicis longus	Interosseous membrane, middle third of posterior surface of radius and ulna	Lateral surface of base of first metacarpal	Radial, deep branch, posterior interosseous nerve C7, C8	Abducts thumb and hand
Articularis cubiti	Distal portion of posterior aspect of shaft of humerus	Posterior fibrous capsule of elbow joint	Radial, C7, C8	Retracts posterior joint capsule during extension of elbow
Brachioradialis	Lateral supracondylar ridge of humerus	Base of radial styloid process	Radial, C5, C6, C7	Flexes forearm
Extensor carpi radialis brevis	Lateral epicondyle of humerus	Posterior base of third metacarpal	Radial, deep branch, C7, C8	Extends fingers and abducts hands at wrist
Extensor carpi radialis longus	Lateral supracondylar ridge of humerus	Dorsum of base of second metacarpal	Radial, C6, C7	Extends and abducts hand at wrist joint
Extensor carpi ulnaris	Lateral epicondyle and posterior surface of ulna	Base of fifth metacarpal	Radial, deep branch, posterior interosseous nerve C7, C8	Extends and adducts hand at wrist joint
Extensor digiti minimi	Common extensor tendon and interosseous membrane	Extensor expansion, base of middle and distal phalanges	Radial, deep branch, posterior interosseous nerve C7, C8	Extends little finger

(continued)

Muscle	Origin	Insertion	Nerve	Action
Extensor digitorum	Lateral epicondyle of humerus	Extensor expansion, base of middle and digital phalanges	Radial, deep branch, posterior interosseous nerve C7, C8	Extends fingers and hand at wrist
Extensor indicis	Posterior surface of ulna and interosseous membrane	Extensor expansion of index finger	Radial, deep branch, posterior interosseous nerve C7	Extends index finger, helps extend hand
Extensor pollicis brevis	Interosseous membrane and posterior surface of middle third of radius	Base of proximal phalanx of thumb	Radial, deep branch, posterior interosseous nerve C7, C8	Extends proximal phalanx of thumb and abducts hand
Extensor pollicis longus	Interosseous membrane, middle third of posterior surface of ulna	Base of distal phalanx of thumb	Radial, deep branch, posterior interosseous nerve C7, C8	Extends distal phalanx of thumb and abducts hand
Supinator	Lateral epicondyle of humerus, radial collateral and anular ligaments, crest of ulna	Lateral side of upper part of radius	Radial, deep branch, C5, C6	Supinates forearm

5. Muscles of the Hand

Muscle	Origin	Insertion	Nerve	Action
Abductor digiti minimi	Pisiform, pisohamate ligament, flexor retinaculum	Medial side of base of proximal phalanx of little finger	Ulnar, deep branch, C8, T1	Abducts little finger
Abductor pollicis brevis	Flexor retinaculum, scaphoid, and trapezium	Lateral side of base of proximal phalanx of thumb	Median, recurrent branch, C8, T1	Abducts thumb

(*continued*)

Muscle	Origin	Insertion	Nerve	Action
Adductor pollicis	Capitate and bases of second and third metacarpals, (oblique head); palmar surface of third metacarpal (transverse head)	Medial side of base of proximal phalanx of the thumb	Ulnar, deep branch, C8, T1	Adducts thumb towards middle digit
Dorsal interossei (4)	Adjacent sides of metacarpal bones	Extensor expansions and bases of phalanges of digits 2–4	Ulnar, deep branch, C8, T1	Abducts fingers; flexes metacarpophalangeal joints; extends interphalangeal joints
Flexor digiti minimi brevis	Flexor retinaculum and hook of hamate	Medial side of base of proximal phalanx of little finger	Ulnar, deep branch, C8, T1	Flexes proximal phalanx of little finger
Flexor pollicis brevis	Flexor retinaculum and trapezium	Base of proximal phalanx of thumb	Median, recurrent branch, C8, T1	Flexes thumb
Lumbricals (4)	1–2 lateral, 3–4 medial side of tendons of flexor digitorum profundus	Lateral side of extensor expansion	Median (two lateral), ulnar (two medial)	Flexes metacarpophalangeal joints, extends interphalangeal joints
Opponens digiti minimi	Flexor retinaculum and hook of hamate	Medial side of fifth metacarpal	Ulnar, deep branch, C8, T1	Opposes little finger with thumb
Opponens pollicis	Flexor retinaculum and tubercles of scaphoid and trapezium	Lateral side of first metacarpal	Median, recurrent branch, C8, T1	Opposes thumb to other digits
Palmar interossei (3)	Palmar surfaces of 2nd, 4th, and 5th metacarpals (unipennate muscles)	Bases of proximal phalanges on same sides as their origins; extensor expansion	Ulnar, deep branch, C8, T1	Adducts fingers; flexes metacarpophalangeal joints; extends interphalangeal joints

(continued)

Muscle	Origin	Insertion	Nerve	Action
Palmaris brevis	Ulnar side of flexor retinaculum, palmar aponeurosis	Skin of ulnar side of hand	Ulnar, superficial, T1	Wrinkles skin on palmar side of hand

6. Anterior Muscles of the Thigh

Muscle	Origin	Insertion	Nerve	Action
Abductor brevis/minimus	Inferior pubic ramus	Pectineal line; uppermost linea aspera of femur	Obturator, L2, L3, L4	Adducts, flexes, rotates thigh laterally
Abductor longus	Body of pubis below its crest	Middle third of linea aspera of femur	Obturator, branch of anterior division, L2, L3, L4	Adducts, flexes, rotates thigh laterally
Adductor magnus	Ischiopubic ramus; ischial tuberosity	Linea aspera; medial supracondylar line; adductor tubercle	Obturator, L2, L3, L4; sciatic L4	Adducts, flexes, rotates, and extends thigh
Gracilis	Body and inferior ramus of pubis	Superior part of medial surface of tibia	Obturator, L2, L3	Adducts and flexes thigh; flexes and rotates leg medially
Iliacus	Iliac crest, iliac fossa; ala of sacrum	Lesser trochanter, psoas major tendon	Femoral, L2, L4	Flexes and rotates thigh medially with psoas major
Obturator externus	Margin of obturator foramen and obturator membrane	Trochanteric fossa of femur	Obturator, L3, L4	Rotates thigh laterally
Pectineus	Pectineal line of pubis	Pectineal line of femur	Femoral, L3, L4; obturator	Adducts and flexes thigh; helps with rotation
Rectus femoris	Anterior inferior iliac spine; ilium rim of acetabulum	Base of patella; tibial tuberosity	Femoral, L2, L3, L4	Extends leg at knee joint; stabilizes hip; helps iliopsoas flex thigh

(continued)

Muscle	Origin	Insertion	Nerve	Action
Sartorius	Anterior superior iliac spine, superior part of notch inferior to it	Upper medial side of tibia	Femoral, L2, L3	Flexes, abducts, rotates thigh at hip laterally; flexes, rotates leg at knee joint
Vastus intermedius	Upper shaft of femur; lower lateral intermuscular septum	Base of patella; by patellar ligament to tibial tuberosity	Femoral	Extends leg at knee joint
Vastus lateralis	Intertrochanteric line; greater trochanter; linea aspera; gluteal tuberosity; lateral intermuscular septum	Lateral side of patella; tibial tuberosity	Femoral, L2, L3, L4	Extends leg at knee joint
Vastus medialis	Intertrochanteric line; linea aspera; medial intermuscular septum	Medial side of patella; tibial tuberosity	Femoral, L2, L3, L4	Extends leg at knee joint

7. Medial Muscles of the Thigh

Muscle	Origin	Insertion	Nerve	Action
Abductor brevis	Body and inferior ramus of pubis	Pectineal line and proximal part of linea aspera of femur	Obturator, L2, L3, L4	Adducts thigh; aids in flexion
Adductor longus	Body of pubis inferior to pubic crest	Middle third of linea aspera of femur	Obturator L2, L3, L4	Adducts thigh
Adductor magnus	Ischiopubic ramus; ischial tuberosity	Linea aspera; medial supracondylar line; adductor tubercle	Obturator and sciatic	Adducts, flexes, and extends thigh

(continued)

Muscle	Origin	Insertion	Nerve	Action
Gracilis	Body of inferior pubic of ramus	Superior part of medial surface of tibia	Obturator, L2, L3	Adducts thigh; flexes leg; helps rotate thigh medially
Obturator externus	Margin of obturator foramen and obturator membrane	Trochanteric fossa of femur	Obturator, L3, L4	Laterally rotates thigh; steadies head of femur in acetabulum
Pectineus	Pectineal line of pubis	Pectineal line of femur	Femoral L2 and L3; branch of obturator	Adducts and flexes thigh; aids in medial rotation of thigh

8. Muscles of the Gluteal Region

Muscle	Origin	Insertion	Nerve	Action
Coccygeus (ischiococcygeus)	Ischial spine	Inferior end of spine	Branches of S4 and S5 nerves	Forms small part of pelvic diaphragm that supports pelvic viscera and flexes coccyx
Gluteus maximus	Ilium; sacrum; coccyx; sacrotuberous ligament	Gluteal tuberosity; iliotibial tract	Inferior gluteal, L5, S1, S2	Extends and rotates thigh laterally
Gluteus medius	Ilium between iliac crest and anterior and posterior gluteal lines	Greater trochanter	Superior gluteal, L5, S1	Abducts and rotates thigh medially; helps keep pelvis level
Gluteus minimus	Ilium between anterior and posterior gluteal lines	Greater trochanter	Superior gluteal, L5, S1	Abducts and rotates thigh medially; helps keep pelvis level
Inferior gemellus	Ischial tuberosity	Obturator internus tendon	Nerve to quadratus femoris	Rotates thigh laterally

(continued)

A71

Muscle	Origin	Insertion	Nerve	Action
Obturator internus	Ischiopubic rami; obturator membrane	Greater trochanter	Nerve to obturator internus, L5, S1	Abducts and rotates thigh laterally
Piriformis	Pelvic surface of sacrum; sacrotuberous ligament	Superior border of greater trochanter	Sacral, S1, S2	Rotates thigh medially
Quadratus femoris	Ischial tuberosity	Inter-trochanteric crest	Nerve to quadratus femoral, L5, S1	Rotates thigh laterally

9. Posterior Muscles of the Thigh *

Muscle	Origin	Insertion	Nerve	Action
Biceps femoris	Long head from ischial tuberosity; short head from linea aspera and upper supracondylar line	Lateral side of head of fibula; tendon split here by fibular collateral ligament of knee	Tibial (long head), common peroneal; division of sciatic nerve, L5, S1, S2	Flexes leg medially; extends thigh
Semimembranosus	Ischial tuberosity	Medial condyle of tibia	Tibial portion of sciatic, L5, S1, S2	Extends thigh; rotates leg medially; helps raise trunk of body against gravity
Semitendinosus	Ischial tuberosity	Medial surface of superior part of tibia	Tibial division of sciatic nerve, L5, S1, S2	Extends thigh; flexes leg; rotates knee medially when flexed

* These three muscles collectively are called hamstrings.

10. Muscles of the Anterior and Lateral Leg

Muscle	Origin	Insertion	Nerve	Action
Anterior				
Articularis genus	Distal portion of anterior aspect of shaft of femur	Synovial membrane of suprapatellar bursa of knee joint	Femoral, L2-L4	Retracts synovial membrane during extension of the knee
Extensor digitorum longus	Lateral tibial condyle; upper two-thirds of fibula	Bases of middle and distal phalanges	Deep peroneal, L5, S1	Extends great toe and dorsiflexes ankle
Extensor hallucis longus	Middle half of anterior surface of fibula; interosseous membrane	Base of distal phalanx of great toe	Deep peroneal, L5, S1	Extends great toe; dorsiflexes and inverts foot
Peroneus tertius	Distal one-third of fibula; interosseous membrane	Base of fifth metatarsal	Deep peroneal	Dorsiflexes and inverts foot
Tibialis anterior	Lateral tibial condyle; interosseous membrane	First cuneiform; first metatarsal	Deep peroneal, L4, L5	Dorsiflexes and inverts foot
Lateral				
Peroneus brevis	Lower lateral side of fibula; interosseous membrane	Base of fifth metatarsal	Superficial peroneal	Everts and plantar flexes foot
Peroneus longus	Lateral tibial condyle; head and upper lateral side of fibula	Base of first metatarsal; medial cuneiform	Superficial peroneal	Everts and plantar flexes foot

11. Posterior Muscles of the Leg

Muscle	Origin	Insertion	Nerve	Action
Superficial group				
Gastrocnemius	Lateral (head) and medial (head) femoral condyle	Posterior aspect of calcaneus via tendo calcaneus	Tibial, S1, S2	Flexes knee; plantar flexes ankle when knee extended
Plantaris	Lower lateral supracondylar line and oblique popliteal ligament	Posterior surface of calcaneus	Tibial, S1, S2	Assist gastrocnemius in plantar flexing ankle and flexing knee
Soleus	Upper fibular head; soleal line on tibia	Posterior aspect of calcaneus via tendo calcaneus	Tibial, S1, S2	Plantar flexes foot and ankle
Deep group				
Flexor digitorum longus	Medial portion of posterior surface of tibia inferior to soleal line	Base of distal phalanges of lateral four digits	Tibial, S2, S3	Flexes lateral four digits; plantar flexes ankle; supports arches of foot
Flexor hallucis longus	Inferior two-thirds of posterior surface of fibula and interior part of interosseous membrane	Base of distal phalanx of great toe	Tibial, S2, S3	Flexes great toe at all joints; weakly plantar flexes ankle; supports medial longitudinal arches of foot
Popliteus	Lateral surface of lateral condyle of femur and lateral meniscus	Posterior surface of tibia, superior to soleal line	Tibial, L4, L5, S1	Weakly flexes knee and unlocks knee
Tibialis posterior	Interosseous membrane; posterior surface of tibia inferior to soleal line; posterior surface of fibula	Tuberosity of navicular cuneiform and cuboid; base of 2nd–4th metatarsals	Tibial, L4, L5	Plantar flexes ankle; inverts foot

12. Muscles of the Foot

Muscle	Origin	Insertion	Nerve	Action
Dorsum of foot				
Extensor digitorum brevis	Dorsal surface of calcaneus	Lateral side of long extensor tendons with slips to proximal phalanges 2nd–4th toes	Deep peroneal, L5, S1	Assists in extending middle three toes
Extensor hallucis brevis	Dorsal surface of calcaneus	Base of proximal phalanx of great toe	Deep peroneal, L5, S1	Extends great toe
Sole of foot				
Abductor digiti minimi	Medial and lateral tubercles of calcaneus, plantar aponeurosis and intermuscular septa	Lateral side of base of proximal phalanx of fifth digit	Lateral plantar, S2, S3	Abducts and flexes fifth digit
Abductor hallucis	Medial tubercle of calcaneus; flexor retinaculum and plantar aponeurosis	Medial side of base of proximal phalanx of first digit	Medial plantar, S2, S3	Abducts and flexes great toe
Adductor hallucis; oblique head	Base of metatarsals 2–4	Proximal phalanx of great toe	Deep branch of lateral plantar, S2, S3	Adducts great toe; assists in maintaining transverse arch
Adductor hallucis; transverse head	Capsule of lateral four metatarsophalangeal joints	Tendon of head attached to lateral sides of base of proximal phalanx of first digit	Deep branch of plantar, S2, S3	Adducts great toe; assists in maintaining transverse arch
Dorsal interossei (4)	Adjacent shafts of metatarsals	Proximal phalanges of second toe medial and lateral sides; third and fourth toes lateral sides	Lateral plantar, S2, S3	Abducts toes; flexes and extends proximal and distal phalanges

(*continued*)

Muscle	Origin	Insertion	Nerve	Action
Flexor digitorum brevis	Medial tubercle of calcaneus, plantar aponeurosis and intermuscular septa	Middle phalanges of lateral four toes	Medial plantar, S2, S3	Flexes middle phalanges of lateral four toes
Flexor digiti minimi brevis	Base of fifth metatarsal	Proximal phalanx of fifth toe	Lateral plantar, S2, S3	Flexes fifth toe
Flexor hallucis brevis	Cuboid; third cuneiform	Proximal phalanx of great toe	Medial plantar, S2, S3	Flexes great toe
Lumbricals (4)	Tendons of flexor digitorum longus	Proximal phalanges; extensor expansion	First by medial plantar nerve; lateral three by lateral plantar nerve, S2, S3	Flexes metatarsophalangeal joints and extends interphalangeal joints
Plantar interossei (3)	Medial sides of metatarsals 3–5	Medial side of base of proximal phalanges 3–5	Lateral plantar, S2, S3	Adducts toes; flexes proximal and extends distal phalanges
Quadratus plantae	Medial and lateral side of calcaneus	Tendons of flexor digitorum longus	Lateral plantar, S2, S3	Assists in flexing toes

13. Muscles of the Posterior Abdominal Wall

Muscle	Origin	Insertion	Nerve	Action
Psoas major	Sides of T12-L5 vertebra and disk; transverse processes	Lesser trochanter of femur	Anterior rami of L1, L2, and L3	Flexes and rotates thigh laterally at hip; flexes lumbar vertebrae anteriorly and laterally
Psoas minor	Sides of T12-L1 vertebra and intervertebral disk	Pectineal line, iliopectineal eminence via iliopectineal arch	Anterior rami of L1, L2	Works conjointly with psoas major to flex thigh at hip; stabilizes joint

(continued)

Muscle	Origin	Insertion	Nerve	Action
Quadratus lumborum	Medial half of inferior border of 12th rib and tips of lumbar transverse processes	Iliolumbar ligament and internal tip of iliac crest	Ventral branches of T12, L1-L4	Extends, laterally flexes vertebral column; flexes 12th rib during inspiration

14. Superficial Muscles of the Back

Muscle	Origin	Insertion	Nerve	Action
Erector spinae	Arises by a broad tendon from posterior part of iliac crest, posterior surface of sacrum, sacral and inferior lumbar spinous processes and supraspinous ligament	Iliocostal—lumborum, thoracis and cervicis; Longissimus—thoracis, cervicis and capitis; spinalis: thoracis, cervicis and capitis	Posterior rami of spinal nerves	Extend vertebral column and head
Interspinales	Superior surface of spinous processes of cervical and lumbar vertebrae	Inferior surface of spinous process of vertebrae superior to vertebrae of origin	Posterior rami of spinal nerves	Assist in extension and rotation of vertebral column
Intertransversarii	Transverse process of cervical and lumbar vertebrae	Transverse process of adjacent vertebrae	Posterior and anterior rami of spinal nerves	Assists in lateral bending of vertebral column; stabilizes vertebral column
Latissimus dorsi	Spines of T5-T12	Floor of bicipital groove	Thoracodorsal	Adducts, extends, and rotates arm medially
Levator scapulae	Transverse process of C1-C4	Superior part of medial border of scapula	Dorsal scapular C5; cervical C3-C4	Elevates scapula

(continued)

Muscle	Origin	Insertion	Nerve	Action
Rhomboid major	Spines of T2-T5	Medial border of scapula	Dorsal scapular, C4, C5	Adducts scapula
Rhomboid minor	Spines of C7-T1	Root of spine of scapula	Dorsal scapular, C4, C5	Adducts scapula
Serratus anterior	External surface of lateral parts of 1–8 ribs	Anterior surface of medial border of scapula	Long thoracic nerve, C5, C6, C7	Protracts and rotates scapula
Serratus posterior inferior	Spinal processes of T11 to L2 vertebrae	Inferior border of 8th–12th ribs near their angles	Anterior thoracic spinal 9–12	Depresses ribs
Serratus posterior superior	Ligamentus nuchae, supraspinal ligament and spines of C7-T3	Superior borders of 2nd–4th ribs	Intercostal, 2–5	Elevates ribs
Transversospinal	Transverse process of C4-T12 vertebrae; multifidus arises from sacrum, ilium, transverse process of T1-T3 and articular process of C4-C7	Thoracis, cervicis, and capitis	Spinal, posterior rami	Extends and rotates vertebral column; stabilizes vertebrae during movement
Trapezius	External occipital protuberance, superior nuchal line, ligamentum nuchae, spines of C7-T12	Lateral third of clavicle, acromion, and spine of scapula	Spinal accessory, C3-C4	Adducts, rotates, elevates, and depresses scapula

15. Prevertebral Muscles

Muscle	Origin	Insertion	Nerve	Action
Lateral vertebral				
Anterior scalene	Transverse process of C4-C6 vertebrae	First rib	Cervical, C4, C5, C6	Elevates first rib; laterally flexes and rotates neck
Middle scalene	Posterior tubercles of transverse processes of C4-C5 vertebrae	Superior surface of first rib, posterior groove for subclavian artery	Cervical spine, anterior rami	Elevates first rib during forced inspiration; flexes neck laterally
Posterior scalene	Posterior tubercles of transverse processes of C4-C5 vertebrae	External border of second rib	Anterior rami of cervical spine, C7, C8	Elevates second rib during forced inspiration; flexes neck laterally
Anterior vertebral				
Longus capitis	Anterior tubercles of C3-C6	Basilar part of occipital bone	Spinal, anterior rami, C1-C3	Flexes or twists neck anteriorly
Longus colli	Anterior tubercle of C2 vertebra; bodies of C1-C3 and transverse processes of C3-C6 vertebrae	Bodies of C5-T3 vertebrae, transverse processes of C3-C5 vertebrae	Spinal, anterior rami, C2-C6	Flexes and rotates head to opposite side
Rectus capitis anterior	Anterior surface of lateral mass of atlas, C1	Base of skull, anterior to occipital condyle	C1 and C2	Flexes head
Rectus capitis lateralis	Transverse processes of C1	Jugular process of occipital bone	C1 and C2	Flexes head; helps stabilize head
Rectus capitis posterior	Spinous processes of C2 vertebra	Middle of inferior nuchal line of occipital bone	Suboccipital	Extends head

(*continued*)

Appendix 3

Muscle	Origin	Insertion	Nerve	Action
Splenius capitis	Inferior half of ligamentum nuchae, spinous processes of C7-T3 of T4 vertebrae	Splenius capitis: superolaterally to mastoid process of temporal bone, lateral third of superior nuchal line of occipital bone Splenius cervicis: posterior tubercles of transverse C1-C3 or C4 vertebrae	Dorsal primary rami, C2–C6	Rotates head and extends neck

From Chung KW. Gross Anatomy, 4th ed. Baltimore: Lippincott Williams & Wilkins, 2000.

Appendix 4

Table of Ligaments and Tendons

Shoulder/Upper Arm

Latin name	English name	Articulation
Lm. acromioclaviculare	acromioclavicular l.	Connects acromion to clavicle; strengthens articular capsule
Lm. anulare radii	anular l. of radius	Connects head of radius in radial notch
Lm. collaterale ulnare	collateral ulnar l.	Connects medial epicondyle to humerus and coronoid process of ulna and olecranon
Lm. conoideum	conoid l.	Connects coracoid process of scapula to clavicle
Lm. coracoacromiale	coracoacromial l.	Connects coracoid process to acromion
Lm. coracoclaviculare	coracoclavicular l.	Connects coracoid process of scapula to clavicle
Lm. coracohumerale	coracohumeral l.	Connects coracoid process of scapula to humerus
Lm. costoclaviculare	costoclavicular l.	Connects 1st costal cartilage to clavicle
La. glenohumeralia	glenohumeral ligs.	Connect articular capsule of humerus to glenoid cavity and anatomical neck of humerus
Lm. interclaviculare	interclavicular l.	Connects clavicle to opposite clavicle
Lm. orbiculare radii	anular l. of radius	Encircles and holds the head of the radius in the radial notch of the ulna
Lm. sternoclaviculare anterius	anterior sternoclavicular l.	Fibrous band that reinforces the sternoclavicular joint anteriorly

(continued)

Abbreviations used: l., ligament; La, ligamenta; Lm, ligamentum; ligs., ligaments.

Shoulder/Upper Arm

Latin name	English name	Articulation
Lm. sternoclavicular posterius	posterior sternoclavicular l.	Fibrous band that reinforces the sternoclavicular joint posteriorly
Lm. suspensorium axillae	suspensory l.	Connects between the clavipectoral fascia downward to the axillary fascia
Lm. transversum humeri	transverse humeral l.	Connects obliquely from the greater to the lesser tuberosity of the humerus
Lm. transversum scapulae inferius	inferior transverse l.	Connects scapula to glenoid cavity; creates foramen of scapula for vessels/nerves
Lm. transversum scapulae superius	superior transverse l.	Connects coracoid process to scapular notch of scapula
Lm. trapezoideum	trapezoid l.	Connects coracoid process to clavicle

Hand/Forearm

Latin name	English name	Articulation
Lm. anulare radii	anular l. of radius	Connects radius to ulna
Lm. carpi radiatum	radiate l. of wrist	Multiple fibrous bands on palmar surface of metacarpal joint
Lm. carpi transversum	transverse carpal l.	Continuous with antebrachial fascia
Lm. carpi volare	transverse carpal l.	Reinforcing fibers in antebrachial fascia, palmar surface of wrist
La. carpometacarpalia dorsalia	dorsal carpometacarpal ligs.	Join carpal bones to bases of metacarpals
La. carpometacarpalia palmaria	palmar carpometacarpal ligs.	Join carpal bones to metacarpal ligs.
La. collateralia articulationum interphalangealium manus	collateral ligs. of interphalangeal articulations	Fibrous bands on each side of interphalangeal joints of fingers

(continued)

Hand/Forearm

Latin name	English name	Articulation
La. collateralia articulationum metacarpophalangealium	collateral ligs. of metacarpophalangeal articulations	Fibrous bands on sides of each metacarpophalangeal joint
Lm. collaterale carpi radiale	radial carpal collateral l.	Connects styloid process of radius to scaphoid
Lm. collaterale carpi ulnare	ulnar carpal collateral l.	Connects styloid process of ulna to triquetral and pisiform bones
Lm. collaterale radiale	collateral radial l.	Connects lateral epicondyle of humerus to anular l. of radius
Lm. intercarpalia dorsalia	dorsal intercarpal ligs.	Connect carpal bones together
Lm. intercarpalia interossea	interosseous intercarpal ligs.	Connect various carpal bones
Lm. intercarpalia palmaria	palmar intercarpal ligs.	Connect various carpal bones
La. metacarpalia dorsalia	dorsal metacarpal ligs.	Interconnect bases of metacarpal bones
La. metacarpalia interossea	interosseous metacarpal ligs.	Interconnect bases of metacarpal bones
La. metacarpalia palmaria	palmar metacarpal ligs.	Interconnect bases of metacarpals
La. metacarpeum transversum profundum	deep transverse metacarpal l.	Interconnects heads of metacarpals
Lm. metacarpale transversum superficiale	superficial transverse metacarpal l.	Between longitudinal bands of palmar aponeurosis
Lm. natatorium	superficial transverse metacarpal l.	Thickening of the deep fascia in most distal part of the base of the triangular palmar aponeurosis

(continued)

Hand/Forearm

Latin name	English name	Articulation
Lm. palmaria	palmar l.	Connects anterior aspect of each metacarpophalangeal and interphalangeal joint of the hand
La. palmaria articulationis interphalangeae manus	palmar ligs. of interphalangeal joints of hand	Interphalangeal articulations of hand between collateral articulations
La. palmaria articulationis metacarpophalangeae	palmar ligs. of metacarpal joints	Connect metacarpophalangeal joints to the collateral ligs.
Lm. pisohamatum	pisohamate l.	Connects pisiform bone to hook of hamate bone
Lm. pisometacarpeum	pisometacarpal l.	Connects pisiform bone to bases of metacarpals
Lm. quadratum	quadrate l.	Connects radial notch of ulna to neck of radius
Lm. radiocarpale dorsale	dorsal radiocarpal l.	Connects radius to carpal bones
Lm. radiocarpale palmare	palmar radiocarpal l.	Connects radius to lunate, triquetral, capitate, and hamate bones
Lm. ulnocarpale palmare	palmar ulnocarpal l.	Connects styloid process of ulna to carpal bones

Spine

Latin name	English name	Articulation
La. alaria	alar l.	Connects axis to occiput; limits rotation of head
Lm. apicis dentis axis	apical dental l.	Connects axis to occiput
La. atlantooccipitale laterale	lateral atlantooccipital l.	Connects occiput to atlas
Lm. capitis costae intra-articulare	interarticular l. of head of rib	Connects crest of rib to intervertebral disk

(continued)

Spine

Latin name	English name	Articulation
Lm. capitis costae radiatum	radiate l. of head of rib	Connects head of rib to adjacent vertebrae/disks
Lm. caudale integumenti communis	caudal retinaculum	Forms coccygeal foveola
Lm. costotransversarium	costotransverse l.	Connects neck of rib to transverse process of corresponding vertebra
Lm. costotransversarium laterale	lateral costotransverse l.	Connects transverse process of vertebra to corresponding rib
Lm. costotransversarium superius	superior costotransverse l.	Connects neck of rib to transverse process of vertebra above
Lm. cruciforme atlantis	cruciform l. of atlas	Connects transverse l. of atlas to longitudinal fascicles
La. flava	yellow ligs.	Join laminae of two adjacent vertebrae
Lm. iliofemorale	iliofemoral l.	Connects anterior/inferior iliac spine and intertrochanteric femur
Lm. iliolumbale	iliolumbar l.	Connects L4-L5 to iliac crest
Lm. interspinale	interspinous l.	Interconnect spinous processes
Lm. intertransversarium	intertransverse l.	Interconnect vertebral transverse processes
Lm. longitudinale anterius	anterior longitudinal l.	Extends from occiput/atlas to sacrum
Lm. longitudinale posterius	posterior longitudinal l.	Extends from occiput to coccyx
Lm. lumbocostale	lumbocostal l.	Connects 12th rib to transverse processes of L1-L2

(continued)

Appendix 4

Spine

Latin name	English name	Articulation
Lm. nuchae	radiate l.	Connects head of each rib to bodies of the two vertebrae with which it articulates
Lm. sacrococcygeum anterius	anterior sacrococcygeal l.	Connects sacrum to coccyx
Lm. sacrococcygeum laterale	lateral sacrococcygeal l.	Connects 1st coccygeal vertebra to sacrum; completes foramen of S5
Lm. sacrococcygeum posterius protundum	deep posterior sacrococcygeal l.	Terminal portion of posterior longitudinal l.; unites S5 and profundum coccyx
Lm. sacrococcygeum posterius superficiale	superficial posterior sacrococcygeal l.	Connects sacral hiatus to coccyx superficiale
La. sacroiliaca anteriora	anterior sacroiliac ligs.	Connect sacrum to ilium
La. sacroiliaca interossea	interosseous sacroiliac ligs.	Numerous bundles connecting tuberosities of sacrum to those of ilium
La. sacroiliaca posteriora	posterior sacroiliac ligs.	Connect ilium and iliac spines to sacrum
Lm. sacrospinale	sacrospinous l.	Connects ischium to lateral margins of sacrum
Lm. sacrotuberale	sacrotuberous l.	Connects ischial tuberosity to sacrum and coccyx and iliac spine
Lm. supraspinale	supraspinous l.	Interconnects tips of spinous processes of vertebrae
Lm. transversum atlantis	transverse l. of atlas	Horizontal portion of cruciform l. of atlas

Abdominal/Pelvic

Latin name	English name	Articulation
Lm. arcuatum laterale	lateral arcuate l.	Connects first lumbar vertebra and 12th rib to diaphragm

(continued)

A86

Abdominal/Pelvic

Latin name	English name	Articulation
Lm. arcuatum mediale	medial arcuate l.	Connects body of first lumbar vertebra to transverse process
Lm. arcuatum pubis	inferior pubic l.	Arches across pubic symphysis
Lm. falciforme	falciform process of sacro-tuberous l.	Passes from ischial tuberosity to ilium, sacrum, and coccyx
Lm. laterale vesicae	lateral bladder l.	Passes from one side of the bladder to blend with the pelvic fascia
Lm. pectineale	pectineal l.	A strong fibrous band that passes laterally from the lacunar l. along the pectineal line of the pubis
Lm. pubicum inferius	inferior pubic l.	Arches across the inferior aspect of the pubic symphysis
Lm. pubicum superius	superior pubic l.	Passes transversely above the pubic symphysis
Lm. pubofemorale	pubofemoral l.	Connects from the superior ramus of the pubis to the intertrochanteric femur
Lm. sacrodurale	sacrodural l.	Connects between the midline of the inferior part of the dorsal sac to the posterior longitudinal l. of the sacrum.
Lm. sacroiliacum posterius	posterior sacroiliac ligs.	Connect from the ilium to the sacrum posterior to the sacroiliac joint
Lm. sacrospinale	sacrospinous l.	Connects between the ischial spine and the sacrum and coccyx

Hip/Thigh

Latin name	English name	Articulation
Lm. capitis femoris	l. of head of femur	Connects femur, acetabular notch, and transverse l. of acetabulum
Lm. inguinale	inguinal l.	Connects ilium to pubis
Lm. ischiofemorale	ischiofemoral l.	Connects ischium to femur
Lm. transversum acetabuli	transverse acetabular l.	Connects acetabular lip of hip joint to acetabular notch

Knee/Calf

Latin name	English name	Articulation
Lm. capitis fibulae anterius	anterior l. of fibular head	Connects head of fibula to lateral condyle of tibia
Lm. capitis fibulae posterius	posterior l. of fibular head	Connects head of fibula to lateral condyle of tibia
Lm. collaterale fibulare	collateral fibular l.	Connects lateral epicondyle of femur to head of fibula
Lm. collateral tibiale	tibial collateral l.	Connects medial epicondyle of femur to medial meniscus and tibia
Lm. cruciatum anterius genus	anterior cruciate l. of knee	Connects lateral condyle of femur to condylar eminence of tibia
La. cruciata genus	cruciate ligs. of knee	Bundles in knee joint between condyles of femur
Lm. cruciatum posterius genus	posterior cruciate l. of knee	Connects medial condyle of femur to intercondylar area of tibia
Lm. menisci lateralis	posterior meniscofemoral l.	Connects between the medial condyle of the femur to the posterior crus of the lateral meniscus
Lm. meniscofemorale anterius	anterior meniscofemoral l.	Connects lateral meniscus to posterior cruciate l.

(continued)

Knee/Calf

Latin name	English name	Articulation
Lm. meniscofemorale posterius	posterior meniscofemoral l.	Connects lateral meniscus to medial condyle of femur
Lm. patellae	patellar l.	Connects patella to tibial tuberosity
Lm. popliteum arcuatum	arcuate popliteal l.	Connects fibula to articular capsule
Lm. popliteum obliquum	oblique popliteal l.	Connects medial condyle of tibia to lateral epicondyle of femur
Lm. teres femoris	head of femur l.	Connects from the fovea in the head of the femur to the borders of the acetabular notch
Lm. tibiofibulare anterius	anterior tibiofibular l.	Connects tibia to fibula
Lm. tibiofibulare posterius	posterior tibiofibular l.	Connects tibia to distal fibula
Lm. tibionaviculare	tibionavicular part of medial l. of ankle joint	Connects from medial malleolus of the tibia downward to the tarsal bones
Lm. transversum genus	transverse l. of knee	Connects lateral meniscus to medial meniscus

Foot and Ankle

Latin name	English name	Articulation
Lm. bifurcatum	bifurcate l.	Dorsum of foot; comprises calcaneonavicular and calcaneocuboid ligs.
Lm. calcaneocuboideum	calcaneocuboid l.	Connects calcaneus to cuboid
Lm. calcaneocuboideum plantare	plantar calcaneocuboid l., short plantar l.	Connects calcaneus to cuboid

(*continued*)

Foot and Ankle

Latin name	English name	Articulation
Lm. calcaneofibulare	calcaneofibular l.	Connects fibula to calcaneus
Lm. calcaneonaviculare	calcaneonavicular l.	Connects calcaneus to navicular bone
Lm. calcaneonaviculare dorsale	dorsal calcaneonavicular l.	Connects calcaneus to navicular bone
Lm. calcaneonaviculare plantare	plantar calcaneonavicular l.	Connects sustentaculum tali to navicular; supports talus
Lm. calcaneotibiale	calcaneotibial l.	Connect medial malleolus to sustentaculum tali of calcaneus
La. collateralia articulationum	collateral ligs. of metatarsophalangeal articulations	Fibrous bands on sides of each metatarsophalangeal joint
Lm. cruciatum cruris	inferior extensor of foot	Joins malleolus to dorsum of foot
Lm. cuboideonaviculare dorsale	dorsal cuboideonavicular l.	Connects cuboid and navicular bones
Lm. cuboideonaviculare plantare	plantar cuboideonavicular l.	Connects cuboid and navicular bones
Lm. cuneocuboideum dorsale	dorsal cuneocuboid l.	Connects cuboid and lateral cuneiform bones
Lm. cuneocuboideum interosseum	interosseus cuneocuboid l.	Connects cuboid and lateral cuneiform bones
Lm. cuneocuboideum plantare	plantar cuneocuboid l.	Connects cuboid and lateral cuneiform bones
La. cuneometatarsalia interossea	cuneometatarsal interosseous ligs.	Connect cuneiform and metatarsal bones
La. cuneonavicularia dorsalia	dorsal cuneonavicular ligs.	Connect navicular and cuneiform bones
La. cuneonavicularia plantaria	plantar cuneonavicular ligs.	Connect navicular to cuneiform bones

(continued)

Foot and Ankle

Latin name	English name	Articulation
La. intercuneiformia dorsalia	dorsal intercuneiform ligs.	Connect dorsal surfaces of cuneiform bones
La. intercuneiformia interossea	interosseous intercuneiform ligs.	Connect adjacent cuneiform bones
La. intercuneiformia plantaria	plantar intercuneiform ligs.	Join plantar surfaces of cuneiform bones
Lm. laterale articulationis talocruralis	lateral l. of ankle joint	Lateral side of ankle joint
Lm. mediale articulationis talocruralis	medial l. of ankle	Connects medial malleolus of tibia to tarsal bones
La. meniscofemoralia	meniscofemoral ligs.	Connect from posterior part of lateral meniscus to the lateral surface of the medial meniscus
Lm. metatarsale transversum profundum	deep transverse metatarsal l.	Joins heads of metatarsals
Lm. metatarsale transversum superficiale	superficial transverse metatarsal l.	Lies on sole of foot beneath heads of metatarsals
La. metatarsalia dorsalia	dorsal metatarsal ligs.	Interconnect bases of metatarsal bones
La. metatarsalia interossea	interosseous metatarsal ligs.	Interconnect bases of metatarsal bones
La. metatarsalia plantaria	plantar metatarsal ligs.	Plantar surface of metatarsal bones
La. plantaria articulationum interphalangealium pedis	plantar ligs. of interphalangeal articulations	Interphalangeal articulations of foot between collateral ligs.
La. plantaria articulationum metatarsophalangeae	plantar ligs. of metatarsophalangeal articulations	Plantar surface of metatarsophalangeal articulations between collateral ligs.
Lm. plantare longum	long plantar l.	Connects calcaneus to bases of metatarsal bones

(continued)

Foot and Ankle

Latin name	English name	Articulation
Lm. talocalcaneum	talocalcaneal l.	Connects talus and the Lm. calcaneus
Lm. talocalcaneum laterale	lateral talocalcaneal l.	Connects talus to calcaneus
Lm. talocalcaneum mediale	medial talocalcaneal l.	Connects tubercle of talus to sustentaculum tali of calcaneus
Lm. talocalcaneum interosseum	talocalcaneal interosseous l.	Connects calcaneus to talus
Lm. talofibulare anterius	anterior talofibular l.	Connects lateral malleolus of fibula to posterior process of talus
Lm. talonaviculare	talonavicular l.	Connects neck of talus to navicular bone
La. talotibiale	medial tibiotalar l.	Connects downward from the medial malleolus of the tibia of the tarsal bones
La. tarsi	tarsal ligs.	Connect bones of tarsus
La. tarsi dorsalia	dorsal ligs. of tarsus	Collectively, bifurcate, dorsal cuboideonavicular, cuneocuboid, cuneonavicular, intercuneiform, and talonavicular ligs.
La. tarsi interossea	interosseous ligs. of tarsus	Collectively, interosseous, cuneocuboid, intercuneiform, and talocalcaneal ligs.
La. tarsi plantaria	plantar ligs. of tarsus	Inferior ligs. of foot (long plantar, plantar calcaneocuboid, calcaneonavicular, cuneonavicular, cuboideonavicular, intercuneiform, cuneocuboid)
La. tarsometatarsalia dorsalia	dorsal tarsometatarsal ligs.	Connect bases of metatarsals to dorsal cuboid and cuneiform bones

(continued)

Foot and Ankle

Latin name	English name	Articulation
La. tarsometatarsalia plantaria	plantar tarsometatarsal ligs.	Connect metatarsal bones to cuboid and cuneiform bones
Lm. transversum cruris	superior extensor retinaculum ligs. of foot	Connect tibia to fibula; holds extensor tendons in place
Tendo calcaneus	Achilles tendon, calcaneal tendon	Connects triceps surae muscle to tuberosity of calcaneus

Style Rules

STAGE, TYPE, AND FRACTURE CLASSIFICATIONS

Lowercase the words "stage" and "type," and use roman numerals. For subdivisions of stages, follow *The AAMT Book of Style* rules for cancer classifications, and add on-line capital letters without spaces or hyphens:

- complex regional pain syndrome stage I
- stage II-III
- type I radioulnar synostosis
- type II open fracture
- type IIIB
- Garden II femoral neck fracture
- Salter VI fracture

GRADE

Lowercase the word "grade" and use arabic numerals:

- grade 1 chondromalacia patellae
- grade 2
- grade 3–4

LEVEL, PHASE, AND CLASS

Lowercase the words "level," "phase," and "class," and use arabic or roman numerals according to the system being referenced:

- Radiation Therapy Oncology phase III
- Haggitt level 4 colorectal adenocarcinoma
- physical status class 2E

WRIST ARTHROSCOPY PORTALS

Use arabic numerals. Two numbers should be hyphenated without spaces; add on-line capital letters with no space:

- 1–2 portal
- portal 3–4
- 6U wrist portal

Appendix 6

Professional Organizations, Associations, and Titles

Professional Organizations and Associations

Academy of Forensic and Industrial Chiropractic Consultants (AFICC)
Agency for Health Care Policy and Research (AHCPR)
American Academy of Neurological and Orthopaedic Surgeons (AANOS)
American Academy of Orthopaedic Surgeons (AAOS)
American Academy of Orthotists and Prosthetists (AAOP)
American Academy of Physical Medicine and Rehabilitation (AAPMR)
American Academy of Podiatric Sports Medicine (AAPSM)
American Association of Hand Surgery (AAHS)
American Association of Hip and Knee Surgeons (AAHKS)
American Association of Orthopaedic Foot and Ankle Surgeons (AAOFAS)
American Association of Tissue Banks (AATB)
American Back Society (ABS)
American Board of Certification of Orthotics and Prosthetics (ABC)
American Board of Orthopaedic Surgery (ABOS)
American Board of Physical Therapy Specialists (ABPTS)
American Chiropractic Association (ACA)
American Chiropractic Association Council on Sports Injuries and Physical Fitness
American College of Chiropractic Consultants (ACCC)
American College of Chiropractic Orthopedists (ACCO)
American College of Foot & Ankle Orthopedics & Medicine (ACFAOM)
American College of Foot and Ankle Surgeons (ACFAS)
American College of Occupational and Environmental Medicine (ACOEM)
American College of Rheumatology (ACR)
American College of Sports Medicine (ACSM)
American Congress of Rehabilitation Medicine (ACRM)
American Health Care Association (AHCA)
American Institute of Orthopaedic and Sports Medicine (AIOSM)
American Occupational Therapy Association (AOTA)
American Orthopaedic Foot and Ankle Society (AOFAS)
American Orthopaedic Society for Sports Medicine (AOSSM)
American Orthotic and Prosthetic Association (AOPA)
American Osteopathic Board of Orthopedic Surgery (AOBOS)
American Physical Therapy Association (APTA)
American Podiatric Medical Association (APMA)
American Rheumatism Association (ARA)
American Shoulder and Elbow Surgeons (ASES)
American Society for Testing and Materials (ASTM)

American Spinal Injury Association (ASIA)
Americans with Disabilities Act (ADA)
Armed Forces Institute of Pain
Arthroscopy Association of North America (AANA)
Association for the Study of Internal Fixation (ASIF)
Association of Bone and Joint Surgeons (ABJS)
Association of Chiropractic Colleges (ACC)
Board of Certification in Orthopedic Surgery
British Orthopaedic Association (BOA)
Canadian Association of Physical Medicine and Rehabilitation (CAPMR)
Canadian Physiotherapy Association (CPA)
Chiropractic Rehabilitation Association (CRA)
Commission on Accreditation of Rehabilitation Facilities (CARF)
Council on Chiropractic Education (CCE)
Council on Chiropractic Education International (CCEI)
European Society of Foot and Ankle Surgeons (ESFAS)
Federation of Chiropractic Licensing Boards (FCLB)
Fellow of the American College of Sports Medicine (FACSM)
Fellow of the American Occupational Therapy Association (FAOTA)
Fellow of the American Physical Therapy Association (FAPTA)
Fitness Safety Standards Committee (FSSC)
Foundation for Chiropractic Education and Research (FCER)
International Cartilage Repair Society (ICRS)
International Chiropractors Association (ICA)
International Headache Society (IHS)
International Knee Documentation Committee (IKDC)
International Society of Arthroscopy, Knee Surgery, and Orthopaedic Sports
    (ISAKOS)
International Society of Prosthetics and Orthotics (ISPO)
Japanese Orthopaedic Association (JOA)
Medical Research Council (MRC)
Musculoskeletal Transplant Foundation (MTF)
National Association of Medical Equipment Suppliers (NAMES)
National Board of Chiropractic Examiners (NBCE)
Occupational Safety and Health Administration (OSHA)
Orthopaedic Trauma Association (OTA)
Policy and Review Committee for Human Research
Sacro Occipital Research Society International (SORSI)
Visiting Nurse Association (VNA)

Professional Titles

Certified Orthotist (CO)
Certified Pedorthist (CPed)
Certified Prosthetist (CP)
Certified Prosthetist/Orthotist (CPO)
Doctor of Chiropractic (DC)
Doctor of Occupational Therapy (OTD)
Doctor of Physical Therapy (DPT)
Doctor of Podiatric Medicine (DPM)
Doctor of Podiatry (DP)
Industrial Physical Therapist (IPT)
Master of Physical Therapy (MPT)
Occupational Therapist (OT)
Occupational Therapist (Canada) (OT-C)
Occupational Therapist, Licensed (OT-L)
Occupational Therapist, Registered (OT-R)
Orthopedic Certified Specialist (OCS)
Physical Therapist (PT)
Physical Therapy Assistant (PTA)
Sports Certified Specialist (SCS)

Sample Reports and Dictation

AUSTIN BUNIONECTOMY

PREOPERATIVE DIAGNOSES
1. Metatarsus primus varus deformity, left foot.
2. Bunion hallux valgus deformity, left foot.

POSTOPERATIVE DIAGNOSES
1. Metatarsus primus varus deformity, left foot.
2. Bunion hallux valgus deformity, left foot.

PROCEDURES
1. Base wedge osteotomy with internal cannulated screw fixation, left first metatarsal.
2. Modified Austin bunionectomy/first metatarsal wedge osteotomy with release of contracted fibular sesamoid ligament, release of contracted adductor hallucis tendon, and internal rigid fixation with 3-mm cannulated screw; medial capsule repair and abductor hallucis tendon repair, left foot; and application of well-padded posterior splint.

ANESTHESIA: IV sedation administered by Versed anesthesia group and Mayo block of left first metatarsal, 2% Xylocaine plain mixed with an equal amount of 0.5% Xylocaine with epinephrine 1:100,000.

FINDINGS: The patient had severe metatarsus primus varus angle of the left foot requiring separate base wedge osteotomy to reduce the intermetatarsal angle. The patient has a bunion hallux valgus deformity with displacement of the sesamoid apparatus, which was not arthritic in appearance. Central articular cartilage was normal in appearance. No osteophyte formation was noted about the first metatarsal head dorsally. Small osteophyte over the area of the bunion prominence was noted. Bone stock was excellent.

DESCRIPTION OF PROCEDURE: With the patient lying supine under suitable IV sedation, 2 g of intravenous Ancef was administered. Local anesthesia was then administered to the left foot. The left foot was prepped and draped in the usual aseptic manner, and no tourniquet was used.

Attention was turned to the dorsal aspect of the left foot where medial to the extensor hallucis longus tendon an incision 5 cm in length was made proximally at the base of the first metatarsal and extending distally. This incision was deepened, small bleeding vessels were clamped and coagulated, and vital structures were retracted. The extensor tendon was released medially and retracted. The periosteum was exposed over the base of the metatarsal. A linear longitudinal periosteal incision was made extending from the metatarsal cuneiform articulation distally with the metatarsal shaft. A Freer elevator was used to separate the periosteum from the planned osteotomy site and, using an oscillating bone saw, an oblique first metatarsal wedge osteotomy was performed extending from the proximal medial to distal lateral with the wedge of bone resected and sent for pathologic examination. A test fit of the osteotomy site indicated good closure of the osteotomy site, and the proximal hinge was preserved. The osteotomy site was lavaged with Betadine saline solution. A single 3-mm cannulated Synthes bone screw, 26 mm in length, was then used to fixate the osteotomy site with excellent approximation of the osteotomy surfaces and slight plantar displacement of the distal fragment indicating no metatarsus primus elevatus. With the internal fixation in place, the osteotomy site was very stable. The wound was lavaged with Betadine saline solution. The periosteum was closed with 3–0 Vicryl. The subcutaneous tissue was approximated and maintained with a suture of 3–0 Vicryl. The skin was closed with interrupted 5–0 nylon suture.

Attention was then turned to the left first metatarsophalangeal joint where a curvilinear longitudinal incision, 6 cm in length, was made underlying the bunion deformity. This incision was deepened, and small bleeding vessels were clamped and coagulated; the vital structures were retracted. Dissection was carried down to the level of the first MP joint. The extensor hallucis longus tendon was identified. The hood ligament was resectioned. The brevis tendon was identified. A medially placed, distally based U-shaped capsular flap was fashioned at the first MTP joint capsule to include the abductor hallucis tendon. The capsular flap was separated from the bunion and reflected distally. The bunion was exposed in the wound and resected with the oscillating bone saw. The first metatarsal head was reflected dorsally. The sesamoid pad was reflected in a plantar direction. The contracted fibular sesamoid ligament was sectioned. An intracapsular approach was used to sever the contracted adductor hallucis tendon. Then, using the oscillating bone saw, modified Austin wedge osteotomy was performed in the first metatarsal head with the wedge being based medially to reduce the proximal articular facet angle. With the osteotomy complete, the wedge of bone was resected and sent for pathologic examination. The osteotomy site was lavaged with Betadine saline solution. The first metatarsal head was then translocated laterally, approximately one-third the width of the metatarsal shaft, to further close down the intermetatarsal angle to 0.

With the osteotomy complete in its new position, the first MTP joint range of motion was tested and found to be excellent, and the tibial sesamoid was positioned in the proper portion underneath the metatarsal condyle. A single 3-mm cannulated Synthes screw, 24 mm in length, was then placed across the osteotomy site from dorsal proximal to distal medial. With this point of fixation in place, the osteotomy stability was excellent. The redundant medial stump of metatarsal was resected with the oscillating bone saw and rasped smooth.

The wound was lavaged with Betadine saline solution. The redundant medial capsule was resected. The medial capsule repair and abductor hallucis tendon repair was afforded with 0 Surgidac and additional capsular closure with 3–0 Vicryl. The subcutaneous tissue was approximated and maintained with suture of 3–0 Vicryl. The skin was closed with an interrupted 5–0 nylon. Postoperatively, 0.25% Marcaine plain was instilled approximately at the operative site for postoperative pain. Vaseline gauze and dry sterile compression dressings were applied. Then, a well-padded posterior splint was applied with the knee bent and the foot at 90 degrees and held in place with two Ace wraps.

The patient tolerated the procedure well, had no untoward intraoperative events. She was discharged awake and in good condition, transferred to the recovery room stable. She will be sent to the surgical day care unit where she will be given medication, wound care, and home care instructions. She will then be discharged to recuperate at home, nonweightbearing on crutches for six weeks which was taught preoperatively. She will see me in one week in the office for surgical redressing.

BACK FUSION WITH BAK CAGES AND ROD INSTRUMENTATION

PREOPERATIVE DIAGNOSIS: Degenerative disk disease, L4–5 and L5-S1.

POSTOPERATIVE DIAGNOSIS: Degenerative disk disease, L4–5 and L5-S1.

OPERATION: Posterior lumbar interbody fusion, L4–5, and L5-S1 using BAK threaded fusion cages and Danek pedicle screws with local autogenous bone graft under fluoroscopy.

ANESTHESIA: General.

PROCEDURE: The patient was identified and taken to the operating room, where he was given general anesthesia. He was given antibiotics, and the Foley catheter was placed as well as sequential compression stockings applied. He was transferred onto the surgical table in the prone position on the spinal frame. The back was prepped and draped in the usual sterile fashion. The initial approach to the spine as well as the decompression at the L4–5 and L5-S1 levels was done by the co-surgeon and will be dictated separately.

The fusion was done using the posterior lumbar interbody technique. BAK instrumentation was used. The L4–5 level was addressed first. The alignment guide was placed over the L4–5 disk space and the disk incised with a knife. The initial drill was used to make a hole into the disk space and then spacers were put in sequentially up to a size #12. The x-ray image intensifier was brought into the operating room and draped in a sterile fashion and introduced over the patient to provide a cross-table lateral x-ray of the lumbar spine. An x-ray was taken at every step of the way to provide optimal positioning of all instruments and implants.

The C-ring retractor was placed over the spacer on the left side, and the locking tube sleeve was inserted into the body of L4 and L5. The hole was then drilled with the hand drill and tapped with the hand tap. Loose fragments were removed with the straight pituitary. The assistant held retraction and protection on the nerve roots and dura at all times. At no time were these structures injured.

The cage was then selected and packed with bone graft. There was an abundant quantity of high-quality cancellous bone from the laminectomy, so no bone graft was needed from the iliac crest. This bone graft was packed into the cage at the distal end and then the cage was inserted. The proximal end of the cage was then packed with bone as well. The same technique was then done on the right-hand side and the same technique was done at the L5-S1 level for a total of four cages.

Because this was a two-level cage procedure, the pedicle screw instrumentation was used to augment the stabilization. The pedicle screw was put into the L4 vertebral body by making a bur hole at the junction of the facet joint and transverse process on the left. The assistant held visual and palpable protection of the pedicle and then the curette was used to make an entry hole into the pedicle. This hole was then replaced with the screw. The same technique was done on the contralateral side and at the S1 level bilaterally. The screw from L4 to S1 was connected to the other S1 screw with a rod on both sides, and then the rods were locked into place with the locking nuts. The rods were then connected with a transverse connector piece. A rigid construct was obtained. Final x-rays were taken and the wound was then closed in anatomic layers using interrupted Vicryl suture for the deep layer and staples for the skin. Sterile dressing was applied and the patient was taken to the recovery room in stable condition.

DUPUYTREN CONTRACTURE RELEASE

PREOPERATIVE DIAGNOSIS: Dupuytren contracture, right palm, involving the middle and ring fingers.

POSTOPERATIVE DIAGNOSIS: Dupuytren contracture, right palm, involving the middle and ring fingers.

PROCEDURE: Palmar fasciectomy with release of the contracture around the middle and ring fingers.

ANESTHESIA: IV Bier block.

INDICATIONS: The patient is a 71-year-old woman who presents with a Dupuytren contracture of the right palm. This contracture has progressively involved the base of the middle and ring fingers with progressive inability to straighten the fingers, which necessitates surgical intervention.

DESCRIPTION OF PROCEDURE: With the patient under IV Bier block and in supine position, the right hand was prepped and draped in a sterile fashion. A Z-shaped incision was made over the hypothenar area of the right hand and carried down to the median crease in the hand. The skin flap was dissected free from the palmar fascia, and the dimpling into the skin was removed. The palmar fascia was then dissected free proximally around the transverse carpal ligament and followed distally, removing the palmar fascia intact. The thickening of the palmar ligament into the metacarpophalangeal joint of the ring and middle fingers was resected. The neurovascular bundle was identified and traced distally. Following this, tourniquet was let down after about an hour and hemostasis was maintained in the operative field. The wound was copiously irrigated with saline. A quarter-inch Penrose drain was inserted in the operative field, and the wound was closed with interrupted 5–0 nylon sutures. Pressure dressing was applied to the hand, supported with 3-inch Kling, and a volar splint was applied which was held in place with a 3-inch Ace wrap.

The patient tolerated the procedure well. Blood loss during the procedure was less than 50 cc. There was good capillary refill to the fingers following the release of the tourniquet. The patient was sent home and will be seen in the office for followup.

ILIZAROV FRAME APPLICATION

PREOPERATIVE DIAGNOSES
1. Malunion, left radius and ulna.
2. Unequal arm lengths.
3. Planned removal of deep implants, left radius and ulna.

POSTOPERATIVE DIAGNOSES
1. Malunion, left radius and ulna.
2. Unequal arm lengths.
3. Planned removal of deep implants, left radius and ulna.

OPERATIVE PROCEDURES
1. Osteotomy/osteoplasty, left radius and ulna.
2. Insertion of prophylactic intramedullary nails, left radius and ulna.
3. Iliac crest bone grafting of osteotomy site, left radius and ulna.
4. Application, Ilizarov multiplanar external fixator, left forearm.

INDICATIONS: The patient has a longstanding malunion of the radius and ulna with dorsal plate on both bones. The deformity is angulation with apex radial on the ulna and apex dorsal on the radius. He has full supination and no pronation. In addition, he has marked shortening of the left forearm. Prior to surgery we discussed treatment options, being correction of deformity with internal fixation using plates or IM rods or a combination of both versus lengthening of the forearm in addition to the deformity correction.

DESCRIPTION OF OPERATION AND FINDINGS: After general anesthesia, the left upper extremity was prepped and draped free in the usual manner. Tourniquet was placed on the left arm. The tourniquet was elevated after the arm was prepped in the usual manner. The dorsal ulnar incision was made and carried down to the ulnar plate. All of the screws were removed and the plate was removed from the ulna. Dorsal radial incision was also made and careful dissection to avoid injury to any neurovascular structures, in particular superficial branch of the radial nerve, was done. We then removed the screws and plate. There was one lag screw that was removed separately on the ulna. With both wounds exposed, it was now time to do the osteotomy. We chose to begin with the ulna.

The ulna was osteotomized by making multiple drill holes and then using an osteotome to complete the osteotomy. The osteotomy had been acutely corrected out of its apex radial bow. We then inserted Foresite nails by Smith & Nephew into the ulna using a 4-mm nail. In order to prepare the bone for this, we reamed the proximal segment first, using a combination of cannulated drills as well as the hand reamers. We then did the distal segment, working from the osteotomy site, in a similar manner but also using the flexible reamer. We then passed a guidewire down to the end and measured the length of the bone, then chose a 24 cm x 4 mm Foresite nail. The distal ulna had a separate bow from another malunion that was present, and in passing the nail we reamed a false channel in that, exiting at the second malunion site. We, therefore, had to bend the tip of the rod in order to negotiate around that malunion site. This allowed the intramedullary nail to pass into the distal ulna. We locked the rod proximally from posterior to anterior in the ulna.

Next, we osteotomized the radius at its apex and acutely corrected its apex dorsal bow. We then inserted Foresite nails into the radius. We straightened out the bow but also straightened out the normal radial bow. We, therefore, extracted the nail and bent the nail so that it had an apex radial bow to it.

While I was inserting the rod, the co-surgeon obtained a bone graft from the iliac crest. We had previously prepped and draped the right iliac crest, and we did a limited exposure on the tuberosity of the ilium in order to get the bone graft. After performing a couple of find holes, we removed sufficient bone for the grafting. The wound was closed in layers at the hip.

The next step was to bone graft the site of the radius and ulnar osteotomies. The bone graft was inserted and packed around the osteotomies, with the most important around the ulnar one because of its distraction. The ulna must have been shorter overall than the radius, since it did distract apart in order to maintain the length of the two bones to each other. The interval was packed with cancellous bone. No cortical bone was used. The radius was also packed.

In neither the ulna nor the radius did we distract the interosseous membrane border of the bone, in order to avoid damaging the vascularity to the bone on that side, as well as to minimize the risk of a crossunion between the bones. At all times this dissection was subperiosteal at most in that region.

After completing the bone grafting with the rod in place for both bones, we were ready to close the wounds. The radius rod was inserted from Lister tubercle and should be noted was reamed in the same manner as described for the ulna, using a combination of cannulated drill, flexible drill, and hand reamers. We reamed this from the fracture site but also from the Lister tubercle. A single locking screw was inserted into the radius from its radial aspect, getting two cortices of fixation. The rods were buried within the bone. At this time we closed the wound, which was done in layers. The two main wounds, as well as the smaller one used for the rod insertion, were closed.

After completing the closure and obtaining radiographs demonstrating that the alignment was corrected with both rods, we proceeded with application of the Ilizarov multiplanar external fixator. This involved putting a transradial ulnar wire distally and proximally. Proximally we inserted one wire from the neck of the radius, through the ulna as well, transfixing the two bones but being careful to avoid injury to the radial nerve and the ulnar nerve. The patient was not paralyzed and we did not see any muscle twitches in passing this wire in what was presumed a safe anatomic plane. In addition to that, a half pin was added to the top ring in the ulna alone. Distally, the two radioulnar wires were used. None of the wires or half pins touched the intramedullary implant.

After completing the fixation of the two-ring frame, which was bent at the elbow to allow for elbow flexion, the procedure was completed. Final radiographs were obtained. Sterile dressing was applied, and the arm was secured to an IV pole for elevation and maintained that way in the postoperative period. A drain was used in both the radial and ulnar wounds to minimize swelling.

The compartments were wide open through the incision in order to allow sufficient room for swelling. In the recovery room, the patient was examined and found to be neurologically completely intact for radial, median, and ulnar nerves, including both the proximal and distal motor branches. I was very satisfied with the final position and outcome.

ILIZAROV FRAME REMOVAL

PREOPERATIVE DIAGNOSIS: Hypertrophic nonunion, right tibia.

POSTOPERATIVE DIAGNOSES
1. Hypertrophic nonunion, right tibia.
2. Status post Ilizarov frame application for nonunion treatment.

PROCEDURES PERFORMED
1. Removal of circular external fixator from right tibia.
2. Debridement of pin tracks, right tibia.
3. Application of long leg cast.

CLINICAL HISTORY: The patient is a 12-year-old boy with a hypertrophic nonunion of the right tibia, following an open tibia fracture, with angulation. Five months ago, I applied a halo fracture frame and gradually distracted the nonunion. Recent x-rays show that he is radiographically united, and he now presents for removal. The x-rays also show some osteolysis around the near cortex of several of the half pins.

DESCRIPTION OF PROCEDURE: Having induced satisfactory anesthesia, the patient was placed supine on the OR table. I sequentially disassembled the components of the frame. The wires were painted with iodine, Betadine, and extracted. The half pins were all removed and noted to be fixed tightly within the bone. The leg was then painted with Betadine, and I then took a sterile curette and curetted out the subcutaneous tissue and a bit of the near cortex of each of the pin sites that showed osteolysis on the x-ray. There really was not much in the way of granulation tissue or debris. I used a syringe with sterile saline to irrigate each of the pin sites, and then applied a dry, sterile dressing and well-molded, well-padded, long leg cast with the ankle in neutral position and the knee then approximately 30 degrees. We plan to have this child come back in seven to ten days for a cast change.

OCCUPATIONAL THERAPY DISCHARGE SUMMARY

HISTORY: This patient participated in the occupational therapy portion of the pain management center program for 24 days. He participated in a graduated activity program of upper extremity flexibility stretches, especially neck musculature and increasing upper extremity endurance, directed toward the following goals:
1. Patient will demonstrate understanding of home exercise program of bilateral upper extremity flexibility, stretching, and strengthening.
2. Patient will increase tolerance for bilateral upper extremity/shoulder activity, as evidenced by increased repetitions and increased resistance in exercises.

3. Patient will understand and utilize self-correcting techniques for appropriate head/neck posture with less guarding throughout the shoulders.
4. Patient will elucidate three changes he can make in his habits, which will improve his quality of life.

GOALS ACHIEVED: All of the above.

PHYSICAL EXAMINATION: Patient's full range of motion is essentially within normal limits, except at discharge the patient continues to experience slight pain with upward gaze in right trapezius, and head rotation continues ⁻20 degrees of full 90 degrees, with pain to the right or left shoulder. Squat balance initially was poor and at discharge had improved to good. Initially the patient rated pain at 10/10 and at discharge 1/10 to occasionally 8/10.

THERAPY COURSE: The patient attended scheduled therapy daily for either one hour or for two 30-minute sessions and came in extra time to work on his activity program. He gave fair effort during therapy. The patient was instructed in body mechanics and pacing, and demonstrated fair ability to carry over techniques learned in the treatment sessions. The patient was able to verbalize three changes he plans to make in his home and work routines to incorporate these principles. They are:
1. Relaxation techniques.
2. Exercise/stretching.
3. Pacing.

The patient's kyphosis remains severe with head thrust noted, but by discharge the patient is monitoring his posture better and recognizes the need to do chin tucks. The patient needed frequent reminders, plus demonstration, to stay focused and retain exercise techniques.

THERAPY RESULTS: At discharge, the patient showed the following improvements

	Initial Evaluation	Discharge Evaluation
Grip Strength:	Right 61 lbs. average Left 62 lbs. average	Right 67 lbs. average Left 59 lbs. average
Bilateral Coordination:	Within functional limits	Within functional limits
Able to Lift:	5 lbs. from knee height to 30″ height	10 lbs. from knee height to 30″ height
Able to Carry:	5 lbs. 400′ with some shortness of breath	10 lbs. 400′ with appropriate pacing and had no problems

DISPOSITION: The patient was given a written copy of his personal exercise and stretching routine and demonstrated activities correctly. The patient also requested two back support pillows to facilitate comfort in his seating.

The patient is discharged from the pain management center program at this time and is scheduled for followup in two months, not the traditional two-week followup, as the patient will be on vacation.

OPEN REDUCTION AND INTERNAL FIXATION OF HIP FRACTURE

PREOPERATIVE DIAGNOSIS: Intertrochanteric fracture, left hip.

POSTOPERATIVE DIAGNOSIS: Intertrochanteric fracture, left hip.

PROCEDURE: Open reduction and internal fixation of intertrochanteric fracture, left hip, with DHS hip screw and four-hole sideplate.

INDICATIONS: This 96-year-old female fell at the boarding home, where she lives, on the day of admission and sustained an intertrochanteric fracture of her left hip.

DESCRIPTION OF PROCEDURE: Under satisfactory spinal anesthesia, the patient was placed on the Telos table, and I was able to do some traction with some manipulation and reduction. This was checked in the AP and lateral position. She was then prepped and draped in this position.

A 6-inch incision was made, beginning at the tip of the greater trochanter and going distally along the lateral thigh. Sharp dissection was used to go through the subcutaneous fat. Hemostasis was achieved with electrocoagulation. The fascia was incised in line with the incision, and the vastus lateralis muscle was split by sharp resection down to the underlying femur, and a Bennett retractor placed. Under C-arm control, I placed a guidewire up into the neck. The greater trochanter had fractured right at the place where the guidewire went, so this made placement rather easy. This was checked on the AP and lateral, and I used the 135-degree angle guide. I then measured and determined I needed a 90-mm compression hip screw. The wire was then driven in a little further, and the drill for the hip screw and sideplate barrel was run over the screw under x-ray control. This was then removed, and the 90-mm compression hip screw was placed over the guidewire and again checked in the AP and lateral. It was found to be in good position, and I had very good purchase in the head.

The 135-degree angle, four-hole sideplate was placed, the barrel of which was slipped over the shaft of the screw and fixed to the femoral shaft. It was held in place with a Jackson bone clamp. A total of four screws were put in place by drilling, measuring, and putting in four tap screws. The four tap screws consisted of one 40-mm, two 38-mm, and one 6-mm screw. Finally, all of them were tightened down. The Jackson clamp was removed, and the wound was irrigated. The vastus lateralis muscle was allowed to fall back together.

The fascia was closed with #1 Vicryl interrupted sutures. The subcutaneous fat was closed with 0 Vicryl interrupted inverted sutures, and the skin was closed with skin staples. A Betadine dressing was applied. The patient left the operating room in satisfactory condition with no drains and no complications. Prior to the procedure, the patient received 1 g IV Ancef.

ORTHOFIX EXTERNAL FIXATOR APPLICATION

PREOPERATIVE DIAGNOSES
1. Achondroplasia.
2. Genu varum.
3. Internal tibial torsion.
4. Short stature.
5. Coxa vara.

POSTOPERATIVE DIAGNOSES
1. Achondroplasia.
2. Genu varum.
3. Internal tibial torsion.
4. Short stature.
5. Coxa vara.

OPERATIVE PROCEDURES
1. Osteoplasty, left femur, with coxa vara correction.
2. Osteotomy, distal femur, with deformity correction.
3. Application of multiplanar external fixator, left thigh.
4. Osteotomy/osteoplasty, left tibia and fibula with correction of rotation and planned lengthening.
5. Application of multiplanar external fixator, left tibia.
6. Anterior compartment fasciotomy.
7. Botox injection, left calf.

INDICATIONS: The patient has achondroplasia and has decided to have deformity correction and stature lengthening for her severe short stature of 4 feet 3 inches in height. We decided on an ipsilateral strategy to lengthen the left femur and tibia at the same time in order to get complete realignment. We plan to correct her slight knee flexion deformity and severe varus distal femur, thus correcting her genu varum, as well as her slight coxa vara and her flexion deformity of the left hip by a subtrochanteric osteotomy of the left proximal femur. The lateral osteotomy will also be used for lengthening. Multiplanar external fixator of the Orthofix variety will be used.

DESCRIPTION OF PROCEDURE: Under general anesthesia, the left lower limb was prepped and draped free with the patient lying on a bump under her buttocks. She was given prophylactic antibiotics and had both an epidural catheter and urinary catheter.

I inserted a half pin by the cannulated drill technique through the quadriceps mechanism into the center of rotation angulation of the distal femur, 2 cm proximal to the knee joint, just proximal to the patella. I then used the focal dome side and marked out the trajectory of the focal dome osteotomy with a radius of 3.5 cm. I then made a small transverse incision, longitudinally split through the quadriceps mechanism, and then made multiple drill holes in the controlled center of patient angulation focal dome guide technique, and osteotomized the femur by connecting the drill holes. We then did an acute angular correction for translating medially and then angulating from varus to valgus. Lastly, we slightly posteriorly translated and extended the distal femur. To stabilize this, I applied an Orthofix device between the proximal and distal pins. Because the proximal pins were at a special angle to correct flexion of the hip, I only used one of the proximal pins and two of the distal pins. Having achieved the correction, I then used the fixator to insert two pins in the mid segment of the femur. I was now able to disconnect the fixator from the proximal two pins. I removed the proximal pin clamps, did multiple drill holes just below the proximal two pins, and did an acute correction into extension and slight valgus. I then connected the proximal pin clamp and these pins to the pin clamp, thus correcting the deformity acutely at the proximal femur. Having achieved this correction, I added one more pin in the proximal femur. With the distal femur, because of tenting of the skin, I temporarily removed one pin and then the other, letting the skin equilibrate, and inserted them through new skin holes. Because of the excellent bone contact and the plan to length proximally and not distally, I did not add a third pin distally.

Having completed this femur fixation and correction with two levels of osteotomy, the proximal one planned for lengthening of the femur, I now proceeded to do the tibial correction. I used the medial size fixator for this. Before applying the fixator, I did a fibular osteotomy through a small lateral incision. Multiple drill holes and an osteotome were used to cut the fibula after careful inspection between the lateral and posterior compartments. I did a fasciotomy of the anterior compartment, used our fasciotome to extend it proximally and distally the full length of the leg. All incisions were closed. I then applied a fixator from the medial side. I put in two pins, one proximal and one distal, at an angle about 30 degrees to each other, in order to correct the rotational deformity of the tibia. These were in different planes. When they were brought into the same plane, this deformity was corrected.

I made a small incision over the mid tibia, made multiple drill holes, and then completed an osteotomy with an osteotome. I then acutely rotated the pins to each other. After doing so, I applied the external fixator. This allowed me to insert a second proximal and second distal pin and ultimately a third proximal and third distal pin.

With the tibial fixation completed and all incisions in the leg closed, the last step of the procedure was to inject Botox into the calf muscle. I used a total of 5 cc into each head of the gastrocnemius muscle, injecting 100 units of Botox into each head of the gastrocnemius.

The procedure was tolerated well. Radiographs were obtained, confirming excellent alignment of the lower limb. I was present and performed the entire surgery. The patient was taken to the operating room with vital signs stable and neurovascularly intact.

OUTPATIENT TOENAIL REMOVAL

SUBJECTIVE: The patient returns today for removal of his left great toenail. PARQ held previously. Patient consented today.

ANESTHESIA: Digital anesthetic block with 2 cc of 1:1 mixture of 2% Xylocaine and 0.5% Marcaine.

PROCEDURE: The patient's foot was sterilely prepped and draped. Nail plate was freed with a curette and bluntly removed with straight Kelly hemostat. Penrose drain was applied, followed by application of phenolic acid. At this point, Penrose drain was released, with the kneecap being refilled. Postoperative dressing was applied.

PLAN: The patient should follow up for any deviation from the anticipated and explained postoperative course.

PAIN MANAGEMENT INITIAL EVALUATION

PRESENTING CHARACTERISTICS: The patient is a 57-year-old married Caucasian female. She presented herself for interview dressed and groomed appropriately and casually. Interpersonal presentation was friendly but somewhat reserved. Eye contact was normal and sustained. Speech and voice quality were unremarkable. The patient appeared obese. Posture was good. Her affect appeared slightly dysphoric.

PRESENTING ISSUES: The patient presents for consultation regarding ongoing back pain. The patient did not appear to be a good historian, generally giving very vague and general answers, even when questioned on specific matters. However, the patient did report that she first injured her back when she was in the sixth grade. She reports that she was always active in school but that her back generally hurt and got worse over the ensuing years. The location of her pain is described as in her lower back, also her left leg and occasionally up in her left shoulder and neck area. She describes the pain as burning. The patient indicates that her pain interferes a great deal with her ongoing activities. However, she generally maintains her household and does all the attendant chores. However, she does not appear to be very active or engaged in any other activities outside the home.

PSYCHOLOGICAL SYMPTOM PATTERN: The patient indicates that she felt somewhat suicidal in the past. When questioned about this, she indicated that she had no active plan for suicide but that sometimes wishes she would die. The patient indicated that she was sometimes quite disgusted with herself because she cannot do what she used to do. When asked to give an example of this, the patient indicated that she cannot sweep or vacuum anymore and that her husband must take on these chores. She indicated that she still does her usual household chores during the day, but gets frustrated with herself and disgusted because she cannot seem to get her chores done many times.

The patient reports that her sleep is not good. She wakes up frequently during the night. She is not sure what to attribute this to, raising the possibility that it could be attributable to a patient-identified ongoing heart problem, to her need to urinate frequently, to her coughing spells from a recent bout of pneumonia, or to her pain. She notes that her sleep is worse since September, primarily, in her mind, due to the onset of the pneumonia.

The patient reports that her appetite is off a bit and that she has lost 20 pounds over the past several months. The patient further reports that she feels tired and rundown every day since her pain has increased over the past few months. She notes that she feels like she cannot change anything and appears somewhat resigned to her life continuing as it has.

The patient reports some reduction in her usual activity level, which she attributes to the pain. There appear to be very few, if any, reinforcing activities in this patient's behavioral repertoire. The patient does not appear to have neglected her personal appearance and denies ongoing crying spells.

Interpersonally, the patient interacts somewhat with her family and children, although she does not appear to be a very socially engaged peson. There appears to be no loss of significant relationships, lack of necessary social skills, or change in life status recently.

Cognitively, the patient reports a low general sense of self-worth and appears to exhibit a great deal of self-criticism and reproach.

SOCIAL/INTERPERSONAL HISTORY: The patient lives with her husband of 38 years. The patient and her husband have produced six children of this marriage and 11 grandchildren. They are currently living with one of their grandchildren, a 16-year-old granddaughter. When questioned about this, the patient reported that this granddaughter's mother had remarried an alcoholic man and could not handle her being at home at this time. The granddaughter has been living with them for one year. The patient's husband has retired and is reported to be suffering from cardiomyopathy. She denies any ongoing marital problems between the two of them.

The patient denies use of alcohol or tobacco. Reinforcing activities include reading or watching TV.

MEDICAL BACKGROUND: Details of the medical background may be found in the physician's report. The patient reported to this interviewer that in addition to the back pain she also has a history of Bell palsy and whiplash. She reported that the whiplash was suffered approximately 27 years ago. She was treated with a cervical collar and at-home traction. The patient reports that the Bell palsy consists of spasms in her face and neck. She notes that if she is able to relax, the spasms will be prevented or will subside. The patient also reports a history of rheumatoid arthritis. The patient had back surgery approximately three years ago. She reported that the pain decreased for several days following the surgery but then increased to its original level.

The patient reports no previous or ongoing psychotherapy.

RESULTS OF PSYCHOMETRIC EXAMINATION: As part of the overall evaluation, the patient took an MMPI, a Beck Depression Inventory, and a Multidimensional Pain Inventory.

The results of the MMPI are invalid. The patient's profile is similar to others who have a strong tendency to exaggerate their symptomatology in an effort to look worse than they actually are on the examination. Thus, the patient's MMPI cannot be interpreted.

The patient was classified in the interpersonally distressed category on the Multidimensional Pain Inventory. Persons with scores in this range generally have higher than average levels of received punishing responses from a significant other, lower than average levels of perceived solicitous responses, and lower than average levels of perceived distracting responses from a significant other. The patient reports a high degree of pain severity and a high degree of interference in her life from the pain. The patient's general activity score is below the average when compared with other pain patients. Persons with scores in the interpersonally distressed area generally indicate that they are not being supported in an appropriate way by significant others, that they are not being taken care of, and that, in fact, significant others may punish them when they exhibit pain behaviors.

The patient obtained a total score of 22 on the BDI. Scores in this range are indicative of persons with a moderate to high level of clinical depression.

DIAGNOSTIC HYPOTHESIS: AXIS I: 311.00, depressive disorder, not otherwise specified.

SUMMARY AND RECOMMENDATIONS: The patient was moderately verbal throughout the course of the interview; however, she gave few details and exhibited little insight into her pain or psychological or psychosocial issues. It does appear from the psychometric testing that the patient is depressed when compared with others and also exhibits a great deal of self-criticism and reproach. The patient also appears to largely lack any reinforcing activities in her life, and the results of the MPI would indicate that her relationship with her significant other, as far as her pain coping, needs further attention. The results of the MMPI are invalid, but they would indicate somebody who may be exaggerating her symptoms as a possible cry for help.

Based on these results, the following recommendations are made
1. That this patient be seen at least on several more occasions in order to assess her motivation to engage in a behavioral self-management program. If the patient is not so motivated, basic motivational interviewing strategies should be undertaken in an effort to increase the patient's motivation.
2. That this patient's husband should be included in at least some of these sessions to ascertain his reactions to his spouse's pain and to encourage their involvement in more reinforcing activities and more positive communication.
3. That this patient be given some basic strategies for managing her moods. This information would be primarily from a cognitive behavioral perspective.
4. To coordinate this patient's care with pain center medical personnel in an effort to increase this patient's activity level and general functioning.

PHYSICAL THERAPY INITIAL EVALUATION

CHIEF COMPLAINT: Pain in the right buttock, extending down the right lateral thigh and into the foot.

HISTORY OF PRESENT ILLNESS: This patient reports that she has had pain in the right buttock that extends down into her right lower extremity, and has had this pain for approximately four to five years. This began after a hemorrhoidectomy. Subsequent to that she has had three other procedures to attempt to remove scar tissue. She states that her pain is aggravated by bowel movements and sitting for prolonged periods of time. The pain is relieved when she lies down and rests.

In the morning her pain is minimal to nonexistent, and she considers it a 0/10 on the pain scale. She states it is consistently 10/10 at the end of a working day. During the interview today, she states her pain is a 7/10 to 8/10 on the pain scale this afternoon. She describes the quality of her pain as aching and very deep, originating in her buttocks. The pain does go down her right leg along the lateral thigh and lateral calf and occasionally extends into her foot. The intensity of the pain does decrease as it goes more distally down her leg.

She describes multiple functional limitations from this chronic pain. She works as a legal secretary and has had to cut her workday from an eight-hour day to a six-hour day, five days a week. She states that she does best at tolerating a four-hour workday, but because of personnel shortages she has been forced to increase this to a six-hour day. Pain at the end of the day is intense, but she will go home and lie down for a while and then be able to continue with some activities at home in the evening. She also feels her recreational activities have been severely curtailed. Sitting for long periods in the automobile is very painful, so she has limited her traveling because of this. She also states that she is unable to go to movies or plan social activities in the evening because she knows the pain will be too severe.

PREVIOUS THERAPY: This patient has received physical therapy for a few sessions in the past for treatment of low back pain. She was given some Mackenzie back exercises, as well as a lumbar roll for sitting.

PHYSICAL EXAMINATION

Pain Behaviors: The patient exhibited no overt pain behaviors, other than an abnormal sitting posture. She sits on her left hip with her right leg crossed over, stretching her right lateral hip muscles. She states that this is the only way she can feel comfortable. We discussed sitting postures at work, etc., and because she is a small woman in stature she has had difficulty getting a chair that fits her comfortably. She states it is difficult for her to sit back in her chair far enough to have any type of lumbar support, so she usually sits on the end of her chair with most weightbearing through the left buttock. During the interview she was asked to sit in the chair properly with her back supported in a normal amount of lordosis and stated that this felt quite comfortable.

Range of Motion: Range of motion of her extremities is within functional limits. Her back range of motion is also within functional limits, with some limitation in lumbar extension. This is limited by a feeling of tightness and does not reproduce any of her pain. Straight leg raising is limited on the right at approximately 75 degrees and on the left at 65 degrees by tight hamstrings.

Posture: Standing posture is good and well balanced. Sitting posture is described previously.

Strength: Overall, strength is 5/5 with manual muscle testing, with the exception of the gluteus medius on the right, which tests at a 4/5 and the left a 5/5.

Gait: The patient appears to have a gluteus medius limp when weightbearing on the right lower extremity. Trendelenburg was negative bilaterally. She is able to correct her gait pattern fairly well when she concentrates on not sagging over the right hip.

Special Tests: Piriformis stretch test did not reproduce the exact pain. However, she is tighter on her left side than her right. She is not tender to palpation on the piriformis on the right side. Iliac crest, ASIS, PSIS, greater trochanter, and gluteal folds appeared equal in height.

IMPRESSION: This patient has a long history of right buttock, right low back, and right lower extremity pain that worsens as her day progresses. She appears to be exacerbating this pain by the posture she has adapted over the years, as well as some weakness in the right hip musculature. She is a very motivated person, and she has continued to do all of her housework and other activities through the pain. She appears willing to try any suggestions and is anxious for education.

TREATMENT PLAN: This patient will be in the day program for one week only. During that time our goals will be to educate her in an aerobic walking program, as well as to educate her in proper sitting posture, especially in the workplace. She will be given ideas on how to improve the fit of her current chair in the workplace, as well as some ideas on other office chairs that may fit her better and improve her sitting posture.

PHYSICAL THERAPY FINAL EVALUATION

PRIMARY DIAGNOSIS: Right basal ganglia, temporal lobe infarct.

TREATMENT DIAGNOSIS: Decreased functional mobility, inability to ambulate.

TREATMENT RECEIVED TODAY: Functional training, sit to stand with left AFO with minimal assistance for left knee extension, hip extension, transfer training, wheelchair to mat, mat to stand, gait training. Patient ambulated 150 feet with minimal assistance from her mother with left AFO and knee immobilizer. Patient was safe ambulating with mother. Patient's mother was also able to don the knee immobilizer properly. Patient has received quad cane from case manager. Patient has an orthotic order for a knee immobilizer for her left lower extremity, which she should receive shortly.

ASSESSMENT: Patient has met her goal of ambulating with minimal assistance for 150 feet with left ankle-foot orthosis, knee immobilizer, and large base quad cane with aid from mother. Patient continues to need contact guard assistance/standby assistance for sit to stand from wheelchair and wheelchair to mat transfers, secondary to decreased safety awareness and impulsivity. Patient and her mother understand home exercise plan and perform properly. Patient and her mother are encouraged to continue home exercise plane and ambulation at home. Patient will be discharged from outpatient physical therapy at this time secondary to meeting long-term goal of ambulation with plateau in progression.

PLATE AND SCREW HARDWARE REMOVAL

PREOPERATIVE DIAGNOSIS: Metatarsalgia, left foot.

POSTOPERATIVE DIAGNOSES
1. Metatarsalgia, left foot.
2. Stable nonunion, left first metatarsophalangeal joint.

OPERATIONS PERFORMED
1. Removal of hardware, left foot.
2. Bone biopsy, left first metatarsal bone.
3. Shortening osteotomies, left second and third metatarsals.

DESCRIPTION OF PROCEDURE: The patient was brought to the operating room and placed on the operating table in a supine position. Following the administration of intravenous sedation, an infiltrative block of 0.5% Marcaine plain was administered to the left foot in ankle block fashion. The left foot was then prepped and draped in the usual sterile manner. A well-padded pneumatic tourniquet was placed on the left ankle and the limb exsanguinated via gravity. Upon adequate exsanguination of the limb, the cuff was inflated to 250 mmHg. Attention was now directed to the left foot where a surgical scar was noted over the dorsal aspect of the first metatarsophalangeal joint.

In the first metatarsophalangeal joint area, a dorsal incision was performed over the previous surgical scar. This incision was deepened in the same plane, taking care to clamp, cauterize, or ligate any superficial bleeders as necessary. Blunt and sharp dissection was utilized to penetrate the soft tissue layers, with care being taken to preserve and retract all vital structures. Moderate scar tissue was noted in the surgical area, consistent with multiple previous surgeries.

Blunt and sharp dissection was utilized to penetrate the soft tissue layers until reaching the level of the internal fixation plate and screws. The hardware was exposed via sharp dissection. Bony growth was noted around the metallic plate overlying the dorsal aspect of the fusion site. The internal fixation screws were removed utilizing the AO screwdriver in the standard AO technique. The periosteal elevator was then utilized to free the plate and remove it from the surgical field in toto. There, overlying the plate and screws, was abnormal-appearing fibrous tissue which was sent for pathology. There was no evidence of abscess formation in the area. Inspection of the plate and screws did not demonstrate any evidence of biocorrosion or infection.

Upon removal of the hardware, the first metatarsophalangeal joint area was manipulated. Inspection demonstrated fibrous tissue at the fusion site at the interface of the proximal phalanx and first metatarsal. The interface of the metatarsal and graft proximally appeared solid and well healed. Motion was noted across the fusion site with manipulation of the area distally.

Wound cultures were also taken in this area due for aerobic and anaerobic bacterial cultures. In addition, a deep bone biopsy was taken for pathology to rule out pseudoarthrosis versus osteomyelitis. The surgical site was flushed copiously with normal saline and closed in a layered fashion utilizing 2–0 and 3–0 Vicryl to reapproximate the deep tissues, 4–0 Vicryl to reapproximate the subcutaneous tissues, and 4–0 nylon to reapproximate the skin margins.

Attention was now directed to the lesser metatarsals where a dorsal incision was performed between the second and third metatarsal bones. This incision was deepened in the same plane, taking care to clamp, cauterize, or ligate any superficial bleeders as necessary. Blunt and sharp dissection was utilized to penetrate soft tissue layers with care being taken to preserve and retract all vital structures. Attention was first directed towards second metatarsal bone, where the extensor tendon and neurovascular structures were retracted from the surgical site. Upon reaching the level of the periosteum and joint capsule, this tissue layer was incised in a linear fashion to provide exposure to the distal aspect of the second metatarsal bone and second metatarsal head. The periosteum was reflected from its underlying bony attachments to facilitate exposure. A 0.045 K-wire was then driven from dorsal to plantar through the metatarsal neck, slightly medial to center point to serve as an axis guide. The power bone saw was then utilized to perform a V-shaped osteotomy with the apex oriented distally and long medial arm through the metatarsal bone. Upon completion of the osteotomy, the axis guide was removed. An approximate 3-mm wedge of bone was then removed from the shorter lateral arm of the osteotomy to provide for shortening of the second metatarsal bone. Temporary fixation was achieved via K-wire and bone clamp fixation. Attention was then directed to the third metatarsal bone where a similar V-shaped osteotomy with long medial arm was performed. A 3-mm wedge of bone was removed from the shorter lateral arm of the osteotomy to also provide for shortening of the metatarsal bone. Temporary fixation was achieved via bone clamps, and intraoperative radiographs were taken. The radiographs demonstrated shortening of the metatarsal bones and rebalancing of the forefoot.

Permanent fixation of the osteotomies was achieved utilizing 2-mm cortical screws inserted parallel from medial to lateral across the metatarsal bone in standard AO fashion. Upon permanent fixation, a second set of intraoperative radiographs was taken. They demonstrated preservation of the metatarsal parabola through the shortening osteotomies of the second and third metatarsal bones. It was not deemed necessary to perform an additional osteotomy beneath the fourth metatarsal bone at this time as this area remained clinically asymptomatic for him. The surgical site was flushed copiously with normal saline, and the wound was closed in a layered fashion utilizing 3–0 Vicryl to reapproximate the periosteal and capsular tissues, 4–0 Vicryl to reapproximate the subcutaneous tissues and 5–0 Vicryl to reapproximate the skin margins in continuous subcuticular fashion.

The patient left the operating room in good condition with all digits warm and viable. The left lower extremity was immobilized in a well-padded fiberglass posterior splint beneath compressive dressings.

Common Terms by Procedure

Austin Bunionectomy

Ace wrap
adductor hallucis tendon
Ancef
approximation
articular cartilage
base wedge osteotomy
Betadine saline solution
bone stock
brevis tendon
bunion deformity
bunion hallux valgus deformity
bunion prominence
cannulated screw
capsular flap
capsule repair
clamped and coagulated
compression dressing
curvilinear longitudinal incision
dry sterile compression dressing
epinephrine 1:100,000
extensor tendon
extensor hallucis longus tendon
fibular sesamoid ligament
Freer elevator
hallux valgus deformity
hood ligament
intermetatarsal angle
internal fixation
internal rigid fixation
interrupted 5–0 nylon suture
intracapsular approach
linear longitudinal periosteal incision
local anesthesia
0.25% Marcaine plain
Mayo block
medial capsule repair
metatarsal condyle
metatarsal cuneiform articulation

metatarsophalangeal (MTP)
metatarsus primus elevatus
metatarsus primus varus angle
metatarsus primus varus deformity
modified Austin bunionectomy
modified Austin wedge osteotomy
oscillating bone saw
osteophyte formation
pathologic examination
periosteum
prepped and draped
sesamoid apparatus
sesamoid pad
subcutaneous tissue
Surgidac suture
Synthes bone screw
usual aseptic manner
Vaseline gauze
Versed
3–0 Vicryl suture
vital structure
wedge osteotomy
well-padded posterior splint
2% Xylocaine plain

Back Fusion With BAK Cages and Rod Instrumentation

alignment guide
autogenous bone graft
BAK instrumentation
BAK threaded fusion cage
bone graft
cancellous bone
contralateral
C-ring retractor
Danek pedicle screw
degenerative disk disease
dura
facet joint

fluoroscopy
Foley catheter
iliac crest
image intensifier
interbody fusion
interbody technique
laminectomy
locking nut
locking tube sleeve
nerve root
pedicle screw instrumentation
posterior lumbar interbody technique
rigid construct
spinal frame
transverse process

Dupuytren Contracture Release

Ace wrap
Bier block
dimpling
Dupuytren contracture
hemostasis
hypothenar area
interrupted 5–0 nylon suture
Kling wrap
median crease
metacarpophalangeal joint
neurovascular bundle
palmar fascia
palmar fasciectomy
Penrose drain
pressure dressing
skin flap
surgical intervention
transverse carpal ligament
volar splint
Z-shaped incision

Ilizarov Frame Application

bone graft
cancellous bone
cannulated drill
crossunion

dorsal plate
dorsal radial incision
dorsal ulnar incision
false channel
flexible drill
flexible reamer
Foresite nail
guidewire
hand reamer
iliac crest bone grafting
Ilizarov multiplanar external fixator
interosseous membrane border
intramedullary implant
intramedullary nail
lag screw
Lister tubercle
locking screw
malunion site
motor branch
multiple drill holes
neurovascular structure
osteotome
osteotomized
osteotomy/osteoplasty
planned removal
pronation
prophylactic
radial bow
radioulnar wire
Smith & Nephew
superficial branch of the radial nerve
supination
transradial ulnar wire
two-ring frame
unequal arm lengths
vascularity

Ilizarov Frame Removal

cast change
circular external fixator
debris
granulation tissue
half pin

halo fracture frame
hypertrophic nonunion
Ilizarov frame application
long leg cast
near cortex
neutral position
operating room (OR)
osteolysis
sterile saline

Occupational Therapy Discharge Summary
kyphosis
self-correcting technique
squat balance
upward gaze

Open Reduction and Internal Fixation of Hip Fracture
Bennett retractor
Betadine dressing
C-arm control
compression hip screw
DHS hip screw
electrocoagulation
femoral shaft
four-hole sideplate
good purchase
greater trochanter
guidewire
intertrochanteric fracture
Jackson clamp
open reduction and internal fixation
sharp dissection
sideplate
sideplate barrel
skin staple
subcutaneous fat
tap screw
Telos table
vastus lateralis muscle
Vicryl interrupted inverted suture
Vicryl interrupted suture

Orthofix External Fixator Application
achondroplasia
anterior compartment fasciotomy
bone contact
Botox injection
cannulated drill technique
coxa vara
distal femur
drill hole
epidural catheter
equilibrate
fasciotome
fasciotomy
fibular osteotomy
flexion deformity
focal dome
gastrocnemius muscle
genu varum
internal tibial torsion
ipsilateral
knee flexion deformity
lateral osteotomy
longitudinal split
multiplanar external fixator
neurovascularly intact
Orthofix device
osteoplasty
osteotome
osteotomized
osteotomy
patella
pin clamp
posterior compartment
prepped and draped free
prophylactic antibiotic
proximal femur
quadriceps mechanism
radiograph
rotation angulation
rotational deformity
stature lengthening
tenting of the skin

tibial fixation
trajectory
transverse incision
urinary catheter
valgus
varus

Outpatient Toenail Removal

curette
digital anesthetic block
Kelly hemostat
0.5% Marcaine
nail plate
Penrose drain
phenolic acid
Physical Activity Readiness
    Questionnaire (PARQ)
sterilely prepped and draped
2% Xylocaine

Pain Management Initial Evaluation

Beck Depression Inventory (BDI)
behavioral self-management program
Bell palsy
cognitive behavioral perspective
depressive disorder
dysphoric
whiplash
Minnesota Multiphasic Personality
    Inventory (MMPI)
Multidimensional Pain Inventory (MPI)
psychosocial issues

Physical Therapy Initial Evaluation

anterior superior iliac spine (ASIS)
functional limitation
gluteal fold
gluteus medius
lumbar roll
overt pain behavior
piriformis stretch test

posterior superior iliac spine (PSIS)
stretch test
Trendelenburg
within functional limits

Physical Therapy Final Evaluation

ankle-foot orthosis (AFO)
basal ganglion
contact guard assistance (CGA)
decreased functional mobility
functional training
home exercise program (HEP)
infarct
knee immobilizer
large base quad cane (LBQC)
quad cane
standby assistance (SBA)
temporal lobe
transfer training

Plate and Screw Hardware Removal

ankle block
AO screwdriver
axis guide
biocorrosion
blunt and sharp dissection
bone clamp
bony growth
cauterize
compressive dressing
cortical screw
exsanguinated
extensor tendon
fiberglass posterior splint
forefoot
infiltrative block
internal fixation plate
internal fixation screw
in toto
joint capsule
K-wire

lesser metatarsal
0.5% Marcaine plain
metatarsal bone
metatarsalgia
metatarsal parabola
metatarsophalangeal joint
neurovascular structure
nonunion
osteomyelitis
osteotomy
periosteal elevator
periosteum
permanent fixation

pneumatic tourniquet
power bone saw
proximal phalanx
pseudoarthrosis
shortening osteotomy
skin margin
subcuticular fashion
superficial bleeder
Vicryl suture
V-shaped osteotomy
wedge of bone
wound culture

Drugs by Indication

ARTHRITIS

Aminoquinoline (Antimalarial)
Aralen® Phosphate
chloroquine phosphate
hydroxychloroquine
Plaquenil®

Analgesic, Topical
Arth Dr®
Arthricare Hand & Body®
Born Again Super Pain Relieving®
Caprex®
Caprex Plus®
Capsagel®
Capsagel Extra Strength®
Capsagel Maximum Strength®
Capsagesic-HP Arthritis Relief®
capsaicin
Capsin® [OTC]
Capzasin-P® [OTC]
D-Care Circulation Stimulator®
Dolorex®
Double Cap®
Icy Hot Arthritis Therapy®
Pain Enz®
Pharmacist's Capsaicin®
Rid-A-Pain®
Rid-A-Pain-HP®
Sloan's Liniment®
Sportsmed®
Theragen®
Theragen HP®
TheraPatch Warm®
Trixaicin®
Trixaicin HP®
Zostrix® [OTC]
Zostrix High Potency®
Zostrix®-HP [OTC]
Zostrix Sports®

Antiinflammatory Agent
Arava™

leflunomide

Antirheumatic, Disease Modifying
Enbrel®
etanercept

Chelating Agent
Cuprimine®
Depen®
penicillamine

Gold Compound
auranofin
Aurolate®
aurothioglucose
gold sodium thiomalate
Ridaura®
Solganal®

Nonsteroidal Antiinflammatory Drug (NSAID)
Aches-N-Pain® [OTC]
Actron® [OTC]
Advil® [OTC]
Albert® Tiafen (Can)
Aleve® [OTC]
Alti-Flurbiprofen (Can)
Alti-Piroxicam (Can)
Amigesic®
Anacin® [OTC]
Anaprox®
Ansaid® Oral
Apo®-Diclo (Can)
Apo®-Diflunisal (Can)
Apo®-Flurbiprofen (Can)
Apo®-Ibuprofen (Can)
Apo®-Indomethacin (Can)
Apo®-Keto (Can)
Apo®-Keto-E (Can)
Apo®-Nabumetone (Can)
Apo®-Napro-Na (Can)
Apo®-Naproxen (Can)
Apo®-Piroxicam (Can)
Apo®-Sulin (Can)

Apo®-Tiaprofenic (Can)
Argesic®-SA
Arthritis Foundation® Pain Reliever
   [OTC]
Arthropan® [OTC]
Ascriptin® [OTC]
aspirin
Asprimox® [OTC]
Back-Ese M (Can)
Bayer® Aspirin [OTC]
Bayer® Buffered Aspirin [OTC]
Bayer® Low Adult Strength [OTC]
Bufferin® [OTC]
Buffex® [OTC]
Cama® Arthritis Pain Reliever [OTC]
Cataflam® Oral
Children's Advil® Suspension
Children's Motrin® Suspension
   [OTC]
choline magnesium trisalicylate
choline salicylate
Clinoril®
Daypro™
diclofenac
diflunisal
Disalcid®
Doan's Backache Pills (Can)
Doan's®, Original [OTC]
Dolobid®
Easprin®
Ecotrin® [OTC]
Ecotrin® Low Adult Strength [OTC]
Empirin® [OTC]
Excedrin® IB [OTC]
Extra Strength Adprin-B® [OTC]
Extra Strength Bayer® Enteric 500
   Aspirin [OTC]
Extra Strength Bayer® Plus [OTC]
Extra Strength Doan's® [OTC]
Feldene®
fenoprofen
Fexicam (Can)
flurbiprofen

Froben® (Can)
Gen-Naproxen EC (Can)
Gen-Piroxicam (Can)
Genpril® [OTC]
Halfprin® 81® [OTC]
Haltran® [OTC]
Heartline® [OTC]
Herbogesic (Can)
Ibuprin® [OTC]
ibuprofen
Ibuprohm® [OTC]
Ibu-Tab®
Indocid® (Can)
Indocin® Oral
Indocin® SR Oral
indomethacin
Indotec® (Can)
Junior Strength Motrin® [OTC]
ketoprofen
Magan®
magnesium salicylate
Magsal®
meclofenamate
Medipren® [OTC]
Menadol® [OTC]
Midol® IB [OTC]
Mobidin®
Mono-Gesic®
Motrin®
Motrin® IB [OTC]
nabumetone
Nalfon®
Naprelan®
Naprosyn®
naproxen
Naxen® (Can)
Novo-Difenac-K (Can)
Novo-Difenac®-SR (Can)
Novo-Diflunisal (Can)
Novo-Flurprofen (Can)
Novo-Keto (Can)
Novo-Keto-EC (Can)
Novo-Methacin (Can)

Novo-Naprox (Can)
Novo-Pirocam (Can)
Novo-Piroxicam (Can)
Novo-Profen® (Can)
Novo-Sundac (Can)
Novo-Tiaprofenic (Can)
Novo-Tolmetin (Can)
Nu-Diclo (Can)
Nu-Diflunisal (Can)
Nu-Flurprofen (Can)
Nu-Ibuprofen (Can)
Nu-Indo (Can)
Nu-Ketoprofen (Can)
Nu-Ketoprofen-E (Can)
Nu-Naprox (Can)
Nu-Pirox (Can)
Nuprin® [OTC]
Nu-Sulindac (Can)
Nu-Tiaprofenic (Can)
Ocufen® Ophthalmic
Orafen (Can)
Orudis®
Orudis® KT [OTC]
Oruvail®
oxaprozin
Pamprin IB® [OTC]
Pedia-Profen™
piroxicam
PMS-Diclofenac (Can)
PMS-Tiaprofenic (Can)
Regular Strength Bayer® Enteric 500
   Aspirin [OTC]
Relafen®
Rhodacine® (Can)
Rhodis™ (Can)
Rhodis-EC™ (Can)
Rhovail® (Can)
Riva-Naproxen (Can)
Saleto-200® [OTC]
Saleto-400®
Salflex®
salsalate

St. Joseph® Adult Chewable Aspirin
   [OTC]
sulindac
Surgam® (Can)
Surgam® SR (Can)
Synflex® (Can)
Synflex® DS (Can)
Teejel® (Can)
tiaprofenic acid (Canada only)
Tolectin®
Tolectin® DS
tolmetin
Trendar® [OTC]
Tricosal®
Trilisate®
Uni-Pro® [OTC]
Vofenal™ (Can)
Voltaren® Ophthalmic
Voltaren® Oral
Voltaren Rapide® (Can)
Voltaren®-XR Oral
ZORprin®
Nonsteroidal Antiinflammatory Drug
   (NSAID), COX-2 Selective
Celebrex™
celecoxib

BACK PAIN (LOW)
Analgesic, Narcotic
   codeine
   Codeine Contin® (Can)
Analgesic, Nonnarcotic
   Anacin® [OTC]
   Arthritis Foundation® Pain Reliever
      [OTC]
   Arthropan® [OTC]
   Ascriptin® [OTC]
   aspirin
   Asprimox® [OTC]
   Bayer® Aspirin [OTC]
   Bayer® Buffered Aspirin [OTC]
   Bayer® Low Adult Strength [OTC]

Bufferin® [OTC]
Buffex® [OTC]
Cama® Arthritis Pain Reliever [OTC]
choline salicylate
Easprin®
Ecotrin® [OTC]
Ecotrin® Low Adult Strength [OTC]
Empirin® [OTC]
Extra Strength Adprin-B® [OTC]
Extra Strength Bayer® Enteric 500
    Aspirin [OTC]
Extra Strength Bayer® Plus [OTC]
Halfprin® 81® [OTC]
Heartline® [OTC]
Regular Strength Bayer® Enteric 500
    Aspirin [OTC]
St. Joseph® Adult Chewable Aspirin
    [OTC]
Teejel® (Can)
ZORprin®
Benzodiazepine
    Apo®-Diazepam (Can)
    diazepam
    Valium® Injection
    Valium® Oral
    Vivol® (Can)
Nonsteroidal Antiinflammatory Drug
    (NSAID)
    Back-Ese M (Can)
    Doan's Backache Pills (Can)
    Doan's®, Original [OTC]
    Extra Strength Doan's® [OTC]
    Herbogesic (Can)
    Magan®
    magnesium salicylate
    Magsal®
    Mobidin®
Skeletal Muscle Relaxant
    Aspirin® Backache (Can)
    methocarbamol
    methocarbamol and aspirin
    Methoxisal (Can)

Robaxin®
Robaxisal®

BURSITIS
Nonsteroidal Antiinflammatory Drug
    (NSAID)
    Aches-N-Pain® [OTC]
    Advil® [OTC]
    Aleve® [OTC]
    Anacin® [OTC]
    Anaprox®
    Apo®-Ibuprofen (Can)
    Apo®-Indomethacin (Can)
    Apo®-Napro-Na (Can)
    Apo®-Naproxen (Can)
    Arthritis Foundation® Pain Reliever
        [OTC]
    Arthropan® [OTC]
    Ascriptin® [OTC]
    aspirin
    Asprimox® [OTC]
    Bayer® Aspirin [OTC]
    Bayer® Buffered Aspirin [OTC]
    Bayer® Low Adult Strength [OTC]
    Bufferin® [OTC]
    Buffex® [OTC]
    Cama® Arthritis Pain Reliever [OTC]
    Children's Advil® Suspension
    Children's Motrin® Suspension [OTC]
    choline magnesium trisalicylate
    choline salicylate
    Easprin®
    Ecotrin® [OTC]
    Ecotrin® Low Adult Strength [OTC]
    Empirin® [OTC]
    Excedrin® IB [OTC]
    Extra Strength Adprin-B® [OTC]
    Extra Strength Bayer® Enteric 500
        Aspirin [OTC]
    Extra Strength Bayer® Plus [OTC]
    Gen-Naproxen EC (Can)
    Genpril® [OTC]

Halfprin® 81® [OTC]
Haltran® [OTC]
Heartline® [OTC]
Ibuprin® [OTC]
ibuprofen
Ibuprohm® [OTC]
Ibu-Tab®
Indocid® (Can)
Indocin® Oral
Indocin® SR Oral
indomethacin
Indotec® (Can)
Junior Strength Motrin® [OTC]
Medipren® [OTC]
Menadol® [OTC]
Midol® IB [OTC]
Motrin®
Motrin® IB [OTC]
Naprelan®
Naprosyn®
naproxen
Naxen® (Can)
Novo-Methacin (Can)
Novo-Naprox (Can)
Novo-Profen® (Can)
Nu-Ibuprofen (Can)
Nu-Indo (Can)
Nu-Naprox (Can)
Nuprin® [OTC]
Pamprin IB® [OTC]
Pedia-Profen™
Regular Strength Bayer® Enteric 500
   Aspirin [OTC]
Rhodacine® (Can)
Riva-Naproxen (Can)
Saleto-200® [OTC]
Saleto-400®
St. Joseph® Adult Chewable Aspirin
   [OTC]
Synflex® (Can)
Synflex® DS (Can)
Teejel® (Can)
Trendar® [OTC]

Tricosal®
Trilisate®
Uni-Pro® [OTC]
ZORprin®

DEBRIDE CALLOUS TISSUE
Keratolytic Agent
   Tri-Chlor®
   trichloroacetic acid

DEBRIDEMENT OF ESCHAR
Protectant, Topical
   Granulex
   trypsin, balsam Peru, and castor oil

DECUBITUS ULCER
Enzyme
   collagenase
   Santyl®
Enzyme, Topical Debridement
   Accuzyme™
   papain and urea
Protectant, Topical
   Granulex
   trypsin, balsam Peru, and castor oil
Topical Skin Product
   Accuzyme™
   Debrisan® [OTC]
   dextranomer
   papain and urea

DEEP VEIN THROMBOSIS (DVT)
Anticoagulant
   Coumadin®
   dalteparin
   danaparoid
   enoxaparin
   Fragmin®
   Fraxiparine™ (Can)
   Hepalean® (Can)
   Hepalean-Lok® (Can)
   heparin

Innohep®
Lovenox®
nadroparin (Canada only)
Orgaran®
tinzaparin
warfarin

EPICONDYLITIS

Nonsteroidal Antiinflammatory Drug
  (NSAID)
  Aches-N-Pain® [OTC]
  Advil® [OTC]
  Aleve® [OTC]
  Anaprox®
  Apo®-Ibuprofen (Can)
  Apo®-Indomethacin (Can)
  Apo®-Napro-Na (Can)
  Apo®-Naproxen (Can)
  Children's Advil® Suspension
  Children's Motrin® Suspension
    [OTC]
  Excedrin® IB [OTC]
  Gen-Naproxen EC (Can)
  Genpril® [OTC]
  Haltran® [OTC]
  Ibuprin® [OTC]
  ibuprofen
  Ibuprohm® [OTC]
  Ibu-Tab®
  Indocid® (Can)
  Indocin® Oral
  Indocin® SR Oral
  indomethacin
  Indotec® (Can)
  Junior Strength Motrin® [OTC]
  Medipren® [OTC]
  Menadol® [OTC]
  Midol® IB [OTC]
  Motrin®
  Motrin® IB [OTC]
  Naprelan®
  Naprosyn®
  naproxen

Naxen® (Can)
Novo-Methacin (Can)
Novo-Naprox (Can)
Novo-Profen® (Can)
Nu-Ibuprofen (Can)
Nu-Indo (Can)
Nu-Naprox (Can)
Nuprin® [OTC]
Pamprin IB® [OTC]
Pedia-Profen™
Rhodacine® (Can)
Riva-Naproxen (Can)
Saleto-200® [OTC]
Saleto-400®
Synflex® (Can)
Synflex® DS (Can)
Trendar® [OTC]
Uni-Pro® [OTC]

GOUT

Antigout Agent
  colchicine
  colchicine and probenecid
Nonsteroidal Antiinflammatory Drug
  (NSAID)
  Aches-N-Pain® [OTC]
  Advil® [OTC]
  Aleve® [OTC]
  Anaprox®
  Apo®-Diclo (Can)
  Apo®-Ibuprofen (Can)
  Apo®-Indomethacin (Can)
  Apo®-Napro-Na (Can)
  Apo®-Naproxen (Can)
  Apo®-Sulin (Can)
  Cataflam® Oral
  Children's Advil® Suspension
  Children's Motrin® Suspension
    [OTC]
  Clinoril®
  diclofenac
  Excedrin® IB [OTC]
  Gen-Naproxen EC (Can)

Genpril® [OTC]
Haltran® [OTC]
Ibuprin® [OTC]
ibuprofen
Ibuprohm® [OTC]
Ibu-Tab®
Indocid® (Can)
Indocin® Oral
Indocin® SR Oral
indomethacin
Indotec® (Can)
Junior Strength Motrin® [OTC]
Medipren® [OTC]
Menadol® [OTC]
Midol® IB [OTC]
Motrin®
Motrin® IB [OTC]
Naprelan®
Naprosyn®
naproxen
Naxen® (Can)
Novo-Difenac-K (Can)
Novo-Difenac®-SR (Can)
Novo-Methacin (Can)
Novo-Naprox (Can)
Novo-Profen® (Can)
Novo-Sundac (Can)
Nu-Diclo (Can)
Nu-Ibuprofen (Can)
Nu-Indo (Can)
Nu-Naprox (Can)
Nuprin® [OTC]
Nu-Sulindac (Can)
Pamprin IB® [OTC]
Pedia-Profen™
PMS-Diclofenac (Can)
Rhodacine® (Can)
Riva-Naproxen (Can)
Saleto-200® [OTC]
Saleto-400®
sulindac
Synflex® (Can)
Synflex® DS (Can)

Trendar® [OTC]
Uni-Pro® [OTC]
Vofenal™ (Can)
Voltaren® Ophthalmic
Voltaren® Oral
Voltaren Rapide® (Can)
Voltaren®-XR Oral
Uricosuric Agent
Anturane®
Apo®-Sulfinpyraz (Can)
Benuryl™ (Can)
Nu-Sulfinpyrazone (Can)
probenecid
sulfinpyrazone
Xanthine Oxidase Inhibitor
allopurinol
Aloprim™ Injection
Apo®-Allopurinol (Can)
Zyloprim®

GUILLAIN-BARRÉ SYNDROME

Immune Globulin
Gamimune® N
Gammagard® S/D
Gammar®-P I.V.
immune globulin (intravenous)
Polygam® S/D
Sandoglobulin®
Venoglobulin®-I
Venoglobulin®-S

INFLAMMATION (NONRHEUMATIC)

Adrenal Corticosteroid
Acthar®
Adlone® Injection
A-hydroCort®
Amcort® Injection
A-methaPred® Injection
Apo®-Prednisone (Can)
Aristocort® Forte Injection
Aristocort® Intralesional Injection

Aristocort® Oral
Aristospan® Intraarticular Injection
Aristospan® Intralesional Injection
Atolone® Oral
betamethasone (systemic)
Celestone® Oral
Celestone® Phosphate Injection
Celestone® Soluspan®
Cel-U-Jec® Injection
corticotropin
cortisone acetate
Decadron® Injection
Decadron®-LA
Decadron® Oral
Decaject®
Decaject-LA®
Delta-Cortef® Oral
Deltasone®
depMedalone® Injection
Depoject® Injection
Depo-Medrol® Injection
Depopred® Injection
dexamethasone (systemic)
Dexasone®
Dexasone® L.A.
Dexone®
Dexone® LA
D-Med® Injection
Duralone® Injection
Hexadrol®
H.P. Acthar® Gel
hydrocortisone (systemic)
Hydrocortone® Acetate
Kenacort® Oral
Kenaject® Injection
Kenalog® Injection
Key-Pred® Injection
Key-Pred-SP® Injection
Medralone® Injection
Medrol® Oral
methylprednisolone
Meticorten®
M-Prednisol® Injection

Pediapred® Oral
PMS-Dexamethasone (Can)
Prednicot®
prednisolone (systemic)
Prednisol® TBA Injection
prednisone
Prelone® Oral
Solu-Cortef®
Solu-Medrol® Injection
Solurex L.A.®
Sterapred®
Tac™-3 Injection
Tac™-40 Injection
Triam-A® Injection
triamcinolone (systemic)
Triam Forte® Injection
Triamonide® Injection
Tri-Kort® Injection
Trilog® Injection
Trilone® Injection
Trisoject® Injection
Winpred™ (Can)

LEG CRAMPS
Blood Viscosity Reducer Agent
  Albert® Pentoxifylline (Can)
  Apo®-Pentoxifylline SR (Can)
  Nu-Pentoxifylline-SR (Can)
  pentoxifylline
  Trental®

MARFAN SYNDROME
Rauwolfia Alkaloid
  reserpine

METABOLIC BONE DISEASE
Vitamin D Analog
  calcifediol
  Calderol®

MUSCLE SPASM
Skeletal Muscle Relaxant
  Antiflex®

Apo®-Cyclobenzaprine (Can)
Aspirin® Backache (Can)
carisoprodol
carisoprodol and aspirin
carisoprodol, aspirin, and codeine
chlorzoxazone
cyclobenzaprine
Flexeril®
Flexitec (Can)
Gen-Cyclobenzaprine (Can)
metaxalone
methocarbamol
methocarbamol and aspirin
Methoxisal (Can)
Mio-Rel®
Mivacron®
mivacurium
Norflex™
Norgesic™
Norgesic™ Forte
Novo-Cycloprine (Can)
Nu-Cyclobenzaprine (Can)
orphenadrine
orphenadrine, aspirin, and caffeine
Orphenate®
Orphengesic®
Parafon Forte™ DSC
Robaxin®
Robaxisal®
Skelaxin®
Soma®
Soma® Compound
Soma® Compound w/Codeine

NERVE BLOCK
Local Anesthetic
  Ametop™ (Can)
  Anestacon® Topical Solution
  bupivacaine
  Carbocaine®
  chloroprocaine
  Citanest® Forte
  Citanest® Plain

Dilocaine® Injection
Duo-Trach® Injection
Duranest®
etidocaine
Isocaine® HCl
lidocaine
lidocaine and epinephrine
Lidodan™ (Can)
LidoPen® I.M. Injection Auto-
  Injector
Marcaine®
mepivacaine
Nervocaine® Injection
Nesacaine®
Nesacaine®-MPF
Novocain®
Polocaine®
Pontocaine®
Pontocaine® With Dextrose
prilocaine
procaine
Sensorcaine®
Sensorcaine®-MPF
tetracaine
tetracaine and dextrose
Xylocaine® Oral
Xylocaine® Topical Ointment
Xylocaine® Topical Solution
Xylocaine® Topical Spray
Xylocaine® With Epinephrine
Xylocard® (Can)

NEURALGIA
Analgesic, Nonnarcotic
  Arthropan® [OTC]
  choline salicylate
  Teejel® (Can)
Analgesic, Topical
  Antiphlogistine Rub A-535 No
    Odour (Can)
  Arth Dr®
  Arthricare Hand & Body®
  Born Again Super Pain Relieving®

Caprex®
Caprex Plus®
Capsagel®
Capsagel Extra Strength®
Capsagel Maximum Strength®
Capsagesic-HP Arthritis Relief®
capsaicin
Capsin® [OTC]
Capzasin-P® [OTC]
D-Care Circulation Stimulator®
Dolorex®
Double Cap®
Icy Hot Arthritis Therapy®
Myoflex® [OTC]
Pain Enz®
Pharmacist's Capsaicin®
Rid-A-Pain®
Rid-A-Pain-HP®
Sloan's Liniment®
Sportscreme® [OTC]
Sportsmed®
Theragen®
Theragen HP®
TheraPatch Warm®
triethanolamine salicylate
Trixaicin®
Trixaicin HP®
Zostrix® [OTC]
Zostrix High Potency®
Zostrix®-HP [OTC]
Zostrix Sports®
Nonsteroidal Antiinflammatory Drug
    (NSAID)
Anacin® [OTC]
Arthritis Foundation® Pain Reliever
    [OTC]
Ascriptin® [OTC]
Aspergum® [OTC]
aspirin
Asprimox® [OTC]
Bayer® Aspirin [OTC]
Bayer® Buffered Aspirin [OTC]
Bayer® Low Adult Strength [OTC]

Bufferin® [OTC]
Buffex® [OTC]
Cama® Arthritis Pain Reliever [OTC]
Easprin®
Ecotrin® [OTC]
Ecotrin® Low Adult Strength [OTC]
Empirin® [OTC]
Extra Strength Adprin-B® [OTC]
Extra Strength Bayer® Enteric 500
    Aspirin [OTC]
Extra Strength Bayer® Plus [OTC]
Halfprin® 81® [OTC]
Heartline® [OTC]
Regular Strength Bayer® Enteric 500
    Aspirin [OTC]
St. Joseph® Adult Chewable Aspirin
    [OTC]
ZORprin®

ONYCHOMYCOSIS
Antifungal Agent
    Fulvicin® P/G
    Fulvicin-U/F®
    Grifulvin® V
    Grisactin®
    griseofulvin
    Gris-PEG®
    Lamisil® Oral
    terbinafine (oral)

OSTEOARTHRITIS
Analgesic, Nonnarcotic
    Arthrotec®
    diclofenac and misoprostol
Analgesic, Topical
    Arth Dr®
    Arthricare Hand & Body®
    Born Again Super Pain Relieving®
    Caprex®
    Caprex Plus®
    Capsagel®
    Capsagel Extra Strength®
    Capsagel Maximum Strength®

Capsagesic-HP Arthritis Relief®
capsaicin
Capsin® [OTC]
Capzasin-P® [OTC]
D-Care Circulation Stimulator®
Dolorex®
Double Cap®
Icy Hot Arthritis Therapy®
Pain Enz®
Pharmacist's Capsaicin®
Rid-A-Pain®
Rid-A-Pain-HP®
Sloan's Liniment®
Sportsmed®
Theragen®
Theragen HP®
TheraPatch Warm®
Trixaicin®
Trixaicin HP®
Zostrix® [OTC]
Zostrix High Potency®
Zostrix®-HP [OTC]
Zostrix Sports®
Nonsteroidal Antiinflammatory Agent
   (NSAID)
   Albert® Tiafen (Can)
   Apo®-Tiaprofenic (Can)
   meloxicam
   Mobic®
   Novo-Tiaprofenic (Can)
   Nu-Tiaprofenic (Can)
   PMS-Tiaprofenic (Can)
   Surgam® (Can)
   Surgam® SR (Can)
   tiaprofenic acid (Canada only)
Nonsteroidal Antiinflammatory Drug
   (NSAID)
   Aches-N-Pain® [OTC]
   Actron® [OTC]
   Advil® [OTC]
   Aleve® [OTC]
   Alti-Piroxicam (Can)
   Amigesic®

Anacin® [OTC]
Anaprox®
Apo®-Diclo (Can)
Apo®-Diflunisal (Can)
Apo®-Etodolac (Can)
Apo®-Ibuprofen (Can)
Apo®-Indomethacin (Can)
Apo®-Keto (Can)
Apo®-Keto-E (Can)
Apo®-Nabumetone (Can)
Apo®-Napro-Na (Can)
Apo®-Naproxen (Can)
Apo®-Piroxicam (Can)
Apo®-Sulin (Can)
Argesic®-SA
Arthritis Foundation® Pain Reliever
   [OTC]
Arthropan® [OTC]
Ascriptin® [OTC]
Aspergum® [OTC]
aspirin
Asprimox® [OTC]
Back-Ese M (Can)
Bayer® Aspirin [OTC]
Bayer® Buffered Aspirin [OTC]
Bayer® Low Adult Strength [OTC]
Bufferin® [OTC]
Buffex® [OTC]
Cama® Arthritis Pain Reliever [OTC]
Cataflam® Oral
Children's Advil® Suspension
Children's Motrin® Suspension
   [OTC]
choline magnesium trisalicylate
choline salicylate
Clinoril®
Daypro™
diclofenac
diflunisal
Disalcid®
Doan's Backache Pills (Can)
Doan's®, Original [OTC]
Dolobid®

Easprin®
Ecotrin® [OTC]
Ecotrin® Low Adult Strength [OTC]
Empirin® [OTC]
etodolac
Excedrin® IB [OTC]
Extra Strength Adprin-B® [OTC]
Extra Strength Bayer® Enteric 500
    Aspirin [OTC]
Extra Strength Bayer® Plus [OTC]
Extra Strength Doan's® [OTC]
Feldene®
fenoprofen
Fexicam (Can)
Gen-Etodolac (Can)
Gen-Naproxen EC (Can)
Gen-Piroxicam (Can)
Genpril® [OTC]
Halfprin® 81® [OTC]
Haltran® [OTC]
Heartline® [OTC]
Herbogesic (Can)
Ibuprin® [OTC]
ibuprofen
Ibuprohm® [OTC]
Ibu-Tab®
Indocid® (Can)
Indocin® Oral
Indocin® SR Oral
indomethacin
Indotec® (Can)
Junior Strength Motrin® [OTC]
ketoprofen
Lodine®
Lodine® XL
Magan®
magnesium salicylate
Magsal®
meclofenamate
Medipren® [OTC]
Menadol® [OTC]
Midol® IB [OTC]
Mobidin®

Mono-Gesic®
Motrin®
Motrin® IB [OTC]
nabumetone
Nalfon®
Naprelan®
Naprosyn®
naproxen
Naxen® (Can)
Novo-Difenac-K (Can)
Novo-Difenac®-SR (Can)
Novo-Diflunisal (Can)
Novo-Keto (Can)
Novo-Keto-EC (Can)
Novo-Methacin (Can)
Novo-Naprox (Can)
Novo-Pirocam (Can)
Novo-Piroxicam (Can)
Novo-Profen® (Can)
Novo-Sundac (Can)
Novo-Tolmetin (Can)
Nu-Diclo (Can)
Nu-Diflunisal (Can)
Nu-Ibuprofen (Can)
Nu-Indo (Can)
Nu-Ketoprofen (Can)
Nu-Ketoprofen-E (Can)
Nu-Naprox (Can)
Nu-Pirox (Can)
Nuprin® [OTC]
Nu-Sulindac (Can)
Orafen (Can)
Orudis®
Orudis® KT [OTC]
Oruvail®
oxaprozin
Pamprin IB® [OTC]
Pedia-Profen™
piroxicam
PMS-Diclofenac (Can)
Regular Strength Bayer® Enteric 500
    Aspirin [OTC]
Relafen®

Rhodacine® (Can)
Rhodis™ (Can)
Rhodis-EC™ (Can)
Rhovail® (Can)
Riva-Naproxen (Can)
Saleto-200® [OTC]
Saleto-400®
Salflex®
salsalate
St. Joseph® Adult Chewable Aspirin
    [OTC]
sulindac
Synflex® (Can)
Synflex® DS (Can)
Teejel® (Can)
Tolectin®
Tolectin® DS
tolmetin
Trendar® [OTC]
Tricosal®
Trilisate®
Ultradol™ (Can)
Uni-Pro® [OTC]
Vofenal™ (Can)
Voltaren® Ophthalmic
Voltaren® Oral
Voltaren Rapide® (Can)
Voltaren®-XR Oral
ZORprin®
Nonsteroidal Antiinflammatory Drug
    (NSAID), COX-2 Selective
Celebrex™
celecoxib
rofecoxib
Vioxx®
Prostaglandin
Arthrotec®
diclofenac and misoprostol

OSTEODYSTROPHY
Vitamin D Analog
calcifediol
Calciferol™

Calcijex™
calcitriol
Calderol®
DHT™
dihydrotachysterol
Drisdol®
ergocalciferol
Ostoforte® (Can)
Rocaltrol®

OSTEOMALACIA
Vitamin D Analog
Calciferol™
Drisdol®
ergocalciferol
Ostoforte® (Can)

OSTEOMYELITIS
Antibiotic, Miscellaneous
Alti-Clindamycin (Can)
Cleocin HCl® Oral
Cleocin Pediatric® Oral
Cleocin Phosphate® Injection
Cleocin T® Topical
Cleocin® Vaginal
Clinda-Derm® Topical
clindamycin
Dalacin® C (Can)
Lyphocin® Injection
Vancocin® Injection
Vancocin® Oral
Vancoled® Injection
vancomycin
Antifungal Agent
Fucidin® I.V. (Can)
Fucidin® Oral Suspension (Can)
Fucidin® Tablet (Can)
fusidic acid (Canada only)
Carbapenem (Antibiotic)
imipenem and cilastatin
meropenem
Merrem® I.V.
Primaxin®

Cephalosporin (First Generation)
  Ancef®
  Cefadyl®
  cefazolin
  cephalothin
  cephapirin
  Ceporacin® (Can)
  Kefzol®
  Zolicef®
Cephalosporin (Second Generation)
  cefonicid
  Cefotan®
  cefotetan
  cefoxitin
  Ceftin® Oral
  cefuroxime
  Kefurox® Injection
  Mefoxin®
  Monocid®
  Zinacef® Injection
Cephalosporin (Third Generation)
  Cefizox®
  Cefobid®
  cefoperazone
  cefotaxime
  ceftazidime
  ceftizoxime
  ceftriaxone
  Ceptaz™
  Claforan®
  Fortaz®
  Rocephin®
  Tazicef®
  Tazidime®
Penicillin
  ampicillin and sulbactam
  dicloxacillin
  Dynapen®
  nafcillin
  oxacillin
  ticarcillin and clavulanate potassium
  Timentin®
  Unasyn®

Quinolone
  Ciloxan™ Ophthalmic
  Cipro®
  ciprofloxacin

OSTEOPOROSIS
Bisphosphonate Derivative
  alendronate
  Aredia™
  Didronel®
  etidronate disodium
  Fosamax®
  pamidronate
Electrolyte Supplement, Oral
  Calbon®
  Calcionate®
  Calciquid®
  calcium glubionate
  calcium lactate
  calcium phosphate (dibasic)
  Cal-Lac®
  Neo-Calglucon® [OTC]
  Posture® [OTC]
  Ridactate®
Estrogen and Progestin Combination
  estrogens and medroxyprogesterone
  Premphase®
  Prempro™
Estrogen Derivative
  Alora® Transdermal
  Cenestin™
  C.E.S.® (Can)
  Climara® Transdermal
  Congest (Can)
  Delestrogen® (Can)
  depGynogen® Injection
  Depo®-Estradiol Injection
  Depogen® Injection
  diethylstilbestrol
  Dioval® Injection
  Esclim® Transdermal
  Estinyl®
  Estrace® Oral

Estraderm® Transdermal
estradiol
Estra-L® Injection
Estratab®
Estring®
Estro-Cyp® Injection
Estrogel® (Can)
estrogens (conjugated A/synthetic)
estrogens (conjugated/equine)
estrogens (esterified)
ethinyl estradiol
Gynodiol™
Gynogen L.A.® Injection
Honvol® (Can)
Menest®
PMS-Conjugated Estrogens (Can)
Premarin®
Stilphostrol®
Vagifem®
Vivelle™ Transdermal
Mineral, Oral
ACT® [OTC]
Fluor-A-Day® (Can)
FluorCare® Neutral
fluoride
Fluorigard® [OTC]
Fluorinse®
Fluoritab®
Fluotic® (Can)
Flura®
Flura-Drops®
Flura-Loz®
Gel-Kam®
Gel-Tin® [OTC]
Karidium®
Karigel®
Karigel®-N
Listermint® with Fluoride [OTC]
Lozi-Tab®
Luride®
Luride®-SF
Minute-Gel®
Pediaflor®

Pharmaflur®
Phos-Flur®
Point-Two®
Prevident®
Stop® [OTC]
Thera-Flur®
Thera-Flur-N®
Polypeptide Hormone
calcitonin
Caltine® (Can)
Miacalcin®
Selective Estrogen Receptor Modulator
   (SERM)
Evista®
raloxifene

PAGET DISEASE OF BONE
Antidote
   Mithracin®
   plicamycin
Bisphosphonate Derivative
   alendronate
   Aredia™
   Didronel®
   etidronate disodium
   Fosamax®
   pamidronate
   Skelid®
   tiludronate
Polypeptide Hormone
   calcitonin
   Caltine® (Can)
   Miacalcin®

PAIN
Analgesic, Narcotic
   acetaminophen and codeine
   Actiq® Oral Transmucosal
   Alfenta®
   alfentanil
   Anexsia®
   Anodynos-DHC®
   aspirin and codeine

Bancap HC®
belladonna and opium
B&O Supprettes®
Buprenex®
buprenorphine
butalbital compound and codeine
butorphanol
Capital® and Codeine
codeine
Codeine Contin® (Can)
Co-Gesic®
Coryphen® Codeine (Can)
Damason-P®
Darvocet-N®
Darvocet-N® 100
Darvon®
Darvon® Compound-65 Pulvules®
Darvon-N®
Demerol®
DHC Plus®
dihydrocodeine compound
Dilaudid® Cough Syrup
Dilaudid-HP® Injection
Dilaudid® Injection
Dilaudid® Oral
Dilaudid® Suppository
Dolacet®
Dolophine®
droperidol and fentanyl
Duocet™
Duradyne DHC®
Duragesic® Transdermal
Duramorph® Injection
Empirin® With Codeine
Endocet®
Endocodone®
Endodan®
fentanyl
Fentanyl Oralet®
Fiorinal®-C (Can)
Fiorinal® With Codeine
Hydrocet®
hydrocodone and acetaminophen

hydrocodone and aspirin
hydrocodone and ibuprofen
Hydrogesic®
Hydromorph Contin® (Can)
hydromorphone
Hy-Phen®
Infumorph™
Innovar®
Kadian™ Oral
Lenoltec No 1, 2, 3, 4 (Can)
Levo-Dromoran®
levorphanol
Lorcet® 10/650
Lorcet®-HD
Lorcet® Plus
Lortab®
Lortab® ASA
Margesic® H
Mepergan®
meperidine
meperidine and promethazine
M-Eslon® (Can)
Metadol™ (Can)
methadone
Methadose® (Can)
morphine sulfate
MS Contin® Oral
MSIR® Oral
nalbuphine
Norcet®
Norco®
Nubain®
Numorphan®
opium tincture
Oramorph SR™ Oral
Oxycocet® (Can)
Oxycodan® (Can)
oxycodone
oxycodone and acetaminophen
oxycodone and aspirin
OxyContin®
OxyIR™
oxymorphone

paregoric
pentazocine
pentazocine compound
Percocet® 2.5/325
Percocet® 5/325
Percocet® 7.5/500
Percocet® 10/650
Percocet®-Demi (Can)
Percodan®
Percodan®-Demi
Percolone®
Phenaphen® With Codeine #3
PMS-Hydromorphone (Can)
Pronap-100®
Propoxacet-N®
propoxyphene
propoxyphene and acetaminophen
propoxyphene and aspirin
Pyregesic-C®
remifentanil
RMS® Rectal
Roxanol™ Oral
Roxanol SR™ Oral
Roxanol-T™
Roxicet® 5/500
Roxicodone™
Roxilox™
Stadol®
Stadol® NS
Stagesic®
Statex® (Can)
Sublimaze® Injection
Sufenta®
sufentanil
Supeudol® (Can)
Synalgos®-DC
222® Tablets (Can)
282® Tablets (Can)
292® Tablets (Can)
624® Tablets (Can)
Talacen®
Talwin®
Talwin® Compound

Talwin® NX
Tecnal C (Can)
T-Gesic®
Triatec-8® (Can)
Triatec-8® Strong (Can)
Triatec-30® (Can)
Tylenol® With Codeine
Tylox®
Ultiva™
Vicodin®
Vicodin® ES
Vicoprofen®
Wygesic®
Zydone®

Analgesic, Nonnarcotic
Abenol® (Can)
Acephen® [OTC]
Aceta® [OTC]
Aceta® Children's [OTC]
Acetagesic® [OTC]
acetaminophen
acetaminophen and diphenhydramine
acetaminophen and
    phenyltoloxamine
acetaminophen, aspirin, and caffeine
Aches-N-Pain® [OTC]
Actamin® [OTC]
Actron® [OTC]
Acular® Ophthalmic
Advil® [OTC]
Aleve® [OTC]
Altenol® [OTC]
Alti-Flurbiprofen (Can)
Alti-Piroxicam (Can)
Amdol 500® [OTC]
Amdol 650® [OTC]
Amdoplus® [OTC]
Amigesic®
Aminofen® [OTC]
Aminofen Plus® [OTC]
Anacin® [OTC]
Anacin® P.M. Aspirin Free [OTC]
Anagesic® [OTC]

Anaprox®
Ansaid® Oral
Apapedyn® Children's [OTC]
Apapedyn® Extra Strength [OTC]
Apaphen® [OTC]
Apo®-Diclo (Can)
Apo®-Diflunisal (Can)
Apo®-Etodolac (Can)
Apo®-Flurbiprofen (Can)
Apo®-Ibuprofen (Can)
Apo®-Indomethacin (Can)
Apo®-Keto (Can)
Apo®-Keto-E (Can)
Apo®-Ketorolac (Can)
Apo®-Mefenamic (Can)
Apo®-Nabumetone (Can)
Apo®-Napro-Na (Can)
Apo®-Naproxen (Can)
Apo®-Piroxicam (Can)
Apo®-Sulin (Can)
Argesic®-SA
Arthritis Foundation® Pain Reliever
    [OTC]
Arthropan® [OTC]
Ascriptin® [OTC]
Aspergum® [OTC]
aspirin
Asprimox® [OTC]
Bayer® Aspirin [OTC]
Bayer® Buffered Aspirin [OTC]
Bayer® Low Adult Strength [OTC]
Bufferin® [OTC]
Buffex® [OTC]
Cama® Arthritis Pain Reliever [OTC]
Cataflam® Oral
Cetafen® [OTC]
Cetafen® Extra [OTC]
Children's Advil® Suspension
Children's Motrin® Suspension
    [OTC]
choline magnesium trisalicylate
choline salicylate
Clinoril®

Daypro™
diclofenac
diflunisal
Disalcid®
Dolobid®
Dolono® [OTC]
Dolono® Infants [OTC]
Double-Action Pain Relief® [OTC]
Easprin®
Eckogesic® [OTC]
Ecotrin® [OTC]
Ecotrin® Low Adult Strength [OTC]
Empirin® [OTC]
etodolac
Excedrin®, Extra Strength [OTC]
Excedrin® IB [OTC]
Excedrin® P.M. [OTC]
Extraprin® [OTC]
Extra Strength Adprin-B® [OTC]
Extra Strength Bayer® Enteric 500
    Aspirin [OTC]
Extra Strength Bayer® Plus [OTC]
Febrol® [OTC]
Feldene®
Fem-Prin® [OTC]
fenoprofen
Feverall™ [OTC]
Fexicam (Can)
Flextra-DS® [OTC]
flurbiprofen
Froben® (Can)
Gelpirin® [OTC]
Genapap® [OTC]
Genapap® Children [OTC]
Genapap® Extra Strength [OTC]
Genapap® Infant [OTC]
Genasec® [OTC]
Genebs® [OTC]
Genebs® Extra Strength [OTC]
Gen-Etodolac (Can)
Gen-Naproxen EC (Can)
Gen-Piroxicam (Can)
Genpril® [OTC]

Goody's® Fast Pain Relief® [OTC]
Goody's® Headache Powders [OTC]
Halenol® [OTC]
Halfprin® 81® [OTC]
Haltran® [OTC]
Headache Formula PM® [OTC]
Headache Relief PM® [OTC]
Headrin® Plus Pain Relief [OTC]
Heartline® [OTC]
Ibuprin® [OTC]
ibuprofen
Ibuprohm® [OTC]
Ibu-Tab®
Indocid® (Can)
Indocin® Oral
Indocin® SR Oral
indomethacin
Indotec® (Can)
Infantaire® [OTC]
Junior Strength Motrin® [OTC]
ketoprofen
ketorolac tromethamine
Legatrin® PM Advanced Formula
    [OTC]
Leg Cramp Relief PM® [OTC]
Lodine®
Lodine® XL
Major-Gesic® [OTC]
Mapap® [OTC]
Mapap® Children's [OTC]
Mapap® Extra Strength [OTC]
Mapap® Infants' [OTC]
Mapap-PM® [OTC]
Mardol® [OTC]
meclofenamate
Meda-Cap® [OTC]
Medipren® [OTC]
mefenamic acid
Menadol® [OTC]
Midol® IB [OTC]
Midol® PM [OTC]
Mono-Gesic®
Motrin®

Motrin® IB [OTC]
nabumetone
Nalfon®
Naprelan®
Naprosyn®
naproxen
Naxen® (Can)
Night-Time Cramp Relief® [OTC]
Night-Time Pain Reliever/Sleep
    [OTC]
Norgesic™
Norgesic™ Forte
Novagesic® [OTC]
Novo-Difenac-K (Can)
Novo-Difenac®-SR (Can)
Novo-Diflunisal (Can)
Novo-Flurprofen (Can)
Novo-Keto (Can)
Novo-Keto-EC (Can)
Novo-Ketorolac (Can)
Novo-Methacin (Can)
Novo-Naprox (Can)
Novo-Pirocam (Can)
Novo-Piroxicam (Can)
Novo-Profen® (Can)
Novo-Sundac (Can)
Novo-Tolmetin (Can)
Nu-Diclo (Can)
Nu-Diflunisal (Can)
Nu-Flurprofen (Can)
Nu-Ibuprofen (Can)
Nu-Indo (Can)
Nu-Ketoprofen (Can)
Nu-Ketoprofen-E (Can)
Nu-Mefenamic (Can)
Nu-Naprox (Can)
Nu-Pirox (Can)
Nuprin® [OTC]
Nu-Sulindac (Can)
Ocufen® Ophthalmic
Ohmni-Gesic® [OTC]
Orafen (Can)
Oraphen PD® [OTC]

orphenadrine, aspirin, and caffeine
Orphengesic®
Orudis®
Orudis® KT [OTC]
Oruvail®
oxaprozin
Pain-Eze® [OTC]
Pain-Gesic® [OTC]
Pain-Off® [OTC]
Pamprin IB® [OTC]
Pedia-Profen™
Pediatrix (Can)
Percogesic® [OTC]
Phenylgesic® [OTC]
piroxicam
piroxicam and cyclodextrin (Canada only)
PMS-Diclofenac (Can)
PMS-Mefenamic Acid (Can)
Ponstan® (Can)
Ponstel®
Pyrecot® [OTC]
Pyregesic® [OTC]
Q-Gesic® [OTC]
Q-Pap® [OTC]
Q-Pap® Children's [OTC]
Redutemp® [OTC]
Regular Strength Bayer® Enteric 500 Aspirin [OTC]
Relafen®
Relagesic® [OTC]
Rhodacine® (Can)
Rhodis™ (Can)
Rhodis-EC™ (Can)
Rhovail® (Can)
Riva-Naproxen (Can)
Saleto-200® [OTC]
Saleto-400®
Salflex®
salsalate
Silapap® Children's [OTC]
Silapap® Infant's [OTC]
sodium salicylate

Sominex® Pain Relief Formula [OTC]
Staflex® [OTC]
St. Joseph® Adult Chewable Aspirin [OTC]
sulindac
Supac® [OTC]
Synflex® (Can)
Synflex® DS (Can)
Tactinal® [OTC]
Tactinal® Children's [OTC]
Tactinal® Extra Strength [OTC]
Teejel® (Can)
Tempra® 1 [OTC]
Tempra® 2 [OTC]
Tension® [OTC]
Tolectin®
Tolectin® DS
tolmetin
Toradol®
T-Painol® [OTC]
T-Painol® Extra Strength [OTC]
tramadol
Trendar® [OTC]
Tricosal®
Trilisate®
Tycolene® [OTC]
Tylenol® [OTC]
Tylenol® Arthritis [OTC]
Tylenol® Children's [OTC]
Tylenol® Extra Strength [OTC]
Tylenol® Infants [OTC]
Tylenol® Infants Original [OTC]
Tylenol® Junior Strength [OTC]
Tylenol® PM Strength [OTC]
Tylenol® Severe Allergy [OTC]
Tylenol® Sore Throat [OTC]
Tylex® [OTC]
Tylex® Extra Strength [OTC]
Tylophen® [OTC]
Tyltabs® [OTC]
Tyltabs® Children's [OTC]
Tyltabs® Extra Strength [OTC]

Tyltabs® PM [OTC]
Ultradol™ (Can)
Ultram®
UniPerr® [OTC]
Uni-Pro® [OTC]
Unison® w/Pain Relief [OTC]
Valorin® [OTC]
Valorin® Extra [OTC]
Vanquish® [OTC]
Vitoxapap® [OTC]
Vofenal™ (Can)
Voltaren® Ophthalmic
Voltaren® Oral
Voltaren Rapide® (Can)
Voltaren®-XR Oral
ZORprin®
Local Anesthetic
    AK-Taine®
    Alcaine®
    Diocaine® (Can)
    ethyl chloride
    ethyl chloride and
        dichlorotetrafluoroethane
    Fluro-Ethyl® Aerosol
    Ocu-Caine®
    Ophthetic®
    Parcaine®
    proparacaine
Neuroleptic Agent
    Apo®-Methoprazine (Can)
    methotrimeprazine (Canada only)
    Novo-Meprazine (Can)
    Nozinan® (Can)
Nonsteroidal Antiinflammatory Drug
    (NSAID)
    Back-Ese M (Can)
    Doan's Backache Pills (Can)
    Doan's®, Original [OTC]
    Extra Strength Doan's® [OTC]
    Herbogesic (Can)
    Magan®
    magnesium salicylate
    Magsal®

Mobidin®
Nonsteroidal Antiinflammatory Drug
    (NSAID), COX-2 Selective
    rofecoxib
    Vioxx®
Nonsteroidal Antiinflammatory Drug
    (NSAID), Oral
    floctafenine (Canada only)
    Idarac® (Can)

PAIN (LUMBAR PUNCTURE)
Analgesic, Topical
    EMLA®
    lidocaine and prilocaine

PAIN (MUSCLE)
Analgesic, Topical
    dichlorodifluoromethane and
        trichloromonofluoromethane
    Fluori-Methane® Topical Spray

PLANTARIS
Keratolytic Agent
    Duofilm® Solution
    Keralyt® Gel
    salicylic acid and lactic acid
    salicylic acid and propylene glycol

PLANTAR WARTS
Keratolytic Agent
    Duofilm® Solution
    salicylic acid and lactic acid
Topical Skin Product
    silver nitrate

POLYMYOSITIS
Antineoplastic Agent
    chlorambucil
    cyclophosphamide
    Cytoxan®
    Leukeran®
    methotrexate
    Neosar®

Procytox® (Can)
Rheumatrex®
Immunosuppressant Agent
  Alti-Azathioprine (Can)
  azathioprine
  Imuran®

PSEUDOGOUT
Antigout Agent
  colchicine
Nonsteroidal Antiinflammatory Drug
  (NSAID)
  Apo®-Indomethacin (Can)
  Indocid® (Can)
  Indocin® Oral
  Indocin® SR Oral
  indomethacin
  Indotec® (Can)
  Novo-Methacin (Can)
  Nu-Indo (Can)
  Rhodacine® (Can)

RHEUMATIC DISORDER
Adrenal Corticosteroid
  Acthar®
  Adlone® Injection
  A-hydroCort®
  Amcort® Injection
  A-methaPred® Injection
  Apo®-Prednisone (Can)
  Aristocort® Forte Injection
  Aristocort® Intralesional Injection
  Aristocort® Oral
  Aristospan® Intraarticular Injection
  Aristospan® Intralesional Injection
  Atolone® Oral
  betamethasone (systemic)
  Celestone® Oral
  Celestone® Phosphate Injection
  Celestone® Soluspan®
  Cel-U-Jec® Injection
  corticotropin
  cortisone acetate

Decadron® Injection
Decadron®-LA
Decadron® Oral
Decaject®
Decaject-LA®
Delta-Cortef® Oral
Deltasone®
depMedalone® Injection
Depoject® Injection
Depo-Medrol® Injection
Depopred® Injection
dexamethasone (systemic)
Dexasone®
Dexasone® L.A.
Dexone®
Dexone® LA
D-Med® Injection
Duralone® Injection
Hexadrol®
H.P. Acthar® Gel
hydrocortisone (systemic)
Hydrocortone® Acetate
Kenacort® Oral
Kenaject® Injection
Kenalog® Injection
Key-Pred® Injection
Key-Pred-SP® Injection
Medralone® Injection
Medrol® Oral
methylprednisolone
Meticorten®
M-Prednisol® Injection
Pediapred® Oral
PMS-Dexamethasone (Can)
Prednicot®
prednisolone (systemic)
Prednisol® TBA Injection
prednisone
Prelone® Oral
Solu-Cortef®
Solu-Medrol® Injection
Solurex L.A.®
Sterapred®

Tac™-3 Injection
Tac™-40 Injection
Triam-A® Injection
triamcinolone (systemic)
Triam Forte® Injection
Triamonide® Injection
Tri-Kort® Injection
Trilog® Injection
Trilone® Injection
Trisoject® Injection
Winpred™ (Can)

RHEUMATOID ARTHRITIS
Analgesic, Nonnarcotic
Arthrotec®
diclofenac and misoprostol
Prostaglandin
Arthrotec®
diclofenac and misoprostol

RICKETS
Vitamin D Analog
Calciferol™
Drisdol®
ergocalciferol
Ostoforte® (Can)

SKIN ULCER
Enzyme
collagenase
Santyl®
Topical Skin Product
Debrisan® [OTC]
dextranomer

SPINAL CORD INJURY
Skeletal Muscle Relaxant
Dantrium®
dantrolene

SPONDYLITIS (ANKYLOSING)
Nonsteroidal Antiinflammatory Drug
(NSAID)

Alti-Piroxicam (Can)
Apo®-Diclo (Can)
Apo®-Piroxicam (Can)
Cataflam® Oral
diclofenac
Feldene®
Fexicam (Can)
Gen-Piroxicam (Can)
Novo-Difenac-K (Can)
Novo-Difenac®-SR (Can)
Novo-Pirocam (Can)
Novo-Piroxicam (Can)
Nu-Diclo (Can)
Nu-Pirox (Can)
piroxicam
PMS-Diclofenac (Can)
Vofenal™ (Can)
Voltaren® Ophthalmic
Voltaren® Oral
Voltaren Rapide® (Can)
Voltaren®-XR Oral

SUDECK ATROPHY
Calcium Channel Blocker
Adalat® CC
Adalat PA® (Can)
Apo®-Nifed (Can)
nifedipine
Novo-Nifedin (Can)
Nu-Nifed (Can)
Nu-Nifedin (Can)
Procardia®
Procardia XL®

TINEA
Antifungal Agent
Absorbine® Antifungal Foot Powder [OTC]
Aftate® [OTC]
Apo®-Ketoconazole (Can)
benzoic acid and salicylic acid
Blis-To-Sol® [OTC]
Breezee® Mist Antifungal [OTC]

butenafine
Canesten® (Can)
carbol-fuchsin solution
ciclopirox
clioquinol
Clotrimaderm (Can)
clotrimazole
D-Care® [OTC]
Desenex® Foot & Sneaker [OTC]
econazole
Ecostatin® (Can)
Exelderm® Topical
Femizol-M® [OTC]
Fulvicin® P/G
Fulvicin-U/F®
Fungi-Gard® [OTC]
Fungoid® Creme
Fungoid® Solution
Fungoid® Tincture
Grifulvin® V
Grisactin®
griseofulvin
Gris-PEG®
Gyne-Lotrimin® [OTC]
Gyne-Lotrimin® 3 [OTC]
ketoconazole
Lamisil® Cream
Loprox®
Lotrimin®
Lotrimin® AF Cream [OTC]
Lotrimin® AF Lotion [OTC]
Lotrimin® AF Powder [OTC]
Lotrimin® AF Solution [OTC]
Lotrimin® AF Spray Liquid [OTC]
Lotrimin® AF Spray Powder [OTC]
Maximum Strength Desenex®
    Antifungal Cream [OTC]
Mentax®
Micatin® Topical [OTC]
miconazole
Mitrazol® [OTC]
Monazole-7® (Can)
Monistat-Derm™ Topical

Monistat i.v.™ Injection
Monistat™ Vaginal
Mycelex®
Mycelex®-7
Mycelex®-G
Myco-Nail® [OTC]
M-Zole® 7 Dual Pack [OTC]
naftifine
Naftin®
Nizoral®
Nizoral® A-D Shampoo [OTC]
Novo-Ketoconazole (Can)
NP-27® [OTC]
oxiconazole
Oxistat® Topical
Penlac™
Pitrex (Can)
Podactin® [OTC]
Prescription Strength Desenex®
    [OTC]
Q-Naftate® [OTC]
sodium thiosulfate
Spectazole™
sulconazole
terbinafine (topical)
Tinactin® [OTC]
Tinamar® [OTC]
Ting® [OTC]
tolnaftate
Tolnaftin® [OTC]
triacetin
Trivagizole 3™ [OTC]
undecylenic acid and derivatives
Undex-25% [OTC]
Versiclear™
Whitfield's Ointment [OTC]
Zeasorb-AF® Powder [OTC]
Antifungal/Corticosteroid
    betamethasone and clotrimazole
    Lotriderm® (Can)
    Lotrisone®
Antiseborrheic Agent, Topical
    Dandrex® [OTC]

Exsel® Shampoo
selenium sulfide
Selsun Blue® Shampoo [OTC]
Selsun® Shampoo

Versel® (Can)
Disinfectant
   sodium hypochlorite solution